Yearbook of Intensive and Emergency Medicine

Edited by J.-L. Vincent

Springer

Berlin
Heidelberg
New York
Barcelona
Hong Kong
London
Milan
Paris
Tokyo

Yearbook
of Intensive Care
and Emergency
Medicine   2002

Edited by J.-L. Vincent

With 170 Figures and 101 Tables

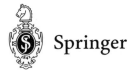 Springer

Prof. Jean-Louis Vincent

Head, Department of Intensive Care
Erasme Hospital, Free University of Brussels
Route de Lennik 808, B-1070 Brussels, Belgium

ISBN 3-540-43149-7 Springer-Verlag Berlin Heidelberg New York

ISSN 0942-5381

Springer-Verlag Berlin Heidelberg New York
a member of BertelsmannSpringer Science+Business Media GmbH

http://www.springer.de

Typesetting: K + V Fotosatz, Beerfelden
Printing: Zechner® Datenservice and Druck
Bookbinding: J. Schäffer, Grünstadt

SPIN: 10863337   21/3130-5 4 3 2 1 0 – Printed on acid-free paper

Contents

Infectious Challenges

Fluid Therapy

Metabolic Support

Cardiorespiratory Monitoring

Oxygen Delivery

Coagulopathies

Head Trauma

Neurological Challenges

Abdominal Crises

Renal Failure

Particular Aspects

Severity of Illness

Quality of Care

List of Contributors

Abella BS
Section of Emergency Medicine
University of Chicago Hospitals
MC 5068
5841 S. Maryland Avenue
Chicago, IL 60637
USA

Adrie C
Dept of Intensive Care
Delafontaine Hospital
2 rue du Dr Delafontaine
93205 Saint Denis
France

Andrews PJD
Dept of Anesthetics
Intensive Care Unit
Western General Hospital
Crew Road South
Edinburgh
Scotland EH4 2XU
UK

Antonelli M
Dept of Intensive Care
and Anesthesiology
Catholic University
Policlinico A. Gemelli
Largo Agostino Gemelli 8
00168 Rome
Italy

Auzinger G
Institute of Liver Studies
LITU
King's College Hospital
Denmark Hill
London SE5 9RJ
UK

Azoulay E
Dept of Medical Intensive Care
Saint-Louis Hospital
1 Ave Claude Vellefaux
75475 Paris Cedex 10
France

Ball JAS
Dept of Anesthesia
and Intensive Care
St. George's Hospital
Cranmer Terrace
London SW17 0RE
UK

Balligand JL
Dept of Internal Medicine
Unit of Pharmacology
and Therapeutics
FATH 5349
University of Louvain Medical
School
53 Ave Mounier
B-1200 Brussels
Belgium

Bates JHT
Dept of Medicine
Vermont Lung Center
University of Vermont
149 Beaumont Ave
Burlington, VT 05405-0075
USA

Beck J
Dept of Medicine
University of Montreal
12750 27th Avenue
Montreal
Quebec H1E 1Z9
Canada

Becker LB
Section of Emergency Medicine
University of Chicago Hospitals
MC 5068
5841 S. Maryland Avenue
Chicago, IL 60637
USA

Bellomo R
Dept of Intensive Care
Austin and Repatriation Center
Studley Road
Heidelberg 3084
Australia

Ben-Abraham R
Surgical Intensive Care Unit
Surasky Tel-Aviv Medical Center
6 Weizman Street
Tel-Aviv
Israel

Berg R
Dept of Pediatric Critical Care
University of Arizona
1501 North Campbell Ave
Tucson, AZ 85724-5073
USA

Berger RP
Safar Center for Resuscitation
Research
3434 Fifth Avenue
Pittsburgh, PA 15260
USA

Bishop G
Division of Critical Care
Liverpool Hospital
Locked Bag 7103
Liverpool, BC
NSW 1871
Australia

Blanch L
Critical Care Center
Hospital de Sabadell
Corporacio Parc Tauli
University Institute
08208 Sabadell
Spain

Bodenham A
Dept of Anaesthesia
Leeds General Infirmary
Great George Street
Leeds LS1 3EX
UK

Boldt J
Dept of Anesthesiology
and Intensive Care Medicine
Klinikum der Stadt Ludwigshafen
Bremerstraße 79
67063 Ludwigshafen
Germany

Bowry R
Dept of Intensive Care
St. Thomas' Hospital
Lambeth Palace Road
London SE1 JEH
UK

Brett SJ
Dept of Anesthesia and Intensive
Care Medicine
Hammersmith Hospital
Du Cane Road
London W12 0HS
UK

Burke-Gaffney A
Unit of Critical Care
Imperial College School of Medicine
Royal Brompton Hospital
Sydney Street
London SW3 6NP
UK

Ceriana P
Respiratory Intensive Care Unit
Fondazione Salvatore Maugeri
Via Ferrata 4
27100 Pavia
Italy

Chaudry IH
Center for Surgical Research
University of Alabama at
Birmingham
G094 Volker Hall
1670 University Blvd
Birmingham, AL 35394-0019
USA

Chiumello D
Instituto di Anestesia e
Rianimazione
Ospedale Maggiore Policlinico-
IRCCS
Via Francesco Sforza 35
20122 Milan
Italy

Citerio G
Dept of Anesthesia
and Intensive Care
Ospedale San Gerardo
Via Donizetti 106
20052 Monza
Italy

Ciurana CLF
Sanquin Research
Dept of Immunopathology
Plesmanlaan 125
1066 CX Amsterdam
The Netherlands

Claassen J
Division of Critical Care Neurology
Neurological Institute
710 West 168th Street, Unit 39
New York
NY 10032
USA

Corwin HL
Dept of Critical Care Medicine
Dartmouth-Hitchcock Medical
Center
1 Medical Center Drive
Lebanon, NH 03756
USA

de Jonge E
Dept of Vascular Medicine/
Internal Medicine
Academic Medical Center F4
University of Amsterdam
Meibergdreef 9
1105 AZ Amsterdam
The Netherlands

Delmastro M
Respiratory Intensive Care Unit
Fondazione Salvatore Maugeri
Via Ferrata 4
27100 Pavia
Italy

Del Turco M
Dept of Surgery
Cattedre di Anestesiologia e
Rianimazione
Ospedale S. Chiara
Università di Pisa
Via Roma 67
56126 Pisa
Italy

Dimopoulos G
Dept of Critical Care Medicine
Sotira Hospital
152 Mesogion Ave
11527 Athens
Greece

Doig CJ
Dept of Critical Care Medicine
Foothills Medical Center
1403 29th Street NW
Calgary, AB T2N 2T9
Canada

dos Santos CC
Dept of Critical Care Medicine
St. Michael's Hospital
Queen St. Wing
30 Bond Street
Toronto
Ontario M5B 1W8
Canada

Dugernier T
Dept of Intensive Care
St. Luc University Hospital
Hippocrate Ave
1200 Brussels
Belgium

Ensinger H
Clinic for Anesthesiology
University of Ulm
D-89070 Ulm
Germany

Evans TW
Unit of Critical Care
Imperial College School of Medicine
Royal Brompton Hospital
Sydney Street
London SW3 6NP
UK

Ferrer M
Dept of Pneumonology
Institut Clinic de Pneumologia i
Chirurgia Toracica
Hospital Clinic Provincial
Villarroel 170
08036 Barcelona
Spain

Fink MP
Dept of Critical Care Medicine
University of Pittsburgh
Medical Center
Room 616 Scaife Hall
3550 Terrace Street
Pittsburgh, PA 15261
USA

Finney SJ
Unit of Critical Care
Imperial College School of Medicine
Royal Brompton Hospital
Sydney Street
London SW3 6NP
UK

Flabouris A
Division of Critical Care
Liverpool Hospital
Locked Bag 7103
Liverpool, BC
NSW 1871
Australia

Foti G
Dept of Anesthesia
and Intensive Care
University of Milano-Bicocca
Ospedale San Gerardo Nuovo
dei Tintori
Via Donizetti 106
20052 Monza
Milan
Italy

Fromm Jr RE
Cardiology, Pulmonary
and Critical Care Section
Baylor College of Medicine
2219 Dorrington
Houston, TX 77030
USA

Gattinoni L
Instituto di Anestesia e
Rianimazione
Ospedale Maggiore Policlinico-
IRCCS
Via Francesco Sforza 35
20122 Milan
Italy

Giles LJ
Dept of Intensive Care
St. Thomas' Hospital
Lambeth Palace Road
London SE1 JEH
UK

Gill V
Depts of Physiology and Biophysics
Foothills Medical Center
1403 29th Street NW
Calgary, AB T2N 2T9
Canada

Giunta F
Dept of Surgery
Cattedre di Anestesiologia
e Rianimazione
Ospedale S. Chiara
Università di Pisa
Via Roma 67
56126 Pisa
Italy

Grounds RM
Dept of Anesthesia
and Intensive Care
St. George's Hospital
Cranmer Terrace
London SW17 0RE
UK

Guery B
Laboratoire de Recherche
en Pathologie Infectieuse
University of Lille II
Hôpital Gustave Dron
59208 Tourcoing Cedex
France

Hack CE
VU Medical Center
Dept of Clinical Chemistry
De Boelelaan 1117
1007 MB Amsterdam
The Netherlands

Harris BA
Dept of Anesthetics
Intensive Care Unit
Western General Hospital
Crew Road South
Edinburgh
Scotland EH4 2XU
UK

Hillman K
Division of Critical Care
Liverpool Hospital
Locked Bag 7103
Liverpool, BC
NSW 1871
Australia

Hirsch LJ
Division of Critical Care Neurology
Neurological Institute
710 West 168th Street, Unit 39
New York
NY 10032
USA

Hopkins RO
Dept of Critical Care Medicine
LDS Hospital
8th Avenue and C Street
Salt Lake City
Utah 84143
USA

Ince C
Dept of Anesthesiology
Academic Medical Center
University of Amsterdam
Meibergdreef 9
1105 AZ Amsterdam
The Netherlands

Ioanas M
Dept of Pneumonology
Institut Clinic de Pneumologia
i Chirurgia Toracica
Hospital Clinic Provincial
Villarroel 170
08036 Barcelona
Spain

Jenkins LW
Safar Center
for Resuscitation Research
3434 Fifth Avenue
Pittsburgh, PA 15260
USA

Jeroukhimov I
Division of Trauma
and Critical Care
Ryder Trauma Center
University of Miami School
of Medicine
1600 NW 10th Ave
Miami, FL 33136
USA

Jonas MM
General Intensive Care Unit
Southampton General Hospital
Tremona Road
Shirley
Southampton SO16 6YD
UK

Jones DWM
Dept of Anesthesia
Leeds General Infirmary
Great George Street
Leeds LS1 3EX
UK

Kapral C
Dept of Internal
and Intensive Care Medicine
Konventhospital Barmherzige Brüder
Seilerstätte 2
4020 Linz
Austria

Karpati P
Dept of Anesthesiology
and Critical Care
Lariboisière Hospital
rue A. Paré 2
75475 Paris Cedex 10
France

Kelbel I
Dept of Postoperative
Intensive Care Medicine
Clinic for Anesthesiology
University of Ulm
D-89070 Ulm
Germany

Kellum JA
Division of Critical Care Medicine
University of Pittsburgh Medical
Center
200 Lothrop Street
Pittsburgh, PA 15213-2582
USA

Klein Y
Division of Trauma
and Critical Care
Ryder Trauma Center
University of Miami School of
Medicine
1600 NW 10th Ave
Miami, FL 33136
USA

Knapp S
Laboratory of Experimental
Internal Medicine
Academic Medical Center
Meibergdreef 9
1105 AZ Amsterdam
The Netherlands

Kochanek PM
Safar Center
for Resuscitation Research
3434 Fifth Avenue
Pittsburgh, PA 15260
USA

Kotanidou A
Critical Care Dept
Evangelismos General Hospital
45–47 Ispilandou Street
10676 Athens
Greece

Koutsoukou A
Critical Care Dept
Evangelismos General Hospital
45–47 Ispilandou Street
10676 Athens
Greece

Kubes P
Depts of Physiology and Biophysics
Foothills Medical Center
1403 29th Street NW
Calgary, AB T2N 2T9
Canada

Kuhlen R
Dept of Anesthesiology
University Hospital
Pauwelsstraße 30
D-52074 Aachen
Germany

Kummer C
Dept of Surgery
Toronto General Hospital
200 Elizabeth Street
Toronto
Ontario M5G 2C4
Canada

Laterre PF
Dept of Intensive Care
St. Luc University Hospital
Hippocrate Ave
1200 Brussels
Belgium

Laureys S
Cyclotron Research Center (B30)
University of Liège-Sart Tilman
Allée du 6 août 8
B-4000 Liège
Belgium

Lebuffe G
Dept of Anesthesiology
and Intensive Care Medicine
Lille University Hospital
Rue Michel Polonowski
F-59037 Lille Cedex
France

Lefering R
Biochemical
and Experimental Division
II.nd Dept of Surgery
University of Cologne
Ostmerheimer Straße 200
51109 Köln
Germany

Lenz K
Dept of Internal
and Intensive Care Medicine
Konventhospital Barmherzige Brüder
Seilerstätte 2
4020 Linz
Austria

Levi M
Dept of Vascular Medicine/
Internal Medicine
Academic Medical Center F4
University of Amsterdam
Meibergdreef 9
1105 AZ Amsterdam
The Netherlands

Levy MM
Medical Intensive Care Unit
Rhode Island Hospital
593 Eddy Street
Providence, RI 02903
USA

Liaudet L
Critical Care Division
Dept of Internal Medicine
University Hospital
1011 Lausanne
Switzerland

Ligtenberg JJM
Intensive and Respiratory Care Unit
Dept of Internal Medicine
University Hospital
PO Box 30.001
NL-9700 RB Groningen
The Netherlands

Liistro G
Service de Pneumonologie
Cliniques Universitaires Saint-Luc
Université Catholique de Louvain
Avenue Hippocrate 10
B-1200 Bruxelles
Belgium

Linz NP
Dept of Internal
and Intensive Care Medicine
Konventhospital Barmherzige Brüder
Seilerstätte 2
4020 Linz
Austria

Lipsett P
Depts of Surgery, Anesthesiology,
and Critical Care Medicine
John Hopkins University School
of Medicine
600 N. Wolfe Street
Blalock 685/683
Baltimore, MD 21287-4685
USA

Lynn M
Division of Trauma
and Critical Care
Ryder Trauma Center
University of Miami School
of Medicine
1600 NW 10th Ave
Miami, FL 33136
USA

Maas AIR
Dept of Neurosurgery
Erasmus MC
PO Box 3000
40 Dr. Molewaterplein
NL-3015 GD Rotterdam
The Netherlands

Majerus S
Dept of Neuropsychology
University of Liège-Sart Tilman
Bvd du Rectorat 3, B33
B-4000 Liège
Belgium

Malbrain M
St. Elisabeth Hospital
Ave DeFré 206
B-1180 Brussels
Belgium

Marchetti P
Unité INSERM 459
University of Lille II
Hôpital Cardiologique
59037 Lille Cedex
France

Marggraf G
Dept of Thoracic
and Cardiovascular Surgery
University of Essen Medical School
Essen
Germany

Marik PE
Dept of Critical Care Medicine
University of Pittsburgh Medical
School
Pittsburgh PA 15219-5166
USA

Marshall JC
Dept of Surgery
Toronto General Hospital
200 Elizabeth Street
Toronto
Ontario M5G 2C4
Canada

Massion PB
Dept of Internal Medicine
Unit of Pharmacology
and Therapeutics FATH 5349
University of Louvain Medical
School
53 Ave Mounier
B-1200 Brussels
Belgium

Matos R
Intensive Care Unit
Hospital de St. António
dos Capuchos
1150 Lisbon
Portugal

Mayer SA
Division of Critical Care Neurology
Neurological Institute
710 West 168th Street, Unit 39
New York, NY 10032
USA

McCloskey BV
Regional Intensive Care Unit
The Royal Group of Hospitals Trust
Grosvenor Road
Belfast BT12 6BA
Northern Ireland

Mebazaa A
Dept of Anesthesiology
and Critical Care
Lariboisière Hospital
rue A. Paré 2
75475 Paris Cedex 10
France

Meduri GU
Memphis Lung Research Program
Dept of Medicine
Division of Pulmonary
and Critical Care Medicine
University of Tennessee
Health Sciences Center
956 Court Avenue, Room H314
Memphis, TN 38163
USA

Mercurio G
Dept of Intensive Care
and Anesthesiology
Catholic University
Policlinico A. Gemelli
Largo Agostino Gemelli 8
00168 Rome
Italy

Metnitz PGH
Dept of Anesthesiology
and Intensive Care Medicine
University Hospital of Vienna
Währinger Gürtel 18–20
1090 Vienna
Austria

Michard F
Medical Intensive Care Unit
CHU de Bicêtre
University of Paris XI
78 rue du Général Leclerc
94275 Le Kremlin Bictre cedex
France

Milic-Emili J
Meakins-Christie Laboratories
McGill University
3626 St. Urbain Street
Montreal
Quebec H2X 2P2
Canada

Moonen G
Dept of Neurology
University of Liège-Sart Tilman
Bvd du Rectorat 3, B33
4000 Liège
Belgium

Moreno R
Intensive Care Unit
Hospital de St. António dos
Capuchos
1150 Lisbon
Portugal

Morgan TJ
Intensive Care Facility
Division of Anesthesiology
and Perioperative Medicine
Royal Brisbane Hospital
Herston
Queensland 4029
Australia

Mullan BA
Regional Intensive Care Unit
The Royal Group of Hospitals Trust
Grosvenor Road
Belfast BT12 6BA
Northern Ireland

Murias G
Catedra de Farmacologia
Facultad de Ciencias Medicas
Universidad Nacional de La Plata
La Plata
Argentina

Nahum A
Dept of Pulmonary
and Critical Care Medicine
University of Minnesota
Regions Hospital
640 Jackson Street
St. Paul, MN 55101
USA

Navelesi P
Respiratory Intensive Care Unit
Fondazione Salvatore Maugeri
Via Ferrata 4
27100 Pavia
Italy

Navickis RJ
Hygeia Associates
17988 Brewer Road
Grass Valley
California 95949
USA

Netto FS
Dept of Surgery
Toronto General Hospital
200 Elizabeth Street
Toronto
Ontario M5G 2C4
Canada

Neugebauer E
Biochemical
and Experimental Division
II.nd Dept of Surgery
University of Cologne
Ostmerheimer Straße 200
51109 Köln
Germany

Odding E
Rehabilitation Center
Rijndam Adriaanstichting
Westersingel 300
NL-3015 LJ Rotterdam
The Netherlands

Orfanos SE
Critical Care Dept
Evangelismos General Hospital
45–47 Ispilandou Street
10676 Athens
Greece

Paterson DL
Infectious Disease Division
University of Pittsburgh
Medical Center
Falk Medical Building
3601 5th Avenue
Pittsburgh PA 15213
USA

Patroniti N
Dept of Anesthesia
and Intensive Care
University of Milano-Bicocca
Ospedale San Gerardo Nuovo
dei Tintori
Via Donizetti 106
20052 Monza
Milan
Italy

Pelosi P
Dipartimento di Scienze Cliniche
e Biologica
Universita' degli Studi dell'Insubria
Varese
Italy

Pennisi MA
Dept of Intensive Care
and Anesthesiology
Catholic University
Policlinico A. Gemelli
Largo Agostino Gemelli 8
00168 Rome
Italy

Pesenti A
Dept of Anesthesia
and Intensive Care
University of Milano-Bicocca
Ospedale San Gerardo Nuovo
dei Tintori
Via Donizetti 106
20052 Monza
Milan
Italy

Pestel G
Dept of Anesthesiology
and Intensive Care Medicine
Leopoldina Hospital
Gustav-Adolf-Straße 8
97422 Schweinfurt
Germany

Pinsky MR
Division of Critical Care Medicine
University of Pittsburgh
Medical Center
606 Scaife Hall
3550 Terrace Street
Pittsburgh, PA 15261
USA

Piper I
Dept of Clinical Physics
Institute of Neurological Sciences
South Glasgow University
Hospitals Trust
1345 Govan Road
Glasgow G51 4TF
UK

Pittet JF
Depts of Anesthesia and Surgery
University of California
505 Parnassus Ave
Box 0624, Rm M917
San Francisco, CA 94143
USA

Poelaert J
Dept of Intensive Care
Ghent University Hospital
De Pintelaan 185
B-9000 Ghent
Belgium

Poeze M
Dept of Surgery
University Hospital Maastricht
P Debyelaan 25
6202 AZ Maastricht
The Netherlands

Preckel B
Dept of Anesthesiology
University Hospital
Postfach 10 10 07
D-40001 Düsseldorf
Germany

Putensen C
Dept of Anesthesiology
and Intensive Care Medicine
Rheinische Friedrich-Wilhelms-
University
Sigmund-Freud-Straße 25
D-53105 Bonn
Germany

Racovitza I
Dept of Anesthesia
and Intensive Care
University Hospital
Spitalstraße 21
CH-4031 Basel
Switzerland

Radermacher PL
Dept of Anesthesiology
University of Ulm
Prittwitzstraße 43
D-89075 Ulm
Germany

Ramsay G
Dept of Surgery
University Hospital Maastricht
P Debyelaan 25
6202 AZ Maastricht
The Netherlands

Ranieri VM
Dept of Medicine
Sezione di Anestesiologica
e Rianimazione
Ospedale S. Giovanni Bosco
Corso Dogliotti 14
10126 Torino
Italy

Redman JW
Dept of Anesthesia
and Intensive Care
St. George's Hospital
Cranmer Terrace
London SW17 0RE
UK

Reinhart K
Dept of Anesthesiology
and Intensive Care Medicine
Friedrich-Schiller-University
Bachstraße 17
D-07740 Jena
Germany

Reiter K
Pediatric Intensive Care Unit
University Children's Hospital
Munich
Germany

Renaud E
Dept of Anesthesiology
and Critical Care
Lariboisière Hospital
rue A. Paré 2
75475 Paris Cedex 10
France

Reynaert MS
Dept of Intensive Care
St. Luc University Hospital
Hippocrate Ave
1200 Brussels
Belgium

Rizoli SB
Dept of Critical Care Medicine
University of Toronto
312 Westlake Ave
Toronto
Ontario M4C 4T9
Canada

Roberts I
Crash Trial Coordinating Center
London School of Hygiene &
Tropical Medicine
49–51 Bedford Square
London WC1B 3DP
United Kingdom

Ronco C
Dept of Nephrology
St. Bortolo Hospital
Via Rodolfi
36100 Vicenza
Italy

Roosens C
Dept of Intensive Care
Ghent University Hospital
De Pintelaan 185
B-9000 Ghent
Belgium

Rossaint R
Dept of Anesthesiology
University Hospital
Pauwelsstraße 30
D-52074 Aachen
Germany

Rotstein OD
Division of General Surgery
Toronto General Hospital
200 Elizabeth Street
Eaton North 9-232
Toronto
Ontario M5G 2C4
Canada

Roussos C
Critical Care Dept
Evangelismos General Hospital
45–47 Ispilandou Street
10676 Athens
Greece

Samy A
Center for Surgical Research
University of Alabama at
Birmingham
G094 Volker Hall
1670 University Blvd
Birmingham, AL 35394-0019
USA

Schlack W
Dept of Anesthesiology
University Hospital
Postfach 10 10 07
D-40001 Düsseldorf
Germany

Schultz MJ
Dept of Intensive Care Medicine
Academic Medical Center
Meibergdreef 9
1105 AZ Amsterdam
The Netherlands

Schwacha MG
Center for Surgical Research
University of Alabama at
Birmingham
G094 Volker Hall
1670 University Blvd
Birmingham, AL 35394-0019
USA

Segers P
Hydraulics Laboratory
Biomedical Technology Institute
Ghent University
St. Pietersnieuwstraat 41
B-9000 Ghent
Belgium

Sherwood ER
Dept of Anesthesiology
University of Texas Medical Branch
301 University Boulevard
Galveston, TX 77555-0591
USA

Sibbald WJ
Dept of Medicine
Sunnybrook and Women's Health
Science Center
2074 Bayview Ave
Room D474
Toronto
Ontario M4N 3N5
Canada

Siegemund M
Dept of Anesthesia
and Intensive Care
University Hospital
Spitalstraße 21
CH-4031 Basel
Switzerland

Sinderby C
Dept of Medicine
University of Montreal
12750 27th Avenue
Montreal
Quebec H1E 1Z9
Canada

Singer M
Bloomsbury Institute
of Intensive Care Medicine
Wolfson Institute of Biomedical
Research
Gower Street
London WC1E 6BT
UK

Slutsky AS
Dept of Critical Care Medicine
St. Michael's Hospital
Queen St. Wing
30 Bond Street
Toronto
Ontario M5B 1W8
Canada

Song M
Division of Critical Care Medicine
University of Pittsburgh
Medical Center
200 Lothrop Street
Pittsburgh, PA 15213-2582
USA

Sorkine P
Surgical Intensive Care Unit
Surasky Tel-Aviv Medical Center
6 Weizman Street
Tel-Aviv
Israel

Spahija J
Dept of Medicine
University of Montreal
12750 27th Avenue
Montreal
Quebec H1E 1Z9
Canada

Subramanian S
Division of Critical Care Medicine
University of Pittsburgh
Medical Center
200 Lothrop Street
Pittsburgh, PA 15213-2582
USA

Suger-Wiedeck H
Dept of Postoperative
Intensive Care Medicine
Clinic for Anesthesiology
University of Ulm
D-89070 Ulm
Germany

Sylvester SL
Division of Infectious Diseases
John Hopkins University
School of Medicine
600 N. Wolfe Street
Blalock 685/683
Baltimore, MD 21287-4685
USA

Szabó C
Inotek Corporation
Suite 419E
100 Cummings Center
Beverly, MA 01915
USA

Szold O
Surgical Intensive Care Unit
Surasky Tel-Aviv Medical Center
6 Weizman Street
Tel-Aviv
Israel

Teboul JL
Medical Intensive Care Unit
CHU de Bicêtre
University of Paris XI
78 rue du Général Leclerc
94275 Le Kremlin Bicêtre cedex
France

Thys F
Services des Urgences
Cliniques Universitaires Saint-Luc
Université Catholique de Louvain
Avenue Hippocrate 10
B-1200 Bruxelles
Belgium

Torres A
Dept of Pneumonology
Institut Clinic de Pneumologia
i Chirurgia Toracica
Hospital Clinic Provincial
Villarroel 170
08036 Barcelona
Spain

Traber DL
Investigative Intensive Care Unit
Dept of Anesthesiology
University of Texas Medical Branch
Galveston, TX 77555-0833
USA

Traber LD
Investigative Intensive Care Unit
Dept of Anesthesiology
University of Texas Medical Branch
Galveston, TX 77555-0833
USA

Träger K
Dept of Postoperative
Intensive Care Medicine
Clinic for Anesthesiology
University of Ulm
Prittwitzstraße 43
D-89075 Ulm
Germany

Uhlig T
Dept of Anesthesiology
and Intensive Care Medicine
Friedrich-Schiller-University
Bachstraße 17
D-07740 Jena
Germany

Vallet B
Dept of Anesthesiology
and Intensive Care Medicine
Lille University Hospital
Rue Michel Polonowski
F-59037 Lille Cedex
France

van Baalen B
Dept of Rehabilitation Medicine
University Hospital
PO Box 3000
Westersingel 300
NL-3015 LJ Rotterdam
The Netherlands

van der Hoeven JG
Dept of Intensive Care
Jeroen Bosch Hospital
PO Box 90153
5200 ME 's-Hertogenbosch
The Netherlands

van der Poll T
Dept of Infectious Diseases,
Tropical Medicine and AIDS
Academic Medical Center
Meibergdreef 9
1105 AZ Amsterdam
The Netherlands

van Haren FMP
Dept of Intensive Care
Jeroen Bosch Hospital
PO Box 90153
5200 ME 's-Hertogenbosch
The Netherlands

Varon J
Pulmonary and Critical Care Section
Baylor College of Medicine
2219 Dorrington
Houston, TX 77030
USA

Venkatesh B
Intensive Care Facility
Division of Anesthesiology
and Perioperative Medicine
Royal Brisbane Hospital
Herston
Queensland 4029
Australia

Verschuren F
Services des Urgences
Cliniques Universitaires Saint-Luc
Université Catholique de Louvain
Avenue Hippocrate 10
B-1200 Bruxelles
Belgium

Vink R
Dept of Vascular Medicine/
Internal Medicine
Academic Medical Center F4
University of Amsterdam
Meibergdreef 9
1105 AZ Amsterdam
The Netherlands

Ward NS
Medical Intensive Care Unit
Rhode Island Hospital
593 Eddy Street
Providence, RI 02903
USA

Wendon J
Institute of Liver Studies
LITU
King's College Hospital
Denmark Hill
London SE5 9RJ
UK

Whitehouse T
Bloomsbury Institute
of Intensive Care Medicine
Wolfson Institute
of Biomedical Research
Gower Street
London WC1E 6BT
UK

Wiel E
Dept of Anesthesiology
and Intensive Care Medicine
Lille University Hospital
Rue Michel Polonowski
F-59037 Lille Cedex
France

Wilkes MM
Hygeia Associates
17988 Brewer Road
Grass Valley, CA 95949
USA

Williams BJ
Dept of Anesthesia
and Intensive Care Medicine
Hammersmith Hospital
Du Cane Road
London W12 0HS
UK

Wolff CB
Dept of Clinical Pharmacology
St. Bartholomew and the London
Hospital medical and Dental Schools
Turner Street
London E1 2AD
UK

Woodson LC
Dept of Anesthesiology
University of Texas Medical Branch
301 University Boulevard
Galveston, TX 77555-0591
USA

Wyncoll DLA
Dept of Intensive Care
St. Thomas' Hospital
Lambeth Palace Road
London SE1 JEH
UK

Young GB
Dept of Clinical
Neurological Sciences
London Health Sciences Center
339 Windermere Road
London
Ontario N6A 5A5
Canada

Zijlstra JG
Intensive and Respiratory Care Unit
Dept of Internal Medicine
University Hospital
PO Box 30.001
NL-9700 RB Groningen
The Netherlands

Zygun DA
Dept of Medicine
Foothills Medical Center
1403 29th Street NW
Calgary, AB T2N 2T9
Canada

Common Abbreviations

AIDS	Acquired immunodeficiency syndrome
ALI	Acute lung injury
APACHE	Acute physiology and chronic health evaluation
APC	Activated protein C
APP	Abdominal perfusion pressure
ARDS	Acute respiratory distress syndrome
ATP	Adenosine triphosphate
BiPAP	Bilevel positive airway pressure
CBF	Cerebral blood flow
CNS	Central nervous system
COPD	Chronic obstructive pulmonary disease
CPAP	Continuous positive airway pressure
CPP	Cerebral perfusion pressure
CSF	Cerebrospinal fluid
CT	Computerized tomography
CVP	Central venous pressure
CVVH	Continuous veno-venous hemofiltration
DIC	Disseminated intravascular coagulation
DNA	Deoxyribonucleic acid
DO_2	Oxygen delivery
ECMO	Extracorporeal membrane oxygenation
EEG	Electroencephalogram
EKG	Electrocardiogram
ELISA	Enzyme-linked immunosorbent assay
EVLW	Extravascular lung water
FRC	Functional residual capacity
GCS	Glasgow coma scale
G-CSF	Granulocyte-colony stimulating factor
HIV	Human immunodeficiency virus
IAH	Intra-abdominal hypertension
IAP	Intra-abdominal pressure
ICAM	Intercellular adhesion molecule

ICH	Intracranial hypertension
ICP	Intracranial pressure
ICU	Intensive care unit
IFN	Interferon
IL	Interleukin
IMV	Intermittent mandatory ventilation
I/R	Ischemia-reperfusion
IV	Intravenous
LPS	Lipopolysaccharide
MAP	Mean arterial pressure
MAPK	Mitogen-activated protein kinase
MOF	Multiple organ failure
MRI	Magnetic resonance imaging
NAD	Nicotinamide adenine dinucleotide
NF-κB	Nuclear factor kappa-B
NIV	Non-invasive ventilation
NO	Nitric oxide
NOS	Nitric oxide synthase
PAI	Plasminogen activator inhibitor
PAOP	Pulmonary artery occlusion pressure
PARS	Poly-ADP ribose synthetase
PEEP	Positive end-expiratory pressure
pHi	Gastric intramucosal pH
PMN	Polymorphonuclear leukocyte
PSV	Pressure support ventilation
RBC	Red blood cell
RNA	Ribonucleic acid
ROS	Reactive oxygen species
SAPS	Simplified acute physiology score
SIRS	Systemic inflammatory response syndrome
SOD	Superoxide dismutase
SVR	Systemic vascular resistance
TBI	Traumatic brain injury
TLC	Total lung capacity
TNF	Tumor necrosis factor
VCAM	Vascular cell adhesion molecule
VILI	Ventilator-induced lung injury
VO_2	Oxygen consumption
WBC	White blood cell
ZEEP	Zero end-expiratory pressure

Cellular Responses

Ischemia-reperfusion and Acute Apoptotic Cell Death

B.S. Abella and L.B. Becker

▌ Introduction

Ischemia, reperfusion, and apoptosis are vital physiological processes that demonstrate fantastic complexity. These processes have stimulated much interest, and even controversy, in part due to the important role they play in determining cell injury and cell death. Both basic scientists and clinicians understand the importance of elucidating these mechanisms. In this chapter, we will discuss the importance of ischemia in human disease, explore the events of reperfusion that may contribute to cell injury following ischemia, review the primary mechanisms of apoptosis, and finally speculate on the mechanisms that link ischemia-reperfusion (I/R) and acute apoptosis.

▌ Ischemia: Scope of the Problem

Ischemic disease, in which blood flow is compromised to a regional vascular bed, whole organ, or globally to the entire organism, is responsible for an enormous degree of morbidity and mortality from such varied conditions as cardiac arrest, cerebrovascular accident, traumatic injury, and myocardial infarction [1]. Ischemia to other organs such as kidney, bowel or liver can also produce severe illness, and can occur as a consequence of clinical situations from septic shock to hypotension during surgery. Numerous clinical observations and laboratory studies support the notion that however deleterious ischemia can be, reperfusion of ischemic tissues may also provoke additional adverse consequences [2–7]. While the treatment of ischemia must eventually reperfuse ischemic tissues, our current techniques for reestablishing blood flow promote a severe inflammatory response as well as production of oxygen free radicals, lipid peroxidation, and accelerated cell death. Recently it has been appreciated that these events are also associated with a marked degree of acute apoptotic cell death, with apoptotic markers appearing far more rapidly (in minutes to hours) than earlier reports of apoptosis where cell death required days to become manifest. The effects of this I/R injury can be experienced beyond the scope of the directly injured tissue. Often, profound I/R results in the systemic inflammatory response syndrome (SIRS) and multi-organ system failure (MOF), a leading cause of death in the intensive care unit (ICU) [8].

Perhaps the most dramatic example of I/R injury is demonstrated by resuscitation from cardiac arrest. Cardiac arrest, which represents global whole body ischemic disease, results in at least 300 000 deaths each year in the United States alone

[9]. Survival from cardiac arrest remains dismal some 40 years after the introduction of cardiac compression and electrical defibrillation, with only 1–11% of patients surviving until hospital discharge after out-of-hospital cardiac arrest [10, 11]. While initial survival from in-hospital cardiac arrest ranges from 25 to over 50%, subsequent survival until hospital discharge is much lower, from 5–22% [12, 13], suggesting that nearly 90% mortality occurs shortly after initial return of spontaneous circulation. Some of this mortality after return of normal circulation may be due to events related to reperfusion injury.

Given the importance of these I/R phenomena, intensive research has examined the various pathophysiologic consequences of I/R, including free radical production, inflammation, and apoptosis (reviewed in [14, 15]). Tissue culture and animal models alike have now been used to demonstrate apoptotic activity after varying degrees of I/R. In this review, we will consider the role of apoptosis, or programmed cell death, after I/R injury. The field of apoptosis has expanded dramatically in recent years, with the importance of cell death mechanisms now recognized to play a role in processes as divergent as nervous system development, immune system regulation, and myocardial infarction (for reviews see [16–18]).

▌ Ischemia-reperfusion

A number of mechanisms have been implicated in the pathophysiology of I/R. The depletion of intracellular energy stores during ischemia results in poor ionic pump function, allowing sodium and calcium influx into ischemic cells. Inflammatory cytokines are produced by endothelium undergoing I/R, and the subsequent inflammation of local tissue can provoke a number of damaging responses [19]. Reactive oxygen species (ROS) such as superoxide, hydrogen peroxide, and hydroxyl radical, produced in small quantities during normal cellular metabolism, are generated in large bursts after I/R, overwhelming scavenging systems such as superoxide dismutase (SOD), catalase, and glutathione peroxidase and leading to tissue damage [20, 21]. Compounding the problem, the preceding ischemia diminishes natural ROS defenses and scavenging mechanisms, leaving tissues even more vulnerable to the burst of ROS associated with reperfusion [22].

A variety of ROS can be produced by cellular mechanisms [14]. These include superoxide radical, hydrogen peroxide, hydroxyl radical, and peroxynitrite. Superoxide can be generated either via the mitochondrial transport chain, as a product of the cyclooxygenase and lipoxygenase pathways, by xanthine oxidase (XO), or by NAD(P)H oxidase within the cell. Superoxide in turn can be metabolized to hydrogen peroxide via the SOD enzymes. Hydrogen peroxide can react with copper and iron atoms via a Fenton reaction to produce the most reactive and destructive ROS, hydroxyl radicals. Finally, the direct reaction of superoxide and nitric oxide (NO) can generate peroxynitrite, another ROS that may have important direct tissue effects (Fig. 1).

ROS production after I/R has been studied in a variety of systems, including tissue culture [7], isolated heart preparations [23], and in intact organisms [24]. ROS can lead to cellular damage via several processes. Direct oxidation of lipid can disrupt both cellular and subcellular membranes [25, 26]. Reperfusion is an essential component of this process, as studies in cardiac tissue show that lipid oxidation is not observed when ROS are inactivated by specific scavengers [27, 28]. Oxidation

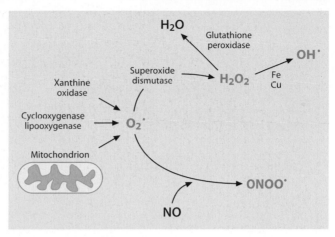

Fig. 1. Cellular generation of reactive oxygen species (ROS). Radicals are noted with a dot, indicating an un-paired electron. The ROS are shown in gray, while other molecules and enzymes are shown in black. $O_2^{\bullet}$: super-oxide; H_2O_2: hydrogen peroxide; $OH^{\bullet}$: hydroxyl radical; $ONOO^{\bullet}$: peroxynitrite; NO: nitric oxide; H_2O: water

of protein sulfhydryl groups can damage cellular structure and enzymatic machin-ery [29]. ROS can also contribute to a specific increase in mitochondrial membrane permeability known as the mitochondrial permeability transition [26], leading to the uncoupling of oxidative phosphorylation and further ROS generation. The physiologic importance of ROS is emphasized by studies showing that transgenic mice which overexpress SOD have a reduction in I/R injury [30]. Similarly, I/R damage was attenuated in hearts from mice containing an additional glutathione peroxidase transgene [31], and I/R injury was increased in heart and brain from mice made homozygous for a glutathione peroxidase gene disruption [31, 32]. Col-lectively, these studies suggest that ROS play an important role within the cell dur-ing ischemia and early moments of reperfusion directly related to cell injury and death.

▌ Apoptosis

The mechanisms by which a cell undergoes programmed cell death, termed apopto-sis in 1972 by Currie and colleagues [33], have been the subject of an enormous body of work over the past two decades (for reviews see [17, 34, 35]). We can only offer a brief summary here. A cell can receive signals to undergo apoptosis either from external sources or from within the cell itself. Extrinsic signals can come in the form of extracellular proteins such as the Fas ligand which binds Fas trans-membrane receptors (members of the tumor necrosis factor [TNF] receptor family) on the surface of the cell and trigger a cascade of intracellular changes leading to apoptosis [36]. Intrinsic signals, produced during hypoxia or reperfusion, can be sensed by a variety of intracellular proteins which can similarly initiate a series of biochemical processes leading to cell death.

Cellular apoptotic machinery can be categorized into three groups: promoters (pro-apoptotic proteins such as bax and bid), inhibitors (anti-apoptotic proteins

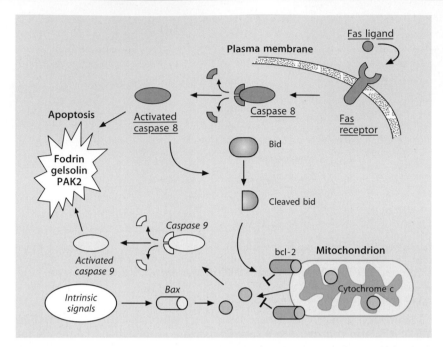

Fig. 2. Mechanisms of apoptosis. In this oversimplified diagram, the intrinsic pathway (sometimes referred to as the 'mitochondrial' pathway) is highlighted in italic, and the extrinsic pathway (sometimes referred to as the 'ligand-mediated' pathway) is underlined. 'Intrinsic signals' may represent a number of cell stresses including DNA damage and ischemia. Note that some interplay between the two pathways does exist, as demonstrated in this figure by the mechanism of bid translocation to the mitochondrion. Both pathways contribute to cytochrome c release from the mitochondrial membrane, a crucial intermediate step in apoptosis. See accompanying text for narrative description of these mechanisms

such as bcl-2 and bcl-xL) and executors of programmed cell death (such as the caspases). Bcl-2, originally identified as a gene involved in B-cell lymphoma [37], is a potent inhibitor of apoptosis found in mitochondrial and nuclear membranes. Interestingly, the cell death inhibitory properties of bcl-2 remain, even when the protein is excluded from mitochondrial localization [38]. Promotors of apoptosis, such as bax, can bind to bcl-2 and block its inhibition of cell death. Other promotors such as bid remain inactive in the cytosol, and when activated can move to mitochondria and promote apoptotic changes [39]. Caspases, cysteine proteases which cleave proteins after aspartic acid residues, are the executors of programmed cell death. The caspases, previously called interleukin (IL)-converting enzyme or ICE proteases [40], cleave a variety of substrate proteins after aspartic acid residues, with target specificity conferred by the four amino acids adjacent to the cleavage site [41]. More than ten human caspase genes have been characterized [42]. The caspases cleave proteins such as fodrin and gelsolin, which are responsible for cytoskeletal structure [43, 44], and p21-activated kinase 2 (PAK2), which in turn seems to activate the 'blebbing' of apoptotic cells seen on histopathology [45]. These mechanisms are summarized in Figure 2.

The apoptotic machinery outlined above plays an important role in a number of cellular insults, such as radiation damage to DNA [46], drug toxicity [47], and hypoxia [48]; it certainly plays a clinically important role in the defense against inappropriate cell division as seen in oncogenesis [46, 49]. Recent work has begun to elucidate the role apoptosis plays after I/R injury. These data have come from tissue culture, isolated organ preparations and whole animal studies of single organ I/R models (reviewed in [14, 26, 34]).

∎ Ischemia-reperfusion: A Trigger of Apoptosis

The expression patterns of both promotors and inhibitors of apoptosis are consistent with a role for programmed cell death in I/R injury. The apoptosis inhibitor bcl-2 is strongly expressed in neurons which survive ischemic insult. Conversely, the apoptosis promotor bax is observed to be upregulated in areas of brain most sensitive to ischemic injury such as the CA1 region of the hippocampus [50, 51]. While largely regulated by post-translational mechanisms, induction of caspase transcription is also seen just hours after ischemic insult [50]. Similar experiments in kidney ischemia models have also shown differential expression of bcl-2 and bax in patterns suggestive of their role in ischemic injury [52].

Cell culture systems have been used to demonstrate apoptotic phenomena after simulated I/R injury [53]. One clear advantage of these *ex vivo* models is the ability to carefully probe molecular mechanisms of cell death. For example, mitochondrial mechanisms play an important role in the apoptotic process in cardiac myocytes, as might be expected [54]. Apoptosis has also been demonstrated after serum starvation in neuronal cell culture [55], and work is underway in our laboratory to establish an I/R injury model in both cardiomyocytes and neuronal culture to assay for markers of apoptosis (K. Hamann et al., unpublished results).

Recent work has demonstrated a direct link between the machinery of apoptosis and injury after ischemic insult. Intraventricular administration of selective caspase inhibitors into the rat brain reduced the extent of injury after ischemia [56]. Armstrong et al. [57] introduced caspase inhibitors into rat hearts undergoing I/R and found a reduction in infarct size. Using a genetic approach, Peng et al. [58] showed that disruption of apoptotic machinery at a variety of targets also decreases infarct size after I/R. Some questions regarding the importance of post-reperfusion apoptosis still remain, however. Tekin et al. [59] found that Fas receptor or ligand knockout hearts undergoing I/R had markedly reduced degrees of apoptosis compared to wild-type controls, but did not show differences in myocardial function or infarct size.

A mechanistic linkage between I/R injury and apoptosis may involve ROS. Augmentation of SOD function in kidney cell culture reduces the degree of apoptosis after I/R injury [60]. Oxidative stress may be sensed by mitochondrial sensors in the form of thiol oxidation, which can trigger apoptotic pathways [61]. Evidence for the role of ROS in the promotion of apoptosis has been provided by transgenic mouse models. Maulik et al. [31] demonstrated that increased apoptotic activity occurred in an isolated mouse heart model of I/R injury when glutathione peroxidase was genetically disrupted. In the same investigation, hearts undergoing I/R had fewer apoptotic nuclei if the cells carried an extra copy of the glutathione peroxidase gene. Mice transgenic for an extra SOD gene showed greatly attenuated apoptosis compared to wild-type animals after pharmacologic injury [62].

▌ Conclusion

Linkage of I/R injury and apoptosis has been suggested by cell culture and targeted organ studies, both in wild-type and transgenic animals. However, an important question regarding the role that humeral and other global factors might play in the triggering of apoptosis after I/R injury still remains poorly understood. The Fas receptor pathway clearly demonstrates the role of extracellular ligands in the initiation of programmed cell death. Fas stimulation has been shown to induce apoptosis after brain ischemia, for example [63]. Whether ligands from distant sources and other soluble factors might modulate apoptotic stimulation can only be answered by whole animal model systems. This is especially important given the context-dependent nature of apoptosis. Signals that promote apoptosis in one model have been shown to suppress cell death in another [34]. An intriguing example of the role distant factors might play in the process of programmed cell death is the evidence that sera from critically ill patients can induce endothelial cell apoptosis [64]. Particularly important to the clinician is the opportunity for therapeutic intervention to save ischemic cells. It is likely that anti-apoptotic agents will be used in the treatment of ischemia in the future. The much sought after cellular 'point of no return' remains elusive and controversial, and may not exist as a single point at all. The development of whole animal models of global ischemia will help further our understanding of this complex and clinically important process.

Acknowledgements. We thank Lynne Harnish and Terry Vanden Hoek for their assistance in the preparation of this manuscript.

References

1. Weil MH, Becker LB, Budinger T, et al (2001) Workshop executive summary report: postresuscitative and initial utility in life saving efforts (PULSE). Circulation 103:1182–1184
2. Parks DA, Granger DN (1986) Contributions of ischemia and reperfusion to mucosal lesion formation. Am J Physiol 250:G749–G753
3. Hearse DJ, Bolli R (1991) Reperfusion induced injury: manifestations, mechanisms, and clinical relevance. Trends Cardiovasc Med 1:233–240
4. Hearse DJ, Humphrey SM, Chain FB (1973) Abrupt reoxygenation of the anoxic potassium-arrested heart: a study of myocardial enzyme release. J Mol Cell Cardiol 5:395–407
5. Opie LH (1989) Reperfusion injury and its pharmacologic modification. Circulation 80:1049–1062
6. Vanden Hoek TL, Shao Z, Li C, Zak R, Schumacker PT, Becker LB (1996) Reperfusion injury in cardiac myocytes after simulated ischemia. Am J Physiol 270:H1334–H1341
7. Vanden Hoek TL, Becker LB, Shao Z, Li C, Schumacker PT (1998) Reactive oxygen species released from mitochondria during brief hypoxia induce preconditioning in cardiomyocytes. J Biol Chem 273:18092–18098
8. Neary P, Redmond HP (1999) Ischaemia-reperfusion injury and the systemic inflammatory response syndrome. In: Grace PA, Mathie RT (eds) Ischemia-Reperfusion Injury. Blackwell Science, London, pp 123–136
9. Thel MC, O'Connor CM (1999) Cardiopulmonary resuscitation: Historical perspective to recent investigations. Am Heart J 137:39–48
10. Gaul GB, Gruska M, Titscher G, et al (1996) Prediction of survival after out-of-hospital cardiac arrest: results of a community-based study in Vienna. Resuscitation 32:169–176
11. Becker LB, Han BH, Meyer PM, et al (1993) CPR Chicago: Racial differences in the incidence of cardiac arrest and subsequent survival. N Engl J Med 329:600–606
12. Saklayen M, Liss H, Markert R (1995) In-hospital cardiopulmonary resuscitation survival in one hospital and literature review. Medicine 74:163–175

13. Cooper S, Cade J (1997) Predicting survival, in-hospital cardiac arrests: resuscitation survival variables and training effectiveness. Resuscitation 35:17–22
14. Collard CDS (2001) Pathophysiology, clinical manifestations, and prevention of ischemia-reperfusion injury. Anesthesiology 94:1133–1138
15. Ambrosio G, Tritto I (1999) Reperfusion injury: experimental evidence and clinical implications. Am Heart J 138:S69–S75
16. Krammer PH (2000) CD95's deadly mission in the immune system. Nature 407:789–795
17. Hengartner MO (2000) The biochemistry of apoptosis. Nature 407:770–776
18. Nicholson DW (2000) From bench to clinic with apoptosis-based therapeutic agents. Nature 407:810–816
19. Beekhuizen H, van de Gevel JS (1998) Endothelial cell adhesion molecules in inflammation and postischemic reperfusion injury. Transplant Proc 30:4251–4256
20. Ambrosio G, Flaherty JT, Duilio C, et al (1991) Oxygen radicals generated at reflow induce peroxidation of membrane lipids in reperfused hearts. J Clin Invest 87:2056–2066
21. Zweier JL, Flaherty JT, Weisfeldt ML (1987) Direct measurement of free radical generation following reperfusion of ischemic myocardium. Proc Natl Acad Sci USA 84:1404–1407
22. Ferrari R, Ceconi C, Curello S, et al (1985) Oxygen-mediated myocardial damage during ischaemia and reperfusion: role of the cellular defences against oxygen toxicity. J Mol Cell Cardiol 17:937–945
23. Weinbroum AA, Hochhauser E, Rudick V, et al (1999) Multiple organ dysfunction after remote circulatory arrest: common pathway of radical oxygen species? J Trauma 47:691–698
24. Bolli R, Jeroudi MO, Patel BS, et al (1989) Direct evidence that oxygen-derived free radicals contribute to postischemic myocardial dysfunction in the intact dog. Proc Natl Acad Sci USA 86:4695–4699
25. Romaschin AD, Wilson GJ, Thomas U, Feitler DA, Tumiati L, Mickle DA (1990) Subcellular distribution of peroxidized lipids in myocardial reperfusion injury. Am J Physiol 259: H116–H123
26. Neumar RW (2000) Molecular mechanisms of ischemic neuronal injury. Ann Emerg Med 36:483–506
27. Becker LC, Ambrosio G (1987) Myocardial consequences of reperfusion. Prog Cardiovasc Dis 30:23–41
28. Ferreira R, Burgos M, Llesuy S, et al (1989) Reduction of reperfusion injury with mannitol cardioplegia. Ann Thorac Surg 48:77–83
29. Oliver CN, Starke-Reed PE, Stadtman ER, Liu GJ, Carney JM, Floyd RA (1990) Oxidative damage to brain proteins, loss of glutamine synthetase activity, and production of free radicals during ischemia/reperfusion-induced injury to gerbil brain. Proc Natl Acad Sci USA 87:5144–5147
30. Wang P, Chen H, Qin H, et al (1998) Overexpression of human copper, zinc-superoxide dismutase (SOD1) prevents postischemic injury. Proc Natl Acad Sci USA 95:4556–4560
31. Maulik N, Yoshida T, Das DK (1999) Regulation of cardiomyocyte apoptosis in ischemic reperfused mouse heart by glutathione peroxidase. Mol Cell Biochem 196:13–21
32. Crack PJ, Taylor JM, Flentjar NJ, et al (2001) Increased infarct size and exacerbated apoptosis in the glutathione peroxidase-1 (Gpx-1) knockout mouse brain in response to ischemia/reperfusion injury. J Neurochem 78:1389–1399
33. Kerr JF, Wyllie AH, Currie AR (1972) Apoptosis: a basic biological phenomenon with wide-ranging implications in tissue kinetics. Br J Cancer 26:239–257
34. MacManus JP, Linnik MD (1997) Gene expression induced by cerebral ischemia: an apoptotic perspective. J Cereb Blood Flow Metab 17:815–832
35. Jacobson MD, Weil M, Raff MC (1997) Programmed cell death in animal development. Cell 88:347–354
36. Hamann KJ, Vieira JE, Halayko AJ, et al (2000) Fas cross-linking induces apoptosis in human airway smooth muscle cells. Am J Physiol 278:L618–L624
37. Tsujimoto Y, Cossman J, Jaffe E, Croce CM (1985) Involvement of the bcl-2 gene in human follicular lymphoma. Science 228:1440–1443
38. Zhu W, Cowie A, Wasfy GW, Penn LZ, Leber B, Andrews DW (1996) Bcl-2 mutants with restricted subcellular location reveal spatially distinct pathways for apoptosis in different cell types. Embo J 15:4130–4141

39. Li H, Zhu H, Xu CJ, Yuan J (1998) Cleavage of BID by caspase 8 mediates the mitochondrial damage in the Fas pathway of apoptosis. Cell 94:491–501
40. Alnemri ES, Livingston DJ, Nicholson DW, et al (1996) Human ICE/CED-3 protease nomenclature. Cell 87:171
41. Thornberry NA, Rano TA, Peterson EP, et al (1997) A combinatorial approach defines specificities of members of the caspase family and granzyme B. Functional relationships established for key mediators of apoptosis. J Biol Chem 272:17907–17911
42. Earnshaw WC, Martins LM, Kaufmann SH (1999) Mammalian caspases: structure, activation, substrates, and functions during apoptosis. Annu Rev Biochem 68:383–424
43. Kothakota S, Azuma T, Reinhard C, et al (1997) Caspase-3-generated fragment of gelsolin: effector of morphological change in apoptosis. Science 278:294–298
44. Nicholson DW (1999) Caspase structure, proteolytic substrates, and function during apoptotic cell death. Cell Death Differ 6:1028–1034
45. Rudel T, Bokoch GM (1997) Membrane and morphological changes in apoptotic cells regulated by caspase-mediated activation of PAK2. Science 276:1571–1574
46. Lowe SW, Schmitt EM, Smith SW, Osborne BA, Jacks T (1993) p53 is required for radiation-induced apoptosis in mouse thymocytes. Nature 362:847–849
47. Bach SP, Renehan AG, Potten CS (2000) Stem cells: the intestinal stem cell as a paradigm. Carcinogenesis 21:469–476
48. Han BH, DeMattos RB, Dugan LL, et al (2001) Clusterin contributes to caspase-3-independent brain injury following neonatal hypoxia-ischemia. Nat Med 7:338–343
49. Knudson CM, Tung KS, Tourtellotte WG, Brown GA, Korsmeyer SJ (1995) Bax-deficient mice with lymphoid hyperplasia and male germ cell death. Science 270:96–99
50. Asahi M, Hoshimaru M, Uemura Y, et al (1997) Expression of interleukin-1 beta converting enzyme gene family and bcl-2 gene family in the rat brain following permanent occlusion of the middle cerebral artery. J Cereb Blood Flow Metab 17:11–18
51. Chen J, Graham SH, Nakayama M, et al (1997) Apoptosis repressor genes Bcl-2 and Bcl-x-long are expressed in the rat brain following global ischemia. J Cereb Blood Flow Metab 17:2–10
52. Gobe G, Zhang XJ, Cuttle L, et al (1999) Bcl-2 genes and growth factors in the pathology of ischaemic acute renal failure. Immunol Cell Biol 77:279–286
53. Xu M, Wang Y, Ayub A, Ashraf M (2001) Mitochondrial K(ATP) channel activation reduces anoxic injury by restoring mitochondrial membrane potential. Am J Physiol 281:H1295–H1303
54. Shiraishi J, Tatsumi T, Keira N, et al (2001) Important role of energy-dependent mitochondrial pathways in cultured rat cardiac myocyte apoptosis. Am J Physiol 281:H1637–H1647
55. Gil-Ad I, Shtaif B, Luria D, Karp L, Fridman Y, Weizman A (1999) Insulin-like-growth-factor-I (IGF-I) antagonizes apoptosis induced by serum deficiency and doxorubicin in neuronal cell culture. Growth Horm IGF Res 9:458–464
56. Loddick SA, MacKenzie A, Rothwell NJ (1996) An ICE inhibitor, z-VAD-DCB attenuates ischaemic brain damage in the rat. Neuroreport 7:1645–1658
57. Armstrong RC, Li F, Smiley R, et al (2001) Caspase inhibitors reduce infarct size when dosed post-reperfusion in a rodent cardiac ischemia/reperfusion model. Circulation 104 (Suppl):II-12 (Abst)
58. Peng CF, Lee P, Deguzman A, et al (2001) Multiple independent mutations in apoptotic signaling pathways markedly decrease infarct size due to myocardial ischemia-reperfusion. Circulation 104 (Suppl):II-187 (Abst)
59. Tekin D, Gursoy E, Xi L, Kukreja R (2001) Genetic disruption of Fas receptor or Fas ligand reduces myocardial apoptosis, but not infarct size caused by ischemia/perfusion injury. Circulation 104 (Suppl):II-12
60. Chien CT, Lee PH, Chen CF, Ma MC, Lai MK, Hsu SM (2001) De novo demonstration and co-localization of free-radical production and apoptosis formation in rat kidney subjected to ischemia/reperfusion. J Am Soc Nephrol 12:973–982
61. Marchetti P, Decaudin D, Macho A, et al (1997) Redox regulation of apoptosis: impact of thiol oxidation status on mitochondrial function. Eur J Immunol 27:289–296
62. Deng X, Cadet JL (2000) Methamphetamine-induced apoptosis is attenuated in the striata of copper-zinc superoxide dismutase transgenic mice. Brain Res Mol Brain Res 83:121–124

63. Felderhoff-Mueser U, Taylor DL, Greenwood K, et al (2000) Fas/CD95/APO-1 can function as a death receptor for neuronal cells in vitro and in vivo and is upregulated following cerebral hypoxic-ischemic injury to the developing rat brain. Brain Pathol 10:17–29

64. Assaly R, Olson D, Hammersley J, et al (2001) Initial evidence of endothelial cell apoptosis as a mechanism of systemic capillary leak syndrome. Chest 120:1301–1308

Alpha-4 Integrin:
A Novel Mechanism for Neutrophil-endothelial Interaction

V. Gill, P. Kubes, and C.J. Doig

▌ Introduction

The systemic inflammatory response syndrome (SIRS) is a ubiquitous characteristic of critically ill, intensive care unit (ICU) patients. The most commonly studied condition that results in SIRS is septic shock. In septic shock, a microbial agent causes a localized tissue injury resulting in a systemic inflammatory response leading to secondary injury to organs not primarily infected by the microbial agent. The consequence of secondary organ injury is often serious morbidity or death from multisystem organ failure (MOF). Severe sepsis syndrome/septic shock continues to be associated with a mortality rate of 20–50% in most tertiary care ICUs [1, 2] Despite advances in the physiologic support of these patients, and multiple studies assessing the activation of the inflammatory cascade and therapeutic interventions with immunomodulatory therapy, consistently effective treatment remains elusive [3]. In fact, the only therapy recently demonstrated to be effective, recombinant human activated protein C, targets the coagulation cascade rather than acting as a specific 'anti-inflammatory' agent [4]. Although the inflammatory and coagulation cascades are related, the pathophysiology of the association, including neutrophil activation and endothelial interactions, remains poorly understood. Activation and migration of leukocytes, specifically neutrophils, to sites of primary and secondary tissue injury is the basis of the pathogenesis of inflammatory conditions including septic shock [5–7].

For neutrophils to localize at the site of injury, the cells must move from the circulating vascular pool through the vascular endothelium to the extravascular space. The process of neutrophil recruitment occurs in three sequential phases, each dependent on the preceding phase. First, neutrophils flowing through the vascular compartment make initial contact with the vascular endothelium by tethering and rolling. Second, the neutrophils migrate and become firmly adherent to the endothelium. Finally, the adherent neutrophils migrate through the endothelium to the extravascular interstitial space and to the site of tissue injury (Fig. 1).

Convention has attributed all neutrophil-endothelial cell interactions as mediated by the selectins and the β_2 integrins. Initial tethering and rolling of neutrophils is thought to be dependent on L-selectin, P-selectin ligand 1, and an E-selectin ligand expressed on the surface membrane of neutrophils [8–10]. These neutrophil receptors interact with ligands expressed on the surface of endothelial cells, including P-selectin, which is rapidly mobilized, E-selectin, which is expressed subsequent to endothelial stimulation with inflammatory cytokines, and L-selectin ligands yet to be fully identified [11–15]. Firm adhesion is mediated by β_2-integrins (CD11/CD18) on the neutrophil surface interacting with multiple endothelial ligands (such as intercellular adhesion molecule [ICAM]-1) [16–19].

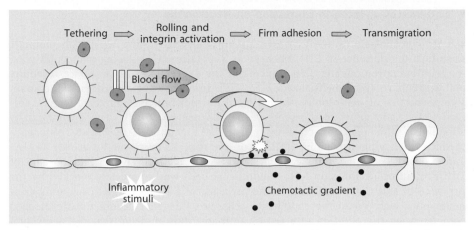

Fig. 1. The leukocyte recruitment cascade. Fast-moving leukocytes in the blood stream tether and roll on activated endothelium via interactions between selectins and their ligands, or in some cases integrin (very late antigen [VLA]-4)-immunoglobulin superfamily (vascular cell adhesion molecule [VCAM]-1) interactions. Chemokines or other pro-adhesive mediators released by various sources are presented to rolling leukocytes on the endothelium resulting in integrin activation and firm adhesion. Firm adhesion permits leukocyte transmigration across the endothelium and entry into inflamed tissue

The importance of β_2-integrins in this process was in part initially identified by clinical observations of individuals who congenitally lack β_2-integrins (leukocyte adhesion deficiency type 1). These individuals cannot accumulate neutrophils at inflammatory sites as the cells are unable to adhere to biological substratum [20].

Leukocytes interact with the vascular endothelium and migrate to sites of tissue injury in response to inflammatory stimuli [21–23]. Peripheral blood mononuclear cells (PBMCs) such as circulating monocytes, eosinophils and lymphocytes, express α_4-integrin. Via interaction with VCAM-1 (vascular cell adhesion molecule-1), PBMCs can utilize this pathway to mediate tethering, rolling and firm adhesion to the endothelium. In the tissue matrix, α_4-integrin is important as a mechanism to mediate mononuclear cell attachment by interacting with ligands such as fibronectin, and has been implicated in several diseases including contact hypersensitivity, allergic asthma, inflammatory bowel disease, and cardiac allograft failure [24–27].

Despite the premise that PBMCs and neutrophils interact and migrate to sites of tissue injury by different processes, there are recent important clinical observations that suggest that this may not be correct. Specifically, there is evidence that neutrophils may infiltrate tissues, including lungs, joints, and retroperitoneum, via a pathway independent of β_2-integrins [28–31]. We will review evidence that has demonstrated the presence of α_4-integrins *in vitro* on the surface of neutrophils, their functional expression following chemotactic stimuli, and the possible role of α_4-integrin in tissue injury. Finally, we will summarize recent evidence utilizing whole blood from septic patients to suggest a functional role for α_4-integrin in neutrophil adhesion in sepsis.

▮ Evidence of α_4-integrin Expression on Neutrophils

Dihydrocytochalasin B (DHCB) is a microtubule disrupting agent. Chemotactic stimuli in the presence of DHCB behave as 'superstimuli', inducing neutrophil plasma membrane remodeling. DHCB increases the expression of cell surface receptors and prevents receptor internalization [32, 33]. In a series of experiments, the adhesive properties of neutrophils isolated from normal human volunteers were examined [34]. Neutrophils in the presence or absence of DHCB were chemotactially stimulated with platelet activating factor (PAF), interleukin (IL)-8, N-formyl-methionyl-leucylphenylalanine (fMLP), or phorbol 12-myristate 13-acetate (PMA) and exposed to human umbilical vein endothelial cells (HUVEC). In the absence of DHCB, neutrophil adhesion to the endothelial cells was completely blocked by the presence of anti-CD18 antibody. In the presence of DHCB, a significant number of neutrophils adhered to the endothelial cells and this effect could not be blocked completely by the addition of a CD-18 antibody thus showing that the neutrophil adhesion was β_2-integrin dependent. Furthermore, neutrophils incubated with DHCB and exposed to tumor necrosis factor (TNF)-α-stimulated HUVEC demonstrated avid neutrophil-endothelial adhesion independent of a CD18 pathway.

CD18 deficient bovine neutrophils (which are essentially identical to human deficient CD18 deficient neutrophils) did not bind to HUVEC in the presence of fMLP (in the absence of DHCB), but did so avidly following concomitant stimulation with DHCB. This experiment provides convincing evidence that the observed neutrophil-endothelial interactions were β_2-integrin independent and not due to an insufficient quantity or proteolytic destruction of the anti-CD18 antibody. Similar adhesion of neutrophils was demonstrated when the neutrophils were exposed to plastic coverslips coated with a protein such as VCAM-1; therefore, the neutrophil adhesion was not due to an E-selectin or P-selectin dependent process.

Administration of an antibody against L-selectin did not have any effect on adhesion of neutrophils stimulated with DHCB and fMLP, and there is evidence that L-selectin had been completely shed from the surface of the neutrophils. Assessment of the neutrophils by flow cytometry following DHCB and fMLP stimulation revealed positive staining for both α_4-integrin and $\beta1$-integrin. Anti-α_4-integrin antibody and anti-$\beta1$-integrin antibody both significantly reduced neutrophil adhesion to HUVEC and the protein coated plastic.

The results from this seminal series of experiments describe a novel pathway of neutrophil-endothelial adhesion independent of β_2-integrin. Although DHCB is an artificial, non-physiological stimulus, these experiments nonetheless provide evidence that mature neutrophils can express α_4-integrin and that α_4-integrin can mediate endothelial-neutrophil interactions in the presence of chemoattractants. The expression of α_4-integrin appears to occur in a manner consistent with membrane expression from a cytoplasmic storage of granules, rather than from upregulated synthesis.

In a separate series of experiments, neutrophils which had been stimulated with various concentrations of fMLP and induced to transmigrate across endothelium or deendothelialized membrane also demonstrated expression of α_4-integrin. The expression of α_4-integrin on the surface of transmigrated neutrophils suggests α_4-integrin expression is not simply a response to a non-physiologic artificial pharmacological stimulus.

▌ Evidence of α_4-integrin Mediated Neutrophil–myocyte Interaction

A consequence of systemic inflammation in sepsis is the secondary damage and consequent dysfunction or failure of organs not primarily injured by the infecting microbes. Examples of secondary organ damage include the acute respiratory distress syndrome (ARDS), acute renal failure, and myocardial dysfunction. In two separate series of experiments, the importance of α_4-integrin in mediating neutrophil-cardiac myocyte interactions was studied [35, 36]. In the first set of observations, two populations of neutrophils were obtained from rats: circulating cells obtained from venipuncture, and emigrated neutrophils from the peritoneal space collected four hours following intraperitoneal injection with 1% oyster glycogen [35]. Interactions were observed by phase contrast microscopy.

Freshly isolated, non-stimulated, circulating neutrophils demonstrated minimal adherence to non stimulated myocytes showing that the model itself was not responsible for any observed neutrophil-myocyte interactions. Circulating neutrophils stimulated with fMLP or IL-8 demonstrated significant adhesion to myocytes that could be completely blocked by anti-CD18 antibody. Unstimulated and fMLP stimulated neutrophils from the emigrated neutrophil population demonstrated dramatic interaction with myocytes in a manner that was only partially inhibited by anti-CD18 antibody. The neutrophil myocyte injury caused by the neutrophil adhesion was inhibited by an antibody against α_4-integrin and an antibody against CS-1 (which is an alternately spliced fibronectin fragment), but was not inhibited by an anti-VCAM-1 antibody.

In this model, neutrophil-endothelial interactions that occur with stimulated circulating neutrophils were found to be CD18 dependent while emigrated neutrophils interacted in a manner independent of a CD18 pathway. In the clinical circumstance of myocardial dysfunction associated with sepsis, emigrated neutrophils must migrate from the vasculature and to the heart. It is of particular interest that α_4-integrin expression on emigrated neutrophils plays a role in regulating myocyte dysfunction during acute systemic inflammatory states. This conclusion is in contrast to previous work that demonstrated CD18 mediated neutrophil-myocyte interaction as the necessary precursor to the release of cytotoxic molecules implicated in myocardial injury [37–40].

To test this hypothesis, murine ventricular myocytes and emigrated neutrophils were isolated in a manner previously described for rat myocytes and neutrophils [36]. Prior to the introduction of neutrophils, myocytes were stimulated in order to cause shortening and isoproterenol was added in order to confirm normal contraction. When neutrophils were added to the myocytes, there was a 50% reduction in myocyte cell shortening on those myocytes that demonstrated neutrophil adhesion. This effect was not attenuated by the addition of an anti-CD18 antibody, but neutrophil-myocyte interaction and myocyte dysfunction was reduced by α_4-integrin antibody. Myocyte death was common when a CD18 antibody was added to the emigrated neutrophils, this effect was absent when anti-α_4-integrin antibody was added to the preparation involving emigrated neutrophils. This study illustrated for the first time that an anti-CD18 antibody was unable to protect against neutrophil mediated cytotoxic cell shortening, myocyte dysrhythmia and myocyte contracture.

Recent data from the same model have demonstrated that the addition of anti-α_4-integrin antibody, but not anti-CD18 antibody, prevents oxidant production in emigrated neutrophils [41]. This suggests that in acute inflammation, α_4-integrin is the predominant molecule in neutrophil-myocyte dysfunction rather than CD-18 as previously believed, and that in emigrated neutrophils the NADPH oxidative system becomes uncoupled from CD18 yet activated by α_4-integrin. If correct, it is not unreasonable to assume that α_4-integrin may play a similar role in (remote) tissue injury caused by emigrated neutrophils in other sites, though this hypothesis remains unproven.

▌ The Function of α_4-integrin during Physiological Flow

These previous studies are intriguing, but the role of α_4-integrin in neutrophil adhesion in the circulation is unclear. An examination of neutrophil-endothelial interactions is possible using intravital microscopy in animal models of disease, but there are difficulties in extrapolating results from animal models to the human condition. Therefore, biological interactions using human substrate have been developed using flow chambers (Fig. 2). The flow chamber design was originally described by Lawrence and Springer, and permits the examination of leukocyte interactions with various biological substrata at defined shear forces. Biological substrata, for example HUVEC, are seeded onto glass coverslips and allowed to grow to form confluent monolayers at a density of 1×10^7 cells/coverslip. The coverslips are then mounted into a polycarbonate flow chamber with parallel plate geometry mounted on an inverted microscope. A syringe pump permits control of flow across the coverslips at a defined shear force [42]. All images are obtained using phase contrast microscopy and are videotaped.

In a series of experiments, we examined whether neutrophil-endothelial interactions could be mediated by α_4-integrin under flow conditions [43]. Coverslips with the biological substrates of HUVEC or murine L-cell transfectants expressing ICAM-1 or VCAM-1 were developed. Freshly isolated human neutrophils from healthy volunteers were observed to tether, roll and adhere on TNF-α stimulated HUVEC at a shear of 2 dynes/cm^2. The tethering and rolling neutrophil-endothelial interactions were inhibited by an antibody against both L-selectin and E-selectin, whereas the firm adhesion of neutrophils to the endothelium was inhibited by an anti CD18 antibody. These results are consistent with the classic understanding of neutrophil-endothelial interactions. The addition of DHCB resulted in a two-fold

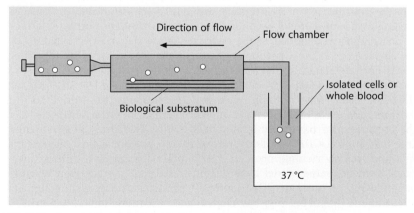

Fig. 2. The flow chamber design used in flow experiments

increase in neutrophil adhesion which was only partially attenuated by the addition of anti-CD18 antibody but could be further decreased by the addition of an antibody against α_4-integrin. When these neutrophils were perfused over VCAM-1-transfected L cells at 2 dynes/cm^2, no endothelial interactions were observed. These results are consistent with an understanding of the importance of the selectins in initiating leukocyte recruitment. When shear forces were decreased α_4-integrin dependent neutrophil-endothelial interactions were observed and similar results were observed when the model was examined with Ramos cells that express exclusively α_4-integrin. In conditions associated with decreased flow (or low shear forces), such as in venules of septic patients, tethering, rolling, and adhesion are dependent upon α_4-integrin, and independent of both selectins and β_2-integrins. These results lend credence to the observations of Doerschuk and colleagues demonstrating that neutrophil migration in response to tissue injury caused by *Streptococcus pneumoniae* or hydrochloric acid was not blocked by the use of a CD18 antibody [29].

More recently, two studies have reported that animals with induced lung inflammation will recruit neutrophils via α_4-integrin. The addition of an anti-α_4-integrin antibody could inhibit neutrophil recruitment into the lung [44, 45]. There are also a number of animal studies that have reported that, in chronic inflammation, α_4-integrin may support neutrophil adhesion. Furthermore, this neutrophil adhesion was found to occur independent of VCAM-1 [46].

Although DHCB has been used in concert with endogenous or exogenous chemotactic stimuli to maximally activate neutrophils, it is reasonable to consider that systemic chemoattractants in the environment of circulating whole blood can also maximally stimulate neutrophils in clinical situations such as bacteremia, sepsis or MOF.

▋ Evidence of α_4-integrin Mediated Adhesion in Septic Patients

The previous experiments provide convincing evidence that α_4-integrin is expressed on activated neutrophils, and that this ligand can mediate neutrophil-endothelial interaction. However, there are important limitations in generalizing these finding to the clinical condition of septic shock. First, the cells were examined when isolated from the inflammatory mileau of plasma. Second, whole blood flow within microvasculature consists of leukocytes and red blood cells. The red blood cells can push leukocytes to the vessel wall thus enhancing leukocyte interactions. Third, there is no single mediator likely to represent the septic situation.

In a series of experiments, we examined the role of α_4-integrin on the neutrophils of patients with documented severe sepsis syndrome (n=6) or septic shock (n=22) [47]. These patients were all adults, and met the criteria for SIRS with a confirmed source of infection [48]. The sources of infection in these patients included pneumonia, intra-abdominal sepsis, bacteremia, and necrotizing fasciitis. All infections were diagnosed based on accepted standards [49–50] and all patients had either hypotension requiring vasopressor support or the presence of at least two organ dysfunctions. The definitions for both hypotension and organ failure were rigorous, consistent with the definitions used for many recent clinical trials on immunomodulatory therapies in sepsis. Patients with leukopenia or classic causes of severe immunosuppression were excluded. There were three cohorts of controls: 1) patients with a source of infection but without concomitant severe sepsis syndrome or septic shock (all of these patients had either pneumonia or urosepsis); 2) patients undergoing major surgery (including laparotomy, thoracotomy, or mediastinoscopy); and 3) healthy volunteers. Whole blood was drawn from both the experimental and control patients. All septic patients met criteria within a consecutive 24-hour period and were enrolled within 36 hours of presenting to the ICU. For the surgical control patients, the blood was drawn within 24 hours after the operation in an attempt to coincide with the timing of blood drawn from septic patients.

These patients had an average APACHE II score of 23.7 ± 3.0 and a mean age of 59.3 years. Of the 28 patients, eight had community-acquired pneumonia, eight had nosocomial pneumonia (of which five were diagnosed after 48 hours of mechanical ventilation), ten had intra-abdominal sepsis, and two had necrotizing fasciitis. Concomitant bacteremia was present in eight of the cases of pneumonia, four of the cases of intra-abdominal sepsis and in both cases of necrotizing fasciitis. Of the patients enrolled with pneumonia, 11 were caused by Gram-positive organisms and all cases of intra-abdominal sepsis were polymicrobial infections although four grew Gram-negative organisms from blood cultures. Both cases of necrotizing fasciitis were caused by Group A streptococcus. These patients represented a reasonable cross-section of sources of infection, causative organism and severity of illness. The non-operative infected group had either pneumonia or a urinary tract source of infection. The post-operative control patients were of a similar age and gender distribution as patients in the septic group.

Leukocyte interactions were examined on two biological substrata: platelet monolayer immobilized to collagen, which is the most consistent method for examining P-selectin and CD18 ligand-dependent neutrophil interactions, and VCAM-1 which is the endothelial ligand for α_4-integrin. The whole blood was perfused following dilution at a shear force of 4 dynes/cm^2. Whole blood perfused over the platelet monolayer demonstrated no increase in rolling between neutrophils from the control and experimental cohorts. However, the number of adherent calls was greatly increased in the septic patients. Therefore, leukocytes from the septic patients had a greater propensity to adhere than leukocytes from the controls. This difference can be expressed by looking at the adhesion/rolling ratio, which was four-fold greater in the septic patients compared to the control patients.

In examining leukocyte interactions on VCAM-1, leukocytes from all groups demonstrated rolling and adhesion; however, from healthy controls, $\sim 8\%$ of the interacting cells were neutrophils, whereas from septic patients $\sim 60\%$ of cells were neutrophils. This seven-fold increase could not be accounted for by simple differences in circulating neutrophil numbers. All interactions with VCAM-1 were blocked by the addition of an α_4-integrin antibody.

A subset of patients underwent 'plasma switch' studies where the cells and plasma from septic patients were separated, and replaced with the respective plasma or cells separated from healthy volunteers. When leukocytes from controls were incubated with plasma from septic patients, there was a substantial increase in neutrophil recruitment on VCAM-1 to levels similar to those seen using whole blood from septic patients. However, the addition of septic leukocytes to plasma from healthy controls caused a decrease in neutrophil recruitment to only $\sim 30\%$. Flow cytometry measurements, performed by adding primary antibodies directed against α_4-integrin, identified surface expression on the membranes of neutrophils from septic patients. These switching experiments suggest that the rapidity of α_4-integrin expression is consistent with release from a cytoplasmic pool, and that the rapid loss of the α_4-integrin from neutrophil surfaces is either due to shedding, or we believe more likely due to reinternalization of the ligand.

These experiments have demonstrated for the first time that in a human disease state, neutrophils express an alternate ligand to β_2-integrin, and this new pathway may mediate neutrophil-endothelial interactions. The expression of α_4-integrin on neutrophils associated with systemic inflammation is unique since localized infections such as pneumonia or physiological stress such as major surgery were not sufficient to activate α_4-integrin expression. Furthermore, this effect is transferable as plasma incubated with neutrophils from healthy controls also expressed and interacted with endothelium via the α_4-integrin pathway. The rapid effect of 'septic' plasma on the neutrophils of healthy controls supports the contention that α_4-integrin is likely to be released from cytoplasmic stores, rather than requiring gene activation and protein transcription. Finally, the neutrophils activated in healthy controls were mature neutrophils, not immature neutrophil precursors that have recently been demonstrated to express α_4-integrin while within the environment of the marrow.

The flow chamber, as used in our studies, provides a novel way to examine leukocyte-endothelial interactions in a system that mimics the shear conditions found in the human microvasculature. It also permits the examination of cells without removing them from their natural milieu. This work does not identify whether there is a single mediator or multiple mediators in septic plasma that activate α_4-integrin expression on neutrophils from healthy donors. What remains uncertain is whether α_4-integrin expression is unique to conditions associated with systemic inflammation related to septic shock, or if other conditions of systemic inflammation related to shock, such as hemorrhagic shock, can result in α_4-integrin expression. An understanding of what conditions activate α_4-integrin expression could assist in identifying the responsible inflammatory mediators. Finally, there is an absence of data to guide an understanding of whether selectins, β_2-integrin and α_4-integrins are complementary – such as redundant systems to ensure neutrophil migration – or if one system plays a unique role in normal or abnormal neutrophil migration.

▋ Conclusion

We have demonstrated that mature neutrophils can express α_4-integrin, which was previously thought to be unique to PBMCs, and immature myeloid lineage cells within the bone marrow. *In vitro*, α_4-integrin can be expressed secondary to non-physiologic stimuli, and as a consequence of neutrophil migration from the vascular space to sites of tissue inflammation. We have demonstrated that the expression of the α_4-integrin ligand on neutrophils can result in tethering, rolling, and firm adherence on vascular endothelium. It has been shown also that α_4-integrin binds to myocytes and results in classic myocyte dysfunction and death (as a model of end-organ damage). Finally, in septic shock, α_4-integrin expression on neutrophils mediates neutrophil-endothelial interactions. This α_4-integrin expression is dependent on unidentified mediators within the plasma. To understand systemic inflammatory states, it is first necessary to elucidate the mechanisms by which neutrophils and endothelium interact. Our data suggest that the previous hypothesis based on selectin and β_2-integrin-dependent mediated neutrophil recruitment on vascular endothelium is not correct in all circumstances. Further work on neutrophil-endothelial interactions in septic shock and other acute inflammatory states is necessary prior to pursuing clinical trials at agents directed against this component of the inflammatory cascade.

References

1. Centers for Disease Control and Prevention, National Center for Health Statistics (1993) Mortality pattern – United States 1990. Monthly Vital Stat Rep 41:5
2. Bone R (1991) Sepsis, the sepsis syndrome, multi organ failure: a plea for comparable definitions. Ann Intern Med 114:332–333
3. Abraham E (1999) Why immunomodulatory therapies have not worked in sepsis. Intensive Care Med 25:556–566
4. Bernard G, Vincent J-L, Laterre P-F, et al (2001) Efficacy and safety of recombinant human activated protein C for severe sepsis. N Engl J Med 344:699–709
5. Lush C, Kvietys P (2000) Microvascular dysfunction in sepsis. Microcirculation 7:83–101
6. Menger M, Vollmar B (1996) Adhesion molecules as determinants of disease: from molecular biology to surgical research. Br J Surg 83:588–601
7. Parent C, Eichacker P (1999) Neutrophil and endothelial cell interactions in sepsis: the role of adhesion molecules. Infect Dis Clin N Am 13:427–447
8. Moore K, Patel K, Brehl R, et al (1995) P-selectin glycoprotein ligand mediates rolling of human neutrophils on P-selectins. J Cell Biol 128:661–671
9. Ley K, Tedder T, Kansas G (1993) L-selectin can mediate leukocyte rolling in untreated mesenteric venules in vivo independent of E- or P-selectin. Blood 82:1632–1638
10. Von Andrian U, Hansell P, Chambers J, et al (1992) L-selectin function is required for beta-2-integrin mediated neutrophil adhesion at physiological shear rates in vivo. Am J Physiol 263:H1034–H1044
11. Kanwar S, Woodman R, Poon MC, et al (1995) Desmopressin induces endothelial P-selectin expression and leukocyte rolling in post-capillary venules. Blood 86:2760–2766
12. Dore M, Korthius R, Granger D, Entman M, Smith C (1993) P-selectin mediates spontaneous leukocyte rolling in vivo. Blood 82:1308–1316
13. Abbassi O, Kishimoto T, Anderson D (1993) E-selectin supports neutrophil rolling in vitro under conditions of flow. J Clin Invest 92:2719–2730
14. Kubes P, Kanwar S (1994) Histamine induces leukocyte rolling in post-capillary venules: a P-selectin mediated event. J Immunol 152:3570–3577
15. Jones D, Abbassi O, McIntire L, McEver R, Smith C (1993) P-selectin mediates neutrophil rolling on histamine stimulated endothelial cells. Biophys J 65:1560–1569
16. Kubes P, Suzuki M, Granger D (1990) Platelet-activating factor-induced microvascular dysfunction: the role of adherent leukocytes. Am J Physiol 258:G158–G163
17. Arfors K, Lundberg C, Lindbom L, Lundberg K, Beatty P, Harlan J (1987) A monoclonal antibody to the membrane glycoprotein CD 18 inhibits polymorphonuclear leukocytes accumulation and plasma leakage in vivo. Blood 69:338–340
18. Smith C, Rothlein R, Hughes B, et al (1988) Recognition of an endothelial determinant for CD18-dependent human neutrophil adherence and transendothelial migration. J Clin Invest 82:1746–1756
19. Tonneson M, Anderson D, Springer T, Knelder A, Avdi N, Henson P (1989) Adherence of neutrophils to cultured human microvasculature endothelial cells. Stimulation by chemotactic peptides and lipid mediators and dependence upon the Mac-1, LFA, p150,95 Glycoprotein family. J Clin Invest 83:637–646
20. Kishimoto T, Anderson D (1992) The role of integrins in inflammation. In: Gallin J, Goldstein I, Snyderman R (eds) Inflammation: Basic Principles and Clinical Correlates. Raven Press, New York, pp 353–406
21. Johnston B, Issekutz T, Kubes P (1996) The alpha-4 integrin supports leukocyte rolling and adhesion in chronically inflamed postcapillary venules in vivo. J Exp Med 183:1995–2006
22. Johnston B, Walter U, Issekutz A, Issekutz T, Anderson D, Kubes P (1997) Differential roles of selectins and the alpha-4 integrin in acute, subacute, and chronic leukocyte recruitment in vivo. J Immunol 159:4514–4523

23. Kanwar S, Bullard D, Hickey M, et al (1997) The association between alpha-4 integrin, P-selectin, and E-selectin in an allergic model of inflammation. J Exp Med 185:1077–1087
24. Molossi S, Elices M, Arrhenius T, Diaz R, Coubler C, Rabinovitch M (1995) Blockade of very late antigen-4 integrin binding to fibronectin with connecting segment-1 peptide reduces accelerated coronary arteriopathy in rabbit cardiac allografts. J Clin Invest 95:2601–2610
25. Podolsky D, Lobb R, King N, et al (1993) Attenuation of colitis in the cotton-top tamarin by anti-a4 integrin monoclonal antibody. J Clin Invest 92:372–380
26. Abraham W, Sielczak M, Ahmed A, et al (1994) Alpha-4 integrins mediate antigen-induced late bronchial responses and prolong airway hyperresponsiveness in sheep. J Clin Invest 93:776–787
27. Chisholm P, Williams C, Lobb R (1996) Monoclonal antibodies to the integrin alpha-4 subunit inhibit the murine contact hypersensitivity response. Eur J Immunol 23:682–688
28. Arndt H, Kubes P, Grisham M, Gonzalez E, Granger D (1992) Granulocyte turnover in the feline intestine. Inflammation 16:549–559
29. Doerschuk C, Winn R, Coxson H, Harlan J (1990) CD-18 dependent and independent mechanisms of neutrophil emigration in the pulmonary and systemic microcirculation of rabbits. J Immunol 144:2327–2333
30. Issekutz A, Issekutz T (1993) A major portion of polymorphonuclear leukocyte and T-lymphocyte migration to arthritic joints in the rat is via LFA-1/MAC-1 independent mechanisms. Clin Immunol Immunopathol 67:257–263
31. Winn R, Harlan J (1993) CD-18 independent neutrophil and mononuclear leukocyte emigration into the peritoneum of rabbits. J Clin Invest; 92:1168–1173
32. Mukherjee G, Quinn M, Linner J, Jesaitis A (1994) Remodeling of the plasma membrane after stimulation of neutrophils with f-Met-Leu-Phe and dihydrocytochalastin B: identification of membrane subdomains containing NADPH oxidase activity. J Leukoc Biol 55:685–694
33. Jesaitis A, Tolley J, Painter R, Sklar R, Cochrane C (1985) Membrane-cytoskeleton interactions and the regulation of chemotactic peptide-induced activation of human granulocytes: the effects of dihydrocytochalasin B. J Cell Biochem 27:241–253
34. Kubes P, Niu X-F, Smith W, Kehrli Jr M, Reinhardt P, Woodman R (1995) A novel beta-1-dependent adhesion pathway on neutrophils: a mechanism invoked by dihydrocytochalasin B or endothelial transmigration. FASEB J 9:1103–1111
35. Reinhardt P, Ward C, Giles W, Kubes P (1997) Emigrated rat neutrophils adhere to cardiac myocytes via alpha-4 integrin. Circ Res 81:196–201
36. Poon B, Ward C, Giles W, Kubes P (1999) Emigrated neutrophils regulate ventricular contractility via alpha-4 integrin. Circ Res 84:1245–1251
37. Shappell S, Toman C, Anderson D, Taylor A, Entman M, Smith C (1990) Mac-1 (CD 11b/CD 18) mediates adherence-dependent hydrogen peroxide production by human and canine neutrophils. J Immunol 144:2702–2711
38. Kraemer R, Smith C, Mullane K (1991) Activated human polymorphonuclear leukocytes reduce rabbit papillary muscle function: role of the CD 18 gylcoprotein adhesion complex. Cardiovasc Res 25:172–175
39. Entman M, Youker K, Shappell S, et al (1990) Neutrophil adherence to isolated adult canine myocytes: evidence for a CD 18 dependent mechanism. J Clin Invest 85:1497–1506
40. Hansen P, Stawski G (1994) Neutrophil mediated damage to isolated myocytes after anoxia and reoxygenation. Cardiovasc Res 28:565–569
41. Poon B, Ward C, Cooper C, Giles W, Burns A, Kubes P (2001) Alpha-4 integrin mediates neutrophil-induced free radical injury to cardiac myocytes. J Cell Biol 152:857–866
42. Lawrence M, Springer T (1991) Leukocytes roll on a selectin at physiologic flow rates: distinction from and prerequisite for adhesion through integrins. Cell 65:859–873
43. Reinhardt P, Elliott J, Kubes P (1997) Neutrophils can adhere via alpha-4 beta-1 integrin under flow conditions. Blood 89:3837–3846
44. Ibbotson G, Doig C, Kaur J, et al (2001) Functional alpha-4 integrin: a newly identified pathway of neutrophil recruitment in critically ill septic patients. Nature Med 7:465–470
45. Burns J, Issekutz T, Yagita H (2001) The $\alpha 4\beta 1$ (very late antigen (VLA)-4, CD49d/CD29) and $\alpha 5\beta 1$ (VLA-5, CD49e/CD29) integrins mediate $\beta 2$ (CD11/CD18) integrin–independent neutrophil recruitment to endotoxin-induced lung inflammation. J Immunol 166:4644–4649

46. Ridger V, Wagner B, Wallace W (2001) Differential effects of CD18, CD29, and CD49 integrin subunit inhibition on neutrophil migration in pulmonary inflammation. J Immunol 166:3484–3490
47. Johnston B, Chee A, Issekutz T (2001) α4 Integrin leukocyte recruitment does not require VCAM-1 in a chronic model of inflammation. J Immunol 164:3337–3344
48. American College of Chest Physicians/Society of Critical Care Medicine Consensus Conference. (1992) Definitions for sepsis and organ failure and guidelines for the use of innovative therapies in sepsis. Crit Care Med 20:864–874
49. Horan T, Emori T (1997) Definitions of key terms used in the NNIS system. Am J Infect Cont 25:112–116
50. Center for Disease Control (1989) CDC definitions for nosocomial infections, 1988. Am Rev Respir Dis 139:1058–1059

Cell Adhesion Molecules and Leukocyte Trafficking in Sepsis

S. J. Finney, T. W. Evans, and A. Burke-Gaffney

▌ Introduction

Histologically, septic foci are characterized by a marked infiltrate of leukocytes, and in particular neutrophils. The movement of leukocytes from the circulation to such foci results from interactions between leukocytes and endothelial cells, controlled by the coordinated expression of cell adhesion molecules (CAM) on both cell types. CAM mediate attachment of cells both to one another and to extracellular matrix. They include the selectins, integrins, cadherins and the immunoglobulin superfamily (Fig. 1). Bacterial products and host pro-inflammatory mediators can initiate changes in CAM expression. CAM are, however, much more than a 'molecular glue' providing structural integrity to tissues and binding leukocytes. Traversing the cell membrane, CAM have intracellular domains linked to signaling proteins and cytoskeletal structures that allow functional responses in cells following binding of CAM to their ligands (so called 'outside-in signaling'). Thus, CAM inform a

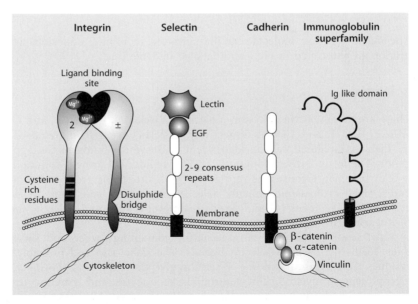

Fig. 1. Basic structural format of the integrins, selectins, and immunoglobulin superfamily cell adhesion molecules. EGF: epidermal growth factor

cell of its position and orientation relative to other cells and matrix components. Cellular responses to ligand binding include altered expression and binding affinity of other CAM (so called 'inside-out signaling'), increased gene expression, exocytosis, and altered structural rigidity promoting locomotion. It is through these mechanisms that specific CAM not only provide adhesive bonds, but also trigger the next stages of the highly regulated leukocyte recruitment process. The importance of CAM in modulating host defense is emphasized by congenital defects in leukocyte adhesive function that render patients more susceptible to infection [1].

If infection overwhelms local host defenses, or the host response is inappropriately excessive, bacteria and bacterial products, or inflammatory mediators may enter the circulation causing systemic inflammation: the clinical syndrome of septic shock with vascular dysfunction, organ failure, and high associated mortality. Widespread upregulation of CAM by pro-inflammatory mediators may promote neutrophil trafficking to non-infected tissues, or excessive movement to sites of infection. Tissue damage from cytotoxic neutrophil products may result, thereby promoting organ dysfunction. Therapies designed to inhibit CAM might be beneficial in septic shock.

This chapter focuses on the role of CAM in mediating leukocyte trafficking in tissues (in this context, however, it should be noted that CAM are also intimately involved in the reparative process, controlling the influx and differentiation of epithelial, stromal, and vascular cells. Manipulation of tissue repair has exciting potential in human sepsis, but is outside the remit of this review). How specific CAM are upregulated in sepsis and mediate neutrophil movement into tissues will be discussed. Finally, experimental and clinical experiences with modulation of CAM function in sepsis are presented.

▌ Adhesion Molecule Families

The major adhesion molecule families involved in rolling, adhesion, and transmigration are illustrated in Fig.1 and detailed in Table 1.

Selectins

There are three selectin adhesion molecules: E-selectin, P-selectin, and L-selectin or CD62E, CD62P, and CD62L respectively. Selectins are glycoproteins characterized by their extracellular, calcium-dependent lectin which binds to the appropriate ligands. The lectin is then bound via an EGF (epidermal growth factor) domain and two to nine short consensus repeats to the hydrophobic trans-membrane portion and a small cytoplasmic domain. Selectin engagement can result in activation of cell signaling moieties [4] and downstream events such as L-selectin shedding and β_2-integrin activation [5].

Sialyl Lewis X (SLe^x), a tetrasaccharide containing fucose and sialic acid residues, forms the basis of selectin ligands. The sialic acid and probably the fucose residues are critical for binding. P-selectin glycoprotein ligand (PSGL-1), a 160 kDa glycoprotein on myeloid cells, neutrophils, monocytes, and lymphocytes [6], binds all three selectins. It constitutes less than 1% of surface SLe^x, and is also expressed on some non-hematopoietic cells such as fallopian tube epithelium and tumor microvascular endothelium. There are few data concerning the regulation of PSGL-1

Table 1. Principal adhesion molecules involved in rolling, adhesion and transmigration. (Adapted from [2, 3])

		Cellular expression			
	Alternate names	Endothelial	Leukocyte	Ligand(s)	Type of expression
▌ Rolling					
P selectin	GMP140	✓		PSGL-1	Inducible
L selectin	Lam1, Leu8		✓	PSGL-1, MADCAM-1, GlyCAM-1, CD34	Constitutive
E selectin	ELAM-1	✓		PSGL-1, ESL-1 (murine), other SLe^x	Inducible
▌ Firm Adhesion					
$a_L\beta_2$	LFA-1		✓	ICAM-1, -2 , and -3	Constitutive/Inducible
$a_M\beta_2$	Mac-1, Mo-1, CR3		✓	ICAM-1, iC3b, factor X, fibrinogen	Constitutive/Inducible
$a_4\beta_1$	VLA-4, LPAM 2		✓	VCAM-1, fibronectin	Constitutive/Inducible
$a_9\beta_1$	VLA-9		✓	Fibronectin, tenascin	Constitutive
ICAM-1		✓	✓	$a_L\beta_2$, $a_L\beta_2$	Constitutive/Inducible
ICAM-2		✓		$a_L\beta_2$	Constitutive
VCAM-1		✓		$a_4\beta_1$	Inducible
▌ Transmigration					
$a_V\beta_3$	VNR	✓	✓	PECAM-1, $a_V\beta_3$	Consitutive
PECAM-1	CD31	✓		$a_V\beta_3$, PECAM-1	Constitutive
VE-cadherin	Cadherin 5	✓		VE-cadherin	Constitutive

PSGL: P-selectin glycoprotein ligand; CAM: cell adhesion molecule; ICAM: intercellular adhesion molecule; VCAM: vascular cell adhesion molecule; PECAM: platelet/endothelial cell adhesion molecule

on the surface of leukocytes, although leukocyte activation with platelet activating factor (PAF) or phorbol myristate acetate causes shedding within minutes [7].

Integrins

The integrin family of cell surface adhesion molecules, first described in 1987 [8], are widely expressed on cells and bind to extracellular matrix, or other CAM. They exist as non-covalently bound heterodimers of a 120–180 kDa a subunit and a 90–110 kDa β subunit (Fig. 1). Thus far, 8β subunits and $17a$ subunits have been described in 23 permutations. Integrins are classified according to their a-β composition. The β_2-integrins are commonly referred to by their cluster differentiation nomenclature as CD18 combined with CD11a, b, c, or d (or a_L, a_M, a_X , and a_D respectively).

All a and β subunits, except β_4, have similar structures: a small cytoplasmic region attached to the actin cytoskeleton; a single trans-membrane domain; and a large extracellular component that binds to the appropriate CAM or matrix component. The β_4 subunit has a much larger cytoplasmic region that binds to intermediate filaments within the cell.

The activity of integrins can be modulated by upregulation of surface expression, alterations in affinity for ligands, or clustering of receptors on the cell surface [9]. For example, neutrophil $a_M\beta_2$ can be upregulated by mobilization from cytoplasmic storage pools [10], or activation to a high affinity state by mediators such as tumor necrosis factor alpha (TNF-a) [11].

Clustering of integrins during ligand binding results in the activation of cytoplasmic tyrosine kinases by an, as yet unidentified, mechanism [12]. The tyrosine kinases modulate a number of intracellular signaling cascades including phosphatidyl inositol, Rho, Jnk, and Erk ('outside-in signaling'), and thereby influence gene transcription, and actin based cytoskeletal rearrangements.

Immunoglobulin Superfamily

The immunoglobulin superfamily is a large cohort of glycoproteins that include the intercellular adhesion molecules (ICAM-1, ICAM-2, and ICAM-3), vascular cell adhesion molecule-1 (VCAM-1), and platelet/endothelial cell adhesion molecule-1 (PECAM-1). They are expressed on many cells including endothelial and epithelial cells. Structurally, they consist of a small cytoplasmic domain, a single trans-membrane region, and repeating extracellular domains with an immunoglobulin-like structure. In general, they bind heterotypically to integrins, although PECAM-1 binds homotypically at inter-endothelial junctions.

Cadherins

The cadherins are a family of calcium dependent cell-cell adhesion molecules including E-cadherin, N-cadherin, P-cadherin, M-cadherin, and VE-cadherin. They bind homotypically between cells in a zipper-like manner, characteristically in tissues exposed to mechanical strain. It is now clear that lateral and heterotypic binding is possible and that they contribute to cell-cell recognition, growth control, and cytoskeletal organization. Research has focused on the role of cadherins in tumor metastasis and neural development. Since cadherins form an intimate part of the endothelial adherens junction, they can influence the paracellular movement of both solutes and leukocytes. Their importance in the pathogenesis of sepsis is not known.

▌ Leukocyte Trafficking to Tissues

In non-pulmonary tissues, circulating leukocytes enter the interstitium from postcapillary venules [13]. By contrast, in the lung, migration occurs through capillaries [14]. The rheological phenomenon of leukocyte margination during inflammation [15] coupled with a lower fluid velocity in the periphery of the vessel lumen allows the possibility of interactions between CAM on leukocytes and endothelial cells lining the vessels. These interactions may be sufficient to transiently tether the leukocyte and decelerate it from the free flowing stream of blood. Shear forces at the blood-endothelial interface act to disrupt these adhesive bonds (Fig. 2). The balance between these disruptive forces and the tendency for new adhesive bonds to form dictates the subsequent behavior of the leukocyte. If shear prevails, the leukocyte breaks away and returns to the circulation. By contrast, if pro-adhesive forces dominate, the leukocyte rolls along the endothelium, adhesive bonds breaking at the trailing edge and new bonds forming at the leading edge. If the equilibrium moves further towards adhesive forces, the leukocyte stops rolling and becomes firmly ad-

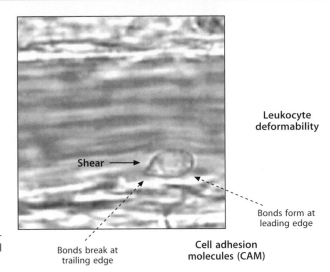

Fig. 2. Photomicrograph of a rolling leukocyte, and the principal factors influencing its behavior

herent to the endothelium. Firm adhesion is usually followed by diapedesis along a chemotactic gradient into the interstitium (transmigration).

Rolling

The selectins play a significant role in modulating rolling. Thus, in mice genetically modified for P-selectin or L-selectin, rolling is reduced (Table 2). In P-selectin null mice, additional deletion of E-selectin reduces rolling further [16]; these mice are particularly prone to mucocutaneous infections. In mesenteric post-capillary venules, early lipopolysaccharide (LPS) induced rolling is dependent on both L-selectin and P-selectin [17]. In the murine cremasteric circulation, TNF-α induces rolling after 2 hours via either E-selectin or P-selectin, which operate in a redundant manner [18]. In triple selectin deficient mice there is surprisingly little tendency to recurrent infection [19], although leukocyte rolling is markedly reduced; residual rolling occurs at 5 hours and is prevented by the blockade of α_4 integrins.

The importance of selectins in mediating rolling is reinforced by data concerning their ligands. PSGL-1 deficiency due to either genetic deletion, genetic disrup-

Table 2. Selection deficient nice have impaired rolling. (Adapted from [4]).

Mutation	Phenotype	Leukocyte count	Rolling	Peritoneal neutrophil accumulation (4 hrs)
P-selectin	Healthy	↑	↓↓	↓
E-selectin	Healthy	Normal	Normal	Normal
L-selectin	Healthy	Normal	↓↓	↓
P-selectin & ICAM-1	Healthy	↑↑	↓↓↓	Absent
P- & E-selectin	Recurrent infections	↑↑↑↑	↓↓↓↓	Absent
P-, E-, & L-selectin	Healthy	↑↑↑↑	↓↓↓↓	↓↓

ICAM: intercellular adhesion molecule

tion of its biosynthesis, or blocking antibodies dramatically reduces P-selectin mediated rolling *in vivo* [20–22]. E-selectin mediated rolling is less affected, suggesting E-selectin can utilize other SLe^x glycoconjugates *in vivo*.

The importance of β_2-integrins/ICAM-1 in mediating rolling is minor. In β_2 integrin null mice, cytokine-induced rolling is normal [18] after correction for the marked leukocytosis. Furthermore, neutrophils from humans deficient in β_2 integrins exhibit normal rolling behavior *in vivo* [23]. However, in P-selectin knockouts, additional deletion of ICAM-1 (a ligand for the β_2-integrins) reduces trauma-induced rolling further [24] demonstrating some redundancy in adhesion molecule function.

Although all three selectins provide the dominant substrates for rolling, their expression varies temporally; L-selectin is expressed constitutively, whist endothelial E- and P-selectins are not. P-selectin from Weibel-Palade bodies [25] is upregulated within minutes of administration of histamine, thrombin, complement fragments, reactive oxygen species (ROS), and cytokines. E-selectin expression occurs following *de novo* protein synthesis after a few hours, and is induced by LPS and cytokines. The role of LPS in P-selectin upregulation is debated; while endothelial upregulation undoubtedly occurs during endotoxemia *in vivo* [26], LPS is not essential in murine peritonitis [27], and results from *in vitro* studies are divergent [17, 26, 28].

L-selectin engagement is an important event, since this triggers both upregulation of the β_2 integrins [29, 30], an important event for the transition to firm adhesion, and also shedding of L-selectin from the leukocyte [31], which may be necessary for subsequent transmigration [32]. L-selectin shedding occurs via an as yet undefined metalloprotease 'sheddase', and is also triggered by phorbol esters and LPS.

Firm Adhesion

Whilst β_2-integrins have little influence on rolling, they are important in mediating firm adhesion. The efficiency of cytokine-induced adhesion relative to the number of leukocytes rolling is reduced in β_2-integrin knockouts by 33% [18], an effect that was amplified with additional E-selectin blockade. Similar observations have been observed in response to C5a [33] and LPS [34]. Human neutrophils deficient in β_2-integrins do not adhere *in vivo* [23], and these patients have recurrent bacterial infections [1]. The ligands for the β_2-integrins include ICAM-1 [35], which is constitutively expressed on endothelial cells. *In vitro*, endothelial surface expression of ICAM-1 is further increased following 24 hours stimulation with LPS, TNF-a, interleukin-1β (IL-1β), and interferon-γ (IFN-γ) [36].

β_2-integrins are upregulated by L-selectin engagement [29, 30], and chemokines [37], such as IL-8 and ENA-78. Indeed, blockade of the rat CXC chemokine, cytokine-induced neutrophil chemoattractant (CINC-1), reduces LPS induced rolling and adhesion in rodent mesenteric vessels [38]. Chemokines are released into the environment as soluble forms, and associated to luminal proteoglycans on the endothelium via a heparin-like binding domain. Therefore, although LPS and pro-inflammatory cytokines can directly upregulate β_2-integrins, local mechanisms may be more important, serving to compartmentalize the immune response and only activating integrins once rolling has commenced. Chemokine-mediated activation of β_2-integrins may explain the significant contribution of E selectin to adhesion. E-selectin mediates rolling at the lowest rolling velocities, approximating leukocytes to local chemokines for a prolonged period of time, thus increasing the likelihood of β_2-integrin upregulation and adhesion [18].

ESM-1 (endothelial specific molecule-1) is a soluble chondroitin/dermatan sulfate proteoglycan molecule that is restricted to the lung and kidney. Recent work has demonstrated it binds to $a_L\beta_2$ [39] competing sterically for ICAM-1 and may thus modulate firm adhesion. Levels of ESM-1 are increased in sepsis, but their physiological relevance is not known [40].

Recently it has become evident that neutrophils express the integrin $a_4\beta_1$ at low levels basally, and that this may increase in septic patients [41]. Upregulation *in vitro* can be induced by C5a, N-formyl-methionyl-leucylphenylalanine (fMLP), and leukotriene B_4 in the presence of cytochalasins; the role of cytochalasin is unclear although it may prevent re-internalization of induced $a_4\beta_1$. The ligand for $a_4\beta_1$ is VCAM-1, which is expressed at low levels basally on endothelial cells, but is upregulated in the presence of IL-1β, TNF-a, LPS, and IL-4 [36]. Triple selectin mice, and *in vitro* studies demonstrate that $a_4\beta_1$ can mediate rolling and transient adhesion [19, 41]. Engagement of $a_4\beta_1$ may be another important mechanism whereby β_2-integrins are upregulated [42, 43].

Transmigration

Although transcytosis through endothelial cells does occur [44], leukocytes tend to pass into the interstitium through inter-endothelial gaps. This typically occurs at tricellular corners where both tight junctions and adherens junctions are discontinuous [45]. Transmigration involves simultaneous 'unzipping' of inter-endothelial junctional proteins whilst the leukocyte moves in the direction of a chemotactic gradient (reviewed [45, 46]).

Neutrophil adhesion disrupts the inter-endothelial catenin-VE-cadherin complex [47], by endothelial-derived proteases [45] activated by leukocyte adhesion and changes in intracellular calcium. Leukocyte-derived elastases also contribute to disruption of the interendothelial junction. These elastases, activated following adhesion, focus on specific interendothelial junctions by virtue of their short range of activity (since they are rapidly degraded in plasma), and their localization to the leading edge of the migrating leukocyte [48].

Directed motility requires polarization of the leukocyte by a chemotactic gradient. A high concentration of the chemoattractant at the leading edge results in the local intracellular accumulation of phosphatidylinositol 3-kinase (PI3K). PI3K activity [49] in conjunction with β_2-integrin engagement during adhesion [50] activate Cdc42 and Rac1, intracellular enzymes of the Rho GTPase family, that cause membrane and cytoskeletal protrusions by actin polymerisation at the leading edge of the cell [51]. As the leukocyte moves, adhesive complexes must break at the rear of the cell whilst new bonds form at the front. Another Rho GTPase, RhoA, appears important in this process, by promoting integrin recycling. β_2-integrin engagement during adhesion increases the activity of RhoA. It is hypothesized that spatial separation of this to the trailing edge of the cell results in relatively increased integrin recycling at the rear with integrin stabilization at the front.

A key integrin at the leading edge is $a_v\beta_3$, which binds to both PECAM-1 and vitronectin. In cultured endothelial cells PECAM-1 accumulates at abluminal cell-cell borders [52], and is required for the passage of leukocytes through the perivascular basement membrane [53]. Indeed, in PECAM-1 deficient mice neutrophils accumulate at the basement membrane of IL-1β stimulated venules [54]. PECAM-1's role in

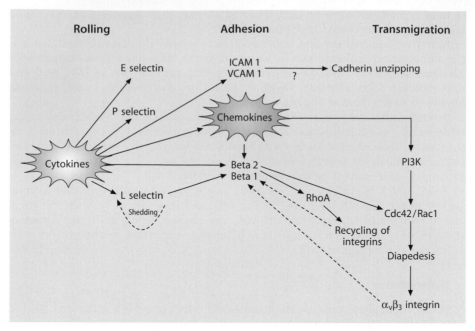

Fig. 3. Schematic diagram of main pathways for regulation of leukocyte adhesion molecules. Bold arrows represent positive relationships, and broken arrows negative feedback. See main text for abbreviations

basement membrane penetration is unclear, but may involve $\alpha_v\beta_3$ engagement once the leukocyte reaches the abluminal border. Additionally, $\alpha_v\beta_3$ engagement decreases the affinity of β_2-integrins for ICAM-1 [55] and $\alpha_4\beta_1$ for VCAM-1 [56], thus promoting the transition from firm adhesion to migration.

Finally, the β_1-integrins also contribute to transmigration, inhibition of both $\alpha_9\beta_1$ and $\alpha_4\beta_1$ preventing *in vitro* neutrophil adhesion to VCAM-1 and transmigration across endothelial monolayers [57]. $\alpha_9\beta_1$ and $\alpha_4\beta_1$ promote cell motility by as yet unclarified mechanisms, although the nature of the α subunit is important, rather than a general β_1 effect [58].

The cascades influencing the ordered regulation of CAM are illustrated in Figure 3.

▌ Evidence for Disordered Leukocyte Trafficking in Septic Shock

Generalized Upregulation of CAM

In vitro, both bacterial products and inflammatory mediators modulate CAM expression on leukocytes and endothelial cells (Table 1).

In animal models of sepsis, there is good evidence for the widespread activation of adhesion molecules. In mice following cecal ligation and puncture, immuno-histochemistry has demonstrated upregulation of P- and E-selectin in remote organs, such as the heart and lung [59]. Further, circulating plasma levels of these CAM are increased in endotoxemic rodents [60], and baboons [61]. Endotoxemic animals demonstrate upregulation of the β_2-integrins and shedding of L-selectin on circulating neutrophils [62].

In septic humans, shedding of L-selectin [63, 64] and upregulation of β_2-integrins and $\alpha_4\beta_1$ [63, 65, 66] has been shown on circulating neutrophils. There are few data regarding endothelial CAM, although pulmonary endothelial E-selectin and ICAM-1 are increased in patients dying from sepsis in comparison to non-septic deaths [66, 67]. Increased levels of soluble plasma CAM are often cited as surrogate evidence for the upregulation of endothelial CAM, and increases in plasma E-selectin, P selectin, VCAM-1, and ICAM-1 have been demonstrated repeatedly [68–70] in human sepsis. One group has demonstrated increased levels of soluble E-cadherin in human sepsis [71].

Generalized Neutrophil Recruitment to Remote Sites

While there is evidence for generalized upregulation of adhesion molecules in sepsis, the consequences for leukocyte trafficking are less clear. Polarization of the leukocyte is a key event in leukocyte trafficking and requires the presence of a chemotactic gradient which will only be present at remote sites if there is tissue damage due to an alternative process; or if epithelial/ stromal cells produce chemokines under the influence of systemic pro-inflammatory mediators such as IL-1β and TNF-α. Apart from the lung, there is little evidence for leukocyte recruitment to remote sites. The susceptibility of the lung may be attributable to the fact that neutrophils (diameter 7–8 µm) must squeeze through 5.5–6 µm diameter pulmonary capillaries. Neutrophil deformability thus influences significantly their retention in the pulmonary circulation. Neutrophil accumulation has been demonstrated in the hearts and livers of septic rodents [72, 73].

▌ Therapeutic Modulation of Adhesion Molecule Function

Many of the molecular pathways described above have been identified through the use of inhibitors of CAM function such as monoclonal antibodies or ligand excess. There have been several studies using these tools *in vivo,* and assessing endpoints such as mortality.

In vivo Experiences

Administration of antibodies against components of the $\alpha_M\beta_2$-ICAM-1 adhesive pathway has had variable benefit [2], depending on the nature of the septic model employed. In general, in endotoxemic models [74–76] or cytokine-induced shock [77], inhibition of this pathway confers a mortality benefit. By contrast, bacteremic models have had varied results; several studies have shown a worsening of mortality [78–81] even with the concomitant administration of antibiotics [82]. This is supported by the increased likelihood of abscesses forming from intradermal bacterial inoculates with inhibition of β_2-integrins [83]. However, others have shown, in rabbits with appendicitis or bacterial meningitis, that blockade of β_2 integrins improves [84, 85], or does not alter [86], mortality. ICAM-1 null mice have unaltered mortality in response to intraperitoneal bacteria [87].

Similar results have been obtained using inhibition of selectin function *in vivo*. In models of inflammation not employing bacteria, such as those following endotoxin administration or ischemia-reperfusion, selectin inhibition is generally beneficial in terms of mortality [88–91] and leukocyte recruitment to the lung [92, 93], although this is not universal [94]. However, L-selectin inhibition is detrimental in rodent bacterial pneumonia [95] and septic baboons [96], although inhibition of L-selectin does not increase the likelihood of abscess formation following intradermal bacterial inoculates [97]. Genetic deletion of E- and P-selectin predispose mice to death from intraperitoneal bacteria [98]. Finally, a truncated form of human PSGL-1 fused to immunoglobulin G (PSGL-1-IgG) does not increase mortality in bacteremic rodents [99]. PSGL-1-IgG inhibits leukocyte rolling and adhesion both *in vitro* and *in vivo* [100] by competition for PSGL-1 receptors, which include all three selectins.

The effects of soluble CAM released in sepsis are unclear. Indeed L-selectin at levels found in human sepsis, inhibits leukocyte binding to endothelial cells [101].

Adhesion molecule function can be altered by other pharmacological agents that have been employed in sepsis, for example corticosteroids [38], anti-cytokine agents, the antioxidant taurine [102] and notably nitric oxide (NO). Inhibition of NO synthase (NOS) increases rolling and adhesion in otherwise unstimulated feline mesenteric venules [103] and rats [104], possibly through inhibition of selectin expression [59]. Promotion of leukocyte rolling and adhesion may explain at least in part the failure of the trials of non-specific NOS inhibition in sepsis.

Clinical Investigations

Therapeutic use of blocking monoclonal antibodies in humans is complicated by the induction of an immune response against the species the antibody was raised in. This makes prolonged or repeated dosing difficult. Although antibodies can be humanized by cleavage or linkage to fusion proteins (such as PSGL-1-Ig) there has been interest in alternative methods of CAM blockade. These include anti-sense nucleotides for specific CAM mRNA, and the use of short peptide sequences that block CAM epitopes.

Inhibition of ICAM-1 has been attempted in patients with successful phase II trials utilizing a humanized antibody in rheumatoid arthritis; and an oligodeoxynucleotide anti-sense drug in inflammatory bowel disease (ISIS 2302). Preliminary results using humanized anti-$\alpha_4\beta_1$ in multiple sclerosis are promising, and a short peptide against $\alpha_4\beta_1$ (BIO 1211) is being developed for trials in asthma.

Data in human sepsis are minimal. Since patients with congenital defects in the β_2-integrins have recurrent infections, and CAM blockade is detrimental in some bacteremic animal models (*vide supra*), there are concerns about the use of such agents in human sepsis. However, humanized anti-β_2-integrins with concomitant antibiotics have been used safely in hemorrhagic shock in a phase II trial [105].

Blockade of E-selectin is an attractive proposition, since P- and L-selectin mediated rolling at sites of sepsis would be preserved whilst systemic upregulation of E-selectin would be abrogated. Indeed, a phase II clinical trail of a single bolus of a murine anti-E-selectin monoclonal antibody in septic shock ($t_{1/2} = 17$ hours) was undertaken following favorable preliminary results in rodents [106]. Only nine patients were studied, and results were encouraging in terms of improved oxygenation, ability to wean vasopressors, and mortality. The antibody was well tolerated, although eight patients developed an anti-murine response making prolonged or repeated dosing difficult. To date, no phase III study has been published, some five years after the results of the phase II trial.

Conclusion

During acute inflammation, neutrophils move from the circulation to the interstitium under the control of cell adhesion molecules, which are regulated in a sequential and highly coordinated manner. In severe human sepsis, there is good evidence for the widespread upregulation of CAM on leukocytes and endothelial cells. Whilst leukocytes do become entrapped in capillaries of the lung and heart, it is not clear whether this results from the systemic upregulation of CAM.

Inhibition of selectins and β_2-integrins has been demonstrated to improve mortality and organ dysfunction in some animal models of systemic inflammation, such as that induced by cytokines, LPS, or ischemia-reperfusion. However, in models of inflammation characterized by bacteremia, the results of CAM have been variable and often characterized by increased mortality, even when antibiotics are given concomitantly. Thus, adhesion molecule function seems to be critical for effective bacterial clearance and inhibition of this process an unfavorable intervention. The role and safety of CAM inhibition in human non-infectious inflammation has yet to be assessed, particularly in critically ill humans who are so susceptible to new nosocomial infection.

Acknowldegements. SJF and ABG are sponsored by the British Heart Foundation.

References

1. Springer TA, Thompson WS, Miller LJ, Schmalstieg FC, Anderson DC (1984) Inherited deficiency of the Mac-1, LFA-1, p150,95 glycoprotein family and its molecular basis. J Exp Med 160:1901–1918
2. Parent C, Eichacker PQ (1999) Neutrophil and endothelial cell interactions in sepsis. The role of adhesion molecules. Infect Dis Clin North Am 13:427–447
3. Hynes RO (1992) Integrins: versatility, modulation, and signaling in cell adhesion. Cell 69:11–25
4. Vestweber D, Blanks JE (1999) Mechanisms that regulate the function of the selectins and their ligands. Physiol Rev 79:181–213
5. Blanks JE, Moll T, Eytner R, Vestweber D (1998) Stimulation of P-selectin glycoprotein ligand-1 on mouse neutrophils activates beta 2-integrin mediated cell attachment to ICAM-1. Eur J Immunol 28:433–443
6. Sako D, Chang XJ, Barone KM, et al (1993) Expression cloning of a functional glycoprotein ligand for P-selectin. Cell 75:1179–1186
7. Davenpeck KL, Brummet ME, Hudson SA, Mayer RJ, Bochner BS (2000) Activation of human leukocytes reduces surface P-selectin glycoprotein ligand-1 (PSGL-1, CD162) and adhesion to P-selectin in vitro. J Immunol 165:2764–2772
8. Hynes RO (1987) Integrins: a family of cell surface receptors. Cell 48:549–554
9. Detmers PA, Wright SD (1988) Adhesion-promoting receptors on leukocytes. Curr Opin Immunol 1:10–15
10. Jones DH, Schmalstieg FC, Dempsey K, et al (1990) Subcellular distribution and mobilization of MAC-1 (CD11b/CD18) in neonatal neutrophils. Blood 75:488–498
11. Harris ES, McIntyre TM, Prescott SM, Zimmerman GA (2000) The leukocyte integrins. J Biol Chem 275:23409–23412
12. Berton G, Lowell CA (1999) Integrin signalling in neutrophils and macrophages. Cell Signal 11:621–635

13. Fiebig E, Ley K, Arfors KE (1991) Rapid leukocyte accumulation by "spontaneous" rolling and adhesion in the exteriorized rabbit mesentery. Int J Microcirc Clin Exp 10:127–144
14. Lien DC, Henson PM, Capen RL, et al (1991) Neutrophil kinetics in the pulmonary microcirculation during acute inflammation. Lab Invest 65:145–159
15. Chien S (1982) Rheology in the microcirculation in normal and low flow states. Adv Shock Res 8:71–80
16. Bullard DC, Kunkel EJ, Kubo H, et al (1996) Infectious susceptibility and severe deficiency of leukocyte rolling and recruitment in E-selectin and P-selectin double mutant mice. J Exp Med 183:2329–2336
17. Davenpeck KL, Steeber DA, Tedder TF, Bochner BS (1997) P- and L-selectin mediate distinct but overlapping functions in endotoxin-induced leukocyte-endothelial interactions in the rat mesenteric microcirculation. J Immunol 159:1977–1986
18. Jung U, Norman KE, Scharffetter-Kochanek K, Beaudet AL, Ley K (1998) Transit time of leukocytes rolling through venules controls cytokine-induced inflammatory cell recruitment in vivo. J Clin Invest 102:1526–1533
19. Collins RG, Jung U, Ramirez M, et al (2001) Dermal and pulmonary inflammatory disease in E-selectin and P-selectin double-null mice is reduced in triple-selectin-null mice. Blood 98:727–735
20. Yang J, Hirata T, Croce K, et al (1999) Targeted gene disruption demonstrates that P-selectin glycoprotein ligand 1 (PSGL-1) is required for P-selectin-mediated but not E-selectin-mediated neutrophil rolling and migration. J Exp Med 190:1769–1782
21. Norman KE, Moore KL, McEver RP, Ley K (1995) Leukocyte rolling in vivo is mediated by P-selectin glycoprotein ligand-1. Blood 86:4417–4421
22. Sperandio M, Forlow SB, Thatte J, Ellies LG, Marth JD, Ley K (2001) Differential requirements for core2 glucosaminyltransferase for endothelial l-selectin ligand function in vivo. J Immunol 167:2268–2274
23. von Andrian UH, Berger EM, Ramezani L, et al (1993) In vivo behavior of neutrophils from two patients with distinct inherited leukocyte adhesion deficiency syndromes. J Clin Invest 91:2893–2897
24. Kunkel EJ, Jung U, Bullard DC, et al (1996) Absence of trauma-induced leukocyte rolling in mice deficient in both P-selectin and intercellular adhesion molecule 1. J Exp Med 183:57–65
25. McEver RP, Beckstead JH, Moore KL, Marshall-Carlson L, Bainton DF (1989) GMP-140, a platelet alpha-granule membrane protein, is also synthesized by vascular endothelial cells and is localized in Weibel-Palade bodies. J Clin Invest 84:92–99
26. Coughlan AF, Hau H, Dunlop LC, Berndt MC, Hancock WW (1994) P-selectin and platelet-activating factor mediate initial endotoxin-induced neutropenia. J Exp Med 179:329–334
27. Bauer P, Lush CW, Kvietys PR, Russell JM, Granger DN (2000) Role of endotoxin in the expression of endothelial selectins after cecal ligation and perforation. Am J Physiol 278:R1140-1147
28. Khew-Goodall Y, Butcher CM, Litwin MS, et al (1996) Chronic expression of P-selectin on endothelial cells stimulated by the T-cell cytokine, interleukin-3. Blood 87:1432–1438
29. Steeber DA, Engel P, Miller AS, Sheetz MP, Tedder TF (1997) Ligation of L-selectin through conserved regions within the lectin domain activates signal transduction pathways and integrin function in human, mouse, and rat leukocytes. J Immunol 159:952–963
30. Hafezi-Moghadam A, Thomas KL, Prorock AJ, Huo Y, Ley K (2001) L-selectin shedding regulates leukocyte recruitment. J Exp Med 193:863–872
31. Palecanda A, Walcheck B, Bishop DK, Jutila MA (1992) Rapid activation-independent shedding of leukocyte L-selectin induced by cross-linking of the surface antigen. Eur J Immunol 22:1279–1286
32. Kishimoto TK, Jutila MA, Berg EL, Butcher EC (1989) Neutrophil Mac-1 and MEL-14 adhesion proteins inversely regulated by chemotactic factors. Science 245:1238–1241
33. Argenbright LW, Letts LG, Rothlein R (1991) Monoclonal antibodies to the leukocyte membrane CD18 glycoprotein complex and to intercellular adhesion molecule-1 inhibit leukocyte-endothelial adhesion in rabbits. J Leukoc Biol 49:253–257
34. Harris NR, Russell JM, Granger DN (1994) Mediators of endotoxin-induced leukocyte adhesion in mesenteric postcapillary venules. Circ Shock 43:155–160

35. van de Stolpe A, van der Saag PT (1996) Intercellular adhesion molecule-1. J Mol Med 74:13–33
36. Haraldsen G, Kvale D, Lien B, Farstad IN, Brandtzaeg P (1996) Cytokine-regulated expression of E-selectin, intercellular adhesion molecule-1 (ICAM-1), and vascular cell adhesion molecule-1 (VCAM-1) in human microvascular endothelial cells. J Immunol 156: 2558–2565
37. Campbell JJ, Hedrick J, Zlotnik A, Siani MA, Thompson DA, Butcher EC (1998) Chemokines and the arrest of lymphocytes rolling under flow conditions. Science 279:381–384
38. Davenpeck KL, Zagorski J, Schleimer RP, Bochner BS (1998) Lipopolysaccharide-induced leukocyte rolling and adhesion in the rat mesenteric microcirculation: regulation by glucocorticoids and role of cytokines. J Immunol 161:6861–6870
39. Bechard D, Scherpereel A, Hammad H, et al (2001) Human endothelial-cell specific molecule-1 binds directly to the integrin CD11a/CD18 (LFA-1) and blocks binding to intercellular adhesion molecule-1. J Immunol 167:3099–3106
40. Bechard D, Meignin V, Scherpereel A, et al (2000) Characterization of the secreted form of endothelial-cell-specific molecule 1 by specific monoclonal antibodies. J Vasc Res 37:417–425
41. Ibbotson GC, Doig C, Kaur J, et al (2001) Functional alpha4-integrin: a newly identified pathway of neutrophil recruitment in critically ill septic patients. Nat Med 7:465–470
42. May AE, Neumann FJ, Schomig A, Preissner KT (2000) VLA-4 (alpha(4)beta(1)) engagement defines a novel activation pathway for beta(2) integrin-dependent leukocyte adhesion involving the urokinase receptor. Blood 96:506–513
43. Chan JR, Hyduk SJ, Cybulsky MI (2000) Alpha 4 beta 1 integrin/VCAM-1 interaction activates alpha L beta 2 integrin-mediated adhesion to ICAM-1 in human T cells. J Immunol 164:746–753
44. Feng D, Nagy JA, Pyne K, Dvorak HF, Dvorak AM (1998) Neutrophils emigrate from venules by a transendothelial cell pathway in response to FMLP. J Exp Med 187:903–915
45. Johnson-Leger C, Aurrand-Lions M, Imhof BA (2000) The parting of the endothelium: miracle, or simply a junctional affair? J Cell Sci 113:921–933
46. Worthylake RA, Burridge K (2001) Leukocyte transendothelial migration: orchestrating the underlying molecular machinery. Curr Opin Cell Biol 13:569–577
47. Del Maschio A, Zanetti A, Corada M, et al (1996) Polymorphonuclear leukocyte adhesion triggers the disorganization of endothelial cell-to-cell adherens junctions. J Cell Biol 135: 497–510
48. Cepinskas G, Sandig M, Kvietys PR (1999) PAF-induced elastase-dependent neutrophil transendothelial migration is associated with the mobilization of elastase to the neutrophil surface and localization to the migrating front. J Cell Sci 112:1937–1945
49. Benard V, Bohl BP, Bokoch GM (1999) Characterization of rac and cdc42 activation in chemoattractant-stimulated human neutrophils using a novel assay for active GTPases. J Biol Chem 274:13198–13204
50. Price LS, Leng J, Schwartz MA, Bokoch GM (1998) Activation of Rac and Cdc42 by integrins mediates cell spreading. Mol Biol Cell 9:1863–1871
51. Wittmann T, Waterman-Storer CM (2001) Cell motility: can Rho GTPases and microtubules point the way? J Cell Sci 114:3795–3803
52. Ayalon O, Sabanai H, Lampugnani MG, Dejana E, Geiger B (1994) Spatial and temporal relationships between cadherins and PECAM-1 in cell-cell junctions of human endothelial cells. J Cell Biol 126:247–258
53. Wakelin MW, Sanz MJ, Dewar A, et al (1996) An anti-platelet-endothelial cell adhesion molecule-1 antibody inhibits leukocyte extravasation from mesenteric microvessels in vivo by blocking the passage through the basement membrane. J Exp Med 184:229–239
54. Duncan GS, Andrew DP, Takimoto H, et al (1999) Genetic evidence for functional redundancy of platelet/endothelial cell adhesion molecule-1 (PECAM-1): CD31-deficient mice reveal PECAM-1-dependent and PECAM-1-independent functions. J Immunol 162:3022–3030
55. Weerasinghe D, McHugh KP, Ross FP, Brown EJ, Gisler RH, Imhof BA (1998) A role for the alpha(v)beta3 integrin in the transmigration of monocytes. J Cell Biol 142:595–607

56. Imhof BA, Weerasinghe D, Brown EJ, et al (1997) Cross talk between alpha(v)beta3 and alpha4beta1 integrins regulates lymphocyte migration on vascular cell adhesion molecule 1. Eur J Immunol 27:3242–3252

57. Taooka Y, Chen J, Yednock T, Sheppard D (1999) The integrin alpha9beta1 mediates adhesion to activated endothelial cells and transendothelial neutrophil migration through interaction with vascular cell adhesion molecule-1. J Cell Biol 145:413–420

58. Young BA, Taooka Y, Liu S, et al (2001) The cytoplasmic domain of the integrin alpha9 subunit requires the adaptor protein paxillin to inhibit cell spreading but promotes cell migration in a paxillin-independent manner. Mol Biol Cell 12:3214–3225

59. Lush CW, Cepinskas G, Sibbald WJ, Kvietys PR (2001) Endothelial E- and P-selectin expression in iNOS-deficient mice exposed to polymicrobial sepsis. Am J Physiol 280:G291–297

60. Misugi E, Tojo SJ, Yasuda T, Kurata Y, Morooka S (1998) Increased plasma P-selectin induced by intravenous administration of endotoxin in rats. Biochem Biophys Res Commun 246:414–417

61. Kneidinger R, Bahrami S, Redl H, Schlag G, Robinson M (1996) Comparison of endothelial activation during endotoxic and posttraumatic conditions by serum analysis of soluble E-selectin in nonhuman primates. J Lab Clin Med 128:515–519

62. Granton JT, Goddard CM, Allard MF, van Eeden S, Walley KR (1997) Leukocytes and decreased left-ventricular contractility during endotoxemia in rabbits. Am J Respir Crit Care Med 155:1977–1983

63. Thiel M, Zourelidis C, Chambers JD, et al (1997) Expression of beta 2-integrins and L-selectin on polymorphonuclear leukocytes in septic patients. Eur Surg Res 29:160–175

64. Ahmed NA, Christou NV (1996) Decreased neutrophil L-selectin expression in patients with systemic inflammatory response syndrome. Clin Invest Med 19:427–434

65. Lin RY, Astiz ME, Saxon JC, Rackow EC (1993) Altered leukocyte immunophenotypes in septic shock. Studies of HLA-DR, CD11b, CD14, and IL-2R expression. Chest 104:847–853

66. Tsokos M, Fehlauer F (2001) Post-mortem markers of sepsis: an immunohistochemical study using VLA-4 (CD49d/CD29) and ICAM-1 (CD54) for the detection of sepsis-induced lung injury. Int J Legal Med 114:291–294

67. Tsokos M, Fehlauer F, Puschel K (2000) Immunohistochemical expression of E-selectin in sepsis-induced lung injury. Int J Legal Med 113:338–342

68. Boldt J, Wollbruck M, Kuhn D, Linke LC, Hempelmann G (1995) Do plasma levels of circulating soluble adhesion molecules differ between surviving and nonsurviving critically ill patients? Chest 107:787–792

69. Newman W, Beall LD, Carson CW, et al (1993) Soluble E-selectin is found in supernatants of activated endothelial cells and is elevated in the serum of patients with septic shock. J Immunol 150:644–654

70. Facer CA, Theodoridou A (1994) Elevated plasma levels of P-selectin (GMP-140/CD62P) in patients with Plasmodium falciparum malaria. Microbiol Immunol 38:727–731

71. Pittard AJ, Banks RE, Galley HF, Webster NR (1996) Soluble E-cadherin concentrations in patients with systemic inflammatory response syndrome and multiorgan dysfunction syndrome. Br J Anaesth 76:629–631

72. Barroso-Aranda J, Schmid-Schonbein GW, Zweifach BW, Mathison JC (1991) Polymorphonuclear neutrophil contribution to induced tolerance to bacterial lipopolysaccharide. Circ Res 69:1196–1206

73. Mercer-Jones MA, Heinzelmann M, Peyton JC, Wickel D, Cook M, Cheadle WG (1997) Inhibition of neutrophil migration at the site of infection increases remote organ neutrophil sequestration and injury. Shock 8:193–199

74. Ikeda N, Mukaida N, Kaneko S, et al (1995) Prevention of endotoxin-induced acute lethality in Propionibacterium acnes-primed rabbits by an antibody to leukocyte integrin beta 2 with concomitant reduction of cytokine production. Infect Immun 63:4812–4817

75. Maeda T, Marubayashi S, Fukuma K, et al (1997) Effect of antileukocyte adhesion molecule antibodies, nitric oxide synthase inhibitor, and corticosteroids on endotoxin shock in mice. Surg Today 27:22–29

76. Xu N, Rahman A, Minshall RD, Tiruppathi C, Malik AB (2000) beta(2)-Integrin blockade driven by E-selectin promoter prevents neutrophil sequestration and lung injury in mice. Circ Res 87:254–260

77. Eichacker PQ, Farese A, Hoffman WD, et al (1992) Leukocyte CD11b/18 antigen-directed monoclonal antibody improves early survival and decreases hypoxemia in dogs challenged with tumor necrosis factor. Am Rev Respir Dis 145:1023–1029

78. Freeman BD, Correa R, Karzai W, et al (1996) Controlled trials of rG-CSF and CD11b-directed MAb during hyperoxia and E. coli pneumonia in rats. J Appl Physiol 80:2066–2076

79. Tomida S, Hasegawa T, Takeuchi M, et al (1994) Intercellular adhesion molecule-1 and leukocyte function-associated antigen-1 are involved in protection mediated by CD3+TCR alpha beta-T cells at the early stage after infection with Listeria monocytogenes in rats. Int Immunol 6:955–961

80. Zeni F, Parent C, Correa R, et al (1999) ICAM-1 and CD11b inhibition worsen outcome in rats with E. coli pneumonia. J Appl Physiol 87:299–307

81. Welty-Wolf KE, Carraway MS, Huang YC, et al (2001) Antibody to intercellular adhesion molecule 1 (CD54) decreases survival and not lung injury in baboons with sepsis. Am J Respir Crit Care Med 163:665–673

82. Eichacker PQ, Hoffman WD, Farese A, et al (1993) Leukocyte CD18 monoclonal antibody worsens endotoxemia and cardiovascular injury in canines with septic shock. J Appl Physiol 74:1885–1892

83. Mileski WJ, Sikes P, Atiles L, Lightfoot E, Lipsky P, Baxter C (1993) Inhibition of leukocyte adherence and susceptibility to infection. J Surg Res 54:349–354

84. Tuomanen EI, Saukkonen K, Sande S, Cioffe C, Wright SD (1989) Reduction of inflammation, tissue damage, and mortality in bacterial meningitis in rabbits treated with monoclonal antibodies against adhesion-promoting receptors of leukocytes. J Exp Med 170: 959–969

85. Thomas JR, Harlan JM, Rice CL, Winn RK (1992) Role of leukocyte CD11/CD18 complex in endotoxic and septic shock in rabbits. J Appl Physiol 73:1510–1516

86. Mileski WJ, Winn RK, Harlan JM, Rice CL (1991) Transient inhibition of neutrophil adherence with the anti-CD18 monoclonal antibody 60.3 does not increase mortality rates in abdominal sepsis. Surgery 109:497–501

87. Sarman G, Shappell SB, Mason EO Jr, Smith CW, Kaplan SL (1995) Susceptibility to local and systemic bacterial infections in intercellular adhesion molecule 1-deficient transgenic mice. J Infect Dis 172:1001–1006

88. Tedder TF, Steeber DA, Pizcueta P (1995) L-selectin-deficient mice have impaired leukocyte recruitment into inflammatory sites. J Exp Med 181:2259–2264

89. Sun X, Rozenfeld RA, Qu X, Huang W, Gonzalez-Crussi F, Hsueh W (1997) P-selectin-deficient mice are protected from PAF-induced shock, intestinal injury, and lethality. Am J Physiol 273:G56–G61

90. Seekamp A, Till GO, Mulligan MS, et al (1994) Role of selectins in local and remote tissue injury following ischemia and reperfusion. Am J Pathol 144:592–598

91. Schlag G, Redl HR, Till GO, Davies J, Martin U, Dumont L (1999) Anti-L-selectin antibody treatment of hemorrhagic-traumatic shock in baboons. Crit Care Med 27:1900–1907

92. Mulligan MS, Watson SR, Fennie C, Ward PA (1993) Protective effects of selectin chimeras in neutrophil-mediated lung injury. J Immunol 151:6410–6417

93. Ridings PC, Bloomfield GL, Holloway S, et al (1995) Sepsis-induced acute lung injury is attenuated by selectin blockade following the onset of sepsis. Arch Surg 130:1199–1208

94. Tasaki O, Goodwin C, Mozingo DW, et al (1999) Selectin blockade worsened lipopolysaccharide-induced lung injury in a swine model. J Trauma 46:1089–1095

95. Parent C, Kalil A, Correa R, et al (1998) L-selectin directed Mab increases or decreases survival dependent on site but not severity of infection in rats. Am J Respir Crit Care Med 25:A30 (Abst)

96. Carraway MS, Welty-Wolf KE, Kantrow SP, et al (1998) Antibody to E- and L-selectin does not prevent lung injury or mortality in septic baboons. Am J Respir Crit Care Med 157:938–949

97. Sharar SR, Chapman NN, Flaherty LC, Harlan JM, Tedder TF, Winn RK (1996) L-selectin (CD62L) blockade does not impair peritoneal neutrophil emigration or subcutaneous host defense to bacteria in rabbits. J Immunol 157:2555–2563

98. Munoz FM, Hawkins EP, Bullard DC, Beaudet AL, Kaplan SL (1997) Host defense against systemic infection with Streptococcus pneumoniae is impaired in E-, P-, and E-/P-selectin-deficient mice. J Clin Invest 100:2099–2106

99.   Opal SM, Sypek JP, Keith JC Jr, Schaub RG, Palardy JE, Parejo NA (2001) Evaluation of the safety of recombinant P-selectin glycoprotein ligand-immunoglobulin G fusion protein in experimental models of localized and systemic infection. Shock 15:285–290

100. Eppihimer MJ, Schaub RG (2001) Soluble P-selectin antagonist mediates rolling velocity and adhesion of leukocytes in acutely inflamed venules. Microcirculation 8:15–24

101. Schleiffenbaum B, Spertini O, Tedder TF (1992) Soluble L-selectin is present in human plasma at high levels and retains functional activity. J Cell Biol 119:229–238

102. Egan BM, Chen G, Kelly CJ, Bouchier-Hayes DJ (2001) Taurine attenuates LPS-induced rolling and adhesion in rat microcirculation. J Surg Res 95:85–91

103. Kubes P, Suzuki M, Granger DN (1991) Nitric oxide: an endogenous modulator of leukocyte adhesion. Proc Natl Acad Sci USA 88:4651–4655

104. Sundrani R, Easington CR, Mattoo A, Parrillo JE, Hollenberg SM (2000) Nitric oxide synthase inhibition increases venular leukocyte rolling and adhesion in septic rats. Crit Care Med 28:2898–2903

105. Vedder N, Harlan J, Winn R, et al (1997) Pilot phase 2 clinical trial of a humanized CD11/CD18 monoclonal antibody in hemorrhagic shock. Shock 7:A659 (Abst)

106. Friedman G, Jankowski S, Shahla M, et al (1996) Administration of an antibody to E-selectin in patients with septic shock. Crit Care Med 24:229–233

Molecular Mechanisms of Complement Activation during Ischemia and Reperfusion

C. L. F. Ciurana and C. E. Hack

▌ Introduction

Ischemia is a frequent clinical problem occurring, amongst others, in myocardial infarction, transplantation, vascular surgery, and thrombo-embolic disease. The obvious treatment of ischemia is reperfusion of the jeopardized organ or tissue. However, when ischemia is too severe, reperfusion may exacerbate rather than limit tissue damage, a phenomenon known as ischemia/reperfusion (I/R)-injury. A number of studies have been performed to unravel the pathophysiology of I/R-injury, and it is now clear that this condition is mainly due to an inflammatory process elicited by reperfusion. Hence, limiting I/R-induced inflammatory reactions is expected to improve the efficacy of reperfusion. Indeed, inhibition of inflammatory mediators improves the beneficial effects of reperfusion of ischemic tissues in animal models. In this chapter we will summarize the role of inflammation in the pathogenesis of I/R-injury, and discuss in more detail that of the complement system, as this plasma cascade system seems to be a key mediator in this condition.

▌ The Inflammatory Cascade

Inflammation is an extremely complex interaction of an array of so-called inflammatory mediators resulting in activation of various cells such as leukocytes, endothelial cells and platelets, and in the generation of aggressive molecules including multispecific proteases, oxygen and nitrogen radicals, and various lipid mediators, which degrade proteins and other biomolecules, and cause dysfunction and death of cells. Clinical manifestations of inflammation may range from the classical signs of rubor, calor, tumor, dolor and functio laesa, to organ dysfunction and severe shock. A simplified scheme describing the inflammatory cascade is given in Fig. 1.

According to the scheme outlined in Fig. 1, cytokines should be considered as primary inflammatory mediators orchestrating a number of down-stream inflammatory effector mechanisms. The pro-inflammatory effects of cytokines are numerous and include activation of various cells such as endothelial cells, leukocytes and platelets. Part of their effects are exerted by activating nuclear factor kappa B (NF-κB), which induces the synthesis of other cytokines and inflammatory proteins. For example, the expression of adhesion molecules, such as intercellular adhesion molecule (ICAM)-1, which increases during I/R [1], is under control of NF κB. As depicted in Fig. 1, plasma cascade systems, such as the coagulation and the complement systems, endothelial cells, polymorphonuclear neutrophils (PMN) and plate-

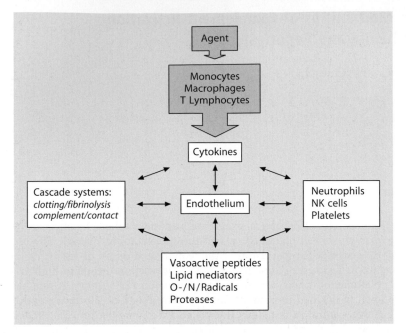

Fig. 1. Inflammatory cascade with various mediators, activators and effectors. NK: natural killer

lets, may be considered as secondary inflammatory mediators. Coagulation is activated when endothelial cells or blood mononuclear cells are stimulated by the cytokines tumor necrosis factor (TNF) or interleukin (IL)-1; the expression of tissue factor, which interacts with coagulation factor VII, is induced whereas anti-coagulant molecules such as thrombomodulin are down-regulated. Finally, tertiary inflammatory mediators such as multispecific proteases, oxygen and nitrogen radicals are generated, which degrade proteins and phospholipid membranes and induce cell damage and death.

Role of Inflammation in I/R-injury

A number of studies have demonstrated the involvement of a variety of inflammatory mediators in I/R-injury. In general, these studies have shown:
- the activation or release of inflammatory mediators following I/R-injury;
- reduction of I/R-injury during treatment with anti-inflammatory drugs; and
- reduced I/R-injury in animals deficient in inflammatory mediators.

Increased plasma levels of cytokines including TNF, IL-6, IL-8 and others, and increased mRNA levels of pro-inflammatory cytokines, support the notion that these mediators play a role in the pathogenesis of I/R-injury. Notably, this increase occurs within hours after reperfusion of ischemic tissues. For example, pro-inflammatory cytokine mRNA is upregulated in parallel with a decreased expression of superoxide dismutase (SOD) and a rise in oxygen radicals in a rat gastrointestinal I/R model [2]. Definite proof for a role in the pathogenesis of I/R-injury was provided in studies showing that inhibition of cytokines, such as TNF, with neutralizing antibodies reduces I/R-injury [3]. Also, in human I/R-injury, cytokines likely play a role. Plasma levels of IL-6 increase in patients undergoing cardiopulmonary bypass [4]. Notably, not only pro-inflammatory cytokines increase during I/R, but also anti-inflammatory cytokines such as IL-10 [5], presumably to off-set inflammation in the later stages of I/R.

Among the multiple effects of pro-inflammatory cytokines is endothelial cell stimulation. Stimulated endothelium actively contributes to inflammatory processes by promoting coagulation, secreting mediators such as cytokines, vasoactive compounds, and chemoattracting agents, and expressing adhesion molecules. These processes orchestrate the infiltration of leukocytes into the inflamed tissues. Adhesion molecules, for example selectins, are upregulated during I/R [6], which allows the transmigration of PMN into the ischemic tissue. These cells exaggerate tissue damage by producing oxygen radicals and other cytotoxic components. Many animal models have shown that the activation of PMN (as well as of complement, see below) during I/R may provoke injury in remote organs particularly the lungs [7, 8]. Both endothelial cells and PMN secrete platelet activating factor (PAF), which activates platelets and PMNs.

As a result of the interaction of the endothelium with activated PMN, the endothelium may become dysfunctional. Indeed, impaired functions of ionic canals with influx of Ca^{2+}, formation of reactive oxygen species (ROS), generation of lipid derived mediators and deregulation of nitric oxide (NO) metabolism are among the features observed with endothelial cells exposed to I/R. Damage to the endothelium may result in enhanced vascular leakage, thrombus formation, and loss of regulation of microcirculatory flow [9–12]. These phenomena may exaggerate hypoxygenation of the tissues upon reperfusion. This phenomenon is also enhanced by another mechanism involving PMN. During I/R these inflammatory cells become activated within the blood vessels. As a consequence of activation, PMN become stiff, and, due to their relatively large diameter, plug capillaries, which have a smaller diameter. This mechanism is thought to explain the so-called 'no reflow' phenomenon, which is often observed when severely ischemic tissues are reperfused. Indeed, evidence for a role of neutrophils in I/R-injury was provided by studies showing that neutropenia is associated with less I/R-related injury [13]. Furthermore, blockade of ICAM-1 also attenuates I/R-injury [14], suggesting that the interaction of activated PMN with the ischemic endothelium, is an important event in the pathogenesis of I/R-injury.

▌ The Complement System

In addition to the mediators briefly discussed above, the complement system constitutes an important mediator of I/R-injury. Complement has a major function in innate immunity but it is also contributes to adaptive immune reactions in particular at low antigen concentrations [15]. The complement system is composed of more than 30 proteins, most of which circulate in peripheral blood as inactive zymogens. During activation, the various complement components are activated by limited proteolysis, in a process in which one component activates the next one in the cascade and so on. Ultimately, the membrane attack complex (MAC) consisting of the components C5, C6, C7, C8 and polymeric C9 is formed, which can induce

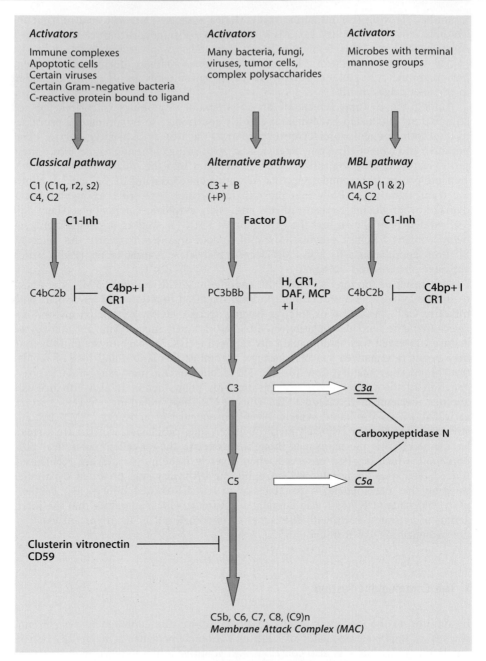

Fig. 2. Complement activation cascades. The three different pathways (classical, alternative and mannan binding lectin [MBL]) are depicted here and inhibitors are also indicated in bold. Inflammatory mediators are indicated in bold, italic, underlined symbols

cell lysis. Upstream to C5, and central in the complement cascade is the third component, C3. C3 can be activated via various pathways: the classical; the alternative; and the mannan binding lectin (MBL) pathways (Fig. 2).

Immune complexes containing IgM or IgG are well known activators of the classical pathway. This pathway is also activated by other agents, including bacterial components and C-reactive protein (CRP) [16]. Activators of the classical pathway bind and activate the first complement protein, C1. C1 consists of three components: C1q, which binds to the activator; and the pro-enzymes C1r and C1s, which both are present as dimers in the C1 complex, and become active enzymes upon activation. Activated C1s activates C4 and C2, which together form the bimolecular C4b2b complex. This complex is a C3-convertase, able to activate C3.

Bacterial products can activate complement in an antibody-independent fashion via at least two different mechanisms. One of these involves alternative pathway activation, which leads to the formation of the C3bBb complex. This bimolecular complex, another C3-convertase, is stabilized by properdin (P). The other mechanism starts with the binding of MBL, a protein resembling C1q, to sugar residues, particularly mannose, in the bacterial wall. Bound MBL then will activate so-called MBL-associated serine proteinase-1 and/or -2 (MASP-1 and MASP-2, respectively), which are homologous to C1r and C1s. Activated MASPs can either activate C3 directly, or indirectly via activation of C4 and C2. Many molecular aspects of this MBL-pathway are not clear yet. There is evidence for the involvement of other collectins (MBL and C1q both belong to this superfamily of proteins) such as ficolin. Furthermore, another MASP, MASP-3, has been identified recently, but its role is far from clear yet.

Inflammatory Effects of Complement Activation Products

All three pathways of complement ultimately lead to the activation of C3 and the formation of MAC, which can penetrate into the cell membrane to form a pore. Insertion of various MAC complexes in the membrane induces lysis of the cells. Smaller amounts of MAC are not necessarily lethal to cells, but rather may signal the cells to produce inflammatory mediators, which in part results from NF-κB activation. Among the effects of sublytic amounts of MAC are adhesion molecule expression and the synthesis of pro-inflammatory cytokines [17, 18]. In addition, C5b-7 and C5b-8, incomplete forms of MAC, can activate intracellular mechanisms [19]. MAC is not the only inflammatory complement product. During activation of C4, C3 and C5, small peptides, C4a, C3a and C5a, respectively, are cleaved off, which, because of their biological effects, are known as the anaphylatoxins. In particular C5a is a potent peptide being able to attract, activate, and degranulate PMN, and to induce bronchoconstriction and vasodilation due to its effects on smooth muscle cells (contraction in the airways, relaxation in the arterioles, respectively). Furthermore, the anaphylatoxins are able to activate and degranulate mast cells and platelets, and have many more inflammatory effects [20–22].

Regulation of Complement Activation

In order to control excessive activation and to overcome unwanted detrimental effects, complement activation is regulated at various levels. Two main classes of regulators exist: fluid phase and membrane-bound regulators. Some regulators act as enzyme inhibitors (C1-inhibitor, C1-Inh), some are protease (factor I) that serve to degrade active complement components into inactive species, whereas others, such as factor H, compete with cofactors of the complement enzymes [15, 23]. Factors H and I are fluid phase inhibitors that regulate amplification and the alternative pathway, whereas C4-binding protein (C4bp), C1-Inh and factor I regulate both the classical and the MBL pathways. Membrane cofactor protein (MCP or CD46), decay accelerating factor (DAF or CD55), and complement receptor 1 (CR1 or CD35) are membrane-bound proteins that inhibit all pathways at the level of the C3 and C5 convertases [24].

The formation of MAC is inhibited by several plasma proteins, including vitronectin S protein and clusterin SP40, 40, apolipoproteins J, AI and AII, and also the membrane-bound complement regulators, C8 binding protein (C8bp), and protectin (CD59). The membrane-bound regulatory proteins are differently expressed depending on the cell type [25]. Endothelial cells in general are well endowed with membrane-bound complement regulatory proteins, presumably to protect these cells from so-called innocent bystander lysis by activation processes induced by complement activators in the neighborhood. This protection may be lost during I/R: glycosyl phosphatidyl inositol (GPI)-anchored regulators CD35 and CD59 are released during inflammation, which renders the cells more sensitive to complement attack. This has been shown both in vitro [26], in a rat model of acute myocardial infarction, as well as in human acute myocardial infarction [27, 28]. Notably, membrane-bound complement regulators also may be upregulated during I/R, though this phenomenon needs more then 24 h, and hence is probably not important for the protection of cells during I/R injury, as this damage occurs within hours after reperfusion [29, 30].

Complement Activation During I/R

Complement involvement in the inflammatory process induced by I/R was proposed more than three decades ago by Hill and Ward [31]. Since then, a number of studies have shown that complement is activated during I/R-injury [24, 32–36]. In general, this activation occurs within minutes after reperfusion, diminishing within 30 to 60 minutes [35]. To assess whether complement activation contributes to the pathophysiology of I/R-injury or constitutes an epiphenomenon, initially the effect of cobra venom factor (CVF) was evaluated in animal models. CVF binds to factor B, which subsequently becomes activated by factor D, and activates native C3 into C3a and C3b, and C5 into C5a and C5b. As it is not regulated by factors I and H, the complex of CVF with factor B constitutes an unregulated C3-convertase that within 1–2 hours depletes circulating complement, an effect that may last up to 24–48 hours. Hence, pretreatment with CVF renders an animal virtually complement-deficient during this period. CVF pretreatment reduced I/R-injury in a number of animal models [37, 38]. As CVF extensively depletes the complement system by activation within the vascular compartment, its application is associated with serious side effects such as dyspnea, hypotension, and others. Hence, this agent cannot be used in clinical practice. Over the last decade a number of complement inhibitors, which do not have this disadvantage of intravascular activation of the system, have been developed and evaluated for their effects in animal models for I/R-injury. All these inhibitors, which include C1-Inh [32, 33], sCD35 or sCR1 [34–36] as well as DAF/MCP hybrid molecules [39] showed beneficial effects in these models. Antibodies against C5 or the MAC complex also showed beneficial effects [40–42]. Final proof for the involvement of complement in I/R-injury came from experiments in complement-deficient mice [43], which showed significantly less I/R-injury than their wild-type littermates. The deficient animals developed normal I/R-injury when supplemented with the lacking protein.

The studies discussed above clearly demonstrated that complement is activated during I/R and contributes to the injury induced by reperfusion. Likely the most toxic complement activation products are generated at the level of C5, since inhibition of C5 activation by monoclonal antibodies, which allows C3 activation, reduces I/R-injury. These activation products likely are C5a and /or MAC, as is discussed in a previous paragraph.

Mechanisms of Complement Activation During I/R

A number of studies have shown that the classical, the alternative, as well as MBL pathways could be involved in the development of I/R-injury depending on the model, the type of tissue and the time course of inflammation [44].

Involvement of IgM. IgG or IgM antibodies bound to antigens are strong activators of the classical complement pathways. Observations in mouse models have revealed that in particular IgM may be involved in the pathogenesis of I/R-injury. In initial experiments it was shown that mice deficient in rag (RAG1-/- (C57BL/6J-RAG $1^{tm\ 1\ Mom}$) and RAG2-/-), and hence unable to form immunoglobulins, had about half the I/R-injury in a hind-limb model as compared to wild-type mice. Deficient mice substituted with polyclonal IgM had I/R-injury comparable with wild-type mice. Finally, it was established that upon reperfusion, IgM bound to the endothelium in the ischemic tissues, although the epitopes for this IgM are not known at present [45]. Similar results were obtained in a mouse model for intestinal I/R [46].

Involvement of C-reactive protein (CRP). CRP is an acute phase protein that, upon binding to a ligand, can activate the classical complement pathway. It also inhibits the activation of the alternative pathway by increasing the binding of regulator factor H to C3b [47]. Lyso-phospholipids generated in the cell membrane may be a ligand for CRP [16, 48]. These lyso-phospholipids may be generated in a membrane by interaction with phospholipase A_2 (PLA$_2$) with a flip-flopped membrane [49], as occurs in damaged cells.

In a post-mortem study of patients with acute myocardial infarction, CRP was found to be co-localized with activated C3 and C4 on cardiomyocytes [50], suggesting this mechanism may be relevant for ischemia of tissues in humans. Human CRP indeed was found to enhance reperfusion-induced cell death in a rat model of myocardial infarction [51]. Pasceri et al. [52] have shown *in vitro* that endothelial cells exposed to I/R, had an increased expression of adhesion molecules (ICAM-1, vascular cell adhesion molecule [VCAM]-1 and E-Selectin) upon binding of CRP in the presence of serum, an effect that is likely complement-mediated [50].

Mitochondrial disturbance. Many *in vitro* data have emphasized a role for mitochondria in the onset of complement activation by I/R injury. In these studies, mitochondria were shown to be able to activate complement when added to normal human serum. Sera deficient in immunoglobulins allowed complement activation to a similar extent as normal sera, ruling out the involvement of immunoglobulins in this activation process [53]. Few candidate proteins able to activate C1, have been purified from mitochondria. Also cardiolipin was described to bind C1q and was detected *in vivo* in cardiac lymph upon reperfusion [54]. In another study from

Giclas et al. [55], both classical and alternative pathways were activated in serum incubated with human heart mitochondrial membrane constituents. Though the molecular mechanism causing complement activation by mitochondria is not completely resolved yet, these studies clearly demonstrate an intriguing mechanism of complement activation. However, whether this mechanism really contributes to complement-mediated damage during I/R is not clear since it requires exposure of mitochondria to extracellular proteins, i.e., complement components. This implies that the cells providing mitochondria for this activation process, are already permeable, and probably dead.

Other mechanisms of activation. Many studies have been undertaken to elucidate the mechanism of activation of complement during I/R. Various activation mechanisms other than those described above, have been suggested, and include activation of the classical, MBL, and alternative pathways.

Since activation of C4 has been observed without apparent involvement of immunoglobulins, the role of the MBL pathway in I/R was studied. Indeed, cultured endothelial cells exposed *in vitro* to hypoxia followed by reoxygenation, bound MBL [56]. Cytokeratin 1, which is upregulated during I/R, was identified as a ligand for MBL [57]. Although a role for MBL was also pointed out in I/R *in vivo* [58], it remains to be established to what extent this mechanism contributes to I/R-injury in man.

Erythrocytes, of which the membranes are disturbed and flip-flopped upon oxidative stress, were shown to activate complement *in vivo* via the alternative pathway; this induced recruitment of neutrophils and amplified the inflammatory process [59–61]. A flip-flop of the cell-membrane likely occurs on endothelial cells upon I/R. Thus, it is conceivable that a similar activation process may take place on these cells, at least during I/R. Subendothelial extracellular matrix, exposed to blood upon endothelial disruption, also has been suggested to activate complement [62]. In addition, oxidized molecules generated by I/R such as oxidized low density lipoproteins (LDL) [17], were found to activate proteases, which in turn activate the alternative pathway of complement. Apoptotic endothelial cells can also activate the classical complement pathway *in vitro*. Among the mechanisms causing this activation, IgM deposition may be involved [63]. On the other hand, evidence is accumulating that apoptotic cells directly or indirectly via adaptor molecules, such as CRP or serum amyloid P component [64], may activate complement.

▌ Conclusion

It is now well accepted that complement plays a role in the initiation of I/R injury in animals. However, whether this occurs in humans as well remains to be established. Inhibition of complement reduces I/R-injury significantly, though not completely. Hence, complement inhibitors constitute an attractive option for therapy in clinical conditions resulting from I/R-injury. Complement is likely activated during I/R via multiple mechanisms. Unraveling the relative contribution of these mechanisms to I/R-injury in man, probably allows for the best therapeutic approach to reduce this injury.

References

1. Li C, Browder W, Kao RL (1999) Early activation of transcription factor NF-κB during ischemia in reperfused rat heart. Am J Physiol 276:H543–H552 (Abst)
2. Konturek PC, Duda A, Brzozowski T, et al (2000) Activation of genes for superoxide dismutase, interleukin-1β, tumor necrosis factor-alpha and intercellular adhesion molecule-1 during healing of ischemia-reperfusion-induced gastric injury. Scand J Gastroenterol 35: 452–463
3. Seekamp A, Warren JS, Remick DG, Till GO, Ward PA (1993) Requirements for tumor necrosis factor-alpha and interleukin-1 in limb ischemia/reperfusion injury and associated lung injury. Am J Pathol 143:453–463
4. Steinberg JB, Kapelanski DP, Olson JD, Weiler JM (1993) Cytokine and complement levels in patients undergoing cardiopulmonary bypass. J Thorac Cardiovasc Surg 106:1008–1016
5. Yang Z, Zingarelli B, Szabo C (2000) Crucial role of endogenous IL-10 production in myocardial ischemia reperfusion injury. Circulation 101:1019–1026
6. Zund G, Nelson DP, Neufeld EJ et al (1996) Hypoxia enhances stimulus-dependent induction of E-selectin on aortic endothelial cells. Proc Natl Acad Sci USA 93:7075–7080
7. Lindsay TF, Hill J, Ortiz F et al (1992) Blockade of complement activation prevents local and pulmonary albumin leak after lower torso ischemia-reperfusion. Ann Surg 216:677–683
8. Seekamp A, Mulligan MS, Till GO, et al (1993) Role of β2 integrins and ICAM-1 in lung injury following ischemia-reperfusion of rat hind limb. Am J Pathol 143:464–472
9. Lucchesi BR, Kilgore KS (1997) Complement inhibitors in myocardial ischemia/reperfusion injury. Immunopharmacology 38:27–42
10. Entman ML, Michael L, Rossen RD, et al (1991) Inflammation in the course of early myocardial ischemia. Faseb J 5:2529–2537
11. Cines DB, Pollak ES, Buck CA, et al (1998) Endothelial Cells in Physiology and in the Pathophysiology of vascular disorders. Blood 91:3527–3561
12. Silverstein RL (1999) The vascular endothelium. In: Gallin JI, Snyderman R, Haynes BF (eds) Inflammation: Basic Principles and Clinical Correlates. 3rd edition, Lipincott Williams & Wilkins, Philadelphia, pp 207–225
13. Iwahori Y, Ishiguro N, Shimizu T, et al (1998) Selective neutrophils depletion with monoclonal antibody attenuates I/R injury in skeletal muscle. J Reconstr Microsurg 14:109–116
14. Zhao ZQ, Lefer DJ, Sato H, Hart KK, Jefforda PR, Vinten-Johansen J (1997) Monoclonal antibody to ICAM-1 preserves postischemic blood flow and reduces infarct size after ischemia-reperfusion in rabbit. J Leukoc Biol 62:292–300
15. Cooper NL (1999) Biology of the complement system. In: Gallin JI, Snyderman R, Haynes BF (eds) Inflammation: Basic Principles and Clinical Correlates. 3rd edition, Lipincott Williams & Wilkins, Philadelphia, pp 281–307
16. Wolbink GJ, Brouwer MC, Buysmann S, Ten Berge IJM, Hack CE (1996) CRP-mediated activation of complement in vivo. J Immunol 157:473–479
17. Vakeva AP, Agah A, Rollins SA, et al (1998) Myocardial infarction and apoptosis after myocardial ischemia and reperfusion. Role of the terminal complement components and inhibition by anti-C5 therapy. Circulation 97:2259–2267
18. Tedesco F, Pausa M, Nardon E, Introna M, Mantovani A, Dobrina A (1997) The cytolytically inactive terminal complement complex activates endothelial cells to express adhesion molecules and tissue factor procoagulant activity. J Exp Med 185:1619–1627
19. Agostoni A, Gardinali M, Frangi D, et al (1994) Thrombolytic treatment and complement activation. Ann Ital Med Int 9:178–179
20. Marks RM, Todd III RF, Ward PA (1989) Rapid induction of neutrophil-endothelial adhesion by endothelial complement fixation. Nature 339:314–317
21. Vakeva A, Meri S (1998) Complement activation and regulator expression after anoxic injury of human endothelial cells. APMIS 106:1149–1156
22. Chenoweth DE, Cooper SW, Hugli TE, Steward RW, Blackstone EH, Kirklin JW (1981) Complement activation during cardio-pulmonary bypass. Evidence for generation of C3a and C5a anaphylatoxins. N Engl J Med 304:497–503

23. Jones J, Morgan BP (1995) Apoptosis is associated with reduced expression of complement regulatory molecules, adhesion molecules and other receptors on polymorphonuclear leucocytes: functional and role in inflammation. Immunology 86:651–660

24. Weisman HF, Bartow T, Leppo MK, et al (1990) Soluble human complement receptor type 1: in vivo inhibitor of complement suppressing post-ischemic myocardial inflammation and necrosis. Science 249:146–151

25. Soarzec JY, Delautier D, Moreau A, et al (1994) Expression of complement-regulatory proteins in normal and UW-preserved human liver. Gastroenterology 107:505–516

26. Brooimans RA, Van der Ark AAJ, Tomita M, Van Es LA, Daha M (1992) CD59 expressed by human endothelial cells functions as a protective molecule against complement-mediated lysis. Eur J Immunol 22:791–797

27. Vakeva A, Morgan BP, Tikkanen I, Helin K, Laurila P, Meri S (1994) Time course of complement activation and inhibitor expression after ischemic injury of rat myocardium. Am J Pathol 144:1357–1368

28. Vakeva A, Lehto T, Takala A, Meri S (2000) Detection of a soluble form of the complement membrane attack complex inhibitor CD59 in plasma after acute myocardial infarction. Scand J Immunol 52:411–414

29. Collard CD, Vakeva A, Bukusoglu C, et al (1997) Reoxygenation of hypoxic human umbilical vein endothelial cells activates the classic complement pathway. Circulation 96:326–333

30. Collard CD, Bukusoglu C, Agah A, et al (1999) Hypoxia-induced expression of complement receptor type 1 (CR1, CD35) in human vascular endothelial cells. Am J Physiol 276:C450–C458

31. Hill JH, Ward PA (1971) The phlogistic role of C3 leukotactic fragments in myocardial infarcts of rats. J Exp Med 133:885–900

32. Horstick G, Heimann A, Götze O, et al (1997) Intracoronary application of c1 esterase inhibitor improves cardiac function and reduces myocardial necrosis in an experimental model of ischemia and reperfusion. Circulation 95:701–708

33. Buerke M, Prüfer D, Dahm M, et al (1998) Blocking of classical complement pathway inhibits endothelial adhesion molecule expression and preserves ischemic myocardium from reperfusion injury. J Pharmacol Exp Ther 286:429–438

34. Lehmann TG, Koeppel TA, Kirschfink M, et al (1998) Complement inhibition by soluble complement receptor type 1 improves microcirculation after rat liver transplantation. Transplantation 66:717–722

35. Eror AT, Stojadinovic A, Starnes BW, et al (1999) Antiinflammatory effects of soluble complement receptor type 1 promote rapid recovery of ischemia/reperfusion injury in rat small intestine. Clin Immunol 90:266–275

36. Lazar HL, Bao Y, Gaudiani J, et al (1999) Total complement inhibition: An effective strategy to limit ischemic injury during coronary revascularization on cardiopulmonary bypass. Circulation 100:1438–1442

37. Maroko PR, Carpenter CB, Chariello M (1978) Reduction by cobra venom factor of myocardial necrosis after coronary artery occlusion. J Clin Invest 61:661–670

38. Ikai M, Itoh M, Joh T, et al (1996) Complement plays an essential role in shock following intestinal ischaemia in rats. Clin Exp Immunol 106:156–159

39. Kroshus TJ, Salerno CT, Yeh CG, et al (2000) A recombinant soluble chimeric complement inhibitor composed of human cd46 and cd55 reduces acute cardiac tissue injury in models of pig-human heart transplantation. Transplantation 69:2282–2289

40. Heller T, Hennecke M, Baumann U et al (1999) Selection of C5a receptor antagonist from phage libraries attenuating the inflammatory response in immune complex disease and ischemia/reperfusion injury. J Immunol 163:985–994

41. Fitch JCK, Rollins S, Matis L, et al (1999) Pharmacology and biological efficacy of recombinant, humanized, single-chain antibody c5 complement inhibitor in patients undergoing coronary artery bypass graft surgery with cardiopulmonary bypass. Circulation 100:2499–2506

42. Collard CD, Agah A, Reenstra W, Buras J, Stahl GL (1999) Endothelial nuclear factor-κb translocation and vascular cell adhesion molecule-1 induction by complement: inhibition with anti-human C5 therapy or cGMP analogues. Arterioscler Thromb Vasc Biol 19:2623–2629

43. Kyriakides C, Austen W, Wang Y, et al (1999) Skeletal muscle reperfusion injury is mediated by neutrophils and the complement membrane attack complex. Am J Physiol 277:1263–1268

44. Collard CD, Lebowski R, Jordan JE, Agah A, Stahl GL (1999) Complement activation following oxidative stress. Mol Immunol 36:941–948

45. Weiser MR, Williams JP, Moore FD, et al (1996) Reperfusion injury of ischemic skeletal muscle is mediated by natural antibody and complement. J Exp Med 183:2343–2348

46. Williams JP, Pechet TTV, Weiser MR, et al (1999) Intestinal reperfusion injury is mediated by IgM and complement. J Appl Physiol 86:938–942

47. Suankratay C, Mold C, Zhang Y, et al (1998) Complement regulation in innate immunity and the acute-phase response: inhibition of mannan-binding lectin-initiated complement cytolysis by C-reactive protein (CRP). Clin Exp Immunol 113:353–359

48. Volanakis JE, Narkates AJ (1981) Interaction of C-reactive protein with artificial phosphatidylcholine bilayers and complement. J Immunol 126:1820–1825

49. Lagrand WK, Visser CA, Hermens WT et al (1999) C-Reactive protein as a cardiovascular risk factor. More than epiphenomenon? Circulation 100:96–102

50. Lagrand WK, Niessen HWM, Wolbink GJ, et al (1997) C-Reactive protein colocalizes with complement in human hearts during acute myocardial infarction. Circulation 95(1):97–103

51. Griselli M, Herbert J, Hutchinson WL, et al (1999) C-reactive protein and complement are important mediators of tissue damage in acute myocardial infarction. J Exp Med 190:1733–1740

52. Pasceri V, Willerson JT, Yeh ETH (2000) Direct proinflammatory effect of c-reactive protein on human endothelial cells. Circulation 102:2165–2168

53. Kagiyama A, Savage HE, Michael LH, Hanson G, Entman ML, Rossen RD (1989) Molecular basis of complement activation in ischemic myocardium: identification of specific molecules of mitochondrial origin that bind human C1q and fix complement. Circ Res 64:607–615

54. Rossen RD, Michael LH, Hawkins HK, et al (1994) Cardiolipin-protein complexes and initiation of complement activation after coronary artery occlusion. Circ Res 75:546–555

55. Giclas PC, Pinckard RN, Olson MS (1979) In vitro activation of complement by isolated human heart subcellular membranes. J Immunol 122:146–151

56. Collard CD, Vakeva A, Morrissey MA, et al (2000) Complement activation after oxidative stress: role of the lectin complement pathway. Am J Pathol 156: 1549–1556

57. Collard CD, Montaldo MC, Reenstra WR, Buras JA, Stahl GL (2001) Endothelial oxidative stress activates the lectin complement pathway; role of cytokeratin 1. Am J Pathol 159:1045–1054

58. Jordan JE, Montaldo MC, Stahl GL (2001) Inhibition of mannose-binding lectin reduces postischemic myocardial reperfusion injury. Circulation 104:1413–1418

59. Salama A, Hugo FH, Heinrich D, et al (1988) Deposition of terminal C5b-9 complement complexes on erythrocytes and leukocytes during cardiopulmonary bypass. N Engl J Med 318:408–414

60. Hostetter MK, Johnson GM (1989) The erythrocytes as instigator of inflammation. J Clin Invest 84:665–671

61. Test ST, Mitsuyoshi J (1997) Activation of the alternative pathway of complement by calcium-loaded erythrocytes resulting from loss of membrane phospholipid asymmetry. J Lab Clin Med 130:169–182

62. Hindsmarsh EJ, Marks RM (1998) Complement activation occurs on subendothelial extracellular matrix in vitro and is initiated by retraction or removal of overlying endothelial cells. J Immunol 160:6128–6136

63. Mold C, Morris CA (2001) Complement activation by apoptotic endothelial cells following hypoxia/reoxygenation. Immunology 102:359–364

64. Familian A, Zwart B, Huisman HG, et al (2001) Chromatin-independent binding of serum amyloid P component to apoptotic cells. J Immunol 167:647–654

Gender and Cell-mediated Immunity Following Trauma, Shock, and Sepsis

M. G. Schwacha, A. Samy, and I. H. Chaudry

▌ Introduction

While improved preventative methods and patient care have decreased patient morbidity and mortality, major traumatic injury remains one of the leading causes of death for young adults (< 30 years of age) in the United States. Trauma represents a severe form of injury including bone fracture, penetrating soft tissue injury, (i.e., gunshot wounds), thermal injury and protracted surgical procedures. Many forms of traumatic injury, such as penetrating soft tissue trauma, are usually associated with a subsequent loss of significant blood volume. During the initial 60-minute post-traumatic period, approximately 50% of the observed mortality is due to exsanguination or central nervous system (CNS) complications. In the subsequent 2 hours, close to 30% of the victims succumb to major internal organ damage. Unfortunately, surviving trauma patient prognosis remains dire, since these patients display a 50% mortality rate from secondary complications that include sepsis, multiple organ failure (MOF), and eventual death [1–3]. Sepsis is the major non-neurological cause of death following trauma. A significant effort in scientific and medical research has been directed towards understanding the relationship between major traumatic injury and/or shock and the predisposition to septic/infectious complications and/or MOF.

Several clinical and experimental studies have demonstrated that trauma and hemorrhage markedly influence cell-mediated immune responses. The observed changes in immune responsiveness following trauma and hemorrhage involve T- and B-lymphocytes, macrophages, and neutrophils. The functional capacity of these immune cells are altered as reflected in suppressed antigen presentation, lymphocyte proliferation, and antibody production as well as altered release of pro- and anti-inflammatory cytokines [4, 5]. Dysfunctional cell-mediated immune response after traumatic injury is believed to be a key factor in the development of sepsis and MOF. In addition, sepsis (independent of an initiating insult such as trauma) has marked deleterious effects on cell-mediated immunity [4]. Similar to the disease states of systemic lupus erythematosus (SLE), Hashimoto's thyroiditis, rheumatoid arthritis [6, 7], gender also plays an important role in the regulation of the immune response following traumatic injury [8]. This chapter will focus on the current state of knowledge regarding the role of gender and sex hormones in the regulation of cell-mediated immune responses following traumatic injury, hemorrhage and sepsis.

▌ Gender and the Post-injury Immune Response

Shock

Gender has been shown to markedly alter the immune response following the induction of hemorrhagic shock. For example, female rats have been reported to be more resistant to lethal circulatory stress induced by trauma or intestinal ischemia [9], and female mice in the proestrus state of the estrus cycle have been found to exhibit maintained or enhanced cell-mediated immune responses as opposed to depressed responses in males following trauma-hemorrhage [10]. Recent studies have been directed towards elucidating the mechanisms responsible for this gender dimorphic response. Castration of male mice prior to the induction of trauma-hemorrhage results in the maintenance of cell-mediated immune responses [11]. Treatment of castrated animals with 5a-dihydrotestosterone induced an immunosuppressed phenotype following trauma-hemorrhage similar to that normally observed in intact male mice. Thus, 5a-dihydrotestosterone appears to be a factor responsible for inducing immunosuppression following trauma-hemorrhage.

The induction of lung injury following hemorrhagic shock also appears to be gender dimorphic, with male rats, but not female rats, subjected to hemorrhage showing evidence of increased lung permeability [12]. Moreover, mesenteric lymph collected from hemorrhaged male rats was toxic to human umbilical vein endothelial cells. Furthermore, shock caused gut injury in males, whereas no such injury was observed in hemorrhaged females. These findings suggest that the resistance of females to hemorrhage-induced lung injury may be due to the lack of gut injury in females under those conditions.

Knöferl and co-workers [13, 14] have recently demonstrated beneficial effects of 17β-estradiol on cell-mediated immune responses following trauma-hemorrhage. In their studies, ovariectomized female mice subjected to trauma-hemorrhage displayed immune responses following trauma-hemorrhage that were similar to those of intact males subjected to trauma-hemorrhage (i.e., suppressed macrophage and T-lymphocyte function). These immune functional parameters were restored by a single treatment of 17β-estradiol during resuscitation [13]. Similarly, the treatment of non-castrated male mice with 17β-estradiol during resuscitation also restored cell-mediated immune responsiveness to pre-hemorrhage levels [14].

Gender dimorphism in thymic responses following trauma-hemorrhage has also been observed [15]. Increased thymic apoptosis (programmed cell death) was observed in males, as compared to proestrus females following trauma-hemorrhage. The increased apoptotic rate in males correlated with decreased release of interleukin (IL)-3. The possibility that the presence of increased apoptosis in T-cell lymphopoietic tissue (i.e., thymus) following trauma-hemorrhage contributes significantly to systemic immune suppression under such conditions remains to be explored.

Aging also influences the gender dimorphism in the immune response following trauma-hemorrhage, in part because circulating levels of androgens in males, and estrogen in females, decline with aging. In parallel with the altered sex steroid levels, aged females become susceptible to the deleterious effects of trauma-hemorrhage on immune function, whereas in aged males cell-mediated immune responses (macrophage and T-lymphocyte) are maintained [16, 17].

These above mentioned experimental studies strongly suggest that gender dimorphism in the cell-mediated immune response to hemorrhage exists; with females having a significant advantage over males. The differences between males and females also appear to be directly related to the suppressive effects of androgens (i.e., 5α-dihydrotestosterone) in males and the enhancing/protective effects of estrogens (i.e., 17β-estradiol) in females.

Sepsis

A number of clinical and epidemiological studies have suggested that gender differences exist in the response to sepsis [18–20]. In general, these studies have concluded that females are at a lower risk than males of developing septic complications and, when sepsis was evident, females had decreased morbidity and mortality as compared to males. Wichmann et al. [19], in a prospective study of 4,218 intensive care patients (2,709 males and 1,509 females), observed that 7.6% of female patients developed sepsis, compared to 10.4% of male patients. In another prospective study, Schroder et al. [18] observed a mortality rate of 70% (23 of 33 patients) in male septic patients, whereas a markedly lower mortality rate (26%; 5 of 19 patients) was observed in septic females. The significantly better outcome for septic women in this study also positively correlated with increased systemic levels of anti-inflammatory mediators. In contrast, a recent retrospective study of 443 patients suggests that female gender is an independent predictor of increased mortality in septic surgical patients [21]. Nonetheless, the preponderance of evidence suggests that pre-menopausal women are more tolerant to sepsis than men of comparable age.

Gender related differences in the immune response following the induction of sepsis or sepsis-like states have also been shown in experimental studies. Proestrus female mice, which have elevated estrogen and prolactin levels, have been shown to tolerate sepsis better than male mice, as demonstrated by markedly increased survival rates following a polymicrobial septic challenge of cecal ligation and puncture [22]. This improved survival rate was associated with maintained splenocyte immune functions in females compared to depressed immune responses in male mice under those conditions. Diodato et al. [23] have recently shown that proestrus female mice have a survival advantage over males in a 'two-hit' model of trauma-hemorrhage and sepsis. Similar to previous findings, mortality following sepsis alone was greater in the male animals as compared to proestrus females. In addition, prior trauma-hemorrhage increased mortality in male animals following the induction of sepsis, whereas no such increase in mortality was observed in the hemorrhaged female group. Analysis of circulating levels of inflammatory mediators (IL-6, tumor necrosis factor [TNF]-α, prostaglandin [PG] E_2) showed that plasma levels of these mediators were significantly higher in males following sepsis and a strong positive correlation ($r^2 > 0.80$) with mortality was observed.

These above mentioned studies suggest that females have a survival advantage following a septic episode. This advantage appears to relate to the presence of female sex hormones, such as estrogen and prolactin, which are elevated during the proestrus stage of the estrus cycle. Additionally, the elevated or maintained immune responses in proestrus females following trauma-hemorrhage would appear to translate into a relevant beneficial outcome when subjected to a secondary lethal challenge such as polymicrobial sepsis.

Trauma and Burn Injury

Clinical studies have also shown that gender dimorphism exists in the response to trauma [24, 25]. Similar to sepsis, these studies suggest that pre-menopausal women have an advantage over age-matched males. Wohltmann et al. [24] in a retrospective study of over 20,000 patients from three separate trauma centers observed that women who were younger than 50 years of age had a significant survival advantage over men of comparable age. Moreover, the study found that this advantage for females was most notable in the more severely injured patients (injury severity score [ISS] >25). Studies have also shown that male trauma patients are at a greater risk of developing infections than female trauma patients [25]. Nonetheless, while males are at a greater risk of serious infection, it appears that female trauma patients infected (e.g., pneumonia) after injuries are at a higher risk for mortality than infected male trauma patients. The reason for these gender differences remains to be elucidated.

Thermal injury appears to provide a unique form of major trauma that exhibits an opposite gender dimorphic response than hemorrhage and sepsis. A recent retrospective study indicates that pre-menopausal women are at a greater risk of mortality following burn injury than age matched male patients [26]. Moreover, this increased risk appears to disappear with aging as female sex steroid levels decline. Additional studies from Panjeshahin et al. [27] also confirm the finding that females are at a greater risk of complications following thermal injury. Initial experimental findings appear to confirm this 'reversed' gender dimorphic immune response following thermal injury as opposed to non-thermal trauma. In these experimental studies, female mice were immunosuppressed (splenocyte proliferation, delayed type hypersensitivity) as compared to males following a 15% total body surface area burn. Other findings suggest that estrogen is causative, since ovariectomy prevented immunosuppression in females under such conditions [28]. Additional studies will hopefully elucidate not only the mechanism responsible for post-burn immune dysfunction, but also the reason as to why the gender dimorphic response is the opposite of that found in other forms of major injury (i.e., hemorrhage, sepsis, and blunt trauma).

▌ Modulation of Cell-mediated Immunity with Sex Hormones and Related Agents

The understanding of sex hormone action has expanded dramatically due to the identification of cognate receptors within the cell and elucidation of the ligand-induced cascade of events leading to cellular differentiation and division. Steroid hormones (i.e., testosterone, 5α-dihydrotestosterone, 17β-estradiol, progesterone) induce biological effects by binding to specific high affinity receptors. With regard to estrogen receptors, both an α and β isoform have been identified. Steroid hormones after binding to their cognate receptors act as nuclear transcription factors and regulate the expression of specific genes. In the absence of ligand (i.e., sex steroid), the receptor is complexed with heat shock proteins (HSP) and is inactive in the cytoplasm. Upon steroid binding, the receptor dimerizes with concomitant release of the HSP. The ligand-receptor dimers are subsequently phosphorylated and translocate to the nucleus where they bind to their own specific response element or other response elements situated in the promoter region of specific genes (i.e., cy-

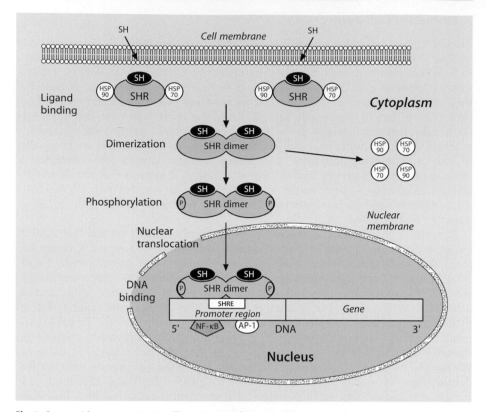

Fig. 1. Sex steroid receptor activation. The activation of sex steroid hormone receptors (SHR) consists of 4 steps:
1) the steroid hormone (SH) crosses the cell membrane and binds to its specific receptor in the cytoplasm that is in an inactive state complexed with heat shock proteins (HSP) 70 and 90;
2) Upon binding of SH, SHR dimerizes with concomitant release of HSP 70 and 90;
3) the SHR dimer is phosphorylated by cytoplasmic kinases and translocates across the nuclear membrane;
4) the activated ligand-receptor complexes bind to their own specific response element (sex hormone response element; SHRE) or other response elements situated in the promoter region of sex steroid sensitive genes.
NF-κB: nuclear factor kappa B; AP-1: activator protein-1

tokines) and regulate gene expression (Fig. 1). Recent findings by Samy et al. [29] have demonstrated that the expression of androgen and estrogen receptors in T lymphocytes is modulated after hemorrhagic shock and these receptors appear to play a critical role in the gender dimorphic immune response under such conditions.

In contrast to the sex steroids testosterone and estrogen, the female sex hormone prolactin acts via more traditional membrane bound receptors belonging to the hemopoietic receptor superfamily. The binding of ligand to this type of receptor leads to the activation of the JAK-STAT (Janus kinase – signal transduction and activators of transcription) family of tyrosine kinases followed by phosphorylation of specific cytosolic proteins and subsequent induction of gene transcriptional activity. While sex steroid receptors are located in the nucleus and prolactin receptors are membrane bound, their ultimate action following activation appears similar, namely gene activation. Thus, the action of sex hormones on cellular functions is

Table 1. Agents/hormones that modulate cell-mediated immune responses following injury

Agent/Hormone	Mode of action	Effects	References
▌ 17β-Estradiol	Receptor-mediated	Nuclear binding and gene expression	[13, 14]
▌ Prolactin	Receptor-mediated	JAK/STAT activation and gene expression	[39–42]
▌ Metoclopramide	Dopamine antagonist	Increase prolactin secretion and suppress glucocorticoid release	[43]
▌ DHEA	Receptor-mediated	Estrogenic agonist and glucocorticoid antagonist	[35–37]
▌ Flutamide	Androgen receptor antagonist	Inhibition of androgen activity and upregulation of estrogen receptors	[29, 45, 46]
▌ 4-OHA	5α reductase inhibitor	Prevent conversion of testosterone to 5α-dihydrotestosterone	[47]

DHEA: dehydroepiandrosterone; 4-OHA: 4-hydroxyandrostenedione

genomic, whether their action is direct (i.e., sex steroids) or indirect (i.e., prolactin).

Recent findings have demonstrated that a number of sex hormones and related compounds can influence cell-mediated immune responses following trauma-hemorrhage. The agents include 17β-estradiol, dehydroepiandrosterone (DHEA), prolactin, flutamide (androgen receptor antagonist) and 4-hydroxyandrostenedione (4-OHA, aromatase inhibitor) and are outlined in Table 1.

Estrogens

Female sex steroids have stimulatory effects on cell-mediated immunity [30]. For example, 17β-estradiol can stimulate macrophage function [31] and T-cell activity has also been reported to be modulated by estrogen therapy by either enhancing helper cell activity or by attenuating suppressor cell activity [32]. Support for the immunoprotective role of estrogens comes from recent studies by Knöferl et al. [14] showing that administration of 17β-estradiol to male mice following trauma-hemorrhage prevented immunosuppression. In this study, T-cell IL-2 and IL-3 production was not suppressed in 17β-estradiol-treated animals under such conditions. In contrast, the production of the immunosuppressive Th-2 cytokine IL-10 by T-cells and macrophages was reduced in the estradiol-treated group following trauma-hemorrhage.

Dehydroepiandrosterone (DHEA)

DHEA is the most abundant steroid produced by the adrenals and is often called an 'adrenal androgen', because it can be converted to testosterone [33]. However, DHEA also is an intermediate in the pathway for the synthesis of both testosterone and estrogen and in the male hormonal environment, has predominantly estrogenic effects [34]. Administration of DHEA to male mice following trauma-hemorrhage normalized various aspects of cell-mediated immunity [35, 36]. DHEA treatment of male mice under such conditions also improved the survival rate of animals sub-jected to subsequent sepsis [36]. With regards to thermal injury, Araneo et al. [37] have demonstrated that DHEA treatment of male mice prevented the suppression of splenic immune functions. Moreover, *in vitro* treatment of splenocytes isolated from burned mice with DHEA restored T-cell responses. Thus, DHEA appears to have salutary effects on immune responses, irrespective of whether it is adminis-tered following trauma-hemorrhage or thermal injury.

Prolactin

Recent studies indicate that the immune system is an important target site for pro-lactin and evidence supports the presence of specific receptors for prolactin on im-mune cells [38]. Treatment of septic male mice with prolactin increased innate and inducible IL-1β, IL-6, and TNF-α gene expression in splenic and peritoneal macro-phages as well as Kupffer cells [39]. The suppression of T-cell responses following severe hemorrhage was also restored by prolactin treatment [40]. Recent findings also indicate that the effect of prolactin under such conditions is likely to be direct, since *in vitro* treatment of immune cells from hemorrhaged mice had a similar ef-fect [41]. Prolactin administration following hemorrhagic shock also decreased mortality from a subsequent polymicrobial septic insult [42].

Prolactin secretion is increased by the administration of the dopamine antago-nist metoclopramide. A single dose of metoclopramide administered following hemorrhage improved cell mediated immune responses [43]. The mechanism by which metoclopramide normalizes cell-mediated immune responses following trau-ma-hemorrhage is likely to be related to its ability to increase plasma prolactin lev-els by blocking the antagonistic effect of dopamine on the anterior pituitary. None-theless, metoclopramide administration following trauma-hemorrhage also normal-ized plasma corticosterone levels [43], suggesting that beneficial immunological effects of metoclopramide may be in part related to suppression of glucocorticoid release.

Flutamide

Flutamide is a non-steroidal agent with potent anti-androgenic activity. This com-pound inhibits androgen uptake and/or nuclear binding of the activated androgen receptor to DNA response elements in the nucleus. The immune enhancing effects of castration on B-lymphocyte function in male mice, as evidenced by acceleration of autoimmune disease processes, can be mimicked by flutamide [44]. Flutamide treatment after trauma-hemorrhage normalized cell-mediated immune responses in intact male mice and decreased the susceptibility of hemorrhaged animals to mor-tality associated with a subsequent septic challenge [45, 46]. The beneficial effects of flutamide appear to be not only due to blockade of androgen receptors, but also due to the upregulation of estrogen receptors in immune cells from male mice sub-jected to trauma-hemorrhage [29].

4-Hydroxyandrostenedione (4-OHA)

Studies have demonstrated that 4-OHA, while classically considered as an aroma-tase inhibitor (the enzyme responsible for the conversion of testosterone to estra-diol), also inhibits 5α-reductase, the enzyme responsible for the conversion of tes-

tosterone to the more potent androgen 5α-dihydrotestosterone. Treatment of hemorrhaged male mice with 4-OHA prevented the suppression of cell-mediated immune
responses [47]. Moreover, the increased mortality following subsequent sepsis normally observed in male was prevented by 4-OHA administration. Thus, inhibition
of 5α-reductase activity appears to produce salutary effects on immune responses
in males following trauma-hemorrhage. Since 4-OHA is capable of inhibiting both
5α-reductase and aromatase activity, a specific 5α-reductase inhibitor may be more
efficacious for restoring immune functions following trauma-hemorrhage.

▌ Steroidogenic Enzymes and Cell-mediated Immunity following Injury

Testosterone and 17β-estradiol are synthesized primarily in the gonads, to a lesser
extent in the adrenals, and exert a broad range of biological effects. These steroids
regulate cellular function through interaction with their cognate receptors that are
found in a number of different tissues. Sex steroid receptor activation requires local
formation of active steroids. The synthesis of biologically active sex steroids depends upon the activity of androgen and estrogen synthesizing enzymes that include 5α reductase, aromatase and 3β- and 17β-hydroxysteroid dehydrogenases
(Fig. 2). A number of studies have shown the presence of these steroidogenic en-

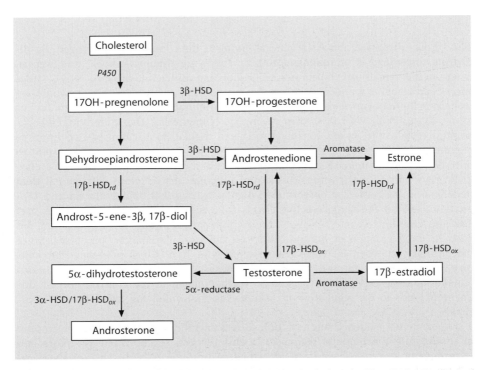

Fig. 2. Sex steroid biosynthesis. The critical steroidogenic enzymes involved in the biosynthesis of androgens
and estrogens. HSD: hydroxysteroid dehydrogenase. 17β-HSD has both oxidative (HSD$_{ox}$) and reductive (HSD$_{rd}$)
activity

zymes not only in the adrenals and gonads but also in peripheral tissues including spleen and T lymphocytes [48, 49].

While previous studies have demonstrated that sex steroids regulate T-cell function [29, 30], it remained unclear whether or not the local synthesis of biologically active sex steroids was required for the regulation of immunological function. Recent findings by Samy et al. [49] demonstrated the presence of these steroidogenic enzymes in the spleen, and more specifically, in T cells. Moreover, following trauma-hemorrhage a gender dimorphic alteration in their activity was observed. Specifically, 5α-reductase activity increased in T cells from hemorrhaged male animals, whereas aromatase activity increased in T cells from hemorrhaged proestrus females. The increase in 5α-reductase activity in T cells from male mice was immunosuppressive because of elevated 5α-dihydrotestosterone synthesis and increased aromatase activity was immunoprotective in females due to elevated 17β-estradiol synthesis (Fig. 2). Since immune cells express receptors for androgen and estrogens, alterations in the activity of these steroidogenic enzymes following hemorrhagic shock affects the availability of biologically active steroids for receptor binding, activation and subsequent modulation of cellular function. These studies confirm the importance of local synthesis of sex steroids within the immune compartment and its influence on cell-mediated immunity in a gender dependent manner following trauma-hemorrhage.

▌ Conclusion

The studies discussed above, in general, point to the concept that androgen, 5α-dihydrotestosterone, is immunosuppressive following trauma, shock and sepsis, whereas the female sex hormones, estradiol and prolactin, are protective under such conditions. A unique exception appears to exist for burn injury in which estrogen is immunosuppressive, pointing to a potential different mechanism of immune dysfunction with this form of injury. Nonetheless, the underlying mechanism(s) responsible for sex hormone mediated regulation of cell-mediated immune responses under these conditions remains to be fully elucidated. It is important to note that the inflammatory cascade/response is homeostatic in principal and pathogenic only when its activation leads to an outcome that is more detrimental than beneficial to the host. The observations demonstrating that both prolactin and 17β-estradiol exhibit immunoprotective effects following trauma and hemorrhage suggest the coordinated interaction of the hypothalamus-pituitary, adrenals, and gonads in the regulation of immune function during inflammatory processes. Since the pituitary has been shown to have receptors for IL-6 (which is elevated after injury), knowledge of the interaction of cytokines with the hypothalamic-pituitary-gonadal-adrenal axis will be needed to further elucidate the contribution of this hormonal axis to the regulation of immune function following trauma and hemorrhage.

Experimental evidence supports both direct and indirect effects of sex hormones in modulating the immune response. In this respect, sex hormone receptors and steroidogenic enzymes have been identified in immune cells. In view of these experimental findings, it can be proposed that clinically relevant therapeutic strategies could be developed using estrogens, DHEA, prolactin and dopamine antagonists which enhance prolactin secretion, androgen receptor antagonists, and steroidogenic enzyme inhibitors (Table 1). These hormones/agents may represent safe, useful, novel, and relatively inexpensive therapeutic adjuncts for the treatment of immune dysfunction in trauma victims.

Acknowledgements. This work was supported by United States Public Health Service grant R01 GM 37127.

References

1. Baue AE, Durham R, Faist E (1998) Systemic inflammatory response syndrome (SIRS), multiple organ dysfunction syndrome (MODS), multiple organ failure (MOF): are we winning the battle? Shock 10:79–89
2. Vincent JL (2000) Update on sepsis: pathophysiology and treatment. Acta Clin Belg 55:79–87
3. Goris RJ (1989) Multiple organ failure: whole body inflammation? Schweiz Med Wochenschr 119:347–353
4. Schwacha MG, Knöferl MW, Samy TSA, Ayala A, Chaudry IH (1999) The immunologic consequences of hemorrhagic shock. Crit Care Shock 2:42–64
5. Napolitano LM, Faist E, Wichmann MW, Coimbra R (1999) Immune dysfunction in trauma. Surg Clin North Am 79:1385–1416
6. Bone RC (1992) Toward an epidemiology and natural history of SIRS (systemic inflammatory response syndrome). JAMA 268:3452–3455
7. Lahita RG, Bradlow HL, Ginzler E, Pang S, New M (1987) Low plasma androgens in women with systemic lupus erythematosus. Arthritis Rheum 30:241–248
8. Angele MK, Schwacha MG, Ayala A, Chaudry IH (2000) Effect of gender and sex hormones on immune responses following shock. Shock 14:81–90
9. Altura BM (1976) Sex and estrogens in protection against circulatory stress reactions. Am J Physiol 231:842–847
10. Wichmann MW, Zellweger R, DeMaso CM, Ayala A, Chaudry IH (1996) Enhanced immune responses in females as opposed to decreased responses in males following haemorrhagic shock. Cytokine 8:853–863
11. Angele MK, Knöferl M, Schwacha MG, Cioffi WG, Bland KI, Chaudry IH (1999) Testosterone and estrogen regulate pro- and antiinflammatory cytokine release by macrophages following trauma-hemorrhage. Am J Physiol 277:C35–C42
12. Adams CAJ, Magnotti LJ, Xu DZ, Lu Q, Deitch EA (2000) Acute lung injury after hemorrhagic shock is dependent on gut injury and sex. Am Surg 66:905–912
13. Knöferl MW, Jarrar D, Angele MK, et al (2001) 17β-estradiol normalizes immune responses in ovariectomized females after trauma-hemorrhage. Am J Physiol 281:C1131–C1138
14. Knöferl MW, Diodato MD, Angele MK, et al (2000) Do female sex steroids adversely or beneficially affect the depressed immune responses in males after trauma-hemorrhage? Arch Surg 135:425–433
15. Angele MK, Xin Xu Y, Ayala A, et al (1999) Gender dimorphism in trauma-hemorrhage-induced thymocyte apoptosis. Shock 12:316–322
16. Kahlke V, Angele MK, Ayala A, et al (2000) Immune dysfunction following trauma-hemorrhage: influence of gender and age. Cytokine 12:69–77
17. Kahlke V, Angele MK, Schwacha MG, et al (2000) Reversal of sexual dimorphism in splenic T-lymphocyte responses following trauma-hemorrhage with aging. Am J Physiol 278:C509–C519
18. Schroder J, Kahlke V, Staubach KH, Zabel P, Stuber F (1998) Gender differences in human sepsis. Arch Surg 133:1200–1205
19. Wichmann MW, Inthorn D, Andress HJ, Schildberg FW (2000) Incidence and mortality of severe sepsis in surgical intensive care patients: the influence of patient gender on disease process and outcome. Intensive Care Med 26:167–172
20. Chernow B (1999) Variables affecting outcome in critically ill patients. Chest 115:71S–76S
21. Eachempati SR, Hydo L, Barie PS (1999) Gender-based differences in outcome in patients with sepsis. Arch Surg 134:1342–1347

22. Zellweger R, Ayala A, Stein S, DeMaso CM, Chaudry IH (1997) Females in proestrus state tolerate sepsis better than males. Crit Care Med 25:106–110

23. Diodato MD, Knöferl MW, Schwacha MG, Bland KI, Chaudry IH (5-7-2001) Gender differences in the inflammatory response and survival following haemorrhage and subsequent sepsis. Cytokine 14:162–169

24. Wohltmann CD, Franklin GA, Boaz PW, et al (2001) A multicenter evaluation of whether gender dimorphism affects survival after trauma. Am J Surg 181:297–300

25. Offner PJ, Moore EE, Biffl WL (1999) Male gender is a risk factor for major infections after surgery. Arch Surg 134:935–938

26. O'Keefe GE, Hunt JL, Purdue GF (2001) An evaluation of risk factors for mortality after burn trauma and the identification of gender-dependent differences in outcomes. J Am Coll Surg 192:153–160

27. Panjeshahin MR, Lari AR, Talei A, Shamsnia J, Alaghehbandan R (2001) Epidemiology and mortality of burns in the South West of Iran. Burns 27:219–226

28. Gregory MS, Duffner LA, Faunce DE, Kovacs EJ (2000) Estrogen mediates the sex difference in post-burn immunosuppression. Endocrinology 164:129–138

29. Samy TS, Schwacha MG, Cioffi WG, Bland KI, Chaudry IH (2000) Androgen and estrogen receptors in splenic T lymphocytes: effects of flutamide and trauma-hemorrhage. Shock 14:465–470

30. Olsen NJ, Kovacs WJ (1996) Gonadal steroids and immunity. Endocrin Rev 17:369-384

31. Hu SK, Mitcho ML, Rath NC (1988) Effect of estradiol on interleukin-1 synthesis by macrophages. Int J Immunopharm 10:247–252

32. Carlsten H, Tarkowski A, Holmdahl R, Nilsson LA (1990) Oestrogen is a potent disease accelerator in SLE-prone MRL 1pr/1pr mice. Clin Exp Immunol 80:467–473

33. Svec F, Porter JR (1998) The actions of exogenous dehydroepiandrosterone in experimental animals and humans. Proc Soc Exp Biol Med 218:174–191

34. Ebeling P, Koivisto VA (1994) Physiological importance of dehydroepiandrosterone. Lancet 343:1479–1481

35. Catania RA, Angele MK, Ayala A, Cioffi WG, Bland KI, Chaudry IH (1999) Dehydroepiandrosterone restores immune function following trauma-haemorrhage by a direct effect on T lymphocytes. Cytokine 11:443–450

36. Angele MK, Catania RA, Ayala A, Cioffi WG, Bland KI, Chaudry IH (1998) Dehydroepiandrosterone: an inexpensive steroid hormone that decreases the mortality due to sepsis following trauma-induced hemorrhage. Arch Surg 133:1281–1288

37. Araneo BA, Shelby J, Li GZ, Ku W, Daynes RA (1993) Administration of dehydroepiandrosterone to burned mice preserves normal immunologic competence. Arch Surg 128:318-325

38. Gala RR (1991) Prolactin and growth hormone in the regulation of the immune system (Mini review). Proc Soc Exp Biol Med 198:513–527

39. Zhu XH, Zellweger R, Wichmann MW, Ayala A, Chaudry IH (1997) Effects of prolactin and metoclopramide on macrophage cytokine gene expression in late sepsis. Cytokine 9:437–446

40. Zellweger R, Wichmann MW, Ayala A, DeMaso CM, Chaudry IH (1996) Prolactin: a novel and safe immunomodulating hormone for the treatment of immunodepression following severe hemorrhage. J Surg Res 63:53–58

41. Knoferl MW, Angele MK, Ayala A, Cioffi WG, Bland KI, Chaudry IH (2000) Insight into the mechanism by which metoclopramide improves immune functions after trauma-hemorrhage. Am J Physiol 279:C72–C80

42. Zellweger R, Zhu XH, Wichmann MW, Ayala A, DeMaso CM, Chaudry IH (1996) Prolactin administration following hemorrhagic shock improves macrophage cytokine release capacity and decreases mortality from subsequent sepsis. J Immunol 157:5748–5754

43. Zellweger R, Wichmann MW, Ayala A, Chaudry IH (1998) Metoclopramide: A novel and safe immunomodulating agent for restoring the depressed macrophage function following trauma-hemorrhage. J Trauma 44:70–77

44. Walker SE, Besch-Williford CL, Keisler DH (1994) Accelerated deaths from systemic lupus erythematosus in NZB × NZW F_1 mice treated with the testosterone-blocking drug flutamide. J Lab Clin Med 124:401–407

45. Angele MK, Wichmann MW, Ayala A, Cioffi WG, Chaudry IH (1997) Testosterone receptor blockade after hemorrhage in males. Restoration of the depressed immune functions and improved survival following subsequent sepsis. Arch Surg 132:1207–1214
46. Wichmann MW, Angele MK, Ayala A, Cioffi WG, Chaudry I (1997) Flutamide: A novel agent for restoring the depressed cell-mediated immunity following soft-tissue trauma and hemorrhagic shock. Shock 8:1–7
47. Schneider CP, Nickel EA, Samy TS, et al (2000) The aromatase inhibitor, 4-hydroxyandros-tenedione, restores immune responses following trauma-hemorrhage in males and decreases mortality from subsequent sepsis. Shock 14:347–353
48. Martel C, Rheaume E, Takahashi M, et al (1992) Distribution of 17 beta-hydroxysteroid dehydrogenase gene expression and activity in rat and human tissues. J Steroid Biochem Mol Biol 41:597–60349
49. Samy TS, Knöferl MW, Zheng R, Schwacha MG, Bland KI, Chaudry IH (2001) Divergent immune responses in male and female mice after trauma-hemorrhage: dimorphic alterations in T lymphocyte steroidogenic enzyme activities. Endocrinology 142:3519–3529

Basic Mechanisms
in Acute Respiratory Failure

Regulatory Role of Alveolar Macrophages and Cytokines in Pulmonary Host Defense

M. J. Schultz, S. Knapp, and T. van der Poll

▌ Introduction

The lungs are repeatedly exposed to respiratory pathogens, either by inhalation or (micro-) aspiration of microorganisms that colonize the oropharynx. Infectious agents that have passed the structural defenses and have entered the terminal airways may cause pneumonia, one of the most common infectious diseases. Both the growing number of immunocompromised patients susceptible to pneumonia, and the widespread use of antibiotics that has led to a rise in antibiotic resistance among microorganisms, have made the treatment of pneumonia more difficult. Hence, there is a need for novel therapeutic approaches for pneumonia. Immunotherapy, aimed at modulating the immune response, is one such approach. Immunotherapy may serve as an important adjuvant to antibiotic therapy in the treatment of infectious diseases. However, before such immunotherapies can become serious tools in the treatment of severe pneumonia, increased knowledge of the immune host defense is needed.

Normal pulmonary host defense includes both innate and acquired immune responses. While innate immune responses are primarily responsible for the elimination of bacterial pathogens from the alveolar spaces, specific immune responses are involved in eradication of encapsulated pathogens, and pathogens that survive after phagocytosis. Innate defenses consist of structural defenses, antimicrobial molecules generated in airways, and phagocytosis by resident alveolar macrophages (alveolar macrophages) and recruited polymorphonuclear cells (PMN). Acquired immune defense is antigen-specific, and includes cell-mediated and antibody-mediated immune responses.

Both alveolar macrophages and PMN play a prominent role in innate immunity. Alveolar macrophages are avidly phagocytic and readily kill ingested microorganisms. In addition, they play an important role in orchestrating inflammatory responses. Alveolar macrophages and PMN need to communicate in mounting an effective host defense against invading pathogens; after their initiation, innate immune responses need to be localized, reinforced and finally resolved. Cytokines play a critical role in these processes by mediating leukocyte recruitment and by serving as important signals in the activation of leukocytes. Numerous cytokines have been implicated in pulmonary host defense (e.g., tumor necrosis factor-α [TNF], interleukin [IL]-6, IL-10, interferon [IFN]-γ and cytokines with chemotactic activities).

In this chapter, the role of alveolar macrophages and cytokines in innate immunity against respiratory pathogens is discussed. Furthermore, we focus on how alveolar macrophages and cytokines are involved in the defense against different respiratory bacterial pathogens under different conditions.

▌ The Cellular Component of Innate Immunity

Infectious agents that have entered the terminal airways are first encountered by alveolar macrophages. These cells play a central role in pulmonary host defense. The recruitment of large numbers of PMN in the alveolar space from the marginated pool of leukocytes in the pulmonary circulation is initiated when the microbial challenge is too large or too virulent to be contained by the alveolar macrophages alone. These recruited neutrophils provide auxiliary phagocytic capacities, critical for the effective eradication of pathogens.

In the respiratory tract alveolar macrophages respond to pathogens by two means: First, alveolar macrophages directly bind, phagocytose, and kill pathogens. Second, alveolar macrophages secrete a large range of mediators, some acting directly on the pathogens, while others such as chemokines exert their effects indirectly by recruiting other components of the host defense system. Therefore, it is suggested that alveolar macrophages or alveolar macrophage-derived substances can play a crucial role in the pathogenesis of acute lung injury (ALI) during pneumonia.

The crucial role of alveolar macrophages or alveolar macrophage-derived substances in the process of recruitment of PMN in response to invading pathogens or their products has become clear from several studies: compared with control rats, PMN numbers were decreased in bronchoalveolar lavage (BAL) fluid from alveolar macrophage-depleted rats after instillation of a sublethal dose of *Pseudomonas aeruginosa* into the airways, concordant with significantly decreased levels of TNF and macrophage inflammatory protein (MIP)-2 mRNA expression in one study [1]. In another study, in which alveolar macrophages from lipopolysaccharide (LPS)-exposed mice were transferred to the lungs of naive recipient mice, nearly a threefold increase in the numbers of neutrophils in BALF was found, compared to instillation of alveolar macrophages from unexposed mice. Transfer of alveolar macrophages from LPS-exposed mice into cutaneous air pouches of naive mice also caused greater local neutrophil accumulation (10-fold) than the transfer of alveolar macrophages from normal mice [2].

Along with the effect of alveolar macrophages on PMN recruitment, the role of alveolar macrophages as regulators of inflammation has been illustrated by studies demonstrating that alveolar macrophages engulf apoptotic PMN and release anti-inflammatory mediators [3, 4]. These data indicate that the role of alveolar macrophages in host defense is not limited to the generation of the initial inflammatory response, but extends to regulation of inflammation, including elimination of phagocytosed pathogens.

Considerable evidence exists for the importance of alveolar macrophages in host defense against different respiratory pathogens. In a murine *Streptococcus pneumoniae* pneumonia model, impaired survival was found in mice depleted of alveolar macrophages. The detrimental outcome was accompanied by pronounced elevations of pro-inflammatory cytokines (TNF, IL-1) and the chemokine KC, enhanced recruitment of PMN and excessive inflammation in the lung as indicated by histopathology. In this model, no difference in bacterial outgrowth could be observed, whereas PMN influx was increased in alveolar macrophage depleted mice [5].

Similarly, in a murine *Mycoplasma* pneumonia model, alveolar macrophage-depletion in mice resulted in elevated outgrowth of *Mycoplasma* from the lungs [6]. In this study, alveolar macrophage-depletion exacerbated the *Mycoplasma* infection in *Mycoplasma*-resistant mice by reducing killing of the pathogen to a level com-

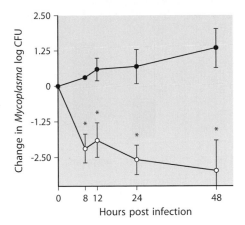

Fig. 1. Effect of alveolar macrophage-depletion on intrapulmonary killing of *Mycoplasma pulmonis*. Alveolar macrophage-depleted *Mycoplasma*-resistant C57BL mice (*closed circles*) and control C57BL mice (*open circles*) were infected with 10^5 CFU of *M. pulmonis* and were sacrificed and analyzed at the specified time intervals. *: p ⩽ 0.05 versus control mice. (Adapted from [6])

parable to that in *Mycoplasma*-susceptible mice without alveolar macrophage-depletion, suggesting that defective alveolar macrophage function is the likely explanation for the difference between susceptible and resistant mice (Fig. 1). Interestingly, higher levels of PMN in lavage fluids were recovered from the alveolar macrophage-depleted mice, indicating that the differences in killing of the invading pathogen could not be explained by an effect on neutrophil recruitment. Furthermore, depletion of alveolar macrophages in a *K. pneumoniae* pneumonia model in mice influenced mortality dramatically, with 100% lethality after three days in alveolar macrophage-depleted mice compared to 100% long-term survival in non-depleted mice [7]. This was accompanied by an increased outgrowth of *K. pneumoniae* from lungs and blood in alveolar macrophage-depleted mice, and, similar to the former study, an increase in PMN influx into the pulmonary compartment, together with elevated levels of TNF and MIP-2. The decreased bacterial clearance seen in this murine *Klebsiella* pneumonia model has been confirmed by others [8].

Similar data have been reported in a murine pneumonia model with *P. aeruginosa* [9]. Alveolar macrophage-depletion resulted in higher local chemokine levels, a prolonged inflammatory PMN recruitment, and a delayed bacterial clearance compared to control mice (Fig. 2). Furthermore, destruction of alveolar structures and thickening of the interstitial spaces were marked in the alveolar macrophage-depleted mice. However, it was also demonstrated that, early after the initiation of pneumonia, compared with control mice, alveolar macrophage-depleted mice had lower concentrations of chemokines and fewer PMN in the BAL fluid, and a significant improvement in lung edema. Importantly, although alveolar macrophage-depletion improved early-phase inflammation, late survival was not altered (Fig. 2). These data illustrate both the beneficial and deleterious effects of alveolar macrophages during the orchestration of inflammation during pneumonia. Depletion of alveolar macrophages in the early phase of *Pseudomonas* pneumonia may initially improve lung injury, but may worsen the eventual outcome, as seen in the models of pneumonia with this pathogen, and other pathogens like *K. pneumoniae*, *Strep. pneumoniae*, and *M. pneumoniae*. It remains unclear why the overzealous PMN infiltration, as seen in the absence of alveolar macrophages, does not lead to a complete clearance of bacteria from the lungs in these models, but again indicates a prominent role of alveolar macrophages in host defense.

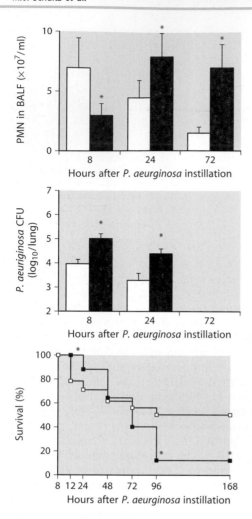

Fig. 2. Polymorphonuclear cells (PMN) in broncho-alveolar lavage fluid (BALF), number of bacteria (CFU) in lung tissue, and survival after an intratracheal challenge with *Pseudomonas aeruginosa*. Alveolar macrophage-depleted mice (*solid bars/symbols*) and control mice (*open bars/symbols*) received 5×10^5 CFU of *P. aeruginosa* and were sacrificed and analyzed at the specified time intervals. *: $p \leq 0.05$ versus control mice. (Adapted from [38])

Alveolar macrophages are regarded as major modulators of pulmonary host defense. Whereas early on alveolar macrophages readily phagocytose and (thereby) eliminate certain inhaled pathogens, they later represent important effector cells in the resolution process [10, 11]. The (above mentioned) observation of overzealous and persistent PMN infiltration in the absence of alveolar macrophages may be related to the equally important function of alveolar macrophages during resolution of inflammation. To restitute tissue homeostasis, all processes involved in the initiation of inflammation must be reversed and one important prerequisite for resolution to occur is the removal of extravasated PMN. Several lines of evidence support the hypothesis that PMN undergo programmed cell death (apoptosis) followed by rapid clearance by alveolar macrophages [11, 12]. Apoptosis thereby provides an injury-limiting mechanism since the PMN membrane remains intact, preventing potentially injurious granule contents from being released. Thus, to prevent the potentially harmful event of secondary necrosis, when membrane integrity gets lost and histotoxic granule contents are exposed to the surrounding tissue, the immediate recognition of apoptotic PMN by alveolar macrophages is required. A variety of recognition mechanisms including phosphatidylserine, exposed on apoptotic cell surfaces, have been described so far [13, 14]. Moreover, it has been nicely demonstrated that the uptake of apoptotic PMN by macrophages not only cleared PMN but also actively induced anti-inflammatory properties in human macrophages, illustrated by the suppressed release of pro-inflammatory cytokines (IL-1β, IL-8, TNF) and increased release of agents with anti-inflammatory properties (like transforming growth factor [TGF]-α and prostaglandin [PG]-E$_2$) [13–16].

▌ The Humoral Component of Innate Immunity

Alveolar macrophages and recruited PMN orchestrate the immune response by initiating a complex network of pro-inflammatory and anti-inflammatory cytokines. Cytokines can be considered to be involved in the early response after the recognition of a pathogen (e.g., TNF and IL-β), to be involved in the recruitment of immune cells to the site of infection (chemokines, such as IL-8), or to be involved in the activation of alveolar macrophages and recruited PMN (e.g., IFN-γ, IL-12, IL-6, and IL-10).

The early response cytokines TNF and IL-1 have both been studied in pulmonary host defense. Increased expression of TNF and IL-1 has been observed in bacterial pneumonia, in humans [17] and in animals [18–22]. TNF activates both alveolar macrophages and PMN, leading to augmented phagocytosis, oxidative burst, protein release and bacterial killing [23, 24]. TNF contributes to the recruitment of PMN by stimulating the expression of adhesion molecules [24, 25], and inducing the production of chemokines [26, 27]. Several lines of evidence suggest that TNF and IL-1 are important components of host defense in bacterial pneumonia: systemic neutralization of TNF attenuated host defense in pulmonary bacterial infections with *Strep. pneumoniae* and *K. pneumoniae*, resulting in decreased survival [18–20, 22], while administration of low doses of exogenous TNF, and augmentation of local expression of TNF in the lungs through gene therapy, significantly diminished mortality and enhanced bacterial clearance from the pulmonary compartment during severe pneumonia with these pathogens [28–30]. Similar data exist for IL-1: after a bacterial challenge, IL-1 receptor type I deficient mice demonstrated an impaired clearance of *Strep. pneumoniae* and a reduced capacity to form inflammatory infiltrates [31]. Of considerable interest, treatment with a neutralizing anti-TNF antibody made IL-1 receptor deficient mice extremely susceptible to pneumococcal pneumonia, more so than IL-1 receptor knockout mice treated with a control antibody and wild type mice treated with anti-TNF [31]. These data indicate that the concurrent action of TNF and IL-1 is required for an adequate host defense against pneumococcal pneumonia.

Chemokines, low molecular weight cytokines, are involved in the recruitment of immune cells to the site of infection. CXC chemokines (e.g., IL-8, epithelial neutrophil activating protein [ENA]-78 in humans; MIP-2, and KC in mice) exhibit chemotactic and activating effects on PMN. Elevated levels of IL-8 have been found in BAL fluid of patients with pneumonia [32, 33], and IL-8 levels correlated with PMN counts in, and PMN chemotactic activity of, pleural fluid [34]. Similarly, elevated chemokine levels have been detected in lungs of mice with pneumonia with *Strep.*

pneumoniae, K. pneumoniae, and *P. aeruginosa* [31, 35–39]. Several studies suggest a regulating role for chemokines in pneumonia. Administration of chemokine neutralizing antibodies resulted in a reduction in PMN influx, which was associated with an attenuation of bacterial clearance from the lung, and an increased incidence of bacteremia in several murine pneumonia models [36, 40, 41], whereas local chemokine over-expression in the lungs of transgenic mice led to an increase in PMN influx after intra-tracheal administration of bacteria, which was associated with a striking improvement in survival, increased bacterial clearance from the lungs, and reduced incidence of bacteremia [37].

Like that of TNF, IL-β and chemokines, the production of the pro-inflammatory cytokine IFN-γ has been found to be enhanced during murine pneumonia [18, 39, 42–46]. Similarly, the expression of another pro-inflammatory cytokine, IL-12, is enhanced in bacterial pneumonia [43, 44]. IFN-γ is a cytokine mainly produced by antigen activated T and natural killer (NK) cells. The secretion of IFN-γ is induced by TNF and IL-12. IFN-γ exerts several immune regulatory activities, including activation of phagocytes, stimulation of antigen presentation by increasing the expression of major histocompatibility complex (MHC) molecules class I and II on antigen presenting cells, orchestration of leukocyte-endothelium interactions, and stimulation of the respiratory burst [47, 48]. Macrophages are stimulated by IFN-γ to secrete TNF and IL-12, setting up a paracrine positive-feedback cycle [48].

The role of IL-12 and IFN-γ in host defense during pneumonia has been demonstrated in different animal studies. Neutralization of IL-12 led to reduced bacterial clearance and increased mortality of mice with *K. pneumoniae* pneumonia, while overexpression of IL-12 reduced mortality [44]. By contrast, IL-12 knockout mice had a normal host defense against *Strep. pneumoniae,* since bacterial outgrowth from lung tissue and survival was similar to wild type mice in a pneumonia model with this pathogen [49]. The role of IFN-γ in the setting of bacterial pneumonia is less clear. Whereas in one study IFN-γ knockout mice demonstrated higher mortality compared to wild type mice [42], and in other studies local overexpression of IFN-γ in rats resulted in increased bacterial clearance from the pulmonary compartment [50–52], other data suggest that endogenous IFN-γ may impair an effective pulmonary defense in pneumonia, since pulmonary clearance of *Strep. pneumoniae* was attenuated in IFN-γ-R knockout mice, as well as in IFN-γ knockout mice compared to wild type mice [43].

IL-17 is a cytokine that induces granulopoiesis via granulocyte colony-stimulating factor (G-CSF) production and stimulates the production of CXC chemokines. The release of IL-17 in the lungs in *K. pneumoniae* pneumonia has been demonstrated recently [53]. IL-17 receptor deficient mice were exquisitely sensitive to intranasal *K. pneumoniae* with 100% lethality after 48 hours compared to 40% mortality in control mice. The IL-17 R deficient mice displayed a significant delay in PMN recruitment into the lungs, associated with significant reduction in local G-CSF and MIP-2 levels [53]. From these data it can be concluded that IL-17 receptor signaling is critical for host defense against *K. pneumoniae.*

IL-18, originally identified in mice during shock as a co-stimulatory factor for the production of IFN-γ, has many pro-inflammatory effects. The role of IL-18 in the host response to pulmonary infection has been studied recently [49]. IL-18 deficient mice demonstrated a reduced clearance of *S. pneumoniae* and were more susceptible for progression to systemic infection at 24 and 48 hours after an intranasal challenge with this pathogen. Although survival was not different between knockout mice and wild type mice, these data suggest that IL-18 plays a protective role in the early host response during pneumococcal pneumonia.

IL-10 is a cytokine that attenuates the production of TNF, IL-1β, chemokines, IFN-γ, and IL-12, and has potent inhibitory effects on PMN resulting in reduced phagocytosis and bactericidal killing [26, 54, 55]. IL-10 is produced in the pulmonary compartment in mice with pneumonia [56, 57]. Considerable evidence exists that the anti-inflammatory cytokine IL-10 plays a detrimental role in the clearance of bacteria during pulmonary infections; administration of exogenous IL-10 reduced survival and increased outgrowth of bacteria in lungs of mice with *Strep. pneumoniae* pneumonia [56]. Conversely, neutralization of endogenous IL-10 led to enhanced clearance of bacteria and improved survival in mice with pulmonary infection with *K. pneumoniae* or *Strep. pneumoniae* [56, 57].

IL-6 is both a pro-inflammatory and an anti-inflammatory cytokine. The production of IL-6 is under the influence of TNF and IL-β. Many cell types, including macrophages, T and B-cells and parenchymal cells, produce IL-6. IL-6 is produced in the lung during pneumonia [32]. Evidence for the importance of IL-6 in host defense during pneumonia was obtained from a study on *Strep. pneumoniae* pneumonia in IL-6 knockout mice [58]. IL-6 knockout mice had more bacteria in their lungs after an intranasal challenge with this pathogen, and died significantly earlier than normal mice (Fig. 3).

In conclusion, while the pro-inflammatory cytokines and chemokines appear to play a protective role in pulmonary host defense by initiating a protective inflam-

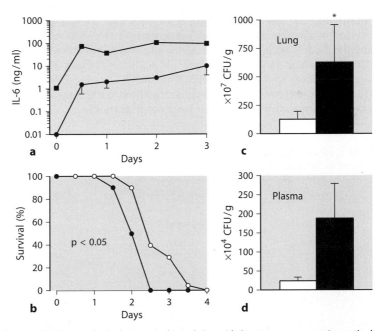

Fig. 3. (a) Induction of pneumonia in normal mice by intranasal inoculation with *Streptococcus pneumoniae* resulted in sustained IL-6 levels in lungs (*filled squares*) and plasma (*filled circles*). **(b)** IL-6 deficient mice (*filled circles*) died significantly earlier from pneumococcal pneumonia than normal mice (*open circles*) after an intranasal bacterial challenge. **(c + d)** Lungs and blood harvested from IL-6 deficient mice (*solid bars*) 40 h after inoculation contained more *Strep. pneumoniae* CFUs, compared to normal mice (*open bars*). *: $p < 0.05$. (Adapted from [58])

matory reaction, the anti-inflammatory cytokines demonstrate a detrimental role in the innate immunity against respiratory pathogens by resolving the immune responses. In this respect, the role of pro-inflammatory and anti-inflammatory cytokines in local inflammation is the opposite of that in systemic inflammation, where excessive production of pro-inflammatory cytokines causes organ failure and death in animal models of fulminate sepsis, and the anti-inflammatory cytokine IL-10 is protective. From the point of view that after the initiation and, if necessary, reinforcement of the inflammatory reaction, there is a need for innate immune responses to be stopped when the invading pathogens have been erased from the pulmonary compartment, it is logical that both pro-inflammatory and anti-inflammatory cytokines are produced locally in an inflammatory reaction. This fine-tuning of inflammation is necessary to protect the host from an overzealous reaction.

▌ Innate Immunity against Different Pathogens under Different Conditions

The majority of the above mentioned models on the role of alveolar macrophages and different cytokines involved infection with *Strep. pneumoniae*, *K. pneumoniae* or *P. aeruginosa*. Alveolar macrophages and cytokines influence host defense during these respiratory tract infections, although their role may vary depending on the pathogen used (Table 1).

We have already emphasized both the beneficial and deleterious effects of alveolar macrophages during the orchestration of inflammation during pneumonia. While depletion of alveolar macrophages in the early phase of *Pseudomonas* pneumonia may initially improve lung injury, yet may worsen the eventual outcome, depletion of alveolar macrophages certainly leads to an increased mortality in pneumonia models with other pathogens, like *Strep. pneumoniae*, *K. pneumoniae*, and *M. pneumoniae* [5–8]. Temporary blockade of alveolar macrophages (-functions) may contribute to decreasing (PMN-mediated) tissue injury early after the start of pneumonia, improving acute survival without compromising the beneficial effects of the inflammatory reaction on bacterial pneumonia.

Table 1. Cytokines influence host defense during respiratory tract infections, although their role may vary depending on the pathogen

Cytokine	*Strep. pneumoniae*	*K. pneumoniae*	*P. aeruginosa*	References
▌ TNF	+	+	+/–	18–20, 22, 28–30
▌ IL-1	+	?	–	31, 60
▌ CXC-chemokines	?	+	+	36, 37, 40, 41
▌ IL-10	–	–	+/–	56, 57
▌ IL-6	+	?	?	58
▌ IL-12	0	+	?	44, 49
▌ IL-17	?	+	?	53
▌ IL-18	+	?	?	49
▌ IFN-γ	+/–	?	+/–	43, 50–52

+, indicates a beneficial role in case of respiratory infection with the specified pathogen; –, indicates a detrimental role in case of respiratory infection with the specified pathogen; +/–, indicates conflicting data; ?, indicates that there are no data on the effect of this cytokine: 0, indicates no effect. See text for details

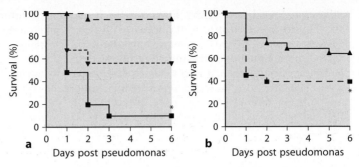

Fig. 4. (**a**) Effect of intratracheal *P. aeruginosa* administration (8×10^5 CFU, 24 *h* post surgery) on survival in cecal ligation + puncture (CLP) (*filled squares*) and sham operated mice (*inverted triangles*); filled triangles: CLP + intratracheal saline. *: $p < 0.01$ compared with other groups. (**b**) Effect of IL-10 neutralization on survival in CLP mice administered *P. aeruginosa* (4×10^5 CFU, 24 *h* post surgery) (filled squares: CLP + control rabbit serum; filled triangles: CLP + rabbit anti-murine IL-10 serum). *: $p < 0.05$ compared with animals receiving control serum. (Adapted from [62])

While endogenous TNF was important for clearance of *Strep. pneumoniae* and *K. pneumoniae* [18, 20] from mouse lungs, TNF impaired host defense mechanisms during pneumonia with *P. aeruginosa* [59]. Similarly, while IL-1 receptor I deficient mice demonstrated an impaired bacterial clearance and a reduced capacity to form inflammatory infiltrates during infection with *Strep. pneumoniae* [31], during infection with *P. aeruginosa*, IL-1 receptor I deficient mice demonstrated an enhanced bacterial clearance [60]. Furthermore, while endogenous IL-10 hampered bacterial clearance in mouse models of *Strep. pneumoniae* and *K. pneumoniae* [56, 57], IL-10 improved host defense in a model of pneumonia caused by *P. aeruginosa* [61]. It is not clear whether the protective role of IL-10 in *P. aeruginosa* pneumonia represented IL-10-mediated protection from systemic endotoxin exposure. These data suggest that in more gradually developing pneumonias, such as caused by *Strep. pneumoniae* and *K. pneumoniae*, a certain pro-inflammatory cytokine response within the pulmonary compartment is required to combat the invading microorganism, while in a more acute form of pneumonia, such as caused by *P. aeruginosa*, an excessive inflammatory response contributes to an adverse outcome.

IL-10 appears to be important in sepsis-induced immunosuppression; mice with abdominal sepsis induced by cecal ligation and puncture were more susceptible to intratracheally administered *P. aeruginosa*, with a higher lethality compared to normal mice or mice undergoing sham abdominal surgery [62]. The development of pneumonia in animals undergoing cecal ligation and puncture was associated with a marked increase in IL-10 expression in lungs, and administration of neutralizing IL-10 antibodies resulted in enhanced bacterial clearance from lungs and reduced mortality (Fig. 4).

▌ Conclusion

We have reviewed the literature on innate immunity against respiratory pathogens. Although manipulation of innate immunity through deletion of alveolar macrophages or modulation of the cytokine cascade occurred before, at, or directly after the time of challenge with a respiratory pathogen in the reviewed animal studies, unlike the clinical setting, this novel approach may in the future serve as an adjuvant therapy in the treatment of patients with severe pneumonia.

Several limitations exist. Targeting only alveolar macrophages or only one cytokine may be too simplistic, as the innate responses are complex, and as cytokines have pleotropic effects, this can lead to unexpected effects when used in an intervention *in vivo*. Furthermore, host responses against different respiratory pathogens differ quite substantially, which may make it necessary to develop different strategies for different pathogens. Additional studies are necessary to overcome these issues.

References

1. Hashimoto S, Pittet JF, Hong K, et al (1996) Depletion of alveolar macrophages decreases neutrophil chemotaxis to Pseudomonas airspace infections. Am J Physiol 270:L819–L828
2. Harmsen AG (1988) Role of alveolar macrophages in lipopolysaccharide-induced neutrophil accumulation. Infect Immun 56:1858–1863
3. Ren Y, Savill J (1995) Proinflammatory cytokines potentiate thrombospondin-mediated phagocytosis of neutrophils undergoing apoptosis. J Immunol 154:2366–2374
4. Cox G (1996) IL-10 enhances resolution of pulmonary inflammation in vivo by promoting apoptosis of neutrophils. Am J Physiol 271:L566–L571
5. Knapp S, Leemans JC, Maris NA, et al (2001) Alveolar macrophages protect mice against lethality during *Streptococcus pneumoniae* pneumonia by attenuating lung inflammation. 41st ICACC Abstract Book. ASM press, Herndon. (Abst, in press)
6. Hickman-Davis JM, Michalek SM, Gibbs-Erwin J, Lindsey JR (1997) Depletion of alveolar macrophages exacerbates respiratory mycoplasmosis in mycoplasma-resistant C57BL mice but not mycoplasma-susceptible C3H mice. Infect Immun 65:2278–2282
7. Broug-Holub E, Kraal G (1997) In vivo study on the immunomodulating effects of OM-85 BV on survival, inflammatory cell recruitment and bacterial clearance in Klebsiella pneumonia. Int J Immunopharmacol 19:559–564
8. Cheung DO, Halsey K, Speert DP (2000) Role of pulmonary alveolar macrophages in defense of the lung against Pseudomonas aeruginosa. Infect Immun 68:4585–4592
9. Kooguchi K, Hashimoto S, Kobayashi A, et al (1998) Role of alveolar macrophages in initiation and regulation of inflammation in Pseudomonas aeruginosa pneumonia. Infect Immun 66:3164–3169
10. Haslett C (1999) Granulocyte apoptosis and its role in the resolution and control of lung inflammation. Am J Respir Crit Care Med 160:S5–S11
11. Cox G, Crossley J, Xing Z (1995) Macrophage engulfment of apoptotic neutrophils contributes to the resolution of acute pulmonary inflammation in vivo. Am J Respir Cell Mol Biol 12:232–237
12. Hussain N, Wu F, Zhu L, Thrall RS, Kresch MJ (1998) Neutrophil apoptosis during the development and resolution of oleic acid-induced acute lung injury in the rat. Am J Respir Cell Mol Biol 19:867–874
13. Fadok VA, Savill JS, Haslett C, et al (1992) Different populations of macrophages use either the vitronectin receptor or the phosphatidylserine receptor to recognize and remove apoptotic cells. J Immunol 149:4029–4035
14. Savill J, Hogg N, Ren Y, Haslett C (1992) Thrombospondin cooperates with CD36 and the vitronectin receptor in macrophage recognition of neutrophils undergoing apoptosis. J Clin Invest 90:1513–1522
15. Fadok VA, Bratton DL, Rose DM, et al (2000) A receptor for phosphatidylserine-specific clearance of apoptotic cells. Nature 405:85–90
16. Fadok VA, Bratton DL, Guthrie L, Henson PM (2001) Differential effects of apoptotic versus lysed cells on macrophage production of cytokines: role of proteases. J Immunol 166:6847–6854
17. Dehoux MS, Boutten A, Ostinelli J, et al (1994) Compartmentalized cytokine production within the human lung in unilateral pneumonia. Am J Respir Crit Care Med 150:710–716

18. van der Poll T, Keogh CV, Buurman WA, Lowry SF (1997) Passive immunization against tumor necrosis factor-alpha impairs host defense during pneumococcal pneumonia in mice. Am J Respir Crit Care Med 155:603–608

19. Takashima K, Tateda K, Matsumoto T, et al (1997) Role of tumor necrosis factor alpha in pathogenesis of pneumococcal pneumonia in mice. Infect Immun 65:257–260

20. Laichalk LL, Kunkel SL, Strieter RM, et al (1996) Tumor necrosis factor mediates lung antibacterial host defense in murine Klebsiella pneumonia. Infect Immun 64:5211–5218

21. Gosselin D, DeSanctis J, Boule M, et al (1995) Role of tumor necrosis factor alpha in innate resistance to mouse pulmonary infection with Pseudomonas aeruginosa. Infect Immun 63:3272–3278

22. Brieland JK, Remick DG, Freeman PT, et al (1995) In vivo regulation of replicative Legionella pneumophila lung infection by endogenous tumor necrosis factor alpha and nitric oxide. Infect Immun 63:3253–3258

23. Beutler B (1995) TNF, immunity and inflammatory disease: lessons of the past decade. J Investig Med 43:227–235

24. Le J, Vilcek J (1987) Tumor necrosis factor and interleukin 1: cytokines with multiple overlapping biological activities. Lab Invest 56:234–248

25. Tan AM, Ferrante A, Goh DH, Roberton DM, Cripps AW (1995) Activation of the neutrophil bactericidal activity for nontypable Haemophilus influenzae by tumor necrosis factor and lymphotoxin. Pediatr Res 37:155–159

26. Oswald IP, Wynn TA, Sher A, James SL (1992) Interleukin 10 inhibits macrophage microbicidal activity by blocking the endogenous production of tumor necrosis factor alpha required as a costimulatory factor for interferon gamma-induced activation. Proc Natl Acad Sci USA 89:8676–8680

27. Huffnagle GB, Toews GB, Burdick MD, et al (1996) Afferent phase production of TNF-alpha is required for the development of protective T cell immunity to Cryptococcus neoformans. J Immunol 157:4529–4536

28. Amura CR, Fontan PA, Sanjuan N, et al (1995) Tumor necrosis factor alpha plus interleukin 1 beta treatment protects granulocytopenic mice from Pseudomonas aeruginosa lung infection: role of an unusual inflammatory response. APMIS 103:447–459

29. Amura CR, Fontan PA, Sanjuan N, Sordelli DO (1994) The effect of treatment with interleukin-1 and tumor necrosis factor on Pseudomonas aeruginosa lung infection in a granulocytopenic mouse model. Clin Immunol Immunopathol 73:261–266

30. Standiford TJ, Wilkowski JM, Sisson TH, et al (1999) Intrapulmonary tumor necrosis factor gene therapy increases bacterial clearance and survival in murine gram-negative pneumonia. Hum Gene Ther 10:899–909

31. Rijneveld AW, Florquin S, Branger J, et al (2001) Tumor necrosis factor-alpha compensates for the impaired host defense of IL-1 type I receptor deficient mice during pneumococcal pneumonia. J Immunol 167:5240–5246

32. Boutten A, Dehoux MS, Seta N, et al (1996) Compartmentalized IL-8 and elastase release within the human lung in unilateral pneumonia. Am J Respir Crit Care Med 153:336–342

33. Rodriguez JL, Miller CG, DeForge LE, et al (1992) Local production of interleukin-8 is associated with nosocomial pneumonia. J Trauma 33:74–81

34. Broaddus VC, Hebert CA, Vitangcol RV, et al (1992) Interleukin-8 is a major neutrophil chemotactic factor in pleural liquid of patients with empyema. Am Rev Respir Dis 146:825–830

35. Schultz MJ, Wijnholds J, Peppelenbosch MP, et al (2001) Mice lacking the multidrug resistance protein 1 are resistant to Streptococcus pneumoniae-Induced pneumonia. J Immunol 166:4059–4064

36. Greenberger MJ, Strieter RM, Kunkel SL, et al (1996) Neutralization of macrophage inflammatory protein-2 attenuates neutrophil recruitment and bacterial clearance in murine Klebsiella pneumonia. J Infect Dis 173:159–165

37. Tsai WC, Strieter RM, Wilkowski JM, et al (1998) Lung-specific transgenic expression of KC enhances resistance to Klebsiella pneumoniae in mice. J Immunol 161:2435–2440

38. Kooguchi K, Hashimoto S, Kobayashi A, et al (1998) Role of alveolar macrophages in initiation and regulation of inflammation in Pseudomonas aeruginosa pneumonia. Infect Immun 66:3164–3169

39. Schultz MJ, Rijneveld AW, Speelman P, Deventer SJ, van der Poll T (2001) Endogenous interferon-gamma impairs bacterial clearance from lungs during Pseudomonas aeruginosa pneumonia. Eur Cytokine Netw 12:39–44

40. Moore TA, Newstead MW, Strieter RM, et al (2000) Bacterial clearance and survival are dependent on CXC chemokine receptor-2 ligands in a murine model of pulmonary Nocardia asteroides infection. J Immunol 164:908–915

41. Tsai WC, Strieter RM, Mehrad B, et al (2000) CXC chemokine receptor CXCR2 is essential for protective innate host response in murine Pseudomonas aeruginosa pneumonia. Infect Immun 68:4289–4296

42. Rubins JB, Pomeroy C (1997) Role of gamma interferon in the pathogenesis of bacteremic pneumococcal pneumonia. Infect Immun 65:2975–2977

43. Rijneveld AW, Lauw FN, Schultz MJ, et al (2002) The role of interferon-gamma in murine pneumococcal pneumonia. J Infect Dis 185:91–97

44. Greenberger MJ, Kunkel SL, Strieter RM, et al (1996) IL-12 gene therapy protects mice in lethal Klebsiella pneumonia. J Immunol 157:3006–3012

45. Tsai WC, Strieter RM, Zisman DA, et al (1997) Nitric oxide is required for effective innate immunity against Klebsiella pneumoniae. Infect Immun 65:1870–1875

46. Zisman DA, Strieter RM, Kunkel SL, et al (1998) Ethanol feeding impairs innate immunity and alters the expression of Th1- and Th2-phenotype cytokines in murine Klebsiella pneumonia. Alcohol Clin Exp Res 22:621–627

47. Murray HW (1988) Interferon-gamma, the activated macrophage, and host defense against microbial challenge. Ann Intern Med 108:595–608

48. Boehm U, Klamp T, Groot M, Howard JC (1997) Cellular responses to interferon-gamma. Annu Rev Immunol 15:749–795

49. Lauw F, Florquin S, Akira S, et al (2001) IL-18 has a protective role in the early antimicrobial host response to pneumococcal pneumonia. J Immunol 69:5949–5952

50. Kolls JK, Lei D, Nelson S, et al (1995) Adenovirus-mediated blockade of tumor necrosis factor in mice protects against endotoxic shock yet impairs pulmonary host defense. J Infect Dis 171:570–575

51. Kolls JK, Lei D, Nelson S, Summer WR, Shellito JE (1997) Pulmonary cytokine gene therapy. Adenoviral-mediated murine interferon gene transfer compartmentally activates alveolar macrophages and enhances bacterial clearance. Chest 111 (suppl 6):104S

52. Kolls JK, Lei D, Stoltz D, et al (1998) Adenoviral-mediated interferon-gamma gene therapy augments pulmonary host defense of ethanol-treated rats. Alcohol Clin Exp Res 22:157–162

53. Ye P, Rodriguez FH, Kanaly S, et al (2001) Requirement of interleukin 17 receptor signaling for lung CXC chemokine and granulocyte colony-stimulating factor expression, neutrophil recruitment, and host defense. J Exp Med 194:519–527

54. Laichalk LL, Danforth JM, Standiford TJ (1996) Interleukin-10 inhibits neutrophil phagocytic and bactericidal activity. FEMS Immunol Med Microbiol 15:181–187

55. Ralph P, Nakoinz I, Sampson-Johannes A, et al (1992) IL-10, T lymphocyte inhibitor of human blood cell production of IL-1 and tumor necrosis factor. J Immunol 148:808–814

56. van der Poll T, Marchant A, Keogh CV, Goldman M, Lowry SF (1996) Interleukin-10 impairs host defense in murine pneumococcal pneumonia. J Infect Dis 174:994–1000

57. Greenberger MJ, Strieter RM, Kunkel SL, et al (1995) Neutralization of IL-10 increases survival in a murine model of Klebsiella pneumonia. J Immunol 155:722–729

58. van der Poll T, Keogh CV, Guirao X, et al (1997) Interleukin-6 gene-deficient mice show impaired defense against pneumococcal pneumonia. J Infect Dis 176:439–444

59. Skerrett SJ, Martin TR, Chi EY, et al (1999) Role of the type 1 TNF receptor in lung inflammation after inhalation of endotoxin or Pseudomonas aeruginosa. Am J Physiol 276:L715–L727

60. Schultz MJ, Speelman P, van Deventer SJH, van der Poll T (1999) The role of IL-1 in inflammation during *Pseudomonas aeruginosa* pneumonia in mice. 39th ICAAC Abstract Book. ASM Press, Herndon, pp 383 (Abst)

61. Sawa T, Corry DB, Gropper MA, et al (1997) IL-10 improves lung injury and survival in Pseudomonas aeruginosa pneumonia. J Immunol 159:2858–2866

62. Steinhauser ML, Hogaboam CM, Kunkel SL, et al (1999) IL-10 is a major mediator of sepsis-induced impairment in lung antibacterial host defense. J Immunol 162:392–399

Apoptosis in Pneumonia

B. Guery, J. F. Pittet, and P. Marchetti

▮ Introduction

In their initial work published in 1972, Kerr and Currie described a new type of cell death characterized by morphological changes distinct from the features observed in necrosis [1]. The term apoptosis, from the Greek word meaning 'falling off', was adopted to describe this highly conserved genetic program leading to regulated cellular self-destruction. Subsequent investigations showed that this programmed cell death was crucial during fetal development and critical for controlling harmful mechanisms triggered by environmental stresses. Recent literature has defined new roles for apoptosis in the normal and injured lung. Apoptosis plays an important role not only during postnatal lung development [2] but also in the remodeling of the lung after acute lung injury (ALI) for both the elimination of excess alveolar epithelial and mesenchymal cells from resolving lesions [3, 4].

With nearly 1 million annual hospitalizations in the United States and 4 million outpatient attendances, respiratory tract infections are the leading cause of death from infectious disease. Both host factors and organism virulence are the main determinants of clinical recovery, however, the role of apoptosis and alterations in cell cycle regulatory proteins, as well as necrosis, could represent a key issue in this disease. In this chapter, we will first summarize the process of apoptosis and its cell signaling regulation; then we will review some of the most exciting data regarding the role of apoptosis in pneumonia.

▮ Features of Apoptosis

Cell death occurs via different pathways; among them, apoptosis is a well defined phenomenon which can be opposed to necrosis. Each has distinctive morphological or biochemical characteristics: necrosis is a spontaneous and unregulated process resulting in the disintegration of the cell membrane. On the contrary, apoptosis is a gene-regulated phenomenon commonly divided into three successive phases (Fig. 1). First, the initiation phase defines the earliest stage corresponding to the induction of apoptosis by various stimuli (such as ligation of death receptors, generation of secondary messengers by stress induction).

In response to these stimuli, the execution phase of apoptosis is activated leading to a change in the permeability of the outer mitochondrial membrane and/or the activation of caspases, enzymes specifically activated in apoptotic cells. Most of the biochemical changes characteristic of apoptotic cells are caused by a set of cysteine proteases that selectively cleave substrates at the level of an aspartate residue.

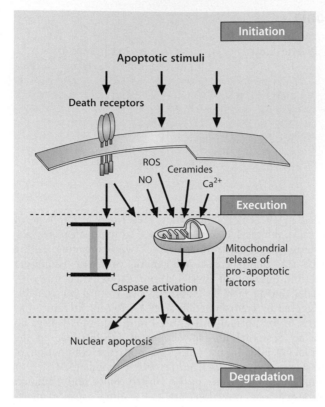

Fig. 1. The biochemical pathways of apoptosis (see text for details). ROS: reactive oxygen species; NO: nitric oxide

Caspases (cysteine ASP aspartate enzymes) are thought to be one of the central executioners of the apoptotic process because, in most of experimental models, elimination of caspase activity will slow down or prevent apoptosis. Schematically, there are two major pathways that trigger caspase proteolytic activity. The first, the death receptor pathway [6], is characterized by the activation of specialized cell surface receptors belonging to the tumor necrosis factor (TNF) receptor (R) gene superfamily (or death receptors). The second, the mitochondrial pathway, is triggered either by extracellular agents like reactive nitrogen species (RNS), oxygen reactive species (ROS) and cytokines, or internal insults, such as DNA damage (e.g., after exposure to ionizing radiation), that results in the release of cytochrome c across the outer membrane of mitochondria into the cytosol. Moreover, cross-talks between death receptor pathways and mitochondria exist in some circumstances (see below and Fig. 3).

It is during the execution phase of apoptosis that members of the bcl-2 family regulate the development of apoptosis mainly at the level of mitochondria whereas caspases are regulated by proteins belonging to the inhibitor of apoptosis (IAP) family. Finally, the apoptotic process enters an irreversible phase of degradation resulting in the morphological and biochemical appearance of typical apoptosis.

Morphology

Apoptosis is well-characterized by the appearance of morphological and biochemical features (Fig. 2). One typical aspect concerns the nucleus which becomes condensed, basophilic, and the chromatin marginates to the periphery forming a crescent halo. The internucleosomic DNA is progressively fragmented by endonucleases responsible for the generation of fragments of 180 to 200 base pairs that may be detected as a ladder on gel electrophoresis (Fig. 2). The changes of the cytoskeleton are more subtle, the cytoplasm is segmented, associated with a global shrinkage of the cell, while the integrity of intracellular organelles is initially maintained. Adherent cells lose their attachment and changes in the plasma membrane are characterized by a loss of the membrane asymmetry and exposure of phosphatidylserine on the extracellular side. The nucleus then breaks up and cytoplasmic blebs appear on the cell surface, followed by the formation of a number of membrane-bound apoptotic bodies. *In vivo*, apoptotic bodies are phagocytosed by neighbor cells. Phagocytosis of apoptotic bodies has commonly been viewed as the clearance of cell corpses by neighbor phagocytes that prevents spilling of cell components into the extracellular space. Apoptosis is therefore a 'clean death' avoiding the initiation of an inflammatory response. However, these clearance events allow scavenger cells to confer meaning upon cell death. For example, recent data indicate that the phagocytosis of apoptotic bodies affects the functions of the phagocytes causing a downregulation of the inflammatory cascade controlled by these cells, a regulation

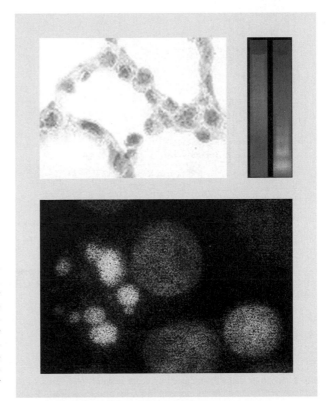

Fig. 2. Morphological and biochemical features of apoptosis. Detection of nuclear apoptosis by the TUNEL (terminal transferase biotinylated-dUTP nick end labeling) method (upper right) and by DNA ladder (upper left). Condensation and fragmentation of the nucleus after DAPI (4′,6-diamino-2-phenylindole) staining (lower panel)

of the immune response via MHC class I and II receptors and a modulation of the cell killing [5].

In contrast to apoptosis, necrosis is described as an unregulated event associated with random DNA breakdown and swelling of cellular components leading to the release of toxic mediators into the surrounding microenvironment.

∎ Cell Signaling by Ligation of Death Receptors

At least, six death receptors have been identified (TNFR1, CD95, DR3, DR4, DR5, DR6) that can activate death caspases within seconds causing an apoptotic demise of the cell within hours. Cysteine-rich extracellular domains and a homologous cytoplasmic sequence named death domain (DD) define them. CD95 (or Fas or Apo1) and TNFR1 (or p55 or CD120a) are well characterized: the death ligand, respectively CD95L (or FasL) and TNF-α, binds to, and causes trimerization of its specific death receptor. The Fas-FasL system is composed of the membrane receptor Fas (CD95), a 45 kDa membrane receptor which belongs to the TNF-α family of proteins, and its natural ligand, FasL [7]. FasL exists as a membrane bound and a

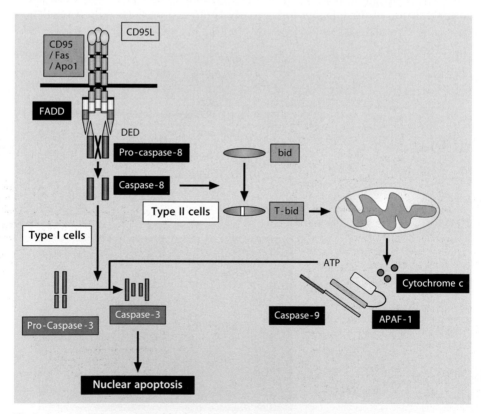

Fig. 3. Apoptotic pathways triggered by death receptors (see text for details). APAF: apoptotic protease activating factor; DED: death effector domain; FADD: Fas-associated death domain

soluble form (sFasL), both can activate Fas [8]. It has also been shown that binding of Fas to FasL could lead to activation of nuclear factor-κB (NF-κB) and release of inflammatory cytokines [9]. Unlike CD95L, TNF-α rarely triggers apoptosis unless protein synthesis is blocked, which suggests the existence of cellular factors that can suppress the apoptotic stimulus generated by TNF-α. Expression of these suppressive proteins is controlled by NF-κB and Jnk/AP1, as inhibition of either pathway sensitizes cells to induction of apoptosis by TNF-α [10]. A similar mechanism has been described for the death receptor DR3 [6].

After binding to its ligand, the death receptor rapidly initiates cell apoptosis through the direct death effector domain (DED)-induced activation of caspase-8 (Fig. 3). In turn, caspase-8 can activate directly caspase-3 in type I cells [6]. However, cross talk between death receptors and mitochondrial pathways are provided by bid protein. Indeed, in some cells (type II cells) caspase-8-mediated cleavage of bid, a proapoptotic member of the bcl-2 member family, promotes its translocation to mitochondria and results in the release of cytochrome c into the cytoplasm [12].

Apoptosis in Acute Lung Injury and Pneumonia

ALI is a syndrome characterized by a major increase in the permeability of the alveolar-capillary membrane, with morphological and physiological evidence of severe epithelial injury in distal airways and alveoli that influences the outcome of the patients with this syndrome. ALI is characterized in its early stage by the association of edema, exudation, and hyaline membrane in the alveolar space. The mechanisms responsible for alveolar epithelial and lung endothelial damage in ALI remain uncertain. Although cell death during ALI has classically been defined as necrosis, there is a growing body of experimental and clinical evidence that apoptosis of parenchymal cells may play an important role in the mechanisms of injury to these cells. In the latter stages, the organizing phase, hyperplasia of type II pneumocytes in the alveoli, is associated with an interstitial proliferation of fibroblasts.

Apoptosis in ALI has been observed in different models. Mantell et al. [13] showed in three distinct models of ALI (hyperoxia, oleic acid, and bacterial pneumonia) that apoptosis was clearly a feature of ALI. The alveolar epithelium forms a tight barrier between the airspaces and the vascular compartment. In addition, alveolar epithelial cells and mostly type II pneumocytes, actively regulate the transport of fluid between the airspaces and the interstitium. A characteristic feature of ALI is a widespread destruction of the alveolar epithelium that affects the outcome of patients with this syndrome, although the exact mechanism of cell death is uncertain [14].

Apoptosis of the Alveolar Epithelium

Among the different factors that may regulate epithelium apoptosis, three factors have to be underlined: Fas/FasL, the renin-angiotensin system, and ROS.

Fas/FasL System: Experimental studies have demonstrated that Fas, originally characterized in lymphocyte T cells as the primary effector molecule of Th1 cytotoxicity, is expressed on the apical surface of a subset of alveolar epithelial type II cells and may trigger apoptosis in these cells [15–17]. Fas and FasL are also expressed on bronchial epithelial cells in primary cultures [18] and it was shown that Fas ligation in bronchiolar cells leads to apoptosis [19]. Matute-Bello et al. [20] recently reported that soluble FasL is released in the airspaces of patients with ALI, but not of those at risk for the syndrome. In addition, bronchoalveolar lavage (BAL) fluid, recovered from patients with ALI, induced apoptosis of distal lung epithelial cells. These results suggest that activation of the Fas/FasL system contributes to the severe epithelial damage that occurs with ALI. Both *in vivo* and *in vitro*, the same authors demonstrated that recombinant human FasL as well as Fas could induce alveolar epithelial cell apoptosis and lung injury [21, 22]. A similar observation has recently been made in patients with ALI from sepsis [23]. Experimental activation of the Fas/FasL system in mice not only induced apoptosis and injury to the alveolar epithelium, but was also associated with the development of lung inflammation characterized by the airspace release of proinflammatory mediators. In bronchial cells, Fas ligation was responsible for apoptosis but also for interleukin (IL)-8 production, which may amplify the inflammatory cascade. Similarly, intranasal instillation of Fas was associated with increased mRNA expression in the lung for TNF-a, macrophage inflammatory protein (MIP)-1a, MIP-2, (MCP)-1, and IL-6 [21], probably related to NF-κB translocation [6]. Interestingly, in this experimental model, damage to the alveolar epithelium occurred before neutrophil recruitment to the alveolar spaces. This observation is of crucial importance because it is still not clear in humans whether the first event leading to lung injury involves neutrophil migration or whether epithelial injury occurs before neutrophils are involved. Answering this question will be a critical step to developing new specific strategies to treat ALI.

Finally, some experimental reports link Fas-induced apoptosis of the alveolar epithelium to development of lung fibrosis. Repeated inhalation of anti-Fas antibody mimicking Fas-FasL cross-linking, induced excessive apoptosis of the alveolar epithelium and an inflammatory response in the airspaces of the lung, which resulted in pulmonary fibrosis in mice [24, 25]. In a classical model of pulmonary-induced fibrosis with bleomycin, Fas-FasL interaction was found to be critical [26]; the administration of a soluble form of Fas antigen or anti-FasL antibody prevented the development of fibrosis. To date, there is no evidence demonstrating a link between excessive apoptosis of the lung epithelium and development of pulmonary fibrosis in patients with ALI. However, it is not unrealistic to hypothesize that excessive apoptosis of the alveolar epithelium may prolong airspace inflammation and interfere with re-epithelialization, which may result in overgrowth of mesenchymal cells and lung fibrosis. To further support this hypothesis, Kazzaz et al. [27] showed in pneumonia models that the location and timing of apoptosis could be a major determinant in the evolution toward fibrosis; in the nonresolving model, apoptosis was persistent. Fas expression was not evaluated in this study. In conclusion, the Fas/FasL system may serve a dual role in the pathogenesis of ALI by causing direct damage to the alveolar epithelial barrier and by initiating the inflammatory cascade, thus perhaps promoting the development of lung fibrosis.

Local Renin-angiotensin System. Recent evidence indicates that a local renin-angiotensin system is expressed in the distal lung parenchyma and plays a central role in the signaling of apoptosis in alveolar type II cells [28–30]. For example, apoptosis in response to Fas activation can be abrogated by antisense oligonucleotides against angiotensinogen, by angiotensin-converting enzyme (ACE) inhibitors or by angiotensin receptor antagonists. These results indicate that the *de novo* synthesis of angiotensin II and receptor interaction are required for the induction of apoptosis of alveolar type II cells by Fas [30]. Moreover, angiotensinogen is also secreted by human lung myofibroblasts isolated from patients suffering from interstitial pulmonary fibrosis [31], and its conversion to angiotensin II by the alveolar epithelium [30] provides a mechanism to explain alveolar epithelial cell death adjacent to underlying myofibroblasts within the fibrotic human lung [32]. Taken together, these data support the hypothesis that a local renin-angiotensin system plays a critical role as a second messenger during the apoptotic process of the alveolar epithelium. They also suggest that therapeutic manipulation of Fas-induced apoptosis *in vivo* should be feasible in the near future with a variety of well-characterized pharmacological antagonists of the renin-angiotensin system.

Reactive Oxygen and Nitrogen Species: The lung is exposed to a variety of ROS and RNS during the acute phase of ALI. Earlier studies showed that both ROS and RNS caused apoptosis of a rat alveolar epithelial cell line [33]. The apoptosis was preceded by upregulation of c-fos and c-jun and the transcription factor activator protein (AP)-1. In contrast, high concentrations of peroxynitrite, a metabolite of nitric oxide (NO), did not lead to c-fos, c-jun and AP-1 activation, and failed to induce apoptosis of lung epithelial cells. Further studies reported that NO may actually inhibit stretch- or hyperoxia-induced alveolar type II cell apoptosis [34, 35]. To explain this discrepancy, recent studies from Dr. Janssen's [16] laboratory suggest that the cellular responses to nitrating species may be different under conditions of injury and repair. Specifically, there was a marked induction of apoptosis in log-phase cultures exposed to peroxynitrite [16]. Similarly, under conditions that mimic wound healing, RNS cause apoptosis selectively in cells that are migrating into the wound, indicating that the response of the lung epithelium under conditions of repair may be different than for quiescent cells. These results indicate that the presence of RNS in the lung may interfere with epithelial repair and contribute to the continuous shedding of epithelial cells in ALI.

Apoptosis and Infectious Agents

We described in the first part of this chapter the different pathways of apoptosis. Infectious agents can trigger the apoptotic cascade by almost any means, both the Fas/FasL system and the mitochondria can be involved (Fig. 4).

Concerning recruited inflammatory cells, a paradox is based on the location of the pathogen: in infections where the pathogen exists within the host macrophage (as in mycobacterial infections) [36], apoptosis of the host defense cell favors the host. On the contrary, for extracellular infections, apoptosis of the host inflammatory cells is advantageous to the pathogen [37]. Apoptosis of parenchymal cells may be protective by promoting pathogen removal and diminishing their infectivity. However, uncontrolled cell apoptosis will induce extensive epithelial injury, increasing the severity of ALI. As we previously reported, Kazzaz et al. [27] used two models of pneumonia with either *Streptococcus sanguis* or *Strep. pneumoniae* in mice; they showed that the pattern and the extent of apoptosis in the acute phase was similar in both models, but after 8 days, apoptosis persisted in the non-resolving model and could explain a progression toward fibrosis through an imbalance between cell death which could be slower than cell division resulting in a steady state of fibro-proliferation.

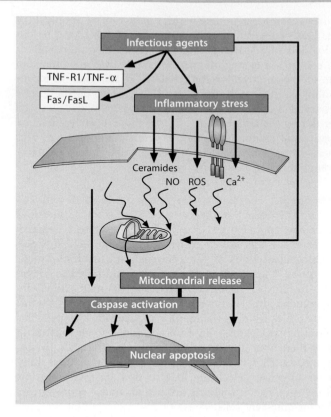

Fig. 4. Hypothetical apoptotic pathways induced by infectious agents. TNF: tumor necrosis factor; NO: nitric oxide; ROS: reactive oxygen species

Apoptosis and Inflammatory Cells. As we previously stated, apoptosis of inflammatory cells can either be beneficial or detrimental for the host. Moreover two phases must be differentiated: the early phase where apoptosis will either enhance or limit the host response, and the resolution of the acute inflammation from which the functional prognosis will depend. Several earlier clinical studies have reported that neutrophils infiltrate the lungs in large numbers after the onset of ALI and their persistence is an important determinant of poor survival [38, 39]. An *in vitro* study has also shown that neutrophils could induce epithelial cell apoptosis mediated by sFasL [40]. Therefore, elucidation of the mechanisms that maintain pulmonary neutrophilia in ALI may be of considerable prognostic and therapeutic significance. Apoptosis and necrosis are the main mechanisms of neutrophil clearance from the alveolar spaces, although apoptosis may be of greater importance because it is a biological process subject to regulatory control, as opposed to necrosis [41]. We have previously discussed the role of the Fas-FasL system in epithelial apoptosis; many experimental data have also shown that this system plays a critical role in the regulation of both T cell and B cell development [42]. Fas is constitutively expressed on human neutrophils, monocytes, and eosinophils, but FasL is restricted to neutrophils and activated lymphocytes [43]. This coexpression of Fas and FasL is probably responsible for the spontaneous apoptosis of human mature neutrophils but also after interaction with FasL expressed on an adjacent cell. Neutrophil Fas-triggered apoptosis can be suppressed by incubation with granulocyte-colony stimulating factor (G-CSF), granulocyte-macrophage colony stimulating factor (GM-CSF), interferon (IFN)-γ, TNF-α, tyrosine kinase inhibitors or dexamethasone [43]. Several studies have recently studied the modulation of neutrophil apoptosis in the airspaces of patients with ALI. The number of apoptotic neutrophils is significantly decreased during the early phase of ALI [44–46]. In contrast, the percentage of apoptotic airspace neutrophils later during the course of the disease appears to be comparable to the one measured in patients without ALI or at risk of developing the syndrome [46]. Moreover, decreased neutrophil apoptosis was associated with increased levels of G-CSF and GM-CSF in the BAL fluid of those patients [44–46]. Although both growth factors prolong the survival of blood neutrophils *in vitro* [47], higher BAL fluid levels of G-CSF were found in non-survivors in one study [45], whereas significantly higher BAL fluid levels of GM-CSF were reported in survivors in another study [46]. Differences between the studies may be explained by the fact that GM-CSF is less specific than G-CSF to induce apoptosis [48]. Moreover, the association between GM-CSF and survival could be independent of the effect of GM-CSF on neutrophil apoptosis and explained by the proliferative effect of this cytokine on alveolar macrophages and epithelial cells [46]. Finally, BAL fluid from patients with early, but not late ALI, inhibited apoptosis of normal blood neutrophils [46]. These findings are important because they show that the inhibitory effect of BAL fluid changed during time in patients with ALI, suggesting that the rate at which neutrophils become apoptotic varies depending on the stage of inflammation.

In pneumonia, neutropenia is often considered as a marker of poor prognosis, it has been shown that sera from infected patients could promote neutrophil apoptosis; whether the pathogen was Gram-positive or Gram-negative did not influence the rate of apoptosis [49]. The same study demonstrated that part of the activity of the sera could be related to FasL. These results may appear to conflict with the previous observation in ALI and acute respiratory distress syndrome (ARDS), however, it could be interesting to separate the fate of systemic and pulmonary neutrophils. In community-acquired pneumonia, Droemann et al. [50] studied systemic and BAL-recovered neutrophils; the rate of apoptosis was significantly decreased in pulmonary neutrophils compared to systemic neutrophils without any changes in Fas expression. This difference is probably critical for the effective control of pulmonary infection.

From these observations, it can be emphasized that besides the massive emigration of neutrophils and the decreased pulmonary neutrophil apoptosis observed in pneumonia, tissue clearance of granulocytes is critical for the resolution of acute inflammation. It has long been assumed that necrosis was the main pathway to neutrophil clearance in pneumonia and ALI, there is now a growing body of evidence that apoptosis provides an injury-limiting, granulocyte clearance mechanism. During apoptosis, neutrophil surface membrane remains intact and neutrophils lose their ability to degranulate on external stimulation [51, 52]. Apoptotic neutrophils are then engulfed in macrophages to be cleared from the lungs [53], peroxidase-positive macrophages are observed very early in the course of the disease, maximal at 24 hours in lipopolysaccharide (LPS)-induced injury [54]. The macrophage recognition mechanism to identify apoptotic granulocytes involves the vitronectin receptor $\alpha_v\beta_3$ and the thrombospondin receptor CD36 [55]. Tissue macrophages are therefore critical in inflammation resolution as scavenger cells; clearance of these cells may also play a pivotal role in inflammation. Human alveolar macrophages undergo apoptosis when stimulated with LPS; a modulation is observed with various cytokines such as IFN-γ, TNF-α, or IL-10 [56].

In summary, although neutrophil apoptosis may be a potential major mechanism in the resolution of airspace inflammation in patients with ALI, it is still unclear whether inhibition of neutrophil apoptosis during the acute phase of inflammation is good or bad for the host, in part because the exact role of neutrophils in the pathogenesis of ALI remains uncertain in humans.

The Pathogen and the Alveoli-capillary Barrier. There is good experimental evidence that various bacteria, including *Staphylococcus aureus* [57–60], *Strep. pneumonia* [61, 62] and *Pseudomonas aeruginosa* [63, 64] cause apoptosis of the lung epithelium *in vitro*. Pathogens such as *Chlamydia* have also been reported to cause apoptosis of epithelial cells and host macrophages [65]. Interestingly, unlike other mucosal surfaces, the lung epithelium is highly resistant to apoptosis induced by *P. aeruginosa*. This response requires a loss of the integrity of the epithelial tight junctions allowing the bacteria to reach the basolateral surface of the cells, and a fully virulent bacteria capable of expressing both adhesins and cytotoxins [64]. The mechanisms by which bacteria induce apoptosis in lung epithelial cells are complex; recent data suggest that *P. aeruginosa* may activate the Fas/FasL pathway in epithelial cells [66]. In fact, deficiency of Fas or FasL on epithelial cells could prevent *P. aeruginosa*-induced apoptosis *in vitro* and *in vivo* and prevented systemic dissemination of bacteria from the lung [66]. Consistent with this hypothesis, a recent study showed that the Fas-FasL system could contribute to the development of permeability changes and tissue injury in Gram-negative sepsis [67]. These authors reported in Fas-deficient mice a less severe change in alveolar permeability after bacterial challenges, this effect was not related to the bacterial count which was similar in both strains of mice. Recently, Jendrossek et al. [68] observed with *P. aeruginosa*, PAO1 strain, a rapid apoptosis of human conjunctiva epithelial cells; in this model apoptosis was mediated by mitochondrial alterations and was dependent on CD95 upregulation in infected cells. A deficiency of CD95 or CD95 ligand prevented mitochondrial changes, the expression of a type III secretion system by the pathogen could also be involved. In fact upregulation of CD95 is largely but not completely dependent on expression of a type III secretion system in *P. aeruginosa* [69]. This system has been shown to be involved in the release of several toxins such as Exo S, T, U or Y. Exo U expression has been shown to correlate with the cytotoxicity of the pathogen *in vitro* and *in vivo* [70, 71]. However, a recent study suggested that Exo U predominantly induced necrosis in macrophages and that a second, yet unidentified, effector protein could trigger apoptosis [63]; in fact, deficiency of the type III system does not completely abrogate apoptosis in epithelial cells [68]. So the upregulation of the Fas-FasL system could be related to multiple factors including type III-dependent toxins, pili, or LPS. Pili can initiate apoptosis [72] and even if this effect was not demonstrated on the Fas-FasL system, LPS can upregulate the TNF factor-related apoptosis-inducing ligand (TRAIL)-APO2 ligand in monocyte and macrophages [73].

Besides the Fas-FasL complex, porins are also involved in *P. aeruginosa*-induced apoptosis; purified porins isolated from the outer membrane of the pathogen induced *in vitro* apoptosis of an epithelial cell line [74]. The effect was P53 independent and associated with a significant decrease in bcl-2 expression; an important role of calcium influx in the cell was underlined. Similar results were obtained with *Neisseria gonorrhoeae*; the infection of cell cultures with this pathogen resulted in apoptosis mediated by the PorB porin with an effect at the mitochondrial voltage-dependent anion channel [75].

Although there is a good amount of literature on bacteria-induced epithelial cell apoptosis, only a few data can be recovered on endothelial cells. Sylte et al. [76] developed a model of endothelial cell culture exposed to *Haemophilus somnus*. This pathogen induced apoptosis within one hour of incubation, the effect was mediated by *H. somnus* lipooligosaccharide. Other pathogens have been shown to induce endothelial cell apoptosis *in vitro* [77–80]. *In vivo*, endothelial cell apoptosis has been studied in LPS or TNF-treated mice; LPS induced a disseminated form of endothelial apoptosis which was mediated sequentially by TNF and ceramide generation [81]. The role of ceramide can, however, be challenged in epithelial cells compared to endothelial cells, TNF-α-induced production of ceramide did not induce type II cell apoptosis [82].

Apoptosis and Lung Function: Lung fluid balance is regulated by alveolar liquid clearance and lung liquid clearance. Alveolar liquid clearance depends on the active sodium transport from the alveoli to the interstitium, this transport relies on sodium channels located on type II cells apical surface, and Na, K-ATPase on the basolateral side. There is actually a solid line of evidence that the capacity of maintaining alveolar fluid transport active is highly correlated with a favorable outcome in patients with ALI [14, 83]. Preliminary data from our laboratory indicate that *P. aeruginosa*-induced apoptosis is associated with a significant decrease in lung liquid clearance in anesthetized rats. We have previously shown that *P. aeruginosa* instillation could decrease lung liquid clearance both at the early phase and after 24 hours [84]; we therefore hypothesized that these changes could be related to apoptotic modifications in the alveoli-capillary barrier. When apoptosis was prevented by pretreatment with keratinocyte growth factor (KGF) or Z-VAD.fmk, a pharmacological inhibitor of the caspases, there was a complete restoration of physiological lung fluid clearance (Fig. 5).

In lung homogenate, the oligonucleosome assay showed an increased oligonucleosomal fragmentation in the PNP group compared to the control group (respectively 26.8 ± 4.6 and 3.2 ± 0.7 OD/mg). Consistent with these data, caspase 3 activity

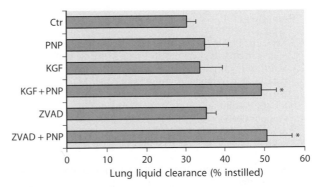

Fig. 5. Lung liquid clearance: intratracheal and intravenous phosphate-buffered saline (PBS) coadministration (Ctr); intratracheal *Pseudomonas aeruginosa* and intravenous PBS coadministration (PNP); intratracheal PBS and intravenous keratinocyte growth factor (KGF) coadministration (KGF); intratracheal *Pseudomonas aeruginosa* and intravenous KGF coadministration (KGF+PNP); intratracheal PBS and intravenous Z-VAD.fmk coadministration (ZVAD); and intratracheal *Pseudomonas aeruginosa* and intravenous Z-VAD.fmk coadministration (ZVAD+PNP). *p<0.05 compared to the pneumonic group (PNP)

in pneumonic lungs was significantly increased compared to controls (respectively 12.9 ± 1.6 and 2.57 ± 1.23 picomol of pNa/µg·min). In KGF-pretreated animals, the oligonucleosome assay showed a decrease to 10.3 ± 2.9 OD/mg of oligonucleosomal fragmentation. Measurement of caspase 3 activity was also significantly decreased to 4.3 ± 1.1 picomol of pNa/µg·min compared to the PNP group.

In conclusion, apoptosis occurs in the early phase of *P. aeruginosa* pneumonia. KGF or Z-VAD.fmk coadministration with the pathogen, can significantly decrease this apoptotic process *in vivo*. The administration of KGF or Z-VAD.fmk can restore lung fluid balance suggesting a link between apoptosis and fluid transport. Apoptosis is an important feature in *P. aeruginosa* pneumonia; further evaluation of blocking factors, such as KGF or Z-VAD.fmk, may represent an interesting pathway of therapeutic research. Nevertheless, the importance of apoptosis of the lung epithelium during pneumonia-induced ALI remains to be demonstrated in humans.

■ Conclusion

Apoptosis of lung parenchymal and inflammatory cells is part of the host response to noxious stimuli during both the acute inflammatory and resolution phases of ALI. There is also limited experimental and clinical evidence that abnormalities in the apoptotic process (i.e., inefficient or excessive apoptosis) may increase damage to the lung parenchyma, prevent resolution of inflammation, and perhaps promote abnormal tissue repair (i.e., lung fibrosis) in ALI. Modulating the apoptotic process with bcl-2 antisense, recombinant TRAIL, caspase inhibitors, and inhibitors of the renin-angiotensin system, could be considered in the future to control abnormal apoptosis in ALI. However, before these new therapeutic strategies can be used in patients with ALI, there is a need for a better understanding of (a) the significance of the apoptotic process in clinically relevant experimental models of ALI and (b) the importance of specific clinical disorders associated with ALI (i.e., pneumonia, trauma, sepsis, aspiration of gastric contents) in modulating the activation of apoptosis in the lung.

References

1. Kerr JF, Wyllie AH, Currie AR (1972) Apoptosis: a basic biological phenomenon with wide-ranging implications in tissue kinetics. Br J Cancer 26:239–257
2. Schittny JC, Djonov V, Fine A, Burri PH (1998) Programmed cell death contributes to postnatal lung development. Am J Respir Cell Mol Biol 18:786–793
3. Bardales RH, Xie SS, Schaefer RF, Hsu SM (1996) Apoptosis is a major pathway responsible for the resolution of type II pneumocytes in acute lung injury. Am J Pathol 149:845–852
4. Polunovsky VA, Chen B, Henke C, et al (1993) Role of mesenchymal cell death in lung remodeling after injury. J Clin Invest 92:388–397
5. Savill J, Fadok V (2000) Corpse clearance defines the meaning of cell death. Nature 407: 784–788
6. Ashkenazi A, Dixit VM (1998) Death receptors: signaling and modulation. Science 281: 1305–1308
7. Itoh N, Yonehara S, Ishii A, et al (1991) The polypeptide encoded by the cDNA for human cell surface antigen Fas can mediate apoptosis. Cell 66:233–243
8. Tanaka M, Suda T, Takahashi T, Nagata S (1995) Expression of the functional soluble form of human fas ligand in activated lymphocytes. EMBO J 14:1129–1135
9. Ponton A, Clement MV, Stamenkovic I (1996) The CD95 (APO-1/Fas) receptor activates NF-kappaB independently of its cytotoxic function. J Biol Chem 271:8991–8995

10. Beg AA, Baltimore D (1996) An essential role for NF-kappaB in preventing TNF-alpha-induced cell death. Science 274:782–784
11. Adams JM, Cory S (1998) The Bcl-2 protein family: arbiters of cell survival. Science 281:1322–1326
12. Hengartner MO (2000) The biochemistry of apoptosis. Nature 407:770–776
13. Mantell L, Kazzaz J, Xu J, et al (1997) Unscheduled apoptosis during acute inflammatory lung injury. Cell Death Diff 4:600–607
14. Matthay MA, Wiener-Kronish JP (1990) Intact epithelial barrier function is critical for the resolution of alveolar edema in humans. Am Rev Respir Dis 142:1250–1257
15. Fine A, Anderson NL, Rothstein TL, Williams MC, Gochuico BR (1997) Fas expression in pulmonary alveolar type II cells. Am J Physiol 273:L64–L71
16. Fine A, Janssen-Heininger Y, Soultanakis RP, Swisher SG, Uhal BD (2000) Apoptosis in lung pathophysiology. Am J Physiol 279:L423–L427
17. Wen LP, Madani K, Fahrni JA, Duncan SR, Rosen GD (1997) Dexamethasone inhibits lung epithelial cell apoptosis induced by IFN-gamma and Fas. Am J Physiol 273:L921–L929
18. Hamann KJ, Dorscheid DR, Ko FD, et al (1998) Expression of Fas (CD95) and FasL (CD95L) in human airway epithelium. Am J Respir Cell Mol Biol 19:537–542
19. Hagimoto N, Kuwano K, Kawasaki M, et al (1999) Induction of interleukin-8 secretion and apoptosis in bronchiolar epithelial cells by Fas ligation. Am J Respir Cell Mol Biol 21:436–445
20. Matute-Bello G, Liles WC, Steinberg KP, et al (1999) Soluble Fas ligand induces epithelial cell apoptosis in humans with acute lung injury (ARDS). J Immunol 163:2217–2225
21. Matute-Bello G, Winn RK, Jonas M, et al (2001) Fas (CD95) Induces alveolar epithelial cell apoptosis in vivo: Implications for acute pulmonary inflammation. Am J Pathol 158:153–161
22. Matute-Bello G, Liles WC, Frevert CW, et al (2001) Recombinant human Fas ligand induces alveolar epithelial cell apoptosis and lung injury in rabbits. Am J Physiol 281:L328–L335
23. Hashimoto S, Kobayashi A, Kooguchi K, Kitamura Y, Onodera H, Nakajima H (2000) Upregulation of two death pathways of perforin/granzyme and FasL/Fas in septic acute respiratory distress syndrome. Am J Respir Crit Care Med 161:237–243
24. Hagimoto N, Kuwano K, Miyazaki H, et al (1997) Induction of apoptosis and pulmonary fibrosis in mice in response to ligation of Fas antigen. Am J Respir Cell Mol Biol 17:272–278
25. Kuwano K, Miyazaki H, Hagimoto N, et al (1999) The involvement of Fas-Fas ligand pathway in fibrosing lung diseases. Am J Respir Cell Mol Biol 20:53–60
26. Kuwano K, Hagimoto N, Kawasaki M, et al (1999) Essential roles of the Fas-Fas ligand pathway in the development of pulmonary fibrosis. J Clin Invest 104:13–19
27. Kazzaz JA, Horowitz S, Xu J, et al (2000) Differential patterns of apoptosis in resolving and nonresolving bacterial pneumonia. Am J Respir Crit Care Med 161:2043–2050
28. Wang R, Alam G, Zagariya A, et al (2000) Apoptosis of lung epithelial cells in response to TNF-alpha requires angiotensin II generation de novo. J Cell Physiol 185:253–259
29. Wang R, Ibarra-Sunga O, Verlinski L, Pick R, Uhal BD (2000) Abrogation of bleomycin-induced epithelial apoptosis and lung fibrosis by captopril or by a caspase inhibitor. Am J Physiol 279:L143–L151
30. Wang R, Zagariya A, Ibarra-Sunga O, et al (1999) Angiotensin II induces apoptosis in human and rat alveolar epithelial cells. Am J Physiol 276:L885–L889
31. Wang R, Ramos C, Joshi I, et al (1999) Human lung myofibroblast-derived inducers of alveolar epithelial apoptosis identified as angiotensin peptides. Am J Physiol 277:L1158–L1164
32. Uhal BD, Joshi I, Hughes WF, Ramos C, Pardo A, Selman M (1998) Alveolar epithelial cell death adjacent to underlying myofibroblasts in advanced fibrotic human lung. Am J Physiol 275:L1192–L1199
33. Janssen YM, Matalon S, Mossman BT (1997) Differential induction of c-fos, c-jun, and apoptosis in lung epithelial cells exposed to ROS or RNS. Am J Physiol 273:L789–L796
34. Edwards YS, Sutherland LM, Murray AW (2000) NO protects alveolar type II cells from stretch-induced apoptosis. A novel role for macrophages in the lung. Am J Physiol 279:L1236–L1242

35. Howlett CE, Hutchison JS, Veinot JP, Chiu A, Merchant P, Fliss H (1999) Inhaled nitric oxide protects against hyperoxia-induced apoptosis in rat lungs. Am J Physiol 277:L596–L605

36. Keane J, Balcewicz-Sablinska MK, Remold HG, et al (1997) Infection by Mycobacterium tuberculosis promotes human alveolar macrophage apoptosis. Infect Immun 65:298–304

37. Hutchison ML, Poxton IR, Govan JR (1998) Burkholderia cepacia produces a hemolysin that is capable of inducing apoptosis and degranulation of mammalian phagocytes. Infect Immun 66:2033–2039

38. Baughman RP, Gunther KL, Rashkin MC, Keeton DA, Pattishall EN (1996) Changes in the inflammatory response of the lung during acute respiratory distress syndrome: prognostic indicators. Am J Respir Crit Care Med 154:76–81

39. Steinberg KP, Milberg JA, Martin TR, Maunder RJ, Cockrill BA, Hudson LD (1994) Evolution of bronchoalveolar cell populations in the adult respiratory distress syndrome. Am J Respir Crit Care Med 150:113–122

40. Serrao KL, Fortenberry JD, Owens ML, Harris FL, Brown LA (2001) Neutrophils induce apoptosis of lung epithelial cells via release of soluble Fas ligand. Am J Physiol 280:L298–L305

41. Haslett C (1999) Granulocyte apoptosis and its role in the resolution and control of lung inflammation. Am J Respir Crit Care Med 160:S5–S11

42. Alderson MR, Tough TW, Davis-Smith T, et al (1995) Fas ligand mediates activation-induced cell death in human T lymphocytes. J Exp Med 181:71–77

43. Liles WC, Kiener PA, Ledbetter JA, Aruffo A, Klebanoff SJ (1996) Differential expression of Fas (CD95) and Fas ligand on normal human phagocytes: implications for the regulation of apoptosis in neutrophils. J Exp Med 184:429–440

44. Matute-Bello G, Liles WC, Radella F, et al (1997) Neutrophil apoptosis in the acute respiratory distress syndrome. Am J Respir Crit Care Med 156:1969–1977

45. Aggarwal A, Baker CS, Evans TW, Haslam PL (2000) G-CSF and IL-8 but not GM-CSF correlate with severity of pulmonary neutrophilia in acute respiratory distress syndrome. Eur Respir J 15:895–901

46. Matute-Bello G, Liles WC, Radella F, et al (2000) Modulation of neutrophil apoptosis by granulocyte colony-stimulating factor and granulocyte/macrophage colony-stimulating factor during the course of acute respiratory distress syndrome. Crit Care Med 28:1–7

47. Brach MA, deVos S, Gruss HJ, Herrmann F (1992) Prolongation of survival of human polymorphonuclear neutrophils by granulocyte-macrophage colony-stimulating factor is caused by inhibition of programmed cell death. Blood 80:2920–2924

48. Aglietta M, Piacibello W, Sanavio F, et al (1989) Kinetics of human hemopoietic cells after in vivo administration of granulocyte-macrophage colony-stimulating factor. J Clin Invest 83:551–557

49. Nwakoby IE, Reddy K, Patel P, et al (2001) Fas-mediated apoptosis of neutrophils in sera of patients with infection. Infect Immun 69:3343–3349

50. Droemann D, Aries SP, Hansen F, et al (2000) Decreased apoptosis and increased activation of alveolar neutrophils in bacterial pneumonia. Chest 117:1679–1684

51. Savill JS, Wyllie AH, Henson JE, Walport MJ, Henson PM, Haslett C (1989) Macrophage phagocytosis of aging neutrophils in inflammation. Programmed cell death in the neutrophil leads to its recognition by macrophages. J Clin Invest 83:865–875

52. Whyte MK, Meagher LC, MacDermot J, Haslett C (1993) Impairment of function in aging neutrophils is associated with apoptosis. J Immunol 150:5124–5134

53. Ishii Y, Hashimoto K, Nomura A, et al (1998) Elimination of neutrophils by apoptosis during the resolution of acute pulmonary inflammation in rats. Lung 176:89–98

54. Cox G, Crossley J, Xing Z (1995) Macrophage engulfment of apoptotic neutrophils contributes to the resolution of acute pulmonary inflammation in vivo. Am J Respir Cell Mol Biol 12:232–237

55. Savill J, Hogg N, Ren Y, Haslett C (1992) Thrombospondin cooperates with CD36 and the vitronectin receptor in macrophage recognition of neutrophils undergoing apoptosis. J Clin Invest 90:1513–1522

56. Bingisser R, Stey C, Weller M, Groscurth P, Russi E, Frei K (1996) Apoptosis in human alveolar macrophages is induced by endotoxin and is modulated by cytokines. Am J Respir Cell Mol Biol 15:64–70
57. Bayles KW, Wesson CA, Liou LE, Fox LK, Bohach GA, Trumble WR (1998) Intracellular Staphylococcus aureus escapes the endosome and induces apoptosis in epithelial cells. Infect Immun 66:336–342
58. Kahl BC, Goulian M, van Wamel W, et al (2000) Staphylococcus aureus RN6390 replicates and induces apoptosis in a pulmonary epithelial cell line. Infect Immun 68:5385–5392
59. Wesson CA, Liou LE, Todd KM, Bohach GA, Trumble WR, Bayles KW (1998) Staphylococcus aureus Agr and Sar global regulators influence internalization and induction of apoptosis. Infect Immun 66:5238–5243
60. Wesson CA, Deringer J, Liou LE, Bayles KW, Bohach GA, Trumble WR (2000) Apoptosis induced by Staphylococcus aureus in epithelial cells utilizes a mechanism involving caspases 8 and 3. Infect Immun 68:2998–3001
61. Kuo CF, Wu JJ, Tsai PJ, et al (1999) Streptococcal pyrogenic exotoxin B induces apoptosis and reduces phagocytic activity in U937 cells. Infect Immun 67:126–130
62. Tsai PJ, Lin YS, Kuo CF, Lei HY, Wu JJ (1999) Group A Streptococcus induces apoptosis in human epithelial cells. Infect Immun 67:4334–4339
63. Hauser AR, Engel JN (1999) Pseudomonas aeruginosa induces type-III-secretion-mediated apoptosis of macrophages and epithelial cells. Infect Immun 67:5530–5537
64. Rajan S, Cacalano G, Bryan R, et al (2000) Pseudomonas aeruginosa induction of apoptosis in respiratory epithelial cells: analysis of the effects of cystic fibrosis transmembrane conductance regulator dysfunction and bacterial virulence factors. Am J Respir Cell Mol Biol 23:304–312
65. Ojcius DM, Souque P, Perfettini JL, Dautry-Varsat A (1998) Apoptosis of epithelial cells and macrophages due to infection with the obligate intracellular pathogen Chlamydia psittaci. J Immunol 161:4220–4226
66. Grassme H, Kirschnek S, Riethmueller J, et al (2000) CD95/CD95 ligand interactions on epithelial cells in host defense to pseudomonas aeruginosa. Science 290:527–530
67. Matute-Bello G, Frevert CW, Liles WC, et al (2001) Fas/Fas ligand system mediates epithelial injury, but not pulmonary host defenses, in response to inhaled bacteria. Infect Immun 69:5768–5776
68. Jendrossek V, Grassme H, Mueller I, Lang F, Gulbins E (2001) Pseudomonas aeruginosa-induced apoptosis involves mitochondria and stress-activated protein kinases. Infect Immun 69:2675–2683
69. Donnenberg MS (2000) Pathogenic strategies of enteric bacteria. Nature 406:768–774
70. Sawa T, Yahr TL, Ohara M, et al (1999) Active and passive immunization with the Pseudomonas V antigen protects against type III intoxication and lung injury. Nat Med 5:392–398
71. Kurahashi K, Kajikawa O, Sawa T, et al (1999) Pathogenesis of septic shock in Pseudomonas aeruginosa pneumonia. J Clin Invest 104:743–750
72. Comolli JC, Waite LL, Mostov KE, Engel JN (1999) Pili binding to asialo-GM1 on epithelial cells can mediate cytotoxicity or bacterial internalization by Pseudomonas aeruginosa. Infect Immun 67:3207–3214
73. Halaas O, Vik R, Ashkenazi A, Espevik T (2000) Lipopolysaccharide induces expression of APO2 ligand/TRAIL in human monocytes and macrophages. Scand J Immunol 51:244–250
74. Buommino E, Morelli F, Metafora S, et al (1999) Porin from Pseudomonas aeruginosa induces apoptosis in an epithelial cell line derived from rat seminal vesicles. Infect Immun 67:4794–4800
75. Müller A, Günther D, Brinkmann V, Hurwitz R, Meyer TF, Rudel T (2000) Targeting of the pro-apoptotic VDAC-like porin (PorB) of Neisseria gonorrhoeae to mitochondria of infected cells. EMBO J 19:5332–5343
76. Sylte MJ, Corbeil LB, Inzana TJ, Czuprynski CJ (2001) Haemophilus somnus induces apoptosis in bovine endothelial cells in vitro. Infect Immun 69:1650–1660
77. Clifton DR, Goss RA, Sahni SK, et al (1998) NF-kappa B-dependent inhibition of apoptosis is essential for host cell survival during Rickettsia rickettsii infection. Proc Natl Acad Sci USA 95:4646–4651

78. Kee SH, Cho KA, Kim MK, Lim BU, Chang WH, Kang JS (1999) Disassembly of focal adhesions during apoptosis of endothelial cell line ECV304 infected with Orientia tsutsugamushi. Microb Pathog 27:265–271
79. Kim MK, Kee SH, Cho KA, et al (1999) Apoptosis of endothelial cell line ECV304 persistently infected with Orientia tsutsugamushi. Microbiol Immunol 43:751–757
80. Menzies BE, Kourteva I (1998) Internalization of Staphylococcus aureus by endothelial cells induces apoptosis. Infect Immun 66:5994–5998
81. Haimovitz-Friedman A, Cordon-Cardo C, Bayoumy S, et al (1997) Lipopolysaccharide induces disseminated endothelial apoptosis requiring ceramide generation. J Exp Med 186: 1831–1841
82. Mallampalli RK, Peterson EJ, Carter AB, Salome RG, Mathur SN, Koretzky GA (1999) TNF-alpha increases ceramide without inducing apoptosis in alveolar type II epithelial cells. Am J Physiol 276:L481–L490
83. Ware LB, Matthay MA (2001) Alveolar fluid clearance is impaired in the majority of patients with acute lung injury and the acute respiratory distress syndrome. Am J Respir Crit Care Med 163:1376–1383
84. Viget N, Guery B, Ader F, et al (2000) Keratinocyte growth factor protects against *Pseudomonas aeruginosa*-induced lung injury. Am J Physiol 279:L1199–L1209

Hypoxic Pulmonary Vasoconstriction and the Pulmonary Microcirculation

D. L. Traber and L. D. Traber

▌ Introduction

In a normal individual, pulmonary arterial blood is diverted from alveoli that are not being ventilated and perfuses the alveoli that are being ventilated [1, 2]. The mechanism that is responsible for this physiological shunt in blood flow is called hypoxic pulmonary vasoconstriction (HPV). When the PaO_2 falls, the smooth muscle of the pulmonary arterioles contracts. The only non-oxygenated blood that enters the pulmonary veins is from the bronchial and thebesian vessels with this perfect match of ventilation and perfusion [3, 4]. With atelectasis, airway obstruction, alveolar edema and abnormalities of nitric oxide (NO) production, there can be a disruption of the pulmonary microcirculation. We will discuss the physiological processes that are responsible for HPV and how they can be disrupted by various pulmonary problems commonly encountered in the intensive care unit (ICU).

▌ Hypoxic Pulmonary Vasoconstriction

The mechanisms responsible for HPV are complex. HPV does not appear to be mediated by nervous mechanisms because HPV can be seen in isolated perfused lungs. Pulmonary vascular smooth muscle will also increase its tone in the presence of a low oxygen tension. Hypoxia inhibits the potassium permeability of the smooth muscle of the pulmonary arteriole [2, 5]. As potassium stays in the cell, the cell depolarizes and calcium enters, causing the smooth muscle to contract. The smooth muscle cells of the pulmonary system contract as a result of the phosphorylation of myosin light chain proteins. Rho-kinase is involved in this process. Rho-kinase is reported to increase in activity during hypoxia [6].

The endothelium of the pulmonary vasculature contains the enzyme endothelial NO synthase (ecNOS or NOS III). This enzyme converts arginine into NO and citrulline. NO diffuses into the pulmonary arteriolar smooth muscle where it combines with the heme group of the enzyme guanylate cyclase. Activation of guanylate cyclase results in the formation of cGMP. cGMP causes calcium to be pumped from the cell resulting in relaxation of the arterioles [7–10]. The degree of pulmonary arteriolar contraction depends on the degree of contractile and relaxing factors. Thus, if the activity of ecNOS were to increase there would be vascular relaxation. Similarly if the activity of ecNOS were to decrease, the muscle would relax. The degree of NO formation is dependent on the concentration of the substrate arginine. Arginine is transported into the cell by a special transport mechanism called the y+ or cationic transporter [11]. Recent data suggest that the activity of the y+ transporter is depressed by hypoxia. If arginine is not pumped into the cell there will be a lack of substrate for the formation of NO. The reduction in ecNOS activity would result in less NO formation and thus pulmonary arteriolar tone would increase. Thus, if alveolar oxygen falls the combination of these various events will lead to increased vascular tone and thus reduced flow of mixed venous pulmonary arterial blood to unventilated alveoli and towards those that are ventilated.

In hypoxic alveoli, reduction in NO formation as a result of ecNOS activity results in pulmonary arteriolar constriction. In ventilated alveoli, NO results in pulmonary arteriolar vasodilation. The airway epithelium also makes NO. The inducible form of NOS (iNOS) is present in these cells [12,13]. NO diffuses into the airway and diffuses into the alveoli that are ventilated. This NO dilates the arterioles of these ventilated alveoli. Thus at the same time that the arterioles of non-ventilated alveoli are being constricted, the arterioles of the ventilated alveoli are being dilated. If the patient is hyperventilated, not only will the $PaCO_2$ drop but also the PaNO and thus there will be an increase in vascular resistance to the ventilated alveoli. This will lead to pulmonary hypertension. Much of the airway epithelium is in the nasal pharynx. If an individual is intubated, this NO does not reach ventilated alveoli.

The amount of blood that perfuses the non-ventilated alveoli is called shunt blood flow. This poorly saturated blood will mix with blood from alveoli that are ventilated resulting in a fall in PaO_2. The amount of shunt is affected by the tone of the microvasculature to the ventilated alveoli. As vascular resistance to the ventilated alveoli increases, pulmonary arterial pressures will increase and more blood will shunt to non-ventilated alveoli. The second component in this relationship will be the pulmonary blood flow or cardiac output. As the cardiac output rises, pulmonary pressure rises and again blood flow to the non-ventilated alveoli will increase. Thus, in a patient with normal cardiac output only the ventilated portion of the lung is perfused. On the other hand, when the cardiac output is increased above normal, the increased pulmonary arterial pressure that results may cause perfusion of unventilated alveoli. By the same token, individuals with large portions of the lung that are unventilated, such as occurs with airway obstruction or atelectasis, may have a normal PaO_2 if the cardiac output is low but a marked fall in arterial saturation when the cardiac output is normalized.

Other factors affect the degree of alveolar ventilation. Airway inflammation leads to the formation of casts in the airway. This leads to blockage of the airway and alveolar hypoxia. Since fewer ventilated alveoli are available for perfusion, the pulmonary pressure rises. This will have two effects: 1) the number of non-ventilated alveoli that are perfused increases reducing arterial saturation, and 2) pulmonary microvascular pressure in the perfused alveoli will increase. Increase in pulmonary microvascular pressure will lead to an increase in pulmonary edema formation. Interstitial edema will reduce oxygen diffusion and further reduces arterial saturation. The reduction in arterial oxygen saturation causes cardiac output to rise further increasing the pulmonary pressures. A positive feedback loop is set into play with the developing pathology causing further pathology. Pulmonary toilet and reduction in airway inflammation will remove the casts and prevent further cast formation. Increasing the inspired oxygen fraction (FiO_2) will overcome the diffusion gradient created by the interstitial edema and restore saturation to the blood perfusing ventilated alveoli. These clinical activities can thus break the positive feedback loop and restore homeostasis.

▌ HPV During Sepsis

Under normal circumstances the alveolar epithelial cells do not make iNOS. However under conditions of trauma or sepsis, cytokines are released that can cause the upregulation of iNOS [14]. Under normal circumstances, in ventilated alveoli, the NO produced by this enzyme in the airway would enter the alveoli and blood and some would be exhaled. In the blood the NO would either be converted into nitrates and nitrites (NOx) by the hemoglobin or combined to the hemoglobin as S-nitrosothiol [15]. Some would diffuse across the epithelium into the efferent arteriole but should not cause much vasodilatation since the vessel is already dilated. In an unventilated alveolus, some of the NO would diffuse into the airway if it were patent and some into the blood, but some would dilate the efferent arteriole. Thus there would be some loss of hypoxic vasoconstriction. In situations in which the airway is blocked by casts or mucous plugs, NO cannot diffuse into the airway and thus higher concentrations can be expected in the alveoli with subsequent loss of HPV. We have previously reported this to be the case in sepsis [16] and acute respiratory distress syndrome (ARDS) [17] and that this loss of HPV can be restored by administration of a NOS inhibitor (Fig. 1).

In sepsis there are several factors that can contribute to the loss of hypoxic pulmonary vascular resistance. This is certainly a situation in which one would expect to see an elevation in cytokines and bacterial products, both of which are inducers of iNOS. We studied this in sheep that were made septic by the continuous infusion of either bacteria [18] or endotoxin [19]. Under these circumstances there is a large increase in shunt blood flow that is markedly reduced by the administration of a NOS inhibitor [19] suggesting that the increase in shunt blood flow is mediated by NO. On the other hand, the NOS inhibitor reduced cardiac output [20] and an increased cardiac output also increases shunt blood flow. With the administration of bacteria there is a marked increase in the up-take of arginine by the lung and an increase in the pulmonary for-

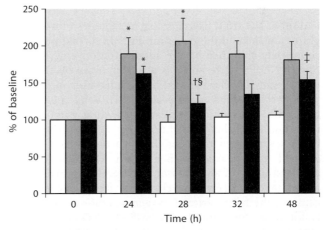

Fig. 1. Intrapulmonary shunt as percent of baseline. Control group (open bars), sepsis group (stippled bars), L-NMMA group (filled bars). * P < 0.05 versus 0 h; † p < 0.05 versus 24 h (sepsis); ‡ p < 0.05 versus 28 h (L-NMMA); § p < 0.05 versus sepsis group. After 24 h of sepsis, shunt was increased; after L-NMMA infusion, shunt decreased. (modified from [16])

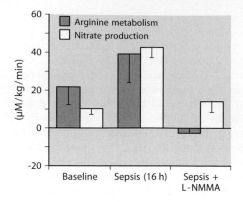

Fig. 2. Uptake of arginine and output of NO_2/NO_3 by the lung with a continuous infusion of *Pseudomonas* bacteria. These are data from sheep that were prepared given 106 kg/h of *Pseudomonas* and infused with the stable isotope [$^{15}N_2$-guanidino]arginine

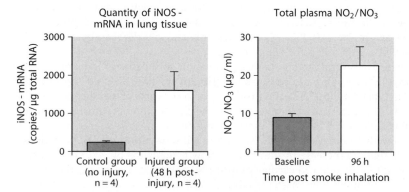

Fig. 3. Changes in iNOS mRNA and NO_2/NO_3 in sheep following a 40% body surface area 3rd degree burn. Data (mean ± standard deviation) are from six animals. mRNA was determined by competitive PCR. NO_2/NO_3 was determined by chemiluminescence

mation of NO_2/NO_3 (NOx), stable metabolites of NO (Fig. 2). The augmentation of arginine uptake and the reduction in NOx formation that is seen with sepsis is almost completely abolished by the administration of L-NMMA, an inhibitor of NOS. The role of NO in the response is also supported by the our finding that the total iNOS mRNA and NOx are elevated in the lung after injury (Fig. 3).

To test this further we evaluated HPV by measuring the blood flow to the left lung with and without ventilating the lung with nitrogen. HPV was manifest by a reduction in left lung blood flow (Fig. 1). The administration of either endotoxin or bacteria prevented much of the vasoconstriction of the left lung, which was seen when it was ventilated with nitrogen. This vasoconstriction was restored with the administration of an inhibitor of NOS. These experiments were performed in a relevant model of sepsis developed in sheep, and support the concept that a major cause of the fall in arterial oxygen saturation that is observed in sepsis may be the result of the formation of the NOS and NO and the loss of HPV. In this model the airways are not damaged and the fall in PaO_2 could be prevented by augmenting the positive end-expiratory pressure (PEEP) and FiO_2. These latter two manipulations of ventilation are not without side effects, such as tissue oxidation and volutrauma. In the future, a specific inhibitor of NOS may be available to aid in the treatment of these patients. In addition newer CO_2 removal devices have been developed that can reduce the need for ventilators [21].

▌ HPV With Acute Lung Injury

Acute lung injury (ALI), such as that seen with the inhalation of smoke or aspiration of acid, will lead to the formation of casts that obstruct the airways. In the terminal bronchioles these casts have a heavy component of neutrophils that enter the airway through the columnar epithelium, and mucus that is formed from the upper airway [22]. We created inhalation injury to the left lung by insufflating it with cotton smoke and determined its blood flow using a flow probe on the left pulmonary artery. Blood flow to the lung gradually decreased following inhalation insult [23]. The decrease in blood flow to the left lung was proportional to the formation of casts in the airway of the damaged lung. Thus, airway obstruction from inflammatory cells, cellular debris, fibrin and mucous occludes the airways and the unventilated alveoli then realize a constriction of their associated pulmonary blood supply. This HPV raises pulmonary arterial pressure that can override some of the vasoconstriction to the non-ventilated alveoli and thus there will be some desaturation of arterial blood. With the increase in blood flow to remaining ventilated alveoli, there is an increase in pulmonary microvascular pressure [24] that can lead to edema formation further decreasing PaO_2.

With both sepsis and ARDS there is an activation of macrophages and neutrophils. A majority of these cells find their way to the pulmonary circulation. Pulmonary capillaries are smaller than those of the systemic circulation [25–27]. The leukocytes are actually larger than the capillaries and cannot go through the pulmonary microcirculation without distortion. This distortion is dependent on the driving pressure [28]. With low driving pressures, the transit time of the leukocytes is prolonged. Thus in the hypo-ventilated areas of the lung, where HPV is in effect, the activated cells are in contact with the pulmonary microvaculature for a longer time period and consequently lung damage in these areas is more likely. A similar situation will occur with under-resuscitation. A low cardiac output will prolong the transit time of the neutrophils through the pulmonary microcirculation [28]. We have previously reported that holding back on fluid in cases of ARDS will make the lung injury worse [29].

In these same instances, the polymorphonuclear (PMN) cells also release oxygen radicals [30]. Unlike many tissues the alveoli have some supply of oxygen. The bronchial circulation, the systemic circulation of the lung, is oxygenated under most situations. The venous drainage of the bronchial circulation drains into the pulmonary microvasculature [31]. Thus there is a source of oxygen for the formation of oxygen radicals. We have determined that following ALI there is a marked increase in bronchial blood flow [32]. The presence of oxygen radicals may be more intense in the areas where there has been hypoxic vasoconstriction. These areas have a greater bronchial blood flow because pulmonary microvascular pressures, and thus bronchial venous pressure, are lower here. In addition, these are areas where more numerous neutrophils might be predicted to be present. Hypoxia is here defined by the low oxygen tension within the alveoli. The presence of cells producing oxygen free radicals such as superoxide and NO creates the possibility for formation of the potent oxidant, peroxynitrite [33]. The recent finding that hypoxia will cause a decrease in the y+ transporter that brings arginine into the cell offers some interesting possibilities for damage [34]. With a deficiency of arginine, NOS forms superoxide and, thus, peroxynitrite [35].

Anesthetics also effect HPV. Most intravenous anesthetics have little effect on the phenomenon, but propofol actually increases it [36]. It is generally accepted that most halogenated anesthetic agents cause a loss of hypoxic vasoconstriction. However, most of the reports dealing with this subject are based on *in vitro* studies. *In vivo* studies do not always support this effect [37, 38]. However, even NO has been reported to reduce HPV [39]. How these agents effect the pulmonary micro-vasculature remains to be seen.

▌ Conclusion

HPV is an important mechanism for the maintenance of normal homeostasis of blood gases. The basic mechanism responsible for the control of this very important physiological function is the level of oxygen in the alveoli. When this variable is low, there is a reduction of blood flow to the alveoli. Hypoxia affects the tone of the pulmonary arterioles through changes in potassium permeability and NO synthesis. Presence of NO in the airway plays an important role in dilation of the arterioles of ventilated alveoli. The basic control mechanisms of HPV are made ineffective in sepsis mainly as a result of excessive NO production as well as formation of airway casts.

References

1. Marshall BE, Hanson CW, Frasch F, Marshall C (1994) Role of hypoxic pulmonary vasoconstriction in pulmonary gas exchange and blood flow distribution. 2. Pathophysiology. Intensive Care Med 20:379–389
2. Sweeney M, Yuan JX (2001) Hypoxic pulmonary vasoconstriction: role of voltage-gated potassium channels. Respir Res 1:40–48
3. Lakshminarayan S, Kowalski TF, Kirk W, Graham MM, Butler J (1990) The drainage routes of the bronchial blood flow in anesthetized dogs. Respir Physiol 82:65–73
4. Agostoni PG, Doria E, Bortone F, Antona C, Moruzzi P (1995) Systemic to pulmonary bronchial blood flow in heart failure. Chest 107:1247–1252
5. Hulme JT, Coppock EA, Felipe A, et al (1999) Oxygen sensitivity of cloned voltage-gated K(+) channels expressed in the pulmonary vasculature. Circ Res 85:489–497
6. Wang Z, Jin N, Ganguli S, et al (2001) Rho-kinase activation is involved in hypoxia-induced pulmonary vasoconstriction. Am J Respir Cell Mol Biol 25: 628–635
7. Moncada S (1999) Nitric oxide: discovery and impact on clinical medicine. JR Soc Med 92:164–169
8. Moncada S (1997) Nitric oxide in the vasculature: physiology and pathophysiology. Ann N Y Acad Sci 811:60–67
9. Furchgott RF (1999) Endothelium-derived relaxing factor: discovery, early studies, and identification as nitric oxide. Biosci Rep 19:235–251
10. Furchgott RF (1996) The 1996 Albert Lasker Medical Research Awards. The discovery of endothelium-derived relaxing factor and its importance in the identification of nitric oxide. JAMA 276:1186–1188
11. Deves R, Angelo S, Rojas AM (1998) System y+L: the broad scope and cation modulated amino acid transporter. Exp Physiol 83:211–220
12. Guo FH, Uetani K, Haque SJ, et al (1997) Interferon gamma and interleukin 4 stimulate prolonged expression of inducible nitric oxide synthase in human airway epithelium through synthesis of soluble mediators. J Clin Invest 100:829–838
13. Lundberg JO, Weitzberg E, Rinder J, et al (1996) Calcium-independent and steroid-resistant nitric oxide synthase activity in human paranasal sinus mucosa. Eur Respir J 9:1344–1347

14. Punjabi CJ, Laskin JD, Pendino KJ, et al (1994) Production of nitric oxide by rat type II pneumocytes: increased expression of inducible nitric oxide synthase following inhalation of a pulmonary irritant. Am J Respir Cell Mol Biol 11:165–172
15. Gow AJ, Stamler JS (1998) Reactions between nitric oxide and haemoglobin under physiological conditions. Nature 391:169–173
16. Fischer SR, Deyo DJ, Bone HG, et al (1997) Nitric oxide synthase inhibition restores hypoxic pulmonary vasoconstriction in sepsis. Am J Respir Crit Care Med 156:833–839
17. Soejima K, McGuire R, Snyder N, et al (2000) The effect of inducible nitric oxide synthase (iNOS) inhibition on smoke inhalation injury in sheep. Shock 13:261–266
18. Lingnau W, McGuire R, Dehring DJ, et al (1996) Change in regional hemodynamics after nitric oxide inhibition during ovine bacteremia. Am J Physiol 39:R207–R216
19. Meyer J, Lentz CW, Stothert JC, et al (1994) Effects of nitric oxide synthesis inhibition in hyperdynamic endotoxemia. Crit Care Med 22:306–312
20. Meyer J, Hinder F, Stothert J Jr, et al (1994) Increased organ blood flow in chronic endotoxemia is reversed by nitric oxide synthase inhibition. J Appl Physiol 76:2785–2793
21. Brunston RL,Jr., Zwischenberger JB, Tao W, et al (1997) Total arteriovenous CO_2 removal: simplifying extracorporeal support for respiratory failure. Ann Thorac Surg 64:1599–1604
22. Cox RA, Murakami K, Katahira J, et al (2001) Measurement of airway obstruction in sheep after smoke inhalation and burn injury. J Burn Care Rehabil 22:S127 (Abst)
23. Theissen JL, Herndon DN, Traber LD, et al (1990) Smoke inhalation and pulmonary blood flow. Prog Respir Res 26:77–84
24. Isago T, Traber LD, Herndon DN, et al (1990) Pulmonary capillary pressure changes following smoke inhalation in sheep. Anesthesiology 73:A1234 (Abst)
25. Doerschuk CM, Allard MF, Martin BA, MacKenzie A, Autor AP, Hogg JC (1987) Marginated pool of neutrophils in rabbit lungs. J Appl Physiol 63:1806–1815
26. Hogg JC, Doerschuk CM (1995) Leukocyte traffic in the lung. Annu Rev Physiol 57:97–114
27. Wiggs BR, English D, Quinlan WM, et al (1994) Contributions of capillary pathway size and neutrophil deformability to neutrophil transit through rabbit lungs. J Appl Physiol 77:463–470
28. Thommasen HV, Martin BA, Wiggs BR, Quiroga M, Baile EM, Hogg JC (1984) Effect of pulmonary blood flow on leukocyte uptake and release by dog lung. J Appl Physiol 56:966–974
29. Herndon DN, Traber DL, Traber LD (1986) The effect of resuscitation on inhalation injury. Surgery 100:248–251
30. Goldman G, Welbourn R, Kobzik L, et al (1992) Reactive oxygen species and elastase mediate lung permeability after acid aspiration. J Appl Physiol 73:571–575
31. Charan NB, Turk GM, Dhand R (1984) Gross and subgross anatomy of bronchial circulation in sheep. J Appl Physiol 57:658–664
32. Abdi S, Herndon D, Mcguire J, Traber L, Traber DL (1990) Time course of alterations in lung lymph and bronchial blood flows after inhalation injury. J Burn Care Rehabil 11:510–515
33. Koppenol WH, Moreno JJ, Pryor WA, et al (1992) Peroxynitrite, a cloaked oxidant formed by nitric oxide and superoxide. Chem Res Toxicol 5:834–842
34. Zharikov SI, Herrera H, Block ER (1997) Role of membrane potential in hypoxic inhibition of L-arginine uptake by lung endothelial cells. Am J Physiol 272:L78–L84
35. Xia Y, Dawson VL, Dawson TM, et al (1996) Nitric oxide synthase generates superoxide and nitric oxide in arginine-depleted cells leading to peroxynitrite-mediated cellular injury. Proc Natl Acad Sci USA 93:6770–6774
36. Nakayama M, Murray PA (1999) Ketamine preserves and propofol potentiates hypoxic pulmonary vasoconstriction compared with the conscious state in chronically instrumented dogs. Anesthesiology 91:760–771
37. Karzai W, Haberstroh J, Priebe HJ (1999) The effects of increasing concentrations of desflurane on systemic oxygenation during one-lung ventilation in pigs. Anesth Analg 89:215–217
38. Satoh D, Sato M, Kaise A, et al (1998) Effects of isoflurane on oxygenation during one-lung ventilation in pulmonary emphysema patients. Acta Anaesthesiol Scand 42:1145–1148
39. Sustronck B, Van Loon G, Deprez P, Muylle, Gasthuys F, Foubert L (1997) Effect of inhaled nitric oxide on the hypoxic pulmonary vasoconstrictor response in anaesthetised calves. Res Vet Sci 63:193–197

Pulmonary Endothelial Angiotensin Converting Enzyme Activity in Lung Injury

S. E. Orfanos, A. Kotanidou, and C. Roussos

▌ Introduction

The intimal lining of all blood vessels is composed of a single continuous layer of simple squamous epithelial cells of mesenchymal origin, which are called endothelial cells. In the past, vascular endothelium was mainly credited for being part of the semi-permeable barrier that separates blood from the surrounding tissues and, in the lungs, blood from air. However, extensive research performed during the last twenty-five years proved that the aforementioned 'static' endothelial feature was false, and that vascular endothelium is instead a 'dynamic' organ possessing numerous physiologic, immunologic, and metabolic functions. In the human lung, endothelial cells occupy an area with a surface of approximately 130 m² [1]. The strategic location of the lungs, and the tremendous surface area of the pulmonary capillary endothelium allows the latter to filter the entire circulating blood volume before it enters the systemic circulation. Thus, pulmonary endothelial functional and structural integrity are essential for adequate pulmonary and systemic cardiovascular homeostasis.

Pulmonary Endothelial Functions

Identification of the various pulmonary endothelial metabolic properties has been obtained using isolated perfused lung preparations, *in vivo* studies of various animal models, and endothelial cell culture techniques. It is well recognized now that the pulmonary endothelium:

- ▌ Synthesizes and releases several vasoactive compounds such as angiotensin II, prostacyclin, thromboxane, nitric oxide (NO), and endothelins;
- ▌ Expresses enzymes such as angiotensin converting enzyme (ACE), nucleotidases, NO synthase (NOS) and lipoprotein lipase;
- ▌ Expresses receptors and signal transduction molecules;
- ▌ Removes and biotransforms several drugs;
- ▌ Regulates coagulation and thrombolysis, mainly through the synthesis and release of procoagulant, anticoagulant, fibrinolytic and antithrombolytic mediators, such as von Willebrand factor (vWF), thromboplastin, thrombomodulin, and tissue plasminogen activator;
- ▌ Participates in immune reactions;
- ▌ Binds immune complexes;
- ▌ Interacts with bacteria (phagocytosis) and blood components such as leukocytes and platelets;

▌ Participates in local vasoregulation;
▌ Expresses adhesion molecules;
▌ Produces growth factors, etc. [2, 3].

Most of these functions are constitutive while others, such as the expression of adhesion molecules and/or receptors to circulating immune complexes, are induced upon endothelial exposure to endotoxin or other inflammatory stimuli [4].

Many of the above-mentioned metabolic functions depend on enzymes that metabolize, secrete or degrade vasoactive substances or other mediators. In this respect, many enzymes are located on the luminal surface area of the endothelial cells, with their catalytic sites exposed to the blood stream. These ectoenzymes interact with blood-borne substrates or inhibitors without the time and energy expenses required for interactions with cytosolic enzymes. One such enzyme is the ACE [4].

Angiotensin Converting Enzyme (ACE)

ACE is a monomeric zinc dipeptidyl carboxypeptidase also known as kininase II. ACE hydrolyzes the conversion of the decapeptide angiotensin I to the octapeptide angiotensin II, as well as the degradation of the nonapeptide bradykinin [5]. Angiotensin II is a potent vasoconstrictor; it acts on vascular smooth muscle cells, interacts with the nervous system and causes volume expansion and fluid retention. At the cellular level, angiotensin II promotes migration, proliferation, and hypertrophy. Bradykinin promotes vasodilation mainly through production of NO, arachidonic acid products and endothelium-derived hyperpolarizing factor. ACE appears thus to regulate the balance between the vasodilatory properties of bradykinin and the vasoconstrictive properties of angiotensin II, promoting vascular tone and acting as a regulator between the renin-angiotensin and the kallikrein-kinin systems. ACE is widely distributed as both a membrane-bound and as a soluble ectoenzyme. The former is mainly found on endothelial cells, the surface of absorptive epithelia (intestinal and renal), and in the central nervous system (CNS) [6]. ACE molecules are uniformly distributed throughout the endothelial plasma membrane, including the membrane caveolae [7]. Due to the tremendous capillary surface and high enzyme concentrations, the pulmonary vasculature appears to be the major site of ACE activity in the body [6].

▌ Assessment of Pulmonary Endothelium-bound ACE Activity, *in vivo*

During the last twenty years, increasing attention has been focused on the monitoring of pulmonary capillary endothelial ectoenzyme activity in several animal models *in vivo* and *in situ* [8]. The pulmonary capillary bed provides an ideal environment for the function of these enzymes because it offers very high enzyme concentrations resulting from the combination of low plasma volume and high surface area (i.e., high enzyme mass available for reaction). Additionally, it accepts the highest possible substrate delivery, since 100% of the cardiac output passes through the lungs. The demonstration that ACE is uniformly distributed along the luminal pulmonary endothelial surface, raised the possibility that in addition to its biological activity, this enzyme may be a useful indicator of endothelial functional integrity and, under physiologic conditions, an indirect but quantifiable measure of the perfused pulmonary vascular bed [6, 9]. As described below, we and others have provided evidence in support of both possibilities, originally in animals, and, more recently, in humans.

Indicator-dilution Technique

The most common assay to estimate *in vivo* the activity of pulmonary endothelium-bound ACE (and/or other ectoenzymes), is a modification of the indicator-dilution technique, originally introduced for cardiac output estimations. Briefly, trace amounts of a radio-labeled substrate are injected as a rapid bolus into a central vein. Simultaneously, arterial blood is withdrawn by means of a peristaltic pump into a fraction collector, for the duration of a single transpulmonary passage. Blood is collected into tubes containing 'stop' solution, to prevent further activity of plasma soluble ACE (sACE). Blood samples are then collected and the amount of radioactivity associated with both the substrate that survived the single transpulmonary passage and the formed product is quantified in each sample [4, 6]. This technique allows estimations of very rapid interactions between substrate and the endothelium-bound enzyme, thus minimizing the contribution of sACE. In addition, capillaries with a diameter of < 20 µm (i.e., alveolar capillaries) appear to be responsible for the great majority of the product formed, due to the very high local enzyme concentration. Thus in this type of study, measurement of pulmonary ACE activity represents, in practical terms, pulmonary capillary endothelium-bound (PCEB) ACE activity [6].

ACE Synthetic Substrates

In the mid-1970s, synthetic radio-labeled substrates highly specific for ACE substrates were introduced by J.W. Ryan [10]. Contrary to the natural ACE substrates, angiotensin I and bradykinin, which are also substrates for other naturally occurring enzymes, these synthetic substrates could be quantified easily and rapidly. Furthermore, they were sufficiently reactive to allow measurable hydrolysis during a single transpulmonary passage *in vivo*. The first, and more widely used to date, synthetic substrate is benzoyl-Phe-Ala-Pro (BPAP). ACE hydrolyzes BPAP to benzoyl-Phe (Bphe). BPAP is pharmacologically inactive, water soluble and readily excreted in the urine. Other synthetic ACE substrates include benzoyl-Ala-Gly-Pro (BAGP), benzoyl-Phe-Gly-Pro (BPGP) and benzoyl-Phe-His-Leu (BPHL). There is a wide range of reactivity (k_{cat}/K_m) among them, with BPAP being more reactive [10].

∎ Calculations of ACE Activity Parameters

When trace amounts of ^{3}H-BPAP are injected, substrate hydrolysis (v) proceeds under first-order reaction conditions. BPAP transpulmonary hydrolysis is then measured by applying the integrated Henri-Michaelis-Menten equation [11], as proposed by Ryan and Catravas [9], and corrected for a 7% non-reactive fraction (nrf = 0.07) of BPAP (*cis* isomer), as proposed by Cziraki et al [12]:

$$v = \ln\{(1 - nrf)/(([S]/[S_o]) - nrf)\} = [E] \times t_c \times k_{cat}/K_m \qquad \text{(Eqn 1)}$$

with [E], t_c, k_{cat} and K_m being the capillary enzyme concentration, reaction time (capillary mean transit time), catalytic rate constant, and Michaelis-Menten constant respectively [11]. [S_o] and [S] reflect the initial and final substrate concentrations in the effluent arterial plasma estimated in dpm/mL, where [S_o] is [^{3}H-BPAP] +[^{3}H-BPhe] and [S] is the surviving substrate concentration, i.e., [^{3}H-BPAP].

3H-BPAP utilization may also be calculated as percent transpulmonary metabolism (%M), also corrected for the *cis* BPAP nonreactive fraction:

$$\%M = 100 \times \{([S_o] - [S])/([S_o] \times (1 - nrf))\} \qquad \text{(Eqn 2)}$$

Both v and %M are reflections of ACE activity per capillary. While v has the advantage of being directly proportional to all three factors that determine product formation (see equation 1), percent substrate metabolism is a term that investigators are more familiar with.

The obtained data may be further analyzed, utilizing the integrated Henri-Michaelis-Menten equation as modified by Catravas and White [13]:

$$A_{max}/K_m = E \times k_{cat}/K_m = F_p \times v \qquad \text{(Eqn 3)}$$

$$\text{where } A_{max} = E \times k_{cat} = V_{max} \times Q_{cap} \qquad \text{(Eqn 4)}$$

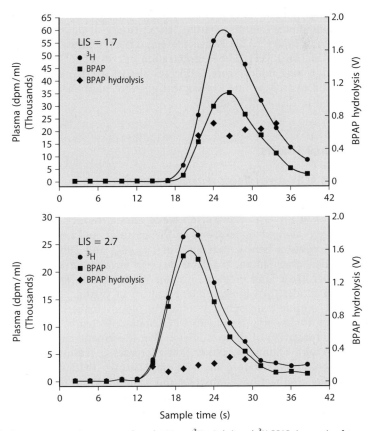

Fig. 1. Effluent arterial plasma concentration curves of total tritium (^{3}H, *circles*) and ^{3}H-BPAP (*squares*), of two critically ill, mechanically ventilated subjects suffering from mild (*top*) and severe lung injury (*bottom*). BPAP hydrolysis (v, diamonds) was estimated from samples where total radioactivity dpm > 10 × background-dpm. (From [15] with permission). LIS: lung injury score.

with E, F_p, V_{max}, and Q_{cap} being total enzyme mass, pulmonary plasma flow, maximal velocity and capillary plasma volume, respectively.

A_{max}/K_m reflects ACE activity per vascular bed. Under physiological (normal) conditions, as long as the catalytic properties of the enzyme remain unchanged, A_{max}/K_m is an index of PCEB-ACE mass (equation 3) and, for ACE that is evenly distributed along the luminal endothelial surface, an index of dynamically perfused (i.e., accessible to substrate) capillary surface area (DPCSA). Under toxic conditions, when alterations of enzyme expression and/or kinetic constants may exist, A_{max}/K_m should be viewed as an index of functional capillary surface area (FCSA) related to the enzyme mass available for reaction (the product of DPCSA and the enzyme mass expressed on the endothelial surface) and the enzyme kinetic constants.

The aforementioned equations apply for any other synthetic ACE substrate, provided that first order-reaction conditions exist (i.e., substrate concentrations $\ll K_m$). (For more detailed information the reader is referred to [14]),

These techniques have been extensively used in various animal models. More recently we introduced similar techniques in humans [14, 15]. Representative arterial outflow concentration curves of total ^3H (i.e., initial BPAP concentrations) and the surviving ^3H-BPAP after a single passage through the lungs, and the corresponding transpulmonary hydrolysis from two critically-ill patients with various degrees of acute lung injury (ALI) and acute respiratory distress syndrome (ARDS) are presented in Fig. 1 [15]. The concentration curves of ^3H and ^3H-BPAP in the patient with high lung injury score (LIS) [16] almost overlap each other denoting minimal substrate hydrolysis and consequently severe pulmonary capillary endothelial dysfunction in this ARDS patient.

▌ Animal Studies

PCEB ACE Activity under Normal Conditions

In vivo assays under normal physiologic conditions have established the normal range of PCEB ACE activity in several animal models. More importantly however, they have allowed estimations of the perfused pulmonary capillary vascular bed. The correlation between changes in A_{max}/K_m and DPCSA has been demonstrated in rabbits, dogs, guinea pigs and sheep *in vivo*, under both anesthesia and exercise, and in isolated lung preparations [6]. When rabbits were placed on total heart bypass, a model that allows precise control of cardiac output [17, 18], increases in cardiac output from sub-physiologic to approximately 2.5-fold the normal values, resulted in similar increases in DPCSA, as reflected by A_{max}/K_m. A prerequisite for the interpretation of these studies is that the kinetic constants of PCEB ACE do not change with pulmonary blood flow increases (equation 3). We have provided evidence that this is indeed the case, at least over the aforementioned cardiac output range, by co-injecting a substrate and an inhibitor at different blood flows and obtaining unchanged catalytic and binding ACE properties [4, 17]. In all these studies, transpulmonary hydrolysis of all substrates used was independent of cardiac output implying that higher pulmonary blood volumes are accommodated mainly through parallel recruitment of capillaries with similar enzyme concentrations and capillary transit times [4, 17, 18]. When pulmonary blood flow was increased beyond full recruitment, no additional changes in A_{max}/K_m were observed, while sub-

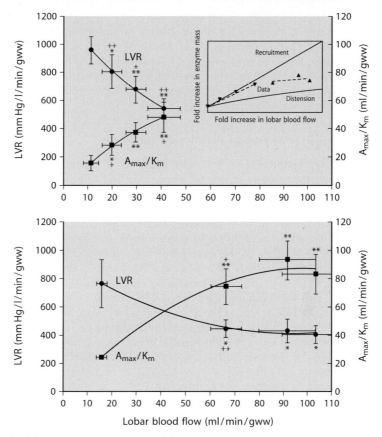

Fig. 2. Effect of lobar blood flow on A_{max}/K_m (*squares*) and lobar vascular resistance (LVR, *circles*) under partial (*top*) and full capillary recruitment (*bottom*). Values are normalized per wet tissue weight. Values are means ± SEM. *$p < 0.05$, **$p < 0.01$ from the initial determination with ANOVA and Dunnet's test; +$p < 0.05$, ++$p < 0.01$ from the previous determination with ANOVA and Newman-Keuls' multiple range test. In the figure insert, a model for the theoretical relationships between blood flow and perfused surface area under recruitment or distension is presented along with the obtained data. Inverted triangles represent data from partially recruited lobes; triangles represent data from fully recruited lobes. (Modified from [19] with permission)

strate hydrolysis decreased mainly due to decreased transit times through the fully recruited capillary bed [4, 18].

A similar situation was more recently demonstrated in isolated dog lungs, where lobar blood flow elevations from normal values to approximately 3.5-fold caused a proportional and parallel increase in A_{max}/K_m and an inversely proportional decrease in lobe vascular resistance (LVR), indicative of increasing perfused vascular bed (Fig. 2, top) [19]. When blood flow was increased to >4-fold the normal, both parameters reached their maximal and minimal values respectively, suggesting that the perfused vascular bed was not further increased, thus confirming the validity of A_{max}/K_m as a DPCSA index (Fig. 2, bottom) [19]. Similar results were obtained by Dupuis et al. [20–22] who studied PCEB ACE activity as well as pulmonary norepinephrine and serotonin uptake during exercise in dogs.

The higher A_{max}/K_m values observed with increasing blood flows could result from either recruitment of non-perfused capillaries or distension of already perfused vessels or a combination of both. When the data obtained were compared with a model for the theoretical relationships between blood flow and perfused surface area under the two extreme conditions, it appears that recruitment of capillaries accounts for most of the increase in DPCSA, while distension occurs mainly near or after full recruitment (Fig. 2, insert).

PCEB ACE Activity under Pathological Conditions

Pulmonary endothelial injury may begin as a subtle metabolic dysfunction and then progress to overt structural alterations and cell death. Numerous studies performed over the last fifteen years have shown that reduction in PCEB ACE activity is among the earliest signs of lung injury, preceding changes in all commonly measured parameters such as acid-base balance, gas exchange, hemodynamic parameters, increased permeability, and morphologic changes at the light and electron-microscopy level. This is the case following administration of bleomycin to rabbits [23], exposure of rabbits to hyperoxia [24], phorbol-ester administration to rabbits and dogs [25, 26], and chest-irradiation in rabbits [27, 28]. PCEB-ACE activity reduction also occurs in an animal model of chronic familiar hyperlipidemia [29].

Assessing PCEB ACE activity in lung injury may help distinguish between abnormalities secondary to endothelial dysfunction *per se* and decreased pulmonary vascular surface area. If endothelial dysfunction is related to either decreased enzyme mass or kinetic constant alterations, then substrate hydrolysis would be altered (equation 1). In such a case, A_{max}/K_m is an index of FCSA, related to both enzyme quantity and functional integrity. If loss of DPCSA occurs with neither endothelial dysfunction nor changes in capillary transit times, substrate hydrolysis would not change, while A_{max}/K_m would decrease, since the enzyme mass available for reaction would be decreased (equation 3). In this respect, acid-base imbalance [30] and changes in alveolar pressure [31] affect PCEB ACE indirectly through changes in DPCSA. Similarly, indomethacin administration appears to protect against PMA-induced PCEB ACE dysfunction by diverting flow to 'healthier' capillaries [25].

▌ Human Studies

PCEB ACE Activity in the Normal Lung

We have recently validated the PCEB ACE activity indicator-dilution technique at the bedside with humans who had no lung disease, and correlated it with pulmonary hemodynamics, in order to identify patterns of enzyme activity under normal lung conditions [14]. These patients received two rapid bolus injections of BPAP through a pulmonary artery catheter: one into the vascular bed of both lungs, the other into the vascular bed of one lung (the right lung in all but one patient). Similar transpulmonary substrate hydrolysis and percentage metabolism were observed in one and both lungs, suggesting homogeneous PCEB ACE concentrations and capillary transit times in both human lungs. As in the animals, BPAP hydrolysis and percentage metabolism were independent of cardiac index (CI), consistent with similar t_c among individuals within the normal range of pulmonary blood flow at rest. A_{max}/K_m in the right lung was 54% of total A_{max}/K_m in both lungs, suggesting that A_{max}/K_m is a reliable and quantifiable index of DPCSA in humans. Repeated PCEB ACE activity determinations performed in brain-dead subjects with LIS=0, at different cardiac outputs in each subject, showed unchanged substrate hydrolysis over a wide range of cardiac output, whereas A_{max}/K_m increased linearly with flow [32]. This pattern is similar to that observed in animal studies and further confirms the validity of A_{max}/K_m as a DPCSA index.

PCEB ACE Activity in ALI

Pulmonary endothelium is severely affected in ALI/ARDS, and a number of endothelium related indices are altered during the disease process [33]. We assessed PCEB ACE activity in 33 critically-ill, mechanically ventilated patients belonging to high-risk groups for ARDS development, and suffering from various degrees of ALI/ARDS, with lung injury scores (LIS) ranging from 0 to 3.7 [15]. Both BPAP transpulmonary hydrolysis and A_{max}/K_m decreased early during the ALI/ARDS con-

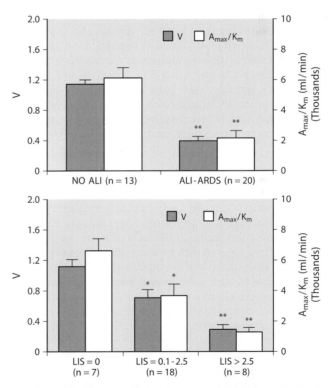

Fig. 3. *Top.* BPAP hydrolysis (v) and A_{max}/K_m in 33 critically ill patients belonging to high risk groups for development of ARDS, divided into those who have no acute lung injury (NoALI) and those with ALI/ARDS according to the American-European Consensus Criteria [36]. Values are mean±SEM. **p<0.01, with Student's t-test. *Bottom.* BPAP hydrolysis (v) and A_{max}/K_m in the same patients divided according to Murray et al [16] as having: no lung injury (lung injury score (LIS)=0), mild-to-moderate lung injury (LIS=0.1–2.5) and severe lung injury (LIS>2.5), *p<0.05, **p<0.01, from LIS=0 with ANOVA and Newman-Keuls' test. (From [15] with permission)

tinuum (Fig. 3) and were inversely related to APACHE II score and LIS. Contrary to the observations made in animals and humans with normal/healthy lungs, substrate hydrolysis decreased with increasing cardiac output, suggesting decreasing t_c at higher cardiac output, probably because of vascular loss occurring from occluded or obliterated vessels.

A_{max}/K_m increased with higher cardiac output in healthier survivors, while no increases occurred in the more severely ill, implying that in the latter higher blood volumes should be accommodated mainly through dysfunctional capillaries, whereas no FCSA reserves are available to be recruited. The fact that in our population high A_{max}/K_m values are associated with better survival raises the interesting possibility that this kinetic parameter might be of value as an outcome predictor in ARDS [15].

PCEB ACE Activity in Systemic Vascular Disease

In order to establish the validity of the PCEB ACE activity indicator-dilution technique in subjects with systemic vascular diseases, we studied patients suffering from systemic sclerosis, an autoimmune multisystem disease with known endothelial dysfunction [34]. The presence of early pulmonary endothelial dysfunction in systemic sclerosis patients has been demonstrated on lung biopsies [35]. Two subsets of disease can be identified: diffuse and the limited systemic sclerosis subset. PCEB ACE activity was found decreased at an early disease stage (absence of pulmonary hypertension or pulmonary interstitial fibrosis) in both subsets, while it appeared to be mostly related to subset (lower in diffuse systemic sclerosis) and pulmonary hemodynamic parameters [34]. We feel that the PCEB ACE activity indicator-dilution technique offers a means of detecting early pulmonary endothelial dysfunction that is less invasive than lung biopsy, and might ultimately assist the clinician in initiating early treatment and monitoring its results.

∎ Conclusion

The pulmonary vascular endothelium participates in various important physiologic and pharmacokinetic processes, essential for the maintenance of cardiovascular homeostasis. Assessing PCEB ACE activity by means of indicator dilution techniques offers accurate information on pulmonary endothelial function and pulmonary metabolism in health and disease. This procedure is relatively simple, highly reproducible in both animals and humans, and can be safely applied at the bedside. Analysis of the obtained data in humans with pulmonary vascular pathologies may help distinguish between enzyme dysfunction (i.e., endothelial cell dysfunction *per se*) and decreased perfused capillary bed. The fact that dynamically perfused capillary surface area increases during exercise in animals raises the intriguing possibility that a failure to increase DPCSA during exercise in humans might prove to be an early marker of subtle pulmonary vascular disease. Future studies should also determine the utility of this method in predicting either the onset or the outcome from pathologies such as ALI and ARDS.

References

1. Simionescu M (1991) Lung endothelium: Structure-function correlates. In: Crystal RG, West JB (eds) The Lung: Scientific Foundations. Raven Press, New York, pp 301–312
2. Hassoun PM, Fanburg BL, Junod AF (1991) Metabolic functions. In: Crystal RG, West JB (eds) The Lung: Scientific Foundations Raven Press, New York, pp 313–327
3. West JB (2001) Pulmonary embolism. In: West JB (ed) Pulmonary Physiology and Pathophysiology: An Integrated, Case-Based Approach. Lippincott Williams & Wilkins, New York, pp 84–99
4. Orfanos SE, Catravas JD (1993) Metabolic functions of the pulmonary endothelium. In: Yacoub M, Pepper J (eds) Annual Review of Cardiac Surgery, 6th edn. Current Science, London, pp 52–59
5. Ryan JW, Ryan US (1982) Processing of endogenous polypeptides by the lung. Annu Rev Physiol 44:241–255
6. Catravas JD, Orfanos SE (1997) Pathophysiologic functions of endothelial angiotensin-converting enzyme. In: Born GVR, Schwartz CJ (eds) Vascular Endothelium: Physiology, Pathology and Therapeutic Opportunities. Schattauer, Stuttgart, pp 193–204
7. Ryan US, Ryan JW, Whitaker C, Chiu A (1976) Localization of angiotensin-converting enzyme (kinase II). Immunocytochemistry and immunofluorescence. Tissue Cell 8:125–146
8. Pitt BR, Lister G, Gillis CN (1987) Hemodynamic effects on lung metabolic function. In: Ryan US (ed) Pulmonary Endothelium in Health and Disease. Marcel Dekker, New York, pp 65–87
9. Ryan JW, Catravas JD (1991) Angiotensin converting-enzyme as an indicator of pulmonary microvascular function In: Hollinger MA (ed) Focus on Pulmonary Pharmacology & Toxicology. CRC Press, Boca Raton, pp 183–210
10. Ryan JW (1987) Assay of pulmonary endothelial surface enzymes in vivo. In: Ryan US (ed) Pulmonary Endothelium in Health and Disease. Marcel Dekker, New York USA, pp 161-188
11. Segel IH (1975) Enzyme Kinetics. Wiley, New York
12. Cziraki A, Ryan JW, Horvarth I, Fisher LE, Parkerson JB, Catravas JD (1995) Comparison of the hydrolyses of 2 synthetic ACE substrates by rabbit lung in vivo. FASEB J 9:A719 (Abst)
13. Catravas JD, White RE (1984) Kinetics of pulmonary angiotensin-converting enzyme and 5′-nucleotidase in vivo. J Appl Physiol 57:1173–1181
14. Orfanos SE, Langleben D, Khoury J, et al (1999) Pulmonary capillary endothelium-bound angiotensin-converting enzyme activity in humans. Circulation 99:1593–1599
15. Orfanos SE, Armaganidis A, Glynos C, et al (2000) Pulmonary capillary endothelium-bound angiotensin converting enzyme activity in acute lung injury. Circulation 102:2011–2018
16. Murray JF, Matthay MA, Luce JM, Flick MR (1988) An expanded definition of the adult respiratory distress syndrome. Am Rev Respir Dis 138:720–723
17. Orfanos SE, Chen XL, Ryan JW, Chung AYK, Burch SE, Catravas JD (1994). Assay of pulmonary microvascular endothelial angiotensin-converting enzyme in vivo: comparison of three probes. Toxicol Appl Pharmacol 124:99–111
18. Toivonen HJ, Catravas JD (1991) Effects of blood flow on lung ACE kinetics: Evidence for microvascular recruitment. J Appl Physiol 71:2244–2254
19. Orfanos SE, Ehrhart IC, Barman S, Hofman WF, Catravas JD (1997) Endothelial ectoenzyme assays estimate perfused capillary surface area in the dog lung. Microvasc Res 54:145–155
20. Dupuis J, Goresky CA, Ryan JW, Rouleau JL, Bach GG (1992) Pulmonary angiotensin-converting enzyme substrate hydrolysis during exercise. J Appl Physiol 72:1868–1886
21. Dupuis J, Goresky CA, Junear C (1990) Use of norepinephrine uptake to measure lung capillary recruitment with exercise. J Appl Physiol 68:700–713
22. Dupuis J, Goresky CA, Rouleau JL, Simard A, Schwab AJ (1996) Kinetics of pulmonary uptake of serotonin during exercise in the dog. J Appl Physiol 80:30–46
23. Lazo JS, Catravas JD, Gillis CN (1981) Reduction in rabbit serum and pulmonary angiotensin converting enzyme after subacute bleomycin treatment Biochem Pharmacol 30:2577–2584

24. Dobuler KJ, Catravas JD, Gillis CN (1982) Early detection of oxygen-induced lung injury in conscious rabbits: reduced in vivo activity of angiotensin converting enzyme and removal of 5-hydoxytryptamine Am Rev Respir Dis 126:534–539

25. Chen XL, Orfanos SE, Catravas JD (1992) Effects of indomethacin on PMA-induced pulmonary endothelial enzyme dysfunction, in vivo. Am J Physiol 262:L153–L162

26. Ehrhart IC, Orfanos SE, McCloud LL, Sickles DW, Hoffman WF, Catravas JD (1999) Vascular recruitment increases evidence of lung injury. Crit Care Med 27:120–129

27. Orfanos SE, Chen XL, Burch SE, Ryan JW, Chunk AYK, Catravas JD (1994) Radiation-induced early pulmonary endothelial ectoenzyme dysfunction in vivo: effect of indomethacin. Toxicol Appl Pharmacol 124:112–122

28. Catravas JD, Burch SE, Sprulock BO, Mills LR (1988) Early effects of ionising radiation on pulmonary endothelial angiotensin converting enzyme and 5'-nucleotidase, in vivo. Toxicol Appl Pharamacol 94:342–355

29. Orfanos SE, Parkerson JB, Chen XL, et al (2000) Reduced lung endothelial angiotensin-converting enzyme activity in Watanabe hyperlipidemic rabbits *in vivo*. Am J Physiol 278: L1280–L1288

30. Toivonen HJ, Catravas JD (1987) Effects of acid-base imbalance on pulmonary angiotensin-converting enzyme, in vivo. J Appl Physiol 63:1629–1637

31. Toivonen HJ, Catravas JD (1986) Effects of alveolar pressure on lung angiotensin-converting enzyme, in vivo. J Appl Physiol 61:1041–1050

32. Orfanos SE, Langleben D, Armaganidis A, et al (1998) Patterns of an angiotensin-converting enzyme substrate hydrolysis by PCEB-ACE in critically-ill patients. In: Catravas JD, Callow AD, Ryan US (eds) Vascular Endothelium Pharmacologic and Genetic Manipulations. Plenum Press, New York, pp 269–271

33. Pittet JF, Mackersie RC, Martin TR, Matthay MA (1997) Biological markers of acute lung injury: prognostic and pathogenic significance. Am J Respir Crit Care Med 155:1187–1205

34. Orfanos SE, Psevdi E, Stratigis N, et al (2001) Pulmonary capillary endothelial dysfunction in early systemic sclerosis. Arthritis Rheum 44:902–911

35. Harisson NK, Myers AR, Corrin B, et al (1991) Structural features of interstitial lung disease in systemic sclerosis. Am Rev Respir Dis 144:706–713

36. Bernard GR, Artigas A, Brigham KL, et al, and the Consensus Committee (1994) The American-European consensus conference on ARDS: definitions, mechanisms, relevant outcomes, and clinical trial coordination. Am J Respir Crit Care Med 49:818–824

Modulating Host Response

Antioxidants and Endothelial Function: Therapeutic Implications

B. A. Mullan and B. V. McCloskey

▌ Introduction

Endothelial function may be impaired in critically ill patients [1]. The endothelium actively regulates vascular tone, platelet aggregation, coagulation, fibrinolysis, and leukocyte activation [2]. Endothelial dysfunction may, therefore, be important in the pathophysiology of some of the conditions encountered in the intensive care unit (ICU).

Critically ill patients may also display oxidative stress [3]. This is a disturbance in the prooxidant-antioxidant balance due to either increased free radical genera-tion or reduced antioxidant defenses or a combination of the two. Tissue damage, whether from trauma, ischemia or infection, can generate reactive oxygen species (ROS) via a number of mechanisms. The redistribution and increased utilization of different antioxidants during critical illness will compromise plasma total antioxi-dant status [4]. Poor nutritional state prior to illness, or inadequate supplementa-tion during illness, will also reduce tissue antioxidant defenses.

Oxidative stress may contribute to the etiology of endothelial dysfunction [5]. Antioxidants have been reported to improve endothelial function in a number of conditions, such as atherosclerosis, hypertension, diabetes, and dyslipidemia [6]. The therapeutic role for antioxidants in critical care medicine is controversial [7]. However this may relate in part to antioxidant therapy being initiated after the es-tablishment of overt organ failure. There is limited research on the use of antioxi-dants as prophylaxis against endothelial dysfunction. If endothelial dysfunction can be targeted at an early stage, then perhaps progression to organ failure could be prevented, or at least attenuated. This chapter will discuss the beneficial effects of anti-oxidants on the endothelium. It will also suggest that future research should be directed at the early use of antioxidants in the ICU.

▌ Endothelial Physiology

The vascular endothelium is a monolayer of cells between the vessel lumen and the vascular smooth muscle. Far from being inert, it is metabolically active, and should be thought of as a complex endocrine and paracrine organ. Various endothelial-de-rived mediators help to regulate vascular homeostasis (Table 1).

Endothelial dysfunction commonly affects nitric oxide (NO) bioactivity. NO has a number of important biological functions. It is a potent vasodilator [8]. The bal-ance between NO, various endothelial-derived vasoconstrictors, and the sympa-thetic nervous system, modulates blood vessel tone. Changes in this balance affect

Table 1. Regulatory functions of the vascular endothelium

Function	Mediators
▌ **Platelet aggregation**	Prostacyclin (−) Nitric oxide (−)
▌ **Coagulation**	Von Willebrand factor (+) Thrombomodulin (−) Heparin-like proteoglycans (−)
▌ **Fibrinolysis**	Tissue plasminogen activator (+) Urokinase (+) Plasminogen activator inhibitor-1 (−)
▌ **Vascular smooth muscle tone**	Prostacyclin (−) Nitric oxide (−) Endothelium-derived hyperpolarising factor (−) Endothelin (+)
▌ **Vascular smooth muscle proliferation**	Nitric oxide (−) Transforming growth factor β (−) Platelet-derived growth factor (+)
▌ **Leukocyte adhesion**	Nitric oxide (−) E-selection (+) Intercellular adhesion molecule-1 (+) Vascular cell adhesion molecule-1 (+)

+, stimulates or increases; −, inhibits or decreases

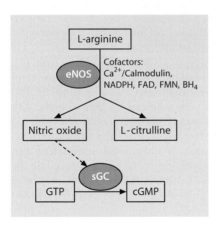

Fig. 1. The endothelial L-arginine nitric oxide (NO) pathway. Endothelial NO synthase (eNOS) catalyzes the conversion of L-arginine to NO and L-citrulline. NO then stimulates soluble guanylate cyclase (sGC) to convert guanylate triphosphate (GTP) to cyclic guanosine-3′,5-monophosphate (cGMP). NADPH, nicotinamide adenine dinucleotide phosphate; FAD, flavin adenine dinucleotide, FMN, flavin mononucleotide; BH_4, tetrahydrobiopterin

peripheral vascular resistance and hence blood pressure [6]. In addition, endothelial NO may be important in the functional regulation of large artery stiffness [9]. Alteration in the stiffness of major arteries, such as the aorta, affects the velocity and amplitude of pulse waves reflected from the peripheral circulation back to the heart [10]. Increased peripheral pulse wave reflection leads to augmentation of central aortic systolic blood pressure [11]. Changes in large artery stiffness may therefore affect central aortic hemodynamics and left ventricular function [9]. Other endothelial NO-mediated biological effects include control of endothelial permeability, inhibition of platelet aggregation, inhibition of vascular smooth muscle cell proliferation, and inhibition of leukocyte adhesion to the endothelium [8].

Endothelial-derived NO is synthesized from the amino acid L-arginine by the endothelial isoform of NO synthase, eNOS (Fig. 1). Several co-factors are required for NO biosynthesis. These include nicotinamide adenine dinucleotide phosphate (NADPH), flavin mononucleotide (FMN), flavin adenine dinucleotide (FAD), tetrahydrobiopterin (BH$_4$), and calmodulin. Once synthesized, the NO diffuses across the endothelial cell membrane and enters the vascular smooth muscle cells where it activates soluble guanylate cyclase (sGC), leading to an increase in intracellular cyclic guanosine-3′,5-monophosphate (cGMP) [8]. cGMP mediates many of the biological effects of NO including the control of vascular tone and platelet function. NO also interacts with heme, DNA and thiols, to alter the function of other key enzymes and ion channels.

▌ Oxidative Stress and Endothelial Dysfunction

Free radicals are atoms or molecules possessing a free umpaired electron. They may be formed by three methods: the loss of a single electron from a nonradical molecule; the addition of a single electron to a nonradical molecule; or the homolytic cleavage of the cofalent bond of a nonradical molecule so that each fragment retains one of the electrons [12]. Examples of free radicals include the hydroxyl radical (OH$^-$) and the superoxide radical (O$_2^-$). Their electron imbalance renders them highly reactive and unstable.

Oxidative stress may arise from a number of sources. In aerobic cells, incomplete reduction of oxygen in the mitochondrial electron transport chain can release superoxide into the cytosol. Neutrophil activation during inflammation will produce a variety of free radicals, which may damage innocent bystander cells as well as intended micro-organisms. Drugs can exert toxic effects if free radical formation occurs during their metabolism, e.g., the hepatotoxicity associated with paracetamol. Finally xanthine oxidase (XO) is capable of generating superoxide during the reperfusion of ischemic tissues.

Free radicals can damage endothelial cells by attacking their lipid membranes, protein, or DNA. They can also degrade endothelial-derived NO, thereby reducing its bioactivity [13]. In addition, oxidative stress may lead to the depletion of the eNOS cofactors NADPH and BH$_4$. Deficiency of BH$_4$ can uncouple oxygen reduction and L-arginine oxidation by eNOS, and lead to the generation of superoxide anions [14]. Studies on isolated canine coronary arteries have shown that BH$_4$ depletion will result in eNOS producing excessive amounts of free radicals [15]. Oxidative stress may also increase the oxidation of low density lipoprotein particles (LDL). Oxidized LDL is directly toxic to endothelial cells and can impair endothelial function [16]. Recent research has suggested that, as well as producing free radicals, the inflammatory cascade may also be stimulated by them. Nuclear factor kappa B (NF-κB) is a ubiquitous rapid response transcription factor involved in the inflammatory activation of endothelial cells [17]. ROS have been shown to increase NF-κB activation [18]. Further inflammatory stimulation of the endothelium by NF-κB will potentiate endothelial dysfunction. Finally, increasing evidence suggests that oxidative stress may regulate endothelial cell apoptosis, i.e., programmed cell death. Free radicals, such as the hydroxyl radical, can induce endothelial cell apoptosis [19]. Thus, the enhancement of apoptosis may be another mechanism whereby oxidative stress can contribute to endothelial dysfunction.

▌ Antioxidants

Antioxidants are substances whose presence in relatively low concentrations can significantly inhibit the rate of oxidation. Natural antioxidants can be classified as enzymatic and non-enzymatic. The enzymatic antioxidants are superoxide dismutase (SOD), catalase and glutathione peroxidase (GPX). A number of trace elements are necessary cofactors for these enzymes (e.g., selenium for GPX, zinc for cytosolic SOD, and manganese for mitochondrial SOD).

The non-enzymatic antioxidants can be subdivided into scavengers and transition metal chelators. Scavenging antioxidants react with free radicals to prevent tissue damage. In scavenging free radicals, these molecules are themselves oxidized. The scavenging antioxidants may be water-soluble (ascorbate, glutathione, urate) or lipid-soluble (a-tocopherol, carotenoids).

a-tocopherol (vitamin E) is the principle antioxidant in the lipid phase of cell membranes. Glutathione, a tripeptide containing a sulfhydryl group, is present in millimolar concentrations intracellularly and acts as both a substrate for glutathione peroxidase and as a direct scavenger of radicals and their metabolites. Ascorbate (vitamin C) is the most effective aqueous phase antioxidant in human plasma. It readily scavenges superoxide, peroxyl and hydroxyl radicals. Ascorbate can also act as a co-antioxidant by regenerating a-tocopherol from the a-tocopheroxyl radical, produced via scavenging of lipid-soluble radicals. This is a potentially important function as *in vitro* experiments have shown that a-tocopherol can act as a pro-oxidant in the absence of co-antioxidants such as ascorbate [20]. Ascorbate has also been shown to regenerate urate, glutathione, and β-carotene *in vitro* from their respective one-electron products [21].

Other potential non-endogenous antioxidants include the XO inhibitors and the lazaroids. XO has been implicated in superoxide formation during the reperfusion of ischemic tissues. There is some experimental evidence to show that allopurinol, a XO inhibitor, can act as an antioxidant in this situation [22]. The lazaroids are 21-aminosteroids which inhibit iron-dependent lipid peroxidation. Their clinical antioxidant role remains uncertain.

▌ Assessment of Endothelial Dysfunction

Endothelial function cannot be measured directly in the clinical setting. Estimates of different types of endothelial dysfunction may be obtained indirectly by measuring endothelium-dependent vasodilatation (i.e., post-ischemic flow-mediated dilatation of the brachial artery, reactive hyperemia of forearm resistance vessels, or direct intra-arterial infusion of endothelial agonists), plasma levels of endothelium-derived regulatory proteins, and microalbuminuria (Table 2).

These markers of endothelial dysfunction have been described in a number of conditions associated with endothelial injury, such as atherosclerosis, pre-eclampsia, vasculitis, hypertension, smoking, and diabetes [23]. The alteration in these markers observed during critical illness may signifiy damage to the endothelium. There is some clinical evidence, from a limited number of studies, to suggest that these indirect markers of endothelial dysfunction may be prognostic for outcome. In one small study on elective aortic surgery, urine albumin excretion four hours after the start of the operation predicted those patients who developed pulmonary

Table 2. Indirect markers of endothelial dysfunction

Marker	Interpretation
▌ Impaired endothelial-dependent vasodilatation	Decreased bioactivity of endothelial-derived vasodilators, e.g., nitric oxide
▌ Von Willebrand factor	Increased thrombotic activity
▌ Plasminogen activator inhibitor-1	Decreased fibrinolytic activity
▌ sE-selectin, sICAM-1, sVCAM-1	Increased leukocyte adhesion to endothelium
▌ Microalbuminuria	Increased endothelial permeability

ICAM: Intercellular adhesion molecule; *VCAM*: Vascular cell adhesion molecule

dysfunction 24 hours later [24]. Microalbuminuria has also been reported to be predictive of complications in acute pancreatitis [25]. In another study in trauma patients, the magnitude of microalbuminuria correlated with the extent of injury [26]. However, it was not sensitive enough to predict outcome. Dysregulation of endothelial-derived products, such as plasminogen activator inhibitor-1 (PAI-1) and soluble cell adhesion molecules, are consistent findings in critical illness and are likely to be important in the pathophysiology of organ dysfunction [27, 28]. A recent study described an association between impaired endothelial-dependent vasodilatation and myocardial perfusion defects [29]. Endothelial dysfunction may therefore pedict those patients at risk of myocardial ischemia.

▌ Anti-oxidant Therapy

There are numerous mechanisms whereby antioxidants may improve endothelial dysfunction. There may be direct beneficial effects on the endothelium or indirect actions in modifying the systemic inflammatory response. Potentially, the biological activity of endothelial-derived NO could be preserved by therapies which:
- ▌ prevent excessive free radical degradation of NO,
- ▌ increase the activity of eNOS (either via modification of the intracellular redox state, or via BH_4),
- ▌ prevent the oxidation of LDL particles,
- ▌ increase target site sensitivity of NO,
- ▌ decrease endothelial cell inflammatory activation,
- ▌ prevent endothelial cell apoptosis.

Anti-oxidants may improve endothelial function by some or all of these mechanisms. The intra-arterial administration of antioxidants has been shown to reverse impaired endothelial-dependent vasodilatation in patients with ischemic heart disease, cardiac failure, hypertension, smoking, dyslipidemia, and diabetes [5, 6]. Oral therapy is also beneficial, with studies reporting an improvement in endothelial function in coronary artery disease [5, 6], a reduction in urinary albumin excretion in diabetes [30], a lowering of blood pressure in hypertension [31], and a suppression of endothelial cell apoptosis in congestive heart failure [32].

The adverse cardiovascular effects of acute hyperglycemia are probably mediated by free radicals [33]. Antioxidants can prevent the impaired endothelial-dependent vasodilatation [34], the systemic hemodynamic changes [35], the elevation in PAI-1 concentrations [36], and the up-regulation of soluble cell adhesion molecules [37], during hyperglycemia. Antioxidant therapy has also been reported to reduce the plasma concentrations of soluble cell adhesion molecules in patients with diabetes, and in post-menopausal women with high cardiovascular risk [38, 39].

The value of antioxidant supplementation in intensive care medicine is currently unclear [7]. While some studies have shown positive effects on outcome, clearly there are other studies which suggest that antioxidants are of no benefit. The problem may be related to the timing of therapy. Those studies where antioxidants were initiated early in the course of illness generally show beneficial effects. Pre-treatment of laboratory rats with N-acetylcysteine, significantly atenuates endotoxin-induced alterations in leukocyte-endothelial cell adhesion and macromolecular leakage [40]. This suggests that antioxidant therapy may prevent endothelial dysfunction if given prophylactically before an injury stimulus. Currently there is some limited clinical evidence to support this hypothesis. A small prospective study in 18 trauma patients examined the effects of prophylactic antioxidant therapy on complications [41]. Compared with the control group, the antioxidant group showed fewer infectious complications (eight versus 18) and less frequent organ dysfunction (zero versus nine). Another prospective study in 37 severely burned patients, reported that adjuvant administration of high-dose ascorbic acid 66 mg/kg/h) during the first 24 hours after injury significantly reduced resuscitation fluid volume requirements, body weight gain, and wound edema [42]. A reduction in the severity of respiratory dysfunction was also apparent. The study did not, however, show a reduction in mortality. Further investigation in larger patient numbers is clearly necessary.

Apart from the timing of therapy, there are other explanations why some antioxidant studies have failed to show a benefit in the critically ill. The rate constant for the reaction of ascorbate and a-tocopherol with superoxide is much slower than the rate constant for the reaction between NO and superoxide. Therefore, in order to scavenge superoxide, antioxidants must be administered in very high concentrations [43]. Recycling processes are also important. When a-tocopherol reacts with a radical, it becomes the a-tocopheroxyl radical, which itself may participate in pro-oxidative events. Adequate concentrations of ascorbate are necessary for the recycling of a-tocopherol. Glutathione is also required for the recycling of ascorbate. It seems likely therefore, that optimal antioxidant therapy may require a combination of different antioxidants.

▌ Conclusion

Endothelial dysfunction in critical illness may be due in part to increaed oxidative stress. Targeting protective therapies at the endothelium may help to prevent the occurrence of infective complications or the progression to multiple organ failure (MOF). Studies in patients with endothelial dysfunction secondary to atherosclerosis, hypertension, dyslipidemia, or diabetes, have shown that antioxidants can improve endothelial function. Antioxidants may exert their beneficial vascular effects via a number of direct and indirect mechanisms. There are currently very few clinical studies in intensive care medicine examining the role of antioxidants as prophylaxis against endothelial dysfunction. Antioxidant modification may be a simple and inexpensive adjunct therapy in critical illness. Further clinical research is urgently warranted to investigate the role of early antioxidant therapy in critical care.

References

1. Cardigan R, McGloin H, Macki I, Machin S, Singer M (1998) Endothelial dysfunction in critically ill patients: the effect of haemofiltration. Intensive Care Med 24:1264–1271
2. De Caterina R (2000) Endothelial dysfunctions: common denominators in vascular disease. Curr Opin Clin Nutr Metab Care 3:453–467
3. Oldham KM, Bowen PE (1998) Oxidative stress in critical care: is antioxidant supplementation beneficial? J Am Diet Assoc 98:1001–1008
4. Goode HF, Webster NR (1993) Anti-oxidants in intensive care medicine. Clin Intensive Care 4:265–270
5. Carr A, Frei B (2000) The role of natural antioxidants in preserving the biological activity of endothelium-derived nitric oxide. Free Radic Biol Med 28:1806–1814
6. Vallance P, Chan N (2001) Endothelial function and nitric oxide: clinical relevance. Heart 85:342–350
7. Haji-Michael PG (2000) Antioxidant therapy in the critically ill. Br J Intensive Care 10:88–93
8. Moncada S, Higgs A (1993) The L-arginine-nitric oxide pathway. N Engl J Med 329:2002–2012
9. Cockcroft JR, Wilkinson IB, Webb DJ (1997) Age, arterial stiffness and the endothelium. Age Ageing 26:53–60
10. Nichols WW, O'Rourke MF (1998) McDonald's Blood Flow in Arteries: Theoretical, Experimental and Clinical Principles. 4th edn. Arnold, London
11. Wilkinson IB, Cockcroft JR, Webb DJ (1998) Pulse wave analysis and arterial stiffness. J Cardiovasc Pharmacol 32 Suppl 3:S33–S37
12. Cheeseman KH, Salter TF (1993) An introduction to free radical biochemistry. Br Med Bull 49:481–493
13. Gryglewski RJ, Palmer RMJ, Moncada S (1986) Superoxide anion is involved in the breakdown of endothelium-derived vascular relaxing factor. Nature 320:454–456
14. Cosentino F, Luscher TF (1998) Tetrahydrobiopterin and endothelial function. Eur Heart J 19(Suppl G):G3–G8
15. Cosentino F, Katusic ZS (1995) Tetrahydrobiopterin and dysfunction of endothelial nitric oxide synthase in coronary arteries. Circulation 91:139–144
16. Keaney JF, Guo Y, Cunningham D, Shwaery GT, Xu AM, Vita JA (1996) Vascular incorporation of α-tocopherol prevents endothelial dysfunction due to oxidised LDL by inhibiting protein kinase C stimulation. J Clin Invest 98:386–394
17. Weber C, Erl W (2000) Modulation of vascular cell activation, function, and apoptosis: role of antioxidants and nuclear factor-kappa B. Curr Topics Cell Regul 36:217–235
18. Altavilla D, Saitta A, Guarini S , et al (2001) Oxidative stress causes nuclear factor-kappa B activation in acute hypovolemic hemorrhagic shock. Free Radic Biol Med 30:1055–1066
19. Abello PA, Fidler SA, Buckley GB, Buchman TG (1994) Antioxidants modulate induction of programmed endothelial cell death (apoptosis) by endotoxin. Arch Surg 129:134–140
20. Browry VW, Mohr D, Clearly J, Stocker R (1995) Prevention of tocopherol-mediated peroxidation in ubiquinol-20-free human low density lipoprotein. J Biol Chem 270:5756–5763
21. Halliwell B (1996) Vitamin C: antioxidant or pro-oxidant in vivo. Free Radic Res 25:439–454
22. Maxwell SRJ (1995) Prospects for the use of antioxidant therapies. Drugs 49:345–361
23. Stehouwer CDA (1999) Is measurement of endothelial dysfunction clinically useful? Eur J Clin Invest 29:459–461
24. Smith FCT, Gosling P, Sanghera K, Green MA, Paterson IS, Shearman CP (1994) Microproteinuria predicts the severity of systemic effects of reperfusion injury following infrarenal aortic aneurysm surgery. Ann Vasc Surg 8:1–5
25. Shearman CP, Gosling P, Walker KJ (1989) Is low proteinuria an early predictor of severity of acute pancreatitis? J Clin Pathol 42:1132–1135

26. De Gaudio AR, Spina R, Di Filippo A, Feri M (1999) Glomerular permeability and trauma: a correlation between microalbuminuria and injury severity score. Crit Care Med 27:2105–2108

27. Hack Ce, Zeerleder S (2001) The endothelium in sepsis: source of and target for inflammation. Crit Care Med 29(Suppl):S21–S27

28. Yamamoto K, Saito H (1998) A pathological role of increased expression of plasminogen activator inhibitor-1 in human or animal disorders. Int J Hematol 68:371–385

29. Hasdai D, Gibbons RJ, Holmes DR, Higano ST, Lerman A (1997) Coronary endothelial dysfunction in humans is associated with myocardial perfusion defects. Circulation 96:3390–3395

30. McAuliffe AV, Brooks BA, Fisher EJ, Molyneaux LM, Yue DK (1998) Administration of ascorbic acid and an aldose reductase inhibitor (tolrestat) in diabetes: effect on urinary albumin excretion. Nephron 80:277–284

31. Duffy SJ, Gokce N, Holbrook M, et al (1999) Treatment of hypertension with ascorbic acid. Lancet 354:2048–2049

32. Rossig L, Hoffmann J, Hugel B, et al (2001) Vitamin C inhibits endothelial cell apoptosis in congestive heart failure. Circulation 104:2182–2187

33. Ceriello A (1997) Acute hyperglycaemia and oxidative stress generation. Diabetic Med 14:S45–S49

34. Beckman JA, Goldfine AB, Gordon MB, Creager MA (2001) Ascorbate restores endothelium-dependent vasodilation impaired by acute hyperglycemia in humans. Circulation 103:1618–1623

35. Marfella R, Verrazzo G, Acampora R, et al (1995) Glutathione reverses systemic hemodynamic changes induced by acute hyperglycemia in healthy subjects. Am J Physiol 268:E1167–E1173

36. Ceriello A, Curcio F, dello Russo P, et al (1995) The defence against free radicals protects endothelial cells from hyperglycemia-induced plasminogen activator inhibitor-1 over-production. Blood Coagul Fibrinolysis 6:133–137

37. Ceriello A, Falleti E, Motz E, et al (1998) Hyperglycemia-induced circulating ICAM-1 increase in diabetes mellitus: the possible role of oxidative stress. Horm Metab Res 30:146–149

38. De Mattia G, Bravi MC, Laurenti O, et al (1998) Reduction of oxidative stress by oral N-acetyl-L-cysteine treatment decreases plasma soluble vascular cell adhesion molecule-1 concentrations in non-obese, non-dyslipidaemic, normotensive patients with non-insulin-dependent diabetes. Diabetologia 41(11):1392–1396

39. Goudev A, Kyurkchiev S, Gergova V, et al (2000) Reduced concentrations of soluble adhesion molecus after antioxidant supplementation in postmenopausal women with high cardiovascular risk profiles – a randomised double-blind study. Cardiology 94:227–232

40. Schmidt H, Schmidt W, Muller T, Bohrer H, Gebhard MM, Martin E (1997) N-acetylcysteine attenuates endotoxin-induced leukocyte-endothelial cell adhesion and macromolecular leakage in vivo. Crit Care Med 25:858–863

41. Porter JM, Ivatury RR, Azimuddin K, Swami R (1999) Antioxidant therapy in the prevention of organ dysfunction syndrome and infections complications after trauma: early results of a prospective randomised study. Am Surg 65:478–483

42. Tanaka H, Matsuda T, Miyagantani Y, Yukioka T, Matsuda H, Shimazaki S (2000) Reduction of resuscitation fluid volumes in severely burned patients using ascrobic acid administration. Arch Surg 135:326–331

43. Jackson TS, Xu A, Vita JA, Keaney JFJ (1998) Ascorbate prevents the interaction of superoxide and nitric oxide only at very high physiological concentrations. Circ Res 83:916–922

Pentoxifylline: A Useful Adjuvant in the Critically Ill?

J. Boldt

▌ Introduction

Sepsis and the systemic inflammatory response syndrome (SIRS) represent an extremely complex biochemical and pathophysiological disorder which still lacks specific effective pharmacological intervention. Infection, trauma, major surgery (e.g., cardiac surgery) or critical illness initiate an inflammatory cascade, which leads to an activation of various regulatory mechanisms. There is a large body of literature implicating that the inflammatory process is initiated and/or maintained by interactions of circulating leukocytes with the endothelium via cell, and organ-specific, adhesion molecules [1–3]. Neutrophils are essential for bacterial killing in infectious disease, but they also are able to injure the host tissue. Neutrophil 'rolling' along the endothelium initiates a cascade of cellular interactions resulting in endothelial damage (e.g., capillary leakage) and subsequent development of (multiple) organ damage [3]. 'Rolling' is defined as deceleration and attachment of neutrophils to the luminal surface of the vascular endothelium. Intercellular adhesion and adhesion to endothelial cells are necessary for the arrest of circulating leukocytes and transendothelial migration [3, 4]. The process of 'rolling', firm adhesion, emigration, and migration in the interstitial space are mediated by adhesion molecules expressed on both the endothelial and the leukocyte surface. Three main families of adhesion molecules have been identified [4, 5]:

▌ The immunoglobulin superfamily (e.g., vascular cell adhesion molecule-1 [VCAM-1]; intercellular adhesion molecule-1 [ICAM-1])
▌ the integrins (e.g., lymphocyte function-associated antigen), and
▌ the selectins (E-selectin = endothelial leukocyte adhesion molecule [ELAM-1]; L-selectin = leukocyte endothelial cell adhesion molecule; P-selectin = granule membrane protein 140 [GMP-140]).

During inflammation, adhesion molecules are up-regulated on the endothelial surface to act with circulating (activated) leukocytes. Tumor necrosis factor (TNF)-a and interleukin (IL)-1 are cytokines which synergistically induce up-regulation of adhesion molecules, thus promoting leukocyte adherence to the endothelium and inducing or maintaining the inflammatory process.

Soluble forms of these adhesion molecules have been detected in the circulating blood under various conditions [6]. They may not only serve as markers of endothelial activation and damage, they may modulate the inflammatory process in many different ways, e.g., by acting as chemotaxins, blocking neutrophil activation or competing with membrane bound forms of cell-cell adhesion [5, 7]. Some clinical trials have reported an extensive increase in some of these adhesion molecules in the critically ill [8]. Other processes are also involved in the initiation or maintenance of SIRS or sepsis, including the activation of the coagulation cascade, release of various cytokines, and enhanced superoxide production.

▌ Pentoxifylline as an Adjunct to Standard Supportive Therapy

In recent years, several immunotherapeutic interventions have been studied, aimed at reducing the still high lethality in septic patients. Pentoxifylline (PTX), chemically: 3,7-dimethyl-1-[5-oxohexyl]-xanthine, is a non-specific phosphodiesterase inhibitor that has gained some interest in this context. A Medline search identified 1,841 papers dealing with PTX in the period from 1990 to 2000 indicating the considerable interest in this substance. The definite mechanisms by which PTX exerts its possible beneficial effects are not fully known (Table 1), but are thought to be attributable, in part, to inhibition of phosphodiesterase (PDE) activity resulting in accumulation of the intracellular signaling molecule cyclic adenosine monophosphate (cAMP) [9]. Possible other mechanisms include blockade of the production and release of proinflammatory cytokines (e.g., TNF-α, IL-6), attenuated lipopolysaccharide (LPS)-induced leukocyte-endothelial adhesion/emigration and macromolecular extravasation, altered polymorphonuclear (PMN) chemotaxis, reduced superoxide production, and microbicidal activity [10–13]. PTX is known to inhibit PDE, thereby increasing cAMP levels, and elevation of cAMP strongly inhibits TNF-α gene transcription [11]. The positive effects of PTX in sepsis may be explained, in part, by decreased endothelial and/or cell-to-cell leukocyte adhesion which may result in improved microperfusion and reduced autoinflammation [14]. Additionally, PTX possesses vasodilatator properties (e.g., by prostaglandin I_2 re-

Table 1. Pharmacological properties of pentoxifylline (PTX)

Antiinflammatory properties
▌ blocking cytokine production (e.g., TNF, IL-6)
▌ leukocyte superoxide anion production
▌ blocking the inflammatory actions of cytokines on neutrophils
▌ inhibition of IL-6 and TNF-alpha secretion
▌ inhibition of TNF-alpha mRNA accumulation in monocytes and T cells
▌ reduced leukocyte adhesion
▌ altered PMN chemotaxis

Effects on fluidity
▌ increased red cell deformability
▌ decreased red blood cell aggregation
▌ decreased platelet adhesion and aggregation
▌ decreased fibrinogen concentration

Effects on systemic hemodynamics
▌ vasodilation by intracellular Ca^{++} accumulation

Effects on microcirculation
▌ improved perfusion by prostaglandin I_2 release

Miscellaneous
▌ stabilization of cell membranes

lease) leading to improved microcirculatory blood flow [15, 16]. The value of administering PTX has not been fully clarified and data regarding the influence of PTX on outcome are conflicting [17].

Animal Experiments

In an endotoxin shock model in sheep, PTX provided protection against the deleterious sequelae of endotoxemia when given prior to endotoxin. PTX was also of benefit when given after hemodynamic and respiratory signs of shock had appeared [18]. In a rat model of subacute bacterial peritonitis, Nelson et al. [19] showed that treatment with PTX (5 mg/kg/day) resulted in improved survival. In another experiment using rats and dogs, pretreatment with PTX prior to LPS injection protected the animals from intestinal damage and bowel hypoperfusion [20]. In septic rats, treatment with PTX (50 mg/kg) was a useful adjunct for maintaining hepatocellular function [21]. The morphological alterations in the liver, small intestine, and kidneys were attenuated by administration of PTX early after the onset of sepsis [22]. Experimental data have demonstrated that PTX is able to attenuate endotoxin-induced acute lung injury (ALI) when given after the septic insult [23]. Similar results were reported by Tighe et al. [13]; even when given after induction of fecal peritonitis in rabbits, PTX administration decreased histopathological changes in the lungs with reduced pulmonary leukostasis and improved capillary patency. Apart from its anti-inflammatory actions, PTX has been shown to influence (micro-) organ perfusion beneficially, maintaining intestinal and renal perfusion after mesenteric ischemia and reperfusion [24].

Human Data

In patients undergoing bone marrow transplantation, PTX (1,200, 1,600 or 2,000 mg given orally) was associated with a reduction in morbidity and mortality [25]. In septic patients, infusion of PTX (5 mg/kg) resulted in a significant improvement in hemodynamic status compared to a non-treated control group [26]. The cytokine response to i.v. endotoxin was altered by PTX in human volunteers [27]. In patients suffering from postoperative sepsis, PTX was administered as an adjunct to standard supportive therapy [28]. An initial bolus of 300 mg of PTX was given followed by a continuous infusion of 1.4 mg/kg/h for the next 5 days. PTX did not decrease elevated plasma levels of circulating soluble ELAM-1, soluble ICAM-1, and soluble VCAM-1, indicating no beneficial effect on endothelial activation or damage in inflammation. Only soluble GMP-140 concentrations did not increase further, in contrast to the untreated control group who showed a significant increase in sGMP-140 over time. These findings may be explained by the antiaggregatory and fibrinolytic properties of PTX that may have limited thrombin generation, an important stimulus for GMP-140 expression. There were no differences in morbidity or mortality [28]. Hoffmann et al. [29] used PTX (300 mg initial bolus followed by a continuous infusion of 1.5 mg/kg/h over the following 7 days) in cardiac surgery patients who were at risk of developing multiple organ failure (MOF) with an APACHE II score of >19 on the first postoperative day. The duration of mechanical ventilation was significantly greater in the untreated control patients, and PTX-patients experienced fewer days on hemofiltration and had a shorter ICU stay compared to the untreated controls. Mortality did not differ between the two groups (PTX: 33%, control: 36%). The authors concluded that supplemental PTX treatment may decrease the incidence of MOF in patients at risk of SIRS after complicated cardiac surgery.

▌ Prophylactic use of PTX in Critically Ill Patients

Administration of PTX has been reported to be useful not only for treating septic (inflammatory) complications, but also for preventing inflammation-related organ disorders. Cardiac surgery using cardiopulmonary bypass (CPB) has been shown to be associated with a considerable risk of perfusion deficits, possibly resulting in the development of post-bypass organ dysfunction. A complex pathophysiological process is activated during CPB which may result in reduced endothelial integrity and marked microvascular injury [30]: The "blood becomes a stew of powerful enzymes and chemicals" [31]. Inflammation appears to be an important component in the pathogenesis of postperfusion organ injury. This inflammatory activation results from stimulation of immune effector cells that subsequently synthesize and release potent mediators of inflammation (e.g., different pro-inflammatory cytokines such as IL-6 or IL-8) as well as different anti-inflammatory cytokines (e.g., IL-10). The function of various organs, including lungs, heart, brain, liver, and kidneys, may be impaired after cardiac surgery, and there is convincing evidence that alterations of endothelial function also play a pivotal role in the pathogenesis of post-bypass organ dysfunction. In the inflammation process and reperfusion injury associated with CPB, adhesion of neutrophils to the vascular endothelium is of importance. Abnormalities in endothelial function in this situation can be triggered and/or modified by circulatory, inflammatory or metabolic disorders.

Pharmacological manipulations to attenuate CPB-associated organ dysfunction have received some attention, and include the use of corticosteroids, proteinase inhibitors (e.g., aprotinin), or specific antagonists of the inflammatory cascade [32, 33]. As biomaterials, surgical techniques, anesthetic and intensive care management have improved, patients with advanced age have become acceptable candidates for cardiac surgery. It is generally accepted that several organ systems are altered in the elderly and age-specific alterations of organ function appear to pave the way for the development of MOF [34, 35]. Elderly patients often show considerable comorbidity and a limited functional reserve. Thus, these patients appear to be particularly prone to developing post-bypass organ dysfunction. Renal function, for example, has often been reported to be disturbed in patients undergoing cardiac surgery. Due to age-related limitations in renal function, the elderly cardiac surgery patient appears to be especially prone to develop renal dysfunction [35]. In 20 cardiac surgery patients aged >80 years, PTX (loading bolus of 300 mg followed by a continuous infusion of 1.5 mg/kg/h until the second postoperative day) was given after induction of anesthesia, another 20 patients received saline solution as placebo [36]. The pretreatment of these patients aged >80 years attenuated the post-bypass deterioration of endothelial, renal, and liver function that was seen in the untreated control group. In PTX-pretreated rats undergoing cardiac transplantation, survival rates, liver enzymes, and postperfusion histology were significantly improved compared to an untreated control group [37]. PTX given orally three days prior to surgery (400 mg/day) in patients undergoing mitral valve surgery, resulted in inhibition of the postoperative increase in pulmonary vascular resistance (PVR) and reduction in leukocyte sequestration in the lung secondary to CPB [38].

▌ Conflicting Data on the use of PTX

In spite of some promising experimental and human data on inflammation and organ function, studies showing no beneficial effects of PTX have also been reported. The dose used in the study may be an important reason for these conflicting results [17]. Some studies showing overall beneficial effects used high doses of PTX (e.g., 1.5 mg/kg/h) which amounted to approximately 3 g of PTX per day [39]. Butler et al. [40] used an infusion of 1 mg/h of PTX only during surgery amounting to approximately 200–250 mg PTX. With this dose, PTX did not show beneficial effects on inflammation. Dose-dependence of the beneficial effects of PTX was also demonstrated in other human studies: plasma levels achievable by oral PTX failed to alter the cardiovascular response to endotoxin in normal human subjects [41]. However, even after high doses of PTX, no beneficial effects have been seen: in an animal experiment, 60 mg/kg of PTX was given over 2.5 hrs after pancreatitis was induced (approximately equivalent to 4.8 g in a 70 kg patient). PTX failed to show any beneficial effects in this study [42]. In rats, gastric mucosal damage secondary to indomethacin was maximally prevented by 200 mg/kg of PTX given intraperitoneally [43] – this would be approximately 16 g of PTX in a 80 kg human!

The timing and duration of PTX administration may be also of interest with regard to interpreting the conflicting data. Prophylactic and continuous administration of PTX, rather than using it only after the injury or insult, may be important. Early use of PTX before cardiac surgery (400 mg one week before surgery) resulted in attenuation of endothelial injury and permeability after CPB [44]. In an experimental endotoxic shock model in animals, PTX provided protection against the deleterious sequelae of endotoxemia when given prior to endotoxin [18]. In rats, PTX given prior to operation improved tissue oxygenation following surgery [15]. Levi et al. [45] administered PTX (1.5 g/3 hrs) in chimpanzees before injection of endotoxin. TNF and IL-6 plasma levels were significantly elevated by endotoxin and this increase was significantly attenuated by PTX-pretreatment.

▌ Possible Side-effects of PTX

Possible side-effects, particularly on coagulation, may limit the use of PTX in the critically ill. PTX is a dimethyl xanthine derivative that acts as a PDE inhibitor, by which intracellular cAMP is increased. In the platelet, cAMP inhibits phospholipase activation, and thus the liberation of arachidonic acid from membrane phospholipids. Additionally, by increasing intracellular cAMP, intracellular Ca^{++} levels are decreased thus impairing Ca^{++}-dependent effects, such as phospholipase activation and microfilament contraction. Thus, various steps may be influenced by increasing cAMP levels in the platelet resulting in alterations in platelet shape change, granule secretion, and prostaglandin synthesis. PDE inhibition by dipyridamole has been shown to result in increased intracellular camp levels subsequently inhibiting *in vitro* platelet aggregation [46]. In an experimental setting, Hammerschmidt et al. [39] reported that PTX was only a modest inhibitor of platelet aggregation: with 1 µmol/l of PTX only a very small decrement in aggregation was seen after ADP (4 mol/l) as the aggregating stimulus. To induce a 50% inhibition of aggregation, 200 µmol/l of PTX were necessary. This quantity represents a tremendously high plasma level of PTX: peak plasma levels after an oral dose of 400 mg of PTX were 3–5 µmol/l [47]. In a study in critically ill intensive care unit (ICU) patients, continuous infusion of 1.4 mg/kg/h of PTX for 5 days did not significantly impair platelet function [48]. The normally observed deterioration of platelet function was even attenuated by PTX, which may be due to the effects of PTX on cytokine release (e.g., reduction in TNF and IL-1), improvement in microcirculation, or additional fibrinolytic effects. In *in vitro* studies, Ohdama et al. [49] found that PTX up-regulated expression of endothelial surface thrombomodulin antigen. Additionally, TNF-induced suppression of thrombomodulin was counterbalanced by PTX. Thus the anticoagulant properties of the endothelium appear to be protected or restored by PTX.

Due to its pharmacological properties, PTX may also have some effects on hemdynamics. As a PDE inhibitor, PTX thus possesses some vasodilating actions by increasing intracellular Ca^{++} concentrations. However, even in patients in whom high doses of PTX were given (e.g., 1.5 mg/kg/h) no relevant reduction in systemic vascular resistance (SVR) was observed [28, 36] and systemic hemodynamics remained stable.

∎ Conclusion

Due to the complex pathophysiologic processes in the critically ill patient, the 'magic bullet' that could solve all our problems in one go cannot exist. Numerous proinflammatory and anti-inflammatory substances are produced. Anti-inflammatory approaches aimed at limiting production of one specific substance (e.g., anti-TNF) must fail because the inflammatory process is much too complex. PTX displays a broad spectrum of pharmacological properties. The possible effects of PTX are comprehensive and include effects on the immune system, on hemodynamics, and on coagulation. With its beneficial rheologic and possible anti-inflammatory effects, prophylactic use of PTX appears to be a promising supportive approach in patients who are at risk of developing organ dysfunction. PTX may also be a promising substance for treating inflammation-related organ dysfunction in the ICU patient. However, the definite value of PTX has not been fully clarified [17]. Even the precise mechanisms by which the drug may improve organ function remain debatable. Early use appears to be as important as the correct dose of PTX. More controlled studies in different patient populations are necessary before any conclusions can be drawn about the therapeutic potential of this substance.

References

1. Ley K (1992) Leukocyte adhesion to vascular endothelium. J Reconstr Microsurg 8:495–503
2. Mariscalco MM (1993) Leukocytes and the inflammatory response. Crit Care Med 21:S347–S348
3. Williams TJ, Hellewell PG (1992) Endothelial cell biology. Am Rev Respir Dis 146:S45–S50
4. Osborn L (1990) Leukocyte adhesion to endothelium in inflammation. Cell 62:3–6
5. McKeating EG, Andrews PJD (1998) Cytokines and adhesion molecules in acute brain injury. Br J Anaesth 80:77–84
6. Gearing AJH, Newman W (1993) Circulating adhesion molecules in disease. Immunol Today 14:506–512
7. Rothlein R, Mainolfi EA, Czajkowski M, Marlin SD (1991) A form of circulating ICAM-1 in human serum. J Immunol 147:3788–3793
8. Paret G, Prince T, Keller N, et al. (2000) Plasma soluble E-selectin after cardiopulmonary bypass in children: is it a marker of the postoperative care? J Cardiothorac Vasc Anesth 14:433–437

9. Semmler J, Gebert U, Eisenhut T, et al (1993) Xanthine derivatives: comparison between suppression of tumor necrosis factor-alpha production and inhibition of cAMP phosphodiesterase activity. Immunolgy 78:520–525
10. Seiffge D, Bissinger T, Kremer E, Laux V, Schleyerbach R (1995) Inhibitory effects of pentoxifylline on LPS-induced leukocyte adhesion and macromolecular extravasation in the microcirculation. Inflamm Res 44:281–286
11. Doherty GM, Jensen JC, Alexander IIR, et al (1991) Pentoxifylline suppression of tumor necrosis factor gene transcription. Surgery 110:192–198
12. Edwards MJ, Abney DL, Miller FN (1991) Pentoxifylline inhibits interleukin-2-induced leukocyte-endothelial adherence and reduces systemic toxicity. Surgery 110:199–204
13. Tighe D, Hynd J, Boghossian S, et al (1990) Pretreatment with pentoxifylline improves the hemodynamic and histologic changes and decreases neutrophil adhesiveness in a pig fecal peritonitis model. Crit Care Med 18:184–189
14. Waxmann K (1990) Pentoxifylline in septic shock. Crit Care Med 18:243–244
15. Soliman HM, O'Neal K, Waxman K (1987) Pentoxifylline improves tissue oxygenation following anesthesia and operation. Crit Care Med 15:93–94
16. Flynn WJ, Cryer HG, Garrison RN (1991) Pentoxifylline restores intestinal microvascular blood flow during resuscitated hemorrhagic shock. Surgery 110:350–356
17. Fink MP (1999) Whither pentoxifylline? Crit Care Med 27:19–20
18. Sigurdsson GH, Youssef H (1993) Effects of pentoxifylline on hemodynamics, gas exchange and multiple organ platelet sequestration in experimental endotoxic shock. Acta Anaesthesiol Scand 37:396–403
19. Nelson JL, Alexander JW, Mao JX, et al (1999) The effects of pentoxifylline on survival and intestinal cytokine mRNA transcription in a rat model of ongoing peritoneal sepsis. Crit Care Med 27:113–119
20. Cardelus I, Gras J, Jauregui J, Llenas J, Palacios JM (1996) Inhibition of lipopolysaccharide-induced bowel erythrocyte extravasation in rats, and of mesenteric hypoperfusion in dogs, by phosphodiesterase inhibitors. Eur J Pharmacol 299:153–159
21. Wang P, Ba ZF, Chaudry IH (1997) Pentoxifylline maintains hepatocellular function and improves cardiac performance during early sepsis. J Trauma 42:429–435
22. Yang S, Zjou M, Koo DJ, Chaudry IH, Wang P (1999) Pentoxifylline prevents the transition from the hyperdynamic to hypodynamic response during sepsis. Am J Physiol 277:H1036–H1044
23. Hoffmann H, Hatherill JJR, Crowley J, et al (1991) Early post-treatment with pentoxifylline or dibutyryl cAMP attenuates Escherichia coli-induced acute lung injury in guinea pigs. Am Rev Respir Dis 143:289–293
24. Myers SI, Horton JW, Hernandez, et al (1994) Pentoxifylline protects splanchnic prostacyclin synthesis during mesenteric ischemia/reperfusion. Prostaglandins 47:137–150
25. Bianco JA, Appelbaum FR, Nemunaitis J, et al (1993) Phase I–II of pentoxifylline for the prevention of transplant-related toxicities following bone marrow transplantation. Blood 78:1205–1211
26. Bacher A, Mayer N, Klimschka W, Oismuller C, Steltzer H, Hammerle A (1997) Effects of pentoxifylline on hemodynamics and oxygenation in septic and nonseptic patients. Crit Care Med 25:795–800
27. Zabel P, Schonharting MM, Wolter DT, Schade UF (1989) Oxpentifylline in endotoxemia. Lancet 2:1474–1477
28. Boldt J, Muller M, Heesen M, Martin K, Hempelmann G (1996) Influence of different volume therapies and pentoxifylline infusion on circulating soluble adhesion molecules in critically ill patients. Crit Care Med 24:385–391
29. Hoffmann H, Markewitz A, Kreuzer E, Reichert, Jochum M, Faist E (1998) Pentoxifylline decreases the incidence of multiple organ failure in patients after major cardio-thoracic surgery. Shock 19:234–240
30. Boyle EM, Pohlman TH, Johnson MC, Verrier ED (1997) Endothelial cell injury in cardiovascular surgery: the systemic inflammatory response. Ann Thorac Surg 63:277–284
31. Edmunds HL Jr (1993) Blood surface interactions during cardiopulmonary bypass. J Card Surg 20:404–410

32. Gott JP, Cooper WA, Schmidt FE, et al (1998) Modifying risk of extracorporeal circulation: trial of four antiinflammatory strategies. Ann Thorac Surg 66:747–754
33. Royston D (1997) The inflammatory response and extracorporeal circulation. J Cardiothorac Vasc Anesth 11:341–354
34. Harris J (1999) Cardiac surgery in the elderly. Heart 82:119–120
35. Christenson JT, Simonet F, Schmuziger M (1999) The influence of age on the outcome of primary coronary artery bypass grafting. J Cardiovasc Surg 40:333–338
36. Boldt J, Brosch C, Piper SN, Suttner S, Lehmann A, Werling C (2001) Influence of prophylactic use of pentoxifylline on postoperative organ function in elderly cardiac surgery patients. Crit Care Med 29:952–958
37. Astarcioglu H, Karademir S, Unek T, et al (2000) Beneficial effects of pentoxifylline pretreatment in non-heart-beating donors in rats. Transplantation 69:93–98
38. Turkoz R, Yorukoglu K, Akcay A, et al (1996) The effect of pentoxifylline on the lung during cardiopulmonary bypass. Eur J Cardiothorac Surg 10:339–346
39. Hammerschmidt DE, Vercellotti GM (1987) Mechanism of action of pentoxifylline (PTX) in peripheral vascular disease: inhibition of platelet and granulocyte responsiveness. Clin Hemorheol 7:529–533
40. Butler J, Baigrie RJ, Parker D, et al (1993) Systemic inflammatory responses to cardiopulmonary bypass: a pilot study of the effects of pentoxifylline. Respir Med 87:285–288
41. Martich GD, Parker MM, Cunnion RE, Suffredini AF (1992) Effects of ibuprofen and pentoxifylline on the cardiovascular response of normal humans to endotoxin. J Appl Physiol 73:925–931
42. Bassi DG, Foitzik T, Rattner DW, Lewandrowski K, Warshaw AL, Castillo CF (1994) Failure of pentoxifylline to ameliorate severe acute pancreatitis in the rat: Results of a prospective, randomized, controlled study. Crit Care Med 22:1960–1963
43. Santucci L, Fiorucci S, Giansanti M, Brunori PM, Di Matteo FM, Morelli A (1994) Pentoxifylline prevents indomethacin induced acute gastric mucosal damage in rats: role of tumour necrosis factor alpha. Gut 35:909–915
44. Tsang GM, Allen S, Pagano D, Wong C, Graham TR, Bonser RS (1996) Pentoxifylline preloading reduces endothelial injury and permeability in cardiopulmonary bypass. ASAIO J 42:M429–434
45. Levi M, ten Cate H, Bauer KE, et al (1994) Inhibition of endotoxin-induced activation of coagulation and fibrinolysis by pentoxifylline or by a monoclonal anti-issue factor antibody in chimpanzees. J Clin Invest 93:114–120
46. Campbell FW, Addonizio VP Jr (1988) Platelet function alterations during cardiac surgery. In: Ellison N, Jobes DR (eds) Effective hemostasis in cardiac surgery. WB Saunders, Philadelphia, pp 85–109
47. Ward A, Clissold SP (1987) Pentoxifylline – A review of its pharmacodynamic and pharmacokinetic properties, and its therapeutic efficacy. Drugs 34:50–97
48. Boldt J, Muller M, Heesen M, Heyn S, Hempelmann G (1996) Does long-term continuous administration of pentoxifylline affect platelet function in the critically ill? Intensive Care Med 22:644–650
49. Ohdama S, Takano S, Ohashi K, Miyake S, Aoki N (1991) Pentoxifylline prevents tumor necrosis factor-induced suppression of endothelial cell surface thrombomodulin. Thromb Res 62:745–755

High Volume Hemofiltration in Sepsis

K. Reiter, R. Bellomo, and C. Ronco

Introduction

Continuous renal replacement therapy (CRRT) in the intensive care unit (ICU) is a common treatment in acute renal failure. CRRT is mainly conceived as merely supportive and as a replacement of the lost kidney function. On the other hand, evidence accumulated over recent years demonstrates that many soluble mediators of the systemic inflammatory (and anti-inflammatory) response syndrome (SIRS) can be removed by CRRT. This has led to the suggestion that CRRT could play a major role in sepsis therapy as an immunomodulatory treatment and not only as a blood purification technique. In this perspective, whereas animal studies yielded encouraging results, early clinical trials showed only minor clinical benefits, mainly dealing with hemodynamic improvements. The question of treatment dose has appropriately been raised as it remains undefined and a matter of controversy. A large-scale clinical trial has clarified issues on treatment dose in acute renal failure but a sufficiently powered study on hemofiltration dose in sepsis is still lacking.

In this chapter, we will review the rationale for application of CRRT in the treatment of the septic syndrome with specific focus on the use of high ultrafiltration rates (i.e., high-volume hemofiltration, HVHF). We will integrate the discussion into the most recent hypothesis proposed to explain some of the clinical results obtained with high efficiency, non-selective removal of mediators of sepsis. Further, we will describe the necessary technical requirements for HVHF and the most recent machine development concurring with these.

The Rationale of CRRT in Sepsis

The sepsis syndrome has been described as a systemic malignant inflammation, where the circulation is invaded by enormous amounts of pro-inflammatory mediators produced by activated mononuclear cells. In fact, sepsis is associated with an overwhelming, systemic overflow of both pro- and anti-inflammatory mediators; this leads to altered immune cellular responsiveness, generalized endothelial damage and multiple organ failure (MOF) derived from a complete disruption of the 'immunological homeostasis' [1, 2].

The characteristics of the mediator network are of fundamental relevance in order to allow selection of the most rational and effective treatment approach. The network is redundant and synergistic; it acts like a cascade modulated by multiple positive and negative feedback loops. A vast array of humoral mediators have been identified as exerting pro-inflammatory effects; on the other hand, a seemingly

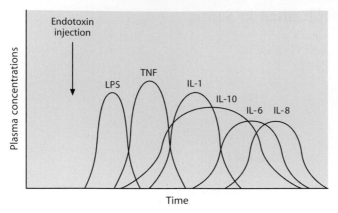

Fig. 1. The sequential appearance of various cytokines in sepsis. LPS: lipopolysaccharide; TNF: tumor necrosis factor; IL: interleukin

equally broad spectrum of molecules with opposite function has been demonstrated to emerge in the time course of the septic syndrome. Both pro- and anti-inflammatory mediators, while designed to mainly act in an autocrine and/or paracrine mode, spill over into the circulation during sepsis and display disastrous systemic effects. In some circumstances, depending on which additional stimuli are present, the same mediator can exert alternatively pro- or anti-inflammatory action. Apart from inciting substances (e.g., endotoxin, products of cell injury) and very early mediators of the septic process (e.g., complement factors, factor XIIa), chemokines and cytokines have a central role in the propagation of the inflammatory process including regulatory effects on immune cells. In fact, mortality in sepsis is correlated with persistently elevated levels of pro-inflammatory cytokines [3, 4] and in a parallel way, persisting immune cellular hypo-responsiveness associated with high levels of anti-inflammatory cytokines [5, 6]. This feature has been similarly observed early in the sequence of effects induced by endotoxin injection in animal models (Fig. 1) [7].

▌ The Peak Concentration Hypothesis

The concept of blocking one mediator has not led to measurable improvement in outcome in patients with sepsis [8]. Possibly more rigidly defined subgroups would profit from tumor necrosis factor (TNF)-antagonizing treatments [9]. On the other hand, it has been shown that antagonizing a cytokine could lead to deleterious consequences encompassing substantially higher mortality [10]. A low-level TNF response seems to be necessary for the host defense to infection [11, 12], and high levels seemingly need to be modulated by an anti-inflammatory feedback; in sepsis, however, failed regulation may cause an excess of the anti-inflammatory response which generates monocyte downregulation and exposes to further infections. Both these processes (inflammation and anti-inflammation) are designed to act in response to specific stimuli in a well-balanced fashion defined as immuno-homeostasis. The excess of one process over the other may produce a deleterious effect either leading to systemic inflammation or immune-cell hypo-responsiveness. In

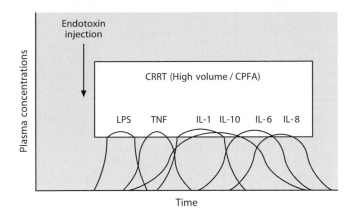

Fig. 2. The peak concentration hypothesis: the sequential appearance of various cytokines in sepsis is schematically depicted. Using continuous renal replacement therapy (CRRT), peak plasma cytokine levels could be nonselectively reduced bringing the organism to a less severe degree of immunological derangement. Lower levels of pro- and anti-inflammatory mediators could allow the restoration of immuno-homeostasis. LPS: lipopolysaccharide; TNF: tumor necrosis factor; IL: interleukin; CPFA: coupled plasma filtration with adsorption

the septic syndrome, it seems that these processes are both exaggerated in the time course of the disease and may put the patient at risk for endothelial dysfunction and shock, or overwhelming infections.

Furthermore, the time point of therapeutic intervention in the septic process seems to be crucial. As the network acts like a cascade, early intervention would seem most beneficial. On the other hand sepsis does not fit a one-hit model but shows complex and varying time courses in mediator levels. Neither single-mediator-directed nor one-time interventions therefore seem appropriate.

One of the major criticisms attributed to continuous blood purification treatments in sepsis – its lack of specificity – could turn out to be a major strength. Nonspecific removal of soluble mediators – be they pro- or anti-inflammatory – without completely eliminating their effect may be the most logical and adequate approach to a complex and long-running process like sepsis. The concept of cutting peaks of soluble mediators, e.g., through continuous hemofiltration (Fig. 2), is a paradigm called by us "the peak concentration hypothesis" [13].

▌ Ultrafiltration Dose and Outcome

Numerous *in vitro* as well as animal and human studies (reviewed in [14]) have shown that synthetic filters in common use in hemofiltration can extract nearly every substance involved in sepsis to a certain degree. Prominent examples are complement factors [15, 16], TNF, interleukin (IL)-1, IL-6 [17–19], IL-8 [20] and platelet activating factor (PAF) [21]. Regarding plasma cytokine levels, the decreases appeared, nevertheless, to be of minor degree. Other studies showed no influence of CRRT on cytokine plasma levels (Cole et al., unpublished data) [22].

On the other hand, significant clinical benefits in terms of hemodynamic improvement have been achieved even without measurable decreases in cytokine plasma levels [23]. Obviously the removal of substances different to the measured cytokines was responsible for the achieved effect. When the response to sepsis is viewed in a network perspective, absolute values would be less relevant than relative ones within an array of interdependent mediators as even small decreases could induce major balance changes. This makes measurement of cytokine plasma levels debatable whilst more local or tissue levels should be measured. These issues are extremely controversial and do not permit a definitive answer in favor or against the use of CRRT as a therapy of sepsis. In this context, a further step in clarifying the immunological impact of CRRT has been taken by measuring a more downstream event integrating the influence of several cytokines: monocyte responsiveness [24, 25].

In spite of some encouraging results as mentioned, the extent of achievable clinical benefit with conventional CRRT (using conventional filters and flow rates) in sepsis has generally been disappointing. Consequently it was sought to improve the efficiency of the methodology regarding removal of soluble mediators of sepsis by increasing the amount of plasma water exchange, i.e., by increasing ultrafiltration rates.

Animal studies provided much support for this concept. Starting in the early nineties, several studies using different septic animal models examined the effect of high ultrafiltration rates (up to 300 ml/kg/h) on physiological parameters and outcome. In a landmark study, a porcine model of septic shock induced by endotoxin infusion was investigated [26]. The animals developed profound arterial hypotension and a decrease in cardiac output, stroke volume, and right ventricular stroke work index. Using HVHF at 6 l/h, right ventricular function, blood pressure, and cardiac output showed a remarkable improvement compared to control and sham-filtered animals [26, 27]. The same group extended their findings in the same model by intravenously administering ultrafiltrate of endotoxin-infused animals into healthy animals. These developed a hemodynamic picture similar to septic shock whereas animals infused with ultrafiltrate from healthy animals showed a moderate blood pressure rise [28]. In a further study by the same group, a bowel ischemia-reperfusion (I/R) model in pigs was investigated. HVHF started before clamping of the superior mesenteric artery significantly diminished bowel damage and prevented hemodynamic deterioration [29].

These classic studies established that a convection-based treatment can remove substances with hemodynamic effects resembling septic shock, when sufficiently high ultrafiltration rates are applied. Several studies have confirmed and refined these results. In three such studies [30–32], the correlation of survival with ultrafiltration rate was specifically examined. A direct correlation could be demonstrated. Significant improvements in cardiac function, systemic and pulmonary vascular resistance, and hepatic perfusion [30] were reported. Another study in lambs showed significant improvements in lung function [33]. Only a minority of the studies identified reduced mediator plasma levels [32, 34].

A very recent study in pigs made septic by induced pancreatitis, compared low-volume continuous veno-venous hemofiltration (CVVH) with HVHF of 100 ml/kg/h. The influence of frequent filter changes on survival, changes in TNF-levels as well as monocyte and polymorphonuclear (PMN) leukocyte-function was analyzed [32]. Early filter change allows to delineate the effect of cytokine removal by adsorption on the filter since membrane capacity saturates after a few hours. By changing filters, adsorption is continued to a certain extent. In this model, a hyperdynamic septic picture was induced through an intervention which approximates underlying conditions encountered in human sepsis. Additionally the intervention started late to simulate real clinical conditions. Hemofiltration was commenced

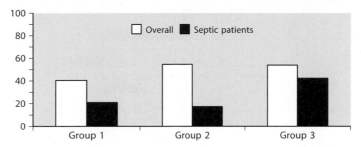

Survival rates stratified by trial group and by presence of sepsis

Group and Uf rates	No sepsis (%)	Sepsis (%)	p-value
Group 1 (20 ml/h/kg)	55/126 (44 %)	5/20 (25 %)	0.90
Group 2 (35 ml/h/kg)	76/122 (62 %)	3/17 (18 %)	0.001
Group 3 (45 ml/h/kg)	74/125 (59 %)	7/15 (47 %)	0.256

Fig. 3. Survival rates observed in patients treated with different hemofiltration doses. While the effect is evident in the overall population from group 1 to group 2 and no further effect is observed in group 3, when patients are stratified for sepsis, a significant effect of higher doses of treatment is observed in group 3. Uf: ultrafiltration

when the animals developed the clinical picture of hyperdynamic septic shock. HVHF was superior in all mentioned endpoints and, importantly, increasing ultrafiltration had more effect than frequency of filter change [32].

Of major influence concerning human sepsis studies has been the finding that ultrafiltration dose is correlated to outcome in critically ill patients with acute renal failure. In a large, randomized, controlled study including 425 patients, an ultrafiltration dose of 35 ml/kg/h increased survival rate from 41 to 57% compared to a dose of 20 ml/kg/h [35]. Eleven to 14% (per randomization group) of the patients had sepsis. In these subgroups there was a trend of direct correlation of treatment dose with survival even above 35 ml/kg/h in contrast to the whole group where a survival plateau was reached (Fig. 3).

This lends support to the concept of a 'sepsis dose' of hemofiltration in septic patients contrasting to a 'renal dose' in critically ill patients without systemic inflammation, the former being probably distinctly higher (without proven upper limit). Of note there was no increase in adverse effects even with the highest ultrafiltration dose.

Over recent years, several human studies have examined the clinical effects of high-volume hemofiltration. In 20 children undergoing cardiac surgery, zero-balanced HVHF was administered with ultrafiltration rates equivalent to 7–9 l/h for a 70 kg adult [36]. Endpoints correlating to the cardiopulmonary-bypass associated delayed inflammatory response were examined. There was a significant reduction in post-operative blood loss and time to extubation, and improvement in the arterial-alveolar oxygen gradient.

In a prospective cohort analysis in 306 critically ill patients with varying underlying diseases a mean ultrafiltration rate of 3.8 l/h was applied [37]. Observed survival rates were significantly higher in the treated population compared to predicted survival by three well validated scores.

A study in 12 critically ill patients with acute renal failure comparing low-volume CVVH (1500 ml/h) with a high-volume technique was performed in a non-

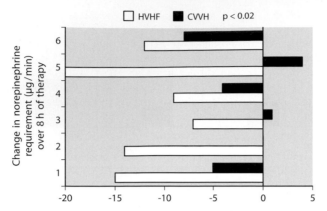

Fig. 4. Significant reduction in norepinephrine requirement is observed in unstable septic patients treated with high volume hemofiltration (HVHF). Less evident is the effect of low volume continuous veno-venous hemofiltration (CVVH)

randomized, comparative fashion [38]. High-flux bicarbonate dialysis amounting to 4200 ml/h was used and the effect on monocyte responsiveness (*ex vivo* endotoxin-stimulated TNF production) was studied. Both techniques resulted in early improvement but persistent effects were only displayed with the high-volume technique. The ultrafiltrate contained monocyte-suppressive activity only with high-flux dialysis.

In another trial in 11 septic patients with shock and MOF, a randomized cross-over design of 6 l/h vs. 1 l/h ultrafiltration was applied [39]. The HVHF group displayed significantly greater reduction in vasopressor requirements (Fig. 4). Both treatment groups showed a decrease in C3a and C5a plasma levels which was significantly greater in the HVHF group.

Impressive clinical results were obtained in an evaluation of short-term HVHF in 20 patients with catecholamine-refractory septic shock [40] comprising a patient cohort with very poor expected survival. A control group was not defined. Only one four-hour session of HVHF removing 35 l of ultrafiltrate replaced by bicarbonate-containing fluid was applied as soon as mean blood pressure could not be stabilized above 70 mmHg with dopamine, norepinephrine, and epinephrine after appropriate volume resuscitation. HVHF was followed by conventional CVVH. Endpoints were an increase in cardiac index, mixed venous oxygen saturation (SvO_2), and arterial pH, and decrease in epinephrine requirements. Eleven patients reached all predefined endpoints and showed impressively good survival (9 of 11) at 28 days. Nine patients did not reach all endpoints and had a 100% mortality rate. Apart from responding to HVHF, only time from ICU admission to start of HVHF and body weight were survival-associated factors in the analysis. Patients with higher body weight did worse possibly because they received a smaller ultrafiltration dose per body weight, as speculated by the authors.

These trials still need cautious interpretation with respect to their limited design but they certainly deliver sound evidence of feasibility and efficacy to set the stage for a large-scale trial on HVHF in sepsis.

▮ Unresolved Issues

Ultrafiltration is associated with loss of a vast array of water-soluble substances. Not all of these losses are desirable and many have not been characterized quantitatively [41] or even qualitatively. HVHF constitutes a major intervention in acid-base balance as many strong ions and, up to now, poorly defined small to middle molecular acids (and bases) of intermediate metabolism are filtered. Furthermore, lactate replacement fluid leads to hyperlactatemia that possibly can be tolerated well even in septic shock (Cole et al., unpublished data) but not in all patient groups [42, 43]. Bicarbonate replacement would appear physiologic but is very expensive and not available in many parts of the world.

Losses of hormones, vitamins, molecules of intermediate metabolism, and amino acids in HVHF have not been studied up to now. As CRRT can be regarded as a powerful metabolic intervention (constituting a continuous plasma water exchange), its intensification by using HVHF may encompass undefined dangers (by loss of specific substances, by high lactate loads). On the other hand, HVHF possibly opens a therapeutic avenue to administer substances with specific metabolic activity without volume restriction (e.g., inosine [44], pyruvate [45]).

Another issue involves the modification of thermal energy balance especially when high volumes of fluid are exchanged. Specific studies have not been carried out, but an increasing consensus exists on the need for a fluid warmer in the newly designed machines.

▮ Methodological Aspects of HVHF

Major methodological details in using a technique which requires a fluid exchange rate of 6 l/h and more (possibly up to 10 l/h that would equal about 140 ml/kg in a 70 kg adult) have to be considered. To avoid excessive hemoconcentration within the filter with consequent clotting problems, high blood flows in the range of 400 to 500 ml/min have to be applied. For the same reason, at least part of the replacement fluid has to be administered in a predilution mode. This may reduce middle molecule clearance proportionally by the dilutional effect at filter entry [46].

Certainly high volumes increase the risks of technical problems (catheter problems, disconnection, dosing errors). Catheters have to be large to tolerate blood flows at least above 300 ml/min. High blood flows must be maintained at all times and in variable patient positions with minimal recirculation. Consequently, the technique needs a high degree of supervision by experienced personnel exclusively devoted to the treated patient. Most practical in this respect seems to be an intermittent technique with HVHF over 4 to 8 hours during daytime embedded in conventional CVVH for the rest of the day. Furthermore, high amounts of replacement fluids are needed which may try financial limits. Systems designed for in-line preparation of fluids by cascade filtration may have to be considered.

Obviously the hemofiltration machine is vital for the safe performance of HVHF. First, machines need to be capable of administering volumes in this range including warming capacity. Further safety regards are appropriate pressure monitoring, exactness in applying high volumes, and calculating balances. Certainly a friendly user interface and ease of use is a must (Fig. 5).

The Aquarius Hemofiltration machine (ELS, Germany) has been developed specifically to reach the above-mentioned goals and serves as a representative of the

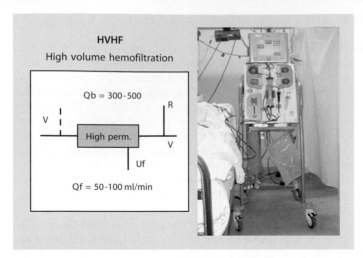

Fig. 5. High volume hemofiltration (HVHF) performed either in pre- or postdilution modes (machine: Aquarius from Edwards Life Sciences GmbH, Unterschleissheim, Germany). Qb: Blood flow; V: venous access; Uf: ultrafiltrate; Qf: ultrafiltrate flow; R: replacement fluid

latest generation of machines in the field. In this machine, HVHF can be performed in addition to all other types of blood purification therapies considered for use in the ICU. Blood flows required for effective HVHF in the range of 300 to 450 ml/min can be programmed. Ultrafiltration rates in the range of 6 l/h (requiring replacement fluid infusion rates of about 100 ml/min) can be prescribed as well. The Aquarius machine delivers pump flow rates up to 450 ml/min for blood, up to 10 l/h for pre- or post-dilution replacement, and up to 2000 ml/h for additional fluid removal.

Volume accuracy as well as sensitive, fast-response pressure monitoring is of utmost importance in these high ranges. This aspect is properly realized with scales ensuring substitution and filtrate volume accuracy with 0.1% precision. Pump accuracy reaches 5%. Only a 50 g deviation of the target value is permitted before alarming will be activated. Precision within this range is obligatory for HVHF. Replacement fluid can be administered in a pre- and post-dilution mode, and concurrently. Pressure monitoring is installed in the access and return line as well as in a prefilter position and in the ultrafiltrate compartment. Sensor accuracy amounts to +/–5 mmHg. The pressure sensors operate without blood-air interface. Air embolism is prevented by an ultrasonic air detector which controls a line clamp. Effective heating capacity is essential when high volumes are processed. Otherwise major energy losses and possibly severe hypothermia could be induced in the patient. For this purpose the machine uses a coil-tubing design which ensures heating up to 39 °C for up to 6 l/h fluid turnover.

HVHF is a high-risk procedure regarding immediate consequences of technical or user errors. In order to minimize the probability of their occurrence, user-friendly properties are of high priority. This need is served by the concept of a one-button machine. A single selector knob guides all functions supported by a self-explanatory screen.

▮ Other Approaches to High Efficiency Blood Purification in Sepsis

Cytokines and other immunomodulating substances generally have molecular weights in the range from 5 to 50 kDa. These substances may be eliminated by diffusion, convection, or adsorption depending on the material and the rather variable cut-off of highly permeable membranes (from 30 to 40 kDa) [17]. As adsorptive processes easily saturate and are therefore transient, the effect of CRRT on sepsis could be limited because of a low convective clearance of many mediators.

Therefore, other approaches to achieve higher mediator clearance in sepsis have been sought. Apart from increasing ultrafiltration rates, higher removal rates of middle molecular weight molecules could be achieved by enlarging membrane pore size. Animal data [47, 48] as well as preliminary clinical data [49] demonstrate feasibility and probable superior removal rates of select cytokines using larger cut-off membranes.

A study in 30 patients with severe sepsis using continuous plasma filtration for 34 h [50] found attenuation of the acute phase response and a trend towards clinical benefit although not significant (fewer failing organs). A further refinement has been achieved with plasma filtration coupled with adsorption and followed by dialysis or filtration (Fig. 6) [51]. This would allow effective removal of mediators in the borderline zone of filtration by hemofilters (40 to 60 kDa) without the need for exogenous plasma replacement. Furthermore, higher plasma clearance rates could be achieved. An animal study [52] and a first clinical trial reported beneficial effects on hemodynamic and immune cell function [25, 53].

Conclusions on efficiency would be premature to draw. Taking the available data together, more studies are required to see a major advantage in laboratory and clinical endpoints with plasma filtration compared to ultrafiltration techniques. Certainly larger pore size membranes and plasma filtration combined with sorbent

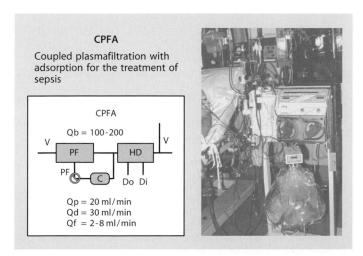

Fig. 6. Coupled plasma filtration with adsorption (CPFA). Plasma filtered in a plasma filtration unit is circulated through an adsorbent cartridge and then returned to the main stream. Reconstituted blood is then dialyzed (machine: Multimat B from Bellco s.p.a. Mirandola, Italy). Qb: Blood flow; V: venous access; Uf: ultrafiltrate; Qf: ultrafiltrate flow rate; R: replacement fluid; PF: plasma filtrate; Do: dialysate outlet; Di: dialysate inlet; Qp: plasma flow rate; Qd: dialysate flow rate

techniques enlarge the therapeutic armamentarium significantly. They constitute a promising adjunctive modality easy to use in combination with hemofiltration.

▌ Conclusion

A vast array of mostly water-soluble mediators play a strategic role in the septic syndrome. Compared to eliminating or completely antagonizing single mediators, therapeutic intervention by non-selective removal of pro- and anti-inflammatory mediators seems a rational and possibly superior concept. A further advantage seems to be gained by having a continuously acting therapy, as in the case of CRRT. Hereby, sequentially appearing peaks of systemic mediator overflow could be curbed as well as reducing persistently high plasma levels. This process is proposed as the underlying biological rationale for a series of innovative therapies in sepsis. The whole story of antagonizing pro- and anti-inflammatory processes by reducing the relative excess of active substances has been termed the 'peak concentration hypothesis'.

Recent animal and human trials have delivered much support to this concept. It has been conclusively shown that treatment dose in CRRT is a major factor concerning survival in acute renal failure in the critically ill patient. There is accumulating evidence of increased efficacy of high volume hemofiltration compared to conventional CVVH in terms of laboratory and clinical improvement including survival. Machines to perform HVHF safely are available on the market.

Yet, the evidence is still not strong enough to recommend HVHF outside clinical studies, taking into account the possible adverse effects of the technique. A large-scale clinical trial is urgently needed to resolve the issue.

Other blood purification techniques using large pore membranes or plasma filtration with sorbent perfusion are in the early stages of clinical testing. They are conceptually promising and possibly constitute an important refinement.

References

1. Pinsky MR (2001) Sepsis: a pro- and anti-inflammatory disequilibrium syndrome. Contrib Nephrol 132:354–366
2. Adrie C, Pinsky MR (2000) The inflammatory balance in human sepsis. Intensive Care Med 26:364–375
3. Casey LC, Balk RA, Bone RC (1993) Plasma cytokine and endotoxin levels correlate with survival in patients with the sepsis syndrome. Ann Intern Med 15:771- 778
4. Pinsky MR, Vincent JL, Deviere J, Alegre M, Kahn RJ, Dupont E (1993) Serum cytokine levels in human septic shock. Relation to multiple-system organ failure and mortality. Chest 103:565–575
5. Adib-Conquy M, Adrie C, Moine P, et al (2000) NF-kB expression in mononuclear cells of septic patients resembles that observed in LPS tolerance. Am J Respir Crit Care Med 162: 1877–1883
6. Van Dissel JT, van Langevelde P, Westendorp RG, Kwappenberg K, Froelich M (1998) Anti-inflammatory cytokine profile and mortality in febrile patients. Lancet 351:950-953
7. Klosterhalfen B, Horstmann-Jungemann K, Vogel P, et al (1991) Hemodynamic variables and plasma levels of PGI2, TXA2 and IL-6 in a porcine model of recurrent endotoxemia. Circ Shock 35:237–244
8. Abraham E, Matthay M, Dinarello CA, et al (2000) Consensus Conference definitions for sepsis, septic shock, acute lung injury, and acute respiratory distress syndrome: time for a reevaluation. Crit Care Med 28:232–235

9. Abraham E, Glauser MP, Butler T, et al (1997) p55 tumor necrosis factor receptor fusion protein in the treatment of patients with severe sepsis and septic shock. A randomized controlled multicenter trial. Ro 45-2081 study group. JAMA 277:1531–1538

10. Fisher CJ, Agosti JM, Opal SM (1996) Treatment of septic shock with the tumor necrosis factor receptor: Fc fusion protein. New Engl J Med 334:1697–1702

11. Echtenacher B, Falk W, Mannel D, Krammer PH (1990) Requirement of endogenous tumour necrosis factor/cachectin for recovery from experimental peritonitis. J Immunol 145:3762–3766

12. Van der Meer JWM (1988) The effects of recombinant interleukin-1 and recombinant tumor necrosis factor on non-specific resistance to infection. Biotherapy 1:19–25

13. Ronco C, Ricci Z, Bellomo R (2001) Importance of increased ultrafiltration volume and impact on mortality: sepsis and cytokine story and the role of continuous veno-venous hemofiltration. Curr Opin Nephrol Hypertens 10:755–761

14. De Vriese AS, Vanholder RC, Pascual M, Lameire NH, Colardyn FA (1999) Can inflammatory cytokines be removed efficiently by continuous renal replacement therapies? Intensive Care Med 25:903–910

15. Hoffmann JN, Hartl WH, Deppisch R, Faist E, Jochum M, Inthorn D (1995) Hemofiltration in human sepsis: evidence for elimination of immunomodulatory substances. Kidney Int 48:1563–1570

16. Gasche Y, Pascual M, Suter PM, Favre H, Chevrolet JC, Schifferli JA (1996) Complement depletion during haemofiltration with polyacetonitrile membranes. Nephrol Dial Transplant 11:117–119

17. Kellum JA, Johnson JP, Kramer D, Palevsky P, Brady JJ, Pinsky MR (1998) Diffusive vs. convective therapy: effects on mediators of inflammation in patients with severe systemic inflammatory response syndrome. Crit Care Med 26:1995–2000

18. Goldfarb J, Golper TA (1994) Proinflammatory cytokines and hemofiltration membranes. Am Soc Nephrol 5:228–232

19. Braun N, Giolai M, Rosenfeld S, et al (1993) Clearance of interleukin-6 during continuous veno-venous hemofiltration in patients with septic shock. A prospective, controlled clinical study. J Am Soc Nephrol 4:336 (Abst)

20. Mariano F, Tetta C, Guida GE, Triolo G, Camussi G (2001) Hemofiltration reduces the priming activity on neutrophil chemiluminescence in septic patients. Kidney Int 60:1598–1605

21. Ronco C, Tetta C, Lupi A, et al (1995) Removal of platelet-activating factor in experimental continuous arteriovenous hemofiltration. Crit Care Med 23:99–107

22. Sander A, Armbruster W, Sander B, Daul AE, Lange R, Peters J (1997) Haemofiltration increases IL-6 clearance in early systemic inflammatory response syndrome but does not alter IL-6 and TNF alpha plasma concentrations. Intensive Care Med 23:878–884

23. Heering P, Morgera S, Schmitz FJ, et al (1997) Cytokine removal and cardiovascular hemodynamics in septic patients with continuous venovenous hemofiltration. Intensive Care Med 23:288–296

24. Munoz C, Carlet J, Fitting C, Misset B, Bleriot JP, Cavaillon JM (1991) Dysregulation of in vitro cytokine production by monocytes during sepsis. J Clin Invest 88:1747–1754

25. Ronco C, Brendolan A, Lonnemann G, et al (2002) A randomized cross-over study on couplet plasma filtration with adsorption in septic shock. Crit Care Med (in press)

26. Grootendorst AF, van Bommel EFH, van der Hoven B, van Leengoed LAM, van Osta ALM (1992) High volume hemofiltration improves hemodynamics of endotoxin-induced shock in the pig. J Crit Care 7:67–75

27. Grootendorst AF, van Bommel EFH, van der Hoven B, van Leengoed LAM, van Osta ALM (1992) High volume hemofiltration improves right ventricular function of endotoxin-induced shock in the pig. Intensive Care Med 18:235–240

28. Grootendorst AF, van Bommel EFH, van Leengoed LAM, van Zanten AR, Huipen HJ, Groeneveld AB (1993) Infusion of ultrafiltrate from endotoxemic pigs depresses myocardial performance in normal pigs. J Crit Care 8:161–169

29. Grootendorst AF, van Bommel EFH, van Leengoed LAM, Naburus M, Bouman CSC, Groeneveld ABJ (1994) High volume hemofiltration improves hemodynamics and survival of pigs exposed to gut ischemia and reperfusion. Shock 2:72–78

30. Lee PA, Matson JR, Pryor RW, Hinshaw LB (1993) Continuous arteriovenous hemofiltration therapy for staphylococcus aureus-induced septicemia in immature swine. Crit Care Med 21:914–924
31. Rogiers P, Zhang H, Smail N, Auwels D, Vincent JL (1999) Continuous venovenous hemofiltration improves cardiac performance by mechanisms other than tumor necrosis factor-alpha attenuation during endotoxic shock. Crit Care Med 27:1848–1855
32. Yekebas EF, Eisenberger CF, Ohnesorge H, et al (2001) Attenuation of sepsis-related immunoparalysis by continuous veno-venous hemofiltration in experimental porcine pancreatitis. Crit Care Med 29:1423–1430
33. Nagashima M, Shin'oka T, Nollert G, Shum-Tim D, Rader CM, Mayer JE Jr (1998) High-volume continuous hemofiltration during cardiopulmonary bypass attenuates pulmonary dysfunction in neonatal lambs after deep hypothermic circulatory arrest. Circulation 98 (Suppl 19):II378–II384
34. Bellomo R, Kellum JA, Gandhi CR, Pinsky MR (2000) The effect of intensive plasma water exchange by hemofiltration on hemodynamics and soluble mediators in canine endotoxemia. Am J Respir Crit Care Med 161:1429–1436
35. Ronco C, Bellomo R, Homel P, et al (2000) Effects of different doses in continuous veno-venous haemofiltration on outcomes of acute renal failure: a prospective randomised trial. Lancet 356:26–30
36. Journois D, Israel Biet D, Pouard P, et al (1996) High-volume, zero-balanced hemofiltration to reduce delayed inflammatory response to cardiopulmonary bypass in children. Anesthesiology 85:965–976
37. Oudemans-van Straaten HM, Bosman RJ, van der Spoe JI, Zandstra DF (1999) Outcome of critically ill patients treated with intermittent high-volume haemofiltration: a prospective cohort analysis. Intensive Care Med 25:814–821
38. Lonnemann G, Bechstein M, Linnenweber S, Burg M, Koch KM (1999) Tumor necrosis factor-alpha during continuous high-flux hemodialysis in sepsis with acute renal failure. Kidney Int 56 (Suppl 72):S84–S87
39. Cole L, Bellomo R, Journois D, Davenport P, Baldwin I, Tipping P (2001) High-volume hemofiltration in human septic shock. Intensive Care Med 27:978–986
40. Honore PM, Jamez J, Wauthier M, et al (2000) Prospective evaluation of short-term, high-volume isovolemic hemofiltration on the hemodynamic course and outcome in patients with intractable circulatory failure resulting from septic shock. Crit Care Med 28:3581–3587
41. Guth HJ, Zschiesche M, Panzig E, Rudolph PE, Jager B, Kraatz G (1999) Which organic acids does hemofiltrate contain in the presence of acute renal failure? Int J Artif Organs 22:805–810
42. Barenbrock M, Hausberg M, Matzkies F, de la Motte S, Schaefer RM (2000) Effects of bicarbonate- and lactate-buffered replacement fluids on cardiovascular outcome in CVVH patients. Kidney Int 58:1751–1757
43. Davenport A, Will EJ, Davison AM (1991) Hyperlactatemia and metabolic acidosis during hemofiltration using lactate-buffered fluids. Nephron 59:461–465
44. Sims CA, Wattanasirichaigoon S, Menconi MJ, Ajami AM, Fink MP (2001) Ringer's ethyl pyruvate solution ameliorates ischemia/reperfusion-induced intestinal mucosal injury in rats. Crit Care Med 29:1513–1518
45. Soriano FG, Liaudet L, Marton A, et al (2001) Inosine improves gut permeability and vascular reactivity in endotoxic shock. Crit Care Med 29:703–708
46. Bellomo R, Baldwin I, Cole L, Ronco C (1998) Preliminary experience with high-volume hemofiltration in human septic shock. Kidney Int 53 (Suppl 66):182–185
47. Lee PA, Weger G, Pryor RW, Matson JR (1998) Effects of filter pore size on efficacy of continuous arteriovenous hemofiltration therapy for staphylococcus aureus-induced septicemia in immature swine. Crit Care Med 26:730–737
48. Kline JA, Gordon BE, Williams C, Blumenthal S, Watts JA, Diaz-Buxo J (1999) Large-pore hemodialysis in acute endotoxin shock. Crit Care Med 27:588–596
49. Morgera S, Buder W, Lehmann C, et al (2000) High cut off membrane haemofiltration in septic patients with multiorgan failure. A preliminary report. Blood Purif 18:61 (Abst)

50. Reeves JH, Butt WW, Shann F, et al (1999) Continuous plasmafiltration in sepsis syndrome. Crit Care Med 27:2096–2104
51. Tetta C, Cavaillon JM, Schulze M, et al (1998) Removal of cytokines and activated complement components in an experimental model of continuous plasma filtration coupled with sorbent adsorption. Nephrol Dial Transplant 13:1458–1464
52. Tetta C, Gianotti L, Cavaillon JM, et al (2000) Coupled plasma filtration-adsorption in a rabbit model of endotoxic shock. Crit Care Med 28:1526–1533
53. Brendolan A, Bellomo R, Tetta C, et al (2001) Coupled plasma filtration adsorption in the treatment of septic shock. Contrib Nephrol 132:383–390

Adjuvant Treatment of Mediastinitis with Immunoglobulins after Cardiac Surgery: The ATMI Trial

E. Neugebauer, G. Marggraf, and R. Lefering

▌ Introduction

Immunoglobulins constitute an innovative product group with a wide spectrum of clinical use. Intravenous immunoglobulin (IVIG) solutions containing IgG in a concentration of 95% or more were introduced in the fifties primarily for the treatment of patients with humoral immunodeficiencies. In primary and secondary humoral immunodeficiencies, intravenously administered immunoglobulins replace the natural immunoglobulins and subsequently maintain the natural function of the humoral immune system. In addition, since 1981, there has been a rapid expansion of use in autoimmune diseases, in particular T-cell- and B-cell-mediated chronic neuroinflammatory diseases. The administration of high-dose IVIG is now accepted for various immune-mediated neuropathies, e.g., in the treatment of Guillain-Barré syndrome, chronic inflammatory demyelinating polyneuropathy, and multifocal motor-neuropathy. Furthermore the National Institutes of Health (NIH) consensus conference in 1990 set up a list of indications for which there was sufficient evidence to justify IVIG application: idiopathic thrombocytopenic purpura, hypogammaglobulinemia in chronic lymphatic leukemia patients, allogenic bone-marrow transplantation, and Kawasaki syndrome. The use of IVIG in the treatment of several inflammatory disorders is a more recent trend. Potential for the clinical use of immunoglobulins has been shown for inflammatory diseases/syndromes such as rheumatoid arthritis, immunovasculitis, dermatomyositis, sepsis, and others.

The mechanisms of action responsible for the efficacy in each of these disorders are, however, not yet fully understood and need further clarification. Potential mechanisms of action of IVIGs are:

- ▌ Interaction of the constant Fc region of IgG with complement activation of Fc-receptors which might result in a clearance of immune complexes.
- ▌ Variable regions of IgG in IVIG may modulate auto-antibody activity and may cause immune regulation through idiotypic network interactions.
- ▌ Antigenic specificities within the IgG pool in IVIG confer additional properties against various microbial antigens, or interact with other network participants such as cytokines and cell surface receptors (induction of anti-inflammatory cytokines, such as interleukin-1 receptor antagonist (IL-1ra)).

Each of the diverse mechanisms of action may be involved to some extent in the beneficial effect of immunoglobulins in different diseases [6].

Concerning the IVIG market in Germany, the Paul-Ehrlich Institute (PEI) has granted marketing authorization for 13 products according to the national procedure. Most of the commercially available preparations are well tolerated, and multiple infusions can be given to patients. The risk of viral transmission has been minimized by careful screening of plasma donors and by single production steps with highly effective viral removal and inactivation. Over recent years, IVIGs have become the most prescribed and administered drugs for off-label treatment (52%). Most off-label uses of IVIG are not yet supported by high quality randomized controlled clinical trials (level 1 evidence, in the notation of evidence-based medicine). It is therefore our duty to translate promising pathophysiological and immunological findings into the justification of clinical use – new indications, however, need good clinical trials.

▌ How Should a Good Clinical Trial in Inflammatory Disorders be Conducted?

The gold standard in the concept of evidence-based medicine is the randomized, controlled clinical trial (RCT level 1 evidence). The objective of a RCT is to find out whether there is a systematic difference in one or more variables, between comparable groups of patients who vary only in their exposure to the treatment being studied. Randomization maximizes the probability that the groups being compared will be similar, while blinding minimizes bias in selection and treatment of patients or evaluation of outcome. The effectiveness of the experimental intervention can be measured by using a control group as a reference. To demonstrate effectiveness it is important that the primary outcome measure in a clinical trial should evaluate clinical benefit and not simply biological activity. This requirement is particularly important in the area of modulation of the host-response, where manipulation of the inflammatory cascade produces both beneficial and detrimental effects in preclinical models [2]. Most studies use mortality as the most important outcome measure. However, if mortality is not frequently observed, measures of morbidity can be used as alternatives, particularly if the morbidity is likely to be associated with increased mortality. The problem, however, is that regulatory agencies such as the FDA have yet to embrace the use of measures other than mortality. For the investigator who is seeking a feasible and reliable marker to evaluate a new treatment, validated organ dysfunction scores such as the multiple organ dysfunction (MOD) score, or the quantification of therapeutic activities (using the therapeutic intervention scoring system, TISS) are alternative approaches to evaluate clinical benefit in such trials [3, 4].

Apart from the discussion about parameters to demonstrate clinical benefit in inflammatory disorders, there is also disagreement about the general conduct of such a study. Do we need large multicenter trials with several hundreds of patients recruited by study centers all over the world using general entry criteria, or do we rather need smaller trials with a specific disease entity and qualified study centers with homogenous treatment algorithms? The Odyssy of clinical trials in the field of sepsis should help us to answer this question. However, previous disappointments have led to different interpretations of the way to go in the future. One group of investigators took as their lesson from the past 30 years of trials of adjunctive immunomodulatory therapies in sepsis, that we need trials that involve 1600–2400 patients to obtain definitive answers for the efficacy of such compounds. The main argument is that trials with less than 400–600 patients show very inconsistent results due to the heterogeneity of sepsis patients regarding the source of sepsis and the underlying concomitant diseases. Only larger trials will show clinical benefit if there is one. Another group of investigators reject this approach but instead favor smaller trials with more homogenous groups of patients and less heterogeneity in treatment algorithms. The authors of this article are in favor of the latter approach.

Complex inflammatory disorders such as sepsis will require a multifaceted therapeutic approach – the chance of establishing the benefit of a single drug is rather small *per se* and may be possible only under standardized and controlled experimental conditions. However, the chance decreases under clinical conditions and even more if the study is performed not as a single center but as a multicenter trial (increase of noise level). To overcome these difficulties, at least two prerequisites have to be fulfilled in the design and the conduct of multicenter trials. The first prerequisite is the concentration on a specific disease entity to control for 'case mix'. The second prerequisite is homogenization of diagnostic and therapeutic treatment algorithms in the participating study centers (control of 'treatment mix'). We tried to fulfill both prerequisites in the adjuvant treatment of mediastinistis with immunoglobulins (ATMI) trial, to demonstrate the clinical benefit of Pentaglobin® for the adjuvant treatment of mediastinitis after cardiac surgery [5].

▌ Mediastinitis and the Concept of the Immunoglobulin Trial

Despite appropriate antibiotic treatment and surgical eradication of the septic focus whenever possible, we still face high mortality rates (up to 40%) after sepsis and septic shock, mostly because of multiple organ failure (MOF) [3]. Such fatal complications are also seen after open cardiac surgical procedures. Mediastinitis, which is the focus of this investigation, is a complication associated with median sternotomy in operations with a heart-lung machine and occurs in 0.4–5% of patients. The mortality under current 'standard treatment' is reported to be between 20 and 40% [7–9] mostly as a consequence of MOF. Mediastinitis usually occurs between day 4 and 30 after operation, with a peak incidence around day 14 [9, 10].

Mediastinitis is an inflammation of the mediastinum caused by pathogenic microorganisms. The bacteriology is highly variable and includes a range of methicillin-restistant staphylococci and streptococci as well as Gram-negative rods and fungi [11]. The clinical symptoms depend on the stage of development of the infection. Locally, sternal instability or dehiscence is considered the most specific and leading symptom [10].

Concerning risk factors for the development of mediastinitis (factors are mostly not differentiated), an array of non-specific variables are described such as obesity, diabetis mellitus, preoperative hypoalbuminemia, and a long operation time. In the ATMI trial, all patients to be included underwent a median sternotomy during an operation with a heart-lung machine. This means that the study population is homogenous, a key prerequisite for showing benefits of novel therapeutic drugs in multicenter trials, as outlined earlier [12]. Lumping together large groups of patients with different diseases (and infecting organisms) has the only advantage of providing a large sample in a short time, but masks any potential therapeutic benefit [13]. In sepsis, we still have to face symptoms rather than a disease and the patients' variability in their underlying health. Preoperative prophylactic antibiotics have been shown to reduce the incidence of mediastinitis after median sternotomy. They should, therefore, be a standard. But is standardization in a multicenter trial possible, necessary, or even counterproductive?

Similar difficulties can be expected in the surgical and adjuvant treatments although removal of any infected tissue is not controversial. The type of sternal closure, the use of a closed irrigation/suction system, and the composition of the solution are only some areas of considerable differences in practice between hospitals. Even if the external evidence from prospective clinical trials is weak for most of the treatments, clinicians are often unwilling to change their daily routine. They persist in their procedures and a clinical trial that needs standardization in certain important areas related to outcome has to try hard to change clinical strategies based on belief or tradition.

Timing of interaction with immunomodulating strategies is critical because in many successful experiments, treatment was given before the onset of sepsis or endotoxiemia. There is consensus that early intervention is more likely to succeed. Relatively low-cost preventive strategies should be evaluated in patients who could easily be assigned to high-risk categories.

The present trial with IgM-enriched IgG immunoglobulin (Pentaglobin®) tries to take advantage of this concept. Only those patients who develop a wound infection (closed or open wound with sternal dehiscence and inflammation) are planned to be included in the study. If sepsis is confirmed preoperatively, or the patient has a closed wound with sternal dehiscence but without inflammation, then the patient is not included. If suspected preoperative sepsis is confirmed microbiologically in the postoperative phase then the patient is withdrawn. This strategy is a further step to making the study population more homogenous and takes advantage of the mode of action of immunoglobulins. When given prophylactically in the intensive care unit (ICU) to patients with high risk of developing severe infections, IVIGs can reduce the incidence and severity of infections.

As discussed earlier, a major subject of considerable controversy in sepsis trials is the choice and the assessment of the primary outcome measure. Currently, most clinical trials use mortality as the primary endpoint. However, this approach has some difficulties because death is both a dichotomous and a non-specific variable. Death as an endpoint is also insensitive, largely regulated by comorbidity, and cause-specific mortality may be prone to bias in interpretation [14]. It has been proposed that sepsis-related morbidity, particularly the degree of organ dysfunction, could be used as surrogate for death in clinical trials. Although a composite score to characterize the degree of organ dysfunction in the course of sepsis may be an attractive alternative to death in the decision about the effect of treatment, difficulties include concerns that clinical relevance may be subjective and multiple comparisons are a problem [14]. This study on immunoglobulins (Pentaglobin®) in patients at risk of mediastinitis uses a novel approach: the primary outcome variable is the cumulative TISS-28 value during the stay in hospital until day 28. Secondary outcome variables are the duration of ICU and hospital stay, the incidence of sepsis, MOF, and mortality. Because mortality in this trial is expected to be less than 5%, it cannot serve as a sensitive primary indicator of treatment effects. The advantage of the cumulative TISS-28 value as an outcome measure is that the score provides an objective quantification of the amount of treatment and hospital care that the patients need during their stay in the ICU.

The study group expected a great number of objections against the use of TISS-28 as primary outcome measure and made this a central topic for discussion with international experts.

❚ Consensus-assisted Protocol Design

Designing clinical trials in complex inflammatory disorders is no longer a matter of only a few days or weeks, or something left to the responsibility of a single researcher or the pharmaceutical industry alone. It requires a group of investigators from various disciplines, including the pharmaceutical industry, as well as experienced clinicians from the participating center. Considerable disagreement between the centers can be expected in diagnostic criteria as well as on the so called 'standard treatment' particularly in the ICU. Hence, consensus has to be developed to create a study protocol that reflects the philosophy of all study centers and that of the scientific community. Lorenz et al. named this a consensus-assisted protocol development [15]. This is a formal process, which compromises consensus methods (e.g., a nominal group process) including all study participants, and a discussion forum with a panel of international experts not involved in the study, for criticism and help. Fulfillment of formal criteria given by the good clinical practice (GCP) guidelines is only one side of the coin – thoughtful discussion of illegibility criteria, the weighing of various clinimetric endpoints, and the analysis and influence of multiple other interventions, are more important. Lorenz and co-workers described this approach as 'the third generation of controlled clinical trial development' [15].

To leave the planning and conduct in the hands of a few, even experienced, enthusiasts (as it was at the beginning of the ATMI trial) is no longer adequate. Even though a benefit from treatment may be shown, the findings will be criticized after publication, whether justified or not. Hence pre-trial criticism is most helpful. Even if we assume that the planning group is omnipotent, the success of a trial depends not only on a good protocol.

In a multicenter trial, the participating departments should have shown previous interest and competence in the management and treatment of the disease under investigation. They should be able to accumulate an adequate number of cases per year [16]. To overcome the obstacles, the planning committee of this immunoglobulin trial in mediastinitis decided to develop a protocol in a formalized consensus-assisted process with prepublication of the protocol. Such a procedure entails important differences from current common practice [15]: changes can be introduced before the study is conducted; reasons for rejecting the criticism can be proposed before the study is published; and the complexity of the trial can be elucidated by a discussion forum published in a journal together with the final protocol. This approach increases the likelihood of results necessary to judge the effectiveness of the intervention. The consensus-assisted process of development of the protocol for the ATMI trial is briefly described in the following paragraph.

The idea comes first – methodology follows the idea [17]. Marggraf and co-workers from the Department of Thoracic and Cardiovascular Surgery of the University of Essen, Germany, set up a draft protocol with only a few pages outlining the rationale of a multicenter study of adjuvant immunoglobulins in patients with suspected mediastinitis. This draft version was sent to all clinics in Germany performing open heart surgery with a heart-lung machine. Ten centers (mostly university hospitals) showed interest and two representatives from each clinic were invited to a first study meeting in Essen in January 1997. They were asked in advance to report the number of operations in cases of mediastinitis in the previous two years and to present their current treatment strategy and outcome to all participants at that meeting. A standardized summary of all reports was prepared and pinned on a poster wall for each clinic (metaplan technique). Huge differences in case numbers, treatment methods and outcome became obvious that would partly be explained by different definitions of mediastinitis. After explanation of the aims of the trial there was unanimous agreement to develop a study protocol together with all centers following the concept of a consensus-assisted process.

After a methodological introduction to the nominal group process (NGP each clinic had one vote [5]) to reach consensus, the second part of the meeting was used to identify areas of agreement and disagreement using the NGP. This method is similar to the technique used in the development of clinical algorithms. The experience with NGP was anonymously evaluated by the participants at the end of the meeting with almost complete agreement. Comments of the participants were collected to be introduced in the second draft of the protocol. The group furthermore set up a list of questions to be discussed by external experts.

The panel of experts was selected, as for a consensus conference [18, 19], on the basis of expertise in different fields: surgeons experienced in open heart surgery, those with special experience in mediastinitis, in performing sepsis trials, in scores, and in outcomes research. There were also statisticians and an immunologist. At a second meeting a few months later, the group met again for agreement on the second draft version of the study protocol which included the points of agreement of the first meeting. Moreover, the group decided that the experts should be invited to criticize the design as a whole, and for specific topics to be covered by different experts. Ten of the eleven invited experts submitted their papers. A third meeting of the same group took place in November 1997 to discuss the comments of the experts, to group and to discuss them in a second NGP. This translated into the third draft version of the protocol and a response paper to the criticism of the experts [5]. After foundation of an independent data monitoring committee, a fourth group meeting took place to discuss further details and criticisms of the Paul-Ehrlich In-

Table 1. Summary of study characteristics of the ATMI trial

▌ Type of study	Phase III
▌ Purpose of study	Investigation of the clinical efficacy of Pentaglobin® when used in conjunction with conventional treatment in patients with wound infection after median sternotomy
▌ Medication	PENTA924
	a) Group A, Active preparation comprising human immunoglobulin as Pentaglobin®
	b) Group B, Placebo: 5% glucose solution containing 1% human albumin
▌ Dosage	5 ml/kg body weight PENTA924 daily for 5 days intravenous infusion
▌ Route	
▌ Study design	prospective, placebo-controlled, double blind, randomized, multicenter
▌ Planned number of patients to be studied	n=120
	60 patients given Pentaglobin®
	60 patients given placebo
▌ Primary endpoint:	the cumulative TISS-28 during stay in hospital (maximum 28 days) will be used as primary outcome measure

TISS: therapeutic intervention scoring system

stitute (responsible for marketing authorization in Germany). Furthermore, as suggested by one of the experts, people were trained to calculate the TISS-28 with sample cases. After the meeting, the final protocol was written and distributed to all study centers.

The whole process of protocol development was well received by all participating centers despite more two years of planning. It can serve as an example of a novel trial design.

In parallel to the consensus-assisted process, the contributions of the experts, the response of the group (agreement and disagreement), and the final study protocol were published in a supplement issue of the European Journal of Surgery [5]. The ATMI study group is convinced that if immunoglobulins (Pentaglobin®) have an adjuvant effect on the clinical course of wound infections after sternotomy, it should be shown in this trial. The first patient was entered in January 1999. A summary of the study characteristics is given in Table 1.

▌ Biometry

The null-hypothesis of the study is that the cumulative TISS-28 during the treatment with the test medication is larger than/or equal to the cumulative TISS-28 score in the placebo group. Thus, if this hypothesis could be rejected it proves that patients given Pentaglobin® need less therapeutic support than placebo patients. It is planned to carry out two interim analysis using an adaptive design. The required number of cases was calculated assuming a difference of at least 28 TISS-28 points which approximately equals one day of ICU care. For group comparison, the nonparametric Mann-Whitney U-Test will be used. For the first interim analysis 2×33 patients are to be randomized in phase 1. If the p-value exceeds $a_0 = 0.4$ the study will be discontinued. On the other hand, if a large effect is observed ($a_1 = 0.0116$) the study will be terminated as well but successfully (rejection of null hypothesis). Only if the calculated p value is between a_1 and a_0 an adjusted calculation of sample size for the second phase will be performed, based on the data of phase one. The decision whether to continue the study or not will be decided by the Independent Data Monitoring Committee (IDMC).

▌ Conclusion

Current clinical management algorithms have not significantly reduced the incidence of infection or mortality of mediastinitis after cardiac surgery over the past 20 years. New therapeutic and prophylactic methods need to be evaluated in the treatment of mediastinitis and sepsis in usually immuno-compromised patients. One promising early therapeutic/prophylactic concept is the 'substitution' of immunoglobulins. A few inconclusive studies have shown that immunoglobulins may be effective in this inflammatory disorder. We are performing a prospective placebo-controlled double blind, randomized, multicenter, phase III trial with a novel approach of study design (consensus-assisted protocol design) using the cumulative TISS-28 score as the primary outcome measure.

References

1. Hures V, Kasatchkine MD, Vassilev T, et al (1997) Pooled normal human polyspecific IgM contains neutralizing anti-idiotypes to IgG autoantibodies of autoimmune patients and protects from experimental autoimmune disease. Blood 90:4004–4013
2. Marshall JC (1994) Infection and the host septic response contribute independently to adverse outcome in critical illness: implications for clinical trials of mediator antagonism. In: Vincent JL (ed) Yearbook of Intensive Care and Emergency Medicine. Springer, Heidelberg, pp 1–13
3. Marshall JC (1999) Organ dysfunction as an outcome measure in clinical trias. Eur J Surg Suppl 584:62–67
4. Lefering R (1999) Biostatistical outcome evaluation using TISS-28. Eur J Surg Suppl 584:56–61
5. Neugebauer E, Marggraf G, Lefering R (1999) Immunoglobulins in inflammation: Consensus-assisted protocol development and discussion forum of the ATMI trial. Eur J Surg Suppl 584
6. Kasatchkine MD, Kaveri SV (2001) Immunomodulation of autoimmune and inflammatory diseases with intravenous immune globulin. N Engl J Med 345:747–755
7. Loop FD, Lytle BW, Cosgrove DM, et al (1990) Sternal wound complications after isolated coronary artery bypass grafting: early and late mortality, morbidity, and cost of care. Ann Thorac Surg 49:179–187
8. Ottino G, DePaulis R, Pansini S, et al (1987) Major sternal wound infection after open-heart surgery: a multivariate analysis of risk factors in 2579 consecutive operative procedures. Ann Thorac Surg 44:173–179
9. Scarr MG, Gott VL, Townsend TR (1984) Mediastinal infection after cardiac surgery. Ann Thorac Surg 38:415–423
10. Marggraf G, Splittgerber FH, Knox M, et al (1999) Mediastinitis after cardiac surgery – epidemiology and current treatment. Eur J Surg 584:12–16
11. Solomkin JS (1999) Microbiology and antibiotic treatment: discussion forum on a study protocol on adjuvant treatment of mediastinitis with immunoglobulin (Pentaglobin®) after cardiac surgery (ATMI). Eur J Surg Suppl 584:43–44
12. Neugebauer E (1994) Multicentre trials in sepsis and septic shock – necessary prerequisites elaborated on the trial of supplement immunoglobulin treatment of Pilz et al. Theor Surg 9:60–62
13. Opal SM (1996) Criticism of clinical trials in sepsis and organ dysfunction. In: Gullo A (ed) Sepsis and Organ Failure, Vol 4. APICE, Trieste, pp 29–41
14. Sibbald WI, Vincent IL (1995) Round table conference on clinical trials for the treatment of sepsis. Intensive Care Med 21:184–189
15. Lorenz W, Neugebauer E, Pilz G, et al (1994) Methodology of clinical trials in sepsis-introduction. Theor Surg 9:10–11
16. Schein M, Assalia A (1994) The role of planned reoperations and laparotomy in severe intraabdominal infection: is a prospective randomized trial possible? Theor Surg 9:38–42
17. Troidl H, McKneally MF, Mulder DS, et al (1997) Surgical Research. Basic Principles and Clinical Practice, 3rd edn. Springer, New York
18. Neugebauer E, Troidl H (1995) Consensus methods as tools to assess medical technologies. Surg Endosc 9:481–482 (Abst)
19. Neugebauer E, Troidl H, Kum CK, et al (1995) The E. A. E. S. Consensus Development Conferences on laparoscopic cholecystectomy, appendectomy, and hernia repair. Consensus statements. Surg Endosc 9:550–563

The Immunomodulatory Effects of Anesthetic and Analgesic Agents

C. Kummer, F. S. Netto, and J. C. Marshall

Introduction

Anesthetic and sedative agents are among the most commonly used medications in critically ill patients. They alleviate pain and anxiety, and facilitate intensive care unit (ICU) care by rendering tolerable interventions that would otherwise be akin to torture – mechanical ventilation, dressing changes, cardioversion, and invasive procedures such as line insertion or bronchoscopy, to name a few. These agents modulate the function of the central and peripheral nervous systems. However they have effects on other organs that are often unanticipated, and occasionally profound.

The possibility that narcotic drugs might also exert immunomodulatory effects arose from the observation that intravenous drug abusers have a higher incidence of infections than non-abusers. In addition to infectious complications resulting directly from inadequate antisepsis, contaminated samples, frequent punctures with consequent thrombophlebitis, or accidents such as arterial embolism, narcotics abusers were also known to develop serious infections that were not acquired by the intravenous route, including tuberculosis, abscesses, bacterial pneumonias, and soft tissue infections [1].

Multiple factors can modulate immune function in critically ill patients, including age- and gender-related variations in immune competence, genetic polymorphisms for cytokines and their receptors, the neuroendocrine stress response to trauma, hypotension, or blood transfusion, and drugs such as steroids, histamine-2 receptor antagonists, and quinolone antibiotics. Anesthetic and sedative agents also interfere with multiple aspects of immune function [2], raising concerns about their prolonged use in critically ill ICU patients.

This brief chapter summarizes the known and potential effects of analgesic and anesthetic agents on immune function in critically ill patients, recognizing that the interplay between immune and neurologic function is extensive, and largely unexplored.

Opiate Alkaloids

A broad range of effects on the function of the immune system has been ascribed to opioid compounds [3]; these are summarized in Table 1. As the prototypical alkaloid opioid, morphine has been the most intensively studied member of this class. The immunomodulatory activity of opioids is both direct and indirect. Their direct influence occurs through an interaction with opioid receptors expressed on immune cells; their indirect effects arise through an influence on the central nervous system (CNS) and the hypothalamic-pituitary-adrenal (HPA) axis. Thus, mor-

Table 1. Effects of opioids on immune cell function

Cell Type	Effect
▪ **Neutrophils**	↓ Phagocytosis ↑ Spontaneous, but ↓ stimulated chemotaxis No effect on adherence or respiratory burst
▪ **Monocytes/Macrophages**	↓ Phagocytosis Altered cytokine production ↑ Apoptosis
▪ **Lymphocytes**	↓ Adherence ↑ Spontaneous, but ↓ stimulated motility ↓ Production of IL-2, interferon γ ↑ Synthesis of TGF-β ↑ CCRC expression ↓ T cell proliferation ↓ Antibody synthesis ↓ NK cell activity

IL: interleukin; TGF: transforming growth factor; NK: natural killer

phine can increase plasma levels of corticotropin releasing hormone (CRH), ACTH, and glucocorticoids [4].

Leukocyte Opioid Receptors

The first evidence for opioid receptors on human peripheral blood T-lymphocytes appeared in 1979 [5]. Pharmacological studies demonstrated μ-, δ- and κ-opioid receptors, as well as non-classical opioid-like receptors, on multiple types of immune cell [6, 7]. It has been proposed, on the basis of binding studies, that the μ receptors on human granulocytes are different from the peptide-opioid binding sites on these cells. The discovery of an opiate alkaloid-selective and opioid peptide-insensitive receptor, designated μ_3 [7], suggested that opiate alkaloids, such as morphine, may have actions that are distinct from those of opioid peptides. The μ_3 receptor is expressed predominantly on macrophages and other immune cells, and is distinguished from the classic neuronal opioid receptor subtypes on the basis of pharmacologic and biochemical properties.

Certain opiate alkaloids, benzomorphanes, and other drugs bind to classic opioid receptors, but not to the μ_3 receptor. The 6-glucuronide, but not the 3-glucuronide metabolite of morphine, binds to the μ_3 receptor. Opiates such as fentanyl, remifentanil and alfentanil had no significant effect *in vitro* on certain human neutrophil functions [8, 9], suggesting that those agents are poor ligands for the μ_3 opiate receptor. The existence of distinct receptor types can explain the divergent effects of the alkaloids and the opioid peptides on immune cell function. In general, the non-peptide opioids (alkaloids) are functionally suppressive, while the peptides (endogenous) are stimulatory.

The intracellular processes activated by engagement of the μ_3 opiate receptor are incompletely understood. It has been suggested that the immunomodulatory effects of morphine result, in part, through stimulation of nitric oxide (NO) production in neutrophils, monocytes, and endothelial cells [10]. Moreover, in human neutrophils and monocytes, morphine can attenuate lipopolysaccharide (LPS)-induced nuclear factor-kappa B (NF-κB) activation by a NO-coupled mechanism, and in a naloxone antagonizable manner [11]. Yet another avenue through which opiates may regulate immune cell function is through the enzyme, neutral endopeptidase 24.11 (NEP). NEP regulates cellular activation by degrading one or more of its neuropeptide substrates, and is itself regulated by the degree of immune cell activation. For example, following cell stimulation by tumor necrosis factor (TNF), the activity of NEP is increased, with the result that the cell's subsequent response to a neuropeptide is downregulated. NEP activation may represent the mechanism responsible for the loss of responsiveness following repetitive cell stimulation during chronic administration of opioids [3]. Morphine can also upregulate NEP in nervous tissue.

Opiate Alkaloids in the Nervous System

The discovery of endogenous morphine-like substances in the nervous system stimulated interest in their functional significance. Dopamine is a precursor in the morphine synthetic pathway, and at least some of morphine's immunomodulatory effects seem to be mediated via the CNS [12]. The exact class of receptor involved within the nervous system is still unclear, however recent studies have suggested that the activation of μ-opioid receptors, but not δ- or κ-receptors, is sufficient to produce immunomodulatory effects [13].

Effects of Opiate Alkaloids on Immune Cell Function

Phagocytosis, Adherence and Motility. Morphine has been reported to inhibit such leukocyte functions as adherence, phagocytosis and motility [3, 14, 15], although the effects are inconsistent [16]. Morphine reduces the phagocytic activity of both monocytes and neutrophils [17], and the capacity of murine macrophages and neutrophils to phagocytose *Candida albicans* is reduced following *in vivo* and *in vitro* administration of morphine [18]. Chronic exposure to morphine, however, results in loss of this inhibitory activity [19]. Interestingly, when morphine was withdrawn following prolonged administration, further inhibition of phagocytosis occurred.

In contrast to their inhibitory effects on phagocytosis, morphine and endogenous opioids have been reported to enhance the chemotaxis of human monocytes and neutrophils [7, 20] when administered alone, although opioid pre-treatment results in inhibition of neutrophil or monocyte chemotaxis in response to complement-derived chemotactic factors, or to chemokines such as interleukin (IL)-8 or monocyte chemoattractant protein (MCP)-1 [20].

Lymphoid Cell Function. μ-, κ- and δ-opioids reduce the capacity of B cells to generate antibodies [21]. Studies in heroin addicts show increased susceptibility to infection in association with decreased T-lymphocyte proliferative responses to mitogenic stimulation [22]. Acute administration of morphine to rats has been shown to suppress T- and B-cell proliferation to mitogen stimulation, to decrease IL-2 and interferon (IFN) production, to suppress primary antibody production, and to alter natural killer (NK) cell activity [23].

The Opioid-cytokine Connection. Opioids share many properties of cytokines, the principal soluble effector molecules of innate immunity. Complex interactions between cytokines and opioids are manifest within the nervous system. Both of these classes of molecule serve roles in intercellular communication, functioning as neurotransmitters or as modulators of neuronal activity. Cytokine effects on the CNS can be modulated by endogenous opioids, and the neural effects of opioids can be altered by cytokines [24]. It has been shown, for example, that μ-, δ- and κ-opioid agonists can alter cytokine levels in macrophage cultures [25], as well as in murine and human microglial cells [26]. Low doses of morphine augment, whereas high doses of morphine inhibit LPS-induced nuclear translocation of the transcription factor, NF-κB [27]. Still other studies have suggested that morphine can stimulate the release of transforming growth factor (TGF)-β by peripheral blood mononuclear cells (PBMC) [28], an activity that may explain the immunosuppressive properties of the drug. A recent study demonstrated that human lymphocytes express the chemokine receptor CCR5 at higher levels when treated with morphine sulphate [29].

Apoptosis of Immune Cells. Morphine induces apoptosis in monocytes, including peritoneal macrophages from rats, the murine macrophage cell line J774.16, and human PBMC [30, 31]. Naloxone inhibits the apoptosis induced by morphine, indicating that this effect is mediated through an interaction with opioid receptors. It has been suggested that morphine activates the apoptotic pathway in macrophages through the generation of NO [32]. Other data suggest that morphine-induced macrophage apoptosis is mediated through the generation of TGF-β [33].

Intravenous Anesthetics

Propofol

Propofol is an intravenous hypnotic agent used in the induction and maintenance of general anesthesia, or for sedation of patents in the ICU. A therapeutic dose of propofol produces hypnosis rapidly and smoothly. This drug also shows a rapid metabolic clearance, leading to fast recovery from anesthesia or sedation. In addition, it exerts multiple effects on normal immunologic function (Table 2).

Effects on Immune Cell Function. At clinically relevant concentrations, propofol suppresses neutrophil chemotaxis, phagocytosis, respiratory burst activity, and bactericidal activity [34–36]. It inhibits cytokine release from cultured mononuclear cells [37], and decreases IL-8 secretion [38]. Production of superoxide anion after N-formylmethionine-leucyl-phenylalanine (fMLP) activation is reduced during propofol anesthesia for elective embolization of cerebral arterio-venous malformations, suggesting that propofol may reduce fMLP receptor expression on the polymorphonuclear leukocyte (PMN) surface [39].

Table 2. Effects of propofol on immune cell function

Cell type	Effect
▮ **Neutrophils**	↓ Chemotaxis
	↓ Phagocytosis
	↓ Production of reactive oxygen species
	No effect on cytokine release
▮ **Lymphocytes**	↓ Cytokine release
	↓ B cell proliferation

Some authors, however, have failed to observe a significant inhibitory effect of propofol on neutrophil function. Larsen and co-workers [40] found only minor effects on spontaneous cytokine release in whole blood, although the ability of mononuclear cells to mount a cytokine response to endotoxin was significantly affected by propofol.

The active component of propofol, 2,6-diisopropylphenol, can inhibit neutrophil superoxide production [35]. However since intravenous propofol is dissolved in 10% Intralipid, it has been suggested that the diluent, rather than the active drug, may be responsible for at least some of the observed effects [41]. Intralipid is composed of long chain triglycerides (LCT), containing unsaturated fatty acids. Moreover parenteral lipid emulsions are known to suppress some leukocyte functions [36, 41], and polyunsaturated fatty acids can be incorporated into cell membranes, increasing membrane rigidity. The proliferative response of lymphocytes from surgical intensive care patients was evaluated *in vitro* following exposure to pure propofol, and to propofol in 10% Intralipid. Both reduced the proliferative response to pokeweed mitogen [42].

The intracellular mechanism underlying the suppressive effect of propofol remains to be elucidated. Propofol interacts with G-proteins, phospholipase C and protein kinase C, and attenuates agonist-induced increases in $[Ca^{2+}]i$ [34, 35]. Other work suggests that the p44/42 mitogen-activated protein kinase (MAPK) pathway may be involved in the inhibitory effects of propofol on neutrophil activity [42].

Benzodiazepines

Benzodiazepines are anxiolytic, anticonvulsant, and sedative drugs whose pharmacological effects are mediated through binding to neuronal post-synaptic γ-aminobutyric acid A receptors (GABAa), that are gated to chloride channels and known as central benzodiazepine receptors (CBR). In addition, peripheral benzodiazepine receptors (PBR) are found in the inner and outer layers of mitochondrial membranes. These receptors have been identified in most mammalian tissues, including the brain [43].

The two classes of benzodiazepine receptors differ in their cellular location, structure and ligand specificity. Diazepam binds with high affinity to both types, while clonazepam has greater affinity for the central type, and chlorodiazepam has high affinity for the peripheral one. PBR function in mitochondrial cholesterol transport and steroidogenesis, in the regulation of physiological responses to stress including cellular metabolism and proliferation, in neuroendocrine activity, and in immune function [44].

Endogenous (natural) ligands for both PBR and CBR have been identified. These include benzodiazepine-like substances, which can act as mixed-type ligands, and porphyrins, which bind selectively to PBR [45]. Another endogenous neuropeptide, called diazepam-binding inhibitor (DBI), has been purified from brain and peripheral tissues. DBI has anxiogenic properties, and binds competitively to the GABAa receptor [45]. Additional evidence indicates that DBI may affect neutrophil function [46], as well as cytokine production by human monocytes [47].

Amongst circulating blood cells, the highest density of benzodiazepine receptors is found on monocytes and neutrophils, with an intermediate density in lymphocytes and low levels in platelets and erythrocytes. It is thought that the PBR must be located on the plasma membrane, since erythrocytes lack mitochondria, while

Table 3. Effects of benzodiazepines on immune cell function

Cell type	Effects
▌ **Neutrophils**	↓ Chemotaxis (↑ in one report) ↓ Adhesion ↓ Phagocytosis ↓ Superoxide production ↓ IL-8
▌ **Monocytes/Macrophages**	↓ Oxidative burst activity ↓ Release of IL-1, IL-6
▌ **Lymphocytes**	↓ Chemotaxis ↓ NK cell activity

IL: interleukin; NK: natural killer

the mitochondrial content of neutrophils reduces during granulocytic differentiation [48]. These plasma membrane receptors might be involved in neuroendocrine-immune function, in contrast to the mitochondrial receptors, which seem to be involved in the transfer of specific molecules into the mitochondria [49].

The presence of PBR in immune cells suggests a potential immunomodulatory role for benzodiazepines, and the observation that PBR binding characteristics and density are altered in neoplastic tissues suggests that they may play a role in cancer [44]. The effects of benzodiazepines on the immune system are summarized in Table 3.

Effects on Immune Cells. Benzodiazepines have contradictory effects on lymphoid cells, promoting growth at nanomolar concentrations, but inhibiting it at micromolar concentrations [43]. Benzodiazepines reduce the oxidative response of murine macrophages *in vivo*, and decrease macrophage secretion of IL-1 and IL-6, and of TNF [50]. Both diazepam, a CBR and PBR ligand, and Ro-5-4864, a PBR ligand only, are able to inhibit neutrophil chemotaxis and superoxide production [51], while benzil-diazepam reduces neutrophil phagocytic capacity [52]. In a rat model of abdominal sepsis, midazolam inhibited hydrogen peroxide production and CD11b expression [53]. *In vitro* studies in human whole blood demonstrated that midazolam reduced *E. coli* clearance, neutrophil and monocyte oxidative burst, and phagocytosis [54]. Midazolam reduces post-ischemic adhesion of human neutrophils to the coronary endothelium of the guinea pig heart, and may attenuate reperfusion injury [55].

Studies of the effects of benzodiazepines on monocyte chemotaxis have yielded divergent results. A report using human monocytes *in vitro* demonstrated reduced chemotaxis when cells were incubated with high doses of midazolam [56]. On the other hand, a separate study showed that peripheral and mixed benzodiazepine agonists induced monocyte chemotaxis, while CBR-selective agonists were without effect [57]. Diazepam stimulates both migration and phagocytosis in neutrophils through activation of PBR [58].

Prenatal exposure to low doses of benzodiazepines can result in long lasting alterations of cytokine levels, with reduced release of TNF-α, IL-1, IL-6, IL-2, and IFN-γ [59]. Midazolam alters IL-8 secretion by human PMN *in vitro* [38]. In another study, PBR density increased in both a dose- and time-dependent manner in cultured astrocytes exposed to TNF-α and IL-1β [60]. Mice subjected to prolonged treatment with benzodiazepines develop an immunodeficiency state and increased susceptibility to infection [61].

Effects on the Stress Response. Anxiolytic benzodiazepines can reverse or attenuate stress-induced immunosuppression. In the brain, benzodiazepine agonists exert positive allosteric modulation at the GABAa receptor and decrease CRH production. On the other hand, the anxiogenic diazepam-binding inhibitor stimulates CRH release, leading to increased ACTH and glucocorticoid secretion in the periphery. Thus in stress situations, peripheral and central benzodiazepine agonists interact with their neuronal receptors and prevent glucocorticoid-induced immunosuppression [44].

Barbiturates

Barbiturates are used less frequently as sedatives in the ICU because agents with shorter half-lives and lower rates of accumulation are readily available. Today their use is primarily for patients who have sustained traumatic brain injury, in whom control of intracranial pressure (ICP) levels is difficult. They, too, are known to possess immunomodulatory activity (Table 4).

Effects on Leukocytes. T helper 1 type cells (Th1) produce IFN-γ and TNF-β and regulate cell-mediated immunity, while T helper 2 type cells (Th2) produce IL-4, and IL-10 and support humoral immunity. Lymphocytes from healthy donors cultured with thiopentone for 48 hours at clinically relevant concentrations showed decreased production of IFN-γ, IL-4, and IL-2, under basal conditions [62].

Thiopentone-inhibited fMLP stimulated neutrophil chemotaxis *in vitro* [63]. In an isolated guinea pig heart model, thiopental reduced neutrophil adhesion under both non-ischemic and post-ischemic conditions [55]. This effect was partially attributed to a direct antioxidant action, reflected in a reduction in the oxidative burst of neutrophils cultured with thiopental in a clinically relevant dose. Others have shown a reduction in the respiratory burst activity, *in vitro,* using higher doses of thiopental [37]. A study of patients undergoing elective surgery found diminished respiratory burst activity in neutrophils after induction with fentanyl, thiopental, isoflurane, and nitrous oxide [64]. Phagocytosis of *Staph. aureus* by PMN is decreased *in vitro* by thiopental at high doses [37].

Table 4. Effects of barbiturates on immune cell function

Cell Type	Effects
▌ **Neutrophils**	↓ Chemotaxis to fMLP ↓ Adhesion ↓ Respiratory burst ↓ Phagocytosis of *Staph. aureus* ↓ Neutrophil count
▌ **Monocytes/Macrophages**	↓ Phagocytosis
▌ **Lymphocytes**	↓ Production of IL-2, IL-4, and interferon γ

IL: interleukin

The influence of thiopental on neutrophil migration through human endothelial cell monolayers was studied *in vitro*. Pretreatment of PMN or endothelial cells with clinically achievable doses of thiopental decreased migration to chemotactic stimuli such as fMLP. When both neutrophils and endothelial cells were pretreated with thiopental, migration was further reduced [65], suggesting that the effects seen in isolated leukocytes *in vitro* might be altered in "*in vivo*" models.

Immunologic Effects of Barbiturates in Severe Head Injury. The beneficial effects of barbiturates for patients with elevated ICP do not result from their analgesic properties, but from their ability to decrease cerebral metabolism and blood flow [66]. Following initial enthusiastic reports about their ability to decrease ICP, concern arose that the resultant hypotension might diminish cerebral perfusion pressure (CPP), and may need to be counteracted with vasoactive drugs [67]. Other complications observed in patients treated with barbiturate coma were hypokalemia, respiratory complications, infections, and hepatic and renal dysfunction [67].

Patients with severe head injury are particularly susceptible to infectious complications. It has been suggested that barbiturate coma might induce reversible bone marrow suppression in these patients [68]. Patients treated with barbiturate coma demonstrated a significantly greater infection rate and 25% developed leukopenia during the use of thiopental, an abnormality that was reversed after the infusion was stopped, raising the possibility that the interaction between thiopental and antibiotics could increase the risk of bone marrow suppression [68]. Other studies of patients with head injury and increased ICP have not observed an increase in infectious complications (pneumonia, meningitis or bacteremia), nor a reduction in leukocyte counts [69].

▌ Local Anesthetics

Local anesthetics relieve pain by interrupting nerve conduction. They bind to a specific receptor site within the Na^+ channels in nerves, blocking ion transport. Their action is restricted to the site of application and is rapidly reversed following diffusion from the site of action in the nerve. Delivery of local anesthetics by axial blockade, particularly by epidural injection, is a common mode of analgesia in ICU patients. The most commonly used local anesthetics are lidocaine, bupivacaine, and ropivacaine.

Table 5. Effects of local anesthetics on immune cell function

Cell type	Effects
▌ **Neutrophils**	↓ Adhesion
	↓ Shedding of L-selectin
	↓ Expression of CD11b/CD18
	↓ Migration
	↓ Release of reactive oxygen intermediates
	↓ Priming by PAF
	↓ Phagocytosis of *Staph. aureus, E. coli*
▌ **Macrophages**	↓ Migration

PAF: Platelet activating factor

In addition to their antinociceptive effects, local anesthetics have a variety of actions, including effects on immune cell function (Table 5). A promising field of research is the potential action of these compounds as anti-inflammatory drugs, based on their effects on PMN. The systemic anti-inflammatory effects of local anesthetic agents are related to their plasma concentration, however, the mechanism of action this effect is unknown.

Effects on Leukocyte Function: Neutrophil adhesion to endothelium is one of the first steps in the response to infectious challenge. Two classes of molecules – the selectins and the integrins – are involved in this process. L-selectin on neutrophils mediates the first interaction between the leukocyte and the endothelium, the rolling process. Subsequently, CD11b/CD18, members of the integrin family, produce firm adhesion between neutrophils and the endothelium.

Ropivacaine and lidocaine decreased the shedding of neutrophil L-selectin, and upregulated CD11b/CD18 expression in response to TNF-a [70], while ropivacaine inhibited the increased leukocyte rolling and adhesion induced by leukotriene B$_4$ (LTB$_4$) in hamster cheek venules by reducing arteriolar diameter and blood flow [70]. The doses of anesthetic used in these studies yield plasma levels similar to those obtained during treatment of patients with inflammatory bowel disease [71, 72]. In other studies, lidocaine, at a dose of 1 mg/ml, inhibited the LPS-mediated adhesion of neutrophils *in vitro* or *in vivo* [73]. Bupivacaine caused a small, but statistically significant, decrease in the expression of CD11b/CD18 in human neutrophils *in vitro*, 10 min of exposure to doses of 1 to 5 µg/ml (119). The inhibitory effects of lidocaine on leukocyte migration are evident at doses between 4–20 µM in neutrophils [74] and 1–100 µM in macrophages, doses that can be readily achieved in peripheral tissues by local injection.

In clinically relevant concentrations, racemic bupivacaine decreased neutrophil phagocytic activity for *Staph. aureus*, and further decreased expression of the Fcγ receptor and CD35, a complement receptor [73]. Lidocaine inhibited *E. coli* ingestion by 50% at an *in vitro* concentration of 1 mg/ml [72]. Lidocaine also inhibited neutrophil priming by platelet activating factor (PAF), but did not modify the activation process. In concentrations between 1 and 100 µM, it inhibited superoxide production after priming with PAF, or activation by fMLP. Ropivacaine and bupivacaine had similar effects [75]. Neutrophil production of reactive oxygen intermediates following the phagocytosis of bacteria was reduced by bupivacaine [73]. Lidocaine also reduced superoxide and hydrogen peroxide production in neutrophils primed by phorbol 12-myristate 13-acetate (PMA). In a clinical study of the effects of anesthesia and tracheal intubation, administration of lidocaine prior to intubation reversed the decreased neutrophil respiratory burst induced by thiopentane and isoflurane [64].

Effects of Local Anesthetics on Systemic Inflammation and Lung Injury. The recognition that local anesthetics can modulate the expression of adhesion molecules has raised the possibility that these agents might favorably modulate pathologic interactions between neutrophils and the endothelium.

Pretreatment of rats with lidocaine infusion in anti-arrhythmic doses prior to endotoxin challenge attenuates the leakage of macromolecules in the mesenteric microcirculation [71]. Similarly, lidocaine pretreatment decreased post-capillary leakage following challenge with LTB$_4$ [70]. Investigators from Kobe University have evaluated the role of local anesthetics in attenuating lung injury induced in rabbits by phospholipase A$_2$ and trypsin, hydrochloric acid aspiration, or hyperoxia. Pretreatment with lidocaine reduced the changes in lung compliance, lung resistance, and wet/dry weight ratio, reduced alveolar/arterial oxygen tension differences, reduced pulmonary neutrophilia and the associated histologic changes of acute lung injury, and improved leukocyte and platelet counts in circulating blood [76, 77]. Improvement occurred even when lidocaine was given 10 min, but not 30 min, after the induction of lung injury [78].

Conclusion

Multiple *in vivo* and *in vitro* studies have shown that anesthetic and analgesic agents commonly used in the care of the critically ill patient can modulate immune cell function. The extent to which these agents contribute to the systemic derangements of critical illness is unknown. Both the adverse and beneficial effects of these agents can be demonstrated using concentrations of the agent that are achieved during normal clinical use, suggesting that greater explicit attention to their potential immunomodulatory activities is a priority for future research.

References

1. Haverkos HW, Lange RW (1990) Serious infections other than human immunodeficiency virus among intravenous drug users. J Infect Dis 161:894–902
2. Stevenson GW, Hall SC, Rudnick S, Seleny FL, Stevenson HC (1990) The effect of anesthetic agents on the human immune response. Anesthesiology 72:542–552
3. Stefano GB, Scharrer B, Smith EM, et al (1996) Opioid and opiate immunoregulatory processes. Crit Rev Immunol 16:109–144
4. Cabot PJ (2001) Immune-derived opioids and peripheral antinociception. Clin Exp Pharmacol Physiol 28:230–232
5. Wybran J, Appelboom T, Famaey J, Govaerts A (1979) Suggestive evidence for receptors for morphine and methionine-enkephalin on normal human blood T-lymphocytes. J Immunol 123:1068–1070
6. Chuang LF, Chuang TK, Killiam KF, et al (1995) Expression of kappa opioid receptors in human and monkey lymphocytes. Biochem Biophys Res Commun 209:1003–1010
7. Sharp BM, Roy S, Bidlack JM (1998) Evidence for opioid receptors on cells involved in host defense and the immune system. J Neuroimmunol 83:45–56
8. Jaeger K, Scheinichen D, Heine J, et al (1998) Remifentanil, fentanyl and alfentanil have no effect on the respiratory burst of neutrophils in vitro. Acta Anaesth Scand 42:1110–1113
9. Krumholz W, Demel C, Jung S, Meuthen G, Hempelmann G (1993) The influence of fentanyl and alfentanil on functions of human polymorphonuclear leukocytes in vitro. Acta Anaesth Scand 37:386–389
10. Stefano GB, Hartman A, Bilfinger TV, et al (1995) Presence of the μ_3 opiate receptor in endothelial cells: coupling to nitric oxide production and vasodilation. J Biol Chem 270: 30290–30293
11. Welters ID, Mezenbach A, Goumon Y, et al (2000) Morphine inhibits NF-κb nuclear binding in human neutrophils and monocytes by a nitric oxide-dependent mechanism. Anesthesiology 92:1677–1684
12. Stefano GB, Scharrer B (1994) Endogenous morphine and related opiates, a new class of chemical messengers. Adv Neuroimmunol 4:57–67
13. Nelson JC, Schneider GM, Lysle DT (2000) Involvement of central μ-, but not δ- or κ-opioid receptors in immunomodulation. Brain Behav Immunity 14:170–184
14. Marcoli M, Ricevuti G, Mazzone A, Bekkering M, Lecchini S, Frigo GM (1988) Opioid-induced modification of granulocyte function. Int J Immunopharmacol 10:425–433
15. Ni X, Gritman KR, Eisenstein TK, Adler MW, Arforks KE, Tuma RF (2000) Morphine attenuates leukocytes/endothelial interactions. Microvasc Res 60:121–130

16. Rud B, Benestad HB, Opdahl H (1988) Dual effect of thiopentone on human granulocyte activation. Non-intervention by ketamine and morphine. Acta Anaesthesiol Scand 32:316–322
17. Luza J (1992) Effect of morphine on phagocytic activity of the polymorphonuclears and monocytes. Acta Univ Palacki Olomuc Fac Me 134:47–57
18. Rojavin M, Szabo I, Bussiere J, et al (1993) Morphine treatment *in vitro* or *in vivo* decreases phagocytic functions of murine macrophages. Life Sci 53:997–1006
19. Pacifi R, Di Carlo S, Bacosi A, Zuccaro P (1993) Macrophage functions in drugs of abuse-treated mice. Int J Immunopharmacol 15:711–716
20. Grimm MC, Ben-Baruch A, Taub DD, et al (1998) Opiates transdeactivate chemokine receptors: delta and mu opiate-receptor mediated heterologous desensitization. J Exp Med 188:317–325
21. Eisenstein TK, Meissler JJ, Rogers TJ, Geller EB, Adler MW (1995) Mouse strain differences in immunosuppression by opioids in vitro. J Pharmacol Exp Ther 275:1484–1489
22. Govitaprong P, Suttitum T, Kotchabhakdi N, Uneklabh T (1998) Alteration of immune functions in heroin addicts and heroin withdrawal subjects. J Pharmacol Exp Ther 286: 883–889
23. Lockwood LL, Silber LH, Fleshner M, Laudenslager ML, Watkins LR, Maier SF (1994) Morphine-induced decreases in *in vivo* antibody responses. Brain Behav Immunol 8:24–36
24. Peterson PK, Molitor TW, Chao CC (1998) The opioid-cytokine connection. J Neuroimmunol 83:63–69
25. Alicea C, Belkowski SM, Eisenstein TK, Adler MW, Rogers TJ (1996) Inhibition of primary murine macrophage cytokine production in vitro following treatment with the κ-opioid agonist U50,488H. J Neuroimmunol 64:83–90
26. Chao CC, Gekker G, Sheng WS, Tsang M, Peterson PK (1994) Priming effect of morphine on the production of tumor necrosis factor-α by microglia: implications in respiratory burst of activity and human immunodeficiency virus-1 expression. J Pharmacol Exp Ther 269:198–203
27. Roy S, Cain KJ, Chapin RB, Charboneau RG (1998) Morphine modulates NF-κB activation in macrophages. Biochem Biophys Res Commun 245:392–396
28. Chao CC, Hu S, Molitor TW (1992) Morphine potentiates transforming growth factor-β release from human peripheral blood mononuclear cell cultures. J Pharmacol Exp Ther 262:19–28
29. Miyagi T, Chuang LF, Doi RH, Carlos MP, Torres JV, Chuang RY (2000) Morphine induces gene expression of CCR5 in human CEM x174 lymphocytes. J Biol Chem 275:31305–31310
30. Hilburger ME, Aldler MW, Roger TJ, Eisenstein TK (1997) Morphine alters macrophage and lymphocyte populations in the spleen and peritoneal cavity. J Neuroimmunol 80:106–114
31. Singhal PC, Reddy K, Franki N, Sanwal V, Gibbons N (1997) Morphine induces splenocyte apoptosis and enhanced mRNA expression of cathepsin-B. Inflammation 21:609–617
32. Singhal PC, Sharma P, Kapase A (1998) Morphine enhances macrophage apoptosis. J Immunol 160:1886–1893
33. Singhal PC, Kapasi AA, Franki N, Reddy K (2000) Morphine-induced macrophage apoptosis: the role of transforming growth factor-beta. Immunology 100:57–62
34. Weiss M, Birkhahn A, Krone M, Schneider EM (1996) Do etomidate and propofol influence oxygen radical production of neutrophils? Immunopharmacol Immunotoxicol 18:291–307
35. Mikawa K, Akamatsu H, Nishina K, et al (1998) Propofol inhibits human neutrophil functions. Anesth Analg 87:695–700
36. Heine J, Jaeger K, Weingaertner N, Scheinichen D, Marx G, Piepenbrock S (2001) Effects of different preparation of propofol, diazepam, and etomidate on human neutrophils *in vitro*. Acta Anaesth Scand 45:213–220
37. Davidson JA, Boom SJ, Pearsall FJ, Shang P, Ramsay G (1995) Comparison of the effects of four i.v. anaesthetic agents on polymorphonuclear leukocyte function. Br J Anaesth 74: 315–318
38. Galley HF, Dubbles AM, Webster NR (1998) The effect of midazolam and propofol on interleukin-8 from human polymorphonuclear leukocytes. Anesth Analg 86:1289–1293
39. Heine J, Jaeger K, Osthaus A, et al (2000) Anaesthesia with propofol decreases FMLP-induced neutrophil respiratory burst but not phagocytosis compared with isoflurane. Br J Anaesth 85:424–430

40. Larsen B, Hoff G, Wilhelm W, Buchinger H, Wanner GA, Bauer M (1998) Effect of intravenous anesthetics on spontaneous and endotoxin-stimulated cytokine response in cultured human whole blood. Anesthesiology 89:1218–1227

41. Heine J, Scheinichen D, Jaeger K, André M, Leuwer M (1999) In vitro influence of parenteral lipid emulsions on the respiratory burst of neutrophils. Nutrition 15:540–545

42. Nagata T, Kansha M, Irita K, Takahashi S (2001) Propofol inhibits FMLP-stimulated phosphorylation of p42 mitogen-activated protein kinase and chemotaxis in human neutrophils. Br J Anesth 86:853–858

43. Gavish M, Bachman I, Shoukrun R, et al (1999) Enigma of the peripheral benzodiazepine receptor. Pharm Rev 51:629–650

44. Zavala F (1997) Benzodiazepines, anxiety and immunity. Pharmacol Ther 75:199–216

45. Barbaccia ML, Berkovich A, Guarnieri P, Slobodyansky E (1990) DBI (diazepam binding inhibitor): the precursor of a family of endogenous modulators of GABAa receptor function: history, perspectives, and clinical implications. Neurochem Res 15:161–168

46. Consentino M, Marino F, Cattaneo S, et al (2000) Diazepam-binding inhibitor-derived peptides induce intracellular calcium changes and modulate human neutrophil function. J Leuk Biol 67:637–643

47. Taupin V, Gogusev J, Descamps-Latscha B, Zavala F (1993) Modulation of tumor necrosis factor-α, interleukin-1β, interleukin-6, interleukin-8 and granulocyte/macrophage colony-stimulating factor expression in human monocytes by an endogenous anxiogenic benzodiazepine ligand, triakontatetraneuropeptide evidence for a role of prostaglandins. Mol Pharmacol 43:64–69

48. Cahard D, Canat X, Carayon P, Roque C, Casellas P, Le Fur G (1994) Subcellular localization of peripheral benzodiazepine receptors on human leukocytes. Lab Invest. 70:23–28

49. Woods MJ, Williams DC (1996) Multiple forms and location for the peripheral-type benzodiazepine receptor. Biochem Pharmacol 52:1805–1814

50. Zavala F, Taupin V, Descamps-Latscha B (1990) In vivo treatment with benzodiazepines inhibits murine phagocyte oxidative metabolism and production of interleukin-1, tumor necrosis factor and interleukin-6. J Pharm Exp Ther 255:442–450

51. Finnerty M, Marczynski TJ, Amirault HJ, Urbancic M, Andersen BR (1991) Benzodiazepines inhibit neutrophil chemotaxis and superoxide production in a stimulus dependent manner, PK-11195 antagonizes these effects. Immunopharmacol 22:185–193

52. Covelli W, Decandia P, Altamura M, Jirillo E (1989) Diazepam inhibits phagocytosis and killing exerted by polymorphonuclear cells and monocytes from healthy donors. In vitro studies. Immunopharmacol Immunotoxicol 11:701–714

53. Inada T, Taniuchi S, Shingu K, Kobayashi Y, Fujisawa J, Nakao S (2001) Propofol depressed neutrophil hydrogen peroxide production more than midazolam, whereas adhesion molecule expression was minimally affected by both anesthetics in rats with abdominal sepsis. Anesth Analg 92:437–441

54. Heller A, Heller S, Blecken S, Urbaschek R, Koch T (1998) Effects of intravenous anesthetics on bacterial elimination in human blood in vitro. Acta Anaesthesiol Scand 42:518–526

55. Szekely A, Heindl B, Zahler S, Conzen PF, Becker BF (2000) Nonuniform behavior of intravenous anesthetics on postischemic adhesion of neutrophils in the guinea pig heart. Anesth Analg 90:1293–1300

56. Ruff MR, Pert CB, Weber RJ, Wahl LM, Wahl SM, Paul SM (1985) Benzodiazepine receptor-mediated chemotaxis of human monocytes. Science 229:1281–1283

57. Krumholz W, Reussner D, Hempelmann G (1999) The influence of several intravenous anaesthetics on the chemotaxis of human monocytes in vitro. Eur J Anaesthesiol 16:547–549

58. Marino F, Cattaneo S, Cosentino M, et al (2001) Diazepam stimulates migration and phagocytosis of human neutrophils: possible contribution of peripheral type benzodiazepine receptors and intracellular calcium. Pharmacology 63:42–49

59. Schlumpf M, Lichtensteiger W, Ramseier H (1993) Diazepam treatment of pregnant rats differentially affects interleukin-1 and interleukin-2 secretion in their offspring during different phases of postnatal development. Pharmacol Toxicol 73:335–340

60. Oh YJ, Francis JW, Markelonis GJ, Oh TH (1992) Interleukin-1β and tumor necrosis factor-α increase peripheral-type benzodiazepine binding sites in cultured polygonal astrocytes. J Neurochem 58:2131–2138

61. Galdiero F, Bentivoglio C, Nuzzo I, et al (1995) Effects of benzodiazepines and resistance in mice. Life Sci 57:2413–2423

62. Salo M, Pirttikangas C-O, Pulkki K (1997) Effects of propofol emulsion and thiopentone on T helper type-1/type-2 balance *in vitro*. Anaesthesia 52:341–344

63. Nishina K, Akamatsu H, Mikakawa K, et al (1998) The inhibitory effects of thiopental, midazolan and ketamine on human neutrophil functions. Anesth Analg 86:159–165

64. Swanton BJ, Iohom G, Wang JH, Redmond HP, Shorten GD (2001) The effect of lidocaine on neutrophil respiratory burst during induction of general anaesthesia and tracheal intubation. Eur J Anaesth 18:524–529

65. Hofbauer R, Moser D, Salfinger H, Frass M, Kapiotis S (1998) Thiopental inhibits migration of human leukocytes through human endothelial cell monolayers *in vitro*. Intensive Care Med 24:973–976

66. Galley HF, DiMatteo MA, Webster NR (2000) Immunomodulation by anaesthetic, sedative and analgesic agents: does it matter? Intensive Care Med 26:267–274

67. Schalen W, Messeter K, Nordstrom C-H (1992) Complications and side effects during thiopentone therapy in patients with severe head injuries. Acta Anaesth Scand 36:369–377

68. Stover JF, Stocker R (1998) Barbiturate coma may promote reversible bone marrow suppression in patients with severe isolated traumatic brain injury. Eur J Clin Pharmacol 54:529–534

69. Ishikawa K, Tanaka H, Shiozaki T, et al (2000) Characteristics of infection and leukocyte count in severely head-injured patients treated with mild hypothermia. J Trauma 49:912–922

70. Martinsson T, Oda T, Fernvik E, Roempke K, Dalsgaard C, Svensjo E (1997) Ropivacaine inhibits leukocyte rolling, adhesion and CD11b/CD18 expression. J Pharm Exp Ther 283:59–65

71. Schmidt W, Schmidt H, Bauer H, Gebhard MM, Martin E (1997) Influence of lidocaine on endotoxin-induced leukocyte-endothelial cell adhesion and macromolecular leakage in vivo. Anaesthesiology 87:617–624

72. Azuma Y, Shinohara M, Wang P, Suese Y, Yasuda H, Ohura K (2000) Comparison of inhibitory effects of local anesthetics on immune functions of neutrophils. Int J Immunopharm 22:789–796

73. Welters ID, Menzebach A, Langefeld TW, Menzebach M, Hempelmann G (2001) Inhibitory effects of S-(–) and R-(+) bupivacaine on neutrophil function. Acta Anaesth Scand 45:570–575

74. Hammer R, Dahlgren C, Stendahl O (1985) Inhibition of human leukocyte metabolism and random mobility by local anaesthesia. Acta Anaesth Scand 29:520–523

75. Hollman MW, Gross A, Jelacin N, Duriex ME (2001) Local anesthetic effects on priming and activation of human neutrophils. Anesthesiology 95:113–122

76. Takao Y, Mikawa K, Nishina K, Maekawa N, Obara H (1996) Lidocaine attenuates hyperoxic lung injury in rabbits. Acta Anaesth Scand 40:318–325

77. Kiyonar Y, Nishina K, Mikawa K, Maekawa N, Obara H (2000) Lidocaine attenuates acute lung injury induced by a combination of phospholipase A_2 and trypsin. Crit Care Med 28:484–489

78. Nishina K, Mikawa K, Takao Y, Shiga M, Maekawa N, Obara H (1998) Intravenous lidocaine attenuates acute lung injury induced by hydrochloric acid aspiration in rabbits. Anesthesiology 88:1300–1309

Myocardial Responses

Myocardial Ischemia-reperfusion Injury: Role of the Peroxynitrite-poly(ADP-ribose) Polymerase Pathway

C. Szabó and L. Liaudet

▌ Introduction

The enzyme poly (ADP-ribose) polymerase (PARP) – also termed poly (ADP-ribose) synthetase (PARS) and poly (ADP-ribose) transferase (pPADPRT) – is an abundant nuclear protein present throughout the phylogenetic spectrum. The precise physiologic roles of PARP remain undefined; its traditional role as a DNA-repair enzyme has been questioned by recent studies. PARP plays diverse roles, participating in DNA repair, chromatin relaxation, cell differentiation, DNA replication, transcriptional regulation, control of cell cycle, p53 expression and apoptosis, and transformation [1].

Based on emerging data in the last decade, PARP activation has been identified as a key pathway of oxidant- and free radical-mediated myocardial reperfusion injury. *In vitro* studies in cardiac myocytes and other cell types demonstrated that when activated in response to DNA single strand breaks, PARP initiates an energy consuming, inefficient cellular metabolic cycle by transferring ADP ribose units to nuclear proteins. This process rapidly depletes the intracellular NAD^+ and ATP pools leading to cellular dysfunction and cell necrosis. This pathway has been well characterized *in vitro*, and is overviewed elsewhere [1–3]. Here, we overview the experimental evidence implicating PARP as a pathophysiological modulator of myocardial injury *in vivo*.

▌ PARP is Activated in the Reperfused Heart

Immunohistochemical detection of poly(ADP-ribose) formation demonstrated that PARP is rapidly activated in the reperfused myocardium [4, 5]. The time course of PARP activation is rather prolonged; it is present at 2 h after the start of reperfusion, and continues to be present as late as 24 h after reperfusion (Fig. 1) [4, 5]. This delayed pattern of PARP activation is likely related to the continuing presence of free radical and oxidant production in the reperfused myocardium. It is also conceivable that a massive, early, DNA single strand breakage, which remains unrepaired for prolonged periods of time, is responsible for the prolonged pattern of PARP activation. The site of the most pronounced PARP activation is the area of necrosis and peri-infarct zone (i.e., the area at risk). Most of the poly(ADP-ribose) staining was seen in cardiac myocytes [4, 5], indicating that the heart tissue itself, rather than the infiltrating mononuclear cells, is the main site of PARP activation. A more diffuse staining pattern can be seen in the area of necrosis; this pattern is

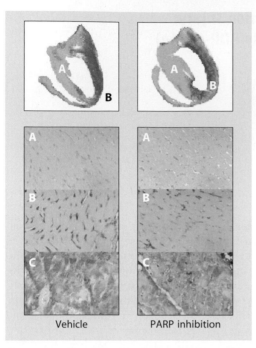

Fig. 1. Immunohistochemical localization of PARP activation in the reperfused myocardium. Poly(ADP-ribose) formation, an indicator of PARP activation, as determined in whole heart sections from rats exposed to 1 h ischemia and 23 hours reperfusion. Massive staining is evident in the left ventricular free wall of control animals, which is clearly reduced in rats treated with the PARP inhibitor 3-aminobenzamide (3-AB). Microscopically, the normal, non-ischemic myocardium from the interventricular septum (zone A) shows no sign of PARP activation, whereas in the ischemic myocardium, PARP activation is mainly located in the nuclei of myocytes in the peri-infarction zone (zone B), a pattern which is reduced by treatment with 3-AB. In the infarcted myocardium, severe architectural alterations coexist with a more diffuse pattern of PAR staining (zone C). (Magnification × 400)

likely to reflect the fact that the cellular content (and thus the poly-ADP-ribosylated proteins) are now more-or-less uniformly distributed in the necrotic area, due to myocardial necrosis and the associated breakdown of the cell membrane permeability. Because PARP activation triggers cellular necrosis due to cellular energetic collapse (see below), the primary mode of action of the cardioprotective effects of PARP inhibitors is related to a direct inhibition of myocyte necrosis. The peri-infarct zone, which contains viable cells, in which PARP is markedly activated, is the likely site of the beneficial effects of PARP inhibitors.

Activation of PARP has also been demonstrated *in vitro*, in an isolated perfused heart system [6]. One of the enzymes that undergoes poly(ADP-ribos)ylation is PARP itself (auto-ribosylation) [6]. Ischemia-reperfusion (I/R)-induced self-ADP-ribosylation of PARP can be attenuated by pharmacological PARP inhibitors [6].

Some information is also available on the activation of PARP in the heart in conditions other than myocardial I/R. In a recent study, 2′,3′-dideoxycytidine, and 3′-azido-3′-deoxythymidine were found to induce PARP activation in the heart, and the PARP pathway has been proposed to play a role in the cardiomyopathy induced by these compounds [7, 8].

We know now that several minor isoforms of PARP exist [1–3]. The original PARP enzyme is now sometimes called PARP–1. In most pathophysiological conditions, it appears that activation of PARP–1 plays the crucial role in modulating intracellular metabolic events. Nevertheless, a significant degree of residual PARP activation was found in the hearts of PARP–1 deficient mice, emphasizing the potential, additional role of the minor PARP isoforms in poly(ADP-ribose) formation [5, 9].

▌ PARP Inhibitors Protect against Myocardial Injury

Various cultured cells, including cultured rat cardiac myoblasts, are protected against hydrogen peroxide and peroxynitrite mediated cell necrosis by PARP inhibitors [10]. We proposed the potential utility of pharmacological inhibition of PARP as a protective agent in myocardial reperfusion injury [11]. We have subsequently evaluated the role of PARP in an acute model of myocardial reperfusion injury in the rat [12]. Peroxynitrite formation was evidenced by plasma oxidation of dihydrorhodamine123 and formation of nitrotyrosine in the reperfused heart [12]. Myocardial reperfusion resulted in marked cellular injury, as measured by an increase of plasma creatine phosphokinase (CPK) activity and development of a large infarcted area. Pharmacological inhibition of PARP with 3-aminobenzamide significantly improved the outcome of myocardial dysfunction, as evidenced by a reduction in CPK levels, diminished infarct size, and preserved the ATP pools [12]. Other investigators have confirmed our results in similar experimental models of myocardial reperfusion. In rabbit and pig models of myocardial infarction, pharmacological inhibitors of PARP, such as nicotinamide and 3-aminobenzamide, dramatically reduced the infarct size [13, 14]. The cardioprotection afforded by the PARP inhibitors was due to a selective inhibition of PARP, since the structurally related but inactive agents, such as 3-aminobenzoic acid and nicotinic acid, did not cause a reduction in infarct size [13]. Over recent years, a multitude of studies have demonstrated the cardioprotective effects of various pharmacological PARP inhibitors in cultured myocytes, in perfused heart systems, and in various *in vivo* models of myocardial reperfusion injury [4–6, 10, 12–24]. Most recently, we have synthesized PJ34, a potent inhibitor of PARP [25, 26], and demonstrated significant cardioprotection with this compound in the rat model (Fig. 2) [4] as well as in a porcine model [20]. Inhibition of PARP activity was found to facilitate energy recovery dur-

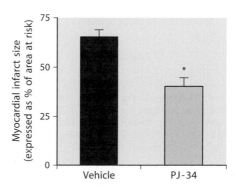

Fig. 2. Effect of the novel potent PARP inhibitor (PJ34, given at 10 mg/kg i.v. 5 min before reperfusion) in a rat model of myocardial ischemia-reperfusion. While the vehicle and the PJ34 treated animals presented with comparable area at risk, PJ34 treatment markedly reduced the area of myocardial necrosis during reperfusion (*p < 0.05). Data presented as mean ± SEM. N = 12 animals per group

Table 1. Protection against myocardial injury by pharmacological inhibition or genetic inactivation of PARP *in vitro* and *in vivo*

Experimental model	Inducer of injury	Mode of PARP inhibition	Effect of PARP inhibition	Refs
▋ Studies in vitro				
Rat cardiomyoblasts	H_2O_2, peroxynitrite H/R	3-AB, Nicam, ISO	Reduction in cell necrosis, improvement in mitochondrial respiration	[10, 16]
Human cardiomyoblasts	H_2O_2	3-AB, Nicam, ISO	Reduction in cell death	[14, 15]
▋ Studies in isolated hearts				
Mouse heart	Global I/R	PARP$^{-/-}$ phenotype	Reduction in NAD$^+$ consumption Suppression in LV dysfunction	[5, 23]
Rat heart	Global I/R	BGP-15, ISO	Reduction in NAD$^+$ and ATP catabolism Reduction in LV dysfunction	[6, 17]
		BGP-15,3-AB, Nicam	Improved ATP and CK recovery	[28]
		Lipoamide (antioxidant)	Reduction in myocardial damage	[19]
	Regional I/R	3-AB	Decrease in infarct size	[16]
Rabbit heart	Global I/R	3-AB	Decrease in infarct size Reduction in LV dysfunction	[13]
▋ Studies in vivo (rodents)				
Mouse	Regional I/R	PARP$^{-/-}$ phenotype	Decrease in infarct size, neutrophil infiltration,and circulating IL-10, TNF-α and nitrate Reduction in P-selectin/ICAM-1 expression	[21, 22]
	IPC	PARP$^{-/-}$ phenotype	Suppression of the benefit of IPC	[24]
Rat	Regional I/R	3-AB GPI6150	Preservation of myocardial ATP stores, decrease in infarct size, reduction in LV dysfunction, reduction in neutrophil infiltration	[4, 5, 12]
	IPC AZT or ddC therapy	3-AB	Suppression of the benefit of IPC Induction of cardiomyopathy through the formation of ROS and PARP activation	[24]
▋ Studies in vivo (large animals)				
Rabbit	Regional I/R	3-AB, Nicam, ISO	Decrease in infarct size	[13]
Pig	Regional I/R	3-AB	Decrease in infarct size,	[14]
		PJ-34	improvement in LV function	[20]

3-AB: 3-aminobenzamide; ATP: adenosine triphosphate; AZT: 3′-azido-3′-deoxythymidine; ddC: 2″,3″-dideoxycytidine; H_2O_2: hydrogen peroxide; H/R: hypoxia/reoxygenation; ICAM-1: intercellular adhesion molecule-1; IL-10: interleukin-10; IPC: ischemic preconditioning; I/R: ischemia/reperfusion; ISO: 1,5 dihydroxyisoquinoline; LV: left ventricle; NAD$^+$: nicotinamide adenine dinucleotide; Nicam: nicotinamide; PARP: poly(ADP-ribose) polymerase; ROS: reactive oxygen species; TNF-α: tumor necrosis factor-α.

ing reperfusion, and reversed some of the functional deterioration caused by reperfusion in isolated hearts. Table 1 overviews the various studies demonstrating myocardial protection in various models of reperfusion injury [4–6, 10, 12–24], and other models of myocardial failure [7, 8].

❚ PARP Deficiency protects against Myocardial Injury

Transgenic mice lacking the functional gene for PARP have recently been developed. These animals provided the unique opportunity to unequivocally define the role of PARP in myocardial injury, and also to investigate some of the cellular mechanisms underlying this disease. Using a murine model of myocardial injury after early reperfusion, we found that absence of a functional PARP gene resulted in a significant prevention of reperfusion injury. Wild-type mice subjected to 1 h ligation and 1 h reperfusion of the left anterior descending branch of the coronary artery developed massive myocardial necrosis and triggered neutrophil infiltration [21]. When the reperfusion after 1h ischemia was prolonged to 24 hours, wild-type mice also developed high mortality [22]. In PARP$^{-/-}$ mice, plasma levels of CPK activity were significantly reduced, the histological features of myocardium were improved, neutrophil infiltration was reduced, and survival was improved [21, 22].

Protective effects of PARP deficiency can also be demonstrated in isolated perfused hearts. We reported that at the end of the reoxygenation, in hearts from wild-type animals, there was a significant suppression in the rate of intraventricular pressure development and in the rate of relaxation [23]. In contrast, in the hearts from PARP knockout animals, no significant suppression of the rate of intraventricular pressure development and relaxation was observed [23]. Our findings, both in isolated perfused hearts, and in the *in vivo* models, have recently been confirmed by Pieper and colleagues, using PARP deficient mice [5]. *In vivo* PARP activation in heart tissue slices was assayed through conversion of [^{33}P]NAD$^+$ into poly(ADP)ribose and also monitored by immunohistochemical staining for poly(ADP-ribose). Cardiac contractility, nitric oxide (NO), production of reactive oxygen species (ROS), NAD$^+$ and ATP levels were measured [5]. I/R augmented formation of NO, oxygen free radicals and PARP activity. I/R decreased cardiac contractility and NAD$^+$ levels, effects that were attenuated in PARP deficient animals [5].

❚ Myocardial Preconditioning: The Essential Role of PARP

Recent work from our laboratory also demonstrates that PARP is necessary for the phenomenon of ischemic myocardial preconditioning. Using a combined approach (pharmacological inhibition of PARP and PARP deficient mice), we have recently observed that the protective effect of preconditioning disappears in PARP$^{-/-}$ mice or in response to the PARP inhibitor 3-aminobenzamide [24]. The protection against reperfusion injury by preconditioning is also associated with partially preserved myocardial NAD$^+$ levels, indicating that PARP activation is attenuated by preconditioning. This conclusion is further strengthened by poly(ADP-ribose) immunohistochemical measurements, demonstrating that ischemic preconditioning markedly inhibits PARP activation during reperfusion [24]. Because ischemic preconditioning itself induces low levels of oxidative stress and a low degree of PARP activation, we proposed that the low level of PARP activation during preconditioning may lead to auto-ribosylation (i.e., auto-inhibition) of PARP. This process could, in turn, protect against the deleterious effects of ischemia and reperfusion, via inhibition of the subsequent, massive activation of PARP, which occurs in naive (non-preconditioned wild-type) animals during reperfusion [24].

Molecular Mechanisms of the Cardioprotection afforded by PARP Inhibition

The Energetic Pathway

It is well known that the myocardial contraction/relaxation process is tightly regulated by an efficient conversion of chemical into mechanical energy. Disruption of cellular energetics in general, or of mitochondrial function in specific, leads to elevated intracellular Na^+ and Ca^{2+} levels, and progressive intracellular acidosis, which will affect myocardial contraction and excitability. Disturbances in the energy generation process and in mitochondrial function severely compromise the myocardial contractile apparatus. Multiple direct measurements demonstrate that NAD^+ and ATP levels are depleted in cells exposed to various forms of oxidative stress, and also in I/R hearts, and these alterations are reversed by PARP deficiency or PARP inhibition (see above). In addition, PARP activation promotes mitochondrial damage and dysfunction. Our *in vitro* studies demonstrated that exposure of cultured cells to oxidants induces a time- and dose-dependent decrease in mitochondrial transmembrane potential ($\Delta\Psi_m$), which is associated with an increase in secondary production of ROS production and a loss of cardiolipin, an indicator of mitochondrial membrane damage [27]. Inhibition or inactivation of PARP attenuates peroxynitrite-induced reduction in mitochondrial transmembrane potential, secondary ROS generation, cardiolipin degradation, and intracellular calcium mobilization [27]. Our studies were subsequently confirmed and extended in studies where cardiac energy metabolism was investigated in a Langendorff heart perfusion system by ^{31}P NMR [28]. It was found that PARP inhibitors (3-aminobenzamide, nicotinamide, BGP-15, and 4-hydroxyquinazoline) improved the recovery of high-energy phosphates (ATP, creatine phosphate) and accelerated the reutilization of inorganic phosphate formed during the ischemic period, showing that PARP inhibitors facilitate the faster and more complete recovery of the energy production. Furthermore, PARP inhibitors significantly decreased the ischemia-reperfusion-induced increase of lipid peroxidation, protein oxidation, and the inactivation of respiratory complexes, which indicates decreased mitochondrial ROS production in the reperfusion period [28]. Although it appears that early nuclear PARP activation rapidly affects a variety of mitochondrial functions, the exact mechanism of this effect is presently unclear. It is possible that rapid cytosolic NAD depletion, coupled with a direct oxidant stress to the mitochondria, regulates early mitochondrial alterations that eventually culminate in mitochondrial energetic breakdown, permeability transition and oxidant generation.

Role of Pro-inflammatory Mediator Production

Inhibition of PARP activation has been shown to exert unexpected actions in regulating the expression, activation, and nuclear translocation of key pro-inflammatory genes and proteins. The absence of PARP or its pharmacological inhibition has been shown to suppress the activation of MAP kinase [29], activator protein (AP)-1 complex [30], and nuclear factor kappa B (NF-κB) [31]. Consequently, PARP inhibition interferes with the expression of pro-inflammatory genes, such as the inducible NO synthase (iNOS) and intercellular adhesion molecule (ICAM)-1 [21, 22]. PARP inhibition blocks ICAM-1 expression in cultured endothelial cells stimulated *in vitro* by a combination of pro-inflammatory cytokines, and in the vascular tissues of hearts subjected to reperfusion [22]. The regulation by PARP of gene expression may involve the poly-ADP ribosylation of transcription factors or the repair of DNA strand breaks which interfere with transcription. PARP may also alter the activation of pro-inflammatory pathways via its influence on the expression of AP-1, a heterodimer composed of c-fos and jun factors. High levels of transcriptional activation of human ICAM-1 and c-fos require AP-1 binding to 5′ flanking regulatory regions. In cultured cells PARP inhibition blocks oxidant-induced c-fos mRNA expression and AP-1 activation [30]. Since the c-fos promoter contains an AP-1 consensus site, c-fos activation could trigger a positive-feedback cycle of gene expression.

The inhibition of PARP, as well as PARP deficiency, also has been shown to suppress tumor necrosis factor (TNF)-a and interleukin (IL)-10 production in myocardial reperfusion injury [22]. Since mitogen-activate protein kinase (MAPK) plays a major role in the pleiotropic transduction of intracellular inflammatory cascades, the anti-inflammatory effects of PARP inhibition may be accounted for at this level of gene regulation. One may also expect that PARP-dependent regulation of NF-κB activation has a pleiotropic effect on the expression of pro-inflammatory genes, given the broad role that NF-κB plays in the transcriptional activation of cytokine and chemokine genes. A microchip analysis study recently completed [32] has investigated the changes in the expression of 15 000 genes in wild-type and PARP deficient fibroblasts. The study has demonstrated that under baseline conditions there is a significant alteration in the expression of a whole host of genes [32]. We believe that even more pronounced differences will be found in immunostimulated cells.

Endothelial Injury and Neutrophil Activation Pathways

Neutrophil invasion is a crucial event for I/R injury. In the early stages of reperfusion after ischemia, neutrophils move out of the circulation into inflamed tissue. Neutrophils augment the reperfusion damage to vascular and parenchymal cellular elements by the release of proteolytic enzymes, free radicals and pro-inflammatory mediators. A growing body of experimental data suggests that activation of PARP is an important modulator of leukocyte-endothelial cell interactions. Inhibition of PARP is frequently associated with a reduction in neutrophil infiltration at the site of injury in various experimental models of inflammation including arthritis and colitis [33–35]. The mechanism of regulation of neutrophil trafficking by PARP may involve: a) the regulation of the expression of adhesion molecules (see above), and b) the maintenance of endothelial integrity. With respect to (b), it is well known that NO derived from the vascular endothelium is a key inhibitor of neutrophil activation, adhesion, and trans-migration. There is also accumulating evidence demonstrating that pharmacological inhibition or genetic inactivation of PARP maintains endothelial integrity under conditions of oxidant stress [25, 36]. We have recently demonstrated that the regulation of endothelium-dependent relaxant ability by PARP is directly related to modulation of intracellular NADPH levels [25] – NADPH being an essential co-factor for NOS. Through the above mechanism, one

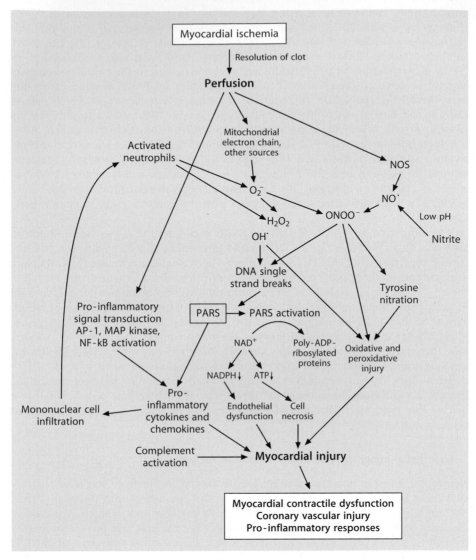

Fig. 3. Proposed pathways related to the poly (ADP-ribose) polymerase (PARP) pathway in the pathogenesis of myocardial ischemia and reperfusion injury. The reduction of oxygen supply during ischemia alters mitochondrial function, leading to the production of reactive oxidant species. Superoxide and nitric oxide (NO) react to yield peroxynitrite. Peroxynitrite and hydroxyl radical induce the single strand breakage in DNA, which, in turn, activates PARP. The activation of PARP rapidly depletes the cellular NAD$^+$ and ATP pools. The cellular energy exhaustion maintains the mitochondria in a reduced state, therefore allowing a further production of reactive oxidants at the reperfusion. Depletion of NAD$^+$ and ATP leads to cellular dysfunction. Depletion of NADPH leads to reduced endothelial NO formation. The cellular dysfunction is further enhanced by promotion of pro-inflammatory gene expression by PARP, via promotion of nuclear factor kappa B (NF-κB), activator protein (AP)-1 and mitogen-activated protein kinase (MAPK) activation. The oxidant-induced pro-inflammatory molecule and adhesion molecule expression, and the endothelial dysfunction induce neutrophil recruitment and neutrophil activation, which initiates a positive feedback cycle of oxidant generation, PARP activation and cellular injury

can hypothesize that, during myocardial injury, free radicals and oxidants injure the vascular endothelium, which reduces NO production, which then leads to neutrophil infiltration and further injury (positive feedback cycle). PARP inhibition, by interrupting this cycle, may both reduce neutrophil infiltration and oxidant and free radical generation.

It is unlikely that PARP directly regulates neutrophil function, since neutrophil granulocytes do not express this enzyme [1]. Also, the regulation of neutrophil infiltration by PARP cannot be the sole or exclusive mechanism of cardioprotection, because PARP inhibition continues to be effective in experimental systems which lack neutrophils (such as studies utilizing cultured cells, and the studies using isolated buffer-perfused heart systems; see above).

Additional Mechanisms

A number of additional mechanisms may contribute to the reduction of myocardial injury in response to PARP inhibition. PARP-related changes in cellular energetics and related processes involving calcium sequestration, biosynthetic processes, and maintenance of the normal cell shape and adherence may be involved. Poly (ADP-ribose) itself may directly play a role in regulating myocardial contractility – as has been shown for ADP-ribose [37] – and/or it may also affect gene expression.

In the literature related to PARP, many studies focus on PARP cleavage (as opposed to PARP activation). PARP cleavage by caspases is a marker of apoptotic cell death, and has been shown to occur in various models of myocardial I/R injury [38, 39]. The pathway proposed herein has no relationship to the PARP cleavage pathway; pharmacological inhibition of PARP inhibits the process of cell necrosis (rather than apoptosis). In fact, the cleaved form of PARP is catalytically inactive; PARP cleavage, in fact, has been considered an endogenous mechanism that serves to prevent PARP-dependent metabolic suppression and necrosis [40, 41].

▌ Conclusion

We conclude that a self-amplifying vicious cycle, regulated by PARP, exists in myocardial I/R (Fig. 3). Early production of oxidants by dysfunctional mitochondria after reperfusion leads to DNA damage and activation of PARP, which in turn causes further derangement of cellular energetic status and induces endothelial injury, production of inflammatory mediators, and expression of adhesion molecules. The loss of the endothelial barrier function is then responsible for the infiltration of neutrophils, which in turn produces additional oxidants. Pharmacological inhibition of PARP ameliorates the endothelial and myocardial dysfunction by interrupting the vicious cycle at various interacting levels (energetic failure, mediator production, neutrophil infiltration and oxidative damage). Further studies, using potent PARP inhibitors with clinically acceptable safety profiles and risk/benefit ratios must determine whether PARP inhibition is a candidate for clinical treatment of myocardial reperfusion injury.

Acknowledgements. This work was supported by a grant from the National Institutes of Health (R01HL59266) to C. S.

References

1. De Murcia G, Shall S (2000) From DNA Damage and Stress Signaling to Cell Death; Poly ADP-ribosylation Reactions. Oxford University Press, Oxford
2. Szabo C (2000) Cell Death: The Role of PARP. CRC Press, Boca Raton
3. Szabó C, Dawson VL (1998) Role of poly(ADP-ribose) synthetase in inflammation and ischaemia-reperfusion. Trends Pharmacol Sci 19:287–298
4. Liaudet L, Szabó E, Timashpolsky L, Virág L, Cziraki A, Szabó C (2001) Localization of poly (ADP-ribose) polymerase (PARP) activation in a rat model of myocardial reperfusion injury: suppression of PARP activation and long-term morphological and functional improvement by 3-aminobenzamide. Br J Pharmacol 133:1424–1430
5. Pieper AA, Walles T, Wei G, Clements EE, Verma A, Snyder SH (2000) Myocardial postischemic injury is reduced by polyADPRibose polymerase–1 gene disruption. Mol Med 6:271–282
6. Szabados E, Literati-Nagy P, Farkas B, Sumegi B (2000) BGP–15, a nicotinic amidoxime derivate protecting heart from ischemia reperfusion injury through modulation of poly(ADP-ribose) polymerase. Biochem Pharmacol 59:937–945
7. Szabados E, Fischer GM, Toth K, Csete B, Nemeti B, Trombitas K (1999) Role of reactive oxygen species and poly-ADP-ribose polymerase in the development of AZT-induced cardiomyopathy in rat. Free Rad Biol Med 26:309–317
8. Skuta G, Fischer GM, Janaky T, Kele Z, Szabo P, Tozser J (1999) Molecular mechanism of the short-term cardiotoxicity caused by 2′,3′-dideoxycytidine (ddC): modulation of reactive oxygen species levels and ADP-ribosylation reactions. Biochem Pharmacol 58:1915–1925
9. Pieper AA, Blackshaw S, Clements EE, Brat DJ, Krug DK, White AJ (2000) Poly(ADP-ribosyl)ation basally activated by DNA strand breaks reflects glutamate-nitric oxide neurotransmission. Proc Natl Acad Sci USA 97:1845–1850
10. Gilad E, Zingarelli B, Salzman AL, Szabo C (1997) Protection by inhibition of poly (ADP-ribose) synthetase against oxidant injury in cardiac myoblasts in vitro. J Mol Cell Cardiol 29:2585–2597
11. Szabó C, Zingarelli B, Salzman AL (1996) Peroxynitrite-mediated activation of poly-ADP ribosyl synthetase contributes to the vascular failure in shock. In: Okada K, Ogata H (ed) Shock: From Molecular and Cellular Level to Whole Body. Excerpta Medica International Congress Series 1102. Elsevier, Amsterdam, pp 3–14
12. Zingarelli B, Cuzzocrea S, Zsengeller Z, Salzman AL, Szabó C (1997) Inhibition of poly (ADP ribose) synthetase protects against myocardial ischemia and reperfusion injury. Cardiovasc Res 36:205–215
13. Thiemermann C, Bowes J, Myint FP, Vane JR (1997) Inhibition of the activity of poly (ADP ribose) synthetase reduces ischemia-reperfusion injury in the heart and skeletal muscle. Proc Natl Acad Sci USA 94:679–683
14. Bowes J, Ruetten H, Martorana PA, Stockhausen H, Thiemermann C (1998) Reduction of myocardial reperfusion injury by an inhibitor of poly (ADP-ribose) synthetase in the pig. Eur J Pharmacol 359:143–150
15. Bowes J, Piper J, Thiemermann C (1998) Inhibitors of the activity of poly (ADP-ribose) synthetase reduce the cell death caused by hydrogen peroxide in human cardiac myoblasts. Br J Pharmacol 124:1760–1766
16. Bowes J, McDonald MC, Piper J, Thiemermann C (1999) Inhibitors of poly (ADP-ribose) synthetase protect rat cardiomyocytes against oxidant stress. Cardiovasc Res 41:126–134
17. Docherty JC, Kuzio B, Silvester JA, Bowes J, Thiemermann C (1999) An inhibitor of poly (ADP-ribose) synthetase activity reduces contractile dysfunction and preserves high energy phosphate levels during reperfusion of the ischaemic rat heart. Br J Pharmacol 127:1518–1524
18. Janero DR, Hreniuk D, Sharif HM, Prout KC (1993) Hydroperoxide-induced oxidative stress alters pyridine nucleotide metabolism in neonatal heart muscle cells. Am J Physiol 264:C1401-C1410
19. Szabados E, Fischer GM, Gallyas F Jr, Kispal G, Sumegi B (1999) Enhanced ADP-ribosylation and its diminution by lipoamide after ischemia-reperfusion in perfused rat heart. Free Rad Biol Med 27:1103–1113

20. Faro R, Toyoda Y, McCully J, et al (2002) Protective effect on regional myocardial function and infarct size induced by PJ34: a novel poly (ADP-ribose) synthetase inhibitor. Ann Thorac Surg (in press)

21. Zingarelli B, Salzman AL, Szabó C (1998) Genetic disruption of poly (ADP-ribose) synthetase inhibits the expression of P-selectin and intercellular adhesion molecule–1 in myocardial ischemia-reperfusion injury. Circ Res 83:85–94

22. Yang Z, Zingarelli B, Szabo C (2000) Effect of genetic disruption of poly (ADP-ribose) synthetase on delayed production of inflammatory mediators and delayed necrosis during myocardial ischemia-reperfusion injury. Shock 13:60–66

23. Grupp IL, Jackson TM, Hake P, Grupp G, Szabó C (1999) Protection against hypoxia-reoxygenation in the absence of poly (ADP-ribose) synthetase in isolated working hearts. J Mol Cell Cardiol 31:297–303

24. Liaudet L, Yang Z, Affar B, Szabó C (2001) Myocardial ischemic preconditioning in rodents is dependent on poly (ADP-ribose) synthetase. Mol Med 7:406–417

25. Garcia Soriano F, Virag L, Jagtap P, et al (2001) Diabetic endothelial dysfunction: the role of poly(ADP-ribose) polymerase activation. Nat Med 7:108–113

26. Jagtap P, Soriano FG, Virag L, Liaudet L, Mabley J, Szabó C (2002) Novel phenanthridinone inhibitors of poly(ADP-ribose) synthetase: potent cytoprotective and anti-shock agents. Crit Care Med (in press)

27. Virag L, Salzman AL, Szabo C (1998) Poly(ADP-ribose) synthetase activation mediates mitochondrial injury during oxidant-induced cell death. J Immunol 161:3753–3759

28. H Halmosi R, Berente Z, Osz E, Toth K, Literati-Nagy P, Sumegi B (2001) Effect of poly-(ADP-ribose) polymerase inhibitors on the ischemia-reperfusion-induced oxidative cell damage and mitochondrial metabolism in Langendorff heart perfusion system. Mol Pharmacol 59:1497–505

29. Szabó C, Wong HR, Bauer PI, Kirsten E, O'Connor M, Zingarelli B (1997) Regulation of components of the inflammatory response by 5-iodo–6-amino–1,2-benzopyrone, and inhibitor of poly (ADP-ribose) synthetase and pleiotropic modifier of cellular signal pathways. Int J Oncol 10:1093–1101

30. Roebuck KA, Rahman A, Lakshminarayanan V, Janakidevi K, Malik AB (1995) H_2O_2 and tumor necrosis factor-activate intercellular adhesion molecule 1 (ICAM–1) gene transcription through distinct cis-regulatory elements within the ICAM–1 promoter. J Biol Chem 270:18966–18974

31. Oliver FJ, Menissier-de Murcia J, Nacci C, Decker P, Andriantsitohaina R, Muller S (1999) Resistance to endotoxic shock as a consequence of defective NF-kappaB activation in poly (ADP-ribose) polymerase–1 deficient mice. EMBO J 18:4446–4454

32. Simbulan-Rosenthal CM, Ly DH, Rosenthal DS, Konopka G, Luo R, Wang ZQ (2000) Misregulation of gene expression in primary fibroblasts lacking poly(ADP-ribose) polymerase. Proc Natl Acad Sci USA 97:11274–11279

33. Szabó C, Lim LHK, Cuzzocrea S, Getting SJ, Zingarelli B, Flower RJ (1997) Inhibition of poly (ADP-ribose) synthetase attenuates neutrophil recruitment and exerts antiinflammatory effects. J Exp Med 186:1041–1049

34. Szabo C, Virag L, Cuzzocrea S, Scott GS, Hake P, O'Connor MP (1998) Protection against peroxynitrite-induced fibroblast injury and arthritis development by inhibition of poly-(ADP-ribose) synthase. Proc Natl Acad Sci USA 95:3867–3872

35. Zingarelli B, Szabó C, Salzman AL (1999) Blockade of poly (ADP-ribose) synthetase inhibits neutrophil recruitment, oxidant generation, and mucosal injury in murine colitis, Gastroenterology 116:335–345

36. Szabo C, Cuzzocrea S, Zingarelli B, O'Connor M, Salzman AL (1997) Endothelial dysfunction in a rat model of endotoxic shock. Importance of the activation of poly (ADP-ribose) synthetase by peroxynitrite. J Clin Invest 100:723–735

37. Sosulina LI, Sukhova GS, Chudnyi MN, Ashmarin IP (1999) The action of ADP ribose on the mechanical and bioelectrical activity of the frog. Ross Fiziol Zh Im I M Sechenova 85:508–514

38. Freude B, Masters TN, Robicsek F, Fokin A, Kostin S, Zimmermann R (2000) Apoptosis is initiated by myocardial ischemia and executed during reperfusion. J Mol Cell Cardiol 32:197–208

39. De Boer RA, van Veldhuisen DJ, van Der Wijk J, Brouwer RM, de Jonge N, Cole GM (2000) Additional use of immunostaining for active caspase 3 and cleaved actin and PARP fragments to detect apoptosis in patients with chronic heart failure. J Cardiac Failure 6:330–337

40. Virag L, Scott GS, Cuzzocrea S, Marmer D, Salzman AL, Szabo C (1998) Peroxynitrite-induced thymocyte apoptosis: the role of caspases and poly (ADP-ribose) synthetase (PARS) activation. Immunology 94:345–355

41. Herceg Z, Wang ZQ (1999) Failure of poly(ADP-ribose) polymerase cleavage by caspases leads to induction of necrosis and enhanced apoptosis. Mol Cell Biol 19:5124–5133

Effects of Anesthetics on Ischemia-reperfusion Injury of the Heart

B. Preckel and W. Schlack

▌ Introduction

Ischemia-reperfusion (I/R) situations may occur in different clinical settings, for example, during percutaneous balloon angioplasty or after coronary artery bypass surgery. Depending on the duration of ischemia, the lack of oxygen supply may result in reversible, or irreversible, damage to the cardiomyocytes. Early restoration of coronary artery blood flow is the main goal in the treatment of patients with acute coronary syndromes and in patients with extracorporal circulation and interruption of coronary perfusion for cardiac surgery. However, reperfusion of temporarily ischemic myocardium can initiate cellular and biochemical changes which reduce the amount of potentially salvageable myocardium. This phenomenon is called 'reperfusion injury' and is – in contrast to the ischemic injury – not the direct result of oxygen deprivation.

Acute myocardial ischemia can also occur during non-cardiac surgery. As anesthetics are an integral part of the perioperative period, these agents have been the subject of close inspection in I/R situations. Several studies showed that the potent inhalational anesthetics particularly can provide protection against the deleterious consequences of I/R injury.

▌ Anti-ischemic Effects

A beneficial role of volatile anesthetics during myocardial ischemia was observed as early as 1969 by Spieckermann and colleagues [1], who found a prolonged tolerance to global ischemia and enhanced preservation of high energy compounds in dog hearts during halothane anesthesia. Several studies have demonstrated that volatile anesthetics reduce myocardial oxygen demand during ischemia, thereby reducing ischemic damage [2–5]. Halothane, enflurane, and isoflurane improved contractile function after cardioplegic arrest [6], after hypoxic perfusion [5] or global ischemia, and reduced infarct size [7]. In patients with coronary heart disease, isoflurane improves the tolerance to pacing-induced myocardial ischemia [8]. Sevoflurane and desflurane also offer anti-ischemic properties [9–11]. The mechanisms behind this protection might be the negative inotropic and negative chronotropic action of the substances. In addition, volatile anesthetics maintain myocardial energy stores [10] and might increase collateral blood flow to the ischemic area [12, 13], thereby reducing the severity of ischemia.

In all these studies, the anesthetics were given before or during ischemia. Therefore, it was not possible to differentiate between anti-ischemic properties or specific actions against the reperfusion injury.

Reperfusion Injury

'Reperfusion injury' has been defined as "metabolic, functional and structural changes after restoration of coronary perfusion, which can be reduced or prohibited by modification of the reperfusion conditions" [14]. An analysis of infarct size development after restoration of myocardial perfusion does not allow to differentiate between the cell death caused by ischemia and the cell death caused by the reperfusion itself.

Reperfusion injury can be divided into non-lethal, reversible cellular damage, and lethal, irreversible damage. Non-lethal reperfusion injury includes myocardial arrhythmias and the post-ischemic reduction of myocardial function. The reversible, but delayed recovery of myocardial function after complete restoration of coronary blood flow is called 'myocardial stunning' [15]. Lethal reperfusion injury is characterized by irreversible cell death (myocardial necrosis) and can be divided into an early (immediately at the beginning of reperfusion), and a late phase of myocardial damage. The different characteristics of the reperfusion injury are caused by distinct patho-mechanisms (Table 1), which can be modified by therapeutic interventions.

The oxygen paradox was first described by Hearse et al. in isolated rat hearts and is characterized by loss of viable tissue due to resupply of oxygen and substrates after myocardial ischemia [16]. The oxygen paradox leads to cellular hypercontracture and subsequent cytolysis at the beginning of reoxygenation. This mechanism is started by the resumption of mitochondrial energy production and therefore, is initiated by the reoxygenation and not by the preceding ischemia [17, 18]. This mechanism is characterized as follows: prolonged energy depletion leads to an increase in cytosolic Ca^{2+} concentration caused by diffusion of Ca^{2+} from the extracellular space. The start of energy resupply leads to: 1) activation of ionic pumps to restore cation homeostasis and 2) to activation of the contractile elements of the myofibrils. During ischemia, cells are overloaded with sodium and calcium. Reoxygenation activates the sarcolemmal Na^+-K^+-ATPase and the Ca^{2+}-ATPase of the sar-

Table 1. Mechanisms of reperfusion injury

Myocardial stunning (sublethal reperfusion injury)
- oxygen radicals
- changes in cellular Ca^{2+}-homeostasis
- reduced Ca^{2+}-sensitivity of the myofilaments
- endogenous mediators (adenosine, K_{ATP}-channels)

Early lethal reperfusion injury
- Ca^{2+}-paradox
- oxygen-paradox
- changes of intracellular pH and osmolarity
- increased sarcolemmal fragility

Delayed lethal reperfusion injury
- adhesion and activation of polymorphonuclear neutrophils
- release of free radicals from activated neutrophils
- adhesion and activation of platelets
- activation of the complement system
- apoptosis

coplasmic reticulum (SR). The activation of the Ca^{2+}-ATPase results in a transient uptake of Ca^{2+} into the SR, subsequently leading to Ca^{2+} overload of the SR. As a result, Ca^{2+} oscillations occur until the intracellular Ca^{2+}-concentration is decreased to normal values by the Na^+-Ca^{2+}-exchanger, which is activated itself by the trans-sarcolemmal Na^+ gradient [17]. At the beginning of reoxygenation, the energy re-supply in the presence of an elevated Ca^{2+}-concentration leads to uncontrolled acti-vation of the myofilaments, followed by cellular hypercontracture. Isolated myo-cytes can regain electrolyte homeostasis without loosing cell integrity [19]; in intact organs, however, the mechanical forces of hypercontracture are mutually exchanged between adjacent cells and result in rupture of the cytoskeleton and finally cell death.

Because the reperfusion injury depends on the severity of the preceding isch-emia, studies in which the volatile anesthetics were given before or during ischemia [1–7, 9–11], cannot differentiate between anti-ischemic effects and specific actions against reperfusion injury. In 1996, a specific protection against myocardial reper-fusion injury by halothane was described [20]. Isolated rat hearts underwent a per-iod of anoxic perfusion and subsequent reperfusion, and halothane was given either during the anoxic perfusion or only during early reperfusion. The recovery of myocardial function (left ventricular developed pressure) was improved only if halothane was present during the early reperfusion period (Fig. 1). In parallel, crea-tine kinase release, an index of cellular damage, was reduced if halothane was given during ischemia, but was nearly abolished if halothane was given during the early reperfusion period. This study demonstrated that modification of the reperfusion conditions by administration of a common volatile anesthetic specifically reduced reperfusion damage. The protection was confirmed for enflurane, sevoflurane and desflurane, while, in contrast, isoflurane did not reduce reperfusion injury in iso-lated rat hearts, suggesting different mechanisms of protection [21]. In addition, enflurane, isoflurane [22], sevoflurane, and desflurane [23] given during early re-perfusion offered additional protection against myocardial reperfusion injury, by protecting the heart against the ischemic damage by HTK (histidine-tryptophan-ke-toglutarate) cardioplegic solution. Protective effects of halothane depended on the Ca^{2+} content of the cardioplegic solution and were absent with the low-calcium HTK solution [22]. This observation indicates that the protection offered by halo-thane depends on changes in Ca^{2+}-homeostasis. Halothane reduces the activity of the Na^+-Ca^{2+} exchanger [24] and blocks the Ca^{2+}-dependent Ca^{2+}-release channel of the SR [25, 26]. At low pH and low ATP concentrations, halothane increases Ca^{2+}-uptake into the SR [27]. In anoxic-reperfused cardiomyocytes, halothane in-hibited the Ca^{2+}-dependent Ca^{2+}-release channel (ryanodine receptor) of the SR, thereby reducing Ca^{2+}-oscillations at the SR and preventing the cells from hyper-contracture (Fig. 2) [28]. This mechanism may explain why halothane offered no protection after application of the low-calcium HTK cardioplegic solution.

Enflurane and isoflurane also reduce intracellular Ca^{2+}-concentration by inhibi-tion of the sarcolemmal Ca^{2+}-channel [29] and the Na^+-Ca^{2+}-exchanger [24]. En-flurane, but not isoflurane, inhibited the Ca^{2+}-dependent Ca^{2+}-channel of the SR [30]; this may explain the lack of protection by isoflurane against cellular damage in isolated rat hearts [21]. Sevoflurane decreased transsarcolemmal Ca^{2+} current [31], increased Ca^{2+} uptake into the SR [32] and reduced transitory release of Ca^{2+} from the SR [33]. These actions result in a decreased cytoplasmic Ca^{2+}-concentra-tion, thereby reducing cellular hypercontracture and myocardial necrosis. The ef-fects of desflurane on cardiac Ca^{2+} homeostasis have not been investigated so far.

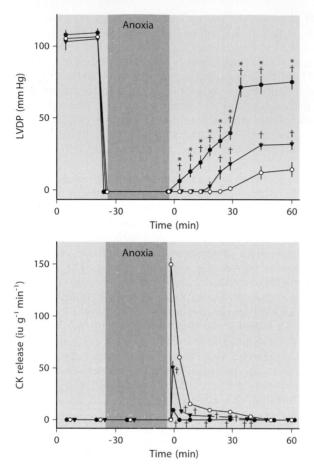

Fig. 1. Influence of halothane on left ventricular developed pressure (LVDP) and creatine kinase (CK) release in isolated rat hearts. Isolated rat hearts were subjected to 30 min anoxic perfusion followed by 60 min of reoxygenation. Halothane was applied during the 30 min anoxic perfusion (▼) or during the first 30 min of reoxygenation (●). †: p<0.05 vs. control (○); *: p<0.05 halothane-anoxia vs. halothane-reoxygenation. The application of halothane during reoxygenation significantly improved post-ischemic functional recovery (upper panel). No CK release was observed during anoxic perfusion but the cell damage occurred during the first minutes of reoxygenation. The CK release was reduced by halothane application during ischemia, but was nearly abolished by halothane application during reoxygenation. (From [20] with permission)

Volatile anesthetics also reduce reperfusion injury *in vivo*. Treatment with 1.0 minimum alveolar concentration (MAC) halothane during the early reperfusion period reduced infarct size in rabbit hearts *in vivo* (Fig. 3) [34]. The reduction in infarct size was similar if negative inotropy and vasodilation were antagonized by infusion of norepinephrine. Therefore, the protection was not caused by the hemodynamic effects of halothane, but by a specific action on the reperfused myocardium [34]. Inhalation of sevoflurane and desflurane during the early reperfusion period also reduced myocardial reperfusion injury after coronary artery occlusion *in vivo*, while enflurane showed only marginal protective effects and isoflurane offered no protection [35]. In addition, sevoflurane and desflurane altered systemic

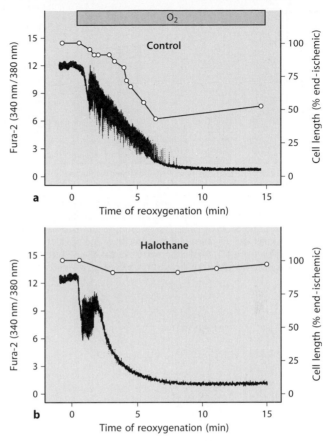

Fig. 2. Time course of fura 2 ratio (continuous trace of original recording) and cell length in percent of end-ischemic cell length (○) in single cardiomyocytes during reoxygenation. The fura 2 ratio (340/380 nm) is an index for changes in cytosolic Ca^{2+} concentration. Cardiomyocytes, superfused with anoxic medium, were allowed to accumulate Ca^{2+} until the saturation of the fura 2 ratio was reached. **a**: Reoxygenation in absence of inhibitors; **b**: reoxygenation in presence of 0.4 mmol/l halothane (equivalent to 1.5 MAC in rats). Untreated cardiomyocytes developed hypercontracture at the start of reoxygenation (reduction in cell length by 50%); simultaneously, reoxygenation induced Ca^{2+} oscillations were observed during the first 7 min of reoxygenation. Halothane reduced reoxygenation induced Ca^{2+} oscillations, thereby preventing cellular hypercontracture (cell length 95%). (From [28] with permission)

hemodynamics less than isoflurane and enflurane [35]. Apart from effects on systemic hemodynamics and intracellular Ca^{2+} homeostasis, other mechanisms have been proposed to offer potential protective effects against reperfusion injury. *In vivo*, the activated leukocyte is an additional potential cause of late lethal reperfusion injury [36]. Although leukocyte activation and accumulation is a consequence of the initial state of tissue injury, leukocytes may cause further injury by synthesizing and releasing a variety of mediators, including oxygen free radicals and oxidants [36]. By plugging capillaries, leukocytes are thought to play an important role in the 'delayed no-reflow phenomenon', resulting in persistent ischemia. Halothane, sevoflurane, and isoflurane reduce post-ischemic adhesion of leukocytes in the cor-

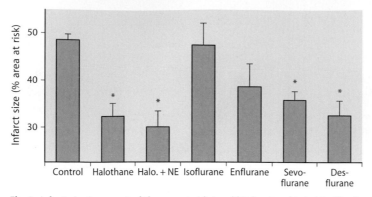

Fig. 3. Infarct size in percent of the area at risk in rabbit hearts subjected to 30 min of coronary artery occlusion followed by 120 min reperfusion *in vivo*. Volatile anesthetics were given only during the first 15 min of the reperfusion period. Mean (SEM); *: $p < 0.05$ vs. control. Halothane significantly reduced infarct size, and this protective action was still observed if the vasodilative and negative inotropic effects were counterbalanced with norepinephrine (Halo+NE). Sevoflurane and desflurane also reduced infarct size, while enflurane had only small effects and isoflurane offered no protection in these experiments

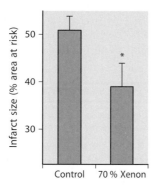

Fig. 4. Infarct size in percent of the area at risk in rabbit hearts subjected to 30 min of coronary artery occlusion followed by 120 min reperfusion *in vivo*. Xenon was administered only during the first 15 min of the reperfusion period and significantly reduced infarct size. Mean (SEM); *: $p < 0.05$ vs. control

onary system [37, 38]. Volatile anesthetics inhibit the release and cytotoxic activity of free radicals [39, 40]. Sevoflurane and isoflurane reduce platelet adhesion as well as release of vasoactive mediators from platelets [41], thereby minimizing the post-ischemic no-reflow phenomenon and reducing reperfusion injury.

In contrast to the clinically available volatile anesthetics, which can all produce marked hemodynamic side effects, the noble gas xenon can be used as an anesthetic agent with minimal cardiovascular side effects. In rabbits subjected to coronary artery occlusion and reperfusion, inhalation of 70% xenon during the early reperfusion period significantly reduced infarct size and protected against reperfusion damage (Fig. 4) [42]. In addition, no significant alterations in hemodynamics could be observed in these experiments. The minimal hemodynamic alterations may make xenon a suitable inhaled anesthetic in a myocardial I/R situation.

As the danger of impending hypercontracture in the reoxygenated myocardial cell is evoked by reactivation of mitochondrial energy production, a protective substance should be present at the onset of reperfusion. In anoxic, reoxygenated rat cardiomyocytes, the intracellular Ca^{2+} homeostasis recovered within 5 min, and after this period administration of halothane could be discontinued without danger of hypercontracture [28]. In rat hearts *in vivo*, the administration of 1.0 MAC sevoflurane for the first two minutes of reperfusion offered marked protection against reperfusion injury. Prolonging the administration time or increasing the concentration did not result in further infarct size reduction, but resulted in more pronounced hemodynamic side effects [43, 44].

At variance with potent inhalation anesthetics, intravenous anesthetics have shown little evidence of cardioprotection during I/R situations. Propofol, for example, is known as a free oxygen radical scavenger [45] and inhibits calcium influx across plasma membranes [46], but does not improve post-ischemic myocardial function [47]. Given only during the reperfusion period, propofol provided no protective effect against cellular damage in isolated rat hearts [48].

▌ Conclusion

Because of the increasing clinical use of thrombolysis, percutaneous balloon angioplasty, and coronary bypass surgery, it is of great practical interest to determine if additional therapeutic interventions during the I/R period can lead to a reduction in I/R injury. Accumulated experimental evidence from *in vitro* and *in vivo* studies for a protective effects of volatile anesthetics suggest that these substances may play a major role in clinical I/R situations.

References

1. Spieckermann PG, Brückner JB, Kübler W, Lohr B, Bretschneider HJ (1969) Preischemic stress and resuscitation time of the heart. Verhandl Dt Ges Herz- Kreislaufforsch 33:358–364
2. Davis RF, DeBoer LW, Rude RE, Lowenstein E, Maroko PR (1983) The effect of halothane anesthesia on myocardial necrosis, hemodynamic performance, and regional myocardial blood flow in dogs following coronary artery occlusion. Anesthesiology 59:402–411
3. Buljubasic N, Stowe DF, Marijic J, Roerig DL, Kampine JP, Bosnjak ZJ (1993) Halothane reduces release of adenosine, inosine, and lactate with ischemia and reperfusion in isolated hearts. Anesth Analg 76:54–62
4. Buljubasic N, Stowe DF, Marijic J, Kampine JP, Bosnjak ZJ (1992) Halothane reduces dysrhythmias and improves contractile function after global hypoperfusion in isolated hearts. Anesth Analg 74:384–394
5. Marijic J, Stowe DF, Turner LA, Kampine JP, Bosnjak ZJ (1990) Differential protective effects of halothane and isoflurane against hypoxic and reoxygenation injury in the isolated guinea pig heart. Anesthesiology 73:976–983
6. Coetzee A, Skein W, Genade S, Lochner A (1993) Enflurane and isoflurane reduce reperfusion dysfunction in the isolated rat heart. Anesth Analg 76:602–608
7. Cope DK, Impastato WK, Cohen MV, Downey JM (1997) Volatile anesthetics protect the ischemic rabbit myocardium from infarction. Anesthesiology 86:699–709
8. Tarnow J, Markschies Hornung A, Schulte Sasse U (1986) Isoflurane improves the tolerance to pacing-induced myocardial ischemia. Anesthesiology 64:147–156
9. Takahata O, Ichihara K, Ogawa H (1995) Effects of sevoflurane on ischaemic myocardium in dogs. Acta Anaesthesiol Scand 39:449–456
10. Oguchi T, Kashimoto S, Yamaguchi T, Nakamura T, Kumazawa T (1995) Comparative effects of halothane, enflurane, isoflurane, and sevoflurane on function and metabolism in the ischaemic rat heart. Br J Anaesth 74:569–575

11. Pagel PS, Hettrick DA, Lowe D, Tessmer JP, Warltier DC (1995) Desflurane and isoflurane exert modest beneficial actions on left ventricular diastolic function during myocardial ischemia in dogs. Anesthesiology 83:1021–1035

12. Takahata O, Ichihara K, Abiko Y, Ogawa H (1998) Sevoflurane preserves endocardial blood flow during coronary ligation in dogs: comparison with adenosine. Acta Anaesthesiol Scand 42:225–231

13. Kersten JR, Schmeling T, Tessmer J, Hettrick DA, Pagel PS, Warltier DC (1999) Sevoflurane selectively increases coronary collateral blood flow independent of K_{ATP} channels in vivo. Anesthesiology 90:246–256

14. Rosenkranz ER, Buckberg GD (1983) Myocardial protection during surgical coronary reperfusion. J Am Coll Cardiol 1:1235–1246

15. Braunwald E, Kloner RA (1982) The stunned myocardium: Prolonged, postischemic ventricular dysfunction. Circulation 66:1146–1149

16. Hearse DJ, Humphrey SM, Chain EB (1973) Abrupt reoxygenation of the anoxic potassium-arrested perfused rat heart: A study of myocardial enzyme release. J Mol Cell Cardiol 5:395–407

17. Siegmund B, Ladilov Y, Piper HM (1994) Importance of Na^+ for the recovery of Ca^{2+} control in reoxygenated cardiomyocytes. Am J Physiol 267:H506–H513

18. Siegmund B, Schlüter KD, Piper HM (1993) Calcium and the oxygen paradox. Cardiovasc Res 27:1778–1783

19. Siegmund B, Koop A, Klietz T, Schwartz P, Piper HM (1990) Sarcolemmal integrity and metabolic competence of cardiomyocytes under anoxia-reoxygenation. Am J Physiol 258:H285–H291

20. Schlack W, Hollmann M, Stunneck J, Thämer V (1996) Effect of halothane on myocardial reoxygenation injury in the isolated rat heart. Br J Anaesth 76:860–867

21. Schlack W, Preckel B, Stunneck D, Thämer V (1998) Effects of halothane, enflurane, isoflurane, sevoflurane and desflurane on myocardial reperfusion injury in the isolated rat heart. Br J Anaesth 81:913–919

22. Preckel B, Schlack W, Thämer V (1998) Enflurane and isoflurane, but not halothane, protect against myocardial reperfusion injury after cardioplegic arrest with HTK solution in the isolated rat heart. Anesth Analg 87:1221–1227

23. Preckel B, Thämer V, Schlack W (1999) Beneficial effects of sevoflurane and desflurane against myocardial reperfusion injury after cardioplegic arrest. Can J Anaesth 46:1076–1081

24. Haworth RA, Goknur AB (1995) Inhibition of sodium/calcium exchange and calcium channels of heart cells by volatile anesthetics. Anesthesiology 82:1255–1265

25. Komai H, Rusy BF (1990) Direct effect of halothane and isoflurane on the function of the sarcoplasmic reticulum. Anesthesiology 72:694–698

26. Lynch C, III, Frazer MJ (1994) Anesthetic alterations of ryanodine binding by cardiac calcium release channels. Biochim Biophys Acta 1194:109–117

27. Blanck TJJ, Thompson M (1981) Calcium transport by cardiac sarcoplasmic reticulum: modulation of halothane action by substrate concentration and pH. Anesth Analg 60:390–394

28. Siegmund B, Schlack W, Ladilov YV, Balser C, Piper HM (1997) Halothane protects cardiomyocytes against reoxygenation-induced hypercontracture. Circulation 96:4372–4379

29. Eskinder H, Rusch NJ, Supan FD, Kampine JP, Bosnjak ZJ (1991) The effects of volatile anesthetics on L- and T-type calcium channel currents in canine cardiac Purkinje cells. Anesthesiology 74:919–926

30. Wheeler DM, Rice RT, DuBell WH, Spurgeon HA (1997) Initial contractile response of isolated rat heart cells to halothane, enflurane, and isoflurane. Anesthesiology 86:137–146

31. Bartunek AE, Housmans PR (2000) Effects of sevoflurane on the intracellular Ca^{2+} transient in ferret cardiac muscle. Anesthesiology 93:1500–1508

32. Azuma M, Matsumura C, Kemmotsu O (1996) The effects of sevoflurane on contractile and electrophysiologic properties in isolated guinea pig papillary muscles. Anesth Analg 82:486–491

33. Davies LA, Gibson CN, Boyett MR, Hopkins PM, Harrison SM (2000) Effects of isoflurane, sevoflurane, and halothane on myofilament Ca^{2+} sensitivity and sarcoplasmic reticulum Ca^{2+} release in rat ventricular myocytes. Anesthesiology 93:1034–1044

34. Schlack W, Preckel B, Barthel H, Obal D, Thämer V (1997) Halothane reduces reperfusion injury after regional ischaemia in the rabbit heart *in vivo*. Br J Anaesth 79:88–96
35. Preckel B, Schlack W, Comfère T, Obal D, Barthel H, Thämer V (1998) Effects of enflurane, isoflurane, sevoflurane and desflurane on reperfusion injury after regional myocardial ischaemia in the rabbit heart *in vivo*. Br J Anaesth 81:905–912
36. Mullane KM, Young M (1992) The contribution of neutrophil activation and changes in endothelial function to myocardial ischemia-reperfusion injury. In: Yellon DM, Jennings RB (eds) The Pathophysiology of Reperfusion and Reperfusion injury. Raven Press, New York, pp 59–83
37. Heindl B, Reichle FM, Zahler S, Conzen PF, Becker BF (1999) Sevoflurane and isoflurane protect the reperfused guinea pig heart by reducing postischemic adhesion of polymorphonuclear neutrophils. Anesthesiology 91:521–530
38. Kowalski C, Zahler S, Becker BF, et al (1997) Halothane, isoflurane, and sevoflurane reduce postischemic adhesion of neutrophils in the coronary system. Anesthesiology 86:188–195
39. Glantz L, Ginosar Y, Chevion M, et al (1997) Halothane prevents postischemic production of hydroxyl radicals in the canine heart. Anesthesiology 86:440–447
40. Nakamura T, Kashimoto S, Oguchi T, Kumazawa T (1999) Hydroxyl radical formation during inhalation anesthesia in the reperfused working rat heart. Can J Anaesth 46:470–475
41. Heindl B, Conzen PF, Becker BF (1999) The volatile anesthetic sevoflurane mitigates cardiodepressive effects of platelets in reperfused hearts. Basic Res Cardiol 94:102–111
42. Preckel B, Müllenheim J, Moloschavij A, Thämer V, Schlack W (2000) Xenon administration during early reperfusion reduces infarct size after regional ischemia in the rabbit heart in vivo. Anesth Analg 91:1327–1332
43. Obal D, Preckel B, Scharbatke H, et al (2001) One MAC of sevoflurane provides protection against reperfusion injury in the rat heart in vivo. Br J Anaesth 87:900–906
44. Obal D, Scharbatke H, Preckel B, et al (2001) Effect of time and concentration of sevoflurane administration on protection against myocardial reperfusion injury in rats *in vivo*. Pflügers Arch 441 (Suppl 2):P31–8 (Abst)
45. Kokita N, Hara A (1996) Propofol attenuates hydrogen peroxide-induced mechanical and metabolic derangements in the isolated rat heart. Anesthesiology 84:117–127
46. Puttick RM, Terrar DA (1993) Differential effects of propofol and enflurane on contractions dependent on calcium derived from the sarcoplasmic reticulum of guinea pig isolated papillary muscles. Anesth Analg 77:55–60
47. Ross S, Muñoz H, Piriou V, Ryder WA, Foëx P (1998) A comparison of the effects of fentanyl and propofol on left ventricular contractility during myocardial stunning. Acta Anaesthesiol Scand 42:23–31
48. Ebel D, Schlack W, Comfère T, Preckel B, Thämer V (1999) Effect of propofol on reperfusion injury after regional ischaemia in the isolated rat heart. Br J Anaesth 83:903–908

Regulatory Role of Nitric Oxide in the Heart of the Critically Ill Patient

P. B. Massion and J. L. Balligand

▍ Introduction

More than two decades ago, Furchgott and Zawadzki [1] discovered that intact endothelium was necessary for acetylcholine-induced vasorelaxation. A substance derived from this endothelium, the so-called 'endothelium-derived relaxing factor' (EDRF), was born. It took until 1988 for this to be identified as nitric oxide (NO) [2]. In addition to its release in the coronary circulation, NO also reduced contractility in cultured cardiomyocytes [3, 4] and was shown to mediate, at least in part, the septic cardiodepression induced by the 'myocardial depressant substance', identified as the combination of tumor necrosis factor (TNF)-α and interleukin (IL)-1 [5]. Since then, this highly diffusable gas has been found to be nearly ubiquitous in the organism in a large variety of cellular types and organs, and implicated in almost all cardiovascular, neuronal, and immune processes.

NO is produced by NO synthase (NOS), when the substrate L-arginine is converted into L-citrulline, in the presence of oxygen and sufficient cofactors. Importantly, three isoforms of NOS have been identified and are all present in the human heart (for a review, see [6]):

▍ neuronal NOS (nNOS, encoded by *NOS1* gene), present in ortho- and parasympathetic nerves terminals of the cardiomyocyte, regulating catecholamine release in the heart;

▍ inducible NOS (iNOS, encoded by *NOS2* gene), expressed under pathophysiological conditions in almost all cell subtypes, including macrophages, neutrophils, but also endothelial cells (endocardial and coronary), fibroblasts, neurons, vascular smooth muscle cells and cardiomyocytes;

▍ endothelial NOS (eNOS, or constitutive NOS, encoded by *NOS3* gene), present in endothelial cells, platelets, and cardiomyocytes. There, besides its mitochondrial localization, eNOS is mainly trapped at the sarcolemma or T-tubules in small (50–100 nm) membrane invaginations called caveolae, where eNOS is tonically inhibited by the caveolar structural protein, caveolin. Caveolin 1 is mainly expressed in endothelial cells, while caveolin 3 is specific to myocytes.

While iNOS is calcium-independent, activated by various inflammatory cytokines and produces high concentrations (hundreds of micromolar) of NO for prolonged periods of time, leading to most of the detrimental – including cardiodepressant – effects of NO, nNOS and eNOS are calcium-dependent and release low concentrations (submicromolar) of NO, responsible for its main beneficial or physiological effects.

After an overview of the different 'fine tuning' effects of NO in the normal heart, including various signaling pathways, we will briefly review the critical role of NO in most relevant heart diseases encountered in intensive care, i.e., acute ischemic syndromes, ischemic cardiomyopathy and dilated cardiomyopathy, as well as septic cardiodepression, cardiac allograft rejection, and myocarditis.

▋ Regulatory Role of NO in the Normal Heart

Before detailing the properties and the mechanisms of action of NO, we will put the specific role of NO as a cardiomodulator in a more global context. Heart function may be considered as a continuous matching balance between myocardial oxygen demand and uptake (VO_2), on one hand, and, on the other hand, myocardial oxygen supply and delivery (DO_2). While the main determinants of myocardial VO_2 (cardiac output times arteriovenous oxygen content difference) correspond to the four factors of cardiac output (i.e., heart rate, preload, afterload, and contractility), DO_2 depends on oxygen carrying capacity (CaO_2) and coronary blood flow [7]. The coronary blood flow itself depends not only on coronary vascular resistance (since coronary blood flow is the coronary perfusion pressure – i.e., mean arterial pressure [MAP] minus left ventricular end-diastolic pressure [LVEDP] – divided by coronary vascular resistance) but also – especially in the subendocardium – on the duration of diastole (because wall contraction together with intracavitary pressure suppresses systolic flow) and on coronary collateral circulation (after coronary occlusion). The main neurotransmitters and hormones involved in the regulation of heart function are listed with their receptor, second messenger, targets and physiological effects in Figure 1 (for review, see [8–10]). Impressively, NO is implicated as second messenger in all processes. NO can be considered as a cardioprotective regulator of intracardiac processes, counterbalancing excessive adrenergic stimulation (mediated by cyclic adenosine monophosphate or cAMP), signaling the parasympathetic pathway (also mediated by cyclic guanosine monophosphate or cGMP), and fine tuning various other pathways.

The predominant myocardial effects of low concentrations of NO (eNOS-generated) are counteracting positive adrenergic inotropic effects, positive lusitropic, negative chronotropic, anti-arrhythmic, oxygen-saving, coronarodilator, anti-hypertrophic, anti-oxidant, anti-apoptotic, anti-aggregant and anti-inflammatory effects (for review, see [11]). In addition, eNOS mediates the increase in excitation-contraction coupling gain in response to cardiomyocyte stretch. NO promotes left ventricular mechanical efficiency, i.e., appropriate matching between cardiac work and myocardial oxygen consumption [12]. In contrast, deleterious effects of NO (or derivatives thereof, such as peroxynitrite), encountered with iNOS-generated high concentrations, are its massively cardiodepressant, negative lusitropic, vasoplegic, pro-oxidant, pro-apoptotic and pro-inflammatory effects.

Figure 2 details the signaling mechanisms whereby NO acts in cardiomyocytes and gives the ultrastructural basis of NO production and NO signaling as well as NO modulation of the main determinants of myocardial function. These different topics are reviewed below.

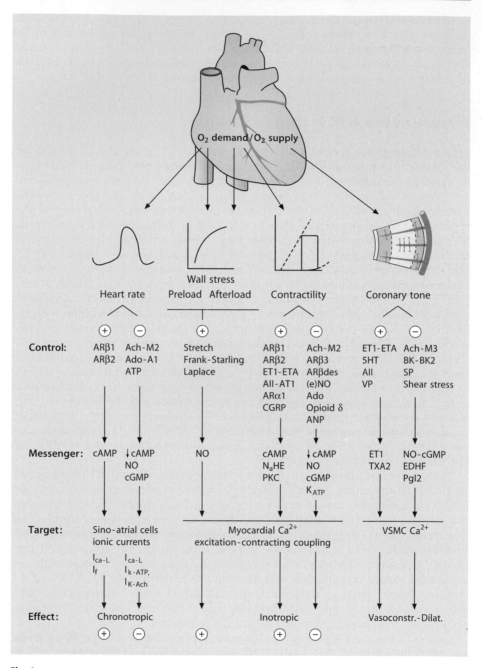

Fig. 1

eNOS-mediated NO Originates from Endothelium or from the Cardiomyocyte

With regard to the coronary endothelium, the stimulation by acetylcholine (M3 muscarinic receptor), bradykinin (B2 receptor) or substance P (NK1 receptor) leads, through the cascade Gq protein-phospholipase C-inositol triphosphate-calcium-calmodulin, to the activation of eNOS [13]. eNOS may also be activated by phosphorylations, as induced by insulin through phosphatidyl-inositol 3 kinase-protein kinase B (PI3K-PKB) signaling [14].

Inside the cardiomyocyte, the caveolar eNOS may be stimulated by M2 muscarinic, β_3 adrenergic, A_1 adenosine or δ opioid receptors as well as by stretch (see infra). Acetylcholine enhances NO production probably through an M2-protein Gi-β,γ-phospholipase C-inositol triphosphate-calcium-calmodulin cascade. Acetylcholine's negative inotropic and chronotropic effects also occur through NO-independent pathways: 1) by direct Ga_{i2}-protein-mediated inhibition of adenylate cyclase and subsequent cAMP reduction (counteracting positive inotropic effect); 2) by Ga_i-protein-mediated stimulation of the K^+current (I_{K-Ach}) in sinoatrial node cells (attenuating the spontaneous pacemaker current I_f) [9]. Of high clinical relevance, the recently identified β_3-adrenoceptor mediates a negative inotropic effect through coupling to a $Ga_{i/o}$-protein and eNOS [15], probably via a PI3K-PKB pathway. Accordingly, β_3-adrenoceptor knockout mice showed increased β-adrenergic-stimulated inotropy [16]. This β_3-adrenoceptor is an important step in the understanding of the altered response to catecholamines in the failing heart (see below).

Note that, in the presence of inflammatory processes, large amounts of iNOS-derived NO may also originate from any cells, e.g., not only endothelial cells and cardiomyocytes but also macrophages and neutrophils, over a long period of time, leading to most of its detrimental effects.

NO Regulates Cardiac Function through cGMP-independent and cGMP-dependent Pathways

First, the gas NO diffuses rapidly through cell membranes in most tissues and may react itself (cGMP-independent pathway) at low concentrations with various atoms or free radicals, such as:

▪ sulfur atoms in thiol residues (S-nitrosylation) of various proteins, e.g., albumin, glutathione, hemoglobin, tissue plasminogen activator (t-PA), glyceraldehyde phosphate dehydrogenase, NADPH oxidase, creatine kinase and ryanodine receptor;

←———————————————————————————————————————

Fig. 1. Regulatory role of nitric oxide (NO) on the response to main neurotransmitters and second messengers regulating myocardial oxygen demand and oxygen supply in human heart. Positive and negative controls for heart rate, preload, afterload, contractility and coronary flow are shown, with respective signaling pathways, second messengers, targets, and final effects. Coronary flow depends on coronary tone but also duration of diastole and density of collateral vessels (not shown). Note the multiple implications of NO in these various processes. AII: angiotensin II; Ach: acetylcholine; Ado: adenosine; ANP: atrial natriuretic peptide; AR: adrenoceptor; AR-des: AR desensitization; ATP: adenosine triphosphate; BK: bradykinin; camp: cyclic adenosine monophosphate; cGMP: cyclic guanosine monophosphate; CGRP: calcitonin gene-related peptide; (e)NO: endothelium-derived NO; ET: endothelin; EDHF: endothelium-derived hyperpolarizing factor; 5-HT: serotonine; I_{Ca-L}: L-type Ca^{2+} current; I_f: spontaneous pacemaker current; I_{K-Ach}: Ach-dependent K^+ current; I_{K-ATP}: ATP-dependent K^+ current; M: muscarinic; NHE: sodium-hydrogen exchanger; PgI$_2$: prostacyclin; SP: substance P; TXA2: thromboxane; VP: vasopressin; VSMC: vascular smooth muscle cells

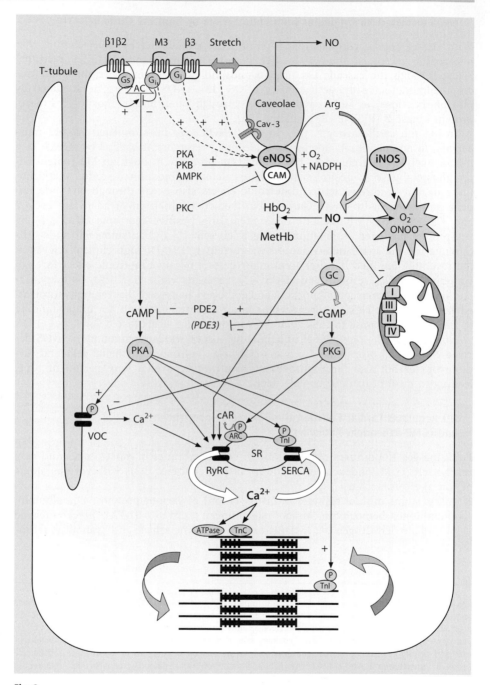

Fig. 2

▌ iron atoms of various proteins, including guanylate cyclase (see cGMP-dependent pathway), mitochondrial respiratory complexes, NOS itself, cyclooxygenase 2, heme-oxygenase and hemoglobin;

▌ radical oxygen species (ROS) such as superoxide anion (O_2^-) (ROS scavenging). High concentrations of iNOS-mediated NO may also combine with equimolar concentrations of O_2^- to produce peroxynitrite (ONOO) or other nitrosative species such as N_2O_3 and S-nitrosoglutathione (GNSO), leading to oxidative and nitrosative stresses (lipid oxidation, tyrosine nitrosylation) (for review, see [6]).

Second, NO activates the soluble isoform of guanylate cyclase to produce cGMP, which in turn activates protein kinase G (PKG) and other cGMP-sensitive molecular targets. This cGMP-dependent pathway provides most of the NO-mediated regulation of heart function (see below).

NO Inhibits Adrenergic-stimulated Contractility but Increases Relaxation

In case of adrenergic stimulation, NO-derived cGMP directly inhibits cAMP through activation of cAMP phosphodiesterase (PDE) 2, responsible for cAMP breakdown (negative inotropic effect). Nevertheless, cGMP may also do the opposite through PDE 3 (positive inotropic effect) depending on the predominant PDE isoform expression. Furthermore, cGMP also activates PKG that phosphorylates three main targets [17]:

▌ a regulatory protein involved in the protein kinase A-dependent phosphorylation of the voltage-operated L-type calcium channel (VOC), resulting in attenuation of Ca^{2+} transsarcolemmal influx and its effect on excitation-contraction coupling (negative inotropic effect);

▌ the adenosine diphosphate (ADP) ribosyl cyclase, producing cyclic ADP ribose that activates the ryanodine-receptor Ca^{2+}-release channels (RyRC) of the sarcoplasmic reticulum (positive inotropic effect);

▌ troponin I, which decreases myofilament sensitivity to calcium and thereby promotes relaxation (positive lusitropic effect). This positive lusitropic effect of NO

Fig. 2. Nitric oxide (NO) signaling into the cardiomyocyte. After muscarinic M2-, β_3-adrenergic receptor or stretch stimulation, caveolar eNOS dissociates from caveolin and generates NO. NO may then: (1) inhibit mitochondrial respiration complexes IV and I (reduction of MVO_2); (2) activate the ryanodine receptor (stretch response); (3) generate toxic peroxynitrite (irreversible inhibition of respiration, oxidative and nitrosative stresses); (4) activate guanylate cyclase to produce cyclic-guanosine monophosphate (cGMP) and to counterbalance the adrenergic drive. Indeed, cGMP activates phosphodiesterase (PDE) 2 to breakdown cyclic adenosine monophosphate (cAMP) (negative inotropic effect, even if a positive inotropic effect is possible via PDE3 depending on the predominant PDE isoform expression), and activates the protein kinase G (PKG), responsible for major effects of NO. PKG modulates the function of key contractile regulatory proteins, such as: (1) the L-type voltage-operated Ca^{2+} channel (VOC) in T-tubules, inhibiting Ca^{2+} entrance (negative inotropic effect); (2) the adenosine diphosphate (ADP) ribosyl cyclase, that activates the ryanodine-receptor Ca^{2+}-release channels (RyRC) of the sarcoplasmic reticulum (SR) through cyclic ADP ribose (positive inotropic effect); (3) the troponin I (TnI), decreasing myofilament sensitivity to calcium and thereby promoting relaxation (positive lusitropic effect). In parallel, β_1-β_2-adrenergic input signals through cAMP and proteine kinase A to stimulate VOC and RyRC, increase Ca^{2+}, stimulate myosin ATPase and troponin C (TnC) and cross-bridge cycling of actin-myosin (positive inotropic effect); on the other hand, the β-adrenergic pathway activates sarcoendoplasmic reticulum Ca^{2+} ATPase (SERCA) by desinhibition from phospholamban (PL) to recapture Ca^{2+} and phosphorylates troponin I (TnI) to desensitize myofilaments to Ca^{2+} (positive lusitropic effects). Full arrows designate stimulation; dashed arrows designate inhibition

is characterized by an earlier onset of left ventricular (LV) relaxation (prolonged duration of diastole) and by a right and downward displacement of the LV end-diastolic pressure-volume relationship [18].

If the negative inotropic effect of NO is not always evident in basal conditions – without adrenergic stimulation – in the normal heart and the failing heart, its effect becomes patent in β-adrenergic-prestimulated conditions, a phenomenon referred to as 'accentuated antagonism' [17].

NO Mediates Stretch Response to Preload and Afterload

Produced by activation of the PI(3)K-PKB-eNOS axis, NO has recently been identified in rats as a second messenger of stretch dependence of Ca^{2+} release in cardio-myocytes, by enhancing ryanodine-receptor Ca^{2+}-release channel activity, probably via their S-nitrosylation [19]. Both preload and afterload generate myocardial wall stress (at the end of diastole and during LV ejection, respectively), according to Laplace's law (wall stress = pressure×radius/2×wall thickness), and subsequent stretching of myofilaments increases their contraction, according to Frank-Starling's law (at any level of the myocardial contractility, cardiac output – stroke volume – is dependent on left ventricular end-diastolic volume (LVEDV)) [8]. NO may now be considered as a biochemical link between cardiac muscle length and excitation-contraction coupling [19].

NO Slows Heart Rate and Prevents Arrhythmias

In sino-atrial node pacemaker cells as well as in atrial and ventricular cells, acetyl-choline exerts its negative chronotropic effects through a M2 muscarinic receptor-Gi-β,γ protein-phospholipase C-inositol triphosphate-Ca^{2+}-calmodulin-eNOS cascade leading to NO production. NO then causes activation of cGMP-activated PDE, enhanced cAMP breakdown and attenuation of L-type Ca^{2+} current (I_{Ca-L}) responsible for phase 0 depolarization and propagation in sinoatrial and auriculoventricular nodal tissue [9]. Accordingly, NO suppresses ouabain-, digoxin- and ischemic-induced arrhythmias and mediates the antiarrhythmic effect of ischemic preconditioning, possibly through endogenous peroxynitrite [20].

eNOS-derived NO Inhibits Mitochondrial Respiration, Reduces Myocardial Oxygen Consumption, Prevents Apoptosis in Glycolytic Cells, and Preserves Ventricular Efficiency

Mitochondria are key organelles in the control of respiration and cell death, at the crossroads of myocardial oxygen demand and supply. Inside the mitochondrial respiratory chain, NO plays a pivotal regulatory role [21], also well documented in cardiac tissue [22]. Indeed, physiological concentrations of NO reversibly inhibit the mitochondrial electron chain complex IV (cytochrome c oxidase), by competition with oxygen. This effect increases as PO_2 falls, and NO may be considered as a mediator of cytochrome c oxidase sensing of hypoxia. Through an as yet unknown mechanism (possibly involving low ATP/ADP ratio-dependent activation of phosphofructokinase 1), NO stimulates glycolysis, thereby maintaining ATP concentrations. Inside the mitochondrion, glycolytically generated ATP is hydrolyzed by the mitochondrial F_1F_0-ATPase (reversal of ATP synthase) and maintains (even hyper-polarizes) the mitochondrial membrane potential ($\Delta\Psi_m$). This prevents cytochrome c release, caspases and subsequent apoptotic cascade activation (antiapoptotic effect of NO). This protective effect of NO requires an intact anaerobic glycolytic machinery, which may determine cellular-specific resistance to ischemia [23]. NO may thereby have a cytoprotective role in myocardial adaptation to ischemia [24] as well as in the development of heart failure [25]. This NO-mediated inhibition of respiratory complex IV dose-dependently reduces myocardial VO_2 [26] with a downward shift of the myocardial VO_2-pressure volume area (PVA, i.e., stroke work plus potential energy) relationship, so that, despite reduced contractility, contractile efficiency is maintained. Accordingly, NOS inhibition increases myocardial VO_2 and, despite increased contractility, does not increase contractile efficiency [12]. This eNOS-mediated reduction in myocardial VO_2, which is lost in eNOS knockout mice, explains the growing interest for endogenous NO releasing drugs such as the angiotensin-converting enzyme (ACE) inhibitor ramaprilat, the calcium antagonist amlodipine, and statins [22] as well as for the angiotensin II type-1 receptor inhibitor losartan [27], the third-generation β_1-blocker nebivolol [28], and new NO donors such as S-nitrosoglutathione or diethylamine/NO. Interestingly, a high load of NO donor inhibits glucose uptake in cardiomyocytes through still unknown cGMP-dependent mechanisms, affecting the traffic of the glucose transporter GLUT 4, decreasing myocardial glucose utilization, and limiting heart work [29], while low concentrations of NO stimulate glycolysis [23].

In contrast, prolonged exposure of NO results in persistent inhibition of complex I by S-nitrosylation [30], thereby producing electron transfer to molecular oxygen to produce superoxide anions. In the presence of high concentrations of NO, subsequent peroxynitrite formation causes irreversible inhibition of multiple respiratory complexes, leading to proton leak, permeability transition pore opening, loss of mitochondrial membrane potential, cytochrome c release and apoptotic cell death [21] as well as reduced contractility [31]. Furthermore, NO may inhibit other energy-related enzymes, such as mitochondrial and cytosolic creatine kinases and mitochondrial aconitase [6], especially when the reducing potential of the cells is impaired, e.g., when the glutathione concentration is decreased [32]. Peroxynitrite is pro-apoptotic, and involves iNOS-derived NO since the phenomenon is lost in iNOS knockout mice [33].

NO Vasodilates Coronary Arteries and Promotes Angiogenesis and Rheology

Once generated in the endothelium, NO diffuses in the abluminal space up to the vascular smooth muscle cells, where it reduces calcium and induces vasorelaxation through soluble guanylate cyclase-cGMP-inositol-triphosphate (IP3) or PKG-Ca^{2+}-dependent K^+ channel pathways. NO itself may also directly modify the Ca^{2+}-dependent K^+ channel [34], leading to hyperpolarization and inhibition of the VOC channel.

NO is a potent *in vivo* coronary vasodilator in normal heart. Accordingly, lack of NO leads to endothelial dysfunction (paradoxal vasoconstrictive response to acetylcholine), as demonstrated in human heart failure, in post-angioplasty restenosis or in arterosclleriosis. Gene therapy by transfecting eNOS- or nNOS-encoding adenoviruses is currently under investigation in animals, with promising results not only in carotid atherosclerosis and peripheral ischemia but also in coronary restenosis [35] and in hypoxia-induced coronary relaxation [36].

Note that NO also prolongs diastole, as mentioned above, and is proangiogenic, since it mediates ischemia-induced coronary collateralization as a second messenger of vascular endothelial growth factor (VEGF) [37] and mediates the pro-angiogenic effects of the statins [38]. Finally, NO rheologically promotes coronary flow by its antiaggregant effects (through increases in platelet cGMP, and also cGMP-independent S-nitrosylation of tissue-plasminogen activator [39]), and its inhibitory properties on leukocyte adhesion (through inhibition of nuclear factor B and subsequent downregulation of adhesion molecules, such as VCAM-1 and intercellular adhesion molecule [ICAM]-1) [40].

▌ Dual Role of NO in Compensated Ischemic Cardiomyopathy

Since NO regulates contractility, heart rate, wall stress, coronary tone, mitochondrial respiration, and apoptosis, NO will participate in various ischemic processes, such as acute ischemia, coronary restenosis, late preconditioning, stunning after ischemia-reperfusion (I/R) and hibernation.

In acute experimental infarction, the iNOS isoform is upregulated, transiently in infarcted tissue but more steadily in non-infarcted tissue [41]. iNOS expression correlates with myocardial dysfunction and mortality since infarcted iNOS knockout mice have improved myocardial contractile function and reduced apoptotic cell death compared with wild type [42, 43]. In contrast to iNOS, the eNOS isoform, albeit not always upregulated [41, 44], seems to have beneficial effects, since infarcted eNOS knockout mice have worse systolodiastolic dysfunction, ventricular remodeling, and increased mortality compared with wild type [45]. Considering coronary restenosis after angioplasty, eNOS also plays a protective role, confirmed by the effect of eNOS gene therapy [35] and of the new NO-releasing aspirin, NCX-4016 [46].

With regard to ischemic preconditioning, iNOS-derived NO plays a protective role in its late phase, lasting 3 to 4 days, protecting against both infarction and stunning, and enhancing the recovery of left ventricular function [47]. The importance of the iNOS isoform was confirmed by the loss of preconditioning protection in iNOS knockout mice [48]. iNOS-released NO acts through PKC-ε and nuclear factor-κB (NF-κB) activation, leading to stimulation of protective tyrosine kinases (Src and Lck) and cytoprotective genes, respectively. NO also mediates *E. coli* endotoxin-induced late preconditioning with improved function recovery after subsequent episode of ischemia [49].

In I/R injury, functional NOS may have beneficial effects. Indeed, NO may scavenge ROS and thereby prevent calcium overload that delays myocardial recovery (stunning), as suggested with by L-arginine infusion during ischemia [29]. Intraoperative eNOS transfection or low-dose peroxynitrite may also reduce leukocyte infiltration through reduction of endothelial vascular cell (ECAM)- and ICAM-1 [50] or P-selectin expression [51]. On the other hand, when adequate substrate and cofactors are lacking, e.g., during ischemia, NOS may produce superoxide anions instead of NO (uncoupled NOS), generate subsequent peroxynitrite, and further increase oxidative stress [52]. This may explain the improvement in postischemic LV function after NOS inhibition with N-monomethyl-L-arginine (L-NMMA) when given before and during ischemia [53].

Finally, the beneficial effect of glucose-insulin-potassium (GIK) infusion in patients with reperfused myocardial infarction [54] and postoperative cardiogenic shock [55] may also involve NO beside its classical metabolic [56] and oxygen-saving [57] effects, although this has not yet been demonstrated directly. Indeed, insulin enhances eNOS expression and activity in human coronary endothelial cells [14] and exerts some of its effects on ICAM through NO production [58]. In addition, the insulin receptor may share the same caveolar compartmentation [59] as eNOS. Conversely, high-glucose extracellular concentrations such as those encountered in diabetes, downregulate eNOS expression [14], arguing for the need to closely monitor glycemic levels in critically-ill patients [60].

▌ eNOS Downregulation and β_3-Adrenoceptor Upregulation in Failing Cardiomyopathy

End-stage ischemic and/or dilated cardiomyopathies are characterized in most studies by a NO imbalance with a progressive downregulation of eNOS expression together with a sustained iNOS expression [10]. In one study, both eNOS and iNOS correlated with LV stroke volume and stroke work [61]. As cited above, NO production is also reduced in the coronary microvessels in such patients.

This lack of eNOS-derived NO is detrimental, and probably plays a causal role in the development of heart failure. In a canine model of rapid pacing-induced heart failure mimicking dilated cardiomyopathy, progressive (after 72 h) impairment of myocardial NO production and eNOS expression indeed paralleled a shift toward decompensated heart failure [62]. Loss of inhibition of myocardial VO_2 by bradykinin and carbachol in these dogs, with substrate switch from fatty acid to glucose utilization, reduced NO-dependent arteriolar dilatation and increased oxygen free radicals in myocardial tissue [63], confirming the importance of NO in the control of respiration and in the development of heart failure [22].

Likewise, treatment with the NOS inhibitor, L-NMMA, is detrimental in heart failure. Despite its short-term safety and efficacy in maintaining MAP and urinary output in intra-aortic balloon pump (IABP) supported patients with refractory cardiogenic shock [64] and its potentiation of dobutamine inotropic responsiveness [65] with increased dobutamine-induced LV contractility and external work, L-NMMA increased myocardial VO_2 so that mechanical efficiency (i.e., external work/ myocardial VO_2) does not increase further [66]. In the absence of adrenergic prestimulation, L-NMMA alone even decreased cardiac output [64] and had a small negative inotropic effect (rightward shift of the LV end-systolic pressure-volume relationship) [67].

In contrast, endogenous NO releasing drugs, such as amlodipine, ramaprilat, or the neutral endopeptidase inhibitor thiorphan, reduced myocardial VO_2 [68]. This is consistent with an oxygen-saving effect of NO through attenuation of the LV contractile responsiveness to β-adrenergic stimulation [66]. Furthermore, despite a negative inotropic effect (rightward displacement of the LV end-systolic pressure-volume relationship) after dobutamine pretreatment – not in basal conditions – [69], intracoronary infusion of substance P has an important lusitropic effect (LV end-diastolic pressure-volume relationship shifted to the right) in patients with elevated LVEDP [61]. This effect is of particular importance in failing hearts, since they depend on the Frank-Starling response to maintain cardiac output. Along the same lines, mechanical unloading with chronic LV assist device (LVAD) implantation augments NO-dependent control of mitochondrial respiration in failing human hearts, potentiates amlodipine- and enalaprilat-induced reduction in myocardial VO_2 [70] and restores β-adrenergic responsiveness through reversing receptor downregulation [71].

Most importantly, while β_1-adrenoceptors are downregulated and β_2-adrenoceptors are unchanged in heart failure [72], the recently identified β_3-adrenoceptors are upregulated in myocardial samples from either ischemic or dilated cardiomyopathic hearts [73]. The imbalance between their inotropic influences may underlie the functional degradation of the human failing heart, with a predominance of negative inotropic adrenergic drive. Furthermore, the β_3-adrenoceptors are mainly expressed in cardiomyocytes, strengthening the paradigm of a direct coupling to eNOS, and are relatively resistant to desensitization by downregulation, reinforcing the imbalance. While the β_3-adrenoceptor should have an adaptive role in early compensated cardiomyopathy, it may have a detrimental effect in end-stage decompensated heart failure. The effects of specific β_3-adrenoceptor antagonists are currently under investigation to resolve this question.

▌ NO Mediates Part of Septic Cardiodepression

The high mortality of septic shock in humans is related to multiple organ failure (MOF), and may involve NO-dependent mechanisms (for review, see [74]). Indeed, the septic shock-induced systolic and diastolic cardiodepression, confirmed by invasive contractility measurements (end-systolic LV pressure-volume relationship) [75], is at least partly mediated by NO [3].

Both eNOS [76] and iNOS [3, 5] isoforms may be upregulated in septic conditions, as well as after TNF-α stimulation [77]. NO mediates septic cardiodepression through:

▌ cGMP-mediated decrease in cAMP [78];
▌ direct inhibition by NO of the mitochondrial respiratory complexes [79]; and
▌ peroxynitrite-induced injury [80].

While iNOS-derived NO plays a deleterious role in sepsis, confirmed by the prevention of hypotension and systolodiastolic dysfunction in iNOS knockout mice [81], eNOS-derived NO seems to play a compensatory protective role [82]. Indeed, the *Staphylococcus aureus* α-toxin induced not only a myocardial depression with thromboxane (TX)A_2-mediated coronary vasoconstriction but also a simultaneous compensatory release of eNOS-derived NO, counteracting its own deleterious effects on myocardial performance [76].

Nevertheless, NO-independent mechanisms also explain sepsis-related cardiodepression, especially in the early phase, such as:

▌ altered β-adrenoceptor coupling to adenylate cyclase;
▌ TNF-α-induced reduction of systolic $[Ca^{2+}]_i$ concentrations;
▌ or increased basal phosphorylation of troponin I, leading to myofilament Ca^{2+} desensitization [83].

Likewise, NO-independent pathways may also explain TNF-α-induced cardiodepression, e.g., activation of the sphingomyelinase, generating ceramide with subsequent ceramide-activated protein kinase cascade. TNF-α is of special interest because it also plays a central role in the pathogenesis of heart failure in animals [84] as well as in patients [85], where its serum levels correlate with New York Heart Association class symptoms, cardiac cachexia, or edematous decompensated heart disease. Similarly, transgenic mice overexpressing TNF-α developed dilated heart failure with myocyte apoptosis, transmural myocarditis and biventricular fibrosis [86].

Of interest, innate immunity after host aggression also involves NO together with IL-1 and TNF-α. Indeed, iNOS-derived NO exerts antimicrobial activities and controls the function of natural killer (NK) cells, on one hand, and suppresses lymphocyte proliferation and may damage host cells, on the other hand. The human Toll-like receptor 4 (TLR4), upstream in the TNF-α and iNOS cascade, seems to play a crucial role in early innate immunity, since this receptor is overexpressed in focal areas of adjacent myocytes from patients with dilated cardiomyopathy [87]. TLR4 deficient mice have delayed and blunted response to lipopolysaccharide (LPS) and lower levels of TNF-α, IL-1β, iNOS and NO [88], confirming the paradigm that heart disease is part of an inflammatory process and opening the possibility for new anti-inflammatory cardiac therapies.

The dual role – deleterious and beneficial, depending on the isoform implicated – of NO may explain why nonselective NOS inhibitors such as L-NMMA [89] or L-NAME [90] failed to be of benefit in septic patients, decreasing their cardiac output, and even increasing their mortality. In addition, non discriminate inhibition of all NOS isoforms also results in weakening of host immune defense by abrogation of the potentiation of cyclo-oxygenase (COX)2 activity by NO [91]. By contrast, relatively selective iNOS inhibitors such as mercaptoethylguanidine, aminoguanidine, S-methylisothiourea sulfate and L-N(6)(1-iminoethyl)-lysine (L-NIL) all prevented LV dysfunction in wild type animals, and accordingly not in iNOS-deficient mice [81]. Nevertheless, iNOS inhibitors may be deleterious in animal models of sepsis induced by low LPS doses because they may abrogate the crosstalk between iNOS and COX1 and subsequent depletion in vasodilatory prostanoids such as prostaglandin (PG)E2 [91].

■ NO Promotes Cardiac Allograft Rejection but Attenuates Allograft Vasculopathy and Myocarditis

With regard to cardiac allograft rejection, iNOS-derived NO has detrimental – mostly peroxynitrite-mediated – effects, since it contributes to rejection and LV dysfunction [92]. Improved coronary flow reserve and cardiac function or even prolonged allograft survival were recently confirmed in iNOS-deficient mice [93] or with selective iNOS inhibitors such as 1400 W or aminoguanidine, with the NO scavenger NOX-100, or with the antioxidant dimethylthiourea [94].

In contrast to cardiac allograft, iNOS-derived NO has beneficial effects in cardiac allograft vasculopathy, as shown with iNOS-deficient mice [95] or by the beneficial adjunction of cAMP in the preservation solution known to increase NO [96].

Finally, iNOS-derived NO attenuates viral and autoimmune myocarditis [97]. Interferon-γ plays a protective role in autoimmune myocarditis by inducing iNOS overexpression [98], while NO itself may inhibit coxsackie viral protease 2 via S-nitrosylation, preventing human and mouse dystrophin proteolysis [99].

▌ Conclusion

Consistent evidence in various models *in vitro* and *in vivo*, including in human patients, now supports a role for NO as the main second messenger counterbalancing adrenergic signaling in the heart. NO modulates both myocardial oxygen uptake and oxygen supply through biochemical regulation of heart rate, preload, afterload, contractility and coronary tone. NO acts directly (mediator for the stretch response, ROS scavenging, inhibition of mitochondrial respiration by competition with oxygen, control of apoptosis), or through cGMP-dependent mechanisms, to inhibit adrenergic input (negative inotropy), hasten diastolic relaxation (positive lusitropy), inhibit pacemaker cell spontaneous depolarization (negative chronotropy), and induce coronary vasorelaxation.

All these beneficial effects of NO are provided by low concentrations of eNOS-derived NO, the production of which is tightly regulated and directed to specific molecular targets through caveolar compartmentation. Nevertheless, high concentrations of iNOS-generated NO may have detrimental effects in the heart – together with its implication in general defense such as innate immunity – attributed either to NO itself (profound cardiodepression, irreversible inhibition of mitochondrial respiration) or derivatives thereof, mainly peroxynitrite (apoptosis, oxidative and nitrosative stresses).

Acute and compensated heart disease usually results in expression of both eNOS and iNOS isoforms, while chronic and decompensated states show progressive eNOS downregulation. Furthermore, heart failure is accompanied by upregulation of the eNOS-coupled β_3-adrenoceptor, that may be adaptive at early stages while probably maladaptive at terminal stages of the disease. Whether the progressive imbalance between β_1-, β_2-, and β_3-adrenoceptors together with eNOS downregulation plays a determinant role in clinical shift towards decompensation will await confirmation in future clinical trials with specific β_3-adrenoceptor antagonists.

This isoform-dependent dual role of NO explains the interest in eNOS-promoting therapies (including ACE inhibitors, amlodipine and angiotensin II type-1 receptor antagonists, but also new NO donors, antioxidants, NO-releasing aspirin or β-blockers, nebivolol, as well as gene therapy), on one hand, and, on the other hand, in selective iNOS inhibitors and β_3-adrenoceptor antagonists, depending on the pathophysiological state of the disease. When properly tested, some of these therapeutic options may open hopeful perspectives for the future management of ischemic, auto-immune, or septic cardiac disease of the critically ill patient.

References

1. Furchgott RF, Zawadzki JV (1980) The obligatory role of endothelial cells in the relaxation of arterial smooth muscle by acetylcholine. Nature 288:373–376
2. Palmer RM, Ashton DS, Moncada S (1988) Vascular endothelial cells synthesize nitric oxide from L-arginine. Nature 333:664–666
3. Balligand JL, Ungureanu D, Kelly RA, et al (1993) Abnormal contractile function due to induction of nitric oxide synthesis in rat cardiac myocytes follows exposure to activated macrophage-conditioned medium. J Clin Invest 91:2314–2319
4. Brady AJ, Poole-Wilson PA, Harding SE, Warren JB (1992) Nitric oxide production within cardiac myocytes reduces their contractility in endotoxemia. Am J Physiol 263:H1963–H1966
5. Kumar A, Thota V, Dee L, Olson J, Uretz E, Parrillo JE (1996) Tumor necrosis factor alpha and interleukin 1 beta are responsible for in vitro myocardial cell depression induced by human septic shock serum. J Exp Med 183:949–958

6. Balligand JL, Cannon PJ (1997) Nitric oxide synthases and cardiac muscle. Autocrine and paracrine influences. Arterioscler Thromb Vasc Biol 17:1846–1858
7. Ardehali A, Ports TA (1990) Myocardial oxygen supply and demand. Chest 98:699–705
8. Opie LH (2001) Mechanisms of cardiac contraction and relaxation. In: Braunwald E, Zipes DP, Libby P (eds) Heart Disease, 6th edn. Saunders Company, Boston, pp 443–478
9. Rubart M, Zipes DP (2001) Genesis of cardiac arrhythmias: electrophysiological considerations. In: Braunwald E, Zipes DP, Libby P (eds) Heart Disease, 6th edn. Saunders Company, Boston, pp 659–699
10. Balligand JL, Feron O, Kelly RA (2000) Role of nitric oxide in myocardial function. In: Ignarro LJ (ed) Nitric oxide: Biology and Pathobiology. Academic Press, San Diego, pp 585–607
11. Massion P, Moniotte S, Balligand J (2001) Nitric oxide: does it play a role in the heart of the critically ill? Curr Opin Crit Care 7:323–336
12. Suto N, Mikuniya A, Okubo T, Hanada H, Shinozaki N, Okumura K (1998) Nitric oxide modulates cardiac contractility and oxygen consumption without changing contractile efficiency. Am J Physiol 275:H41–H49
13. Vanhoutte PM (2000) Say NO to ET. J Auton Nerv Syst 81:271–277
14. Ding Y, Vaziri ND, Coulson R, Kamanna VS, Roh DD (2000) Effects of simulated hyperglycemia, insulin, and glucagon on endothelial nitric oxide synthase expression. Am J Physiol Endocrinol Metab 279:E11–E17
15. Gauthier C, Leblais V, Kobzik L, et al (1998) The negative inotropic effect of beta3-adrenoceptor stimulation is mediated by activation of a nitric oxide synthase pathway in human ventricle. J Clin Invest 102:1377–1384
16. Varghese P, Harrison RW, Lofthouse RA, Georgakopoulos D, Berkowitz DE, Hare JM (2000) Beta(3)-adrenoceptor deficiency blocks nitric oxide-dependent inhibition of myocardial contractility. J Clin Invest 106:697–703
17. Balligand JL (1999) Regulation of cardiac beta-adrenergic response by nitric oxide. Cardiovasc Res 43:607–620
18. Paulus WJ (2001) The role of nitric oxide in the failing heart. Heart Fail Rev 6:105–118
19. Petroff MG, Kim SH, Pepe S, et al (2001) Endogenous nitric oxide mechanisms mediate the stretch dependence of Ca^{2+} release in cardiomyocytes. Nat Cell Biol 3:867–873
20. Altug S, Demiryurek AT, Kane KA, Kanzik I (2000) Evidence for the involvement of peroxynitrite in ischaemic preconditioning in rat isolated hearts. Br J Pharmacol 130:125–131
21. Beltran B, Mathur A, Duchen MR, Erusalimsky JD, Moncada S (2000) The effect of nitric oxide on cell respiration: A key to understanding its role in cell survival or death. Proc Natl Acad Sci USA 97:14602–14607
22. Trochu JN, Bouhour JB, Kaley G, Hintze TH (2000) Role of endothelium-derived nitric oxide in the regulation of cardiac oxygen metabolism: implications in health and disease. Circ Res 87:1108–1117
23. Almeida A, Almeida J, Bolanos J, Moncada S (2001) Different responses of astrocytes and neurons to nitric oxide: the role of glycolytically generated ATP in astrocyte protection. Proc Natl Acad Sci USA 98:15294–15299
24. Heusch G, Post H, Michel MC, Kelm M, Schulz R (2000) Endogenous nitric oxide and myocardial adaptation to ischemia. Circ Res 87:146–152
25. Mital S, Addonizio LJ, Mosca RJ, Quaegebeur JM, Oz MC, Hintze TH (2001) Nitric oxide regulates the apoptotic pathway in explanted failing human hearts. J Heart Lung Transplant 20:220
26. Poderoso JJ, Peralta JG, Lisdero CL, et al (1998) Nitric oxide regulates oxygen uptake and hydrogen peroxide release by the isolated beating rat heart. Am J Physiol 274:C112–C119
27. Hornig B, Landmesser U, Kohler C, et al (2001) Comparative effect of ace inhibition and angiotensin II type 1 receptor antagonism on bioavailability of nitric oxide in patients with coronary artery disease: role of superoxide dismutase. Circulation 103:799–805
28. Broeders MA, Doevendans PA, Bekkers BC, et al (2000) Nebivolol: a third-generation beta-blocker that augments vascular nitric oxide release: endothelial beta(2)-adrenergic receptor-mediated nitric oxide production. Circulation 102:677–684

29. Depre C, Vanoverschelde JL, Taegtmeyer H (1999) Glucose for the heart. Circulation 99:578–588
30. Clementi E, Brown GC, Feelisch M, Moncada S (1998) Persistent inhibition of cell respiration by nitric oxide: crucial role of S-nitrosylation of mitochondrial complex I and protective action of glutathione. Proc Natl Acad Sci USA 95:7631–7636
31. Xie YW, Kaminski PM, Wolin MS (1998) Inhibition of rat cardiac muscle contraction and mitochondrial respiration by endogenous peroxynitrite formation during posthypoxic reoxygenation. Circ Res 82:891–897
32. Beltran B, Orsi A, Clementi E, Moncada S (2000) Oxidative stress and S-nitrosylation of proteins in cells. Br J Pharmacol 129:953–960
33. Virag L, Scott GS, Cuzzocrea S, Marmer D, Salzman AL, Szabo C (1998) Peroxynitrite-induced thymocyte apoptosis: the role of caspases and poly (ADP-ribose) synthetase (PARS) activation. Immunology 94:345–355
34. Bolotina VM, Najibi S, Palacino JJ, Pagano PJ, Cohen RA (1994) Nitric oxide directly activates calcium-dependent potassium channels in vascular smooth muscle. Nature 368:850–853
35. Varenne O, Sinnaeve P, Gillijns H, et al (2000) Percutaneous gene therapy using recombinant adenoviruses encoding human herpes simplex virus thymidine kinase, human PAI-1, and human NOS3 in balloon-injured porcine coronary arteries. Hum Gene Ther 11:1329–1339
36. Cable DG, Pompili VJ, O'Brien T, Schaff HV (1999) Recombinant gene transfer of endothelial nitric oxide synthase augments coronary artery relaxations during hypoxia. Circulation 100:II335–II339
37. Matsunaga T, Warltier DC, Weihrauch DW, Moniz M, Tessmer J, Chilian WM (2000) Ischemia-induced coronary collateral growth is dependent on vascular endothelial growth factor and nitric oxide. Circulation 102:3098–3103
38. Brouet A, Sonveaux P, Dessy C, Moniotte S, Balligand JL, Feron O (2001) Hsp90 and caveolin are key targets for the proangiogenic nitric oxide-mediated effects of statins. Circ Res 89:866–873
39. Stamler JS, Simon DI, Jaraki O, et al (1992) S-nitrosylation of tissue-type plasminogen activator confers vasodilatory and antiplatelet properties on the enzyme. Proc Natl Acad Sci USA 89:8087–8091
40. De Caterina R, Libby P, Peng HB, et al (1995) Nitric oxide decreases cytokine-induced endothelial activation. Nitric oxide selectively reduces endothelial expression of adhesion molecules and proinflammatory cytokines. J Clin Invest 96:60–68
41. Takimoto Y, Aoyama T, Keyamura R, et al (2000) Differential expression of three types of nitric oxide synthase in both infarcted and non-infarcted left ventricles after myocardial infarction in the rat. Int J Cardiol 76:135–145
42. Feng Q, Lu X, Jones DL, Shen J, Arnold JM (2001) Increased inducible nitric oxide synthase expression contributes to myocardial dysfunction and higher mortality after myocardial infarction in mice. Circulation 104:700–704
43. Sam F, Sawyer DB, Xie Z, et al (2001) Mice lacking inducible nitric oxide synthase have improved left ventricular contractile function and reduced apoptotic cell death late after myocardial infarction. Circ Res 89:351–356
44. Valen G, Hansson GK, Dumitrescu A, Vaage J (2000) Unstable angina activates myocardial heat shock protein 72, endothelial nitric oxide synthase, and transcription factors NFkappaB and AP-1. Cardiovasc Res 47:49–56
45. Scherrer-Crosbie M, Ullrich R, Bloch KD, et al (2001) Endothelial nitric oxide synthase limits left ventricular remodeling after myocardial infarction in mice. Circulation 104:1286–1291
46. Priori SG, Napolitano C (2000) From catheters to vectors: the dawn of molecular electrophysiology. Nat Med 6:1316–1318
47. Bolli R (2000) The late phase of preconditioning. Circ Res 87:972–983
48. Zhao T, Xi L, Chelliah J, Levasseur JE, Kukreja RC (2000) Inducible nitric oxide synthase mediates delayed myocardial protection induced by activation of adenosine A(1) receptors: evidence from gene- knockout mice. Circulation 102:902–907

49. Neviere RR, Li FY, Singh T, Myers ML, Sibbald W (2000) Endotoxin induces a dose-dependent myocardial cross-tolerance to ischemia-reperfusion injury. Crit Care Med 28:1439–1444

50. Iwata A, Sai S, Nitta Y, et al (2001) Liposome-mediated gene transfection of endothelial nitric oxide synthase reduces endothelial activation and leukocyte infiltration in transplanted hearts. Circulation 103:2753–2759

51. Lefer DJ, Scalia R, Campbell B, et al (1997) Peroxynitrite inhibits leukocyte-endothelial cell interactions and protects against ischemia-reperfusion injury in rats. J Clin Invest 99:684–691

52. Munzel T, Li H, Mollnau H, et al (2000) Effects of long-term nitroglycerin treatment on endothelial nitric oxide synthase (NOS III) gene expression, NOS III-mediated superoxide production, and vascular NO bioavailability. Circ Res 86:E7–E12

53. Depre C, Vanoverschelde JL, Goudemant JF, Mottet I, Hue L (1995) Protection against ischemic injury by nonvasoactive concentrations of nitric oxide synthase inhibitors in the perfused rabbit heart. Circulation 92:1911–1918

54. Diaz R, Paolasso EA, Piegas LS, et al (1998) Metabolic modulation of acute myocardial infarction. The ECLA (Estudios Cardiologicos Latinoamerica) Collaborative Group. Circulation 98:2227–2234

55. Coleman GM, Gradinac S, Taegtmeyer H, Sweeney M, Frazier OH (1989) Efficacy of metabolic support with glucose-insulin-potassium for left ventricular pump failure after aortocoronary bypass surgery. Circulation 80:I91–I96

56. Apstein CS (2000) Increased glycolytic substrate protection improves ischemic cardiac dysfunction and reduces injury. Am Heart J 139:S107–S114

57. Korvald C, Elvenes OP, Myrmel T (2000) Myocardial substrate metabolism influences left ventricular energetics in vivo. Am J Physiol 278:H1345–H1351

58. Aljada A, Saadeh R, Assian E, Ghanim H, Dandona P (2000) Insulin inhibits the expression of intercellular adhesion molecule-1 by human aortic endothelial cells through stimulation of nitric oxide. J Clin Endocrinol Metab 85:2572–2575

59. Baumann CA, Saltiel AR (2001) Spatial compartmentalization of signal transduction in insulin action. Bioessays 23:215–222

60. Van den Berghe G, Wouters P, et al (2001) Intensive insulin therapy in critically ill patients. N Engl J Med 345:1359–1367

61. Heymes C, Vanderheyden M, Bronzwaer JG, Shah AM, Paulus WJ (1999) Endomyocardial nitric oxide synthase and left ventricular preload reserve in dilated cardiomyopathy. Circulation 99:3009–3016

62. Nikolaidis LA, Hentosz T, Doverspike A, et al (2001) Mechanisms whereby rapid RV pacing causes LV dysfunction: perfusion-contraction matching and NO. Am J Physiol 281:H2270–H2281

63. Nakamura R, Egashira K, Arimura K, et al (2001) Increased inactivation of nitric oxide is involved in impaired coronary flow reserve in heart failure. Am J Physiol 281:H2619–H2625

64. Cotter G, Kaluski E, Blatt A, et al (2000) L-NMMA (a nitric oxide synthase inhibitor) is effective in the treatment of cardiogenic shock. Circulation 101:1358–1361

65. Hare JM, Givertz MM, Creager MA, Colucci WS (1998) Increased sensitivity to nitric oxide synthase inhibition in patients with heart failure: potentiation of beta-adrenergic inotropic responsiveness. Circulation 97:161–166

66. Shinke T, Takaoka H, Takeuchi M, et al (2000) Nitric oxide spares myocardial oxygen consumption through attenuation of contractile response to beta-adrenergic stimulation in patients with idiopathic dilated cardiomyopathy. Circulation 101:1925–1930

67. Harrison RW, Thakkar RN, Senzaki H, et al (2000) Relative contribution of preload and afterload to the reduction in cardiac output caused by nitric oxide synthase inhibition with L-N(G)- methylarginine hydrochloride 546C88. Crit Care Med 28:1263–1268

68. Loke KE, Laycock SK, Mital S, et al (1999) Nitric oxide modulates mitochondrial respiration in failing human heart. Circulation 100:1291–1297

69. Bartunek J, Shah AM, Vanderheyden M, Paulus WJ (1997) Dobutamine enhances cardiodepressant effects of receptor-mediated coronary endothelial stimulation. Circulation 95:90–96

70. Mital S, Loke KE, Addonizio LJ, Oz MC, Hintze TH (2000) Left ventricular assist device implantation augments nitric oxide dependent control of mitochondrial respiration in failing human hearts. J Am Coll Cardiol 36:1897–1902

71. Ogletree-Hughes ML, Stull LB, Sweet WE, Smedira NG, McCarthy PM, Moravec CS (2001) Mechanical unloading restores beta-adrenergic responsiveness and reverses receptor downregulation in the failing human heart. Circulation 104:881–886

72. Bristow MR, Ginsburg R, Minobe W, et al (1982) Decreased catecholamine sensitivity and beta-adrenergic-receptor density in failing human hearts. N Engl J Med 307:205–211

73. Moniotte S, Kobzik L, Feron O, Trochu JN, Gauthier C, Balligand JL (2001) Upregulation of beta(3)-Adrenoceptors and Altered Contractile Response to Inotropic Amines in Human Failing Myocardium. Circulation 103:1649–1655

74. Vincent JL, Zhang H, Szabo C, Preiser JC (2000) Effects of nitric oxide in septic shock. Am J Respir Crit Care Med 161:1781–1785

75. Pinsky MR, Rico P (2000) Cardiac contractility is not depressed in early canine endotoxic shock. Am J Respir Crit Care Med 161:1087–1093

76. Grandel U, Sibelius U, Schrickel J, et al (2001) Biosynthesis of constitutive nitric oxide synthase-derived nitric oxide attenuates coronary vasoconstriction and myocardial depression in a model of septic heart failure induced by Staphylococcus aureus alpha-toxin. Crit Care Med 29:1–7

77. Grandel U, Fink L, Blum A, et al (2000) Endotoxin-induced myocardial tumor necrosis factor-alpha synthesis depresses contractility of isolated rat hearts: Evidence for a role of sphingosine and cyclooxygenase-2-derived thromboxane production. Circulation 102:2758–2764

78. Joe EK, Schussheim AE, Longrois D, et al (1998) Regulation of cardiac myocyte contractile function by inducible nitric oxide synthase (iNOS): mechanisms of contractile depression by nitric oxide. J Mol Cell Cardiol 30:303–315

79. Tatsumi T, Matoba S, Kawahara A, et al (2000) Cytokine-induced nitric oxide production inhibits mitochondrial energy production and impairs contractile function in rat cardiac myocytes. J Am Coll Cardiol 35:1338–1346

80. Ferdinandy P, Danial H, Ambrus I, Rothery RA, Schulz R (2000) Peroxynitrite is a major contributor to cytokine-induced myocardial contractile failure. Circ Res 87:241–247

81. Ullrich R, Scherrer-Crosbie M, Bloch KD, et al (2000) Congenital deficiency of nitric oxide synthase 2 protects against endotoxin-induced myocardial dysfunction in mice. Circulation 102:1440–1446

82. Kumar A, Osman J (2001) Septic myocardial depression: no "no" to no? Crit Care Med 29: 202–203

83. Tavernier B, Li JM, El Omar MM, et al (2001) Cardiac contractile impairment associated with increased phosphorylation of troponin I in endotoxemic rats. FASEB J 15:294–296

84. Bozkurt B, Kribbs SB, Clubb FJ Jr, et al (1998) Pathophysiologically relevant concentrations of tumor necrosis factor-alpha promote progressive left ventricular dysfunction and remodeling in rats. Circulation 97:1382–1391

85. Bolger AP, Anker SD (2000) Tumour necrosis factor in chronic heart failure: a peripheral view on pathogenesis, clinical manifestations and therapeutic implications. Drugs 60:1245–1257

86. Bryant D, Becker L, Richardson J, et al (1998) Cardiac failure in transgenic mice with myocardial expression of tumor necrosis factor-alpha. Circulation 97:1375–1381

87. Frantz S, Kobzik L, Kim YD, et al (1999) Toll4 (TLR4) expression in cardiac myocytes in normal and failing myocardium. J Clin Invest 104:271–280

88. Kalra D, Baumgarten G, Dibbs Z, Seta Y, Sivasubramanian N, Mann DL (2000) Nitric oxide provokes tumor necrosis factor-alpha expression in adult feline myocardium through a cGMP-dependent pathway. Circulation 102:1302–1307

89. Grover R, Zaccardelli D, Colice G, Guntupalli K, Watson D, Vincent JL (1999) An open-label dose escalation study of the nitric oxide synthase inhibitor, N(G)-methyl-L-arginine hydrochloride (546C88), in patients with septic shock. Glaxo Wellcome International Septic Shock Study Group. Crit Care Med 27:913–922

90. Avontuur JA, Tutein Nolthenius RP, Buijk SL, Kanhai KJ, Bruining HA (1998) Effect of L-NAME, an inhibitor of nitric oxide synthesis, on cardiopulmonary function in human septic shock. Chest 113:1640–1646

91. Devaux Y, Seguin C, Grosjean S, et al (2001) Lipopolysaccharide-induced increase of pros-
    taglandin E(2) is mediated by inducible nitric oxide synthase activation of the constitutive
    cyclooxygenase and induction of membrane-associated prostaglandin E synthase. J Immu-
    nol 167:3962–3971
92. Cannon P, Yang X, Szabolcs MJ, Ravalli S, Sciacca RR, Michler RE (1998) The role of indu-
    cible nitric oxide synthase in cardiac allograft rejection. Cardiovasc Res 38:6–15
93. Szabolcs MJ, Ma N, Athan E, et al (2001) Acute cardiac allograft rejection in nitric oxide
    synthase-2(–/–) and nitric oxide synthase-2(+/+) mice: effects of cellular chimeras on myo-
    cardial inflammation and cardiomyocyte damage and apoptosis. Circulation 103:2514–2520
94. Pieper GM, Olds C, Hilton G, Lindholm PF, Adams MB, Roza AM (2001) Antioxidant treat-
    ment inhibits activation of myocardial nuclear factor kappa B and inhibits nitrosylation of
    myocardial heme protein in cardiac transplant rejection. Antioxid Redox Signal 3:81–88
95. Koglin J (2000) Pathogenetic mechanisms of cardiac allograft vasculopathy – impact of
    nitric oxide. Z Kardiol 89 Suppl 9:IX/24–IX/27
96. Wang CY, Aronson I, Takuma S, et al (2000) cAMP pulse during preservation inhibits the
    late development of cardiac isograft and allograft vasculopathy. Circ Res 86:982–988
97. MacMicking J, Xie QW, Nathan C (1997) Nitric oxide and macrophage function. Annu Rev
    Immunol 15:323–350
98. Eriksson U, Kurrer MO, Bingisser R, et al (2001) Lethal autoimmune myocarditis in inter-
    feron-gamma receptor-deficient mice: enhanced disease severity by impaired inducible
    nitric oxide synthase induction. Circulation 103:18–21
99. Badorff C, Fichtlscherer B, Rhoads RE, et al (2000) Nitric oxide inhibits dystrophin proteo-
    lysis by coxsackieviral protease 2A through S-nitrosylation: A protective mechanism against
    enteroviral cardiomyopathy. Circulation 102:2276–2281

TNF as a Mediator of Cardiac Depression following Snakebite

O. Szold, R. Ben-Abraham, and P. Sorkine

▌ Introduction

Snake envenomation is still a major health threat in different parts of the world [1, 2], particularly in rural areas and tropical and subtropical countries [3]. In North America, over 5000 Americans suffer from snakebites annually with as many as a quarter of these being from poisonous species [4]. The incidence of death from snakebites is low in most countries because of the quick availability of medical care, even in rural areas. In the United States, the mortality rate from snakebite is below 1% for victims who receive antivenom [5], while it is 0.5% per 2000 bites in France [6]. Worldwide, some 30,000-to-40,000 persons die every year as a result of venomous snakebite. These numbers seem, however, to underestimate the danger to the population since reports arriving from developing countries are incomplete.

The Viperide family include the Crotalinae snakes (pit vipers) which are found in the New World and Asia, and the Viperinae (vipers) which are abundant in Europe, Asia and Africa. Viper aspis and Viper berus are the two main viper species found in Europe; their venom composition is very similar, and consequently no differences in the clinical features of envenomation have ever been reported. Snake venoms are a complex mixture of enzymes (Table 1), low molecular weight polypeptides, glycoproteins, and metal ions. Clinical manifestations following low-grade envenomation include local and limited edema, necrosis, and marked pain [7], but there can often be systemic effects such as nausea and vomiting, generalized edema, bleeding disorders, cardiovascular instability, renal and respiratory failure, and central nervous system depression that may later result in death [8].

Table 1. A partial list of main venom components

▌ Metalloproteinases	▌ Phospholipase B
▌ Arginine ester hydrolase	▌ Phospholipase C
▌ Collagenase	▌ Acetylcholinesterase
▌ Thrombin-like enzyme	▌ RNAase
▌ Lactate dehydrogenase	▌ DNAase
▌ Phosphomonoesterase	▌ 5'nucleotidase
▌ Phosphodiesterase	▌ NAD nucleotidase
▌ Phospholipase A_2	▌ Myotoxin-α

Cardiac Effects of Snakebite

Myocardial damage following snakebite is observed following envenomation by various species of snake [9–11]. Venom components can injure the heart via different mechanisms, among them direct cardiotoxicity [12]. Several myotoxic components have been identified in snake venoms and they can be categorized into four main groups including:

- presynaptic neurotoxins which are very toxic and possess phospholipase A_2 activity, such as notexin, taipoxin, and crotoxin
- non-neurotoxic basic phospholipase A_2
- myotoxins without detectable phospholipase A_2
- small basic toxins such as crotamine, myotoxin a, peptide c and several other toxins isolated from rattlesnake venom.

The potencies of these myotoxins are very different, and the components of snake venom vary not only with the different species of snake, but also between different members of the same species depending on the location, the season, the age of the snake and nutritional status. Some muscle groups may be less susceptible to the toxic effects of the myotoxin with less histopathological change following exposure to the toxin.

Electrocardiographic abnormalities have been reported following envenomation by a number of different species of snakes including Viper berus, Echis ocellatus, Calloselasma rhodostoma and Oxyuranus scutellatus canni. Venom components can induce coronary vasospasm, thrombosis [13, 14] and myocardial hemorrhage [15]. Envenomation of dog with venom of eastern brown snake resulted in ST elevation and T wave inversion but pretreatment with heparin abolished these changes. Multiple microscopic thrombi within the pulmonary circulation and in the coronary artery were found in animals at post-mortem examination [14]. Moreover, venom-induced hypotension was also shown to compromise coronary circulation, as manifested by electrocardiographic changes following the intravenous infusion of venom in a dog model of snake envenomation [14].

TNF as a Mediator of Hemodynamic Instability
Following Snake Envenomation

Tumor necrosis factor (TNF)-α, a potent pro-inflammatory compound, is synthesized as a 26 kDa-precursor protein that is later cleaved to its mature and active 17 kDa form. The matrix metalloproteinases (MMP) have been implicated in the synthesis of TNF-α [16, 17]. Viper venoms are rich in zinc metalloproteinases, which very closely resemble MMP [18], and have been shown to cleave recombinant pro-TNF-α to form the biologically active mature TNF-α [9]. It was recently suggested that venom-inflicted tissue damage could be partially caused by TNF, which is processed to its active form by the injected venom metalloproteinases (Fig. 1) [17, 19].

In an attempt to characterize the host reactivity to Bothrops asper venom, Lomonte et al. [20] investigated inflammatory responses in a mouse footpad model. After subcutaneous injection of the venom, they observed a rapid increase in serum interleukin (IL)-6 concentration that peaked after 3–6 hours. In contrast, serum TNF and IL-1 were not detectable at any time throughout their study period. In

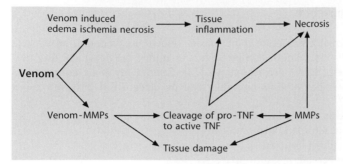

Fig. 1. Venom metalloproteinases (V-MMPs) trigger the cleavage of Pro-TNF to biologically active TNF, which than causes further inflammation and release of human metalloproteinases (MMPs) and the augmentation of local and systemic effects

this study, subcutaneous injection into the footpad was used, inducing local genera-tion of TNF that results only in regional necrosis and not in systemic conse-quences. In a recent study, Viper aspis venom was given by an intramuscular injec-tion, mimicking an actual snakebite [21]. This route of envenomation most likely resulted in systemic absorption of the venom, causing an increase in TNF levels as early as 15 minutes after the venom injection (35.2 ± 1.5 pg/ml, reaching a peak after two hours (485 ± 12.4 pg/ml) in the venom-injected rats, with no increase being detected in the control group. Within 60 minutes of the injection of the ven-om, there was a significant reduction in heart rate (117 ± 3 in the venom group and 155 ± 6 beat/min in the control group) that persisted during the 4 hours of the study. The authors also observed that, 90 minutes following the envenomation, the mean arterial blood pressure was significantly lower in the venom-injected animals (67 ± 2 mmHg) versus the control group (87 ± 18 mmHg). This difference persisted throughout the rest of the experiment. Administration of anti-TNF antibodies or soluble TNF receptor (P55-R) to the venom-injected rats completely blocked the toxic hemodynamic effects of the venom injection [21].

❚ TNF as a Mediator of Cardiac Toxicity following Snake Envenomation

The hypotensive effect of snakebite in humans is well known and was felt to be mainly due to hypovolemia from third-spacing of fluids into the extra-vascular space [22], although already in 1976, Bonilla and Rammel [23] demonstrated the presence of a myocardial depressor protein in Crotalus atrox venom [24]. In a study that investigated whether the hemodynamic instability that was observed fol-lowing venom injection is caused by a possible TNF-mediated cardiac toxicity, a Langendorff perfusion model of isolated rat heart following Viper aspis envenoma-tion was used (Szold et al., unpublished data). Two hours following the IM enven-omation, the rats were anesthetized and their hearts were rapidly excised, im-mersed in ice-cold saline, and mounted on a stainless steel cannula of a modified Langendorff perfusion apparatus. The monitored measurements of cardiac function included: left ventricular peak systolic pressure, time-to-peak systolic pressure, re-laxation time, the first derivative of the rise and fall in left ventricular pressure (dP/dtmax and dP/dtmin), the area calculated under the left ventricular developed pressure curve (pressure-time integral) which correlates with oxygen consumption, and coronary flow. All baseline parameters of cardiac performances were significantly reduced following the venom injection in the experimental group compared to the control group. All the hemodynamic variables exhibited a similar and parallel trend of change during the 60 minutes of the experiment. A maximal depression of the parameters of cardiac performance was observed 40 minutes after the hearts were placed on the Langendorff perfusion apparatus. The venom-induced cardiac depression was significantly attenuated if the animals were given either soluble TNF receptor p55 or anti-TNF antibodies shortly prior to the envenomation.

■ Conclusion

Cardiac and hemodynamic abnormalities, although they are not the main feature following most snakebites, are of significant importance in the event of severe envenomation and can contribute significantly to victims' morbidity and mortality. TNF is a main mediator of inflammation in shock caused by endotoxin and has a pivotal role in the immune response to infection, cancer, trauma, and several chronic inflammatory diseases. TNF also possesses cardiodepressant properties and likely has an important role in patients suffering from cardiac ischemia, heart failure, and those undergoing heart transplantation [25–27]. Until recently the place of TNF as a mediator of cardotoxicity following snakebite was not clear. In a series of experiments Szold et al. have demonstrated a significant increase in serum levels of TNF with parallel depressive hemodynamic effects (bradycardia and hypotension) after IM injection of Viper aspis venom in a rat model of snake envenomation. These deleterious hemodynamic effects were completely blocked by the pre-envenomation administration of anti-TNF antibodies or of TNF surface receptor (p55-R) that mediates the effects of TNF on cell function [21]. Further investigation revealed that an IM injection of Vipera aspis venom can cause cardiac depression, which is probably mediated by systemic TNF release, since these deleterious effects were also attenuated by blockade of TNF activity. Further investigation of the role of TNF as a mediator of venom toxicity is warranted.

References

1. Downy DJ (1991) New Mexico Rattlesnake bites. Demographic review and guidelines for treatment. J Trauma 31:1380–1386
2. Holstege CP, Miller MB, Wermuth M, et al (1997) Crotalid snake envenomation. Med Toxicol 13:889–921
3. Pugh RN, Theakston RD (1980) The incidence and mortality of snake bites in Nigerian savanna. Lancet 29:1181–1183
4. Litovitz TL, Felberg L, White S (1996) 1995 annual report of the American Association of Poison Control Centers Toxic Exposure Surveillance System. Am J Emerg Med 14:487
5. Kunkle DB, Curry SC, Vance MV, et al (1983–1984) Reptile envenomations. J Toxicol Clin 21:503–526
6. Chippaux JP, Goyffon M (1989) Les morsures accidentelles de serpents en France metropolitaine. Presse Med 18:794–795
7. Cardoso JL, Pan HW, Franca FO, et al (1993) Randomized comparative trail of three antivenoms in the treatment of envenoming by lance-headed viper (Bothrops jararaca) in Sao Paulo. Q J Med 86:315–325
8. Audebert F, Sorkine M, Robbe-Vincent A, et al (1994) Viper bites in France: Clinical and biological evaluation of kinetics of envenomations. Hum Exp Toxicol 13:685–688

9. Lalloo DG, Trevett AJ, Nwokolo N, et al (1997) Electrocardiographic abnormalities in patients bitten by taipans (Oxyuranus scutellatus canni) and other elapid snakes in Papua New Guinea. Trans R Soc Trop Med Hyg 91:53–56

10. Reid HA (1976) Adder bites in Britain. Br Med J 2:153–156

11. Warrell DA, Davidson NM, Omerod LD, et al (1974) Bites by the saw-scaled or carpet viper (Echis carinatus): trial of two specific antivenoms. Br Med J 4:437–440

12. Nayler WG, Sullivan AT, Dunnet J, et al (1976) The effects of a cardiotoxic component of the venom of the indian cobra (Naja nigricollis) on the subcellular structure and function of heart muscle. J Mol Cell Cardiol 8:341–360

13. Wollberg Z, Shabo-Shina R, Intrator N, et al (1988) A novel cardiotoxic peptide from the venom of Atractaspis engaddensis (burrowing asp): cardiac effects in mice and isolated rat and human heart preparations. Toxicon 26:525–534

14. Tibballs J, Sutherland SK, Rivera RA, et al (1989) The cardiovascular and haematological effects of purified prothrombin activator from the common brown snake (Pseudonaja textiles) and their antagonism with heparin. Anaesth Intensive Care 20:28–32

15. Than-Than, Francis N, Tin-Nu-Swe, et al (1989) Contribution of focal haemorrhage and microvascular fibrin deposition to fatal envenoming by Russell's viper (vipera russelli siamensis) species in Burma. Acta Trop 46:23–38

16. Gearing AJ, Beckett P, Christodoulou M, et al (1994) Processing of tumor necrosis factor-alpha precursor by metalloproteinases. Nature 370:555–557

17. McGeehan GM, Becherer JD, Bast RC, et al (1994) Regulation of tumor necrosis factor-alpha processing by a metalloproteinase inhibitor. Nature 370:558–561

18. Paine MJI, Moura-da-Silva AM, Theakston RDG, et al (1994) Cloning of metalloprotease genes in the carpet viper (Echis pyramidum leakeyi). Further members of the metalloprotease/disintegrin gene family. Eur J Biochem 224:483–488

19. Moura-da-Silva AM, Laing GD, Paine MJ, et al (1996) Processing of pro-tumor necrosis factor-alpha by venom metalloproteinases: A hypothesis explaining local tissue damage following snakebite. Eur J Immunol 26: 2000–2005

20. Lomonte B, Tarkowski A, Hanson LA (1993) Host response to Bothrops asper snake venom. Analysis of edema formation, inflammatory cells, and cytokine release in a mouse model. Inflammation 17:93–105

21. Szold O, Ben Abraham R, Weinbroum AA, et al (2001) Antagonization of TNF attenuates systemic hemodynamic manifestations of envenomation in a rat model of Vipera aspis snakebite. Intensive Care Med 27:884–888

22. Curry SC, Kunkel DB (1985) Death from a rattlesnake bite. Am J Emerg Med 3:227

23. Bonilla CA, Rammel OJ (1976) Comparative biochemistry and pharmacology of salivary gland secretion. Chromatographic isolation of a myocardial depressor protein (MDP) from the venom of Crotalus atrox. J Chromatogr 124:303–314

24. De Mesquita LC, Selistre H, Giglio JR (1991) The hypotensive activity of Crotalus atrox (western diamondback rattlesnake) venom: Identification of its origin. Am J Trop Med Hyg 44:345–353

25. Gurevitch J, Frolkins I, Yuhas Y, et al (1997) Anti-tumor necrosis factor-alpha improves myocardial recovery after ischemia and reperfusion. J Am Coll Cardiol 30:1554–1561

26. Riemsdijk-van Overbreeke C, Baan C, et al (1999) The TNF-in heart failure and after heart transplantation. Eur Heart J 20:833–840

27. Grossman GB, Rohdle LE, Clausell N (2001) Evidence for increased peripheral production of tumor necrosis factor-alpha in advanced congestive heart failure. Am J Cardiol 88:578–581

Acute Right Ventricular Failure: Physiology and Therapy

E. Renaud, P. Karpati, and A. Mebazaa

Introduction

The right ventricle (RV) has long been considered as a negligible entity, a simple passive passageway between the systemic venous and pulmonary circulations. As far back as 1943, physiologists were studying the hemodynamic effects following destruction of the RV free wall. As long as the conditions of ventricular filling were physiologic, there was no observed change in cardiac output. Subsequently, for the ensuing decades, little research into the RV and its physiologic role was conducted [1]. Progress in the comprehension of cardiovascular physiologic mechanisms paved the way for the discovery of the RV's fundamental role in maintaining right atrial pressure (RAP) as low as possible, with the aim of assuring an optimal venous return.

In general, isolated acute RV dysfunction is a less frequently recognized pathology than left ventricular (LV) failure. Despite this fact, in intensive care, due to the alterations in RV pre- and afterload (mechanical ventilation, sepsis), the frequency of RV failure probably approaches, if not equals, that of LV failure, but is often not recognized as such. Commonly, RV failure is first suspected and treated when pulmonary artery hypertension is present. Our case report will demonstrate that RV failure can be seen with normal pulmonary artery pressures (PAPs), and above all, that ischemic RV failure is very sensible to afterload even when unaltered. Therefore, even a minor reduction of physiologic PAP values will improve RV function, and cardiac output. This is why the ensuing case report is so interesting as it emphasizes the pathophysiologic mechanisms involved in RV failure within the framework of applied therapy. It also demonstrates the therapeutic efficiency of inhaled nitric oxide (NO), a selective pulmonary vasodilator, in acute RV failure.

Case Report

A 30-year-old male patient was undergoing surgery for aortic valve replacement coupled with the insertion of an ascendant aortic prosthesis with re-implantation of the coronary arteries. The diagnostic work up revealed severe aortic insufficiency (4/4), already associated with major dilatation of the initial segment of the aorta. Cardiac echocardiography also showed a dilated left atrium (46 mm), LV hypertrophy, and grade I mitral insufficiency. The whole picture seemed to fit as secondary to Marfan syndrome. Indication for surgery is established.

Under general anesthesia, the patient receives a Stenless homograft aortic valve, together with the implantation of a Bentall prosthesis. The right and left coronary arteries are re-implanted into the prosthesis. The surgery is successfully accomplished in 2 hours of aortic clamping, during which a cardiopulmonary bypass pump is used. The pump is removed at 2 hours 48 minutes with inotropic support of 5 µg/kg/min dobutamine, which is rapidly weaned.

The immediate postoperative period is relatively smooth, with the patient being admitted in a hemodynamically stable condition, without catecholamines, into the surgical intensive care unit (ICU) (arterial blood pressure (BP) 120/80/95 mmHg [systolic/diastolic/mean], RAP 12/6/9 mmHg).

The patient's condition unexpectedly and rapidly deteriorates, with the apparition in a few hours of arterial hypotension (BP 70/40/52 mmHg) while RAP increases to 21/17/19 mmHg, requiring the re-introduction of 10 µg/kg/min dobutamine, rapidly followed by the introduction of 1 mg/h epinephrine in order to restore an acceptable coronary perfusion pressure. Simultaneously, a pulmonary artery catheter is inserted, which shows a physiologic PAP 20/8/13 mmHg, a low pulmonary capillary wedge pressure (PCWP) of 2 mmHg (for a patient under positive pressure mechanical ventilation with a positive end-expiratory pressure (PEEP) of 5 cmH$_2$O), a diminished cardiac output of 2.3 l/min and a mixed venous oxygen saturation (SvO$_2$) of 45%. In this phase of extreme instability the patient also presents severe arrhythmias in the form of ventricular ectopics, followed by ventricular tachycardia, treated by intravenous lidocaine. The electrocardiogram (EKG) also shows a complete right bundle branch block, a 4 mm ST-elevation in the inferior leads (II, III, aVF), and a mirror image in the lateral leads (I, aVL, V$_5$,V$_6$). The metabolic state is characterized by major tissue hypoxia and hepatic hypoperfusion underscored by elevated lactate (8.5 IU/l), and acute hepatocellular failure with hepatic cytolysis (elevated transaminases: ASAT from 48 to 354 IU/l, ALAT 47 to 73 IU/l), thromboplastin (TP) 40%, Factor V 35%. Furthermore, the myocardial iso-enzyme of creatine phosphokinase (CPK-MB) increased from 88 to 546 µg/l (physiologic <10 µg/l), cardiac troponin I (cTnI) 48.1 µg/l (normal <0.4 µg/l), and in a couple of hours the condition rapidly progressed into an acute oligo-anuric renal failure (plasma creatinine 74 to 94 µmol/l). This multiorgan failure (MOF) can be explained not only as the consequence of the severe shock with organ hypoperfusion, but also due to hepatic and renal venous congestion. The analysis of this picture of severe hemodynamic instability with a reduced cardiac output, and greatly elevated RAP, and organ perfusion pressures restored and maintained by vasoconstrictor and inotropic catecholamines, point to acute RV dysfunction. This is poorly tolerated.

An emergency diagnostic coronarography is performed which shows a complete obstruction of the proximal end of the re-implanted right coronary artery. Despite the patient being taken to the operating room for a right coronary bypass using the saphenous vein, there is no immediate hemodynamic improvement postoperatively, due to the already apparent myocardial necrosis. On his return to ICU, the EKG showed Q waves in leads I, II, and aVF.

It is decided to introduce inhaled NO in an attempt to reduce, to the greatest possible degree, the afterload of the failing RV. At a rate of 8 particles per minute (ppm), hemodynamics are restored: BP 90/40/55 mmHg, RAP 10/6/8 mmHg, and cardiac output 5 l/min, while the PCWP remains at 4 mmHg. The reduction in PAP is minimal, going from 24/11/16 to 20/9/13 mmHg. This proves the RV failure and its dependence on the afterload even with a low or normal PAP. Indeed stopping in-

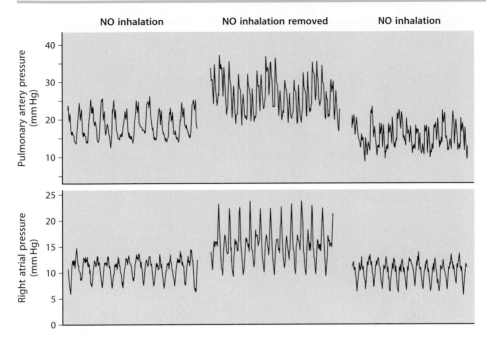

Fig. 1. Hemodynamics with and without inhaled NO. Inhaled NO withdrawal, in this patient with ischemia-induced RV failure, increased mean pulmonary artery pressure (PAP) from 18 to 25 mmHg. Although PAP remained in the normal range, its slight increase deteriorated RV function and dilated RV (Fig. 2). A tricuspid insufficiency emerged (positive waves above mean right atrial pressure, RAP) that worsened cardiac output

haled NO provokes an instant drop in arterial BP (70/25/40 mmHg) and cardiac output (3 l/min), while the RAP rises sharply (16/11/14 mmHg) with the emergence of a tricuspid insufficiency wave (Fig. 1). During this period without NO, echocardiography shows a severe dilatation of the right heart cavities in an already hypokinetic RV, in both systole and diastole (Fig. 2). The inferior vena cava is dilated at 30 mm, and a worsening of the pre-existent tricuspid insufficiency is also visible. This is the beginning of a vicious cycle, which results in the decrease in cardiac output, as the dilatation of the RV worsens the tricuspid insufficiency, which in turn worsens the right heart dilatation.

The patient could be weaned from inhaled NO only on the seventh postoperative day, and was discharged from ICU at day 30.

In summary, this patient presented with an acute RV failure with severe hemodynamic intolerance. Inhaled NO, in association with inotropic support, was an essential therapeutic component necessary to restore hemodynamic stability. The efficiency of NO demonstrates to what extent an ischemic RV is dependant on afterload even if PAPs are low.

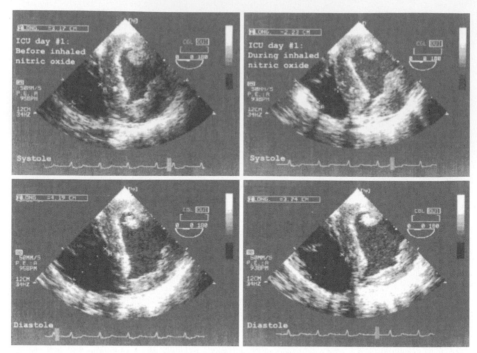

Fig. 2. Therapeutic effect of inhaled NO on RV diameter in ischemia-induced acute RV failure. Systole and diastole both before and during inhaled NO administration (8 ppm) (*left and right panels*, respectively), a couple of hours after coronary artery bypass

Physiology of RV Function

RV Contraction

The Peristaltic Motion. The RV is shaped like a pyramid on a triangular base. The RV cavity comprises both anatomically and functionally distinctly separated chambers [2]:

- the sinus or admission chamber, which has the role of output generator, determining the driving pressure necessary for the ejection of blood into the pulmonary artery
- the cone or ejection chamber that absorbs and dissipates the pressures generated by the sinus, by emulating a resistance, inhibiting the direct transmission of these pressures into the pulmonary circulation.

This anatomic compartmentalization cone/sinus has functional consequences as RV ejection transpires in two phases:

- a primary phase where the ejection is directly the result of RV wall contraction, in conjunction with a peristaltic motion from the admission chamber towards the ejection chamber
- a secondary phase, once the contraction is finished, when the blood already in the ejection chamber continues to flow into the pulmonary circulation, allowing the RV to complete its emptying.

These combined effects result in a more steady increase in pulmonary artery velocity, a delayed peak, and a more gradual decline as compared to the aorta RV failure with dilatation of the cavities causes the loss of peristaltic motion, due to which there will initially be a more sudden rise in the velocity profile of pulmonary artery flow. The resulting higher peak pressure may increase RV afterload, and further compromise RV function.

Differences between the Right and Left Ventricles. The fundamental determinants of RV function are the same as for the LV: pre- and afterload, and the RV's intrinsic contractility. However the pericardium is a major restraining factor for the RV, but not for the LV [3, 4].

The purpose of the RV is to maintain the lowest possible pressures in the right heart cavities to optimize the venous return. To do so, the RV generates flow. It ejects blood into a low resistance, high compliance circuit, as the pressures and resistance in the pulmonary circulation are six times less than those of the systemic circulation. Also, the distension of the pulmonary vascular bed is greater, and pulmonary vessel rigidity is not altered within the lungs. A pressure gradient of 5 mmHg is sufficient for the blood to perfuse across the pulmonary vascular bed [5].

In contrast, the LV's main function is to generate pressure. Additionally, the LV has a weak parietal compliance, a result of its wall thickness, and also ejects into a systemic vascular network with a low compliance and high degree of reflection. Indeed, the diameter of the arterial blood vessels decreases as we progress along the arterial branch, which has important effects on blood flow characteristics.

Right Coronary Perfusion

The muscular mass of the RV corresponds to one sixth that of the LV. The right coronary artery assures the vascularization of the posterior, lateral, anterior region of the RV wall. While in animals, e.g., the dog, the right and left coronary arteries supply the RV and LV respectively, in humans numerous anatomic variations exist. Sometimes the right coronary artery is dominant, in which case it also supplies the base of the LV. Therefore, for example, a stenosis of the right coronary artery will have more significant functional consequences than a stenosis of the anterior interventricular artery.

The specifics of right coronary perfusion are:
- systolo-diastolic perfusion in the right coronary artery, while that of the left coronary artery is mainly diastolic. In the case of acute, or more importantly, chronic pulmonary arterial hypertension, right coronary perfusion becomes primarily diastolic corresponding to that of the left coronary artery.
- as the RV is not pressure driven, its oxygen consumption per 100 g tissue is half that of the LV.

RV Preload

RV end-diastolic volume (RVEDV) is directly dependent on venous return and atrial contraction. Guyton [6] developed the concept that the heart is a motor with the sole aim of maintaining pressures as low as possible in the right atrium (and in the left atrium too) in order to generate the maximal amount of venous return. Therefore, an inverse relationship exists between the pressure in the right atrium and venous return. Venous return depends on both the pressure gradient and the resistance to it.

When preload or end-diastolic pressures are physiologic, the work of ejection of the RV is negligible, and cardiac output depends on venous return. The RV adapts to variations in venous return, without modifying its intracavital pressures. However, if the end-diastolic pressure increases (as is the case in ischemia), the RV dilates, increasing its end-diastolic volume. This residual end-diastolic volume will be added to that of venous return, which further enhances RV dilatation, and leads to increased pressures in the right heart cavity.

RV Afterload

Any increase in RV afterload will increase the right coronary blood flow, when coronary arteries are normal [7]. Indeed increased RV afterload prolongs the isovolemic contraction phase and therefore myocardial oxygen consumption. Similarly, disturbances in right coronary artery perfusion may remain asymptomatic, as long as the PAPs remain normal. By contrast, in pulmonary artery hypertension, the RV exerts its work under pressure, increases wall tension, and subsequently its oxygen consumption. In such a scenario, even a partial occlusion of the right coronary artery hinders the RV in adjusting to its altered oxygen consumption. This demonstrates the crucial role of reducing RV afterload in an effort to improve the right coronary artery oxygen supply/demand ratio.

Ventricular Interdependence

The heart cavities are positioned in an inflexible pericardic sac, with the change in the actual load of a ventricle dependent on the passive filling of the contralateral ventricle. This is so called ventricular coupling. Goto et al. [8] underscore this phenomenon in their study of left systolic and diastolic performance during ischemic RV dysfunction in the dog. They demonstrated that ischemic RV dysfunction induced by right coronary artery occlusion resulted in a significant leftward shift of the LV end-diastolic pressure-volume relation, which was markedly exaggerated by the presence of an intact pericardium. More importantly, when comparing the indexes of LV systolic performance (i.e., cardiac output, LV systolic pressure, peak LV dP/dt, and percent systolic shortening) during right coronary artery occlusion with those during inferior vena caval occlusion at a matched LV end-diastolic volume (LVEDV), they were the same. This indicates that the primary mechanism of decreased cardiac output during right coronary artery occlusion is caused by decreased LV preload (i.e., end-diastolic volume) due to decreased LV chamber compliance rather than by decreased LV contractility. These findings, concluding that opening the pericardium restores right coronary occlusion-induced LV dysfunction, were recently confirmed in a study by Brookes et al. [9] in pigs.

▌ Acute RV Failure: the Vicious Cycle of Auto-aggravation

One of the major differences between acute right and left ventricular failure is that acute RV failure further degenerates into a vicious cycle of auto-aggravation. In addition to its own effect on cardiac output, RV failure induces tricuspic insufficiency and a decrease in LV preload that both aggravate the deterioration in cardiac output.

In acute RV failure, right atrial and ventricular end-diastolic pressures increase causing RV dilatation and subsequent tricuspid insufficiency. The appearance of tricuspid insufficiency is not only important because of its additive deleterious effect on cardiac output. More importantly, it signifies the moment where, due to sudden rise in hepatic congestion and further decrease in cardiac output, the heart can no longer keep pace, and the auto-aggravation turns into an irreversible vicious cycle.

In addition, a decrease in LV preload results in a further drop in cardiac output, a reduction in systemic arterial BP, and, therefore, impairment in organ perfusion pressure, including that of the coronary arteries. This aggravates ventricular ischemia, underscoring the irreversibility of the vicious cycle.

▮ Acute RV Failure: Diagnostics

The diagnosis of acute RV failure is not an easy one to make, particularly if it presents in a patient already on the ICU with other apparent organ dysfunctions.

First, clinically distended jugular veins, hepatomegaly, hepato-jugular reflux, superior vena cava syndrome associated with impaired venous return, or signs of peripheral circulatory failure are more or less manifest. On the ICU, certain hemodynamic alterations such as a decrease in arterial BP, increase in RAP, decrease in cardiac output and mixed venous oxygen saturation despite a usually preserved PAP and PCWP, can point in favor of acute RV failure. However, none of the above signs are specific.

Other associated symptoms indicative of RV injury are:
▮ hepatic congestion characterized by the apparition of cytolysis can be compounded by serious hepatocellular insufficiency, and hemostatic disturbances, with the total protein (TP) rapidly falling, and an early and significant rise in lactate levels, reaching unanticipated levels
▮ renal congestion with diuresis diminishing very early, with an alteration in renal function.

Evaluating RV function is possible by pulmonary catheterization, although it poses difficulties in the interpretation of mean pressure values, above all in the context of large variations of transmural load and pressure associated with the interaction of the circulatory and respiratory system. Similarly, depending on the position of the Swan-Ganz catheter's tip (West zones) obtained pressure values can fluctuate greatly. Despite these difficulties, it is safe to say that in almost all cases, the trend or rather relative change of the values obtained over a period of time, during which different treatments are undertaken, are representative of the underlying hemodynamic alterations. Dembitsky et al. [10] define acute RV failure in terms of an end-diastolic RV pressure (or CVP) > 20 mmHg, a central venous pressure (CVP) superior to that of left atrial pressure, a cardiac index < 2 l/min/m^2 not adjusted to the oxygen consumption (VO$_2$), and a diminished S$_v$O$_2$. Meanwhile the cautious interpretation of the results of the Swan-Ganz catheter take into count the almost constant reflux due to the tricuspid insufficiency.

Transthoracic and transesophageal echocardiography not only provide an essential aid in the diagnosis of acute RV failure, especially in an ischemic setting, but also in the evaluation of its severity, and its response to implemented therapy. Echocardiography is useful in the detection of signs indicating acute RV failure, (which include: compressive pericardial effusion around the RV or atrium, the volume and geometry of the RV, the function of the free wall of the RV and septum, the absence or presence of tricuspid insufficiency, distension and size of the inferior vena cava), as well as in the evaluation of LV function. The ability to monitor the response to administered treatment (volume loading, catecholamines, NO) is an enormous advantage of this imaging technique. In conjunction with the pulmonary artery catheter, the latter can be used to follow the patient's evolution continuously, as well as to monitor the late effects of the given drugs.

■ Acute RV Failure: Therapeutic Approach

The therapeutic approach depends on the etiology of the RV failure, or the status of myocardial contractility, and the level of the RV afterload.

Treatment According to Etiology

In the context of RV infarction, maintaining atrio-ventricular synchronization represents an important aspect of the treatment of hypotension and hemodynamic shock. In the case of pulmonary embolus, anticoagulation with eventual thrombolysis, retains an important role. In acute respiratory distress syndrome (ARDS), etiologic treatment is an essential element in the management of these patients.

Optimization of Preload: Beneficial or Harmful?

Although optimization of preload is usually an objective in the management of ventricular failure, caution is advised in the presence of RV failure, especially in case of reduced RV compliance (ischemia or tamponade) and/or tricuspid insufficiency. Under these circumstances, volume loading will worsen RV failure that may lead to a great deterioration in hepatic and renal congestion. This chain of events may precipitate the vicious cycle of auto-aggravation described above. Even in the absence of these compounding factors, volume loading alone rarely suffices in the treatment of RV failure.

Influence on Contractility

Based on the participation of LV contraction in that of the RV, use of inotropic support seems logical. One can use sympathomimetics such as dobutamine, to improve contractility of both ventricles by increasing intramyocytic calcium influx. Dobutamine also poses a danger as it increases myocardial oxygen consumption without increasing the supply of oxygen to the myocardium. A good alternative would be to use a calcium-sensitizing agent, such as levosimendan. Increasing evidence is currently showing beneficial effects of levosimendan on RV failure.

In a similar fashion, the struggle to prevent myocardial ischemia, beneficial effects on RV performance have been shown by introducing vasopressor treatment with the goal of increasing aortic and coronary perfusion pressure. This is why a sympathomimetic with an almost selectively vasopressor effect (e.g., norepinephrine) can be used to increase arterial BP, and to restore adequate coronary artery perfusion, all the while knowing that these agents too are likely to increase RV afterload.

Reducing RV Afterload: the Most Efficient Means of Improving RV Failure

Inhalation of certain pulmonary arterial vasodilator agents, like NO has greatly improved the prognosis of acute RV failure. NO allows the selective dilatation of pulmonary arterial vessels, without modifying systemic arterial vessel tone. Hence, decreasing PAP, allows for diminution of the RV afterload, and improvement in the ventricle's contractility without modifying systemic arterial BP. After a reduction in RV afterload, and an improved cardiac output, one can observe a decrease in RAP. This in turn reduces hepatic and renal congestion, allowing for an improvement in the function of these organs highlighted by the reappearance of urinary output (Fig. 3 [11]).

Limiting Congestion

Certain medical teams prefer hemofiltration, although no irrefutable evidence of the above mentioned technique has yet been published. However, it appears that hemofiltration allows for the reduction of congestion in organs like the liver and kidneys, by diminishing total circulating blood volume.

∎ Conclusion

Acute RV failure is a pathology that we are likely to be confronted with more frequently than imagined in cardiac, general surgical and medical ICU. The diagnosis of RV failure is demanding, and relies on the combination of hemodynamic, biologic, and echocardiographic signs.

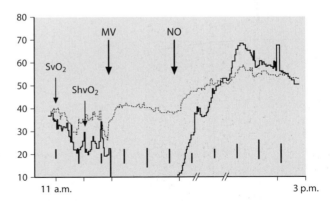

Fig. 3. Mixed venous oxygen saturation (SvO_2) and hepatic venous oxygen saturation ($ShvO_2$) recordings before and after NO inhalation. Mechanical ventilation worsened hepatic perfusion ($ShvO_2$ down to zero = no flow in the liver) while it improved SvO_2 from 28 to 40%, in a patient with severe hepatic and liver congestion due to congestive heart failure. Liver perfusion was subsequently restored by inhaled NO that decreased RV afterload, improved RV function, reduced liver and renal congestion and improved these organ's perfusion pressure. MV = start of mechanical ventilation; NO = start of NO inhalation (18 ppm). (From [11] with permission)

The presented case report illustrates the fact that vital prognosis can be rapidly underscored by the hemodynamic failure. The therapeutic approach is fundamentally based upon the etiology, the reduction in RV afterload, the reinforcement of ventricular contractility, and the maintenance of a sufficient arterial pressure for adequate coronary perfusion.

References

1. Starr I, Jeffers WA, Meade RH (1943) The absence of conspicuous increments of venous pressure after severe damage to the RV of the dog, with discussion of the relation between clinical congestive heart failure and heart disease. Am Heart J 26:291–301
2. Farb A, Burke AP, Virmani R (1992) Anatomy and pathology of the RV. Cardiol Clin 10:1–21
3. Sibbald WJ, Driedger AA (1983) Right ventricular function in acute disease states: pathophysiological conditions. Crit Care Med 11:339–345
4. Weber KT, Janicki JS, Schroff SG, et al (1983) The RV: physiologic and pathophysiologic considerations. Crit Care Med 11:323–328
5. Lee FA (1992) Hemodynamics of the RV in normal and disease states. Cardiol Clin 10:59–67
6. Guyton AC (1955) Determination of cardiac output by equating venous return curves with cardiac response curve. Physiol Rev 35:123–129
7. Konstam MA, Levine HJ (1988) Effects of afterload and preload on RV systolic performance. In: Konstam MA, Isner JM (ed) The Right Ventricle. Kluwer, New York, pp 17–35
8. Goto Y, Yamamoto J, Saito M, et al (1985) Effects of RV ischemia on LV geometry and the end-diastolic pressure-volume relationship in the dog. Circulation 72:1104–1114
9. Brookes C, Ravn H, White P, et al (1999) Acute RV dilatation in response to ischemia significantly impairs LV systolic performance. Circulation 100:761–767
10. Dembitsky WP, Daily PO, Raney AA (1986) Temporary extracorporeal support of the right ventricle. J Thorac Cardiovasc Surg 91:518–525
11. Gatecel C, Mebazaa A, Kong R, et al (1995) Inhaled nitric oxide improves hepatic tissue oxygenation in RV failure: value of hepatic venous oxygen saturation monitoring. Anesthesiology 82:588–590

Cardiovascular Management

The Rationale for Vasodilator Therapy in Sepsis

M. Siegemund, I. Racovitza, and C. Ince

▌ Introduction

In 1969, Joly and Weil showed a direct correlation between toe skin temperature, cardiac output and survival [1]. Since that time many hemodynamic studies in sepsis and septic shock have evaluated therapeutic strategies to increase cardiac output, blood pressure and organ blood flow. Their effect on the skin and other microcirculatory areas has been neglected for the most part, probably because no monitoring techniques were available. Initial studies showed improved survival after the optimization of oxygen delivery (DO_2) [2, 3]. However, controlled clinical trials establishing normal or even supra-normal DO_2 values failed to show any survival benefits [4, 5]. A therapeutic increase in blood pressure did not significantly affect surrogate markers of microcirculatory tissue perfusion and function [6]. In addition, the non-selective inhibition of the endothelial vasodilator nitric oxide (NO), acting primarily in the microcirculation, by L-NG-methylarginine increased mortality in patients with septic shock [7]. One possible cause of this increased mortality is that unselective blockade of NO synthase (NOS) further harms the microcirculatory blood flow and aggravates the already existing impaired tissue oxygenation [8]. This tissue dysoxia, a primary feature of endotoxemia and sepsis, may result from disturbed tissue DO_2 and/or a defect in cellular oxygen utilization resulting in a cellular oxygen extraction deficit [9, 10]. This extraction deficit could be causally related to a shut down of vulnerable microcirculatory units in organ beds promoting shunt flow of oxygen from the microcirculation to the venous system [10]. This effect could be aggravated in sepsis where normally available autoregulatory mechanisms are disturbed leaving these weak microcirculatory units dysoxic [11–15]. In the present chapter, we will address pathophysiologic changes in the microcirculation in sepsis regarding a possible role of vasodilator drugs or selective inducible NOS (iNOS) blocking drugs to improve microcirculatory blood flow and oxygenation.

▌ Altered Microvascular Blood Flow

Sepsis and endotoxemia attenuate arteriolar response to vasoconstrictors in a variety of vascular beds [12, 15, 16]. Despite the decreased peripheral vascular resistance and systemic hypotension there are several studies showing vasoconstricted next to vasodilated vessels in the microcirculation [17–19]. In an intravital microscopy model in rats suffering from peritonitis, impaired microvascular perfusion due to decreased density, increased heterogeneity, and an increased proportion of widely spaced perfused capillaries has been shown. Although the authors could not prove cellular hypoxia, they speculated that these changes may lead to the development of microregional areas of hypoxia, which in turn could cause parenchymal cell injury [18]. Apart from impaired tissue oxygenation, the increased microcirculatory heterogeneity [20] may have an influence on conventional sepsis therapy, since it takes several hours for antibiotic concentrations in the small vessels to reach the same levels as in central veins [12]. This factor may be a reason why antibiotic administration is ineffective in protecting the host during the early phase of shock.

NO, a vasodilator naturally occurring in the body, is overproduced in sepsis and endotoxemia by iNOS and may be responsible for hypotension and vascular hyporeactivity [11, 21, 22]. Beside the influence on vascular homeostasis, the increased amount of iNOS generated NO also has possible advantages. NO is part of the physiologic defense of leukocytes against invading pathogens and works as an oxygen radical scavenger to prevent protein and lipid peroxidation [14, 23]. Pharmacological inhibition of NOS in animal and human studies restores reactivity and tone of resistance vessels as well as the arterial pressure [24, 25], but has not improved outcome [7, 23, 26, 27]. The total blockade of NO production by iNOS and the physiological constitutive NOS (cNOS) could be responsible for the negative outcome, because a total blockade of NO production reduces microcirculatory blood flow, enhances coagulation, and increases cell adhesion in the microcirculation [22, 28]. In addition to the increased expression of iNOS, an impaired endothelium-dependent vascular relaxation after endotoxin could be shown in animals and human volunteers [29, 30]. This decreased reactivity to intravascular mediated vasodilatation may remain for a long period and leave vasoconstricting mechanisms unopposed, with an increased risk of tissue hypoperfusion and organ injury [28].

Since the rheologic properties of blood flow in capillary networks are mainly passive, the increased supply due to vasodilator therapy will decrease microcirculatory heterogeneity [13, 37]. The application of an NO donor for vasodilating properties may work as a surrogate for the decreased endothelial NO release in early phase of sepsis, where vasoconstriction is prominent [28].

Blood Cell Aggregation and Coagulation

Rheologic changes, including impaired red blood cell (RBC) deformability, increased leukocyte aggregation and endothelial adherence, as well as intracapillary coagulation may contribute to the decreased capillary density in sepsis [12, 32]. Recent studies showed a higher degree of adhesion of human erythrocytes on endothelial cells after an inflammatory stimulus and a significantly decreased deformability of RBCs in animal models as well as from septic patients [33–35]. The decreased deformability of erythrocytes seemed to be modulated by NO generated from polymorphonuclear leukocytes (PMN) [36]. Deformability of the erythrocytes could be increased by the vasodilators and NO donors, SIN-1 and sodium nitroprusside, and decreased by the NOS inhibitor, NG-monomethyl-L-arginine.

Activated PMN roll and adhere on the endothelium of venules and capillaries due to endotoxin and inflammatory mediators [37]. In addition to this classical adhesion and migration pathway, a simple plugging of PMN in precapillary vessels occurs, a process that may be facilitated by a decrease in PMN deformability [38]. Concomitantly, there is swelling of endothelial cells that, together with adhering leukocytes, narrows the lumina of venules and capillaries, thereby impairing nutritive blood flow to tissue [37].

In addition to the increased plugging of cells in the microcirculation, there is extensive intravascular coagulation involving cellular and fibrin components as well as severe damage to the endothelial cells with an exposure of the basal lamina to the blood [37]. In a recent study, Bernard et al. [39] showed that activated protein C (APC), a potent antithrombotic and anti-inflammatory enzyme reduced mortality in patients with severe sepsis. APC decreases formation of thrombin and activates fibrinolysis by reducing the concentration of plasminogen-activator inhibitor (PAI) type 1 [40]. These anticoagulant properties of APC may lead to an increased number of perfused capillaries and improved nutritive microvascular blood flow.

The increased rigidity and adhesion of cells together with the activated intravascular coagulation may be the cause of arterio-venous shunting of blood, decreasing microcirculatory flow during septic shock [12]. The therapeutic use of vasodilators may influence the rheologic microcirculatory changes in sepsis and endotoxemia in different ways. Vasodilators will increase the inflow pressure to the microcirculation [41], thereby enhancing flow through microvascular weak units at risk of cell plugging, coagulation, and functional shunting. Increased flow, higher capillary diameter, and increased erythrocyte deformability, if NO donors are used, may have a favorable influence on microcirculatory blood flow and reduce heterogeneity.

Functional Microvascular Oxygen Shunting and Cytopathic Hypoxia

The above mentioned pathophysiologic changes show that an adequate distribution of RBCs, and consequently oxygen, is altered in the septic microcirculation [42]. Capillary recruitment and reactive hyperemia, the physiologic protective mechanisms of the microcirculation against hypoxia cannot work under these conditions [12, 14]. This implies that a minor additional decrease in local DO_2 like hypovolemia or aggravated vasoconstriction, can jeopardize microcirculatory units at risk.

In a study using NADH videofluorimetry to identify hypoxic areas we found in rat hearts the presence of weak microcirculatory units, anatomically defined for a given heart, which were first to become dysoxic during tachycardia and the last to recover from a period of ischemia or hypoxia [43]. We termed these units *microcirculatory weak units* because they are first to become dysoxic during stress and, therefore, are the initially shunted microcirculatory units during distress such as occurs during sepsis [10]. In hearts of endotoxemic rats showing increased coronary flow rates and oxygen consumptions, the non-selective blockade of NO production induced dysoxia in the same microcirculatory weak units whereas control hearts were left unaffected [8, 44]. Microcirculatory units susceptible to ischemia also exist in other organs, e.g., the kidney and the gut. In the kidney, the cortex glomeruli can be regarded as weak microcirculatory units, because they are susceptible to thromboembolic occlusion during sepsis and endotoxemia [45–47]. The special anatomy of the intestinal villi predisposes them to direct arterial-venous shunting from the central artery to the effluent veins in a so-called counter current fashion [10, 48].

The presence of weak microcirculatory units makes a number of different mechanisms promoting functional shunting conceivable (Fig. 1). Under normal physiologic conditions the microcirculatory oxygenation (μPO_2) is related to the PO_2 in the venous outflow of an organ bed. Increased metabolic state of a tissue will increase the VO_2, decrease the μPO_2 and concomitantly lower the venous PO_2. A high or normal venous PO_2 with a simultaneous decrease in μPO_2 is indicative of the presence of functional oxygen shunting [49]. We termed this increased difference

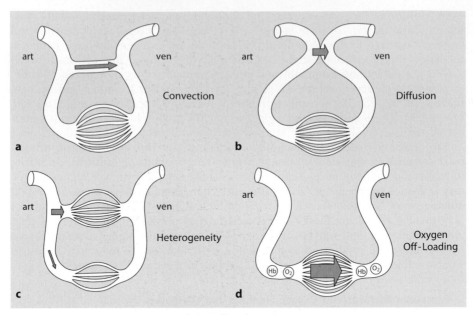

Fig. 1. Mechanisms resulting in functional shunting of the microcirculatory oxygen transport. (**a**) *Convection:* Physiologic shunts through direct anastomoses between arterioles and veins. (**b**) *Diffusion:* The close proximity between arterioles and veins (mucosal villi) allows diffusion of oxygen, especially in low flow states. (**c**) *Heterogeneity:* Different flow rates due to unequal distribution of microcirculatory blood flow. (**d**) *Oxygen off-loading:* High velocity of blood flow in the microcirculation (hyperdynamic state) together with increased intercapillary distance prohibits adequate tissue oxygenation. Art, arteriol; ven, venule; Hb, hemoglobin. (Adapted from [10])

the PO_2-gap and hypothesized that it reflects the severity of oxygen shunting of the microcirculation [10, 50]. Studies from our group showed an increased PO_2-gap in the ileum during hemorrhagic and endotoxic shock. Venous PO_2 showed only a minor decrease during shock while serosal and mucosal μPO_2 decreased significantly [49–51]. This increased PO_2 gap was positively correlated with the intestinal to arterial PCO_2 difference, the PCO_2-gap [52], measured by tonometry. In hemorrhagic shock, resuscitation with crystalloid solutions restores the PO_2-gap to baseline [49]. Fluid resuscitation for endotoxic shock restores the mucosal μPO_2, but not the serosal μPO_2, to baseline resulting in an increased PO_2-gap (Fig. 2). Our results agree with microsphere studies in pigs during continuous endotoxemia where it was found that the mucosa is preferentially perfused above the muscularis during shock and resuscitation [53–55].

Impaired mitochondrial oxygen utilization is an alternative explanation for tissue dysoxia in sepsis. Van der Meer and colleagues [56] showed in a canine model of endotoxic shock, that resuscitation with colloids improved mucosal PO_2 above baseline while the tonometrically measured ileal PCO_2 remained high. They interpreted these findings as indicative for cytopathic hypoxia of the mucosa, whereby decreased oxygen utilization due to mitochondrial dysfunction was the cause of the increased mucosal tissue PO_2 [9, 56]. Although NO has a physiologic role as a scavenger for free oxygen radicals it can affect mitochondrial respiration due to an interaction with superoxide to form the highly reactive peroxynitrite [57]. Peroxynitrite can induce DNA single strand breakage which can lead to activation of the nu-

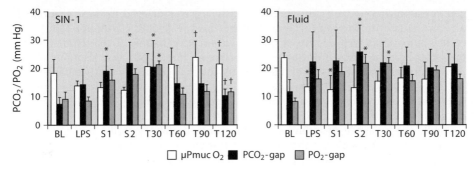

Fig. 2. Relation between mucosal microvascular PO_2 ($\mu PmucO_2$), PO_2-gap, and PCO_2 gap in the ileum of 12 pigs during endotoxemia (LPS) (1 $\mu g/kg/h$ until MAP < 60 mmHg) (S1), endotoxic shock (S2) and therapy with fluid alone or with an additional infusion of 2 $\mu g/kg/min$ SIN-1 for 2 h (T30–T120). While SIN-1 restored the $\mu PmucO_2$ and the PO_2-gap as well as the PCO_2-gap, fluid resuscitation alone only restored the mucosal μPO_2. $* = p < 0.05$ vs BL, $\dagger = p < 0.01$ vs shock, $\dagger\dagger = p < 0.01$ vs shock

clear enzyme poly (ADP-ribose) synthase (PARS) [14, 23]. The extensive ADP ribosylation of nuclear proteins by PARS results in energy depletion and cellular injury. The depression of mitochondrial respiration is blunted in the presence of iNOS, peroxynitrite and PARS inhibitors [23, 57]. In this case also, unselective blockade of NOS would be expected to be inappropriate since NO plays an important role as a physiologic regulator of tissue mitochondrial respiration [58].

According to the presently available data, we believe that functional microvascular oxygen shunting as well as cytopathic hypoxia contributes to tissue dysoxia seen in sepsis. In agreement with Vallet [28], who proposed a differential role for NO in early and late sepsis, we think both mechanisms play a different role during the progress of sepsis. NO modulating drugs and vasodilators may possibly influence both mechanisms leading to dysoxia.

Vasodilators in Sepsis and Endotoxemia

Prostacyclin is the vasodilator drug that has been subject to most research regarding beneficial effects in sepsis. Prostacyclin is formed by the enzyme cyclooxygenase and has vasodilator and anticoagulant properties [59]. Early human and animal studies showed that prostacyclin may improve tissue oxygenation in sepsis [60, 61]. Bihari et al. [60] infused prostacyclin in patients with respiratory failure and sepsis and found an increased oxygen extraction in patients who died. For the patients surviving, a possible recruitment of the microcirculation was suggested as a contributory mechanism. Despite the beneficial effects on the microcirculation [62, 63], prostacyclin has not been evaluated for its influence on outcome of patients with sepsis and septic shock.

NO donors are rarely used for studies in sepsis or endotoxic shock. Two studies in rodents showed an improved hepatic microcirculatory blood flow with either sodium nitroprusside or linsidomine [64, 65]. Zhang and coworkers [66, 67] found in two consecutive studies that the infusion of 2 $\mu g/kg/min$ of the molsidomine metabolite SIN-1 in endotoxemic dogs improved cardiac index, oxygen extraction, and superior mesenteric blood flow. The occurrence of supply dependency, when oxygen consumption becomes dependent on delivery was delayed in these animals. In a recent study, we showed that vasodilatory therapy by the NO-donor SIN-1, corrected mucosal as well as serosal microvascular oxygenation of the ileum to baseline after being depressed during endotoxic shock [68]. SIN-1 was also able to correct microvascular shunting of the serosal microcirculation and normalized the $PiCO_2$-gap (Fig. 2). Fluid resuscitation alone, however, while restoring mucosal μPO_2 above control levels, was not able to improve the lipopolysaccharide-(LPS) induced shunting of the serosal microcirculation and the $PiCO_2$-gap. This observation supports the presence of vulnerable weak microcirculatory units in the serosa or subserosa (e.g., muscularis) that are more difficult to resuscitate than the mucosa and can only be opened up by increasing the input pressure to the microcirculation by vasodilatation, such as provided by the NO donor SIN-1. This study further suggests that these weak microcirculatory units could be the source of tonometrically measured intestinal PCO_2.

Since NO generated from iNOS, in contrast to the endothelium-generated physiologic NO, has detrimental effects on the microcirculation a selective blockade of the iNOS pathway should have positive effects. Indeed improved perfusion of the kidney cortex and reduced glomerular plugging after the application of a selective iNOS blocker was shown to occur in a study in rats [69]. Two other studies showed an improved hemodynamic profile, decreased liver injury, and a protective effect against deterioration in intestinal and hepatocellular energy metabolism [70, 71]. In a recent study in pigs, we found that infusion of the highly selective iNOS inhibitor 1400 W, restored μPO_2 of the serosal and mucosal side of the ileum in an endotoxic shock model comparable to the SIN-1 experiment (Fig. 3) [72]. 1400 W corrected the intestinal PO_2-gap and hereby the functional shunting of oxygen and normalized the PCO_2-gap. According to the SIN-1 study cited above, the control group was resuscitated with fluid alone and showed persistent signs of functional shunting. 1400 W restored global hemodynamic parameters after endotoxic shock

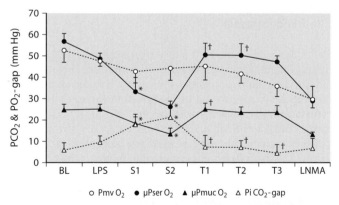

Fig. 3. Time course of mesenteric venous PO_2 (PmvO$_2$), μPO_2 of ileal serosa and mucosa (PserO$_2$, PmucO$_2$) and the arterial to intestinal PCO_2 difference (PiCO$_2$-gap) in the ileum of 12 pigs during endotoxemia (1 μg/kg/h until MAP < 60 mmHg). Therapy with fluid alone or with an additional infusion of 0.5 μg/k/h 1400 W for 3 hours (T1–T3) and a final infusion of 5 mg/kg LNMA over 20 min. 1400 W corrected functional shunting of oxygen in the microcirculation of the ileum. LNMA decreased intestinal blood flow and microcirculatory oxygenation. * = p < 0.05 vs BL, † = p < 0.05 vs S2

to baseline and corrected the epicardial μPO_2 [44]. Injection of 5 mg/kg N^G-mono-methyl-L-arginine at the end of the experiment increased blood pressure and decreased the myocardial μPO_2 below shock values. Beside the possible influence on the heterogeneity of microvascular blood flow and cell deformability, decreased NO production could also blunt cellular and mitochondrial damage due to oxygen radicals, since most iNOS mRNA is found on the tip of the villi [73].

We recently introduced [50, 74], validated and applied clinically a new method called orthogonal polarization spectral (OPS) imaging to observe the microcirculation in patients [75–77]. This technique, based on the use of polarized light, is implemented in a hand-type microscope and has allowed us the first observations of the microcirculation of human internal organs during surgery [74, 76]. For intensive care patients, the technique can be applied easily to the sublingual microcirculation to observe microcirculatory morphology as well as blood flow kinetics [50]. In particular, it allows observation of the easily accessible sublingual microcirculation in great detail, allowing even leukocytes to be observed as they role and stick in the venular part of the microcirculation [75]. Based on our experiments demonstrating improved microcirculatory recruitment using NO donor drugs [68], we performed an observational study in patients being resuscitated from septic and cardiogenic shock. After standard pressure-guided hemodynamic resuscitation, a nitroglycerin infusion was started. OPS imaging showed that sublingual microcirculatory flow is severely impaired following pressure-guided resuscitation in septic and cardiogenic shock [78, 79]. The application of nitroglycerin increased microcirculatory blood flow remarkably, although arterial and central venous pressure decreased slightly. It must be pointed out that these effects may only hold for the specific, entire, clinical therapy applied at that time in the institution. The results from this study should not yet be used as the basis for the standard introduction of nitroglycerin in the treatment of septic shock. Our study does, however, indicate that restoration of blood pressure as a resuscitation end-point alone may be flawed since this can leave the microcirculation ischemic. Whether the vasodilator therapy as applied in these conditions leads to an improvement in outcome still needs to be demonstrated, although it does lead to the intriguing idea that monitoring the microcirculation with techniques such as OPS imaging may provide new resuscitation end-points.

∎ Conclusion

From the data cited above, it seems evident that the application of vasodilators and selective iNOS blockers during sepsis and endotoxemia needs further investigation. The pharmacological properties of these drugs may have a favorable effect on microcirculatory heterogeneity, cell plugging and intravascular coagulation, and ultimately oxygen transport to tissue. An improved microcirculatory blood flow could, however, also affect the generation of oxygen radicals and impact mitochondrial function. Finally it is expected that the development of new monitoring techniques, like OPS imaging, will change resuscitation endpoints from global parameters to those of the tissue cells and their microcirculation.

References

1. Joly HR, Weil MH (1969) Temperature of the great toe as an indication of the severity of shock. Circulation 39:131–138
2. Boyd O, Grounds RM, Bennett ED (1993) The beneficial effect of supranormalization of oxygen delivery with dopexamine hydrochloride on perioperative mortality. JAMA 270:2699–2707
3. Shoemaker WC, Appel PL, Kram HB (1993) Hemodynamic and oxygen transport responses in survivors and nonsurvivors of high-risk surgery. Crit Care Med 21:56–63
4. Gattinoni L, Brazzi L, Pelosi P, et al (1995) A trial of goal-oriented hemodynamic therapy in critically ill patients. N Engl J Med 333:1025–1032
5. Hayes MA, Timmins AC, Yau EHS, Palazzo M, Hinds CJ, Watson D (1994) Elevation of systemic oxygen delivery in the treatment of critically ill patients. N Engl J Med 330:1717–1722
6. LeDoux D, Astiz ME, Carpati CM, Rackow EC (2000) Effects of perfusion pressure on tissue perfusion in septic shock. Crit Care Med 28:2729–2732
7. Grover R, Lopez A, Lorente J, et al (1999) Multi-center, randomized, placebo-controlled, double blind study of the nitric oxide synthase inhibitor 546C88: effect on survival in patients with septic shock (Abstr). Crit Care Med 27(Suppl.):A33
8. Avontuur JA, Bruining HA, Ince C (1995) Inhibition of nitric oxide synthesis causes myocardial ischemia in endotoxemic rats. Circ Res 76:418–425
9. Fink MP (1997) Cytopathic hypoxia in sepsis. Acta Anaesthesiol Scand (Suppl 110):87–95
10. Ince C, Sinaasappel M (1999) Microcirculatory oxygenation and shunting in sepsis and shock. Crit Care Med 27:1369–1377
11. Avontuur JAM, Bruining HA, Ince C (1997) Nitric oxide causes dysfunction of coronary autoregulation in endotoxemic rats. Cardiovasc Res 35:368–376
12. Hinshaw LB (1996) Sepsis/septic shock: participation of the microcirculation: an abbreviated review. Crit Care Med 24:1072–1078
13. Ince C (2000) Microcirculatory weak units – an alternative explanation: In reply (letter). Crit Care Med 28:3127–3129
14. Lush CW, Kvietys PR (2000) Microvascular dysfunction in sepsis. Microcirculation 7:83–101
15. Vallet B (1998) Vascular reactivity and tissue oxygenation. Intensive Care Med 24:3–11
16. Spain DA, Wilson MA, Krysztopik RJ, Matheson PJ, Garrison RN (1997) Differential intestinal microvascular dysfunction occurs during bacteremia. J Surg Res 67:67–71
17. Baker CH, Sutton ET (1993) Arteriolar endothelium-dependent vasodilation occurs during endotoxin shock. Am J Physiol 264:H1118–H1123
18. Lam C, Tyml K, Martin C, Sibbald W (1994) Microvascular perfusion is impaired in a rat model of normotensive sepsis. J Clin Invest 94:2077–2083
19. Spain DA, Wilson MA, Bar-Natan MF, Garrison RN (1994) Nitric oxide synthase inhibition aggravates intestinal microvascular vasoconstriction and hypoperfusion of bacteremia. J Trauma 36:720–725
20. Hiltebrand LB, Krejci V, Banic A, Erni D, Wheatly AM, Sigurdsson GH (2000) Dynamic study of the distribution of microcirculatory blood flow in multiple splanchnic organs in septic shock. Crit Care Med 28:3233–3241
21. Hollenberg SM, Broussard M, Osman J, Parillo JE (2000) Increased microvascular reactivity and improved mortality in septic mice lacking inducible nitric oxide synthase. Circ Res 86:774–779
22. Murray PT, Wylam ME, Umans JG (2000) Nitirc oxide and septic vascular dysfunction. Anesth Analg 90:89–101
23. Liaudet L, Soriano FG, Szabo C (2000) Biology of nitric oxide signaling. Crit Care Med 28:N37–N52
24. Grover R, Zaccardelli D, Colice G, Guntupalli K, Watson D, Vincent JL (1999) An open-label dose escalation study of the nitric oxide synthase inhibitor, N^G-methyl-L-arginine hydrochloride (546C88), in patients with septic shock. Crit Care Med 27:913–922
25. Träger K, Rademacher P, Rieger KM, et al (1999) Norepinephrine and N^G-monomethyl-L-arginine in porcine sepitc shock. Am J Respir Crit Care Med 159:1758–1765

26. Cobb JP, Natanson C, Hoffman WD, et al (1992) N omega-amino-L-arginine, an inhibitor of nitric oxide synthase, raises vascular resistance but increases mortality rates in awake canines challenged with endotoxin. J Exp Med 176:1175–1182

27. Pastor C, Teisseire B, Vicaut E, Payen D (1994) Effects of L-arginine and L-nitro-arginine treatment on blood pressure and cardiac output in a rabbit endotoxin shock model. Crit Care Med 22:465–469

28. Vallet B (2001) Vascular nitric oxide during sepsis: From deficiency to overproduction. Advances in Sepsis 1:52–57

29. Bhagat K, Moss R, Collier J, Vallance P (1996) Endothelial "stunning" following a brief exposure to endotoxin: a mechanism to link infection and infarction? Cardiovasc Res 32:822–829

30. Leclerc J, Pu Q, Corseaux D, et al (2000) A single endotoxin injection in the rabbit causes prolonged blood vessel dysfunction and a procoagulant state. Crit Care Med 28:3672–368

31. Ellis CG, Wrigley SM, Groom AC (1994) Heterogeneity of red blood cell perfusion in capillary networks supplied by a single arteriole in resting skeletal muscle. Circ Res 75:357–368

32. Astiz ME, DeGent GE, Lin RY, Rackow EC (1995) Microvascular function and rheologic changes in hyperdynamic sepsis. Crit Care Med 23:265–271

33. Baskurt OK, Gelmont D, Meiselman HJ (1998) Red blood cell deformability in sepsis. Am J Respir Crit Care Med 157:421–427

34. Eichelbrönner O, Sielenkämper A, Cepinskas G, Sibbald WJ, Chin-Yee IH (2000) Endotoxin promotes adhesion of human erythrocytes to human vascular endothelial cells under conditions of flow. Crit Care Med 28:1865–1870

35. Siegemund M, Hardeman MR, van Bommel J, Stegenga ME, Lind A, Ince C (1999) Red blood cell deformabillity in two different doses of LPS in a porcine model of endotoxemia. Intensive Care Med 25:S21 (Abst)

36. Korbut R, Gryglewski RJ (1993) Nitric oxide from polymorphonuclear leukocytes modulates red blood cell deformability in vitro. Eur J Pharmacol 234:17–22

37. McCuskey RS, Urbaschek R, Urbaschek B (1996) The microcirculation during endotoxemia. Cardiovasc Res 32:752–763

38. Worthen GS, Schwab B, 3rd, Elson EL, Downey GP (1989) Mechanics of stimulated neutrophils: cell stiffening induces retention in capillaries. Science 245:183–186

39. Bernard GR, Vincent JL, Laterre PF, et al. (2001) Efficacy and safety of recombinant human activated protein C for severe sepsis. N Engl J Med 344:699–709

40. Matthay MA (2001) Severe Sepsis – A new treatment with both anticoagulant and antiinflammatory properties. N Engl J Med 344:759–762

41. Taylor AE, Moore TM (1999) Capillary fluid exchange. Am J Physiol 277:S203–S210

42. Groeneveld AB, van Lambalgen AA, van den Bos GC, Bronsveld W, Nauta JJ, Thijs LG (1991) Maldistribution of heterogeneous coronary blood flow during canine endotoxin shock. Cardiovasc Res 25:80–88

43. Ince C, Ashruf JF, Avontuur JA, Wieringa PA, Spaan JA, Bruining HA (1993) Heterogeneity of the hypoxic state in rat heart is determined at capillary level. Am J Physiol 264:H294–H301

44. Siegemund M, van Bommel J, Schwarte LA, Emons M, Ince C (2001) Selective blockade of iNOS by 1400W, but not by LNMA, is beneficial to myocardial oxygenation after endotoxaemia. Intensive Care Med 27:S180 (Abst)

45. Pastor CM (1999) Vascular hyporesponsiveness of the renal circulation during endotoxemia in anesthetized pigs. Crit Care Med 27:2735–2740

46. Shultz PJ, Raij L (1992) Endogenously synthesized nitiric oxide prevents endotoxine-induced glomerular thrombosis. J Clin Invest 90:1718–1725

47. Siegemund M, van Bommel J, Stegenga ME, Ince C (2000) Effect of dopexamine and dopamine on kidney cortex tissue PO_2 in a porcine model of low-dose endotoxemia. Intensive Care Med 26:S258 (Abst)

48. Haglund U (1994) Gut ischaemia. Gut 35:S73–S76

49. Sinaasappel M, van Iterson M, Ince C (1999) Microvascular oxygen pressure in the pig intestine during haemorrhagic shock and resuscitation. J Physiol 514:245–253

50. Siegemund M, van Bommel J, Ince C (1999) Assessment of tissue oxygenation. Intensive Care Med 25:1044–1060

51. Siegemund M, van Bommel J, Stegenga ME, Ince C (1999) Influence of dopexamine on the gut oxygenation in a porcine model of low-dose endotoxaemia. Intensive Care Med 25:S115
52. Russel JA (1997) Gastric tonometry: does it work? Intensive Care Med 23:3–6
53. Revelly JP, Ayuse T, Brienza N, Fessler HE, Robotham JL (1996) Endotoxic shock alters distribution of blood flow within the intestinal wall. Crit Care Med 24:1345–1351
54. Revelly J-P, Liaudet L, Frascarolo P, Joseph J-M, Martinet O, Markert M (2000) Effects of norepinephrine on the distribution of intestinal blood flow and tissue adenosine triphosphate content in endotoxic shock. Crit Care Med 28:2500–2506
55. Neviere RR, Pitt-Hyde ML, Piper RD, Sibbald WJ, Potter RF (1999) Microvascular perfusion deficits are not a prerequisite for mucosal injury in septic rats. Am J Physiol 276:G933–G940
56. van der Meer JT, Wang H, Fink MP (1995) Endotoxemia causes ileal mucosal acidosis in the absence of mucosal hypoxia in a normodynamic porcine model of septic shock. Crit Care Med 23:1217–1226
57. Szabo C, Cuzzocrea S, Zingarelli B, O'Connor M, Salzman AL (1997) Endothelial dysfunction in a rat model of endotoxic shock. Importance of the activation of poly (ADP-ribose) synthetase by peroxynitrite. J Clin Invest 100:723–735
58. Shen W, Hintze TH, Wolin MS (1995) Nitric oxide. An important signaling mechanism between vascular endothelium and parenchymal cells in the regulation of oxygen consumption. Circulation 92:3505–512
59. Scheeren T, Radermacher P (1997) Prostacyclin (PGI2): new aspects of an old substance in the treatment of critically ill patients. Intensive Care Med 23:146–158
60. Bihari D, Smithies M, Gimson A, Tinker J (1987) The effects of vasodilation with prostacyclin on oxygen delivery and uptake in critically ill patients. N Engl J Med 317:397–403
61. Pittet JF, Lacroix JS, Gunning K, Laverriere MC, Morel DR, Suter PM (1990) Prostacyclin but not phentolamine increases oxygen consumption and skin microvascular blood flow in patients with sepsis and respiratory failure. Chest 98:1467–1472
62. Eichelbronner O, Reinelt H, Wiedeck H, et al (1996) Aerosolized prostacyclin and inhaled nitric oxide in septic shock – different effects on splanchnic oxygenation? Intensive Care Med 22:880–887
63. Radermacher P, Buhl R, Santak B, et al (1995) The effects of prostacyclin on gastric intramucosal pH in patients with septic shock. Intensive Care Med 21:414–421
64. Gundersen Y, Corso CO, Leiderer R, et al (1998) The nitric oxide donor sodium nitroprusside protects against hepatic microcirculatory dysfunction in early endotoxaemia. Intensive Care Med 24:1257–1263
65. Pastor CM, Losser MR, Payen D (1995) Nitirc oxide donor prevents hepatic and systemic perfusion decrease induced by endotoxin in anesthetized rabbits. Hepatology 22:1547–1553
66. Zhang H, Rogiers P, Friedman G, et al (1996) Effects of nitric oxide donor SIN-1 on oxygen availability and regional blood flow during endotoxic shock. Arch Surg 131:767–774
67. Zhang H, Rogiers P, Smail N, et al (1997) Effects of nitric oxide on blood flow distribution and extraction capabilities during endotoxic shock. J Appl Physiol 83:1164–1173
68. Siegemund M, van Bommel J, Vollebregt K, Dries J, Ince C (2000) Influence of the NO-donor SIN-1 on the gut oxygenation in a normodynamic, porcine model of endotoxaemia. Intensive Care Med 26:S344 (Abst)
69. Schwartz D, Mendonca M, Schwartz I, et al (1997) Inhibition of constitutive nitric oxide synthase (NOS) by nitric oxide generated by inducible NOS after lipopolysaccharide administration provokes renal dysfunction in rats. J Clin Invest 100:439–448
70. Liaudet L, Rosselet A, Schaller MD, Markert M, Perret C, Feihl F (1998) Nonselective versus selective inhibition of inducible nitric oxide synthase in experimental endotoxic shock. J Infect Dis 177:127–132
71. Matejovic M, Radermacher P, Tugtekin I, et al (2001) Effects of selective iNOS inhibition on gut and liver O2-exchange and energy metabolism during hyperdynamic porcine endotoxemia. Shock 16:203–210
72. Siegemund M, van Bommel J, Schwarte LA, Emons M, Ince C (2001) Selective blockade of iNOS by 1400W restores the gut oxygenation in a pig model of low-dose endotoxemia. Intensive Care Med 27:S147 (Abst)

73. Morin M, J, Unno N, Hodin RA, Fink MP (1998) Differential experession of inducible ni-
    tric oxide synthase messenger RNA along the longitudinal and crypt-villus axes of the in-
    testine in endotoxemic rats. Crit Care Med 26:1258–1264
74. Groner W, Winkelman JW, Harris AG, et al (1999) Orthogonal polarization spectral ima-
    ging: a new method for study of the microcirculation. Nat Med 5:1209–1212
75. Mathura KR, Alic L, Ince C (2001) Initial clinical experience with OPS imaging for obser-
    vation of the human microcirculation. In: Vincent J-L (ed) Yearbook of Intensive Care and
    Emergency Medicine 2001. Springer-Verlag, Berlin, pp 233–244
76. Mathura KR, Bouma GJ, Ince C (2001) Abnormal microcirculation in brain tumours during
    surgery. Lancet 358:1698–1699
77. Mathura KR, Vollebregt KC, Boer K, De Graaff JC, Ubbink DT, Ince C (2001) Comparison
    of OPS imaging and conventional capillary microscopy to study the human microcircula-
    tion. J Appl Physiol 91:74–78
78. Gardien MJ, Spronk PE, Ince C, Oudemans-van Straaten HM, Zandstra DF (2001) Optimiz-
    ing microvascular flow during resuscitation of patients in cardiogenic shock with nitrogly-
    cerin: visualisation by sublingual capillaroscopy. Intensive Care Med 27:S236 (Abst)
79. Spronk PE, Gardien MJ, Ince C, Oudemans-van Straaten HM, Zandstra DF (2001) Micro-
    vascular recruitment by nitroglycerin during resuscitation of patients in septic shock:
    visualisation by sublingual capillaroscopy. Intensive Care Med 27:S251 (Abst)

Vasopressin and its Analogs

G. Auzinger and J. Wendon

Introduction

Hypotension due to peripheral vasodilation and reduced responsiveness to vasopressor therapy are cardinal features of septic, and other forms of vasodilatory, shock. The nonosmotic release of the peptide hormone arginine–vasopressin in response to hypotension and hypovolemia, is an important defense mechanism to counteract systemic hypotension and maintain adequate tissue perfusion. Despite an initial appropriate response, vasopressin plasma levels fall and are inappropriately low in later stages of septic shock [1].

Low dose vasopressin 'replacement' therapy has recently been shown to have significant pressor effects and sometimes enables catecholamine withdrawal in patients with severe vasopressor resistant vasodilatory shock [1–3]. In this chapter we give an overview of the evidence supporting the use of vasopressin or its analogs in patients with vasodilatory shock.

Pathophysiology of Vasodilatory Shock

Despite high levels of endogenous plasma catecholamines and activation of the renin-angiotensin axis, vascular smooth muscles fail to constrict in septic shock; three main mechanisms have recently been implicated as being of pathogenetic importance.

Nitric Oxide (NO)

NO is an endogenous vasodilator synthesized from L-arginine by the enzyme NO synthase (NOS). Endothelial NOS-derived NO is a key regulator of arterial blood pressure, regional vascular tone and is involved in the inhibition of adhesion and aggregation of circulating blood cells to the endothelium. Inducible NOS (iNOS) is not present under physiological conditions, but is induced by proinflammatory stimuli such as bacterial endotoxins or cytokines [4]. Excess production of NO by iNOS leads to marked vasodilation, myocardial depression, and decreased vascular reactivity to vasopressor agents [5]. Recent studies show that treatment with nonselective NOS inhibitors such as L-NMMA or methylene blue improves vascular reactivity and blood pressure in experimental and human septic shock [6, 7]. However a large randomized prospective trial of L-NMMA in septic shock patients was terminated early because of increased mortality in the treatment group [8]. A possible explanation for the negative study outcome is excessive vasoconstriction and tissue hypoxia induced by non selective inhibition of all different NOS isoforms.

ATP-sensitive K$^+$ Channel

The ATP-sensitive K$^+$ (K$_{ATP}$) channel is an important modulator of arterial smooth muscle tone [9]. Activation of the channel hyperpolarizes vascular smooth muscle cells, reduces Ca^{2+} entry into the cell and induces smooth muscle relaxation. Activation of K$_{ATP}$ channels occurs under conditions of impaired tissue oxygenation stimulated by a decrease in ATP, cytosolic acidosis and increased cellular lactate concentrations [10, 11]. In addition, an increase in NO levels as encountered during septic shock can activate K$_{ATP}$ channels through a cGMP dependent mechanism.

Vasopressin

Vasopressin is a peptide hormone synthesized in the paraventricular and supraoptic nuclei of the thalamus. Its release from the posterior pituitary gland is regulated by osmotic and non-osmotic stimuli. Increased plasma osmolarity and baroreceptor-mediated hormone release in response to hypotension and hypovolemia are the most potent stimulants for vasopressin release. Other non-osmotic stimuli include pain, hypoxia and acidosis as frequently encountered in the postoperative patient.

Stimulation of vasopressin V$_2$-receptors in the collecting ducts of the kidney leads to increased water resorption at vasopressin concentrations of 1–7 pg/ml. Stimulation of vasopressin V$_1$-receptors in the vascular smooth muscle have potent vasoconstrictor effects at 10–20-fold higher concentrations (10–200 pg/ml). V$_1$-receptors are coupled to phospholipase C and increase intracellular Ca^{2+} concentration. Plasma vasopressin levels are normally < 4 pg/ml, but in response to hypotension caused by hemorrhagic or septic shock, plasma concentration will increase to more than 300 pg/ml [12]. This increase contributes substantially to the maintenance of arterial blood pressure and the defense of vital organ perfusion in the early phases of shock. However, despite this initial appropriate response, vasopressin plasma levels fall as shock worsens. In a dog model of hemorrhagic shock, plasma vasopressin levels fell from 319 to 29 pg/ml after 60 min of severe hypotension (MAP ≤ 40 mmHg) [12]. Landry and co-workers [1] were the first to show that plasma vasopressin levels failed to rise in advanced septic shock. In 19 patients with vasodilatory septic shock (systolic blood pressure of 92 mmHg on catecholamine support) and persistent hypotension for a duration of 1 to 2 days, vasopressin levels were inappropriately low (3.1 pg/ml). In fact the vasopressin levels measured, equaled levels seen under physiological conditions in patients without shock (< 5 pg/ml). Similar findings have been reported during vasodilatory shock following cardiopulmonary bypass [13] and after implantation of left ventricular assist devices [2]. Several mechanisms have been proposed in order to explain these inappropriately low levels. Stores of vasopressin in the neurohypophysis may become depleted by profound osmotic stimulation [14] or following sustained baroreceptor stimulation due to severe and prolonged hypotension. NOS is present in the supraoptic and paraventricular nuclei of the hypothalamus and in the pituitary gland. NOS activity in these areas is increased in situations of vasopressin stimulation. Administration of L-arginine or NO donors most commonly inhibits central vasopressin secretion [15].

∎ Pressor Effect of Vasopressin in Vasodilatory Shock

Patients with septic shock are very sensitive to low dose vasopressin infusions (0.01–0.04 U/min) and respond with an increase in vasopressin plasma levels to ~30–100 pg/ml [16]. At these dose ranges, vasopressin has no blood pressure effect in normal subjects [17]. Various mechanisms have been proposed to explain the exquisite pressor hypersensitivity to vasopressin in vasodilatory shock.

In contrast to catecholamine receptor down-regulation due to high endogenous and/or exogenous catecholamine levels, the plasma concentration of vasopressin is low in late stages of shock, and exogenous vasopressin can readily bind to free, sensitized receptors. Vasopressin potentiates the vasopressor effects of norepinephrine [18], inactivates K_{ATP} channels in vascular smooth muscle [19], and decreases the synthesis of inducible NO via inhibition of iNOS mRNA transcription and protein kinase C activation [20]. Dogs with baroreceptor denervation show a marked increase in the pressor response to vasopressin [21], and deficient baroreflex mediated secretion of vasopressin has been documented in patients with autonomic failure [17]. There is also evidence for a significantly impaired activity of the sympathetic nervous system during sepsis, reflected by a decrease in heart rate variability [22].

∎ Clinical Trials in Humans

Vasopressin use in various forms of vasodilatory shock has been reported in a total of 272 adult and pediatric patients over the last 5 years including two randomized controlled trials (RCT) [2, 3], three prospective cohort studies [1, 23, 24], six retrospective case series [25–30] and one case report [31]. Patients were treated for septic shock, vasodilatory shock following cardiopulmonary bypass, left ventricular assist device (LVAD) insertion, cardiac transplantation. Brain dead organ donors have also been studied. In one small case series vasopressin was used for reversal of milrinone-induced hypotension.

Randomized Controlled Trials

Malay et al. [2] performed a placebo controlled pilot trial in septic shock patients admitted to a trauma intensive care unit (ICU). Ten patients were studied and randomized to treatment with a low dose vasopressin infusion (0.04 U/min) or placebo. At study entry, all patients were receiving moderate to high dose catecholamine support (norepinephrine 12 and 6.8 μg/min, phenylephrine 170 and 180 μg/min). The study duration was for a period of 24 h after drug initiation. Systolic arterial pressure increased significantly in the vasopressin group from 98 to 125 mmHg (p < 0.008), but remained unchanged in patients receiving placebo. Furthermore all vasopressor medication was withdrawn in the treatment group and all patients survived to 24 h. Two patients in the placebo group died of refractory hypotension before 24 h. Due to the small sample size (only three patients alive in the placebo group) no valid statistical testing could be performed in order to assess the secondary endpoint of withdrawal of catecholamine support. The increase in blood pressure in the treatment group was due to a rise in systemic vascular resistance (SVR), there being no change in heart rate and cardiac index. No clinically obvious adverse effects such as cardiac or mesenteric ischemia were observed during drug administration.

Two years earlier, Argenziano et al. [3] had studied the use of vasopressin in patients with vasodilatory shock necessitating catecholamine support following placement of a left ventricular assist device. Ten patients reached entry criteria: mean arterial pressure (MAP) <70 mmHg despite norepinephrine administration at a dose of 12.8–26.7 µg/min and a cardiac index (CI) on left ventricular assist device support >2.5 l/min/m². They were then randomized to vasopressin infusion of 0.1 U/min or placebo. Within 15 minutes, vasopressin significantly increased MAP by the virtue of an increase in SVR and all patients in the active therapy limb were successfully weaned off catecholamine support. Norepinephrine was discontinued in four patients during the initial 15 minutes of vasopressin therapy, one patient was weaned off over several hours. The median duration of vasopressin treatment was 36 h (1 h to 7 days). Pulmonary artery pressures and CI remained unchanged during study-drug infusion. Placebo patients showed no beneficial hemodynamic response, however three patients in the placebo group were crossed over to vasopressin with significant hemodynamic improvement. Baseline vasopressin levels were inappropriately low in seven patients (mean of 8.8 pg/ml). These patients had a greater rise in MAP following vasopressin therapy compared to the remaining three patients in whom moderately elevated plasma levels were seen prior to randomization (33.7 pg/ml).

Prospective Studies

Donald Landry and colleagues [1] were the first to describe low vasopressin plasma levels (3.1 pg/ml) in 19 patients with established septic shock. In 12 patients who acted as a control group with cardiogenic shock, similar degrees of hypotension and catecholamine dependency, vasopressin levels were significantly higher at 22.7 pg/ml. In two patients with septic shock, a continuous infusion of vasopressin at a dose of 0.01 U/min resulted in an expected plasma concentration of 27 and 34 pg/ml, suggesting impaired hormone secretion rather than increased catabolism of vasopressin as the main cause for the observed plasma levels. In the remaining ten patients in the septic shock group, vasopressin was given at a dose of 0.04 U/min resulting in a significant increase in arterial pressure and SVR and a concomitant reduction in cardiac output.

Similar hemodynamic effects at a similar dose range have been found in unstable organ donors [23]. Ten organ donors with arterial hypotension (MAP<70 mmHg, despite vasopressor support), received vasopressin as a continuous infusion (0.04–0.1 U/min) and responded with a significant increase in MAP and a reduction in catecholamine requirements (40%), or discontinuation of vasopressor therapy (40%). Plasma vasopressin levels were again measured and found to be inappropriately low (2.8 pg/ml) prior to institution of therapy.

In the third prospective trial, Tsuneyoshi et al. [4] studied the hemodynamic and metabolic effects of vasopressin infusions in 16 patients with septic shock. A dose of 0.04 U/min was infused over a study period of 16 h. As in previous trials, MAP and SVR increased significantly. No adverse cardiac or metabolic effects were noted and the urine output increased significantly during vasopressin infusion. The serum lactate levels fell but this was not significant. As a word of caution, the authors add that there was no indication of a clear benefit of vasopressin beyond an increase in blood pressure. The overall mortality rate of 44% was similar to that reported in previous studies with conventional therapy.

Retrospective Case Series

Three sizeable retrospective case series report on the use of vasopressin in septic shock (n=50) [29], vasodilatory shock following left ventricular assist device insertion (n=50) [28], and in a total cohort of 60 patients with vasodilatory shock due to sepsis or following cardiopulmonary bypass [30]. The patients' response to vasopressin was monitored for periods of 24 to 72 h. Indication for vasopressin administration was catecholamine refractory vasodilatory shock. All three studies showed a significant and prompt increase in blood pressure following vasopressin administration and catecholamine requirements decreased significantly during the observation period. The vasopressin doses administered ranged between 0.01–0.6 U/min. In the study of Holmes et al. [29] in septic shock patients, doses above 0.04 U/min did not show any added benefit in terms of further reduction in pressor dose. This may indicate that higher doses could be avoided hence reducing the risk of side effects. In fact, Duenser et al. [30] reported a significant increase in liver enzymes and bilirubin levels in septic shock or post cardio-pulmonary bypass patients during vasopressin infusion. It was proposed that this may have been related to impaired splanchnic perfusion. Mortality in the latter two studies was very high, 85% [29] and 67% [30], respectively, raising concerns of the overall outcome benefit of this treatment beyond improvement in blood pressure. The vasoconstrictive effect of vasopressin in the splanchnic, and especially mesenteric, circulation is mediated via V_1 receptors. This effect is used therapeutically in the treatment of acute variceal hemorrhage and portal hypertension, but can lead to severe unwanted side effects in the septic shock patient. In an endotoxin model, endogenous vasopressin release caused gastrointestinal mucosal injury which was reduced with V_1 receptor antagonist therapy and less pronounced in vasopressin deficient animals [32] and in normovolemic humans, vasopressin infused at 5 IU/70 kg reduced superior mesenteric vein flow by 38% [33]. Various case report of ischemic colitis induced by vasopressin or terlipressin therapy [34–36] emphasize the importance of these experimental findings although the vasopressin doses used for the treatment of variceal hemorrhage are 10 to 20 times higher than the doses administered in septic shock (20 U bolus or 2–4 U/min as an infusion).

Table 1. Change in parameters over time following terlipressin administration. All variables compared to baseline levels. * denotes significant change compared to baseline levels ($p < 0.05$), n=number of patients. NE: norepinephrine dose (µg/kg/min); SVI: stroke volume index; SOFA: sequential organ failure assessment

	Pre n=14	1 h post n=14	4 h n=14	24 h n=12	48 h n=11	72 h n=10
MAP mmHg	68±5	76±13*	77±15*	71±6	72±11	73±10
NE	0.56±0.39	0.56±0.43	0.48±0.39	0.33±0.28*	0.25±0.26*	0.19±0.31*
SVI ml/m²	61±19	60±22	59±19	63±23	60±16	66±27
Lactate mmol/l	4±2.6	4.3±2.7	4.5±3	3.2±2.7	3.6±2.8	3.7±3
SOFA	18±4			18±2	18±3	17±3

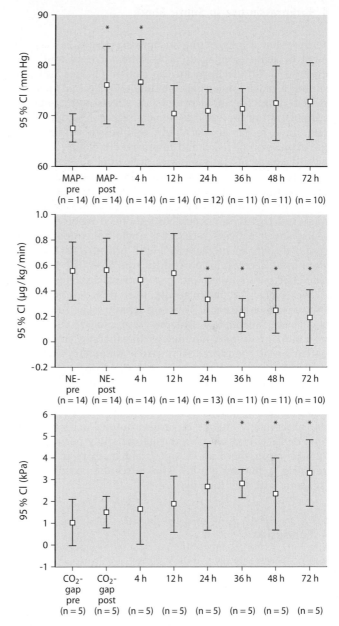

Fig. 1. The top two graphs show changes in mean arterial pressure (MAP) and norepinephrine dose (NE µg/kg/min) over time. * Denotes significant changes compared to baseline ($p < 0.05$). n = patients alive at various time points. The lower graph shows gastric mucosal-to-arterial PCO_2 gap in patients with tonometry surviving to 72 h (n = 5). CI: confidence interval

▌ Terlipressin use in Septic Shock

Terlipressin, a long acting vasopressin-analog is commonly used for the management of acute esophageal variceal hemorrhage and treatment of hepatorenal syndrome [37, 38]. Terlipressin has similar pharmacodynamic properties to vasopressin but a much longer half-life time (50 vs 6 min) permitting intermittent bolus administration. The incidence of side effects and complications related to terlipressin administration for variceal hemorrhage is less than that reported with vasopressin [39]. In a recent animal study, terlipressin administration significantly decreased the expression of iNOS and improved circulatory and liver dysfunction, as reflected by a decrease in transaminases, following an endotoxin-challenge in cirrhotic rats [40]. In a second trial performed in endotoxemic sheep, terlipressin significantly increased MAP and SVR index [41]; this was accompanied by a decrease in CI and heart rate. The efficacy of terlipressin as a pressor agent in humans with catecholamine resistant septic shock has only been reported in abstract form so far [42]. Six septic shock patients received a single bolus dose of terlipressin (1–2 mg) and responded with an increase in blood pressure (MAP 53 vs >70 mmHg) enabling a significant decrease in norepinephrine dose (0.7 vs 0.14 µg/kg/min). No deleterious side effects were noted and three patients survived to ICU discharge.

We treated 14 patients with liver disease and norepinephrine resistant septic shock with terlipressin. We considered 'rescue therapy' with terlipressin if patients had been adequately volume resuscitated and remained hypotensive (MAP <70 mmHg) despite norepinephrine therapy (mean dose 0.55 µg/kg/min). Seven patients were monitored with gastric tonometry during terlipressin treatment.

One to 3 mg of terlipressin in divided doses were administered over a period of 24 h. All patients responded with a significant increase in blood pressure (+13%, $p < 0.05$, Table 1 and Fig. 1) which was accompanied by a significant reduction in norepinephrine requirements (–66% at 72 h, $p < 0.05$, Table 1 and Fig. 1). We did not observe any change in cardiac output, oxygenation indices, metabolic parameters, or liver function tests during the study period. In those patients who survived 72 h or more, there was a significant increase in the gastric mucosal-arterial PCO_2 gap (Fig. 1, bottom graph). This raises the possibility of splanchnic and end organ ischemia with this therapy.

▌ Conclusion

Vasopressin levels are low in advanced stages of vasodilatory shock. A significant body of evidence from small randomized controlled trials, prospective cohort studies, as well as retrospective case series, indicates beneficial hemodynamic effects of low dose 'replacement' therapy with vasopressin or its analog. However, despite reversal of catecholamine resistance, no obvious improvement in outcome can be derived from the available data, partly due to the small sample size of the two randomized controlled trials. The currently available data on the side effects of vasopressin treatment for septic shock especially regarding the splanchnic circulation are very limited, and detrimental changes in splanchnic perfusion and metabolism cannot be predicted by markers of global tissue oxygenation.

Therefore, we recommend judicious use of these compounds ideally inside randomized controlled trials and with adequate monitoring of regional perfusion.

References

1. Landry DW, Levin HR, Gallant EM, et al (1997) Vasopressin deficiency contributes to the vasodilation of septic shock. Circulation 95:1122–1125
2. Malay MB, Ashton RC, Landry DW, Townsend RN (1999) Low-dose vasopressin in the treatment of vasodilatory septic shock. J Trauma 47:699–703
3. Argenziano M, Choudhri AF, Oz MC, Rose EA, Smith CR, Landry DW (1997) A prospective randomized trial of arginine vasopressin in the treatment of vasodilatory shock after left ventricular assist device placement. Circulation 96:II 286–290
4. Moncada S, Higgs A (1993) The L-arginine-nitric oxide pathway. N Engl J Med 329:2002–2012
5. Cobb JP, Danner RJ (1996) Nitric oxide and septic shock. JAMA 275:1192–1196
6. Grover R, Zaccardelli D, Colice G, Guntupalli K, Watson D, Vincent JL (1999) An open label dose escalation study of the nitric oxide synthase inhibitor, N(G)-methyl-arginine hydrochloride (546C88), in patients with septic shock. Crit Care Med 27:913–922
7. Kirov MY, Evgenov OV, Evgenov NV, et al (2001) Infusion of methylene blue in human septic shock: A pilot, randomized, controlled study. Crit Care Med 29:1860–1867
8. Grover R, Lopez A, Lorente J, et al (1999) Multicenter, randomized, placebo-controlled, double blind study of the nitric oxide synthase inhibitor 546C88: Effect on survival in patients in septic shock. Crit Care Med 27:A33 (Abst)
9. Landry DW, Oliver JA (1992) The ATP-sensitive K+ channel mediates hypotension in endotoxemia and hypoxic lactic acidosis in dog. J Clin Invest 89:2071–2074
10. Davies NW (1990) Modulation of ATP-sensitive K+ channels in skeletal muscle by intracellular protons. Nature 343:375–377
11. Keung EC, Li Q (1991) Lactate activates ATP-sensitive potassium channels in guinea pig ventricular myocytes. J Clin Invest 88:1772–1777
12. Morales D, Madigan J, Cullinane, et al (1999) Reversal by vasopressin of intractable hypotension in the late phase of hemorrhagic shock. Circulation 100:226–229
13. Morales DL, Gregg D, Helman DN, et al (2000) Arginine vasopressin in the treatment of 50 patients with postcardiotomy vasodilatory shock. Ann Thorac Surg 69:102–106
14. Cooke CR, Wall BM, Jones GV, Presley DN, Share L (1993) Reversible vasopressin deficiency in severe hypernatremia. Am J Kidney Dis 22:44–52
15. Reid IA (1994) Role of nitric oxide in the regulation of renin and vasopressin secretion. Front Neuroendocrinol 15:351–383
16. Mohring J, Glanzer K, Maciel JA Jr, et al (1980) Greatly enhanced pressor response to antidiuretic hormone in patients with impaired cardiovascular reflexes due to idiopathic orthostatic hypotension. J Cardiovasc Pharmacol 2:367–376
17. Wagner HN Jr, Braunwald E (1956) The pressor effect of the antidiuretic principle of the posterior pituitary in orthostatic hypotension. J Clin Invest 35:1412–1418
18. Bartelstone HJ, Nasmyth PA (1965) Vasopressin potentiation of catecholamine actions in dog, rat, cat and rat aortic strip. Am J Physiol 208:754–762
19. Wakatsuki T, Nakaya Y, Inoue I (1992) Vasopressin modulates K+-channel activities of cultured smooth muscle cells from porcine coronary artery. Am J Physiol 263:H491–H496
20. Umino T, Kusano E, Muto S, et al (1999) AVP inhibits LPS- and IL- 1β- stimulated NO and cGMP via V1 receptor in cultured rat mesangial cells. Am J Physiol 276:F433–F441
21. Cowley AW Jr, Monos E, Guyton AC (1974) Interaction of vasopressin and the baroreceptor reflex system in the regulation of arterial blood pressure in the dog. Circ Res 34:505–514
22. Garrard CS, Kontoyannis DA, Piepoli M (1993) Spectral analysis of heart rate variability in the sepsis syndrome. Clin Auton Res 3:5–13
23. Chen JM, Cullinane S, Spanier TB, et al (1999) Vasopressin deficiency and pressor hypersensitivity in hemodynamically unstable organ donors. Circulation 100:II 244–246
24. Tsuneyoshi I, Yamada H, Kakihana Y, Nakamura M, Nakano Y, Boyle WA (2001) Hemodynamic and metabolic effects of low-dose vasopressin infusion in vasodilatory septic shock. Crit Care Med 29:487–493
25. Landry DW, Levin Hr, Gallant EM, et al (1997) Vasopressin pressor hypersensitivity in vasodilatory septic shock. Crit Care Med 25:1279–1282

26. Rosenzweig EB, Starc TJ, Chen JM, et al (1999) Intravenous arginine-vasopressin in children with vasodilatory shock after cardiac surgery. Circulation 100:II 182–186
27. Gold JA, Cullinane S, Chen J, Oz MC, Oliver JA, Landry DW (2000) Vasopressin as an alternative to norepinephrine in the treatment of milrinone-induced hypotension. Crit Care Med 28:249–252
28. Argenziano M, Chen JM, Cullinane S, et al (1999) Arginine vasopressin in the management of vasodilatory hypotension after cardiac transplantation. J Heart Lung Transplant 18:814–817
29. Holmes CL, Walley KR, Chittock DR, Lehman T, Russell JA (2001) The effects of vasopressin on hemodynamics and renal function in severe septic shock: a case series. Intensive Care Med 27:1416–1421
30. Duenser MW, Mayr AJ, Ulmer H, et al (2001) The effects of vasopressin on systemic hemodynamics in catecholamine-resistant septic and postcardiotomy shock: a retrospective analysis. Anesth Analg 93:7–13
31. Lamarre P, Perreault B, Lesur O (2001) Vasopressin and blood pressure support for pancreatitis-induced systemic inflammatory response syndrome with circulatory shock. Pharmacotherapy 21:506–508
32. Varga C, Pavo I, Lamarque D, et al (1998) Endogenous vasopressin increases acute endotoxin provoked gastrointestinal mucosal injury in the rat. Eur J Pharmacol 352:257–261
33. Erwald R, Wiechel KL, Strandell T (1976) Effect of vasopressin on regional splanchnic blood flows in conscious man. Acta Chir Scand 142:36–42
34. Lambert M, de Peyer R, Muller AF (1982) Reversible ischemic colitis after intravenous vasopressin therapy. JAMA 247:666–667
35. Willems MG, Schoenemann J, Rey C, Schafer H, Lindecken KD (1985) Ischemia of the cecum caused by glycylpressin. Leber Magen Darm 15:165–168
36. Schmitt W, Wagner-Thiessen E, Lux G (1987) Ischemic colitis in a patient treated with glypressin for bleeding oesophageal varices. Hepatogastroenterology 34:134–136
37. Escorsell A, Del Arbol LR, Planas R, et al (2000) Multicenter randomized controlled trial of terlipressin versus sclerotherapy in the treatment of acute variceal bleeding: The TEST study. Hepatology 32:471–476
38. Uriz J, Gines P, Cardenas A, et al (2000) Terlipressin plus albumin infusion: an effective and safe therapy of hepatorenal syndrome. J Hepatol 33:43–48
39. D'Amico G, Traina M, Vizzini G, et al (1994) Terlipressin or vasopressin plus transdermal nitroglycerin in a treatment strategy for digestive bleeding in cirrhosis. A randomized clinical trial. J Hepatol 20:206–212
40. Barriere E, Tazi KA, Poirel O, Lebrec D, Moreau R (2001) Terlipressin administration decreases iNOS expression and improves circulatory and liver dysfunction in endotoxin-challenged rats with cirrhosis. J Heptol 34 (Suppl 1):A519 (Abst)
41. Scharte M, Meyer J, Van Aken H, Bone HG (2001) Hemodynamic effects of terlipressin (a synthetic analog of vasopressin) in healthy and endotoxemic sheep. Crit Care Med 29:1756–1760
42. O'Brian AJ, Clapp LH, Singer M (2001) The use of glypressin in norepinephrine-resistant septic shock. Intensive Care Med 27 (Suppl 2):A110 (Abst)

Mechanical Ventilation

The Use of Ventilatory Modes allowing Spontaneous Breathing during Mechanical Ventilation

R. Kuhlen, C. Putensen, and R. Rossaint

∎ Introduction

The primary goal of mechanical ventilation is to restore gas exchange and to limit patients with acute respiratory failure from an elevated breathing workload. To achieve these goals a variety of different ventilatory modalities are already in clinical use. The development of microprocessor-driven mechanical ventilators has facilitated enormous progress in the implementation of different new modes of ventilatory support into standard ventilators. Most of the newer ventilatory modes are designed for partial ventilatory support reflecting that different technical approaches might be used for patient/ventilator interaction during assisted mechanical ventilation. However, the increasing use of partial support modalities is not only due to technological improvements but also to data showing that avoiding controlled mechanical ventilation by preserving some spontaneous breathing activity by the diaphragm might be beneficial for gas exchange, hemodynamics, and the clinical course of acute lung injury (ALI). In this chapter, we will review the role of preserved spontaneous breathing activity during mechanical ventilation in patients with acute respiratory failure.

∎ Advantages of Maintaining Spontaneous Breathing Efforts during Mechanical Ventilation

Hemodynamics and Organ Perfusion

It is well known that positive thoracic pressure induced by mechanical ventilation might compromise venous return and cardiac output, which may lead to a decrease in organ perfusion. In contrast, spontaneous breathing efforts generate a negative pressure in the thoracic cavity that improves venous return and thereby might increase cardiac output [1]. In accordance with this principle of pathophysiology, it has been found that mechanical ventilation with positive pressure can cause impaired renal function. Steinhoff and colleagues were the first to demonstrate that during intermittent mandatory ventilation (IMV) with some degree of spontaneous breathing activity, the renal water and sodium excretion was improved compared to controlled mechanical ventilation (CMV) [2]. Obviously, a small superimposed spontaneous breathing activity resulted in such a decrease in thoracic pressure, that the renal perfusion as well as the excretion function was better than during CMV [3]. Also, other forms of partial ventilatory support such as airway pressure release ventilation (APRV) [4, 5] or biphasic positive airway pressure (BiPAP) [6–9] have been found to have no negative effect on cardiac output compared to the detrimental effects of CMV. However, for ventilation modes supporting each individual breathing effort, such as pressure support (PSV), the effects on hemodynamics have been reported to be more complex. In cardiac surgery patients, pressure support as high as 30 mbar has been found to have no negative effect on cardiac output [10]. On the other hand in a clinical investigation in patients with acute respiratory distress syndrome (ARDS), Putensen et al. [7] directly compared PSV to CMV and Bi-PAP/APRV but they could only demonstrate beneficial effects on cardiac output for BiPAP/APRV, not for PSV. From these data, it might be speculated that only unassisted spontaneous breaths might effectively decrease intrathoracic pressure thereby increasing venous return and cardiac output. In a clinical study in patients with ALI who were transferred from CMV to PSV as soon as possible after the installation of mechanical ventilation, no major differences in hemodynamics were found between CMV and PSV [11]. However, in this study of 48 patients, 10 failed the transition to PSV and three out of these 10 failures were due to hemodynamic impairment. In all three cases, a history of severe chronic heart disease was present [11] suggesting that the resumption of spontaneous breathing activity during mechanical ventilation might impose an additional workload on the heart eventually leading to left ventricular dysfunction in predisposed patients.

Atelectasis Formation

Atelectasis formation during mechanical ventilation might not only be interpreted as a symptom of the underlying disease, but also as a result of CMV itself, since physiological studies have clearly shown that a different pattern of ventilation distribution is found during controlled ventilation compared to spontaneous breathing. During spontaneous respiration, the most pronounced excursions of the diaphragm are to be found in the dorsal part resulting in a distribution of ventilation mainly towards the dorsal lung regions thereby perfectly matching perfusion which is also high in these areas. During CMV the inactive diaphragm shifts in cranial direction following the force exerted by the intraabdominal pressure (IAP) and hence, the ventilation is mainly distributed to anterior lung regions [12] resulting in some degree of inhomogeneous ventilation-perfusion (V/Q) distribution [13, 14] (Fig. 1). Accordingly, atelectasis formation is a predominant finding during CMV even without preexisting lung disease [15] and it is clearly related to the extent of V/Q mismatching [16]. It has been shown that some, but not all, of this atelectasis might be counterbalanced by the application of positive end-expiratory pressure (PEEP) [17]. Moreover, very elegant physiological experiments have shown that the atelectasis formation in the dependent lung zones during general anesthesia can be effectively decreased when the phrenic nerves are stimulated electrically [18]. Obviously, preserved muscular activity of the diaphragm is an efficient measure to act against lung collapse in the dependent lung areas since it actively opens these zones whereas the application of positive pressure alone might not be sufficient to keep these lung areas open.

It is well known that ALI is characterized by severe lung collapse and atelectasis formation predominately in the dependent zones of the lung [19]. Intrapulmonary shunting has been shown to correlate directly to the amount of non-aerated lung tissue observed by computed tomography (CT) in the dependent lung zones adjacent to the diaphragm. This finding was attributed to alveolar collapse caused by the superimposed pressure on the lung and the cephaled shift of the diaphragm

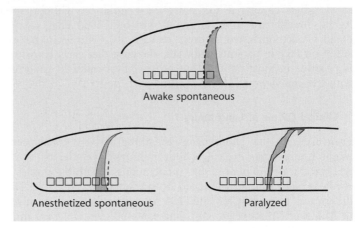

Fig. 1. Diaphragmatic position during spontaneous breathing in awake state, during general anesthesia, and during muscle paralysis in anesthesia. During anesthesia, especially when muscle relaxants are used, a profound shift of the diaphragm into the thoracic cavity accompanied by a loss of excursion of the dorsal parts can be found. Due to this shift of the diaphragm, expiratory lung volumes decrease and atelectasis formation is likely to develop in the dorsal posterior lung regions adjacent to the diaphragm. (Modified from [12])

most evident in the posterior lung units during mechanical ventilation [20]. Accordingly, it might be hypothesized that preserving some degree of spontaneous breathing activity during mechanical ventilation helps to avoid lung collapse and improves V/Q distribution in ALI.

In a dog model of oleic acid-induced lung injury, small spontaneous breathing activity (10% of total minute ventilation) caused a 15% reduction in intrapulmonary shunting of blood and consequently an improvement in oxygenation [6]. Since dead space ventilation was reduced and respiratory system compliance increased in those experiments it was concluded that diaphragmatic activity recruited otherwise collapsed lung areas. However, interfacing between spontaneous breathing and mechanical ventilation seems to have a critical effect on the observed effects of partial ventilatory support on V/Q matching. Whereas uncoupling between spontaneous breaths and mechanical cycles during APRV/BiPAP showed beneficial effects on V/Q matching, mechanical assistance of each inspiratory effort did not counteract the V/Q maldistribution in this model of ALI [9] nor in a model of bronchoconstriction [8].

Sydow et al. [21] found in ARDS patients, that spontaneous breathing with APRV led to a decrease in low V/Q which was more pronounced than the effects of CMV without spontaneous activity. Since the effect was not immediate but occurred after hours, the investigators concluded that a certain time period is necessary until recruitment, and thereby improvements in gas exchange due to spontaneous breathing activity, takes place. In extension of these results, Hörmann et al. [22] reported that very small superimposed spontaneous breaths of 70–150 ml during mechanical ventilation using BiPAP might improve oxygenation as well as CO_2 removal. This finding could be elegantly explained by a study of Putensen and colleagues [7], again showing a clear redistribution of low V/Q towards normal V/Q regions during superimposed spontaneous breathing in ARDS patients. These findings were reported for equal minute ventilation as well as for equal airway pressures when compared to controlled ventilation without spontaneous breathing. Again, in contrast to BiPAP/APRV no beneficial effect of PSV on gas exchange could be demonstrated in these patients [7]. This is in accordance with a clinical study on PSV in patients with ALI, showing that early transition from CMV to PSV is possible in most patients but no specific benefit in gas exchange was associated with the changeover [11].

Clinical Course of Lung Injury

Even allowing that spontaneous breathing activity during acute respiratory failure might improve gas exchange, little is known whether or not the clinical course of ALI might be influenced by spontaneous breathing modes. In an experimental study in pigs with ALI induced by surfactant washout, we did not find any major differences between CMV and PSV in gas exchange, hemodynamics, or the course of ALI over 12 hours [23–25]. These preliminary data are in accordance with a report that PSV is clinically feasible in patients with ALI, although it did not prove any better than CMV on a short term basis [11]. No clinical outcome data using PSV as the initial form of ventilatory assist in ALI have been reported yet.

However, for BiPAP/APRV one study reporting on the clinical outcome of trauma patients at high risk for the development of ARDS has been published [26]. In this investigation, patients with a high trauma score were randomly assigned to undergo CMV or BiPAP/APRV for the first three days. Earlier reports on the beneficial effects of this strategy on gas exchange were confirmed since the group of patients with BiPAP/APRV had a consistently better oxygenation as well as better hemodynamics over the time of the investigation when compared to CMV. Interestingly, BiPAP/APRV was also associated with a shorter duration of mechanical ventilation and a shorter length of stay in the ICU compared to CMV. Furthermore, total cost for analgo-sedation and circulatory support were clearly lower for BIPAP/APRV [26]. These preliminary data suggest that not only gas exchange and hemodynamics but also the clinical course of ALI might be positively affected when allowing some unrestricted spontaneous breathing activity during mechanical ventilation. Obviously, these promising results should be tested in large scale clinical studies focusing primarily on outcome measures in patients with ALI.

Analgo-sedation

It is quiet obvious that the management of patients with assisted modes of ventilation is completely different when compared to the patient mechanically ventilated in a controlled mode. The advantage is that no deep sedation or even muscle relaxation must be applied when a mode allowing spontaneous breathing is used. Since the potential side effects of deep sedation and muscle blocking agents are well known, this should be beneficial for the patient although it has to be admitted that no clinical outcome study has ever addressed this question.

On the other side, it has to be stated clearly that patient monitoring must be somewhat closer and more vigilant when spontaneous breathing is allowed in patients with acute respiratory failure. The patient-ventilator interaction becomes an issue during all forms of assisted spontaneous breathing and few data are available today in order to give clear guidelines how to handle this problem.

Ventilator-associated Lung Injury

During recent years it has become evident that mechanical ventilation is associated with severe risks since it can contribute to the progress of lung injury [27] and might promote non pulmonary organ failure [28]. Therefore, the avoidance of ventilator associated lung injury has become a major goal when setting any mode of ventilator support. Two major factors contributing to the progress of lung injury have been identified: overdistension of the lungs using tidal volumes which are too big for the diseased lung [27] as well as recurrent expiratory lung collapse leading to relevant sheer stress when these collapsed areas are reopened during the next inspiration [29, 30]. According to these findings, it has been clearly demonstrated that the reduction of tidal volumes to 6 ml/kg body weight results in an improved outcome in patients with ALI [31]. Smaller clinical studies suggest that the use of PEEP values avoiding expiratory collapse might result in better outcome [32, 33]. Based on these data it seems reasonable to hypothesize that during ventilatory modes allowing spontaneous breathing the resulting tidal volume should also be limited and the PEEP levels should be set to avoid expiratory lung collapse. Clearly designed studies to address the question of ventilator associated lung injury during assisted spontaneous breathing are warranted before large scale implementation of these modes can be advocated.

▌ Ventilatory Modes allowing Spontaneous Breathing during Mechanical Ventilation

Assist Control (A/C, AMV)

Assist control is a classical form of assisted spontaneous breathing offering the possibility to trigger a breath that is then applied by the machine according to the settings on the ventilator. From a technical point of view this form of assistance appears not to be particularly beneficial since it does not allow any modulation of the breathing pattern other than the frequency with which a preset machine breath will be applied. Nevertheless, it is most widely used in clinical practice since it clearly results in a very effective unloading of the respiratory muscles [34].

Synchronized Intermittent Ventilation (SIMV)

During SIMV, machine cycles are adjusted and, in-between these preset cycles, intermittent spontaneous breathing is possible by applying a demand gas flow. As already mentioned above, this form of assisted spontaneous breathing activity was found to be beneficial on organ function during mechanical ventilation [2, 3]. However, one of the problems with SIMV is that the spontaneously breathing patient is not necessarily unloaded from the elevated workload. During the inspiration of a preset breath, the tidal volume is delivered independent of patient activity and during spontaneous breathing a certain amount of additional workload is imposed by the resistance of the endotracheal tube and the gas delivery system. Combination with pressure support for the intervening breaths during SIMV has, therefore, been widely used in clinical practice. It has been found to result in more efficient unloading not only for the intervening breaths but also for the activity during the preset SIMV breath [34]. However, SIMV has been advocated as a convenient and easy weaning mode since the SIMV frequency could be decreased in a stepwise fashion, thereby allowing a gradual withdrawal of ventilatory support. In clear contrast to this theoretical benefit, SIMV in the clinical setting has been shown to be of little use for weaning, as, compared to other weaning modalities like T-piece trials of pressure support, it was associated with the longest time necessary for weaning and the lowest success rates [35, 36].

Pressure Support Ventilation (PSV)

Pressure support was designed to support each inspiratory effort with flow to reach a preset pressure level. Originally, it was implemented in mechanical ventilators to compensate for a certain pressure drop during demand flow regulation due to non-ideal ventilator properties in the early 1980s. It was further applied as a real mode of ventilation that augmented each inspiratory effort of the patient. As a function of the applied level of pressure support, it is possible to progressively release a patient from an increased breathing workload. In a classical paper, PSV has been found to prevent the development of diaphragmatic fatigue [37] and therefore, it is frequently applied as a weaning mode when the patient is recovering from respiratory failure. Depending on the way it is applied, PSV may facilitate fast and safe weaning [35]. A particular use of PSV might be the potential to unload the intubated patient from external sources of work of breathing [38–40]. However, although it is a widely accepted weaning tool that has been extensively investigated, it is not clear whether or not PSV should be applied early in the course of acute respiratory failure [11]. No long term data are available on the effects of PSV on gas exchange and V/Q relations. There is only preliminary data showing that PSV might be more beneficial for V/Q than CMV [41] but less efficient than BiPAP/APRV [7].

Biphasic Positive Airway Pressure (BiPAP)
and Airway Pressure Release Ventilation (APRV)

These modes of ventilatory support were introduced more than ten years ago by two groups [42, 43]. In concept, BIPAP might be viewed as the cyclic change from a lower to a higher continuous positive airways pressure (CPAP) level with spontaneous breathing being possible on both levels using an active flow regulation. The machine part of ventilation is due to the cyclic shift from the lower level to the higher level and back, whereas the patient might breath spontaneously throughout the whole respiratory cycle. APRV is essentially characterized by spontaneous breathing on a rather high level of CPAP with this pressure released to ambient pressure for short periods to facilitate exhalation.

As already discussed, BiPAP/APRV has been found to result in an improved gas exchange compared to CMV in ALI [7, 26]. It has to be stressed that the setting of the two pressure levels during BiPAP follows the principal rules of a protective ventilation strategy: the lower pressure level should be set to keep a minimal lung volume in order to avoid repetitive lung collapse and reopening. Whenever an inflection point on the static pressure-volume (PV) curve can be found, the lower BiPAP level should be set above this point whereas the upper level should be set below any upper deflection point to avoid lung overdistension. Since a limited tidal volume of 6 ml/kg body weight has been found to produce a better outcome than 12 ml/kg, the resulting tidal volume during BiPAP/APRV should also be around

6 ml/kg body weight. Hence, the pressure amplitude between lower and higher CPAP levels has to be adjusted properly.

APRV is comparable to the BiPAP setting in the sense that it can be accomplished by the same circuit. However, by concept APRV means that a rather high mean airway pressure is kept for almost all the respiratory cycle where spontaneous breathing is warranted followed by a very short release to near ambient pressure which should facilitate CO_2 removal. When the release time becomes so short that the lung cannot be completely emptied, a certain amount of auto-PEEP will be generated with this form of ventilation. This approach in ARDS patients has been found to improve gas exchange due to recruitment over some time [21]. Large scale clinical outcome studies are warranted to prove whether or not theses modes should be implemented in the routine clinical care of patients with ALI.

Proportional Assist Ventilation (PAV)

PAV is a mode which was introduced in 1992 by Younes et al. who described a new approach to unload the respiratory muscles by applying pressure in proportion to patient effort [44, 45]. Such a regulation would allow the patient to be unloaded for a certain percentage of the breathing workload independent from effort. In this view, the original idea of PAV was to make the ventilator act as an additional respiratory muscle fully under the control of patient effort. Since this effort is not readily measurable, flow and volume are taken as the input signal of the PAV regulation. When pressure is applied as a function of flow (flow assist, FA), it might be used to overtake a defined portion of the resistive work of breathing, whereas the application of pressure in proportion to the generated volume (volume assist, VA) should unload from elastic work of breathing. Since FA and VA have to be set as a function of respiratory system mechanics, a fair estimate of the respiratory mechanics during assisted spontaneous breathing is needed to adjust PAV properly. However, since such a measurement is not yet clinically available, the clinical use of PAV remains difficult at the moment. Ongoing studies on measurements of respiratory system mechanics during assisted breathing will show whether or not a sufficiently precise estimate of the necessary input variables for PAV is clinically feasible.

Automatic Tube Compensation (ATC)

For the intubated patient, the endotracheal (ET) tube imposes some additional breathing workload since it acts as an external resistor to the respiratory system. It is clear that the resistance of the ET tube is related to its size, but in addition, it has been found that ET tube resistance is a highly non-linear function of flow especially for higher flow rates [46]. Since during any form of spontaneous breathing flow is variable, it is obvious that any fixed pressure support or linear proportionality between pressure assist and flow rate might not be used to accurately compensate for the ET tube resistance and hence, the imposed work of breathing. Therefore, the mode ATC was introduced as an algorithm that is designed to overtake exactly the amount of pressure which is necessary to overcome the ET tube resistance for each instantaneous flow rate [47]. This mode has been found to work in laboratory models and in patients [48–50]. However, clinical trials on ATC implemented in standard ventilators are necessary to further clarify the role of ATC for the spontaneously breathing patient. It must be investigated as a stand alone mode that, by concept, should be very useful for spontaneous breathing trials during weaning from mechanical ventilation as well as for use in combination with other spontaneous breathing modes.

▌ Conclusions

Physiological studies show that maintaining spontaneous breathing activity during mechanical ventilation might result in improved gas exchange compared to controlled mechanical ventilation. Furthermore, the reduction in intrathoracic pressure with spontaneous breathing can help to avoid hemodynamic and other side effects of controlled mechanical ventilation. With modern types of microprocessor-driven ventilators, the tools to adapt machine assistance to patient demands are clinically available providing the possibility to investigate the clinical effects of assisted spontaneous breathing modes in acute respiratory failure. Some very promising data have been reported in favor of this approach using BiPAP/APRV but no clear cut guidelines on the large scale use of the different forms of partial ventilatory assist are available. Clinical studies on the concept itself and the different modifications to allow spontaneous breathing early in the course of mechanical ventilation for acute respiratory failure are needed to clarify the roles of all the different modes in the clinical setting.

References

1. Downs JB, Douglas ME, Sanfelippo PM, Stanford W, Hodges MR (1977) Ventilatory pattern, intrapleural pressure, and cardiac output. Anesth Analg 56:88–96
2. Steinhoff H, Falke K, Schwarzhoff W (1982) Enhanced renal function associated with intermittend mandatory ventilation in acute respiratory failure. Intensive Care Med 8:69–74
3. Steinhoff H, Kohlhoff R, Falke K (1984) Facilitation of renal function by intermittent mandatory ventilation. Intensive Care Med 10:59–65
4. Valentine DD, Hammond MD, Downs JB, Sears NJ, Sims WR (1991) Distribution of ventilation and perfusion with different modes of mechanical ventilation. Am Rev Respir Dis 143:1262–1266
5. Rasanen J, Downs JB, Stock MC (1988) Cardiovascular effects of conventional positive pressure ventilation and airway pressure release ventilation. Chest 93:911–915
6. Putensen C, Rasanen J, Lopez FA (1994) Ventilation-perfusion distributions during mechanical ventilation with superimposed spontaneous breathing in canine lung injury. Am J Respir Crit Care Med 150:101–108
7. Putensen C, Mutz NJ, Putensen-Himmer G, Zinserling J (1999) Spontaneous breathing during ventilatory support improves ventilation- perfusion distributions in patients with acute respiratory distress syndrome. Am J Respir Crit Care Med 159:1241–1248
8. Putensen C, Rasanen J, Lopez FA (1995) Interfacing between spontaneous breathing and mechanical ventilation affects ventilation-perfusion distributions in experimental bronchoconstriction. Am J Respir Crit Care Med 151:993–999
9. Putensen C, Rasanen J, Lopez FA, Downs JB (1994) Effect of interfacing between spontaneous breathing and mechanical cycles on the ventilation-perfusion distribution in canine lung injury. Anesthesiology 81:921–930
10. Dries DJ, Kumar P, Mathru M, et al (1991) Hemodynamic effects of pressure support ventilation in cardiac surgery patients. Am Surg 57:122–125
11. Cereda M, Foti G, Marcora B, et al (2000) Pressure support ventilation in patients with acute lung injury. Crit Care Med 28:1269–1275
12. Froese AB, Bryan AC (1974) Effects of anesthesia and paralysis on diaphragmatic mechanics in man. Anesthesiology 41:242–255

13. Rehder K, Knopp TJ, Sessler AD, Didier EP (1979) Ventilation perfusion relationship in young healthy awake and anethsetized paralyzed man. J Appl Physiol 47:745–753
14. Gea J, Roca J, Torres A, Agusti AG, Wagner PD, Rodriguez-Roisin R (1991) Mechanisms of abnormal gas exchange in patients with pneumonia. Anesthesiology 75:782–789
15. Reber A, Nylund U, Hedenstierna G (1998) Position and shape of the diaphragm: implications for atelectasis formation. Anaesthesia 53:1054–1061
16. Tokics L, Hedenstierna G, Svensson L, Brismar B, Cederlund T, Lundquist H (1996) V/Q distribution and correlation to gas atelectasis in anesthetized paralyzed humans. J Appl Physiol 81:1822–1833
17. Neumann P, Rothen HU, Berglund JE, Valtysson J, Magnusson A, Hedenstierna G (1999) Positive end-expiratory pressure prevents atelectasis during general anaesthesia even in the presence of a high inspired oxygen concentration. Acta Anaesthesiol Scand 43:295–301
18. Hedenstierna G, Tokics L, Lundquist H, Andersson T, Strandberg A, Brismar B (1994) Phrenic nerve stimulation during halothane anesthesia. Effects of atelectasis. Anesthesiology 80:751–760
19. Gattinoni L, Pesenti A, Bombino M, et al (1988) Relationships between lung computed tomographic density, gas exchange, and PEEP in acute respiratory failure. Anesthesiology 69:824–832
20. Gattinoni L, Bombino M, Pelosi P, et al (1994) Lung function and structure in different stages of severe adult respiratory distress syndrome. JAMA 271:1772–1779
21. Sydow M, Burchardi H, Ephraim E, Zielmann S, Crozier TA (1994) Long term effects of two different ventilatory modes on oxygenation in acute lung injury. Comparison of airway pressure release ventilation and volume controlled inverse ratio ventilation. Am J Respir Crit Care Med 149:1550–1556
22. Hormann C, Baum M, Putensen C, Kleinsasser A, Benzer H (1997) Effects of spontaneous breathing with BIPAP on pulmonary gas exchange in patients with ARDS. Acta Anaesthesiol Scand Suppl 111:152–155
23. Dembinski R, Kuhlen R, Max M, Bensberg R, Kißler J, Rossaint R (2000) Gas exchange and hemodynamics during controlled and mechanical ventilation (CMV) and pressure support (PS) in experimental lung injury. Am J Respir Crit Care Med 161:A391 (Abst)
24. Bensberg R, Kuhlen R, Max M, Dembinski R, Kißler J, Rossaint R (2000) Pressure support versus controlled mechanical ventilation in experimental lung injury. Intensive Care Med 26 (suppl 3):S273 (Abst)
25. Dembinski R, Kuhlen R, Lopez F, et al (2000) Ventilation-perfusion distribution during controlled mechanical ventilation (CMV) and pressure support (PS). Intensive Care Med 26 (suppl 3):S284 (Abst)
26. Putensen C, Zech S, Wrigge H, et al (2001) Long-term effects of spontaneous breathing during ventilatory support in patients with acute lung injury. Am J Respir Crit Care Med 164:43–49
27. Dreyfuss D, Saumon G (1998) Ventilator-induced lung injury: lessons from experimental studies. Am J Respir Crit Care Med 157:294–323
28. Slutsky AS, Tremblay L (1998) Multiple system organ failure: is mechanical ventilation a contributing factor? Am J Respir Crit Care Med 157:1721–1725
29. Chiumello D, Pristine G, Slutsky AS (1999) Mechanical ventilation affects local and systemic cytokines in an animal model of acute respiratory distress syndrome. Am J Respir Crit Care Med 160:109–116
30. Muscedere JG, Mullen JB, Gan K, Slutsky AS (1994) Tidal ventilation at low airway pressures can augment lung injury. Am J Respir Crit Care Med 149:1327–1334
31. The Acute Respiratory Distress Syndrome Network. (2000) Ventilation with lower tidal volumes as compared with traditional tidal volumes for acute lung injury and the acute respiratory distress syndrome. N Engl J Med 342:1301–1308
32. Amato MB, Barbas CS, Medeiros DM, et al (1998) Effect of a protective-ventilation strategy on mortality in the acute respiratory distress syndrome. N Engl J Med 338:347–354
33. Ranieri VM, Suter PM, Tortorella C, et al (1999) Effect of mechanical ventilation on inflammatory mediators in patients with acute respiratory distress syndrome: a randomized controlled trial. JAMA 282:54–61

34. Leung P, Jubran A, Tobin MJ (1997) Comparison of assisted ventilator modes on triggering, patient effort, and dyspnea. Am J Respir Crit Care Med 155:1940–1948
35. Brochard L, Rauss A, Benito S, et al (1994) Comparison of three methods of gradual withdrawal from ventilatory support during weaning from mechanical ventilation. Am J Respir Crit Care Med 150:896–903
36. Esteban A, Frutos F, Tobin MJ, et al (1995) A comparison of four methods of weaning patients from mechanical ventilation. Spanish Lung Failure Collaborative Group. N Engl J Med 332:345–350
37. Brochard L, Harf A, Lorino H, Lemaire F (1989) Inspiratory pressure support prevents diaphragmatic fatigue during weaning from mechanical ventilation. Am Rev Respir Dis 139:513–521
38. Brochard L, Rua F, Lorini H, Lemaire F, Harf A (1991) Inspiratory pressure support compensates for the additional work of breathing caused by the endotracheal tube. Anesthesiology 75:739–745
39. Bersten AD, Rutten AJ, Vedig AE, Skowronski GA (1989) Additional work of breathing imposed by endotracheal tubes, breathing circuits, and intensive care ventilators. Crit Care Med 17:671–677
40. Bersten AD, Rutten AJ, Vedig AE (1993) Efficacy of pressure support in compensating for apparatus work. Anaesth Intensive Care 21:67–71
41. Santak B, Radermacher P, Sandmann W, Falke KJ (1991) Influence of SIMV plus inspiratory pressure support on VA/Q distributions during postoperative weaning. Intensive Care Med 17:136–140
42. Baum M, Benzer H, Putensen C, Koller W, Putz G (1989) [Biphasic positive airway pressure (BIPAP) – a new form of augmented ventilation]. Anaesthesist 38:452–458
43. Stock MC, Downs JB, Frolicher DA (1987) Airway pressure release ventilation. Crit Care Med 15:462–466
44. Younes M (1992) Proportional assist ventilation, a new approach to ventilatory support. Theory. Am Rev Respir Dis 145:114–120
45. Younes M, Puddy A, Roberts D, et al (1992) Proportional assist ventilation. Results of an initial clinical trial. Am Rev Respir Dis 145:121–129
46. Guttmann J, Eberhard L, Fabry B, Bertschmann W, Wolff G (1993) Continuous calculation of intratracheal pressure in tracheally intubated patients. Anesthesiology 73:503–513
47. Fabry B, Guttmann J, Eberhard L, Wolff G (1994) Automatic compensation of endotracheal tube resitance in spontaneously breathing patients. Technol Health Care 1:281–291
48. Kuhlen R, Guttmann J, Nibbe L, et al (1997) Proportional pressure support and automatic tube compensation: new options for assisted spontaneous breathing. Acta Anaesthesiol Scand Suppl 111:155–159
49. Fabry B, Haberthur C, Zappe D, Guttmann J, Kuhlen R, Stocker R (1997) Breathing pattern and additional work of breathing in spontaneously breathing patients with different ventilatory demands during inspiratory pressure support and automatic tube compensation. Intensive Care Med 23:545–552
50. Kuhlen R, Max M, Nibbe L, et al (1999) Atemmuster und Atemanstrengung bei Automatischer Tubuskompensation und inspiratorischer Druckunterstützung. Anaesthesist 48:871–875

Neural Control of Mechanical Ventilation: A New Approach to Improve Patient-Ventilator Interaction

J. Spahija, J. Beck, and C. Sinderby

Introduction

Mechanical ventilation is used to treat acute respiratory failure. In its most conservative form, mechanical ventilation completely replaces the breathing function of the patient. These so-called 'controlled' modes of mechanical ventilation usually require that the patient be sedated or even paralyzed. In non-sedated and spontaneously breathing patients, mechanical ventilation can be delivered by modes of partial ventilatory assist, where mechanical ventilation assists breathing in such a way that ventilation is maintained and that respiratory muscle failure is avoided by unloading the respiratory muscles. Preferably, the ventilatory assist should be delivered in response to the output from respiratory centers, i.e., respond to changes in respiratory demand. Since the respiratory center output is not constant within a given breath, and its duration, shape, and amplitude vary from one breath to the next, a challenge for the application of partial ventilatory assist is therefore to accurately determine:

- when to cycle-on and cycle-off the assist during each breath (triggering)
- the profile of assist delivered within a breath (intra-breath assist profile)
- the level of assist during each breath (level of assist)

To make these decisions, one must be able to accurately measure the timing and magnitude of the patients' inspiratory efforts. In this chapter we will discuss these points and give some new insights on how neural control of mechanical ventilation may be an improvement over current technologies.

Measurement of Neural Inspiratory Effort

In order to discuss how to properly detect and quantify the patient's inspiratory (or expiratory) efforts, it is important to first clarify the use of the word 'effort'. With respect to breathing, the term effort is used to characterize the patient's neural inspiratory drive, although it is routinely quantified as a mechanical output, i.e., measured as pressure. The effectiveness with which the neural activation of the respiratory muscles is transformed into a mechanical force (e.g., pleural pressure) is referred to as the neuro-mechanical coupling. Neuro-mechanical coupling is affected by changes in muscle length, which means that it varies within and between each breath, due to changes in tidal volume and changes in end-expiratory lung-volume, respectively [1]. The neuro-mechanical coupling may also be affected by factors that alter the contractile properties of the respiratory muscles, e.g., muscle fatigue. In practice, this means that for a given neural motor output, increased weakness or neuro-mechanical uncoupling of the respiratory muscles will result in a decreased mechanical output.

Ideally, measurements of neural effort should be made at the level of the brain or the motor nerves. Given that this is not possible in humans, if neuro-muscular transmission to the respiratory muscles is present, measurement of the electrical activity of the inspiratory muscles can be used as an index of the inspiratory neural drive [2]. The electrical activity of a muscle results from the asynchronous propagation of motor unit action potentials along the muscle fibers, and is the signal that activates the muscle contraction. To date, measurement and processing of the electrical activity of the crural diaphragm (EAdi) with esophageal electrodes represents the only technology that has been validated for quantification of neural inspiratory effort in humans [3–6]. Crural EAdi has been demonstrated to accurately express global diaphragm activation in healthy individuals [1], stable patients with chronic obstructive lung disease (COPD) [6] and in patients with acute respiratory failure breathing on mechanical ventilation [7]. The use of esophageal electrodes offers certain important advantages. Different from skin surface electrodes, esophageal electrodes are not affected by electrical activity elicited by expiratory or postural muscles (muscle cross-talk) and thickness of subcutaneous fat. For practical applications, the micro-electrodes used to measure EAdi in the esophagus can be mounted either on the patient's naso-gastric tube, which is routinely introduced in critically ill patients, or on a 'thin and soft' catheter which could minimize discomfort of the positioned catheter.

▌ Triggering

In order to initiate and terminate the ventilator-assisted breaths, today's ventilators use pressure, flow, or volume sensors, which are located in the ventilator's respiratory circuit [8]. These types of trigger systems will subsequently be referred to as pneumatic trigger systems. In patients with altered muscle function and altered respiratory mechanics, there can be considerable limitations in maintaining the timing between onset of inspiratory attempts and the onset of the ventilatory assist with the use of such triggers [9]. Also with respect to cycling-off ventilatory assist, existing triggers are limited in terms of ability to synchronize the end of neural inspiration and end of ventilatory assist [10]. If the timing between the patient's inspiratory attempts and the ventilator assist is asynchronous, patients may experience discomfort, ventilation may be impaired, and inspiratory and/or expiratory work of breathing may be increased [11, 12], which, in the most severe situations may require the use of controlled mechanical ventilation, sedation and even paralysis of the patient [13]. When applying ventilatory assist in spontaneously breathing patients, one goal would, therefore, be to ensure that the onset and end of the patient's neural inspiratory effort are properly detected and that the ventilatory assist is initiated and terminated in synchrony with the patient.

Cycling-on Ventilatory Assist

There are at least three major factors that negatively affect the performance of cycling-on ventilatory assist with pneumatic trigger systems: 1) weakness of inspiratory muscles, 2) intrinsic positive end-expiratory pressure (PEEPi), 3) leaks in the respiratory circuit.

Inspiratory muscle weakness has a major impact on pneumatic triggers because it diminishes the patient's ability to generate force/pressure and requires increased diaphragm activation to obtain the necessary force/pressure to cycle-on ventilatory assist [6]. With neural triggering, cycling-on of ventilatory assist occurs as soon as inspiratory muscle electrical activity is detected, independent of the presence or absence or inspiratory muscle weakness.

Intrinsic PEEP constitutes a threshold load, which, during pneumatic triggering, increases the amount of pleural pressure that must be generated and leads to delays in cycling-on of ventilatory assist [14]. The effects of intrinsic PEEP may be overcome by the application of an extrinsic PEEP, which when applied properly, will reduce patient neural effort, work of breathing, and triggering delays [14]. However, if excessive extrinsic PEEP is applied, it may result in dynamic hyperinflation [14]. Currently, there is no easy and accurate method for determining the optimal level of extrinsic PEEP that should be applied in order to compensate for intrinsic PEEP. With respect to the neural effort (measured as EAdi), the neural onset of inspiration can be detected and the ventilatory assist can be cycled on without delays regardless of the level of intrinsic PEEP [15, 16] (Fig. 1). Neural triggering can therefore minimize the need and side effects associated with external PEEP application [14].

Leaks in the respiratory circuit may cause problems of initiating assist as well as auto-triggering depending on the pneumatic trigger used and the external PEEP applied [17]. In contrast, neural triggering is, by definition, not affected by leaks. As a result, neural triggering may be useful for delivery of ventilatory assist via mask or uncuffed tubes (in infants), where respiratory circuit leaks often pose significant problems [18, 19].

One should keep in mind that, in situations when the neuro-mechanical coupling is normal, the ability to cycle-on with a pneumatic trigger may be just as effective as with neural triggering. Moreover, a pneumatic on-trigger may be more effective in situations where inspiration is initiated by inspiratory muscles other than the diaphragm. Ideally, the combined use of neural and pneumatic on-trigger systems would ensure the earliest possible on-triggering and patient-ventilator synchrony.

Cycling-off Ventilatory Assist

Mechanical ventilators conventionally use algorithms based on either time or pneumatic signals to cycle-off ventilatory assist. With pneumatic signals, one can cycle-off the assist when a certain volume has been reached, when the flow has dropped to a certain level (in absolute or relative terms), or when a given reference pressure limit is exceeded. Since time and volume-cycled breath termination algorithms do not ensure that end-inspiration coincides with the end of a patient's inspiratory effort, these criteria will not be discussed in the present chapter.

Flow is the most common pneumatic variable used to determine the cessation of a patient's inspiratory attempt (i.e., relaxation of inspiratory muscles). However, the accuracy of flow to determine the end of the patient's neural inspiratory effort is imprecise and is influenced by the elastic and resistive properties of the respiratory

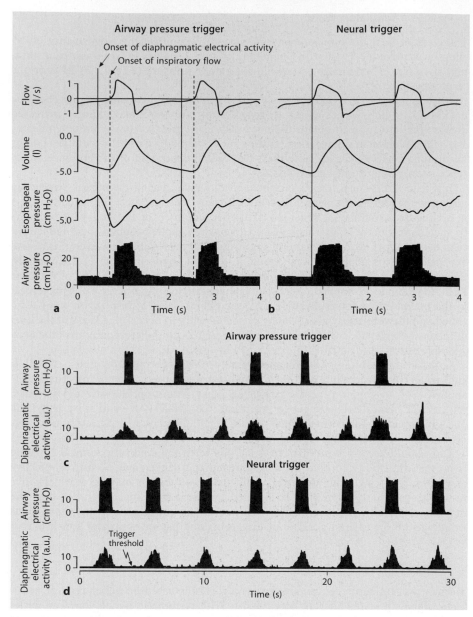

Fig. 1. Partial ventilatory support in two subjects with severe chronic obstructive pulmonary disease and acute respiratory failure. **a** Conventional pressure trigger: Mechanical ventilatory assistance starts when airway pressure decreases by a preset amount. The beginning of inspiratory effort (solid vertical line) precedes inspiratory flow by several hundred milliseconds. This delay is due to intrinsic PEEP and occurs despite externally applied PEEP. A further delay from the onset of inspiratory flow (vertical dashed line) to the rise in positive airway pressure is present, due to the mechanical limitation of the ventilator trigger. **b** Neural triggering. The ventilator provides support as soon as diaphragmatic electrical activity exceeds a threshold level. The delay to onset of inspiratory flow and increase in airway pressure is almost eliminated. **c** Poor patient–ventilator interaction with conventional pressure triggering. Diaphragmatic electrical activity (shaded areas) is poorly coordinated with the ventilatory support (indicated by increased airway pressure) and often results in completely wasted inspiratory efforts. **d** Implementation of the neural trigger (same patient and identical ventilatory settings, except for the trigger system, as in **c** can restore the interaction between the patient's neural drive and the ventilatory support. a. u., arbitrary units (**c** and **d**). (From [15] with permission)

system [20, 21]. In the presence of respiratory circuit leaks, a flow off-trigger would cause ventilatory assist to persist, despite the fact that the patient has terminated his neural inspiratory effort [22]. Such poor cycling-off promotes inefficient respiratory muscle work [23]. Furthermore, poor cycling-off, which causes ventilatory assistance to persist into the neural expiration, may promote delayed on-triggering of subsequent breaths [24].

Generally, with neural cycling-off of mechanical ventilation, the ventilatory assist is terminated when neural inspiratory effort (EAdi) ceases, and, thus, is not affected by factors such as respiratory system elastance, resistance, or presence of leaks in the respiratory circuit. Consequently, neural cycling-off of ventilatory assist has the potential to improve expiratory synchrony, which may in turn reduce complications associated with mechanical ventilation [25] and improve patient comfort [22]. This is especially relevant in the pediatric population, where it has been shown that asynchrony between the infant and the ventilator can cause excess morbidity including decreased oxygenation [26, 27], increased use of sedation or muscle paralysis [28], barotrauma [28, 29], and cerebral blood flow fluctuations, which can be associated with intraventricular hemorrhage [30].

▌ Control of Intrabreath Assist Profile

Modes of partial ventilatory assist have until recently delivered assist in a predetermined fixed intrabreath assist profile. One approach to implement intrabreath adjustment of ventilatory assist is automatic tube compensation, which offers the ability to compensate for the additional work of breathing due to the endtracheal tube [31]. To improve patient-ventilator interaction, it has been suggested that the ventilatory assist delivery within a given breath should parallel the patient's inspiratory neural effort [15, 32]. Consequently, the patient would, within the same inspiration, receive more assist when demand is high and less assist when demand is low. To date, two strategies, proportional assist ventilation (PAV) and a new experimental mode of mechanical ventilation called neurally adjusted ventilatory assist (NAVA), have attempted to acheive such intrabreath control of the intrabreath assist profile. To compare PAV with NAVA it is necessary to return to the discussion of neuro-mechanical coupling.

During an inspiratory attempt, the neural inspiratory output normally increases as a function of time. If the inspiratory attempt is performed under conditions of quasi-isometric muscle contraction, i.e., with occluded airways, where the neuro-mechanical coupling is relatively well maintained, then the neural (EAdi) and mechanical (pleural/transdiaphragmatic pressures) outputs are usually related in a quasi-linear fashion up to about 75% of maximal activation [1]. On the other hand, if an unassisted inspiration is performed, such that the inspiratory muscles shorten as tidal volume increases, the relationship between neural (EAdi) and mechanical (transdiaphragmatic pressure) output becomes alinear and the mechanical output (i.e., pressure) will result in a progressively increasing underestimation of the patient's neural inspiratory effort [1, 33].

PAV is a mode of mechanical ventilation that continuously readjusts the level of assist (assist profile) within each breath in proportion to the predicted pressure generated by the inspiratory muscles (Pmus). Pmus is calculated using the 'equation of motion' and instantaneous measurements of flow and volume as well as constants of resistance and elastance, the latter assumed to be linear within a breath [32]. However, the equation of motion does not correct for neuro-mechanical uncoupling, which, based on the above discussions, is not maintained throughout an inspiration. Although PAV delivers assist in proportion to Pmus, i.e., the mechanical inspiratory effort, how closely Pmus reflects the actual neural inspiratory effort within a breath has yet to be evaluated. When elastance and resistance are overestimated, or if leaks are present, PAV may exhibit 'run away', a situation where the timing and magnitude of the ventilatory assist are no longer controlled [32, 34].

A more recent experimental mode of mechanical ventilation, NAVA, uses inspiratory neural effort to control the intrabreath assist profile. With NAVA, the EAdi determines the intra-breath assist profile by a function where ventilatory assist simply equals EAdi times a constant [15]. The intra-breath assist profile is continuously adjusted throughout each inspiration in response to the inspiratory neural effort, which, in turn, is a reflection of the instantaneous demand regardless of the factors that contribute to altering respiratory drive (Fig. 2). Since the level of assist delivered during NAVA is controlled by the neural inspiratory effort, the servo of the ventilator will automatically act to compensate for leaks in the respiratory circuit while maintaining synchrony between inspiratory neural effort and ventilatory assist.

▌ Controlling the Level of Assist

The act of breathing regulates ventilation by adjusting frequency and tidal volume. Respiratory drive or central motor output is modulated by sensory information arising from numerous sources (chemoreceptors, chest wall/muscle mechanoreceptors, lung/airway receptors and others) and can also be modified by inputs from other parts of the brain (voluntary control of breathing, talking). Electrical impulses, which originate centrally, activate the main 'engines' used to adjust ventilation: the diaphragm, inspiratory rib cage, and accessory muscles. With acute respiratory failure, due to weak inspiratory muscles, increased inspiratory load, and/or increased ventilatory demand, ventilatory assist is applied in order to aid these 'engines' to maintain adequate ventilation while preventing inspiratory muscle fatigue. As the patient's ventilatory status improves or deteriorates, assist levels must be readjusted in order to meet the patient's altered needs. Traditionally, adjustment of ventilatory assist has been performed manually. Recently, however, there has been an increased interest in continuous adjustment of the ventilatory assist, referred to as 'closed-loop control of mechanical ventilation', whereby the patient's own physiological parameter(s) is/are used to automatically adjust ventilatory assist [35, 36].

In addition to the control of the intra-breath assist profile, modes like PAV and NAVA potentially offer a means to compensate for changes in demand, by changing ventilatory assist on a breath-to-breath basis. Both modes deliver assist with a preset 'fixed' proportionality to inspiratory neural effort (NAVA) and an estimated Pmus (PAV). By using repeated measurements of elastance and resistance in order to adjust the constants in the equation of motion, PAV can thereby compensate for changes in inspiratory load [37]. With NAVA also, any adjustment of the 'gain' factor, which determines the level of ventilatory assist that is delivered for a given level of neural activation, must be performed manually. Moreover, because NAVA and PAV provide ventilatory assist in proportion to increased inspiratory neural effort

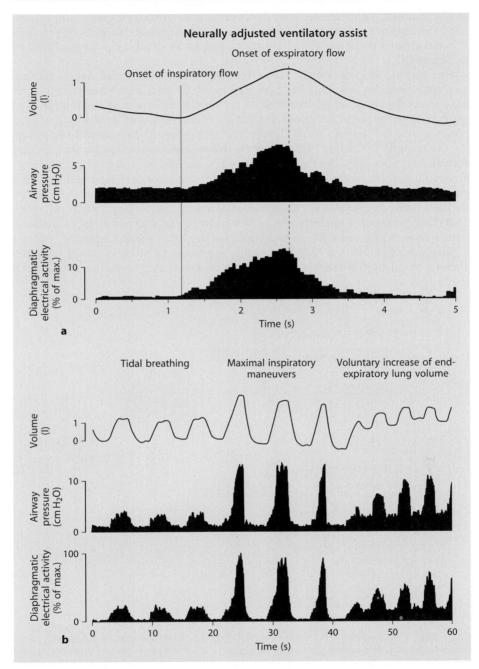

Fig. 2. Neurally adjusted ventilatory assist during a single breath (**a**) and during various breathing maneuvers (**b**). There are continuous proportional adjustments of airway pressure (reflecting ventilatory assist) with changes in diaphragmatic electrical activity (reflecting neural drive) during changes in tidal and end-expiratory lung volumes. (From [15] with permission)

and mechanical output, respectively, by definition, activation or motor output cannot be maintained at a given level or within a predetermined range. In other words it is not clear if these modes can maintain optimal levels of assist from admission to weaning.

One method to continuously adjust ventilatory assist, such that neural inspiratory effort remains constant, has been developed by Iotti and Braschi [38]. Their method continuously adjusts the level of ventilatory assist according to a function using changes in predicted neural inspiratory effort, measured as airway occlusion pressure over 0.1 seconds ($P_{0.1}$), a pneumatic technology simply obtained by delaying the opening of the inspiratory valve by 100 ms., in conjunction with an alveolar volume controller [39]. The measurement of $P_{0.1}$ involves occlusion of the respiratory circuit, and is incompatible with leaks in the respiratory circuit and flow-based trigger systems. Although $P_{0.1}$ has been demonstrated to reflect pleural pressure deflections well, $P_{0.1}$ is affected by neuro-mechanical uncoupling (weakness) [40]. Therefore, progressive respiratory muscle weakness, e.g., due to fatigue or dynamic hyperinflation, may cause $P_{0.1}$ to underestimate the 'true' neural inspiratory effort.

Target drive ventilation (TDV) is another experimental mode of closed-loop mechanical ventilation. It uses the average EAdi observed over several breaths to keep

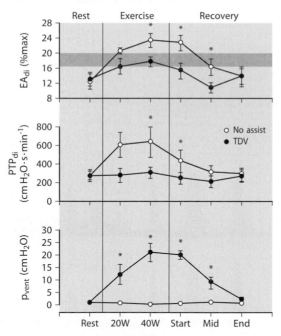

Fig. 3. Target drive ventilation (TDV) versus unassisted breathing during rest, exercise and recovery in six healthy subjects breathing continuously through an inspiratory and Starling-type expiratory resistance in order to simulate airflow limitation. Graph showing group mean values (± SE) averaged over the last minute of control breathing (no assist) and TDV, during conditions of rest, exercise and three phases of recovery following exercise. By automatically increasing ventilatory assist (Pvent) during exercise, TDV suppressed and maintained diaphragm electrical activation (EAdi) within the targeted range, and promoted a significantly lower transdiaphragmatic pressure time product (PTPdi) compared to exercise without any ventilatory assist. Immediately after exercise cessation, EAdi dropped below the target range, which lead to the gradual automatic removal of the ventilatory assist. *: $p < 0.05$

the neural inspiratory effort within a predetermined target range by automatically incrementing/decrementing ventilatory assist [41]. Practically this means that if EAdi exceeds the targeted upper limit, the ventilatory assist will be increased, and if EAdi drops below the targeted lower limit, the ventilatory assist will be decreased, whereas if the EAdi remains within these limits, assist will not be altered. The purpose of the target range is to allow for the normal variability of the neural inspiratory activation pattern, while preventing neural inspiratory effort and pressure output from reaching levels that might otherwise exceed the fatigue threshold or cause over-support of the respiratory muscles. When neural inspiratory activity reaches above the upper limit of the target range, then TDV applies fixed, stepwise increases in ventilatory assist until neural inspiratory activity returns within the target range, whereas, if neural inspiratory activity drops below the lower limit, assist will be reduced until no more assist is delivered. That EAdi can be maintained within a target range has recently been shown in healthy individuals performing constant workload bicycle exercise (Fig. 3). When ventilatory demand increased, automatic increases in the ventilatory assist during TDV proceeded to unload the diaphragm. Moreover, when exercise was stopped, EAdi dropped below target range suggesting that TDV may have the potential to automatically adjust ventilatory assist during weaning from mechanical ventilation.

▌ Conclusion

The use of neural control of mechanical ventilation is anticipated to add new possibilities to better integrate mechanical ventilation with the patient's own respiratory effort, improving patient-ventilator synchrony, patient comfort, and offering possibilities to auto-regulate the level of assist.

References

1. Beck J, Sinderby C, Lindström L, Grassino A (1998) Effects of lung volume on diaphragm EMG signal strength during voluntary contractions. J Appl Physiol 85:1123–1134
2. Lourenco RV, Cherniack NS, Malm JR, Fishman NP (1966) Nervous output from the respiratory center during obstructed breathing. J Appl Physiol 21:527–533
3. Beck J, Sinderby C, Weinberg J, Grassino A (1995) Effects of muscle-to-electrode distance on the human diaphragm electromyogram. J Appl Physiol 79:975–985
4. Beck J, Sinderby C, Lindström L, Grassino A (1996) Influence of bipolar esophageal electrode positioning on measurements of human crural diaphragm EMG. J Appl Physiol 81:1434–1449
5. Sinderby C, Beck J, Lindström L, Grassino A (1997) Enhancement of signal quality in esophageal recordings of diaphragm EMG. J Appl Physiol 82:1370–1377
6. Sinderby C, Beck J, Weinberg J, Spahija J, Grassino A (1998) Voluntary activation of the human diaphragm in health and disease. J Appl Physiol 85:2146–2158
7. Beck J, Gottfried SB, Navalesi P, et al (2001) Electrical activity of the diaphragm during pressure support ventilation in acute respiratory failure. Am J Respir Care Med 164:419–424
8. Sassoon CSH, Gruer SE (1995) Characteristics of the ventilator pressure- and flow-trigger variables. Intensive Care Med 21:159-168
9. Sassoon CSH, Foster GT (2001) Patient-ventilator asynchrony. Curr Opin Crit Care 7:28–33
10. Yamada Y, Du HL (1998) Effects of different pressure support termination on patient-ventilator synchrony. Respir Care 43:1048–1057

11. Jubran A, Van de Graaff WB, Tobin MJ (1995) Variability of patient-ventilator interaction with pressure support ventilation in patients with chronic obstructive pulmonary disease. Am J Respir Crit Care Med 152:129–136
12. MacIntyre NR (1988) Weaning from mechanical ventilator support: volume assisting intermittent breaths versus pressure assiting every breath. Respir Care 33:121-125
13. Brochard L (1994) Pressure Support Ventilation. In: Tobin MJ (ed) Principles and Practice of Mechanical Ventilation. 1st edition. McGraw Hill, New York, pp 239–257
14. Rossi A, Ranieri MV (1994) Positive end-expiratory pressure. In: Tobin MJ (ed) Principles and Practice of Mechanical Ventilation. 1st edition. McGraw Hill, New York, pp 259–303
15. Sinderby C, Navalesi P, Beck J, et al (1999) Neural control of mechanical ventilation. Nature Med 5:1433–1436
16. Leung P, Jubran A, Tobin MJ (1997) Comparison of assisted ventilator modes on triggering, patient effort, and dyspnea. Am J Respir Crit Care Med 155:1940–148
17. Hill L (2001) Flow triggering, pressure triggering, and autotriggering during mechanical ventilation. Crit Care Med 28:579–581
18. Bernstein G, Knodel E, Heldt GP (1995) Airway leak size in neonates and autocycling of three flow-triggered ventilators. Crit Care Med 23:1739–1744
19. Mehta S, McCool FD, Hill NS (2001) Leak compensation in positive pressure ventilators: a lung model study. Eur Respir J 17:259–267
20. Younes M (1993) Patient-ventilator interaction with pressure-assisted modalities of ventilatory support. Sem Resp Med 14:299–322
21. Yamada Y, Du HL (2000) Analysis of the mechanisms of expiratory asynchrony in pressure support ventilation: a mathematical approach. J Appl Physiol 88:2143–2150
22. Calderini E, Confalonieri M, Puccio PG, Francavilla N, Stella L, Gregoretti C (1999) Patient-ventilator asynchrony during noninvasive ventilation: the role of expiratory trigger. Intensive Care Med 25:662–667
23. Van de Graaff WB, Gordey K, Dornseif SE, et al (1991) Pressure support: changes in ventilatory pattern and components of the work of breathing. Chest 100:1082–1089
24. Parthasarathy S, Jubran A, Tobin MJ (1998) Cycling of inspiratory and expiratory muscle groups with the ventilator in airflow limitation. Am J Respir Crit Care Med 158:1471–1478
25. Slutsky AS (1999) Lung injury caused by mechanical ventilation. Chest 116:9S–15S
26. Henry GW, Stevens CS, Schreiner RL, Grosfeld JL, Ballantine TVN (1979) Respiratory paralysis to improve oxygenation and mortality in large newborn infants with respiratory distress. J Pediatr Surg 14:761–766
27. Stark AR, Bascom R, Frantz ID (1978) Muscle relaxation in mechanically ventilated infants. J Pediatr 94:439–434
28. Greenough A, Wood S, Morley CJ, Davis JA (1984) Pancuronium prevents pneumothoraces in ventilated premature babies who actively expire against positive pressure ventilation. Lancet 1:1–13
29. Greenough A, Morley CJ, Davis JA (1983) Interaction of spontaneous breathing with artificial ventilation in pre-term babies. J Pediatr 103:769–773
30. Lipscomb AP, Reynolds EOR, Blackwell RJ, et al (1981) Pneumothorax and cerebral haemorrhage in preterm infants. Lancet 414–416
31. Guttman J, Haberthur, Mols G (2001) Automatic tube compensation. Respir Care Clin N Am 7:503–517
32. Younes M (1992) Proportional assist ventilation, a new approach to ventilatory support. Theory. Am Rev Respir Dis 145:114–120
33. Beck J, Sinderby C, Lindström L, Grassino A (1998) Crural diaphragm activation during dynamic contractions at various inspiratory flow rates. J Appl Physiol 85:451–458
34. Grasso S, Puntillo F, Mascia L, et al (2000) Compensation for increase in respiratory workload during mechanical ventilation: Pressure support (PSV) vs. proportional assist ventilation. Am J Respir Crit Care Med 161:819–826
35. Brunner JX (2001) Principles and history of closed-loop controlled ventilation. Respir Care Clin N Am 7:341–362
36. Ranieri VM (1997) Optimization of patient-ventilator interactions: closed-loop technology to turn the century. Intensive Care Med 23:936–939

37. Grasso S, Ranieri VM, Brochard L, et al (2001) Closed loop proportional assist ventilation (PAV): results of a phase II multicenter trial. Am J Respir Crit Care Med 163:A303 (Abst)
38. Iotti GA, Braschi A (2001) Closed-loop support of ventilatory workload: The pO-1 controller. Respir Care Clin N Am 7:441–464
39. Iotti GA, Brunner JX, Braschi A, et al (1996) Closed-loop control of airway occlusion pressure at 0.1 second (P0.1) applied to pressure-support ventilation: Algorithm and application in intubated patients. Crit Care Med 24:771–779
40. Whitelaw WA, Derenne JP, Milic Emili J (1975) Occlusion pressure as a measure of respiratory center output in conscious man. Respir Physiol 23:181–199
41. Spahija J, Beck J, Gottfried S, Comtois N, Comtois A, Sinderby C (2001) Target drive ventilation (TDV): Automatic regulation of ventilatory assist using diaphragm electrical activity. Am J Respir Crit Care Med 163:A303 (Abst)

Assisting Ventilation by Pressure Support: More than a Weaning Tool

N. Patroniti, G. Foti, and A. Pesenti

▌ Introduction

Since its introduction [1, 2], pressure support ventilation (PSV) has become one of the most frequently used partial ventilatory support techniques [3]. Despite its popularity, PSV in intubated patients is commonly seen as a weaning mode; therefore it comes as no surprise that information on the use of PSV in patients with acute lung injury (ALI) and acute respiratory distress syndrome (ARDS) is rather limited. It is our contention that in patients with ALI/ARDS, PSV could be applied not only safely, but also more broadly than commonly thought. The purpose of this brief chapter is to discuss some of the recent evidence on the use of PSV in patients with ALI/ARDS, which could justify and extend its application in the intensive care unit (ICU).

▌ Selected Technical Aspects of PSV

PSV is classified as a patient triggered, pressure limited, flow cycled mode of ventilation [4]. The patient's own inspiratory effort triggers the ventilator to provide a fixed preset airway pressure level, which normally results in a decelerating gas flow. Depending on the type of ventilator, cycling from the inspiratory to the expiratory phase is determined by the inspiratory flow reaching a low threshold value. Paralleling the fading off of the inspiratory muscle activity, flow decreases from an early inspiratory peak to a low end expiratory value indicating the patient's desire to expire.

During PSV therefore, the respiratory pattern is mainly regulated by the patient, who determines not only the start but also the end of each assisted inspiration. Two of the essential aspects of PSV are indeed the inspiratory and the expiratory trigger functions.

Recognition of Inspiration or Trigger Phase

A major goal in the technology of PSV is to decrease the time lag between the activation of inspiratory muscles by the patient and the beginning of pressurization by the ventilator. A short trigger time lag improves the patient-ventilator synchrony, and minimizes the inspiratory trigger effort, which is an additional load for the patient [5]. Most modern ventilators are fitted with pressure or flow trigger systems [6]. Beyond the possibility offered by the setting of the trigger sensitivity knob, the effort required by the patient is greatly affected by the ventilator's performance and technology [6, 7].

Recognition of the End of Inspiration

The low flow threshold criterion is the primary method to terminate inspiration and flow delivery on most ventilators [4]. A high pressure back up criterion is often present. Trigger sensitivity and pressurization time are the main ventilator settings affecting work of breathing and patient-ventilator synchrony [7, 8]; in selected patients, particularly in those with a long time constant, the inspiration-expiration cycling criterion also may be important to improve patient-ventilator interaction and synchrony [9, 10]. For this reason some of the modern ventilators offer the opportunity of selecting appropriate criteria to start expiration.

▌ Respiratory Function Monitoring During PSV

Respiratory Drive

Since during PSV the patient is in charge of the control of respiratory rate, integrity of the patient control of breathing function, and preservation of spontaneous neural activity are essential. The level of pressure support and the patient-ventilator synchrony may greatly affect the patient's respiratory drive [11]. Conversely, monitoring the respiratory drive may be very useful in setting PSV.

The pressure developed 100 ms after the onset of an expiratory occlusion pressure ($P_{0.1}$) has been widely used as a clinical index of respiratory drive [11, 12], and many authors have used it to investigate the effect of PSV on respiratory drive. It is important to remember that the neural drive and $P_{0.1}$ are affected also by other factors such as drugs, gas exchange, respiratory muscles function [13], and lung volume [14]. Formal measurements of $P_{0.1}$ have been limited by the need of dedicated equipment; however simplified techniques have been proposed [15] and some modern ventilators provide an automatic measurement [16]. A normal $P_{0.1}$ value is suggested as a useful target in setting the level of pressure support [11, 17].

Simple determinants of respiratory pattern, such as tidal volume (VT), respiratory rate (f) and mean respiratory flow, may be a valuable index of the patient respiratory drive and control of breathing. The ratio of breathing frequency to tidal volume (f/VT, shallow breathing index) has been shown to be an accurate predictor of weaning outcome [18]. The product $P_{0.1} \times f/VT$ has shown a sensitivity comparable to $P_{0.1}$ and f/VT in predicting weaning success, but a better specificity [19].

Muscle Function

By varying the level of pressure support, it is possible to change the relative contribution of patient and machine to the total work of breathing (WOB) [20]. The patient potential to contribute to WOB is strictly dependent on the muscle function. The maximal absolute pressure that can be generated against an occluded airway (maximal inspiratory pressure, MIP) [21] is routinely used as an index of global respiratory muscle strength.

Though MIP *per se* is not a sensitive predictive index of successful weaning, integration of $P_{0.1}$ with MIP has been suggested as a more reliable index than $P_{0.1}$

alone, to detect the need for ventilatory support, mainly in patients with low respiratory drive determined by ineffective respiratory muscle function [13].

Respiratory Mechanics

Measurement of respiratory mechanics during partial ventilatory support (assisted breathing) has been limited by the fact that a complete relaxation of respiratory muscle is not always achievable in spontaneously breathing patients. However, the compliance (Crs) and resistance (Rrs) of the respiratory system are the major determinants of respiratory muscle mechanical load, and their measurements are possibly more important during assisted, than during controlled, breathing.

Moreover, in ALI/ARDS patients, Crs may be very valuable in monitoring clinical evolution. While the measurement of Rrs during PSV requires a complex approach and dedicated instrumentation [22, 23], the measurement of Crs could be easily obtained applying to PSV the classical occlusion technique commonly used during controlled mechanical ventilation [24]. Most modern ventilators provide end-inspiratory and end-expiratory maneuvers during partial ventilatory support modes.

The end-expiratory occlusion provides the measurements of $P_{0.1}$, MIP, and intrinsic auto positive end-expiratory pressure (PEEPi), both during continuous positive airway pressure (CPAP) and during PSV [25, 26]. Moreover, we have shown that during PSV the plateau pressure following an inspiratory occlusion is a good estimate of the relaxed elastic recoil pressure of the respiratory system (Pel,rsi) [24].

Therefore, Crs can be computed according to the following equation:

$$\text{Crs} = \text{VT}/(\text{Pel, rsi} - (\text{PEEP} + \text{PEEPi})) \qquad \text{(Eqn 1)}$$

Assessment of the occlusion method in ALI patients who were being weaned from continuous positive pressure ventilation (CPPV) by PSV, showed that Crs measured during PSV was highly correlated with Crs measured during CPPV ($\text{Crs}_{\text{PSV}} = 1.4 + 0.98 \times \text{Cpl}_{\text{CPPV}}$, ml/cm H_2O, n = 31, r = 0.945, p < 0.001) (Fig. 1) [27].

It is, however, important to underline that patients with high respiratory drive may not allow enough time to achieve muscle relaxation, and the occlusion method in these patients should not be held as reliable. In our clinical practise, when the inspection of the occluded airway pressure indicates that muscle relaxation cannot

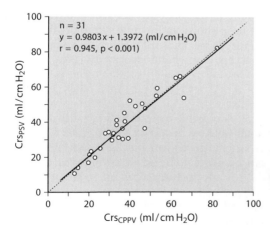

Fig. 1. Correlation between respiratory system compliance (Crs) measurements obtained during pressure support ventilation (Crs$_{PSV}$) and during controlled mechanical ventilation (Crs$_{CPPV}$). Regression line (*solid line*) and identity line (*dotted line*) are represented

be achieved, we usually increase the pressure support level to reduce the respiratory drive, and to obtain a long enough plateau time to provide a reliable elastic recoil pressure measurement.

An alternative approach based on a least square fitting technique, which does not require any airway occlusion, has been proposed by Iotti et al. [23]. This elegant technique provides the simultaneous measurement of Rrs, Crs, and total PEEP.

Respiratory Effort and Work of Breathing

The assessment of respiratory muscle activity during PSV is commonly performed by computing the WOB [28] or the pressure time product [29], both of which require the measurement of esophageal pressure.

Although extensively used in clinical and physiological research, the measurement of esophageal pressure is not yet common in the clinical setting. Once again, $P_{0.1}$ proves a very useful measurement, having shown a very good correlation with WOB during PSV [30].

We have described an index of muscular activity (PMI: P_{musc}), developed specifically to monitor end-inspiratory muscle activity in ALI/ARDS patients undergoing PSV. The measurement is obtained directly from the airway pressure tracing or display by an end-inspiratory occlusion [24]. PMI is computed as the difference between the end-inspiratory occlusion plateau pressure and the airway pressure before the occlusion (PMI = Pel,rsi−[PEEP + PS]); it represents an index of the pressure applied to the respiratory system by the inspiratory muscles at end-inspiration (the estimate contains an intrinsic approximation due to the resistive pressure drop at end-inspiration, which is not taken into account).

When we compared the pressure generated by the inspiratory muscles (directly measured by the use of an esophageal balloon) with PMI obtained by a simple end inspiratory occlusion, we found a very good correlation. Moreover, PMI was correlated to the pressure time product ($p < 0.01$).

In spite of the many assumptions and limitations required, PMI appears to be a sensitive estimation of respiratory effort and could be a useful parameter in setting the level of pressure support, at least in non-obstructive patients.

▮ Common Application of PSV

The most common application of PSV in intubated patients has been in the weaning phase. The main features of PSV, which may explain its popularity as a weaning technique, are the important effects of varying the pressure support level on the respiratory pattern and WOB. In most patients, increased levels of pressure support effect a decrease in respiratory rate and an increase in tidal volume [2, 31]. These changes are commonly associated with decrease of respiratory neural drive and $P_{0.1}$ [11, 30]. At the same time as the pressure support level is increased, the inspiratory muscles are unloaded and the patient inspiratory WOB and pressure time product decrease [20, 30, 31]. This means that by observing the changes in the respiratory pattern and/or in respiratory effort, the amount of assistance can be modulated by simply regulating the level of pressure support.

Another important claimed feature of PSV is better patient-ventilator synchrony and patient comfort, particularly when compared to other popular weaning modes, such as synchronized intermittent mandatory ventilation (SIMV) [2, 32]. Despite these advantages, PSV has not been shown to be more effective than other weaning strategies [33, 34].

The coming of age of new ventilatory modes, which could improve patient-ventilator matching [35] and comfort [36, 37], has partially overshadowed some of the features that made PSV so popular. A recent survey on ventilator use in ICUs from North America, South America, Portugal and Spain, shows however that PSV alone (36% of patients) or in combination with SIMV (28% of patients) is still the most used ventilator mode for weaning [3].

Another frequent application of PSV is in non-invasive ventilation [38, 39]. PSV has been successfully used by face [38, 39] or nasal mask, in acute respiratory failure with [39] or without chronic obstructive pulmonary disease (COPD) [38].

▌ PSV in ALI/ARDS

In the last 10 years, an increasing number of studies have investigated the beneficial effects of maintaining spontaneous breathing activity during mechanical ventilation. Maintenance of spontaneous breathing preserves diaphragmatic activity [40], prevents muscle atrophy, decreases the need for sedative drugs [41], and obviously avoids the use of muscle relaxants [42].

During partial ventilatory support, spontaneous inspiration decreases the intrathoracic pressure, increasing venous return, stroke volume, and cardiac output [43–45]. Both in animals [43] and in ARDS patients [44], Putensen et al. showed a better V_A/Q distribution during spontaneous breathing superimposed to airway pressure release ventilation (APRV) compared to APRV without spontaneous breathing. These findings are justified, at least in part, by the reported [46] better ventilation of non-dependent lung regions obtained during spontaneous inspiration by diaphragmatic contraction. In ALI/ARDS patients these regions are perfused but poorly ventilated, and particularly so during controlled mechanical ventilation when the diaphragm is passive. Finally, in patients with multiple trauma at risk for ALI/ARDS, maintaining spontaneous breathing during APRV resulted in better cardiopulmonary function, shorter duration of ventilatory support and shorter ICU stay [47].

Though the reported beneficial effects of promoting spontaneous breathing should apply also to PSV, there have been very few studies investigating PSV during ALI/ARDS [44, 48, 49]. Surprisingly, Putensen et al. [44] reported no significant improvements in cardiovascular function and ventilation-perfusion distribution in ARDS patients during PSV compared to APRV without spontaneous breathing, at variance with the advantages of adding spontaneous breathing to APRV. The study comprised two groups: one group received PSV and APRV at equal pressure limits, the other at equal minute ventilation (V_E). The authors concluded that the spontaneous activity associated to PSV was not sufficient to reverse the V_A/Q maldistribution caused by the alveolar collapse in ARDS patients. However the way the pressure support level was set raises the possibility that, during PSV patients were somehow overassisted, thus limiting the potential effectiveness of PSV. Unfortunately, though the authors measured Pes, no information about patient effort was reported. In a study in ALI patients with COPD by Viale et al. [50] where PSV and APRV were applied at equal pressure limits, institution of APRV did not result in a decrease in patient WOB or in diaphragm electromyographic activity, while PSV caused a stable reduction in the patient effort. These results suggest that interfacing of spontaneous breathing during PSV and APRV is somehow different and not of simple interpretation.

We have recently explored how PSV can be safely used in ALI patients [49]. In 48 ALI patients receiving CPPV for 24 hours, PSV was started after muscle relaxants were withdrawn and sedative drugs were reduced. The initial pressure support level was chosen to totally unload the patient respiratory muscle. The level of pressure support was then adjusted to maintain respiratory rate and $PaCO_2$ within preset limits. The change to PSV was characterized by a decrease in $PaCO_2$ with a corresponding increase in pH, with no substantial changes in PaO_2/FiO_2 despite a significantly lower mean airway pressure (Table 1). As judged by predetermined criteria, PSV failed in 10 patients (21%), and CPPV was reinstituted. The decision to return to CPPV was based on one or more of the following conditions: high respiratory rate in seven patients, increased $PaCO_2$ in three, decreased PaO_2 in one, and hemodynamic instability in three. Patients who failed PSV showed lower Crs, higher V_E, and longer time of intubation during CPPV (Fig. 2). Though PSV seems more likely to fail in sicker patients, most ALI patients could be successfully managed by PSV (79%), even if the average CPPV PaO_2/FiO_2 ratio was barely higher than 200 mmHg. In this study, as in that by Putensen et al. [44], PSV may not have been exploited to full advantage, since the pressure support level was not targeted to enhance the patient respiratory activity, but rather to maintain predefined $PaCO_2$ and respiratory rate levels. Moreover, since the prolonged use of CPPV might cause respiratory muscle atrophy [40], some degree of muscular dysfunction could have contributed to PSV failure, particularly in patients who had been ventilated longer.

Extended and early use of PSV results in rather high ventilatory rates (> 30 bpm) and low VT. In fact, while the use of ventilation at low VT is now a consolidated part of the ARDS ventilatory strategy [51], during PSV such an approach might lead to an unacceptable increase in the patient cost of breathing. At the same time, the alveolar collapse that may result from low VT ventilation, can further impair gas exchange and respiratory mechanics [52, 53].

Table 1. Effects of transition from continuous positive pressure ventilation (CPPV) to pressure support ventilation (PSV) on gas exchange and ventilatory variables in the general population (mean ± SD). (Modified from [49] with permission)

	CPPV	PSV
PaO_2/FiO_2 (mmHg)	210.3 ± 69.6	219.3 ± 74.2
FiO_2	0.59 ± 0.14	0.55 ± 0.13 [a]
$PaCO_2$ (mmHg)	49.2 ± 10.9	44.4 ± 7.2 [a]
pH	7.405 ± 0.054	7.435 ± 0.064 [a]
V_E (l/min)	9.0 ± 2.3	12.0 ± 4.0 [a]
f (bpm)	16.3 ± 4.1	24.5 ± 9.7 [a]
VT (l)	0.562 ± 0.095	0.492 ± 0.104 [a]
PEEP (cm H_2O)	9.3 ± 3.0	9.2 ± 3.0
MAP (cm H_2O)	15.3 ± 3.9	13.4 ± 3.6 [a]

VE: minute volume; f: respiratory frequency; bpm: breaths per minute; VT: tidal volume; PEEP: positive end-expiratory pressure; MAP: mean airway pressure.
[a] $p < 0.05$ PSV vs. CPPV

PSV may however be combined with other ventilatory modes such as SIMV [54] or biphasic positive airway pressure (BiPAP). It is surprising that despite the relatively limited evidence on the topic [54], the combination PSV + SIMV is one of the most commonly used ventilatory strategies in ICU [4].

We recently studied a ventilatory strategy consisting of the combination of PSV with BiPAP [55]. In order to improve the efficacy of PSV and counteract the derecruitment effect of low VT and low PEEP we added periodical recruitment maneu-

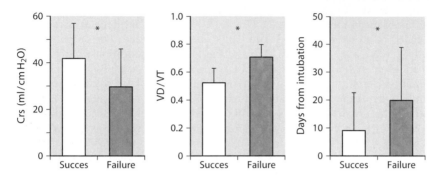

Fig. 2. Compliance of the respiratory system (Crs), physiologic dead space volume to tidal volume ratio (VD/VT), and days from intubation, of patients who were successfully weaned from CPPV to PSV (*white bars*) and of those in whom the trial failed (*gray bars*). Values are expressed as mean ± SD. * Failure vs. success p < 0.05

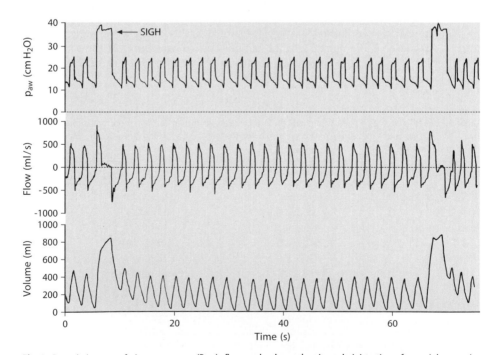

Fig. 3. Recorded traces of airway pressure (Paw), flow, and volume showing administration of one sigh per minute (*arrow*) during PSV

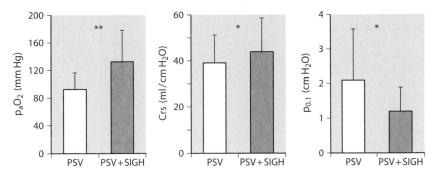

Fig. 4. Oxygen arterial tension (PaO_2), compliance of the respiratory system (Crs), and occlusion pressure ($P_{0.1}$) during 'genuine' PSV (*white bars*) and during PSV with the addition of one sigh per minute (*gray bars*). Values

vers (Sighs) to PSV. In ARDS patients, sighs have been shown to be effective during CPPV [56, 57] in inducing alveolar recruitment and improving gas exchange. We tested this strategy on gas exchange, respiratory mechanics, and respiratory pattern in 13 ARDS patients. We compared PSV alone, with PSV associated to sighs administered once per minute by adding to baseline PSV a 3–5 s CPAP period, set at a level 20% higher than the peak airway pressure of the PSV breaths or at least 35 cm H_2O (Fig. 3). The adjunct of sigh improved PaO_2 in all patients (Fig. 4). We also observed a significant increase in Crs (Fig. 4) and end-expiratory lung volume [EELV]. Finally, this strategy resulted in a decreased $P_{0.1}$ (Fig. 4), suggesting a normalization of the respiratory drive.

Further investigations are needed to explore the long-term benefit of this strategy.

Conclusion

Several different approaches have been proposed to improve matching between the start of a patient's inspiratory effort and the machine start. Innovative solutions which move the trigger signal from the airway closer to the muscles have been proposed by using the esophageal pressure signal [58], or diaphragm electrical activity [59]. This last approach is particularly interesting because it is not affected by PEEPi. On the other hand, attention is being paid to the start of expiration, and to technological improvements in the inspiration to expiration cycling [9, 10]. Yamada and Du [10] proposed an automatic system of expiratory trigger sensitivity regulation, which is based on a mathematical model description of the PSV inspiratory flow profile. It is worth noting that most of these innovations could improve and extend the application of PSV as a weaning mode, particularly in COPD patients.

Last, closed loop automated systems are being developed to control PSV. Iotti et al. [17] proposed a close-loop control which automatically adjusts PSV to control $P_{0.1}$, thus targeting ventilation on patient inspiratory activity and comfort. Dojat et al. [60] have designed a closed-loop control of pressure support level based on f, VT, and end-tidal CO_2 pressure. A fascinating recent approach has been applied by Nemoto et al. [61] using fuzzy logic to automatically control pressure support ventilation on physiologic parameters of the patient. The main application field of these methods is again weaning from the ventilator and faster adaptability of the pressure support level to patient comfort.

New promising possibilities could come from the use of ventilatory strategies, which combine different modes and may integrate the different advantages and benefits within a single approach [55, 62].

References

1. Fahey PJ, Vanderwarf C, David A (1985) Comparison of oxygen costs of breathing during weaning with continuous positive airway pressure versus pressure support ventilation. Am Rev Respir Dis 131 (suppl):A130 (Abst)
2. MacIntyre NR (1986) Respiratory function during pressure support ventilation. Chest 89:677–683
3. Esteban A, Anzueto A, Alia I, et al (2000) How is mechanical ventilation employed in the intensive care unit? Am J Respir Crit Care Med 161:1450–1458
4. Brochard L (1994) Pressure support ventilation. In: Tobin MJ (ed) Principles and Practice of Mechanical Ventilation, 1st edn. McGraw-Hill, New York, pp 239–257
5. Nava S, Bruschi C, Fracchia C, Braschi A, Rubini F (1997) Patient-ventilator interaction and inspiratory effort during pressure support ventilation in patients with different pathologies. Eur Respir J 10:177–183
6. Holbrook PJ, Guiles SP (1997) Response time of four support ventilators: effect of triggering method and bias flow. Respir Care 42:952–959
7. Chatmongkolchart S, Williams P, Hess DR, Kacmarek RM (2001) Evaluation of inspiratory rise time and inspiration termination criteria in new-generation mechanical ventilators: a lung model study. Respir Care 46:666–677
8. MacIntyre NR, Ho L (1991) Effects of initial flow rate and breath termination criteria on pressure support ventilation. Chest 99:134–138
9. Yamada Y, Du H (1998) Effects of different pressure support termination on patient-ventilator synchrony. Respir Care 43:1048–1057
10. Yamada Y, Du H (2000) Analysis of the mechanisms of expiratory asynchrony in pressure support ventilation: a mathematical approach. J Appl Physiol 88:2143–2150
11. Alberti A, Gallo F, Fongaro A, Valenti S, Rossi A (1995) P0.1 is a useful parameter in setting the level of pressure support ventilation. Intensive Care Med 21:547–553
12. Whitelaw WA, Derenne JP, Milic-Emili J (1975) Occlusion pressure as a measure of respiratory centers output in conscious man. Respir Physiol 23:181–199
13. Fernandez R, Cabrera J, Calaf N, Benito S (1990) P0.1/PIMax an index for assessing respiratory capacity in acute respiratory failure. Intensive Care Med 16:175–179
14. Marshall R (1962) Relationship between stimulus and work of breathing at different lung volumes. J Appl Physiol 17:917–919
15. Conti G, Cinnella G, Barboni E, Lemaire F, Harf A, Brochard L (1996) Estimation of occlusion pressure during assisted ventilation in patients with intrinsic PEEP. Am J Respir Crit Care Med 154:907–912
16. Kuhlen R, Hausmann S, Pappert D, Slama K, Roissant R, Falke K (1995) A new method for P0.1 measurement using standard respiratory equipment. Intensive Care Med 21:554–560
17. Iotti GA, Brunner JX, Braschi A, et al (1996) Closed-loop control of airway pressure at 0.1 second (P0.1) applied to pressure support ventilation: Algorithm and application in intubated patients. Crit Care Med 24:771–779
18. Yang KL, Tobin MJ (1991) A prospective study of indexes predicting the outcome of trials of weaning from mechanical ventilation. N Engl J Med 324:1445–1450
19. Sassoon CSH, Mahutte CK (1993) Airway occlusion pressure and breathing pattern as predictors of weaning outcome. Am Rev Respir Dis 148:860–866
20. Brochard L, Harf A, Lorino H, Lemaire F (1989) Inspiratory pressure support prevents diaphragmatic fatigue during weaning from mechanical ventilation. Am Rev Respir Dis 139:513–521
21. Marini JJ, Smith TC, Lamb V (1986) Estimation of inspiratory muscle strength in mechanically ventilated patients: the measurement of maximal inspiratory pressure. J Crit Care 1:32–38

22. Pesenti A, Pelosi P, Foti G, D'Andrea L, Rossi N (1992) An interrupter technique for measuring respiratory mechanics and the pressure generated by respiratory muscles during partial ventilatory support. Chest 102:918–923

23. Iotti GA, Braschi A, Brunner JX, et al (1995) Respiratory mechanics by least squares fitting in mechanically ventilated patients: applications during paralysis and during pressure support ventilation. Intensive Care Med 21:406–413

24. Foti G, Cereda M, Banfi G, Pelosi P, Fumagalli R, Pesenti A (1997) End-inspiratory airway occlusion: a method to assess the pressure developed by inspiratory muscles in patients with acute lung injury undergoing pressure support. Am J Respir Crit Care Med 156:1210–1216

25. Smith TC, Marini JJ (1988) Impact of PEEP on lung mechanics and work of beathing in severe airflow obstruction. J Appl Physiol 65:1488–1499

26. Petrof BJ, Legare M, Goldberg P, Milic-Emili J, Gottfried SB (1990) Continuous positive airway pressure reduces work of breathing and dyspnea during weaning from mechanical ventilation in severe chronic obstructive pulmonary disease. Am Rev Respir Dis 141:281–289

27. Foti G, Patroniti N, Cereda M, Sparacino ME, Giacomini M, Pesenti A (1995) Assessment of the airway occlusion method to estimate respiratory system compliance (Cpl,rs) during pressure support ventilation. Intensive Care Med 21 (suppl 1):S133 (Abst)

28. Kacmarek RM (1988) The role of pressure support ventilation in reducing work of breathing. Respir Care 33:99–120

29. Sassoon CSH, Light RW, Lodia R, Sieck GC, Mahutte K (1991) Pressure-time product during continuous positive airway pressure, pressure support ventilation, and T-Piece during weaning from mechanical ventilation. Am Rev Respir Dis 143:469–475

30. Berger KI, Sorkin B, Norman RG (1996) Mechanism of relief of tachypnea during pressure support ventilation. Chest 109:1320–1327

31. Van de Graaff WB, Gordey K, Dornseif SE, et al (1991) Pressure support : changes in ventilatory pattern and components of the work of breathing. Chest 100:1082–1089

32. Fleury B, Murciano D, Talamo C, Aubier M, Pariente R, Milic-Emily J (1985) Work of breathing in patients with chronic obstructive pulmonary disease in acute respiratory failure. Am Rev Respir Dis 131:822–827

33. Brochard L, Rauss A, Benito S, et al (1994) Comparison of three methods of gradual withdrawal from ventilatory support during weaning from mechanical ventilation. Am J Respir Crit Care Med 150:896–903

34. Esteban A, Frutos F, Tobin MJ, et al (1995) A comparison of four methods of weaning patients from mechanical ventilation. N Engl J Med 332:345–350

35. Younes M, Puddy A, Roberts D, et al (1992) Proportional assist ventilation: results of an initial critical trial. Am Rev Respir Dis 145:121–129

36. Mols G, von Ungern-Stenberg B, Rohr E, Haberthur C, Geiger K, Guttmann J (2000) Respiratory comfort and breathing pattern during volume proportional assist ventilation and pressure support ventilation: A study on volunteers with artificially reduced compliance. Crit Care Med 28:1940–1946

37. Mols G, Rohr E, Benzing A, Haberthur C, Geiger K, Guttmann J (2000) Breathing pattern associated with respiratory comfort during automatic tube compensation and pressure support ventilation in normal subjects. Acta Anaesthesiol Scand 44:223–230

38. Kramer N, Meyer TJ, Meharg J, et al (1995) Randomized prospective trial of non-invasive positive pressure ventilation in acute respiratory failure. Am J Respir Crit Care Med 151:1799–1806

39. Brochard L, Mancebo J, Wysocki M, et al (1995) Noninvasive ventilation for acute exacerbations of chronic obstructive pulmonary disease. N Engl J Med 333:817–822

40. Le Bourdelles G, Viires N, Boczkowski J, Seta N, Pavlovic D, Aubier M (1994) Effects of mechanical ventilation on diaphragmatic contractile properties in rats. Am J Respir Crit Care Med 149:1539–1544

41. Stewart KG (1989) Clinical evaluation of pressure support ventilation. Br J Anaesth 63:362–364

42. Rossiter A, Souney PF, McGowan S (1991) Pancuronium induced prolonged neuromuscular blockade. Crit Care Med 19:1583–1587

43. Putensen C, Räsänen J, Lopez FA (1994) Ventilation-perfusion distributions during mechanically ventilation with superimposed spontaneous breathing in canine lung injury. Am J Respir Crit Care Med 150:101–108

44. Putensen C, Mutz N, PutensenHimmer G, Zinserling J (1999) Spontaneous breathing during ventilatory support improves ventilation-perfusion distributions in patients with acute respiratory distress syndrome. Am J Respir Crit Care Med 159:1241–1248.

45. Downs JB, Douglas ME, Sanfelippo PM, et al (1977) Ventilatory pattern, intrapleural pressure, and cardiac output. Anesth Analg 56:88–96

46. Froese AB, Bryan AC (1974) Effects of anesthesia and paralysis on diaphragmatic mechanics in man. Anesthesiology 38:242–255

47. Putensen C, Zech S, Wrigge H, et al (2001) Long-term effects of spontaneous breathing during ventilatory support in patients with acute lung injury. Am J Respir Crit Care Med 164:43–49

48. Tejeda M, Boix JH, Alvarez F, Balanza R, Morales M (1997) Comparison of pressure support ventilation and assist-control ventilation in the treatment of respiratory failure. Chest 111:1322–1325

49. Cereda M, Foti G, Marcora B, et al (2000) Pressure support ventilation in patients with acute lung injury. Crit Care Med 28:1269–1275

50. Viale JP, Duperret S, Mahul P, et al (1998) Time course evolution of ventilatory responses to inspiratory unloading in patients. Am J Respir Crit Care Med 157:428–434

51. The acute respiratory distress syndrome network (2000) Ventilation with lower tidal volumes as compared with traditional tidal volumes for acute lung injury and the acute respiratory distress syndrome. N Engl J Med 342:1301–1308

52. Pesenti A, Rossi N, Calori A, Foti G, Rossi GP (1993) Effects of short oxygenation on acute lung injury patients undergoing pressure support ventilation. Chest 103:1185–1189

53. Cereda M, Foti G, Mush G, Sparacino ME, Pesenti A (1996) Positive end-expiratory pressure prevents the loss of respiratory compliance during low tidal volume ventilation in acute lung injury patients. Chest 109:480–485

54. Leung P, Jubran A, Tobin MJ (1997) Comparison of assisted ventilator modes on triggering, patient effort, and dyspnea. Am J Respir Crit Care Med 155:1940–1948

55. Patroniti N, Foti G, Cortinovis B, et al (2002) Sigh improves gas exchange and lung volume in ARDS patients undergoing pressure support ventilation. Anesthesiology (in press)

56. Pelosi P, Cadringher P, Bottino N, et al (1999) Sigh in acute respiratory distress syndrome. Am J Respir Crit Care Med 159:872–880

57. Foti G, Cereda M, Sparacino ME, De Marchi L, Villa F, Pesenti A (2000) Effects of periodic lung recruitment maneuvers on gas exchange and respiratory mechanics in mechanically ventilated acute respiratory distress syndrome patients. Intensive Care Med 26:501–507

58. Barnard M, Shukla A, Lowell T, Goldstone J (1999) Esophageal-directed pressure support ventilation in normal volunteers. Chest 115:482–489

59. Sinderby C, Navalesi P, Skrobik Y, et al (1999) Neural control of mechanical ventilation. Nat Med 5:1433–1436

60. Dojat M, Harf A, Touchard D, Lemaire F, Brochard L (2000) Clinical evaluation of a computer-controlled pressure support mode. Am J Respir Crit Care Med 161:1161–1166

61. Nemoto T, Hatzakis GE, Thorpe CW, Olivenstein R, Dial S, Bates JHT (1999) Automatic control of pressure support mechanical ventilation using fuzzy logic. Am J Respir Crit Care Med 160:550–556

62. Takeda S, Nakanishi K, Takano T, et al (1997) The combination of external high-frequency oscillation and pressure support ventilation in acute respiratory failure. Acta Anesthesiol Scand 41:670–674

Conditioning of Inspired Gases
in Mechanically Ventilated Patients

D. Chiumello, P. Pelosi, and L. Gattinoni

▮ Introduction

When the nose and the upper airways are bypassed due to a tracheostomy or endo-tracheal tube, their normal function of heating and humidifying the inspired gases is altered. Therefore, in these situations artificial heating and humification of in-spired gases is mandatory. The goal of any heating and humidification system is to provide inspired gases with a water content similar to that usually provided by the nose or the upper airways. In this chapter we will discuss:
- The physical and physiological background
- The effects of inadequate and excessive conditioning
- The optimal conditioning
- The humidifier equipment
- New devices for conditioning the inspired gases.

▮ Physical Background

The water present as vapor in a gas mixture is defined as the humidity. The maxi-mal amount of water vapor that can be present in a gas mixture depends directly on the temperature of the gas. When a gas mixture holds all the water vapor that it is capable of holding, the term 'saturated' is employed. The amount of water vapor contained in a gas mixture can be estimated as the absolute humidity (absolute hu-midity) or relative humidity (relative humidity) related to that temperature [1].

Absolute humidity (mg/l or g/m^3) is the mass of water vapor held in a given vol-ume of gas at a particular temperature (e.g., at 100% of relative humidity for 32 °C the absolute humidity is 36 mg/l, while for 37 °C the absolute humidity is 44 mg/l).

The relative humidity is the ratio between the actual amount of water vapor and the maximal capacity of water vapor for the same temperature (i.e., at 32 °C with 50% of relative humidity, the absolute humidity is 18 mg/l).

▮ Physiological Background

Non-intubated Patients Breathing Ambient Air

Standard ambient air presents a temperature of 22 °C, with a relative humidity of 50% and an absolute humidity of 10 mg/l, while the alveolar air usually presents a temperature of 37 °C, with a relative humidity of 100% and an absolute humidity of

Table 1. Values of temperature, relative humidity and absolute humidity of the inspired (I) and expired gases (E) at different anatomic points in non-intubated patients breathing ambient air

Site	Temperature °C		Relative humidity (%)		Absolute humidity (mg/l)	
	I	E	I	E	I	E
▌Airway opening	22	33	50	100	10	37
▌Pharynx	30	34	90	100	30	40
▌Upper trachea	33	35	92	100	36	41
▌Lower trachea (carina)	35	37	95	100	37	44
▌Alveoli	37	37	100	100	44	44

44 mg/l. During inspiration the inspired gases are progressively heated and humidified along the nose and the upper airways until they are fully saturated at the body temperature. Table 1 presents the different values of temperature, relative and absolute humidity of inspired and expired gases in non-intubated patients breathing ambient air.

The point in the airways at which the inspired gases reach body temperature (i.e., 37 °C) and 100% relative humidity is called the isothermic saturation boundary (ISB) [1]. Normally the ISB is 5–6 cm below the carina and after this point inspired gases do not change further in temperature or humidity.

Normally the ISB can change in position according to the volume, temperature, and absolute humidity of the inspired gases [2]. The ISB never reaches the bronchioles or alveoli in physiological conditions [3]. However, during severe hyperventilation in extreme cold or dry conditions the ISB can shift towards the alveoli [4].

The difference between the alveolar and ambient air water content is called the humidity deficit [1]. Usually the humidity deficit above the carina (i.e., carina absolute humidity minus airway opening absolute humidity) is around 27 mg/l while the humidity deficit below the carina (i.e., alveolar absolute humidity minus carina absolute humidity) is around 7 mg/l. This suggests that the majority of humidification during inspiration is provided by the upper airways.

During expiration, the gases leaving the alveoli are cooled and lose heat and humidity until they reach a temperature of 33 °C, maintaining 100% relative humidity (i.e., absolute humidity of 37 mg/l). Since the physiological minute ventilation is 7 l/m, in 24 hours there is a net loss of water of around 270 ml through pulmonary ventilation.

Respiratory heat losses are around 5–10 W per day. Since the basal metabolic rate in adult humans is around 100 W per day (1 W = 0.86 Kcal per hour, specific heat for humans = 0.83 Kcal/Kg/°C), the respiratory losses account for only 5–10% of the total balance [5].

Intubated Patients Breathing Medical Gases

Contrary to common knowledge, inspired medical gases are not cold and fully dry. In fact we have evidence that the temperature of the medical gases delivered by mechanical ventilation is normally around 20–25 °C. However, the absolute humidity ranges between 3 and 10 mg/l and is inversely dependent on the inspired oxygen concentration (F_iO_2: i.e., for F_iO_2 of 21%, the absolute humidity is 5.2 ± 1.2 mg/l,

Table 2. Values of temperature, relative humidity and absolute humidity of the inspired (I) and the expired gases (E) at different anatomic points in intubated patients breathing medical gases

Site	Temperature °C		Relative humidity (%)		Absolute humidity (mg/l)	
	I	E	I	E	I	E
Airway opening	22	33	24	100	5	37
End of endotracheal tube	34	36	26	100	9	42
Lower trachea (carina)	35	37	30	100	10	44
Alveoli	37	37	100	100	44	44

for F_iO_2 of 50%, the absolute humidity is 4.1 ± 0.9 mg/l, and for F_iO_2 of 100% the absolute humidity is 3.6 ± 0.6 mg/l). Thus the real problem with medical gases is not the temperature but the inadequate humidification, strongly dependent on the F_iO_2 used [4].

In intubated patients breathing non-conditioned medical gases, similar levels of temperature are present at the carina compared to physiological conditions but with a marked reduction in relative humidity (Table 2). This is due to the fact that the endotracheal tube does not completely avoid heat exchange but is not able to provide more than 3–4 mg/l of the condensed water on the tube surface that occurred in the previous expiratory phase.

In this condition, the ISB is markedly shifted towards the alveoli and can even be absent. In fact, in intubated patients there is a reverse in the humidity deficit compared to non-intubated patients. The upper carina humidity (i.e., endotracheal tube plus lower trachea) deficit is around 5 mg/l, while the lower carina humidity deficit is around 34 mg/l. This suggests that the majority of humidification during inspiration is provided by the lower airways, which are not physiologically adapted to conditioning the gases.

Since the inspired absolute humidity of the ambient air is slightly higher compared to that of medical gases (10 vs 5 mg/l) and the expired gases present the same temperature and absolute humidity as in non-intubated patients, the water losses in a day are only slightly higher compared to non-intubated patients (322 ml vs 270 ml).

A physiological loss of heat and humidity is not a problem unless the body is not able to compensate for this loss, as in conditions when the theromoregulatory response is blunted (i.e., deep sedation or anesthesia) [5]. Thus, the most important problem in intubated patients breathing non-conditioned medical gases is not the heat and water losses, but on the contrary, the shift of ISB towards an anatomical zone not adapted to condition the inspired gases.

Inadequate Conditioning

A typical situation of incorrect conditioning is the administration of cold and dry gases during mechanical ventilation without the use of a humidifier. In this case, the principle negative effects are heat and moisture loss.

Heat loss

The heat loss from the upper airways is due to the increase in temperature and humidity of the inspired gases passing through the airways. The air has a low specific heat (1998 J/Kg) compared to the heat of vaporization for water (2450 J/Kg), so most of the heat lost from the upper airways is used to humidify the inspired gases [6]. This heat loss can cause a decrease in body temperature. Thus, in all situations where there is impaired body thermoregulation, such as prolonged surgery [7, 8], and critically ill patients [9], adequate conditioning is essential to avoid further heat loss.

Moisture loss

Moisture loss, besides causing substantial loss of water from the airways [10], causes dehydration of the nasal and the tracheobronchial mucosa [11]. The tracheobronchial mucosa is more sensitive than the nasal mucosa to dehydration and just 10 minutes of ventilation with dry gases is sufficient to damage the cilia function [10]. The most important damage is the impairment and destruction of mucociliary activity [12], the reduction of mucous production with an increase in viscosity [13] and difficulty in coughing or expectorating [14].

▌ Execessive Conditioning

When the inspired gases are heated and humidified above the body temperature, heat and moisture can be added to the body, causing patient discomfort.

Heat Gain

Besides the heat gain due to the higher inspired gas temperature compared to the body temperature, side effects such as thermal injury [15] or airway burns can develop [16]. It has been shown that thermal injury develops when the tracheal temperature is above 40 °C [17]. It is therefore suggested, to always deliver gases at a temperature less than 40 °C. However, this high temperature is above the standard limit imposed on humidifiers by international committees, so only in cases of malfunction or misuse is it possible to reach this temperature [18].

Moisture Gain

Breathing room air, approximately 6% of the subject's water turnover is given up by the lung during the humidification of the inspired gas. However, breathing over-humidified gases will cause water deposition in the airways, and can induce cellular damage [6]. Furthermore, this water deposition may mechanically obstruct the small airways leading to alveolar collapse [17], and inactivate the pulmonary surfactant [19].

All these side effects can be due to acute or chronic alterations in temperature and moisture delivery. Acute alterations are rare and can be caused by technical problems or by clinical misuse. In our opinion, the most important negative effects are due to minimal changes in temperature and moisture delivery over prolonged periods of time, as occur in mechanically ventilated critically ill patients.

Optimal Conditioning

The heat and humidity of any gas delivered to a patient should have the same inspiratory characteristics occurring at its point of entry into the respiratory system, to correct the humidity deficit and to avoid the risk of inadequate or excessive conditioning [18].

There are different humidification standards both for non-intubated and intubated patients breathing medical gases. In non-intubated patients, a minimum absolute humidity level of 10 mg/l has been suggested [20] while a minimum absolute humidity of 30 [20] to 33 mg/l [21] has been proposed for intubated patients.

In order to choose the adequate conditioning of the inspired gases, we reasoned according to the physiological data of the inspiratory and expiratory phase (Tables 1, 2). As shown above, in intubated patients the absolute humidity delivered by the tube itself is around 3–4 mg/l and the remaining part of the trachea up to the carina can deliver another 1 mg/l. Thus, the absolute humidity delivered by the endotracheal tube and the lower trachea up to carina, is around 5 mg/l. In order to reach the physiological absolute humidity of 37 mg/l at the carina (Table 1), around 32 mg/l of H_2O should be reached at the tip of the tube (27 mg/l directly by water from the humidifier and 5 mg/l by the medical gases). This means that a mixture of gases with a temperature of 31–32 °C with a relative humidity of 100% (i.e., absolute humidity of around 32 mg/l) should be given at the tip of the tube. The amount of water given by the humidifier inversely depends on the absolute humidity of the medical gases (i.e., if the medical gases have an absolute humidity of 3 mg/l the humidifier will provide 29 mg/l while if the medical gases have an absolute humidity of 10 mg/l the humidifier will provide 22 mg/l).

Since the catheter mount causes a drop in gas temperature, between 1–2 °C, the temperature at the Y piece of the ventilator circuit should be around 33–34 °C with a relative humidity of 100%. Using this setting (endotracheal tube plus the humidifier) the absolute humidity that we give to the patient (i.e., 37 mg/l) is comparable to the amount of absolute humidity expired (i.e., 37 mg/l). No water loss is allowed using this method, when compared to physiologic conditions, but it remains to be clarified if this strategy is indeed clinically correct.

In our opinion, heating and humidifying the inspired gas to 37 °C and 100% relative humidity (absolute humidity 44 mg/l) as recently proposed [22], is absolutely incorrect and possibly dangerous, because a greater amount of absolute humidity is given than really needed [18]. In other words, with this proposed setting there is a fluid overload in the airways of about 70–100 ml per day, which could cause epithelial or alveolar damage, or bronchial irritation [17].

In non-intubated patients breathing medical gases, the inspired gases should be humidified until they reach a minimum of 10 mg/l of absolute humidity at room temperature.

Humidifier Equipment

Many different humidifiers (passive and active) are now available to condition the inspired gases. The ideal humidifier should include the properties listed in Table 3.

Table 3. Properties of an ideal humidifier

▌ Adequate levels of humidification	▌ Low dead space
▌ Maintenance of body temperature	▌ Economy
▌ Microbiological safety	▌ Easy to use
▌ Low resistance	

Heat and Moisture Exchangers

Passive humidifiers include the heat and moisture exchanger (HME) and the HME plus an antimicrobiological filter (HMEF) [1]. HME-HMEF, by collecting the heat and moisture of the expired gases, 'passively' heat and humidify the inspired gases at the following inspiration.

Several factors may influence the gas conditioning performance of HME-HMEF during mechanical ventilation:

▌ the type of HME-HMEF (hydrophobic or hygroscopic-hydrophobic);
▌ patient temperature and ambient temperature;
▌ ventilatory settings (tidal volume, minute ventilation, and inspiratory flow).

Type of HME. The first models of HME were purely 'hydrophobic' filters; in other words the water retention was only a physical phenomenon. The expired gases passing through the filter cool, which provokes a condensation on the HME surface. A gradient of temperature is created between the two sides of the filter, determined by the temperature of the expired gases and the ambient temperature. The water retention in the filter depends on the thermal gradient between the two sides.

The effectiveness of this type of HME is quite good for heating the inspired gases but not for providing optimal humidification (absolute humidity between 22–25 mg/l) [23, 24].

A new version of HME, 'hygroscopic-hydrophobic', has been developed in which a hygroscopic unit actively binds the water molecules present in the expired gases, increasing the water content of the inspired gases and ameliorating the humidity added to the inspired gases (absolute humidity 28–32 mg/l) [25].

Many studies have evaluated the performance of HMEs in critically ill patients. The first studies reported an increase in tracheal tube occlusions using hydrophobic HME [26, 27]. Subsequently several studies showed no significant differences in tube occlusions between HME and conventional humidifiers when hygroscopic-hydrophobic HMEs were used [23, 24, 28, 29].

Patient Temperature. HME are not recommended in hypothermic patients (i.e., less than 34°C). Our group found a significant correlation between absolute humidity and esophageal temperature; absolute humidity increased with patient temperature [30]. However, the hygroscopic-hydrophobic HME can adequately humidify also at low body temperature.

Ambient Temperature. The high ambient temperature present in the intensive care unit (ICU) may reduce the difference in temperature between the two sides of the HME and so reduce the conditioning performance [27].

Ventilatory Setting. Many studies have clearly showed that the hygroscopic-hydrophobic HME provided better humidification compared to hydrophobic HME [23, 24, 28, 29]. Moreover, several studies have demonstrated that the hygroscopic-hydrophobic HME maintained adequate humidification of the inspired gases at high tidal volume and minute ventilation (up to 10 l/m) [26, 31]. On the contrary, hydrophobic HMEs have markedly worse performance at high minute ventilation.

HME and Respiratory Mechanics. Because the HME is placed between the Y piece of the ventilator circuit and the endotracheal tube or tracheostomy, it can affect the airflow resistance [32] and increase the dead space [33]. The resistances of the HME are usually low (i.e., range 1–3 cm H_2O for a flow of 60 l/min) [31] and do not induce dynamic hyperinflation [34]. However, airflow resistances can increase with clinical use [32] and in the presence of copious amounts of secretions [35]. The additional dead space (range 50–100 ml) can increase the minute ventilation [33] and the respiratory work [36].

The use of an HME, by increasing the inspiratory work, could affect the outcome of weaning trials in weak patients [37]. So, when choosing a HME we should take into account the volume (i.e., dead space) and the resistance. However, it is possible to reduce the added respiratory work by the HME simply increasing the level of mechanical assistance [36].

HME and Antimicrobiological Activity. An HME with a bacterial barrier effect (efficiency >99.99%) keeps the ventilator circuit clean and free of condensate and reduces the incidence of ventilator circuit colonization [38]. However, the HME does not reduce tracheal colonization or ventilator associated pneumonia [38–40].

The manufacturers recommend that the HME be changed every 24 h, although many studies showed that the hygroscopic-hydrophobic HME could be changed every 48 h without any adverse mechanical or bacterial effects [41, 42]. Moreover, a recent study demonstrated that a HME could be safely used for 7 continuous days of mechanical ventilation in all ICU patients except those with chronic obstructive pulmonary disease (COPD) [43].

However, we believe that the addition of the antimicrobical filter to the HME is not absolutely necessary, at least in ICU patients. This is because the antimicrobical filter further increases the resistance and the dead space of the HME thus increasing the respiratory load [37]. Moreover, while the antimicrobiological activity can play a favorable role during mechanical ventilation in the operating room (prevention of ventilator contamination), this does not seem necessary in the ICU, since there is no evidence of microbial release from the expiratory line to the atmosphere (except when open tuberculosis is present).

Hot Humidifiers

Hot high flow humidifiers (HH) are able to condition the inspired gases with a relative humidity of 100% at temperatures similar to body temperature by heating a water bath [1]. Because the HH is actively heated it is important to monitor the temperature at the patient's airways to avoid thermal injury.

At the present, commercially available HH are the passover, cascade, wick, and vapor phase humidifiers. The simplest HH is the passover, in which the inspired gases pass over a heated water bath. The cascade is a 'bubble humidifier', in which the inspired gases pass beneath the surface of the water reservoir and bubble upward through a grid. The wick is similar to the cascade humidifier, but the inspired gases pass through a cylinder that is lined with a wick of blotting paper. The base of the wick is inserted in the water. The moisture-heated wick increases the relative humidity of the inspired gases. With the vapor phase humidifier, the water is heated and the water vapor penetrates through a hydrophobic filter to humidify the inspired gases.

With all these devices it is very important to have a stable and adequate level of water in the reservoir, to minimize the compressible gas volume and avoid temperature fluctuations. To overcome these problems and also to reduce the risk of contamination, new HH have a closed system that maintains the level of water in the reservoir stable. However, the water supply can significantly increase ICU costs.

A thermistor is usually placed at the end of the inspiratory limb, to measure the temperature of the inspired gases. The thermistor has a slow response and reflects the mean temperature of the inspired gases. So, during mechanical ventilation, the temperature of the inspired gases reaching the patient fluctuates around the preselected value.

During continuous flow continuous positive airway pressure (CPAP), because a bias flow rate up to 100 l/m is used, the time of contact between the inspired dry gases and the humidifying elements is reduced, making it difficult to reach a good level of conditioning [44].

Due to the higher temperature of inspired gases leaving the HH when passing through the ventilator circuit, condensation can occur. This condensate in the circuit can be a reservoir for nosocomial infection [38]. It is important to collect the condensate in the water trap. The water trap must be regularly emptied to avoid the risk of transmitting contamination to the patient's airways.

▌ New Devices for Conditioning the Inspired Gases

Both HME and HH have advantages and disadvantages (Table 4). Recently, new solutions have been developed in order to produce new humidifiers combining the advantages of HME and HH and limiting their disadvantages. In other words, the goals were:
▌ to limit the water air contact,
▌ to avoid condensation in the ventilator circuit,
▌ to reduce costs.

Table 4. Comparison between hot humidifiers (HH) and heat and moisture exchangers (HME-HMEF)

	HH	HME-HMEF
▌ **Performance**	Good	Reduced in low body temperature, low ambient temperature, and high minute ventilation
▌ **Microbiological safety**	Circuit contamination Reservoir contamination	No circuit contamination Microbiological filtration
▌ **Respiratory mechanics**	Limited effects	Increase in airflow resistance and dead space
▌ **Cost**	High	Low

The possible, commercially available solutions are: a cartridge with a new air-water interface (Dar HC 2000); the heated ventilator circuit; the passive-active humidifier.

Dar HC 2000

This system is an active humidifier that differs from the HH humidifier because the inspired gases are conditioned by using the water vaporization principle instead of passing them over a heated water bath. A hydrophobic Gore-Tex membrane is the interface between the water and the vapor dividing the cartridge into two spaces. The inspired gas flows in the inner space, while in the outlet there is the water bath. The main advantages with this system are: no direct contact between water and air, likely reducing contamination, and the reduction in gas compressible volume which makes this system very reliable in pediatric settings. The main disadvantages are that it can reduce its efficiency especially when high minute volumes (greater than 15 l/m) are delivered, and the high cost.

Heated-ventilator Circuit

To prevent the collection of condensation and give more stable conditioning, a heated ventilator circuit (HC) was developed [45]. There are two available heated ventilator circuits. The first heats by using an internal resistance in direct contact with the inspired gases. The main problems are possible electrical shock to the patients, and the not completely uniform heating of the gases resulting in a minimal condensate in the ventilator circuit. The second system heats the inspired gases indirectly by a wire inserted inside the wall of the ventilator circuit without any direct contact with the inspired gases. Both of these systems seem not to be particularly affected by the ventilatory settings. However, if the gases passing through the HC are over heated, i.e., above the temperature of the gases leaving the HH, the relative humidity is reduced and secretions in the endotracheal tube and in the airways can be dried causing dangerous obstruction.

New Passive-active Humidifier

The most effective passive system can deliver a maximum of 80–85% of the expired humidity and heat. Thus, as discussed above, their performance is markedly reduced by patient temperature, ambient temperature and ventilatory setting. Recently a new passive-active humidifier has been proposed (Humid-Heat Gibeck, HME-BOOSTER Tomtec). This consists of a conventional HME with an additional heating element and water supply. Thus, the system combines the efficiency of a HH with the simplicity of a HME [46]. The possible advantages are the stability of gas conditioning independent of patient temperature, ambient temperature, and ventilatory setting, the absence of condensation and, thus, the possible decrease of ventilator associated pneumonia. In addition,the reduction in water supplies can decrease the ICU cost. The possible disadvantages are the fixed inspiratory temperature at 37 °C and 100% relative humidity (Humid-Heat) or the fixed amount of water supply between 2–5 ml per hour (HME-Booster).

Recently a new passive-active humidifier has been developed (Performer StarMed). With this system, it is possible to modify the temperature of the heating element and the water supply to obtain an adequate conditioning of the inspired gases in every condition (patient, ambient, ventilatory setting).

We believe that all these systems need further development, but they will probably prove useful in particular clinical settings such as prolonged anesthesia, in the post-operative period and in neurologically injured patients.

Conclusion

Adequate gas conditioning is mandatory in the clinical management of mechanically ventilated patients. Different humidifiers are commercially available with different advantages and disadvantages. A correct knowledge of the basic physiological principles regulating heat and moisture exchange, is required to choose the appropriate humidifier system for each individual patient.

References

1. Shelly MP, Lloyd GM, Park GR (1988) A review of the mechanisms and methods of humidification of inspired gases. Intensive Care Med 14:1–9
2. Dery R, Pelletier J, Jacques A, Clovet M, Houde JJ (1967) Humidity in anesthesiology III: Heat and moisture patterns in the respiratory procedure during anesthesia with semiclosed system. Can Anaes Soc J 14:287–298
3. Dery R (1971) Humidity in anaesthesiology. Part IV: Determination of the alveolar humidity and temperature in the dog. Can Anaest Soc J 18:145–151
4. Primiano FP, Moranz ME, Montague FW, Miller RB, Sachs DPL (1984) Conditioning of inspired air by a hyroscopic condenser humidifier. Crit Care Med 8:675–678
5. Sessler DI, Moayeri A (1990) Skin surface warming: Heat flux and central temperature. Anesthesiology 73:218–224
6. Graff TD, Benson DW (1968) Systemic and pulmonary changes with inhaled humid atmospheres. Anesthesiology 30:199–207
7. Bissonnette B, Sessler DI, LaFlamme P (1989) Intraoperative temperature monitoring sites in infants and children and the effect of inspired gas warming on esophageal temperature. Anesth Analg 69:192–196
8. Stone DR, Downs JB, Paul WL, Perkins HM (1981) Adult body temperature and heated humidification of anesthetic gases during general anesthesia. Anesth Analg 60:736–741
9. Gentilello LM, Pierson DJ (2001) Trauma critical care. Am J Respir Crit Care 163:604–607
10. Marfatia S, Donahue PK, Hendren WH (1975) Effect of dry and humidified gases on the respiratory epithelium in rabbits. J Paediatr Surg 10:583–592
11. Fonkalsrud EW, Calmes S, Barciff LT, Borret CT (1980) Reduction of operative heat loss and pulmonary secretions in neonates by use of heated and humidified anesthetic gases. J Thorac Cardiovasc Surg 80:718–723
12. Kleeman PP (1994) Humidity of anaesthetic gases with respect to low flow anesthesia. Anaesth Intensive Care 22:396–408
13. Sleigh MA, Blake JR, Liron N (1988) State of the art: the propulsion of mucus by cilia. Am Rev Respir Dis 137:726–741
14. Gawley TH, Dundee W (1981) Attempts to reduce respiratory complications following upper abdominal operations. Br J Anaesth 53:1073–1077
15. Williams RB (1998) The effects of excessive humidity. Respir Care Clin North Am 2:215–228
16. Klein EF, Groves SA (1974) A hot pot tracheitis. Chest 65:225–226
17. Tsuda T, Noguchi H, Takumi Y, Aochi O (1977) Optimum humidification of air administered to a tracheostomy in dogs. Scanning electron microscopy and surfactant studies. Br J Anaesth 49:965–977
18. Chatburn RRT, Primiano FP (1987) A rational basis for humidity therapy. Respiratory Care 4:249–254
19. Johnson JW, Permutt S, Sipple JH, Salem ES (1963) Effect of intra-alveolar fluid on pulmonary surface tension properties. J Appl Physiol 19:769–785

20. American National Standards Institute (1979) Z79.9: Humidifiers and Nebulizers for Medical Use. ANSI, Washington
21. British Standards Institution (1970) BS 4494: Specifications for Humidifiers for Use with Breathing Machines. BSI, London
22. Kanute PR, Youtsey JW (1981) Respiratory Patient Care. Prentice Hall, Englewood Cliffs, pp 46–60
23. Martin C, Papazian L, Perrin G, Bantz P, Gouin F (1992) Performance evaluation of three vaporizing humidifiers and two heat and moisture exchangers in patients with minute ventilation >10 L/min. Chest 102:1347–1350
24. Unal N, Kanhai JKK, Buijk SLCE, et al (1988) A novel method of evaluation of three heat-moisture exchangers in six different ventilator settings. Intensive Care Med 24:138–146
25. Stoutenbeek CH, Miranda D, Zandstra D (1982) A new hygroscopic condenser humidifier. Intensive Care Med 8:231–234
26. Cohen IL, Weinberg PF, Fein A, Rowinski GS (1988) Endotracheal tube occlusion associated with the use of heat and moisture exchangers in the intensive care unit. Crit Care Med 3:277–279
27. Roustan JP, Kienlen J, Aubas P, Aubas S, Cailar J (1992) Comparison of hydrophobic heat and moisture exchangers with heated humidifier during prolonged mechanical ventilation. Intensive Care Med 18:97–100
28. Martin C, Thomachot L, Quinio B, Viviand X, Albanese J (1995) Comparing two heat and moisture exchangers with one vaporizing humidifier in patients with minute ventilation greater than 10 L/min. Chest 107:1411–1415
29. Jackson C, Webb AR (1992) An evaluation of the heat and moisture exchange performance of four ventilator circuit filters. Intensive Care Med 18:264–268
30. Pelosi P, Croci M, Solca M (1994) Use of heat and moisture exchangers in mechanically ventilated patients. In: Vincent JL (ed) Yearbook of Intensive Care and Emergency Medicine, Springer, Heidelberg, pp 545–553
31. Mebius C (1983) A comparative evaluation of disposable humidifiers. Acta Anesthesiol Scand 27:403–409
32. Chiaranda M, Verona L, Pinamonti O, Dominioni L, Minoja G, Conti G (1993) Use of heat and moisture (HME) filters in mechanically ventilated ICU patients: influence on airway flow-resistance. Intensive Care Med 19:462–466
33. Le Bourdelles G, Mier L, Fiquet B, et al (1996) Comparison of the effects of heat and moisture exchangers and heated humidifiers on ventilation and gas exchange during weaning trials from mechanical ventilation. Chest 110:1294–1298
34. Conti G, De Blasi A, Rocco M, et al (1990) Effect of heat-moisture exchangers on dynamic hyperinflation of mechanically ventilated COPD patients. Intensive Care Med 16:441–443
35. Tobin M (1994) Technical aspects of the patient ventilator interface. In: Tobin MJ (ed) Principles and Practice of Mechanical Ventilation. McGraw-Hill, New York, pp 1039–1065
36. Pelosi P, Solca M, Ravagnan I, Tubiolo D, Ferrario L, Gattinoni L (1996) Effects of heat and moisture exchangers on minute ventilation, ventilatory drive, and work of breathing during pressure support ventilation in acute respiratory failure. Crit Care Med 24:1184–1188
37. Iotti GA, Olivei MC, Braschi A (1999) Mechanical effects of heat moisture exchangers in ventilated patients. Crit Care 3:R77–R82
38. Dreyfuss D, Djedaini K, Gros I, et al (1995) Mechanical ventilation with heated humidifiers or heat and moisture exchangers: effects on patients colonization and incidence of nosocomial pneumonia. Am J Respir Crit Care Med 151:986–992
39. Thomachot L, Vialter R, Arnaud S, Barberon B, Nguyen AM, Martin C (1999) Do the components of heat and moisture exchangers filters affect their humidifying efficacy and the incidence of nosocomial pneumonia. Crit Care Med 27:923–928
40. Boots RJ, Howe S, George N, Harris FM, Faoagali J (1997) Clinical utility of hygroscopic heat and moisture exchangers in intensive care patients. Crit Care Med 25:1707–1712
41. Markowics P, Ricard JD, Dreyfuss D, et al (2000) Safety, efficacy, and cost effectiveness of mechanical ventilation with humidifying filters changed every 48 hours: a prospective, randomized study. Crit Care Med 28:665–671

42. Djedaini, Billiard M, Mier L, et al (1995) Changing heat and moisture exchangers every 48 hours rather than 24 hours does not affect their efficacy and the incidence of nosocomial pneumonia. Am J Respir Crit Care Med 152:1562–1569
43. Ricard JD, Le Miere E, Markowics P, et al (2000) Efficiency and safety of mechanical ventilation with a heat and moisture exchanger changed only once a week. Am J Respir Crit Care Med 161:104–109
44. Poulton TJ, Downs JB (1981) Humidification of rapidly flowing gas. Crit Care Med 9:59–63
45. Miyao H, Hirokawa T, Miyasaka K, Kawazoe T (1992) Relative humidity, not absolute humidity, is of great importance when using a humidifier with a heating wire. Crit Care Med 20:674–679
46. Kapadio F, Shelly MP, Anthony JM, Park GR (1992) An active heat and moisture exchanger. B J Anaesth 69:640–642

Bronchodilator Therapy in Mechanically Ventilated Patients

P. Navelesi, P. Ceriana, and M. Delmastro

▌ Introduction

Inhaled bronchodilators are a primary component of the treatment of airway obstruction [1, 2]. During acute respiratory failure due to airway obstruction (asthma attacks and exacerbations of chronic obstructive pulmonary disease [COPD]) their dosage and frequency of administration are increased up to the maximum [3, 4].

Nevertheless, when acute respiratory failure ensues despite aggressive medical therapy, spontaneous breathing may no longer be sustainable and mechanical ventilation may become necessary. Should we keep on delivering aerosolized bronchodilators?

In a recent editorial commenting on a study about aerosol delivery of bronchodilators in mechanically ventilated COPD patients, the authors conclude "Evidence suggests that the COPD patient is very likely to benefit. You just have to do it" [5]. However, in an equally recent systematic review taken from the Cochrane database, it is otherwise stated that "There are no data from well designed randomized controlled trials to provide evidence for or against the current practice regarding use of inhaled beta-agonists in intubated patients". The discrepancy between these statements is probably only apparent and in fact the authors of the review extend their conclusions defining that, in view of the lack of evidence, this practice should not be abandoned until large randomized controlled trials are conducted [6].

▌ What is the Rationale for the Use of Bronchodilators in COPD Patients Requiring Mechanical Ventilation?

Ventilatory failure is consequent to an altered force-load balance (Fig. 1a). While mechanical ventilation relieves the patient by assuming entirely or in part the work of breathing, bronchodilators should, in principle, reduce the load faced by the respiratory muscles by decreasing airway resistance and intrinsic positive end-expiratory pressure (PEEPi) [7]. In addition, by reducing hyperinflation and thus improving the diaphragm force-length relationship, bronchodilators may also enhance the ability of this muscle to generate force [8, 9] (Fig. 1b).

Reviewing some of the physiologic studies performed in the last 10 years in this field, we found reductions in inspiratory resistance [10–17] and in PEEPi [10, 11, 15–17] averaging 15% and 25%, respectively (Table 1). At first sight this effect may appear rather small and of little clinical impact, but is this true?

In ventilator-dependent COPD patients, Appendini et al. [18] found that the amount of inspiratory effort due to airway resistance and PEEPi accounted for al-

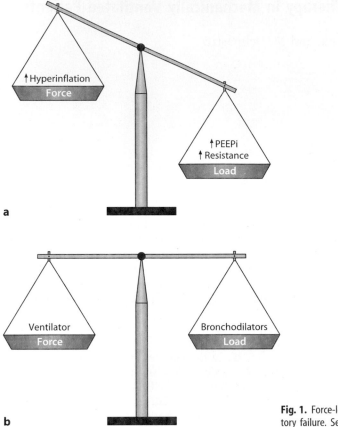

Fig. 1. Force-load balance in acute respiratory failure. See text for explanation

Table 1. Effect of bronchodilator therapy on inspiratory resistance and intrinsic positive end-expiratory pressure (PEEPi)

Authors	Year	Drug	Resistance	PEEPi
Bernasconi et al. [10]	1990	Fenoterol	−28%	−30%
Fernandez et al. [11]	1990	Ipratropium	−15%	−25%
Mancebo et al. [12]	1991	Albuterol	−18%	/
Manthous et al. [13]	1995	Albuterol	−20%	/
Dhand et al. [14]	1996	Albuterol	−17%	/
Guerin et al. [15]	1999	Ipratropium/Fenoterol	−10%	−17%
Mouloudi et al. [16]	1999	Salbutamol	−14%	−25%
Mouloudi et al. [17]	2001	Salbutamol	−15%	−23%

most 80% of the global respiratory muscle effort. Investigating the pathophysiologic determinants of weaning failure and success, Vassilakopoulos et al. [19] showed slightly, but significantly lower values of airway resistance and PEEPi in the group of patients successfully weaned, compared to the failed to-wean group [19]. Interestingly, the differences in airway resistance and PEEPi between the two groups had the same order of magnitude as the effects produced by the bronchodilators in the previously mentioned studies.

Other than for stable COPD patients, who show a positive response to bronchodilators (defined as an increase in the forced expiratory volume in one second [FEV$_1$] >12% and >200 ml [1, 2]) only in a limited number of cases [20], it is interesting to observe that, despite a wide variability [14], the large majority of mechanically ventilated COPD patients have a positive response (i.e., reduction in airway resistance and PEEPi) to the administration of β_2-agonists and anticholinergics [10–17]. Since in most of the studies performed in intensive care unit (ICU) patients, the patients were evaluated within 72 hours from institution of mechanical ventilation, this discrepancy might be due to a more pronounced response to the drug during the exacerbation [7]. However, the ability of FEV$_1$ to assess functional improvement after a reversibility test in COPD patients has been questioned recently by Maesen and coworkers [20] who found that measurements of airway resistance and work of breathing were more appropriate to detect changes in airway caliber than FEV$_1$. Likewise, in stable ventilator-dependent COPD patients, Nava et al. [21] showed that variations in FEV$_1$ following administration of aerosolized steroids by metered-dose inhaler (MDI) significantly underestimated the degree of response (7.6±6.7%) compared to resistance measured using the interrupter technique (19.9±7.8%).

Route of Administration

Bronchodilators may be administered intravenously or via aerosol. Surprisingly, there is no study comparing efficacy and side effects of these two routes of administration in intubated and mechanically ventilated patients. However, in a randomized, multicenter, double blind study performed on spontaneously breathing patients with severe hypercapnic acute asthma, salbutamol was more effective when aerosolized rather than given intravenously [22]. Likewise in non-intubated patients, aerosol therapy may be administered by means of small volume nebulizers (SVN) or MDI. While early studies comparing these two approaches resulted in contrasting results [23, 24], both techniques subsequently have proved effective [3, 15, 25], without any evidence, based on clinical or physiologic results, favoring one over the other.

For various reasons, including reduced risk of contamination and flow sensor damage, ease of administration, dose reliability, and cost containment, the use of MDIs is becoming increasingly popular in the ICU setting [25].

Nevertheless, MDI efficacy can be influenced by several factors [25–27]. The use of a spacer inserted in the inspiratory limb side of the ventilator circuit is mandatory, since many studies have found that connecting the MDI to a spacer chamber device produces a 4- to 6-fold greater delivery of aerosol than MDI directed into a connector attached directly to the tube or into an in-line device without a chamber. A tight fit between the MDI canister and spacer is also necessary [26]. In this regard, it should be kept in mind that the orifices of the actuators for chlorofluoro-carbon (CFC) and hydrofluoroalkane (HFA) propelled MDI have different sizes [26] and that a combination of MDI and actuator different from that originally provided by the manufacturer should be avoided. Regardless of this aspect, aerosol delivery is also significantly reduced when HFA-propelled MDIs are utilized instead of CFC-propelled MDIs [26]. While the duration of the intervals between puffs does not seem to affect aerosol delivery, canister shaking between deliveries has been shown to have a negative effect on MDI delivery [26].

Aerosol deposition has been demonstrated to be reduced when the inhaled air is humidified [26]. Recent work has indicated that the mole fraction of water vapor of the inhaled air, rather than the relative humidity, represents the major determinant of the drop in drug delivered to the lung and that the use of a larger spacer over-comes this problem by allowing longer times for the aerosol to evaporate [27].

Bronchodilator Dose

Even though nebulized ipratropium has also been shown to be effective [11], β_2-agonists have been utilized in the majority of the studies [25]. It has been sug-gested that, during mechanical ventilation, the MDI bronchodilator doses should be increased up to 2–3 times those given to spontaneously breathing subjects [13]. Re-cent work, however, has shown that four puffs of albuterol, corresponding to the maximal dose utilized in stable spontaneously breathing subjects, achieves maximal bronchodilator effect while avoiding side effects [14]. In fact, Dhand et al. deter-mined the bronchodilator response and side effects induced by increasing doses of albuterol delivered by MDI. Four, eight and 16 puffs were delivered at intervals of 15 min in 12 COPD patients sedated and mechanically ventilated in controlled mode for treatment of acute respiratory failure. Measurements of inspiratory resis-tance were obtained by end-inspiratory airway occlusions before, and repeatedly after, albuterol administration. The authors [14] found a significant reduction in in-spiratory resistance after the delivery of four puffs of albuterol. The rate of reduc-tion was quite wide, ranging from 4.6 to 43%, but it exceeded 15% for eight of the 12 patients. The additional eight and 16 puffs did not produce any further im-provement. Heart rate significantly increased at a cumulative dose of 28 puffs. In a second set of experiments performed on seven patients with similar characteristics, the decrease in airway resistance was shown to remain significant 60 min after the administration of four puffs of albuterol.

Is there a Role for Inhaled Steroids
in Mechanically Ventilated Patients with Airway Obstruction?

A randomized, controlled study recently showed that inhaled steroids cause long-term improvement in airway reactivity and respiratory symptoms in patients with stable COPD [28], while another clinical trial demonstrated that in patients hospitalized for exacerbations, systemic steroids moderately ameliorated clinical outcomes, but caused hyperglycemia of sufficient severity to warrant treatment [29]. No large clinical trial is available to assess the role of steroids in such pa-tients, however, a recent study in 12 stable hypercapnic COPD patients tracheostomized for long-term mechanical ventilation using a randomized cross-over design evaluated the physiologic response to fluticasone propionate aerosolized via a MDI connected to a spacer chamber placed on the inspiratory limb side of the ventilator circuit [21]. Even though a few patients did not respond at all to the administration of aerosolized fluticasone, overall the authors found a significant reduction in both airway resistance (29%) and PEEPi (28%) after six days in the treatment group, while no change was detected after 6 days in the placebo group and 2 hours after the first administration in both groups [21].

▌ Effect of Mode of Ventilatory Support

In *in vitro* studies several ventilator settings have been proposed as important determinants of the amount of drug actually delivered to the lung. In a bench study, Fink et al. [30] ascertained that, while spontaneous breathing with continuous positive airway pressure (CPAP) offers the best results, there are no differences between total, conventional mechanical ventilation and partial (assist/control [A/C] and pressure support ventilation [PSV]) forms of mechanical ventilatory assistance, when the breathing pattern is equivalent. In the same study, lung deposition of bronchodilator was not affected by the mode of partial support (A/C vs. PSV) and the type of trigger (pressure vs flow), but increased with tidal volume and both inspiratory time (Ti) and inspiratory duty cycle (Ti/Ttot) [30].

Subsequently, a series of studies performed on mechanically ventilated COPD patients, by Mouloudi and coworkers, suggested that end-inspiratory pause, tidal volume manipulations above 500 ml, inspiratory duty cycle, inspiratory flow rate and pattern had little or no impact on salbutamol delivery by MDI in the clinical setting [16, 17, 31, 32]. These studies indirectly support the concept that the efficacy of the bronchodilators administered via MDI can be extended to the assisted ventilatory modes [7].

Non-invasive mechanical ventilation (NIV) is becoming more and more popular in the treatment of episodes of acute respiratory failure due to exacerbation of COPD since it has proved extremely effective in avoiding endotracheal intubation [33]. Recent work showed comparable results when salbutamol was delivered by MDI during unassisted spontaneous breathing or during NIV in stable asthma patients receiving non-invasive CPAP [34] and COPD patients receiving non-invasive pressure support [35]. These two studies, keeping in mind that both were performed in stable patients not needing NIV to treat respiratory failure, suggest that delivering bronchodilators during NIV is possible.

In COPD patients with acute respiratory failure, the use of helium-oxygen (He-O_2) mixtures can effectively decrease inspiratory effort and dyspnea, while improving gas exchange [36, 37]. Goode and coworkers [38] recently evaluated the impact of gas density on aerosol deposition with SVN and MDI. Interestingly they found that He-O_2 mixtures in the ventilator circuit enhanced aerosol delivery for both devices, however, when SVN was operated by He-O_2 rather than O_2, drug delivery was significantly reduced [38]. In fact, the use of He-O_2 mixtures do not decrease, but actually improve, β_2-agonist delivery during mechanical ventilation. The combination of these two therapeutic strategies in association with NIV is likely to represent the new frontier for the treatment of acute respiratory failure due to airway obstruction.

▌ Conclusion

Although data from well designed randomized controlled trials are lacking, physiologic evidence supports the use of bronchodilator agents in mechanically ventilated COPD patients, provided that several elements are considered. This holds particularly true for MDI, an approach that potentially offers various advantages. So, should we administer aerosolized bronchodilators in mechanically ventilated patients? Paraphrasing the title of the editorial by Bauer and Torres [5] we might suggest: "Just do it well".

References

1. American Thoracic Society (1995) ATS standards for the diagnosis and care of patients with chronic obstructive pulmonary disease. Am J Respir Crit Care Med 152:S78–S121
2. British Thoracic Society (1997) The BTS guidelines for the management of chronic obstructive pulmonary disease. Thorax 52 (suppl 5):S1–S28
3. Raimondi AC, Schottlender J, Lombardi D, Molfino NA (1997) Treatment of acute severe asthma with inhaled albuterol delivered via jet nebulizer, metered dose inhaler with spacer, or dry powder. Chest 112:24–28
4. Rodrigo G, Rodrigo C (1996) Metered dose inhaler salbutamol treatment of asthma in the Emergency Department: comparison of two doses with plasma levels. Am J Emerg Med 14:144–155
5. Bauer TT, Torres A (2001) Aerosolized β_2-agonists in the intensive care unit: just do it. Intensive Care Med 27:3–5
6. Jones A, Rowe B, Peters J, Camargo C, Hammarquist C (2000) Inhaled beta-agonists for asthma in mechanically ventilated patients. Cochrane Database Syst Rev 2:CD001493
7. Nava S, Navalesi P (1999) Bronchodilators and mechanical ventilation in COPD patients. Emptying, pumping or both? Intensive Care Med 25:1206–1208
8. Macklem PT (1984) Hyperinflation. Am Rev Respir Dis 129:1–2
9. Similowski T, Yan S, Gauthier AP, Macklem PT, Bellemare F (1991) Contractile properties of the human diaphragm during chronic hyperinflation. N Engl J Med 325:917–923
10. Bernasconi M, Brandolese R, Poggi R, Manzini E, Rossi A (1990) Dose-response effects and time course of effects of inhaled fenoterol on respiratory mechanics and arterial oxygen tension in mechanically ventilated patients with chronic obstructive pulmonary disease. Intensive Care Med 16:108–114
11. Fernandez A, Lazaro A, Garcia A, Aragon C, Cerda E (1990) Bronchodilators in patients with chronic obstructive pulmonary disease on mechanical ventilation: utilisation of metered-dose inhalers. Am Rev Respir Dis 141:164–168
12. Mancebo J, Amaro P, Lorino H, Lemaire F, Harf A, Brochard L (1991) Effects of albuterol inhalation on the work of breathing during weaning from mechanical ventilation. Am Rev Respir Dis 144:95–100
13. Manthous CA, Chatila W, Schmidt GA, Hall JB (1995) Treatment of bronchospasm by metered-dose inhaler albuterol in mechanically ventilated patients. Chest 107:210–213
14. Dhand R, Duarte AG, Jubran A, et al (1996) Dose-response to bronchodilator delivery by metered-dose inhaler in ventilator-supported patients. Am J Respir Crit Care Med 154:388–393
15. Guerin C, Chevre A, Dessirier P, et al (1999) Inhaled fenoterol-ipratropium bromide in mechanically ventilated patients with chronic obstructive pulmonary disease. Am J Respir Crit Care Med 159:1036–1042
16. Mouloudi E, Katsanoulas K, Anastasaki M, Hoing S, Georgopoulos D (1999) Bronchodilator delivery by metered dose inhaler in mechanically ventilated COPD patients: influence of tidal volume. Intensive Care Med 25:1215–1221
17. Mouloudi E, Prinianakis G, Kondili E, Georgopoulos D (2001) Effect of inspiratory flow rate on beta2-agonist induced bronchodilation in mechanically ventilated COPD patients. Intensive Care Med 27:42–46

18. Appendini L, Purro A, Patessio A, et al (1996) Partitioning of inspiratory muscle workload and pressure assistance in ventilator-dependent COPD. Am J Respir Crit Care Med 154:1301–1309
19. Vassilakopoulos T, Zakynthinos S, Roussos C (1998) The tension-time index and the frequency/tidal volume ratio are the major pathophysiologic determinants of weaning failure and success. Am J Respir Crit Care Med 158:378–385
20. Maesen BLP, Westermann CJJ, Duurkens VAM, Van den Bosch JMM (1999) Effects of formeterol in apparently poory reversible chronic obstructive pulmonary disease. Eur Respir J 13:1103–1108
21. Nava S, Compagnoni ML (2000) Controlled short-term trial of fluticasone propionate in ventilator-dependent patients with COPD. Chest 118:990–999
22. Salmeron S, Brochard L, Mal H, et al (1994) Nebulized versus intravenous albuterol in hypercapnic acute asthma. A multicenter, double-blind, randomized study. Am J Respir Crit Care Med 149:1466–1470
23. Fuller HD, Dolovich MB, Posmituck G, Wong Pack W, Newhouse MT (1990) Pressurized aerosol versus jet aerosol delivery to mechanically ventilated patients. Am Rev Respir Dis 141:440–444
24. Manthous CA, Hall JB, Schmidt GA, Wood LDH (1993) Metered dose inhaler versus nebulized albuterol in mechanically ventilated patients. Am Rev Respir Dis 148:1567–1570
25. Dhand R, Tobin M (1997) Inhaled bronchodilator therapy in mechanically ventilated patients. Am J Respir Crit Care Med 156:3–10
26. Fink JB, Dhand R, Grychowski J, Fahey PJ, Tobin MJ (1999) Reconciling in vitro and in vivo measurements of aerosol delivery from a metered-dose inhaler during mechanical ventilation and defining efficiency-enhancing factors. Am J Respir Crit Care Med 159:63–68
27. Lange CF, Finlay WH (2000) Overcoming the adverse effect of humidity in aerosol delivery via pressurized metered-dose inhalers during mechanical ventilation. Am J Respir Crit Care Med 161:1614–1618
28. The Lung Health Study Research Group (2000) Effect of inhaled triamcinolone on the decline in pulmonary function in chronic obstructive pulmonary disease. N Engl J Med 343:1902–1909
29. Niewoehner DE, Erbland ML, Deupree RH, et al (1999) Effect of systemic glucocorticoids on exacerbations of chronic obstructive pulmonary disease. N Engl J Med 340:1941–1947
30. Fink JB, Dhand R, Duarte AG, Jenne JW, Tobin MJ (1996) Aerosol delivery from a metered-dose inhaler during mechanical ventilation. An in vitro model. Am J Respir Crit Care Med 154:382–387
31. Mouloudi E, Katsanoulas K, Anastasaki M, Askitopoulou E, Georgopoulos D (1998) Bronchodilator delivery by metered-dose inhaler in mechanically ventilated COPD patients: influence of end-inspiratory pause. Eur Respir J 12:165–169
32. Mouloudi E, Prinianakis G, Kondili E, Georgopoulos D (2000) Bronchodilator delivery by metered-dose inhaler in mechanically ventilated COPD patients: influence of flow pattern. Eur Respir J 16:263–268
33. Brochard L, Mancebo J, Wysocki M (1995) Noninvasive ventilation for acute exacerbations of chronic obstructive pulmonary disease. N Engl J Med 333:817–822
34. Parkers SN, Bersten AD (1997) Aerosol kinetics and bronchodilator efficacy during continuous positive airway pressure delivered by face mask. Thorax 52:171–175
35. Nava S, Karakurt S, Rampulla C, Braschi A, Fanfulla F (2001) Salbutamol delivery during non invasive mechanical ventilation in patients with chronic obstructive pulmonary disease: a randomized controlled study. Intensive Care Med 27:1627–1635
36. Jolliet P, Tassaux D, Thouret JM, Chevrolet JC (1999) Beneficial effects of helium:oxygen versus air:oxygen noninvasive pressure support in patients with decompensated chronic obstructive pulmonary disease. Crit Care Med 27:2422–2429
37. Jaber S, Redouane F, Carlucci A (2000) Noninvasive ventilation with helium–oxygen in acute exacerbations of chronic obstructive pulmonary disease. Am J Respir Crit Care Med 161:1191–1200
38. Goode ML, Fink JB, Dhand R, Tobin MJ (2001) Improvement in aerosol delivery with heliumoxygen mixtures during mechanical ventilation. Am J Respir Crit Care Med 163:109–114

Management
of Acute Respiratory Failure

Titrating Optimal PEEP at the Bedside

N. S. Ward and M. M. Levy

▌ Introduction

Determining what is the optimal positive end-expiratory pressure (PEEP) to use in a given patent with acute respiratory distress syndrome (ARDS) has been a controversial topic for several decades now. This controversy, no doubt, exists for two main reasons. One is that there has never been a good 'gold-standard' by which to judge success. The other, and more important reason, is that in all likelihood, finding optimal PEEP is an impossible task. All levels of PEEP carry both benefits and detriments. High levels of PEEP have been shown to prevent end-expiratory collapse of lung units and open previously closed units, but come at the expense of potential hemodynamic compromise and overdistention of the lungs. Lower levels of PEEP can avoid these problems but may not be sufficient to recruit or maintain open lung. Added to these difficulties is the fact that the physiology of a patient's lung with ARDS is constantly changing with fluid shifts, inflammatory responses, body position, and even the effect of the ventilator itself.

In the last two years, there has been much in the medical literature on lung recruitment and determining optimal PEEP that has significantly changed our thinking about these topics. Unfortunately, these studies raise as many questions as they answer and still leave us, as clinicians, with some confusion about how to determine a given patient's 'optimum PEEP' at the bedside with commonly available tools and training. In this chapter, we will discuss some of the newest studies regarding this topic as well as show some data from our intensive care unit (ICU) that we feel are helpful in determining a patient's optimal PEEP at the bedside in every day practice.

▌ Determining a Lower Inflection Point

Since the mid 1980s the lower inflexion point (LIP) on the inspiratory pressure-volume (PV) curve has been used as a tool in setting PEEP in patients with ARDS [1]. The theory behind its use was that there was a critical opening pressure that could be detected as a sharp inflection of the PV curve that corresponded to the recruitment of large amounts of previously collapsed lung units. However, controversy has existed over the use of PV curves in clinical practice almost since its inception. An early finding that directly impacted on the clinician's use of the PV curve was that a clear LIP could not always be detected in all patients. Matamis et al. [2] in 1984 found four distinct types of PV curves in patients with ARDS that correlated with different stages of the disease. Only two of the four categories had a definable LIP.

In another study by Vieira et al. [3] using computerized analysis of the PV curves of patients with ARDS, only 57% had a discernable LIP. In both these studies, the authors use the presence or absence of a LIP to suggest that it may discriminate between patients at different stages of ARDS [2] or patients with some other intrinsically different physiologic state of their lung such as recruitability [3].

In contradiction to those theories, however, a more recent study using pigs, under very controlled and identical conditions, also found that LIPs were identifiable only 50% of the time [4]. This casts doubt on any theory that inability to find a LIP is secondary only to stage or state of disease. It has been our experience that even under optimal conditions we are only able to determine a clear LIP in 68% of our ARDS patients [5].

Perhaps of more obvious concern to physicians trying to use the PV curve are the technical difficulties involved with performing it accurately. In the medical literature, most PV curves were obtained by using the super-syringe or occlusion methods which required full paralysis, lowering a patient's PEEP to zero, and (in the case of a super-syringe) using a piece of equipment not commonly found in an ICU. In addition, anyone who has performed these maneuvers on a human patient knows there is a level of technical expertise required to make accurate measurements in the short (and therefore safe) period of time required.

Finally, several investigators have shown poor physician-to-physician correlation in determining the LIP [6, 7]. Harris et al. [6] showed that human (as opposed to computer) determination of LIP had poor correlation with values on the same patient, differing by as much as 17 cmH_2O. In a recent study in our medical ICU, when three physicians evaluated the same PV curve we found agreement (± 3 cmH_2O) only 64% of the time [5]. These, and other problems associated with PV curves can be found in Table 1.

Table 1. Problems with using a pressure/volume curve to set PEEP

▌**Technical difficulties**
- Extra equipment
- Training of personnel
- Time consuming
- Gas resorbtion may affect values
- Alterations in chest wall compliance affect values
- Poor inter- and intra-observer agreement
- Not always present

▌**Safety concerns**
- Massive derecruitment may be detrimental
- Paralytics usually necessary
- Hypoxia common

▌**Theoretical concerns**
- May not maximize recruitment
- May overestimate pressures needed to prevent collapse/hysteresis

■ Decremental PEEP Trials

Not soon after the introduction of inspiratory PV curves being used to set optimal PEEP, many began to question their validity. The presence of hysteresis on full inspiratory/expiratory PV curves (i.e., a shift between the inspiratory and expiratory curve) seemed to indicate that the pressure necessary to open large numbers of lung units was not necessarily the pressure needed to keep them open during tidal ventilation. In the last year, three studies have been published that suggest that evaluating derecruitment (as opposed to recruitment) during the expiratory limb of a PV curve or other PEEP trial may be superior. Hickling studied this phenomenon using a mathematical model of a lung with ARDS that incorporated such factors as heterogeneous opening pressures and the gravitational effects of surrounding lung. He found that during an incremental PEEP trial evaluating maximal mean compliances these values did not correlate with maximal recruitment whereas there was good correlation with a decremental PEEP trial [8].

Further support for this idea came from a recent human clinical trial by Crotti et al. [9] in which they used CT imaging to determine percentages of aerated and non-aerated lung during ventilation with various levels of PEEP and tidal volume. The authors determined there was a considerable gap between estimated opening and closing threshold pressures (Fig. 1) and found that for a given pressure there was considerably more open lung during the deflation limb of a PV curve than on the inflation limb. For example, at 10 cmH$_2$O pressure only 15% of previously collapsed lung (at PEEP=0) had been opened but on the expiratory limb 50% was open at the same pressure. The authors point out how this fact casts doubt on the ability of an inspiratory maneuver to set optimal PEEP which is an expiratory phenomenon [9].

In yet another recent human clinical trial, Maggiore et al. [10] used a technique of measuring low-flow quasi-static PV curves at different PEEP levels which were then aligned on a common volume axis to determine changes in derecruited lung as the PEEP levels were decreased from a high level to zero. The authors found that derecruitment occurred in a linear correlation with decreasing levels of PEEP, in

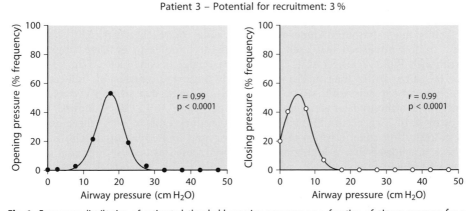

Fig. 1. Frequency distribution of estimated threshold opening pressures as a function of airway pressure for a single patient with ARDS (*left panel*) in contrast to estimated threshold closing pressures (*right panel*). (From [9] with permission)

other words there was no inflection point. Furthermore, they showed that derecruitment paralleled oxygenation changes closely.

Pan-inspiratory Recruitment

The previously mentioned study by Maggiore et al. [10] is one of a growing number of studies that seems to indicate that recruitment does not end with inflation to the LIP. This concept has its foundation in a host of other studies that have also helped to bring criticism to the use of the LIP to set PEEP. Jonson et al. [11] in 1999 analyzed the PV curves from zero end-expiratory pressure (ZEEP) and compared them with those derived from some applied PEEP to show that there is evidence for lung being recruited during a single breath above the LIP. Another study by Svantesson et al. [12] also showed this effect. In addition to these, two complimentary studies were published in 2001 that further clarified this issue. In a study of six dogs with chemically-induced ARDS, Pelosi et al. [13] used computerized tomography (CT) imaging to showed that given enough pressure virtually all of the lung was recruitable but that only about 20% was recruited by inflation to the LIP. In a similar study, evaluating humans with ARDS, Crotti et al. [9] used the same CT imaging techniques to study recruitment. These authors found no evidence of any inflection zone wherein large amounts of lung open up. In their words, "recruitment occurs along the entire VP curve" and is a "pan-inspiratory phenomenon [9]."

CT Imaging to Set PEEP

Perhaps one of the greatest tools available to set optimal PEEP is the use of CT imaging of the lungs. This is not a new tool and its use dates back at least to 1987 when Gattinoni et al. [14] used CT imaging and PV curves to study the effects of various levels of applied PEEP on lung recruitment. CT imaging is unlike most other methods for evaluating the effects of PEEP in that it can 'directly' measure recruitment as opposed to inferring recruitment by indirect measurements like lung pressures and volumes. However, some CT imaging techniques may be more accurate than others.

While much has been done with CT imaging in recent years, 2001 saw three new studies published that used CT imaging techniques to evaluate lung recruitment with PEEP. Pelosi et al. [13] and Crotti et al. [9] combined CT imaging with the measurement of lung mechanics to study dogs with chemically induced ARDS and human subjects with ARDS. Both studies showed that using PV curves is an unreliable technique for determining the 'open lung' PEEP. They showed that recruitment of lung occurs throughout the inspiratory limb of a PV curve and there is no inflection zone in which the majority of lung units open up. Interestingly, Pelosi et al. showed that if high enough inflation pressures are used (54 ± 4.3 cmH$_2$O) almost the entire lung (96%) could be opened up. This suggests that non-aeration in ARDS is mostly a phenomenon of collapse and not alveolar filling.

Another important study done using CT imaging with ARDS came from Malbouisson et al. [15]. This group used a new technique for evaluating the CT images taken during inflation of the lung in patients with ARDS. Instead of using just one cross-sectional image as was done by prior investigators, Malbuisson et al. [15]

used spiral CT imaging to obtain data from the entire lung. The images were then analyzed to determine percentages of non-aerated, poorly aerated, and normally aerated lung for a given PEEP. This technology was also able to assess alveolar distention and alveolar overdistention as evidenced by lower than normal Hounsfield Units (HU). As part of the study, the authors compared their method to the previously used methods and found theirs to be more accurate.

The authors then showed that while going from ZEEP to a PEEP of 15 cmH$_2$O they were able to increase functional residual capacity by 119%. Unfortunately, only half of this increase represented alveolar recruitment, the other half was overdistention of previously open lung units. This is important for two reasons. One is that it reaffirms that PEEP-induced recruitment can come at a cost. The other is that it shows how indirect measurements of recruitment like lung volumes and pressures can be misleading about the true state of the lung.

Maximum Compliance or Best PEEP

The first use of the maximum compliance curve to set PEEP goes back to Suter et al. [16] in 1975, who were able to show that in patients with ARDS the lowest PEEP that yielded the maximum lung compliance correlated with maximum oxygen delivery (DO$_2$). This was called by the authors 'Best PEEP'. Several studies since have supported its use. Recently, Lichtwarck-Aschoff et al. [4] used a pig model of ARDS to look for determinants of recruitment. They, like others, found that recruitment can occur almost continually as the lung is inflated, yielding no 'inflection zone.' Their data also showed evidence that both recruitment and overdistention can occur simultaneously in the same breath. Like the work of Suter et al. [16] they also found that a PEEP that yielded maximum compliance corresponded with a zone in which oxygenation was improved and DO$_2$ had not yet begun to decrease (with higher levels of PEEP). This is illustrated in Fig. 2.

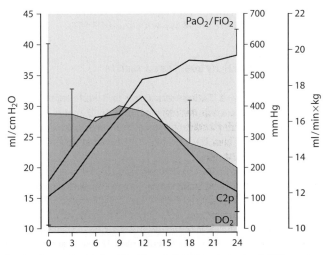

Fig. 2. Oxygen delivery (DO$_2$, shaded area), C2p (static compliance), and PaO$_2$/FiO$_2$ at levels of PEEP ranging from 0 to 24 cm H$_2$O indicated on X axis. (From [4] with permission)

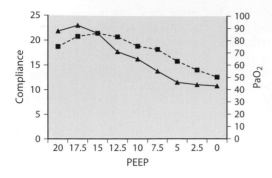

Fig. 3. Decremental PEEP trial results showing maximal compliance curve (squares) plotted against continuous PaO_2 measurements (triangles). The PaO_2 shows an accelerated decline between the highest PEEP yielding maximal compliance (12) and the lowest (7)

Schmitt et al. [17] recently published a study in which PV and maximum compliance curves were calculated on 16 patients with ARDS. They then compared the effects of various levels of PEEP on right ventricular (RV) outflow impedance. They found that impedance was highest at ZEEP and decreased as PEEP was increased. The lowest impedance corresponded with 'Best PEEP' while the impedance at the LIP was as high as ZEEP.

One question that remains about the use of maximal compliance curves is whether one should use the lowest PEEP yielding the maximum compliance or higher PEEP. As several of the above mentioned studies have shown, recruitment seems to increase continually along a PEEP titration curve. Recently, we have used continuous PaO_2 measurements during a decremental PEEP trial to study this issue. In some patients there is an accelerated decline in oxygenation that occurs between the highest PEEP yielding maximum compliance and the lowest PEEP (unpublished data) (Fig. 3).

Many physicians continue to use Best PEEP both for clinical and research purposes as it requires little training or risk to the patient. In addition it can be obtained with a high frequency. In a recent study of 28 patients with ARDS in our ICU we were able to get a Best PEEP 86% of the time, compared with 68% for a LIP. In addition, there was agreement among three observers 93% of the time with Best PEEP compared to 64% with the LIP [5].

▌ Titrating PEEP in Everyday Practise

In addition to the parameters used to titrate optimal PEEP described so far, there are many others such as oxygenation, DO_2, and shunt fraction (Table 2). Unfortunately, none so far have stood out as superior. Perhaps the most accurate method described to date is the use of CT scan imaging. This method, however, is not practical for everyday use.

In trying to decide the optimal PEEP for a given patient the clinician should remember the following. First, many of the described methods for choosing optimal PEEP in the medical literature are too imprecise, lengthy, or technically difficult to be used in common practice. Second, optimal PEEP is likely a moving target that is altered by other factors such as fluid shifts, inflammatory responses, and other ventilator settings such as tidal volumes. Indeed, several studies have shown that tidal volume alone can impact recruitment independently of PEEP [16, 18, 19]. Third, it is unlikely that any PEEP exists that will enable a large amount of lung recruitment

Table 2. Parameters used in determining optimal PEEP

▌**Commonly used**
- PaO_2/FiO_2 ratio
- Maximum compliance (Best PEEP)
- Lower inflection point on a PV curve
- Oxygen delivery (DO_2)
- Shunt fraction

▌**Other strategies**
- Decremental Best PEEP
- CT imaging
- Right ventricular outflow impedance
- Dead space fraction
- Chord compliances
- Multiple inert gas elimination technique (MIGET)

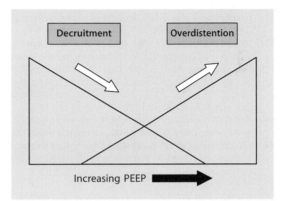

Fig. 4. A graphic representation of the factors affecting optimal PEEP. With increasing PEEP there is less derecruitment but more overdistention. The optimal PEEP would be that which coincides with the intersection of the two curves

and not lead to some overdistention. As illustrated in Fig. 4, an optimal PEEP would be one that has the least derecruitment and the least overdistention but it is unlikely there is point at which there are neither of these. Fourth, while the short term affects of lung recruitment are apparent immediately, the long term harmful effects of using either too little (repetitive opening injury) or too much PEEP (overdistention and volutrauma) are more subtle and impossible to analyze for a given patient at the bedside. While it is possible that some optimal combination of PEEP, tidal volume, and perhaps recruitment maneuvers exists, it will likely require one or more large outcomes study to prove.

References

1. Gattinoni L, Pesenti A, Caspani ML, et al (1984) The role of total static lung compliance in the management of severe ARDS unresponsive to conventional treatment. Intensive Care Med 10:121–126
2. Matamis D, Lemaire F, Harf A, Brun-Buisson C, Ansquer JC, Atlan G (1984) Total respiratory pressure-volume curves in the adult respiratory distress syndrome. Chest 86:58–66
3. Vieira SR, Puybasset L, Lu Q, et al (1999) A scanographic assessment of pulmonary morphology in acute lung injury. Significance of the lower inflection point detected on the lung pressure-volume curve. Am J Respir Crit Care Med 159:1612–1623

4. Lichtwarck-Aschoff M, Mols G, Hedlund AJ, et al (2000) Compliance is nonlinear over tidal volume irrespective of positive end-expiratory pressure level in surfactant-depleted piglets. Am J Respir Crit Care Med 162:2125–2133

5. Ward NS, Lin D, Houtchens J, et al (2002) Successful determination of lower inflection point and maximal compliance in a population of patients with ARDS. Crit Care Med (in press)

6. Harris RS, Hess DR, Venegas JG (2000) An objective analysis of the pressure-volume curve in the acute respiratory distress syndrome. Am J Respir Crit Care Med 161:432–439

7. O'Keefe GE, Gentilello LM, Erford S, Maier RV (1998) Imprecision in lower "inflection point" estimation from static pressure-volume curves in patients at risk for acute respiratory distress syndrome. J Trauma 44:1064–1068

8. Hickling KG. Best compliance during a decremental, but not incremental, positive end-expiratory pressure trial is related to open-lung positive end-expiratory pressure: a mathematical model of acute respiratory distress syndrome lungs. Am J Respir Crit Care Med 163:69–78

9. Crotti S, Mascheroni D, Caironi P, et al (2001) Recruitment and derecruitment during acute respiratory failure: a clinical study. Am J Respir Crit Care Med 164:131–140

10. Maggiore SM, Jonson B, Richard JC, Jaber S, Lemaire F, Brochard L (2001) Alveolar derecruitment at decremental positive end-expiratory pressure levels in acute lung injury. Comparison with the lower inflection point, oxygenation, and compliance. Am J Respir Crit Care Med 164:795–801

11. Jonson B, Richard JC, Straus C, Mancebo J, Lemaire F, Brochard L (1999) Pressure-volume curves and compliance in acute lung injury: evidence of recruitment above the lower inflection point. Am J Respir Crit Care Med 159:1172–1178

12. Svantesson C, Sigurdsson S, Larsson A, Jonson B (1998) Effects of recruitment of collapsed lung units on the elastic pressure-volume relationship in anaesthetised healthy adults. Acta Anaesthesiol Scand 42:1149–1156

13. Pelosi P, Goldner M, McKibben A, et al (2001) Recruitment and derecruitment during acute respiratory failure: an experimental study. Am J Respir Crit Care Med 164:122–130

14. Gattinoni L, Pesenti A, Avalli L, Rossi F, Bombino M (1987) Pressure-volume curve of total respiratory system in acute respiratory failure. Computed tomographic scan study. Am Rev Respir Dis 136:730–736

15. Malbouisson LM, Muller JC, Constantin JM, Lu Q, Puybasset L, Rouby JJ (2001) Computed tomography assessment of positive end-expiratory pressure-induced alveolar recruitment in patients with acute respiratory distress syndrome. Am J Respir Crit Care Med 163:1444–1450

16. Suter PM, Fairley B, Isenberg MD (1975) Optimum end-expiratory airway pressure in patients with acute pulmonary failure. N Engl J Med 292:284–289

17. Schmitt JM, Vieillard-Baron A, Augarde R, Prin S, Page B, Jardin F (2001) Positive end-expiratory pressure titration in acute respiratory distress syndrome patients: impact on right ventricular outflow impedance evaluated by pulmonary artery Doppler flow velocity measurements. Crit Care Med 29:1154–1158

18. Blanch L, Fernandez R, Valles J, Sole J, Roussos C, Artigas A (1994) Effect of two tidal volumes on oxygenation and respiratory system mechanics during the early stage of adult respiratory distress syndrome. J Crit Care 9:151–158

19. Richard JC, Maggiore SM, Jonson B, Mancebo J, Lemaire F, Brochard L (2001) Influence of tidal volume on alveolar recruitment. Respective role of PEEP and a recruitment maneuver. Am J Respir Crit Care Med 163:1609–1613

Effect of PEEP and Targets during Mechanical Ventilation in ARDS

A. Koutsoukou, C. Roussos, and J. Milic-Emili

Introduction

The acute respiratory distress syndrome (ARDS) is characterized pathologically by alveolar edema, consolidation, atelectasis, hyaline membranes, and, in later stages, fibrosis [1]. These findings vary in severity throughout the involved lungs. The loss of lung units through atelectasis and small airway closure (trapping) has two important physiological consequences: decreased lung compliance (stiff lungs) and small lung volume [2].

Among ventilated patients, those with ARDS are at greatest risk of ventilator induced lung injury (VILI) which can delay lung healing, prolong the duration of mechanical support, and enhance intensive care unit (ICU) morbidity, nosocomial pneumonia, and multiple organ failure (MOF) [3, 4].

Mechanical ventilation is merely supportive, allowing time for treatment of the underlying cause of ARDS and for healing of the lungs. The particular mode of ventilation is probably less important than the 'lung protection' goals and principles that should guide ventilatory management. The criteria for selecting the 'optimal respiratory settings' in ARDS are still under debate. In general, however, five main targets should be achieved;

- good oxygenation,
- recruitment of lung units,
- limited end-inspiratory pressures and volumes,
- absence of cyclic compression and re-expansion of peripheral airways, and
- limited negative effects on hemodynamics.

General Considerations

Refractory hypoxemia can be enhanced by supplementing inspired oxygen and by raising mean and end-expiratory alveolar pressures. Each of these interventions, however, has associated risks and benefits. Oxygen toxicity occurs when clinicians are forced to use very high inspired oxygen fractions (FiO_2) (>0.6). In addition to microscopic lung injury, oxygen toxicity results in specific physiologic impairments, including absorption atelectasis, decreased cardiac output, and pulmonary vasodilatation [5, 6]. In general, the increase in FiO_2 is not enough to correct hypoxia and reopening of atelectatic lung units has been advocated as the main way to improve gas exchange. While it is difficult or impossible to reopen consolidated zones, the recruitment of the atelectatic lung units represents a specific therapeutic goal.

▌ Recruitment of Atelectatic Alveoli

In most species a static transpulmonary pressure (P_L) of 20 cmH$_2$O or more is required to reverse significantly atelectasis. Since in the ICU the transthoracic instead of transpulmonary pressure is commonly measured, a static P_L of 20 cmH$_2$O should correspond to a plateau pressure (Pplat) of about 25 cmH$_2$O [7]. Indeed, Crotti and coworkers [8] have recently shown that in patients with ARDS and acute lung injury (ALI), a Pplat of about 25 cmH$_2$O is required to reverse most atelectasis, though some alveoli require higher Pplat. Indeed, in 1991 Ranieri et al. [9] concluded that Pplat rather than positive end-expiratory pressure (PEEP) is useful to predict recruitment and that the recruited volume (V_{rec}) is essentially maximal only at Pplat values of about 32 cmH$_2$O. Further recruitment can probably be achieved with recruitment maneuvers such as that proposed by Marini et al. [10].

▌ High Lung Volume Injury

The Pplat values required to reverse atelectasis closely correspond to the values of Pplat that are regarded as potentially hazardous in terms of 'high lung volume' injury [11]. In recent years it has been recognized that the use of large inflation pressures and volumes, which are often needed to normalize arterial blood gases, may aggravate lung injury [12, 13]. Since the normal lung reaches its maximum volume at a static P_L of 30–35 cmH$_2$O, relatively normal alveoli dispersed among the ARDS lung can be injured by such high pressures. Regional over-distension is probably produced in ARDS patients by static airway pressures >30 cmH$_2$O [7], a pressure level known to cause damage in sheep when sustained for more than a few hours [14]. In addition to microscopic lung damage [15], over-distension can cause macroscopic damage including pulmonary interstitial emphysema, lung cysts, and major air leaks [16].

Thus, the benefits of alveolar recruitment with Pplat of 30–35 cmH$_2$O have to be balanced against the potential hazards of concurrent lung injury. Further studies are required to resolve these conflicting requirements.

Recruitment of Lung Units with Closed Airways

The decrease in lung compliance in the early stages of ARDS was originally attributed to small airway closure [17]. In fact, the 'knee' (lower inflection point [LIP]) on the static inflation pressure-volume (PV) curve of the respiratory system probably mainly reflects the point at which there is a 'massive' reopening of small airways rather than alveoli. Indeed, the values of the LIP are usually much smaller (<15 cmH$_2$O) than the values of Pplat required to reverse atelectasis. Nonetheless, a common approach to selecting the therapeutic level PEEP is based on PEEP$_{IDEAL}$, which is obtained by adding 1–2 cmH$_2$O to LIP [7, 18]. This approach is based on the assumption that the LIP reflects the pressure beyond which there is 'massive' alveolar recruitment: hence, there should be a sudden increase in PaO$_2$ and V_{rec} when PEEP$_{total}$ exceeds PEEP$_{IDEAL}$. Koutsoukou et al. [19], however, have shown that this is not the case in ARDS patients: indeed V_{rec} and PaO$_2$ increased monotonically with increasing PEEP$_{total}$ without a distinct 'knee' in either V_{rec} or PaO$_2$ when PEEP$_{total}$ exceeded PEEP$_{IDEAL}$. This may reflect the fact that, at the onset of the baseline constant flow inflation, the inspiratory driving pressure increases rapidly above the LIP, with a consequent reopening of collapsed peripheral airways from the onset of inspiration. This is consistent with the results of Robertson and coworkers [20] in normal erect subjects. Indeed, boluses of xenon-133 inhaled from residual volume at low flow rates (<0.3 l/s) were distributed preferentially to apical lung regions because of presence of peripheral small airway closure in the dependent lung zones. In contrast, during rapid inspiration with a concurrent rapid increase in transpulmonary pressure, the dependent airways reopened early and, as a result, the boluses of xenon-133 were distributed preferentially to the lower lung zones. In this connection it should be noted that, in presence of peripheral airway closure, the rapid increase in airway pressure (Paw) at the onset of constant flow inflation by snapping open the closed airways, may contribute to 'low lung volume' injury because of the generation of high shear forces within the pulmonary parenchyma. Additional arguments against the use of $PEEP_{IDEAL}$ have been recently provided by Crotti et al. [8].

Low Lung Volume Injury

In 1984, Robertson [21] suggested that ventilation at low lung volumes may cause lung injury as a result of shear stresses caused by cyclic opening and closing of peripheral airways. Using an *ex vivo* model of lavaged rat lung, Muscedere et al. [22] showed that ventilation with physiologic tidal volumes from zero end-expiratory pressure (ZEEP) resulted in a significant increase of injury scores in the respiratory (RIS) and membranous bronchioles (MIS) relative to ventilation from PEEP above the LIP on the static inflation PV curve of the lung. Significant increases in RIS and MIS, as well as increased airway resistance, have been found recently in normal open-chest rabbits ventilated at ZEEP for 3-4 hours [23]. Since in these rabbits there was no evidence of atelectasis, the airway injury was probably due to cyclic opening and closing of peripheral airways. Cyclic peripheral airway closure and reopening probably also occurs in ARDS patients because they breathe at low lung volume. This, together with the reduction in functional lung units ('baby lung'), promotes expiratory flow-limitation which implies cyclic compression and re-expansion of the peripheral airways with risk of peripheral airway injury [24]. Shear forces associated with this phenomenon may be responsible for an important component of VILI and can explain the observed benefits of high frequency ventilation in animal models of ARDS [25].

The PEEP required to avert atelectasis, cyclic small airway closure and dynamic collapse of the peripheral airways due to expiratory flow limitation, varies with the hydrostatic forces applied to the lung. In ARDS there is an enhanced vertical gradient of transpulmonary pressure, due to the weight of the edematous lung and heart [26, 27], which accentuates the tendency for collapse in dependent regions. However, tidal expiratory flow limitation can be assessed on-line during mechanical ventilation and PEEP can be increased progressively until this phenomenon is no longer present [24]. With PEEP of 10 cmH$_2$O tidal flow limitation is abolished in most ARDS patients [19, 24] and atelectasis avoided [8].

▌ Current Practice

Understanding the mechanisms of VILI, prevention strategies should be targeted at reducing over-distension, shearing injury, while ensuring sufficient oxygenation ($SaO_2 > 90\%$). On this basis, pressure limited lung protective mechanical ventilatory strategies have been proposed for ARDS [28] emphasizing the need to 'open the lung and keep it open' [29]. The approach to selecting the therapeutic level of PEEP has been commonly based on assessment of the static pressure-volume curve of the respiratory system. Usually, in patients with ARDS, the inflation limb of the static volume-pressure curve of the respiratory system has a sigmoidal shape, with a lower (LIP) and upper (UIP) inflection point [30]. It has been proposed that these two points identify a safe range of pressures during mechanical ventilation. Animal, and human, studies indicate that ventilation with pressures kept within this range may reduce the so called the VILI, an important factor of increased morbidity and mortality [18]. Recently, it has been shown that ventilating ARDS patients with PEEP above LIP, and end-inspiratory static pressure below UIP, significantly reduced the pulmonary and systemic inflammatory responses, as suggested by the decrease in cytokine levels in bronchoalveolar lavage (BAL) and plasma [31]. According to these studies it follows that determination of LIP and UIP should be an integral part of a lung protective strategy in mechanically ventilated patients with ARDS. This, however, assumes that LIP reflects the pressure beyond which there is a 'massive' alveolar recruitment, which is not the case [8, 19]. Furthermore, obtaining PV curves is a time consuming and cumbersome bedside technique. It should also be noted that assessment of LIP from the static PV curves of the total respiratory system is problematic since it does not take into account the contribution of the mechanical properties of the chest wall (chest wall compliance is markedly reduced in patients with secondary ARDS). In fact, LIP should be determined from static PV curves of the lung [9, 32]. This approach however, is also problematic in the decubitus position because of artifacts in esophageal pressure measurements [33].

In order to avoid large inflation pressures and volumes and thus 'high lung volume' injury, current recommendations include the use of the smallest possible tidal volume compatible with adequate PaO_2, without necessarily attempting to normalize $PaCO_2$ (permissive hypercapnia). In this way, however, Pplat may be kept too low to effectively reverse atelectasis (see above). A recent study [34], however, showed a significant difference in mortality between a group with lung protective ventilation (30%) receiving 6 ml/kg tidal volume and a more conventionally ventilated group of patients (40%) receiving 12 ml/kg tidal volume.

During the early phase of ARDS, apart from the application of external PEEP in order to maximize lung recruitment, large volume recruitment maneuvers have been proposed as ventilatory techniques. Large tidal volumes used either during mechanical ventilation [35] or applied as sighs [36] have been shown to improve oxygenation. Other investigators have used sustained inflation coupled with conventional or high frequency ventilation to recruit the lung.

Prone position is another adjunct to a lung protective strategy, that may promote lung recruitment by decreasing regional pleural pressure gradient [37].

Limitations

Ventilation with low tidal volume, apart from hypercapnia, involves a potential for alveolar de-recruitment and enhanced atelectasis. During mechanical ventilation when the diaphragm is inactive, regional compliance of dependent areas decreases and tidal volume is preferentially distributed in non-dependent parts of the lung. These regions receive the first bulk of air with a potential risk of over-distention. This effect is greatly accentuated by dependent small airways and alveolar collapse occurring in ARDS situations. Increases in lung volume with PEEP may prevent alveolar collapse during expiration, but the application of PEEP can produce an increase in volume preferentially in the non-dependent areas (over-distension of already inflated alveoli) and may not recruit collapsed units. This has been shown in a study [38] where the authors assessed the relationship between the shape of the PV curve and lung morphology (by high-resolution spiral computerized tomography [CT] scan) at different PEEP levels. They found that in patients with predominant consolidation of basal zones, there is a serious risk of over-distention at high PEEP levels. The alveolar recruitment induced by PEEP is not an 'all or-nothing' phenomenon, but a continuous process in which different lung zones open successively according to their respective critical opening pressures, as originally advocated by Ranieri et al. [9]. Furthermore, at end-expiration, peripheral airway closure and atelectasis can occur if the end-expiratory pressure becomes lower than a critical value of about 10 cmH_2O [8, 39].

New Findings

In recent studies [19, 24], using the negative expiratory pressure technique, we have shown that at zero end-expiratory pressure (ZEEP) many ARDS patients exhibit expiratory flow limitation with concurrent intrinsic PEEP (PEEPi) ranging up to 12 cmH_2O. Presence of flow limitation implies cyclic dynamic compression and re-expansion of the peripheral airways with concurrent inhomogeneous filling of airspaces. In non-homogeneous ARDS lungs, this should entail development of high shear forces with risk of 'low lung volume' injury [22, 35, 40]. To avoid this, external PEEP has to be applied in order to increase the end-expiratory lung volume above the 'flow limitation volume'. Such therapeutic levels of PEEP can be readily determined by on-line inspection of the effect of negative expiratory pressure on the expiratory flow-volume ($\dot{V}$-V) loops: PEEP should be increased until tidal flow limitation disappears. Figure 1 shows $\dot{V}$-V loops of an ARDS patient during ventilation on ZEEP (including the negative expiratory pressure test breath) and after the application of 10 cmH_2O of PEEP. On ZEEP, the patient was flow limited, (Fig 1, left) while with PEEP of 10 cmH_2O, flow limitation disappeared (Fig. 1, right). In this connection it should be noted that assessment of flow limitation in ARDS patients provides for the first time an objective assessment of cyclic compression and re-expansion of peripheral airways which has been advocated as a potential hazard for 'low lung volume' injury [21, 22].

The presence of tidal flow limitation, implies sequential dynamic compression of peripheral airways during expiration [41], promoting non-homogeneous lung emptying (the dependent zones achieving flow limitation earlier because of the vertical pleural pressure gradient) and hence regional inequality of PEEPi within the lung.

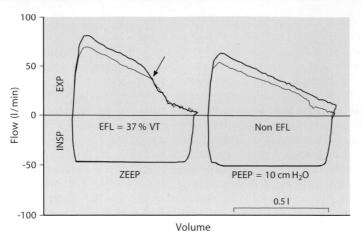

Fig. 1. Flow-volume loops of control and negative expiratory pressure (NEP) test breaths of an ARDS patient on zero end-expiratory pressure (ZEEP) (left) and PEEP of 10 cmH₂O (right). [Thin lines=control breaths; heavy lines=NEP]. On ZEEP, the application of NEP did not induce an increase in expiratory flow (EFL) over 36% tidal volume (VT), indicating presence of flow-limitation over this tidal volume range. With PEEP there was no EFL, since flow with NEP exceeded the reference flow throughout expiration

In this case, application of PEEP may produce an improvement in PaO₂, due to reduced PEEPi inhomogeneity within the lung. This has been recently shown in a group of 13 early ARDS patients under controlled mechanical ventilation [19]. In these patients we assessed the effects of different levels of PEEP on tidal expiratory flow limitation, regional PEEPi inhomogeneity, alveolar recruited volume, respiratory mechanics and arterial blood gases. On ZEEP seven patients exhibited flow limitation. These patients had higher static PEEPi and greater PEEPi inhomogeneity (as assessed by the ratio of total dynamic PEEP to total static PEEP) than the six non-flow limitation patients. With PEEP of 10 cmH₂O, flow limitation was abolished in all patients. In the flow limitation group, PaO₂ correlated with PEEPi inequality index (p=0.002), while in the non-flow limitation patients, PaO₂ correlated with V_{rec} (p=0.0001). Thus, in flow limitation patients, application of PEEP is beneficial because it abolishes tidal flow limitation, with risk of 'low lung volume injury' and improves PaO₂ through reduction of PEEPi inhomogeneity within the lung. In contrast, in non-flow limitation patients, PEEP improves gas exchange mainly through alveolar recruitment.

▌ Conclusion

Ensuring adequate oxygenation and avoiding VILI are the main goals for the management of mechanically ventilated ARDS patients.

Improvement in PaO₂ can be achieved with PEEP by alveolar recruitment, which implies increased lung volume, and/or reduced PEEPi inequality within the lung, which can occur in the absence of changes in lung volume. Applying external PEEP based on the LIP does not result in 'massive' alveolar recruitment nor improvement in PaO₂. Significant alveolar recruitment requires relatively high pressures, and hence should be monitored in terms of Pplat rather than PEEP. The values of Pplat required to reverse atelectasis are close to those eliciting 'high lung volume' injury, and hence should be closely monitored. Detection of tidal flow limitation by expiratory flow volume loops with and without negative expiratory pressure is a potentially useful approach to avoid development of high shear forces within the peripheral airways and risk of 'low lung volume' injury.

References

1. Bachofen M, Weibel ER (1982) Structural alterations of lung parenchyma in the adult respiratory distress syndrome (ARDS). Clin Chest Med 3:35–56
2. Malo J, Ali J, Wood LD H (1984) How does end-expiratory positive pressure reduce intrapulmonary shunt in canine pulmonary edema?. J Appl Physiol 57:1002–1010
3. Cook DJ, Walter S, Cook RJ, et al (1998) Incidence of and risk factors for ventilator-associated pneumonia in critically ill patients. Ann Intern Med 129:433–440
4. Slutsky AS, Tremblay LN (1998) Multiple system organ failure. Is mechanical ventilation a contributing factor? Am J Respir Crit Care Med 175:1721–1725
5. Bryan CL, Jenkinson SG (1998) Oxygen toxicity. Clin Chest Med 9:141–152
6. Nash G, Blennerhasset JB, Pontoppidan H (1967) Pulmonary lesions associated with oxygen therapy and artificial ventilation. N Engl J Med 276:368–374
7. Roupie E, Dambrosio M, Servillo, et al (1995) Titration of tidal volume reduction and induced hypercapnia in adult respiratory distress syndrome (ARDS). Am J Respir Crit Care Med 152:121–128
8. Crotti S, Mascheroni D, Caironi P, et al (2001) Recruitment and corecruitment during acute respiratory failure. Am J Respir Crit Care Med 164:131–140
9. Ranieri VM, Eissa T, Corbeil C, et al (1991) Effects of positive end-expiratory pressure on alveolar recruitment and gas exchange in patients with the adult respiratory distress syndrome. Am Rev Respir Dis 144:355–360
10. Marini JJ, Amato MB (1998) Lung recruitment during ARDS. In: Marini JJ, Amato MB (eds) Acute Lung Injury. Springer, Berlin, pp 236–257
11. Slutsky AS (1993) Mechanical ventilation. American College of Chest Physicians' Consensus Conference. Chest 104:1833–1859
12. Dreyfuss D, Soler P, Basset F, Saumon G (1988) High inflation pressure pulmonary edema. Respective effects of high airway pressure, tidal volume, and positive end-expiratory pressure Am Rev Respir Dis 137:1159–1164
13. Dreyfuss D, Basset F, Soler P, Saumon G (1985) Intermittent positive-pressure hyperventilation with high inflation pressures produces pulmonary microvascular injury in rats. Am Rev Respir Dis 132:880–884
14. Colobow T, Morreti MP, Fumagalli R, et al (1987) Severe impairement in lung function induced by high peak airway pressure during mechanical ventilation. Am Rev Respir Dis 135:312–315
15. Pratt Pc, Vollmer RT, Shelburne JD, Crapo JD (1979) Pulmonary morphology in a multihospital collaborative extracorporeal membrane oxygenation project I. Light microscopy. Am J Pathol 95:191–214
16. Pingleton S (1988) Complications of acute respiratory failure. Am Rev Respir Dis 137:1463-1493
17. Slutsky AS, Scharf SM, Brown R, et al (1980) The effects of oleic-acid-induced pulmonary edema and chest wall mechanics in dogs. Am Rev Respir Dis 121:91–96
18. Amato MB, Barbas CS, Medeiros DM, et al (1995) Beneficial effects of the 'open lung' approach with low distending pressures in acute respiratory distress syndrome. A prospective randomized study on mechanical ventilation. Am J Respir Crit Care Med 152:1835–1846
19. Koutsoukou A, Bekos V, Sotiropoulou CH, et al (2001) Effect of PEEP in mechanically ventilated ARDS patients. Eur Respir J 18:480s (Abst)
20. Robertson PC, Antonishen NR, Ross D (1969) Effect of inspiratory flow rate on regional distribution of inspired gas. J Appl Physiol 26:438–443
21. Robertson B (1984) Lung surfactant. In: Robertson B, Van Golde L, Batenburg J (eds) Pulmonary Surfactant. Elsevier, Amsterdam, pp 549–564

22. Muscedere JG, Mullen JB, Gan K, Slutsky AS (1994) Tidal ventilation at low airway pressures can augment lung injury. Am J Respir Crit Care Med 149:1327–1334
23. D'Angelo E, Pecchiarii M, Baraggia P, Saetta M, Balesiro E, Milic-Emili J (2002) Low-volume ventilation induces peropheral airways injury and increased airway resistance in normal open-chest rabbits. J Appl Physiol (in press)
24. Koutsoukou A, Armaganidis A, Stavrakaki-Kallergi K, et al (2000) Expiratory flow limitation and intrinsic positive end-expiratory pressure at zere positive end-expiratory pressure in patients with adult respiratory distress syndrome. Am J Respir Crit Care Med 161:1590–1596
25. Hamilton PP, Onayemi A, Smith JA, et al (1983) Comparison of conventional and high frequency jet ventilation: oxygenation and lung pathology. J Appl Physiol 55:131–138
26. Gattinoni L, D'Andrea L, Pelosi P, et al (1993) Regional effects and mechanism of positive end-expiratory pressure in early respiratory distress syndrome. JAMA 269:2122–2127
27. Albert RK, Hubmayr RD (2000) The prone position eliminates compression of the lungs by the heart. Am J Respir Crit Care Med 161:1660–1665
28. Artigas A, Bernard GR, Carlet J, et al (1998) The American-European Consensus Conference on ARDS, Part 2. Intensive Care Med 24:378–398
29. Lanchmann B (1992) Open up the lung and keep the lung open. Intensive Care Med 24:319–321
30. Matamis D, Lemire F, Harf A, Brun-Buisson C, Ansqer JC, Atlan G (1984) Total respiratory system pressure-volume curves in the adult respiratory distress syndrome. Chest 86:58–66
31. Ranieri M, Giunto F, Suter PM, Slutsky AS (2000) Mechanical ventilation as a mediator of multisystem organ failure in acute respiratory distress syndrome. JAMA 284:43–44
32. Rossi A, Gottfried SB, Zocch L, Lennox S, Carlverly P (1985) Measurement of static compliance of the total respiratory system in patients with acute respiratory failure. Am Rev Respir Dis 131:672–677
33. Milic-Emili J, Mead J, Turner M (1964) Topography of esophageal pressure as a function of posture in man. J Appl Physiol 19:212–216
34. The Acute Respiratory Distress Syndrome Network (2000) The acute respiratory distress syndrome. Ventilation with lower tidal volumes as compared with traditional tidal volumes for acute lung injury and the acute respiratory distress syndrome. N Engl J Med 342:1301–1308
35. Blanch LR, Fernandez R, Valles J, Solle C, Roussos C, Artigas A (1994) Effect of two tidal volumes on oxygenation and respiratory system mechanics during the early stage of the adult respiratory distress syndrome. J Crit Care 9:151–158
36. Pelosi P, Candringher P, Bottini N, et al (1999) Sigh in acute respiratory distress syndrome. Am J Respir Crit Care Med 159:872–880
37. Mutoh T, Guest J, Lamm WJ, Albert RK (1992) Prone position alters the effect of volume overload on regional pleural pressure and improves hypoxemia in pigs in vivo. Am Rev Respir Dis 146:300–306
38. Vieira S S, Puibasset L, Lu Q, et al (1999) A scanographic assessment of pulmonary morphology in acute lung injury. Am J Respir Crit Care Med 159:1612–1613
39. Milic-Emili J (1974) Pulmonary statics. In: Widdicombe JG (ed) 'MTP' International Review of Science, Vol 2. Respiratory Physiology. Butterworth Ltd, London, pp 105–137
40. Ranieri VM, Zhang H, Mascia L, et al (2000) Pressure time curve predicts minimally injurious ventilatory strategy in an isolated rat lung model. Anesthesiology 93:1833–1859
41. Rodarte J R, Hyatt R E, Cortese DA (1975) Influence of expiratory flow on closing capacity at low expiratory flow rates. J Appl Physiol 39:60–65

Lung Recruitment in Localized Lung Injury

L. Blanch, G. Murias, and A. Nahum

▌ Introduction

Acute respiratory distress syndrome (ARDS) is characterized by diffuse pulmonary infiltrates, severe hypoxemia at high breathing oxygen concentrations, the presence of a precipitating underlying disease, acute onset, and absence of left ventricular failure. The pathophysiology of ARDS includes increased membrane permeability, decreased oncotic pressure, and augmented transvascular hydrostatic pressure gradients that cause non-cardiogenic pulmonary edema, atelectasis and loss of lung volume. As a result of these alterations, ventilation/perfusion (V/Q) heterogeneity and intrapulmonary shunt increase, and oxygenation is severely impaired. Although acute lung injury (ALI) does not have a unilateral distribution, some degree of inhomogeneity generally exits. In clinical practice, lobar or one lung pneumonia or atelectasis, and lung contusion are common findings. In this scenario, application of positive intrathoracic pressure may over-inflate the uninvolved more compliant lung and divert pulmonary blood flow to the injured lung, thereby worsening V/Q mismatch and decreasing oxygenation [1–7].

▌ Lung Recruitment in Acute Non-homogeneous Lung Injury

Studies on unilateral lung injury (lobar pneumonia in dogs or lung contusion with flail chest) demonstrated that the consolidated lung regions did not expand fully during inflation to total lung capacity [2, 6]. Impaired mechanical properties of the consolidated lung were associated with very poor ventilation. Moreover, hypoxemia was due to both increased shunt and V/Q mismatch in the infected regions, and local hypoxic vasoconstriction was in most instances ineffective in directing blood flow away from the consolidated lobe [1, 2]. In such specific circumstances, the effect of global positive end-expiratory pressure (PEEP) on regional lung volume may be unfavorably distributed; normal lung regions with normal compliance will tend to hyperinflate, whereas affected lung regions with decreased compliance will tend to remain collapsed [3, 8].

In the setting of unilateral lung injury, measurement of global respiratory system mechanics does not provide clinically useful information to set ventilator parameters (PEEP or tidal volume) because the mechanical impairment of the injured parts of the lung cannot be specifically assessed [1–3, 9]. In fact, some patients with ARDS presenting with consolidated lower lung lobes that cannot be recruited exhibit a gas exchange response to increasing levels of PEEP similar to that described in patients with unilateral lung injury. In this context, application of PEEP usually does not improve oxygenation as it may cause overdistension of compliant lung regions and redistribute blood flow to collapsed or fluid filled alveoli [10, 11].

Imaging studies using chest computerized tomography (CT) scan provided some answers about the mechanisms of recruitment. Using chest CT scan during a progressive increase in PEEP from 0 to 20 cmH$_2$O, Gattinoni et al. [12] showed that tidal volume distribution decreased significantly in the upper lung level, did not change in the middle levels, and increased significantly in the lower levels. In other words, PEEP reduces the reopening-collapsing tissue, keeping open the lung tissue recruited at end-inspiration. If a moderate/high PEEP level is used in an attempt to keep all alveoli open, the level of tidal volume should not reach high end-inspiratory plateau pressures (>35 cmH$_2$O) because lung recruitment is non-significant and further hyperinflation might be caused as demonstrated by CT scan [10, 13]. When factors influencing PEEP-induced alveolar recruitment were studied using continuous thoracic CT sections from the apex to the diaphragm with and without PEEP, Puybasset et al. [11] found that a cephalocaudal gradient of alveolar recruitment with PEEP, but de-recruitment (increase in non-aerated tissue) was also observed in the lung areas closest to the diaphragm cupola. In fact, non-recruiters with PEEP showed a marked reduction in the volume of left lower lobes and no improvement in oxygenation. It has been shown also in patients with ARDS, that alveolar recruitment and lung overdistension can be observed in different parts of the lung parenchyma after PEEP application [14]. Interestingly, this mechanism is similar to that described in studies of unilateral lung injury [1–3] and suggests that ARDS is a very non-homogeneous disease.

The response to PEEP, and possibly tidal volume, on recruitment might also depend on the cause of the lung injury, or in differences in lung morphology. Gattinoni et al. [15] observed that the response of PEEP on end-expiratory lung volume and estimated recruitment was less in patients suffering from pulmonary ARDS (pneumonia, hemorrhagic alveolitis) compared with patients with extrapulmonary ARDS (peritonitis, polytrauma). Direct insult to the lung parenchyma may produce more severe alveolar damage with a higher derangement of lung mechanics compared with an indirect insult. On the contrary, Puybasset et al. [14] found that the regional distribution of the loss of aeration and the type of atelectasis ('mechanical' with a massive loss of lung volume versus 'inflammatory' with a preservation of lung volume) present in the lower lobes were the main determinants of the cardiorespiratory effects of PEEP. Because the setting of the ventilator (PEEP and tidal volume) has dramatically changed in recent years, appropriate levels of PEEP and tidal volume for patients with unilateral lung disease remain to be elucidated.

▌ Mechanical Ventilation: Tidal Volume and PEEP

Mechanical ventilation is a supportive life-saving therapy but it can produce further lung damage and, more importantly, these can be indistinguishable from the pulmonary alterations attributable to ARDS. Increasing evidence has implicated both cyclical closing and reopening of alveolar units, and elevated alveolar pressures associated with overdistension of lung units, in ventilator-associated lung injury [16, 17]. Based on this work, lung protective mechanical ventilatory strategies have been proposed for ARDS [18, 19]. These strategies typically involve the use of small tidal volumes to avoid high alveolar pressures at end-inspiration and alveolar overdistension, and the use of high PEEP levels to keep alveoli open at end-expiration thus maintaining alveolar recruitment. Recommendations for tidal volume and PEEP application during mechanical ventilation have been made in clinical practice primarily for patients with diffuse lung injury. Consequently, it is difficult to adjust tidal volume and PEEP to avoid ventilator-associated lung injury in unilateral lung injury. Preferential distribution of ventilation promotes overdistension of the normal lung, whereas attempts to minimize it by decreasing PEEP may then lead to repetitive closure and opening of lung units in the injured lung. Currently, differential ventilation with selective PEEP [8, 20] and positioning the patient with the 'good lung down' [4, 9] are the two accepted treatment strategies to improve oxygenation in severe unilateral lung injury although both have serious limitations in clinical practice.

▌ Adjuncts to Mechanical Ventilation: Tracheal Gas Insufflation

Tracheal gas insufflation (TGI) applied together with conventional mechanical ventilation, effectively reduces the size of the dead space compartment and improves overall carbon dioxide (CO_2) elimination by replacing the anatomic dead space normally laden with CO_2 during expiration with fresh gas. As a consequence, less CO_2 is recycled to the alveoli during the next inspiration and the ventilatory efficiency of each tidal respiration is improved. Therefore, TGI reduces anatomic dead space and increases alveolar ventilation for a given frequency and tidal volume combination [21–23]. The main effect of TGI is to flush the dead space from the carina to the Y of the ventilator circuit. However, TGI also has a distal effect that contributes to remove CO_2. Although the distal effect enhances CO_2 removal, the presence of the catheter and the jet effect oppose expiratory flow favoring auto PEEP [24, 25]. A number of studies have been published on the effect of TGI in patients receiving mechanical ventilation. The majority of the studies have been performed in patients with ARDS and focused on demonstrating a reduction in tidal volume and subsequently on airway pressure while $PaCO_2$ was maintained constant, or a reduction in $PaCO_2$ during permissive hypercapnia [23, 26–28].

Selective application of TGI can potentially improve gas exchange and lung mechanics by creating selective autoPEEP only in the injured lung. Selective TGI can be successfully applied during a short time interval using an endotracheal tube with a movable bronchial blocker (Univent®) [29, 30]. In a recent study, we hypothesized that selective application of TGI will recruit the injured lung without causing overdistension of the normal lung [31]. In eight anesthetized dogs, left lung saline lavage was performed until PaO_2/FiO_2 fell below 100 mmHg. Then, the dogs were reintubated with a Univent® single lumen endotracheal tube which incorporates an internal catheter to provide TGI. After injury, increasing PEEP from 3 to 10 cmH_2O did not change gas exchange, hemodynamics, or lung compliance. Selective TGI, while keeping end-expiratory lung volume (EELV) constant, improved PaO_2/FiO_2 from 212 ± 43 to 301 ± 38 mmHg (p<0.01) while $PaCO_2$ and airway pressures decreased (p<0.01). During selective TGI, reducing tidal volume to 5.2 ml/kg while keeping EELV constant, normalized $PaCO_2$, did not affect PaO_2/FiO_2, and decreased end-inspiratory plateau pressure from 16.6 ± 1.0 to 11.9 ± 0.5 cmH_2O, p<0.01 (Fig. 1). In unilateral lung injury, we conclude that selective TGI could improve oxygenation at a lower pressure cost as compared to conventional mechanical ventilation, while allowing a reduction in tidal volume without a change in alveolar ventilation. Although TGI improved pulmonary function without any side effects, it is hazardous to extrapolate experimental data to the clinical setting since it is not known whether high TGI flows could be maintained for a long period. Severe unilateral lung pathology such as lung contusion, unilateral pneumonia, or refractory atelectasis are common diseases in the intensive care setting, often requiring mechanical ventilation with high FiO_2. In this context, regional recruitment with selective TGI may be a useful clinical tool although clinical studies are warranted to assess the safety and validity of this novel treatment.

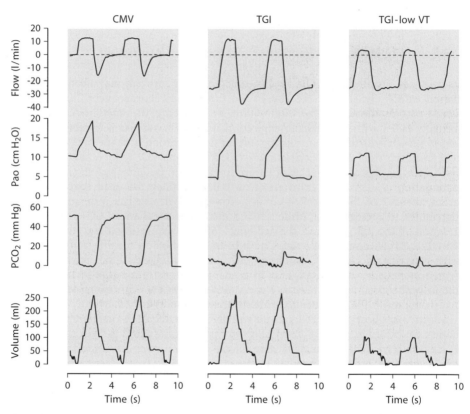

Fig. 1. Tracings of airflow (Flow), airway opening pressure (Pao), exhaled PCO_2 (PCO_2) and lung volume (Volume) estimated with inductive plethysmography obtained during controlled mechanical ventilation (CMV) at PEEP = 10 cmH_2O, selective TGI (TGI), and selective TGI with low tidal volume (TGI-Low VT) in one representative animal. Application of TGI decreased Pao and increased CO_2 clearance when compared with CMV at the same tidal volume and end-expiratory lung volume. Application of TGI with low VT further reduced Pao while end-expiratory lung volume remained constant. At this stage (TGI-Low VT) lung compliance was maximal, indicating better distribution of tidal ventilation between the right (healthy) and left (injured) lung. (From [31] with permission)

▮ Combination of Partial Liquid Ventilation and TGI

Partial liquid ventilation (PLV) [32–34] has been proposed as a new modality to recruit lung units in ALI. Perflubron, due to its low surface tension and high density (1.91 gm/cm^3) may facilitate opening of collapsed, noncompliant dependent lung segments. Consequently, perflubron may function as 'liquid PEEP', preventing complete collapse of unstable alveoli even at low airway pressures, thereby improving oxygenation, and decreasing shear forces acting on the lung parenchyma. The amount of PEEP needed to optimize gas exchange during PLV in a lung lavage model of ALI has been found to be approximately 10 cmH_2O [35]. Previous studies in experimental animals [36, 37] have shown that TGI superimposed on PLV provided better gas exchange compared with PLV alone at similar levels of minute ventilation.

In unilateral injury, selective PLV with perflubron to the diseased lung may act as a local PEEP, recruiting atelectatic lung regions and maintaining their patency, and global lung function may be improved by applying selective TGI and PLV to the injured lung. To test this hypothesis, we [38] have studied six anesthetized dogs in whom left saline lung lavage was performed until PaO_2/FiO_2 fell below 100 mmHg. The dogs were then reintubated with a Univent® single lumen endotracheal tube which incorporates an internal catheter to provide TGI. In a consecutive manner, we studied: 1) the application of 10 cmH_2O of PEEP; 2) instillation of 10 ml/kg of perflubron (Liquivent®) to the left lung (PLV + PEEP) at a PEEP level of 10 cm H_2O; 3) application of selective TGI (PLV + TGI) while maintaining EELV constant; 4) PLV + TGI at reduced tidal volume and 5) PLV + PEEP bracketed. Application of PLV + PEEP did not change gas exchange, lung mechanics or hemodynamics. PLV + TGI improved PaO_2/FiO_2 from 189 ± 13 to 383 ± 44 mmHg (p < 0.01) and decreased $PaCO_2$ from 55 ± 5 to 30 ± 2 mmHg (p < 0.01). During ventilation with PLV + TGI, reducing tidal volume from 15 ml/kg to 3.5 ml/kg while keeping EELV constant decreased PaO_2/FiO_2 to 288 ± 49 mmHg (p = NS) and normalized $PaCO_2$. At this stage, end-inspiratory plateau pressure decreased from 19.2 ± 0.7 to 13.6 ± 0.7 cmH_2O (p < 0.01). With PLV + PEEP bracketed, measurements returned to those observed at previous baseline stage (PLV + PEEP). Therefore, during unilateral lung injury, PLV with a moderate PEEP did not improve oxygenation. The combination of TGI superimposed on PLV improved gas exchange and allowed a 77% reduction in tidal volume without any adverse effect on $PaCO_2$.

The effect of perflubron on arterial oxygenation in ALI appears to depend on PEEP-induced alveolar recruitment. Conceivably, the oxygenation response to PLV during acute severe unilateral injury is dependent on the ability of perflubron to reach and remain in the injured lung units. In the setting of unilateral lung injury, PLV confined to the diseased lung does not protect against the deleterious effects of moderate PEEP (overdistension of normal lung regions). Selective TGI superimposed on PLV allowed decompression of the compliant normal lung while maintaining alveolar recruitment of the diseased lung, thus improving global lung function.

▌ Conclusion

The treatment of unilateral lung injury is largely supportive. Currently, positioning the patient with the 'good lung down' and differential ventilation with selective PEEP in selected patients are the two accepted treatment strategies to improve oxygenation in severe unilateral lung injury although both have serious limitations in clinical practice. Basic research has shown that the application of selective TGI and the combination of selective TGI and PLV permitts a reduction in tidal volume with resultant decrease in airway pressures and improvement in lung compliance, without any adverse effects on CO_2 elimination [31, 38]. Experimental models have shown that the use of selective TGI and PLV at low tidal volume is a simple method to provide regional recruitment, enhancing gas exchange while reducing cyclic lung stretch and shear stresses associated with mechanical ventilation. Further studies are needed to determine the clinical importance and application of these novel therapies.

References

1. Kanarek DJ, Shannon DC (1975) Adverse effect of positive end-expiratory pressure on pulmonary perfusion and arterial oxygenation. Am Rev Respir Dis 112:457–459
2. Mink SN, Light RB, Wood LHD (1981) Effect of PEEP on gas exchange and pulmonary perfusion in canine lobar pneumonia. J Appl Physiol 50:517–523
3. Blanch L, Roussos C, Brotherton S, Michel RP, Angle MR (1992) Effect of tidal volume and PEEP in ethchlorvynol-induced asymmetric lung injury. J Appl Physiol 73:108–116
4. Remolina C, Khan AU, Santiago TV, Edelman NH (1981) Positional hypoxemia in unilateral lung disease. N Engl J Med 304:523–525
5. Marini JJ (1984) Postoperative atelectasis: pathophysiology, clinical importance, and principles of management. Respir Care 29:516–528
6. Craven KD, Oppenheimer L, Wood LDH (1979) Effects of contusion and flail chest on pulmonary perfusion and oxygen exchange. J Appl Physiol 47:729–737
7. Cohn SM (1997) Pulmonary contusion: review of the clinical entity. J Trauma 42:973–979
8. Carlon GC, Ray C, Klein R, Goldiner PL, Miodownik S (1978) Criteria for selective positive end-expiratory pressure and independent synchronized ventilation of each lung. Chest 74:501–507
9. Blanch L, Fernandez R, Baigorri F, Valles J, Bonsoms N, Artigas A (1992) Efecto del volumen corriente y de la posición sobre la oxigenación y la mecánica pulmonar en pacientes afectos de neumonia unilateral ventilados mecanicamente. Med Intensiva 16:318–323
10. Vieira SRR, Puybasset L, Lu Q, et al (1999) A scanographic assessment of pulmonary morphology in acute lung injury. Significance of the lower inflection point detected on the lung pressure-volume curve. Am J Respir Crit Care Med 159:1612–1623
11. Puybasset L, Cluzel P, Chao N, Slutsky AS, Coriat P, Rouby JJ, and the CT scan study group (1998) A computed tomography scan assessment of regional lung volume in acute lung injury. Am J Respir Crit Care Med 158:1644–1654
12. Gattinoni L, Pelosi P, Crotti S, Valenza F (1995) Effects of positive end-expiratory pressure on regional distribution of tidal volume and recruitment in adult respiratory distress syndrome. Am J Respir Crit Care Med 151:1807–1814
13. Crotti S, Mascheroni D, Caironi P, et al (2001) Recruitment and derecruitment during acute respiratory failure. A clinical study. Am J Respir Crit Care Med 164:131–140
14. Puybasset L, Gusman P, Muller JC, Cluzel P, Coriat P, Rouby JJ, and the CT Scan ARDS Study Group (2000) Regional distribution of gas and tissue in acute respiratory distress syndrome. III. Consequences for the effects of positive end-expiratory pressure. Intensive Care Med 26:1215–1227
15. Gattinoni L, Pelosi P, Suter PM, Pedoto A, Vercesi P, Lissoni A (1998) Acute respiratory distress syndrome caused by pulmonary and extrapulmonary disease. Different syndromes? Am J Respir Crit Care Med 158:3–11

16. Dreyfuss D, Saumon G (1998) Ventilator induced lung injury. Lessons from experimental studies. Am J Respir Crit Care Med 157:294–323
17. International Consensus Conferences in Intensive Care Medicine (1999) Ventilator-associated lung injury in ARDS. Am J Respir Crit Care Med 160:2118–2124
18. Amato MBP, Barbas CS, Medeiros DM, et al (1998) Effect of a protective-ventilation strategy on mortality in the acute respiratory distress syndrome. N Engl J Med 338:347–354
19. The Acute Respiratory Distress Syndrome Network (2000) Ventilation with lower tidal volumes as compared with traditional tidal volumes for acute lung injury and the acute respiratory distress syndrome. N Engl J Med 342:1301–1308
20. Light RB, Mink SN, Wood LHD (1981) The effect of unilateral PEEP on gas exchange and pulmonary perfusion in canine lobar pneumonia. Anesthesiology 55:251–255
21. Nahum A, Burke WC, Ravenscraft SA, et al (1992) Lung mechanics and gas exchange during pressure-control ventilation in dogs. Augmentation of CO_2 elimination by an intratracheal catether. Am Rev Respir Dis 146:965–973
22. Nahum A, Ravenscraft SA, Nakos G, et al (1992) Tracheal gas insufflation during pressure-control ventilation. Effect of catheter position, diameter, and flow rate. Am Rev Respir Dis 146:1411–1418
23. Ravenscraft SA, Burke WC, Nahum A, et al (1993) Tracheal gas insufflation augments CO_2 clearence during mechanical ventilation. Am Rev Respir Dis 148:345–351
24. Kalfon P, Umamaheswara GS, Gallart L, Puybasset L, Coriat P, Rouby JJ (1997) Permissive hypercapnia with and without expiratory washout in patients with severe acute respiratory distress syndrome. Anesthesiology 87:6–17
25. Burke WC, Nahum A, Ravenscraft SA, et al (1993) Modes of tracheal gas insufflation. Comparison of continuous and phase-specific gas injection in normal dogs. Am Rev Respir Dis 148:562–568
26. Nakos G, Zakinthinos S, Kotanidou A, Roussos C (1994) Tracheal gas insufflation reduces the tidal volume while $PaCO_2$ is maintained constant. Intensive Care Med 20:407–413
27. Richecoeur J, Lu Q, Vieira SRR, et al (1999) Expiratory washout versus optimization of mechanical ventilation during permissive hypercapnia in patients with severe acute respiratory distress syndrome. Am J Respir Crit Care Med 160:77–85
28. Blanch L (2001) Clinical studies of tracheal gas insufflation. Respir Care 46:158–166
29. Karwande SV (1987) A new tube for single lung ventilation. Chest 92:761–763
30. Kamaya H, Krishna PR (1985) New endotracheal tube (Univent tube®) for selective blockade of one lung. Anesthesiology 63:342–343
31. Blanch L, Van der Kloot TE, Youngblood AM, et al (2001) Application of tracheal gas insufflation to acute unilateral lung injury in an experimental model. Am J Respir Crit Care Med 164:642–647
32. Tutuncü AS, Faithfull NS, Lachmann B (1993) Intratracheal perfluorocarbon administration combined with mechanical ventilation in experimental respiratory distress syndrome: dose-dependent improvement of gas exchange. Crit Care Med 21:962–969
33. Tutuncü AS, Faithfull NS, Lachmann B (1993) Comparison of ventilatory support with intratracheal perfluorocarbon administration and conventional mechanical ventilation in animals with acute respiratory failure. Am Rev Respir Dis 148:785–792
34. Hirschl RB, Pranikoff T, Wise C, et al (1996) Initial experience with partial liquid ventilation in adult patients with the acute respiratory distress syndrome. JAMA 275:383–389
35. Kirmse M, Fujino Y, Hess D, Kacmarek RM (1998) Positive end-expiratory pressure improves gas exchange and pulmonary mechanics during partial liquid ventilation. Am J Respir Crit Care Med 158:1550–1556
36. Meszaros E, Ogawa R (1997) Continuous low-flow tracheal gas insufflation during partial liquid ventilation in rabbits. Acta Anesthesiol Scand 41:861–867
37. Moomey CB, Fabian TC, Croce MA, Melton SM, Proctor KG (1998) Cardiopulmonary function after pulmonary contusion and partial liquid ventilation. J Trauma 45:283–290
38. Blanch L, Van der Kloot TE, Youngblood AM, et al (2002) Selective tracheal gas insufflation during partial liquid ventilation improve lung function in an animal model of unilateral acute lung injury. Crit Care Med (in press)

Advances in ARDS: How do they Impact Bedside Management?

C. C. dos Santos and A. S. Slutsky

▌ Introduction

Since its description 30 years ago [1], the acute respiratory distress syndrome (ARDS) has remained a very topical issue for intensivists, with a large literature ranging from the molecular basis of the disease and underlying physiology to the quality of life of survivors. Despite recent advances, the mortality of this syndrome remains 40 to 50% [2, 3]. Part of the difficulty in developing effective therapies is the heterogeneous nature of the disease and its complex pathophysiology. For the most part, the literature on the management of ARDS seems to converge on two basic principles: 1) preventing further injury improves outcomes; and 2) basic initial management strategies have a larger impact on outcome than 'salvage' therapies. To a certain extent, these concepts are reflected in the results of all the trials carried out to date. This is not surprising. ARDS is not a disease but a syndrome, characterized by a severe localized inflammatory reaction. Most patients who die with this syndrome do not die from their local disease (pulmonary hypoxemia), but rather they succumb to a systemic inflammatory reaction that ultimately leads to diffuse organ failure. Consequently, it makes sense conceptually that all the approaches directed towards preventing loss of pulmonary compartmentalization of the inflammatory reaction could improve patient outcome, versus salvage therapies that are instituted later in the course of the disease – the proverbial "horse is out of the barn" concept. This idea underscores the fundamental importance of early recognition and appropriate aggressive management of the ARDS patient.

In this chapter, we will review some of the recent advances in the ventilatory management of the ARDS patient and how these impact on the bedside management of these patients. The idea is to provide the bedside intensivist with a critical approach to address acute hypoxemia in the ARDS patient. Many recent reviews dealing with therapies for ARDS have been published and we will not duplicate the excellent information published previously [4–10]. In this chapter we will discuss important controversies in the identification and bedside ventilatory management of the ARDS patient. This review is not designed to address the more advanced management of ARDS (high frequency oscillation, partial liquid ventilation, extracorporeal membrane, etc) or pharmacotherapy for ARDS (ketoconazole, steroids, surfactants, etc) and the reader is directed to other sources for further information [4–10].

Defining the Problem

It was only recently that the American-European Consensus Conference (AECC) on ARDS addressed the lack of a uniform definition of the syndrome [11]. The criteria proposed by the AECC are shown in Table 1.

Although these criteria provide us with the rudimentary tools to recognize the syndrome, concerns have been raised about their sensibility. It has been felt that the AECC criteria are vague and therefore unreliable. The sensibility of any clinical index encompasses face validity and content validity as well as other qualitative aspects of an instrument. Appropriate measurement evaluation of this important component has not been formally performed on the standard ARDS definition put forth by the AECC. Ferguson et al. [12] have recently developed a modified clinical definition of ARDS derived using the Delphi technique (Table 2).

A comparison testing of the sensibility of the two clinical ARDS criteria was presented at the American Thoracic Society meeting this year and the authors concluded that the revised criteria might have improved sensibility [12].

Since the AECC, a number of reports have used the AECC definition to look at the incidence and prevalence of ARDS in the intensive care unit (ICU). Luhr et al. [13] published an 8 week prospective cohort trial including 132 ICUs in Denmark, Sweden and Iceland (11.74 million people over the age of 15). This group reviewed all the admissions (n=13 346) and found that the incidence of ARDS was 13.5 patients per 100 000/year, representing 18% of the entire ventilated population. The 90-day mortality of the ARDS patients in this study was 41.2%. In the same year, Roupie et al. [14] evaluated the prevalence of ARDS among hypoxemic patients requiring mechanical ventilation. All patients entering 36 ICUs during a 14-day period were screened prospectively. Hypoxemic patients, defined as having a PaO_2/FiO_2 ratio of 300 mmHg or less and receiving mechanical ventilation were assessed. ARDS accounted for 6.9% of all ICU admissions (n=976 patients) and was present in 31.5% of all hypoxemic ventilated patients. The mortality of these ARDS patients was 60%.

Table 1. ARDS criteria proposed by the American-European Consensus Conference [11]

1. Onset	Acute
2. Clinical Setting	Predisposing condition
3. Gas exchange	$PaO_2/FiO_2 < 200$ mmHg (< 26.7 kPa) regardless of the positive end-expiratory pressure (PEEP) level
4. Chest X-ray	Bilateral Infiltrates
5. Wedge pressure	≤ 18 mmHg

Table 2. ARDS criteria derived by Delphi technique [12]

1. $PaO_2/FiO_2 < 200$ mmHg (< 26.7 kPa) with PEEP ≥ 10 cmH$_2$O
2. Onset < 72 h
3. Airspace disease in ≥ 2 quadrants on chest X-ray
4. Non-cardiogenic origin AND
5. Static lung compliance < 50 ml/cm OR
6. Recognized predisposing factor

▌ The Ventilatory Management of the ARDS Patient

The primary objective of conventional strategies of mechanical ventilation is to maintain normal levels of oxygen and carbon dioxide in the blood, and/or to decrease the energy costs of breathing. Traditionally, this was achieved through the delivery of supra-physiologic tidal volumes (VT) (10–15 ml/kg, which contrasts with the normal resting volume of 4–7 ml/kg). Over the past two decades, evidence from animal and human studies has made it clear that this approach to the management of ARDS contributes to the unacceptably high mortality rates of patients with this syndrome. This seems to be mostly secondary to the iatrogenic complications of ventilation *per se*. In this chapter, we will focus on the clinical evidence in support for lung protective approaches in the management of the ARDS patient.

There are two main approaches to lung protective ventilatory strategies. The first is based on 'permissive hypercapnia'. This strategy was introduced in 1990 and involves limiting tidal volume and airway pressures while disregarding hypercapnia to avoid lung injury. The second is an 'open lung' strategy, which focuses on the use of recruitment maneuvers and positive end-expiratory pressure (PEEP) to open alveoli and keep them opened at a safe level – thus avoiding both overdistention and shear stress from repeated opening and closing of the alveoli. Numerous excellent reviews have been written on this topic over the past few years [4, 5]. We will limit our discussion to highlighting some important points regarding the current state of the evidence.

Strategies for improving hypoxemia in the ventilated patient have generally relied on increasing the inspired oxygen fraction (FiO_2), increasing PEEP, changing the inspiratory to expiratory time ratio (I:E ratio) and optimizing oxygen carrying capacity (hemoglobin level). In this review, we will not discuss these previously well understood approaches (except for the use of PEEP) but will rather look at the more current approaches to the management of the hypoxemic patient including the use of recruitment maneuvers, inhaled nitric oxide (NO), and the prone position. For a review of inverse ratio ventilation, fluid management and vaso-agonist use in the resuscitation of the ARDS patient please see [4, 5].

Over the past decade, major changes in thinking in relation to ventilatory strategies for ARDS patients have occurred. Knowledge that ARDS was not a homogeneous process, but rather an inhomogeneous phenomenon characterized by a reduction in functional alveolar units has shed new light into the concept of ventilator induced lung injury (VILI) [15]. The principals of limiting VILI are illustrated by the examination of the pressure-volume curve (PV curve) of the lung. Matamis et al. [16] used bedside determinations of the PV curve to characterize the abnormalities in pulmonary mechanics in patients with ARDS. With pressure plotted on the x-axis and volume on the y-axis the curve has a sigmoidal shape, which tends to flatten above and below the bends – defining the upper and lower inflection points, respectively. Initial concepts were that end-inspiratory stretch above the upper inflection point (UIP) might lead to alveolar over-distention. As well, allowing end-expiratory pressure to fall below the lower inflection point (LIP) would cause alveoli to collapse and re-open repeatedly. However, there are many caveats to this simple model of recruitment since it is clear that recruitment continues to take place all along the linear portion of the PV curve beyond the upper and lower inflection points. Nevertheless, what seems to be apparent is that volutrauma and atelectrauma play a major role in VILI.

Pressure Control versus Volume Control

Once patients with ARDS are intubated, the first question that arises is which mode of ventilation should be used? A decade ago an editorial by Marini and Kelsen [17] emphasized the need for prospective control trials comparing pressure control (PC) and volume control (VC) ventilation at fixed transalveolar pressures in ARDS patients. Since then, three prospective randomized trails comparing PCV and VCV have been published. Lessard et al. [18] compared nine patients with ARDS treated with either PCV or VCV – while keeping both the level of ventilation and PEEP constant. This group found no difference in respiratory mechanics, hemodynamics, or gas exchange parameters between the two groups. Rappaport et al. [19] prospectively compared early application of PCV and VCV in 27 patients with acute hypoxic respiratory failure and found that PCV was associated with a more rapid increase in static compliance and fewer days of mechanical ventilation in patients who survived and were extubated.

Esteban et al. [20] carried out a multicenter randomized trail of seventy-nine ARDS patients ventilated with either PCV (n=37) or VCV (n=42). In both instances, inspiratory plateau pressures were limited to ≤35 cmH$_2$O. The main finding of this study was that, in ARDS patients, decreasing either tidal volume on VCV or inspiratory pressure on PCV, to reduce inspiratory plateau pressures, did not independently influence mortality. Moreover, this group found that the mortality of ARDS patients is strongly associated with the development of multi-organ failure (MOF) and that neither strategy is particularly better at preventing this complication. One of the key issues in these trials is that they were underpowered; consequently no definitive conclusions regarding the significance of controlling pressure versus volume may be drawn.

Pressure and/or Volume Limited Ventilation (PVLV) in ARDS

Conflicting results have been obtained from five randomized controlled trials (RCTs) evaluating similar PVLV strategies in ALI patients where mortality was the primary end-point [21–25]. Of these, the best powered study was the ARDS network trial that examined 861 patients randomly assigned to PVLV (VT 6 ml/kg predicted body weight; plateau pressure <30 cmH$_2$O) or conventional ventilation (VT 12 ml/kg predicted body weight; plateau pressure <50 cmH$_2$O). In this study, PVLV was associated with a mortality reduction from 39.8% in the control group to 31% in the experimental group (RR 0.75; 95% CI 0.62–0.91). Pooled results of all four published RCTs (Brower et al.'s trial [24] is in abstract form only) yield a relative risk (RR) of mortality associated with PVLV of 0.87 (95% CI 0.75–1.01). Based on the data reported in the NIH trial [21] – the attributable mortality of VILI is approximately 22% (relative risk reduction in mortality between the high and low volume ventilatory strategies). This sobering thought underscores both the vital importance of VILI in determining patient outcome and the importance of current and future research in determining the clinically appropriate choice of ventilatory strategy in the management of ventilated patients. A summary of the five trials is presented in Table 3.

It is difficult to reconcile the discrepancies in the results of the ARDS/Net study with earlier clinical trials evaluating a lung volume restriction strategy because the ARDS/Net study differed in several ways making a direct comparison difficult: (i) the method of determining predicted body weight (and hence tidal volume) was

Table 3. Clinical trials of lung-protective ventilation in acute respiratory distress syndrome (ARDS)

Study	Number of patients	Target VT PLV	Target VT CMV	Mean VT achieved (ml/kg) PLV	Mean VT achieved (ml/kg) CMV	Adjusted[h] VT in CMV group[g] MBW[c]	Adjusted[h] VT in CMV group[g] PBW[d]	Target pressure (cmH2O) PLV	Target pressure (cmH2O) CMV	Mean pressure achieved (cmH2O) PLV	Mean pressure achieved (cmH2O) CMV	PEEP (cmH2O) PLV	PEEP (cmH2O) CMV	Primary outcome measures	Results PLV	Results CMV
Stewart et al. [22]	120	≤8 IBW[e] ml/kg	10–15 ml/kg	6.8	10.1[a]	10.2	12.2	P_{peak} ≤30	P_{peak} 50	P_{peak} 24.3 / $P_{plateau}$ 20.0	P_{peak} 33.5 / $P_{plateau}$ 28.6[a]	9.6	8.0[a]	In-hospital mortality	50%	47%
Brower et al. [24]	52	5–8 PBW ml/kg	10–12 PBW ml/kg	7.3	10.2	8.2	10.2	$P_{plateau}$ <30	45–55	24.9	$P_{plateau}$ 30.6[b]	Numbers not given	Numbers not given	Several	50%	46%
Brochard et al. [23]	116	6–10 DBW[f] ml/kg	10–15 ml/kg	7.4	10.7[a]	9.4	11.3	$P_{plateau}$ ≤25	≤60	24.5	30.5[a]	9.6	8.5[a]	60 day mortality	46.6%	37.9%
Amato et al. [25]	53	≤6 MBW ml/kg	12 MBW ml/kg	387 ml	738 ml	–	–	P_{peak} 20–40 / $P_{plateau}$ 23.9	no limit / $P_{plateau}$ 37.8	P_{peak} 24.0	P_{peak} 45.5	13.2	9.3	28 day mortality	38% (p<0.001)	71%
ARDS Net [21]	861	6 PBW ml/kg	12 PBW ml/kg	6.5	11.4	9.8	11.8	P_{peak} <30	50	26 vs. 37	26 vs. 37	8.1	9.1	Death	31.0% (p=0.007)	39.8%

VT: tidal volume; PLV: protective lung strategy; CMV: conventional mechanical ventilation
a Mean values at day 7
b Average daily mean values
c MBW: measured body weight
d PBW: predicted body weight: male PBW (kg)=50+2.3 [(height in inches)−60]; female PBW (kg)=45+2.3 [(height in inches)−60]
e IBW: IBW=25×[(height in meters)²]
f DBW: DBW=measured weight minus estimated gain from water and salt retention
g Values based on mean VT as reported
h Adjusted VT: please see Thompson BT et al (2001) Chest 120(5):1622−1627

different from earlier trials; (ii) patients in the low tidal volume groups had high respiratory rates which may have contributed to significant auto-PEEP – in turn leading to improved alveolar patency or recruitment; (iii) the use of bicarbonate to correct respiratory acidosis may have reduced the need for dialysis and/or potential detrimental effects of hypercapnic acidosis; and (iv) the difference in tidal volume (and airway pressures) between control and the treatment groups was greater than in the other trials, hence increasing the signal/noise ratio.

The study by Amato et al. [25] evaluating PVLV strategies in the management of ARDS has opened the door to a variety of interesting questions about the ventilatory management of ARDS patients. Specifically, this study alludes to the importance of maintaining an 'open lung' strategy. This group randomly assigned 53 patients to an experimental intervention that combined a strategy employing high PEEP based on the use of the pressure-volume group, and a lung recruitment maneuver, to conventional ventilation. The lung-recruitment maneuver consisted of a 40 second sustained inflation at 35 to 40 cmH_2O. To determine the level of PEEP for patients in the experimental arm, they constructed static PV curves, identified the LIP on the inflation limb, and set PEEP at 2 cmH_2O above this point, using, on average, 16 cmH_2O. This procedure was performed once per patient on the day of randomization to determine PEEP for the duration of mechanical ventilation. Investigators observed quicker recovery of lung function (PaO_2/FiO_2 ratio; lung compliance) and a statistically significant reduction in 28-day mortality (11/29 deaths in experimental patients, 17/74 in controls, RR 0.53; 95% CI 0.31–0.91) for patients exposed to the experimental strategy. Although the positive results associated with this experimental ventilation strategy may be attributed in part to PVLV, given what we know about the alveolar mechanics of the injured lungs, Amato's additional use of liberal PEEP and periodic lung recruitment maneuvers offered additional benefit to study patients in the experimental arm This study however has been criticized for the high mortality rate (exceeding 60%) in the control arm, and the high rate of pneumothoraces in the treatment arm (42%).

Of note, PVLV is not devoid of complications. Limiting tidal volumes can result in progressive alveolar collapse, a reduction in FRC, higher oxygen requirements, and elevation in PCO_2. Thus, the gains achieved by avoiding over-distention injury must be balanced by an increase in shearing injury (if more lung units collapse and re-open) and oxygen toxicity, in addition to potential adverse effects of hypercapnia. One possible deleterious effect of hypercapnia in acute lung injury (ALI) is acute renal failure as suggested by laboratory studies as well as a significant increase in the use of dialysis in an RCT of PVLV conducted by our group (22 versus 8%; relative risk [RR] 2.75; p=0.05) [26].

Based on the physiologic rationale, the results of experimental animal studies, and the positive findings reported by Amato et al. [25] there is a suggestion that additional strategies can overcome the adverse effects of PVLV. For this reason, recent trials have tried to incorporate an open lung strategy to the ventilatory management of ARDS. Strategies that recruit the lung (PEEP, lung recruitment maneuvers and prone position) have been shown, in animal models, to be effective in limiting VILI. Presumably, this is because they aid in achieving oxygenation/ventilation in the 'safe-zone' of the PV curve and hence reduce exposure to injurious mechanical forces [27].

The Role of PEEP

One of the first studies to examine the role of PEEP in effectively 'splinting' open the lung was described in 1963 [28]. This approach involves applying PEEP above an ill-defined, and ever-changing 'critical closing pressure' thus maintaining the lung open. Gattinoni et al. [15] have provided direct evidence of alveolar recruitment with PEEP in patients with ARDS using CT scans. Controlled animal studies show that PEEP can prevent VILI. The results of clinical case series [29] and physiologic studies [30] support a role for high PEEP to maintain lung volumes and reduce VILI. In these studies high PEEP increased lung volumes and improved lung compliance, allowing ventilation at lower airway pressures. Clinically, one of the major problems is how best to evaluate alveolar recruitment at the bedside (see [31]).

Two RCTs have evaluated a role for PEEP, alone, in patients with early ALI. In one study 92 patients were assigned to conventional ventilation using PEEP of zero or 10 cmH$_2$O [32]. There was no apparent effect on the rate of progression of ALI to ARDS (RR 0.92; 95% CI 0.43–2.0), but there were trends toward greater 72 hour recovery from ALI (RR 1.6; 95% CI 0.91–3.0), a lower incidence of major air leaks in patients ventilated with PEEP (RR 0.86; 95% CI 0.53–1.4), and lower mortality (RR 0.79; 95% CI 0.41–1.5). In a related study, Weigelt et al. [33] randomly assigned patients with high risk of ARDS to 'early' PEEP (immediate PEEP at 5 cmH$_2$O) or 'late' PEEP (applied only when required to correct hypoxemia of PaO$_2$ <60 mmHg) [33]. Investigators reported a lower incidence of ARDS (RR 0.38; 95% CI 0.18–0.77) and fewer pulmonary deaths (RR 0.37; 95% CI 0.12–1.1) with early PEEP. Therefore, both studies support the use of PEEP in ALI, however, the relevance of these RCTs to this discussion is limited by what are now considered low levels of PEEP in the 'high' PEEP groups.

Not all PEEP is good however. In a study involving six patients with ALI, the use of PEEP of 13 cmH$_2$O resulted in the recruitment of non-aerated portions of the lung, with a gain of 320 ml in volume, but three patients were believed to have overdistention of already aerated portions of lung, with excess volume of 288 ml [34]. It has been suggested that about 30% of patients with ALI do not benefit from PEEP or have a fall in the partial pressure of oxygen [35–37]. With the patient in the supine position, PEEP generally recruits the regions of the lung closest to the apex and sternum (as opposed to the dependent zones most affected by ARDS) [35]. Moreover, patients who have a primary etiology for their ARDS (pulmonary cause) do not seem to respond to lung recruitment maneuvers as well, when compared with patients with secondary ARDS (non-pulmonary cause) [38].

Moreover, there is no consensus as to what level of PEEP should be used. Some experts have recommended bedside calculations of the PV curve prior to setting PEEP – once the LIP is known, PEEP is set at least 2 cmH$_2$O above that value. This may not necessarily be the best strategy for a variety of reasons: (1) recruitment occurs through the length of the PV curve (including above and below the upper and lower inflection points), (2) the static measurement of the PV curve may not reflect its dynamic variations (over the course of time), and (3) calculating the PV curve is logistically difficult, technically demanding, and may be associated with risks to the patient. The basic point is that the notion that the lower bend in the PV curve signals the level of PEEP necessary to prevent end-expiratory collapse and that pressures above the upper bend signal alveolar overdistension is a gross oversimplification. The relationship between the shape of the PV curve and events at the alveolar level is confounded by numerous factors and is the subject of on-going research and debate. In spite of this controversy, in practice, the common denominator of the results of all studies of PV curve and lung compliance analyses suggest the use of PEEP. What is more, a level of PEEP higher than what is used in conventional strategies, and perhaps as high as 20 cmH$_2$O is believed to help maintain alveolar recruitment for the vast majority of patients with severe ALI [39].

Lung Recruitment Maneuvers

Another strategy to increase FRC is to use periodic lung recruitment maneuvers. The idea is that without periodic inflations there is a progressive fall in compliance during prolonged mechanical ventilation (please see [40, 41] for a comprehensive physiologic review of alveolar recruitment). A common approach to performing recruitment maneuvers involves the application of moderately increased levels of pressure for relatively short periods of time (in the range of 40 seconds), the goal being to open atelectatic alveoli and to stabilize those alveoli that open and close with each respiratory cycle – thus reversing derecruitment and the deterioration in compliance [42]. Shorter inspiratory times do not seem to be enough to recruit more alveolar units [43]. Theoretically, once these units are open, their mechanical properties change so that they may remain open for an undetermined period of time. A key issue, however, is that sufficient PEEP is required to maintain the lung recruited.

Animal studies seem to support the use of lung recruitment maneuvers for the prevention of VILI [44]. Lung recruitment maneuvers have been found to produce physiologic benefits in anesthesia-induced atelectasis [45], and in the setting of high frequency oscillation in pediatric respiratory failure [46]. Moreover, Engelmann et al. [47] observed significant improvements in oxygenation in 13 patients with ARDS by increasing the peak inspiratory pressure by 10 cmH$_2$O every 3 minutes to a mean pressure of 61 cmH$_2$O. Complications during the procedure included transient mild oxyhemoglobin desaturation and hypotension.

In a recent study in humans, the effect of a lung recruitment maneuver on oxygenation over four hours in 12 critically ill patients with severe ALI was evaluated. In this study, Lapinsky and colleagues [26] individualized the inflation pressure by utilizing the lesser of: i) 45 cmH$_2$O, or ii) the peak pressure while ventilated at 12 ml/kg tidal volume, and maintained inflation pressures, which varied from 30 to 45 mmH$_2$O, for 20 seconds. In these patients, there was a modest fall in arterial oxygen saturation (SaO$_2$) (mean 2%) and a modest fall in blood pressure at the end of the lung recruitment maneuver, followed by a mean rise in SaO$_2$ by 6% within 5 minutes (p < 0.001). In eight of the 12 patients, this improvement lasted for at least 4 hours. In the remaining four patients, a repeat lung recruitment maneuver increased SaO$_2$ again, and the effect was sustained in three patients with the use of higher PEEP.

Prone Positioning in ARDS

Most patients with ARDS have an increase in the partial pressure of oxygen when they are changed from the supine to the prone position. In the prone position, there is a decrease in the vertical gradient of lung inflation. By decreasing the compressive force acting on the dorsal lung area, prone position decreases dependent pleural pressure, increases dependent transpulmonary pressure, and consequently, may recruit the dorsal lung into participating in gas exchange [48]. Pappert et al. [49] confirmed the effect of prone position on lung recruitment in patients with ARDS. Using the multiple inert gas elimination technique they demonstrated that the improvement in PaO_2 in the prone position was the result of a reduction in pulmonary shunt blood flow and an increase in blood flow to normal ventilation-perfusion regions. Other theories regarding the mechanism of improved oxygenation in the prone position include increase in end-expiratory lung volume [50] and alterations in chest wall mechanics [51].

Renewed interest in prone position for lung recruitment in ARDS has come about due to observations made by Gattinoni et al. [52] and Langer et al. [53] that in some patients with ARDS proning resulted in a decrease in CT scan densities in dorsal lung regions and improvements in oxygenation. The most recent studies on proning however, have shown that not all patients respond to proning. Response rates in these recent studies range from 60 to 100%. The large variation in response rates may relate to the amount of recruitable tissue or the etiology of the ARDS. In general, responders show an immediate improvement in oxygenation (within the first 10 min). Gattinoni et al. [54] have recently published the results of a large multicenter controlled trial of the effects of prone position in patients with ARDS. This study showed that there was no significant difference in mortality between patients randomly assigned to placement in the prone position and those assigned to conventional treatment. The authors studied more than 300 patients, yet this may still have been an underpowered study. Other explanations for why this trial did not show a benefit in the treatment arm despite the improved oxygenation in the prone position arm of the study may relate to the duration of therapy. Patients were placed prone for 7.0 hours per day. Thus patients may have been exposed to the deleterious effects of injurious ventilation the other 70% of their time each day [55]. The authors also limited the study to 10 days, which may be too short a period for any significant long-term benefit to occur. Despite these discouraging results, *post hoc* analysis showed that placing patients in the prone position reduces mortality at day 10 in the quartile of patients who were the most ill [54].

The results of Gattinoni's trial underscore the need for further investigation of the role of prone position for longer periods of time in the most severely affected ARDS patients.

▍Nitric Oxide in ARDS

The hope that NO would not only improve oxygenation, but also allow for less intense mechanical ventilation and a reduction in FiO_2, both effects potentially leading to a reduction in VILI, originated with Rossaint et al.'s [56] description of a reduction in venous admixture inhalation in nine patients with ARDS. Unfortunately, clinical trials of NO in adults have illustrated how the response to therapy may be only transient or not present at all.

In the pediatric literature NO has been shown to reduce the need for extracorporeal membrane oxygenation (ECMO) in both persistent pulmonary hypertension of the newborn [57] and respiratory failure of the newborn [58]. In contrast, a large adult RCT was not able to show an added benefit to survival or reduction in the duration of mechanical ventilation with inhaled NO therapy. Dellinger et al. [59] studied 177 patients with ARDS who were randomized to placebo or one of five doses of inhaled NO. Despite initial improvement in venous admixture in the inhaled NO group, no benefits were observed after 72 h compared to placebo. Moreover, only 60% of the patients in the inhaled NO group actually responded to the therapy (defined as a >20% increase in PaO_2). Surprisingly, 25% of the patients had a positive response to the placebo. Because perhaps only the subgroup of patients that respond to inhaled NO are likely to benefit from the therapy, Lundin et al. [61] performed a large randomized multicenter control trial enrolling only patients who had ARDS and who responded acutely to inhaled NO [60]. A total of 180 patients were randomized to either inhaled NO or placebo. There was no difference in 30-day mortality (40% in controls and 44% for inhaled NO), nor did inhaled NO significantly reverse ALI. Analysis of the data from this trial did suggest that the likelihood of developing severe ARDS was smaller in the inhaled NO group.

At present, most ICUs use inhaled NO in patients with refractory hypoxemia and who are *in extremis*. There is no current evidence to support the use of inhaled NO as 'salvage' therapy. Dupont et al. [61] recently performed a 2-year multicenter retrospective analysis of all consecutive ARDS patients in whom inhaled NO was tried – to determine if the response to inhaled NO as salvage therapy was an independent factor for survival. This group found that the efficacy of inhaled NO in improving oxygenation was moderate and difficult to predict, response to NO inhalation was not associated with prognosis, and treatment of ARDS with inhaled NO did not influence ICU survival.

One possible explanation for the failure of recent studies to demonstrate a mortality benefit with inhaled NO – despite clear evidence of improved physiological parameters – is that NO has no effect on the underlying pathophysiology driving the acute respiratory inflammatory reaction. Cuthbertson et al. [62] randomized 32 ARDS patients who where responsive to inhaled NO (increase in their PaO_2/FiO_2 ratio ≥25%) to receive mechanical ventilation with or without inhaled NO. Patients were followed for 30 days or until death, and bronchoalveolar lavage (BAL) was performed at 0, 24 and 72 hours. NO activity was measured spectrophotometrically, and myeloperoxidase, elastase, interleukin (IL)-8, and leukotrienes were measured in the BAL fluid by enzyme immunoassay. NO synthase (NOS) activity decreased significantly and total nitrite increased in patients on inhaled NO. Other markers of inflammation in BAL fluid did not change, suggesting that inhaled NO has no effect on several markers of the inflammatory response system [62]. It is also important to note that addressing hypoxemia may not necessarily improve outcome. This again likely reflects the fact that treatment of hypoxemia does not address the underlying pathology in ARDS or VILI – which is inflammation. In fact, in the ARDS Net trial the higher tidal volume group had higher PaO_2/FiO_2 ratios in the first few days of treatment [21].

Recent evidence suggests that there may be a potential role for NO as an adjunct to other therapies for ARDS in those patients with right heart functional impairment. Rialp et al. [63] studied eight primary and seven secondary ARDS patients and compared their response to NO. This group found that only the patients that had a primarily pulmonary cause for their ARDS responded to NO. This study was not designed to look at morbidity and mortality outcomes.

▌ Primary versus Secondary ARDS – Does it Alter Management?

The American-European consensus conference [11] defined two pathogenic processes leading to ARDS: a *direct* ('primary' or 'pulmonary') insult that directly affects lung parenchyma and an *indirect* ('secondary' or 'extra-pulmonary') insult, which results from an acute systemic inflammatory reaction. The distinction was mostly speculative until Gattinoni et al. [38] reported possible differences in the underlying pathology, respiratory mechanics, and response to PEEP.

In a recent review, Gattinoni et al. [38] discuss the possible differences between primary and secondary ARDS. In terms of the pathophysiology, the current hypothesis is that a direct insult would primarily affect the pulmonary epithelium, causing activation of macrophages and subsequently the inflammatory network. Conversely, in the case of an indirect stimulus, endothelial damage predominates. Changes in the integrity of the endothelial cell membrane cause vasoactive pulmonary edema and consolidation with the generation of an inflammatory response. This putative difference in injury mechanisms may explain some of the difference in findings of primary and secondary ARDS. First, radiological studies suggest that primary ARDS is characterized by diffuse interstitial and alveolar infiltration without evidence of atelectasis, while in secondary ARDS dependent atelectasis seems to be the norm. Second, while pulmonary elastance remains within the normal range in primary ARDS, it is markedly increased in secondary ARDS. However, for the same increase in respiratory system elastance in primary ARDS, 80% is due to lung elastance, while increased intra-abdominal pressure (IAP) accounts for 55% of elastance increase in secondary ARDS [38].

The most important consequences of the different respiratory mechanics in intra-pulmonary versus extra-pulmonary ARDS is that, for a given applied airway pressure, i.e., the distending pressure of the lungs, is higher in intra-pulmonary as compared to extrapulmonary ARDS. Moreover, the potential for recruitment is greater in extra-pulmonary causes of ARDS. The finding supports the hypothesis that in primary ARDS, increasing PEEP mainly induces overstretching, while in secondary ARDS this results in recruitment. It also follows that the beneficial effects of recruitment maneuvers on oxygenation are restricted to the secondary ARDS group, since these are the patients more likely to attain a transpulmonary pressure sufficient for lung opening.

These observations seem to be supported by animal experiments. Kloot et al. [64] compared three different experimental models of lung injury during recruitment maneuvers and found that greater alveolar recruitment occurred in models of secondary ARDS as compared to primary ARDS. In contrast, Puybasset et al. [65] found a similar response to PEEP in alveolar recruitment and oxygenation in patients with intra-pulmonary or extra-pulmonary ARDS. This finding could be explained by the existence of specific differences in the study population and/or the ventilatory and clinical management through the course of the study. Another explanation is that they may simply reflect the coexistence of two insults, i.e., direct injury to the lung (for example pneumonia) and secondary inflammatory mediator induced injury as an extrapulmonary stimulus (for example, sepsis).

Two recent trials have attempted to divide patients according to the etiology of their ARDS. Rialp et al. [63] looked at eight primary pulmonary and seven secondary ARDS patients and their response to NO and prone position. Lim et al. [66] looked at 31 primary pulmonary, and 16 secondary, ARDS patients and their response to the prone position. Both studies confirmed that primary pulmonary

ARDS patients do not respond to recruitment maneuvers as markedly (but they have a more pronounced response to NO). Moreover, Desai et al. [67] have attempted to reproduce Gattinoni's findings that primary and secondary ARDS have different CT scan patterns. What this group found, however, is that typical appearances at CT were independently related to the cause of ARDS (odds ratio, 8.9; 95% CI: 1.8, 44.2; p < 0.01) but were dependent on the time from intubation. Foci of non-dependent intense parenchymal opacification were more extensive in primary ARDS than in secondary ARDS, but this finding was ascribable to differences in time to CT (after intubation) between pulmonary and extrapulmonary ARDS. These authors concluded that the differentiation between primary and secondary ARDS can, with some caveats, be based on whether the CT appearances are typical or atypical of ARDS, but not on any individual CT pattern in isolation [67].

To understand whether clinically differentiating primary versus secondary ARDS made a difference in terms of the ventilatory strategy of choice, Eisner et al. [68] examined the relative efficacy of low VT mechanical ventilation among 902 patients with different clinical risk factors for ALI/ARDS who participated in ARDS Network randomized controlled trials [67]. This group found that the clinical risk factor for ALI/ARDS was associated with substantial variation in mortality. Despite these differences in mortality, there was no evidence that the efficacy of the low VT strategy varied by clinical risk factor (p = 0.76, for interaction between ventilator group and risk factor). Visual inspection of the data suggested that only individuals with ARDS secondary to aspiration may not have benefited from low VT ventilation (this was not statistically significant). There was also no evidence of differential efficacy of low VT ventilation in the other study outcomes: proportion of patients achieving unassisted breathing, ventilator-free days, or development of non-pulmonary organ failure. Controlling for demographic and clinical covariates did not appreciably affect these results. After reclassifying the clinical risk factors as pulmonary versus non-pulmonary predisposing conditions and infection-related versus non-infection-related conditions, there was still no evidence that the efficacy of low VT ventilation differed among clinical risk factor subgroups. They thus concluded that there was no evidence that the efficacy of the low VT ventilation strategy differed among clinical risk factor subgroups for ALI/ARDS [68]. However, the study was not designed or powered to detect a difference between primary or secondary ARDS. Given the methodological concerns, the more clinically relevant question is what is the likelihood that this strategy would benefit any ARDS patient. Using Bayesian subset analysis this group calculated that there is a 75% chance that this strategy should benefit patients in different ARDS risk factor groups. Again, this finding may reflect the pathophysiology of the syndrome (how the lung responds to injury) or its complications (VILI).

■ Understanding the Development of MOF in ARDS Patients

Because patients who die with ARDS do not die from hypoxemia, but rather from MOF, it was initially unclear why strategies that reduce the severity of hypoxemia and VILI could lead to a reduction in mortality. Over the past decade, it has become clear that even in the absence of overt structural damage, the lung responds to mechanical stretch/stress by producing pro-inflammatory mediators [69]. Recent work also suggests that in addition to acting locally, these pro-inflammatory mediators may escape the confines of the lung to either generate or propagate the systemic inflammatory reaction characteristic of VILI [70, 71]. Chiumello et al. [72] examined the hypothesis that injurious ventilatory strategies (large VT and/or low PEEP) would increase release of inflammatory mediators into the lung and into the systemic circulation in a lung injury model. Using an *in vivo* lung injury model this group showed that injurious ventilatory strategies are associated with the release of cytokines into the systemic circulation, a finding that may have relevance for the development of MOF in patients with ARDS [72].

In a prospective randomized trial, Ranieri et al. [73] randomized patients with ARDS to receive a conventional ventilation strategy (to keep $PaCO_2$ between 35–40 mmHg) or a lung protective strategy using a VT and PEEP level based on individual PV curves. Patients in the conventional group had an increase in both systemic and lung lavage concentrations of inflammatory cytokines. After 36 hours randomization, the inflammatory mediators were significantly lower in the lung-protection group. In further studies the same group showed that the level of inflammatory mediators correlated with the incidence of MOF in ARDS patients [74]. Further evidence in support of biotrauma comes from the ARDS Net trial. In this study the plasma level of IL-6 was noted to be lower in the intervention arm in comparison with the control group [21]. Consequently, lung protection strategies may achieve their benefit through reduction in the systemic release of inflammatory mediators and the frequency and severity of MOF.

▌Conclusions

So much is still to be learned in the field of critical care. The future abounds with exciting questions and new tools and strategies to help us answer them. We have already learned a number of lessons. First, our patients are critically ill and they require prompt and expeditious institution of appropriate care. This is more than ever true for the ARDS patient. An interesting study would be to randomize patients to a strategy of 'immediate care' versus 'conventional medical care'. Early recognition and intervention may be the best way to reduce morbidity and mortality in these patients. Second, strategies that minimize further injury tend to protect patients from the loss of pulmonary compartmentalization and subsequent systemic complications. Third, no one single approach will prove sufficient in the care of these patients. Combination approaches, tailored to the needs of each individual patient, based on sound pathophysiological basis, will probably emerge as a consequence of our increased understanding of this complex syndrome.

References

1. Ashbaugh DG, Bigelow DB, Petty TL, Levine BE (1967) Acute respiratory distress in adults. Lancet 2:319–323
2. Zilberberg MD, Epstein SK (1998) Acute lung injury in the medical ICU: comorbid conditions, age, etiology, and hospital outcome. Am J Respir Crit Care Med 157:1159–1164
3. Doyle RL, Szaflarski N, Modin GW, Wiener-Kronish JP, Matthay MA (1995) Identification of patients with acute lung injury. Predictors of mortality. Am J Respir Crit Care Med 152:1818–1824
4. Brower RG, Ware LB, Berthiaume Y, Matthay MA (2001) Treatment of ARDS. Chest 120:1347–1367
5. McIntyre RC, Jr., Pulido EJ, Bensard DD, Shames BD, Abraham E (2000) Thirty years of clinical trials in acute respiratory distress syndrome. Crit Care Med 28:3314–3331

6. Lee WL, Detsky AS, Stewart TE (2000) Lung-protective mechanical ventilation strategies in ARDS. Intensive Care Med 26:1151–1155
7. Marini JJ, Amato MB (2000) Lung recruitment during ARDS. Minerva Anestesiol 66:314–319
8. Brochard L, Brun-Buisson C (1999) Clinical trials in acute respiratory distress syndrome: what is ARDS? Crit Care Med 27:1657–1658
9. Nerlich S (1998) Critical care management of the patient with acute respiratory distress syndrome (ARDS). Part 2 – A review of modes and strategies for ventilating the patient with poorly compliant lungs. Aust Crit Care 11:93–98
10. Nerlich S (1997) Critical care management of the patient with acute respiratory distress syndrome (ARDS). Part 1: Pathophysiology and implications for mechanical ventilation. Aust Crit Care 10:49–54
11. Bernard GR, Artigas A, Brigham KL, et al (1994) The American-European Consensus Conference on ARDS. Definitions, mechanisms, relevant outcomes, and clinical trial coordination. Am J Respir Crit Care Med 149:818–824
12. Ferguson ND, Davis AM, Chan CK, Slutsky AS, Detsky AS, Stewart TE (2001) Comparison testing of the sensibility of two clinical definitions of the acute respiratory distress syndrome. Am J Respir Crit Care Med 163:A449 (Abst)
13. Luhr OR, Antonsen K, Karlsson M, et al (1999) Incidence and mortality after acute respiratory failure and acute respiratory distress syndrome in Sweden, Denmark, and Iceland. The ARF Study Group. Am J Respir Crit Care Med 159:1849–1861
14. Roupie E, Lepage E, Wysocki M, et al (1999) Prevalence, etiologies and outcome of the acute respiratory distress syndrome among hypoxemic ventilated patients. SRLF Collaborative Group on Mechanical Ventilation. Societe de Reanimation de Langue Francaise. Intensive Care Med 25:920–929
15. Gattinoni L, Presenti A, Torresin A, et al (1986) Adult respiratory distress syndrome profiles by computed tomography. J Thorac Imaging 1:25–30
16. Matamis D, Lemaire F, Harf A, Brun-Buisson C, Ansquer JC, Atlan G (1984) Total respiratory pressure-volume curves in the adult respiratory distress syndrome. Chest 86:58–66
17. Marini JJ, Kelsen SG (1992) Re-targeting ventilatory objectives in adult respiratory distress syndrome. New treatment prospects–persistent questions. Am Rev Respir Dis 146:2–3
18. Lessard MR, Guerot E, Lorino H, Lemaire F, Brochard L (1994) Effects of pressure-controlled with different I:E ratios versus volume- controlled ventilation on respiratory mechanics, gas exchange, and hemodynamics in patients with adult respiratory distress syndrome. Anesthesiology 80:983–991
19. Rappaport SH, Shpiner R, Yoshihara G, Wright J, Chang P, Abraham E (1994) Randomized, prospective trial of pressure-limited versus volume- controlled ventilation in severe respiratory failure. Crit Care Med 22:22–32
20. Esteban A, Alia I, Gordo F, et al (2000) Prospective randomized trial comparing pressure-controlled ventilation and volume-controlled ventilation in ARDS. For the Spanish Lung Failure Collaborative Group. Chest 117:1690–1696
21. Acute Respiratory Distress Syndrome Network (2000) Ventilation with lower tidal volumes as compared with traditional tidal volumes for acute lung injury and the acute respiratory distress syndrome. N Engl J Med 342:1301–1308
22. Stewart TE, Meade MO, Cook DJ, et al (1998) Evaluation of a ventilation strategy to prevent barotrauma in patients at high risk for acute respiratory distress syndrome. Pressure- and Volume-Limited Ventilation Strategy Group. N Engl J Med 338:355–361
23. Brochard L, Roudot-Thoraval F, Roupie E, et al (1998) Tidal volume reduction for prevention of ventilator-induced lung injury in acute respiratory distress syndrome. The Multicenter Trail Group on Tidal Volume reduction in ARDS. Am J Respir Crit Care Med 158:1831–1838
24. Brower R, Shanholtz C, Shade D, et al. (2001) Randomized trial of small tidal volume ventilation (STV) in ARDS. Am J Respir Crit Care Med 155:A93 (Abst)
25. Amato MB, Barbas CS, Medeiros DM, et al (1998) Effect of a protective-ventilation strategy on mortality in the acute respiratory distress syndrome. N Engl J Med 338:347–354

26. Lapinsky SE, Aubin M, Mehta S, Boiteau P, Slutsky AS (1999) Safety and efficacy of a sustained inflation for alveolar recruitment in adults with respiratory failure. Intensive Care Med 25:1297–1301

27. Froese AB (1997) High-frequency oscillatory ventilation for adult respiratory distress syndrome: let's get it right this time! Crit Care Med 25:906–908

28. Bendixen HH, Hedley-Whyre J, Laver MB (1963) Improved oxygenation in surgical patients during general anesthesia with controlled ventilation. N Engl J Med 263:991–996

29. DiRusso SM, Nelson LD, Safcsak K, Miller RS (1995) Survival in patients with severe adult respiratory distress syndrome treated with high-level positive end-expiratory pressure. Crit Care Med 23:1485–1496

30. Ranieri VM, Mascia L, Fiore T, Bruno F, Brienza A, Giuliani R (1995) Cardiorespiratory effects of positive end-expiratory pressure during progressive tidal volume reduction (permissive hypercapnia) in patients with acute respiratory distress syndrome. Anesthesiology 83:710–720

31. Brochard L (2001) Watching what PEEP really does. Am J Respir Crit Care Med 163:1291–1292

32. Pepe PE, Hudson LD, Carrico CJ (1984) Early application of positive end-expiratory pressure in patients at risk for the adult respiratory-distress syndrome. N Engl J Med 311:281–286

33. Weigelt JA, Mitchell RA, Snyder WH, III (1979) Early positive end-expiratory pressure in the adult respiratory distress syndrome. Arch Surg 114:497–501

34. Vieira SR, Puybasset L, Richecoeur J, et al (1998) A lung computed tomographic assessment of positive end-expiratory pressure-induced lung overdistension. Am J Respir Crit Care Med 158:1571–1577

35. Puybasset L, Cluzel P, Chao N, Slutsky AS, Coriat P, Rouby JJ (1998) A computed tomography scan assessment of regional lung volume in acute lung injury. The CT Scan ARDS Study Group. Am J Respir Crit Care Med 158:1644–1655

36. Horton WG, Cheney FW (1975) Variability of effect of positive end expiratory pressure. Arch Surg 110:395–398

37. Kanarek DJ, Shannon DC (1975) Adverse effect of positive end-expiratory pressure on pulmonary perfusion and arterial oxygenation. Am Rev Respir Dis 112:457–459

38. Gattinoni L, Pelosi P, Suter PM, Pedoto A, Vercesi P, Lissoni A (1998) Acute respiratory distress syndrome caused by pulmonary and extrapulmonary disease. Different syndromes? Am J Respir Crit Care Med 158:3–11

39. Cereda M, Foti G, Musch G, Sparacino ME, Pesenti A (1996) Positive end-expiratory pressure prevents the loss of respiratory compliance during low tidal volume ventilation in acute lung injury patients. Chest 109:480–485

40. Kacmarek RM (2001) Strategies to optimize alveolar recruitment. Curr Opin Crit Care 7:15–20

41. Mehta S, Slutsky AS (1998) Mechanical ventilation in acute respiratory distress syndrome: evolving concepts. Monaldi Arch Chest Dis 53:647–653

42. Bond DM, Froese AB (1993) Volume recruitment maneuvers are less deleterious than persistent low lung volumes in the atelectasis-prone rabbit lung during high-frequency oscillation. Crit Care Med 21:402–412

43. Pelosi P, Bottino N, Panigada M, Eccher G, Gattinoni L (1999) [The sigh in ARDS (acute respiratory distress syndrome)]. Minerva Anestesiol 65:313–317

44. Rimensberger PC, Pristine G, Mullen BM, Cox PN, Slutsky AS (1999) Lung recruitment during small tidal volume ventilation allows minimal positive end-expiratory pressure without augmenting lung injury. Crit Care Med 27:1940–1945

45. Rothen HU, Sporre B, Engberg G, Wegenius G, Hedenstierna G (1993) Re-expansion of atelectasis during general anaesthesia: a computed tomography study. Br J Anaesth 71:788–795

46. McCulloch PR, Forkert PG, Froese AB (1988) Lung volume maintenance prevents lung injury during high frequency oscillatory ventilation in surfactant-deficient rabbits. Am Rev Respir Dis 137:1185–1192

47. Engelmann L, Lachmann B, Petros S, Bohm S, Pilz U (1997) ARDS: dramatic rise in arterial PO_2 with the "open lung" approach. Crit Care 1 (Suppl):P54 (Abst)

48. Albert RK, Leasa D, Sanderson M, Robertson HT, Hlastala MP (1987) The prone position improves arterial oxygenation and reduces shunt in oleic-acid-induced acute lung injury. Am Rev Respir Dis 135:628–633
49. Pappert D, Rossaint R, Slama K, Gruning T, Falke KJ (1994) Influence of positioning on ventilation-perfusion relationships in severe adult respiratory distress syndrome. Chest 106:1511–1516
50. Douglas WW, Rehder K, Beynen FM, Sessler AD, Marsh HM (1977) Improved oxygenation in patients with acute respiratory failure: the prone position. Am Rev Respir Dis 115:559–566
51. Pelosi P, Tubiolo D, Mascheroni D, et al (1998) Effects of the prone position on respiratory mechanics and gas exchange during acute lung injury. Am J Respir Crit Care Med 157:387–393
52. Gattinoni L, Pelosi P, Vitale G, Pesenti A, D'Andrea L, Mascheroni D (1991) Body position changes redistribute lung computed-tomographic density in patients with acute respiratory failure. Anesthesiology 74:15–23
53. Langer M, Mascheroni D, Marcolin R, Gattinoni L (1988) The prone position in ARDS patients. A clinical study. Chest 94:103–107
54. Gattinoni L, Tognoni G, Pesenti A, et al (2001) Effect of prone positioning on the survival of patients with acute respiratory failure. N Engl J Med 345:568–573
55. Slutsky AS (2001) The acute respiratory distress syndrome, mechanical ventilation, and the prone position. N Engl J Med 345:610–612
56. Rossaint R, Falke KJ, Lopez, F, Slama K, Pison U, Zapol WM (1993) Inhaled nitric oxide for the ault respiratory distress syndrome. N Engl J Med 328:399–405
57. Roberts JD, Polaner DM, Lang P, Zapol WM (1992) Inhaled nitric oxide in persistent pulmonary hypertension of the newborn. Lancet 340:818–819
58. The Neonatal Inhaled Nitric Oxide Study Group (1997) Inhaled nitric oxide in full-term and nearly full-term infants with hypoxic respiratory failure. N Engl J Med 336:597–604
59. Dellinger RP, Zimmerman JL, Taylor RW, et al (1998) Effects of inhaled nitric oxide in patients with acute respiratory distress syndrome: results of a randomized phase II trial. Inhaled Nitric Oxide in ARDS Study Group. Crit Care Med 26:15–23
60. Lundin S, Mang H, Smithies M, Stenqvist O, Frostell C (1999) Inhalation of nitric oxide in acute lung injury: results of a European multicentre study. The European Study Group of Inhaled Nitric Oxide. Intensive Care Med 25:911–919
61. Dupont H, Le Corre F, Fierobe L, Cheval C, Moine P, Timsit JF (1999) Efficiency of inhaled nitric oxide as rescue therapy during severe ARDS: survival and factors associated with the first response. J Crit Care 14:107–113
62. Cuthbertson BH, Galley HF, Webster NR (2000) Effect of inhaled nitric oxide on key mediators of the inflammatory response in patients with acute lung injury. Crit Care Med 28:1736–1741
63. Rialp G, Betbese AJ, Perez-Marquez M, Mancebo J (2001) Short-term effects of inhaled nitric oxide and prone position in pulmonary and extrapulmonary acute respiratory distress syndrome. Am J Respir Crit Care Med 164:243–249
64. Kloot TE, Blanch L, Melynne YA, et al (2000) Recruitment maneuvers in three experimental models of acute lung injury. Effect on lung volume and gas exchange. Am J Respir Crit Care Med 161:1485–1494
65. Puybasset L, Cluzel P, Gusman P, Grenier P, Preteux F, Rouby JJ (2000) Regional distribution of gas and tissue in acute respiratory distress syndrome. I. Consequences for lung morphology. CT Scan ARDS Study Group. Intensive Care Med 26:857–869
66. Lim CM, Kim EK, Lee JS, et al (2001) Comparison of the response to the prone position between pulmonary and extrapulmonary acute respiratory distress syndrome. Intensive Care Med 27:477–485
67. Desai SR, Wells AU, Suntharalingam G, Rubens MB, Evans TW, Hansell DM (2001) Acute respiratory distress syndrome caused by pulmonary and extrapulmonary injury: a comparative CT study. Radiology 218:689–693
68. Eisner MD, Thompson T, Hudson LD, et al (2001) Efficacy of low tidal volume ventilation in patients with different clinical risk factors for acute lung injury and the acute respiratory distress syndrome. Am J Respir Crit Care Med 164:231–236

69. Tremblay L, Valenza F, Ribeiro SP, Li J, Slutsky AS (1997) Injurious ventilatory strategies increase cytokines and c-fos m-RNA expression in an isolated rat lung model. J Clin Invest 99:944–952
70. Slutsky AS, Tremblay LN (1998) Multiple system organ failure. Is mechanical ventilation a contributing factor? Am J Respir Crit Care Med 157:1721–1725
71. Tremblay LN, Slutsky AS (1998) Ventilator-induced injury: from barotrauma to biotrauma. Proc Assoc Am Physicians 110:482–488
72. Chiumello D, Pristine G, Slutsky AS (1999) Mechanical ventilation affects local and systemic cytokines in an animal model of acute respiratory distress syndrome. Am J Respir Crit Care Med 160:109–116
73. Ranieri VM, Suter PM, Tortorella C, et al (1999) Effect of mechanical ventilation on inflammatory mediators in patients with acute respiratory distress syndrome: a randomized controlled trial. JAMA 282:54–61
74. Ranieri VM, Giunta F, Suter PM, Slutsky AS (2000) Mechanical ventilation as a mediator of multisystem organ failure in acute respiratory distress syndrome. JAMA 284:43–44

Non-invasive Mechanical Ventilation

Methodology of Non-invasive Mechanical Ventilation in Acute Respiratory Failure

G. U. Meduri

▌ Introduction

The term acute respiratory failure refers to a severe deterioration in gas exchange that may require mechanical ventilation for life support. Instituted when conservative treatment fails, mechanical ventilation aims to correct the pathophysiology of acute respiratory failure and gas exchange abnormalities, reduce the work of breathing (WOB), and ameliorate dyspnea, while concomitant pharmacologic intervention is directed at correcting the condition that resulted in acute respiratory failure. The delivery of positive pressure ventilation (PPV) from the ventilator to the patient's lungs requires the presence of an interface. Traditionally, an endotracheal (ET) tube is inserted into the trachea to deliver PPV. Endotracheal intubation is an invasive procedure associated with potential complications and discomfort and has confined the use of mechanical ventilation to the most severe forms of acute respiratory failure.

In the late 1970s and early 1980s, two methods of non-invasive PPV (NPPV), using a facial or nasal mask, were introduced into clinical practice. These modalities included continuous positive airway pressure (CPAP) to improve oxygen exchange in patients with hypoxemic acute respiratory failure, and intermittent PPV (IPPV) with or without CPAP to augment ventilation and rest the respiratory muscles of patients with chronic respiratory failure due to neuromuscular disease and chronic obstructive pulmonary disease (COPD). In the early 1990s, the encouraging results of a pilot study in ten patients with hypercapnic or hypoxemic acute respiratory failure stimulated investigation of non-invasive ventilation (NIV) with IPPV in patients with acute respiratory failure [1]. In this chapter, clinical application of NIV using CPAP alone is referred to as mask CPAP, and NIV using IPPV with or without CPAP as non-invasive (intermittent) positive-pressure ventilation (NPPV).

When correctly applied, both interfaces – ET and mask – have an important complementary role in the delivery of PPV in patients with acute respiratory failure; they do not exclude each other. In early acute respiratory failure, the mask has a definite advantage, and the ET tube may be used if NPPV fails. In resolving acute respiratory failure, the mask can take the place of the ET tube to accelerate liberation from mechanical ventilation, while removing the imposed WOB and potential complications of ET intubation. Both interfaces, however, can be applied incorrectly or inappropriately. Improper use of a mask or inappropriate application of PPV with NIV cannot be used as criteria to define its usefulness. One of the most frequent problems encountered with NPPV is the under-utilization of PPV when a mask is applied. It is important to recognize that use of a non-invasive interface does not change the severity of acute respiratory failure, and clinicians should be equally aggressive in achieving the full benefits of PPV. Two studies have shown that in patients with postextubation acute respiratory failure, a face mask is as effective as an endotracheal tube for delivering positive pressure and correcting gas exchange abnormality [2, 3]. One randomized study has shown that the mask and the ET are equally effective in correcting gas exchange abnormality in patients with severe hypoxemic acute respiratory failure [4].

The correct implementation of PPV by mask has opened new opportunities for the management of acute respiratory failure. When effective, NPPV avoids the complications associated with ET intubation, improves patient comfort, and preserves airway defense mechanisms, speech, and swallowing. Furthermore, NPPV provides greater flexibility in instituting and removing mechanical ventilation. Randomized studies in homogeneous patient populations with acute respiratory failure have provided supporting evidence for the early application of NPPV in hypercapnic acute respiratory failure due to acute exacerbation of COPD [5–12], and in hypoxemic acute respiratory failure due to cardiogenic pulmonary edema [13–17], severe community-acquired pneumonia [18], and following solid organ transplantation [19]. In these studies, the early application of NPPV in patients not yet meeting criteria for mechanical ventilation was associated with a significant reduction in the rate of ET intubation. Compelling data indicate that avoidance of intubation reduces the morbidity and mortality associated with mechanical ventilation [4]. The effectiveness of NIV was also investigated in patients with severe hypoxemic acute respiratory failure, meeting preselected criteria for mechanical ventilation and randomized to receive mechanical ventilation via a face mask or an ET tube [4]. In this randomized study, mechanical ventilation delivered via a face mask was found to be equally effective to conventional ventilation in improving gas exchange, and intubation was avoided in 69% of the patients [4]. A recent randomized study [11] found that hypoxemic patients without COPD were less likely to require intubation if randomized to NPPV.

Hypercapnic and hypoxemic acute respiratory failure have different pathophysiological abnormalities, and each group is composed of a variety of lung pathologies that benefit in different ways from the application of PPV. Table 1 summarizes the effects of CPAP and IPPV (usually in the form of pressure support ventilation, PSV) delivered by a mask, alone and in combination, on gas exchange and transdiaphragmatic pressure, in patients with obstructive and restrictive lung disease [20–25]. In both conditions, the combination of CPAP and IPPV appears superior to either one alone in reducing transdiaphragmatic pressure, while the combination appears superior for improvement in arterial blood gases only in patients with hypoxemic acute respiratory failure.

Table 1. Effects of continuous positive airway pressure (CPAP) and pressure support ventilation (PSV) delivered by a mask, alone and in combination, on gas exchange and transdiaphragmatic pressure, in patients with obstructive and restrictive lung disease

	Obstructive		Restrictive	
	gas exchange	transdiaphragmatic pressure	gas exchange	transdiaphragmatic pressure
CPAP	$\neq$ or $\uparrow$	$\downarrow$	$\uparrow$	$\downarrow$
PSV	$\uparrow$	$\downarrow$	$\uparrow$	$\downarrow$
CPAP + PSV	$\uparrow$	$\downarrow\downarrow$	$\uparrow\uparrow$	$\downarrow\downarrow$

$\neq$ = no effect; $\uparrow$ = improved or increased; $\downarrow$ = worsen or decreased. Data from [20–25]

Table 2. Methodology for non-invasive positive-pressure ventilation in patients with acute respiratory failure (University of Tennessee, Memphis)

- Position the head of the bed at a 45° angle.
- Choose the correct size mask and connect the mask to the ventilator.
- Turn the ventilator on and silence the alarms. The initial ventilatory settings are CPAP 0 cmH_2O with pressure support 10 cmH_2O. FiO_2 is titrated to achieve an oxygen saturation over 90%.
- Explain the modality to the patient and provide reassurance.
- Hold the mask gently on the patient's face until the patient is comfortable and in full synchrony with the ventilator.
- Apply wound care dressing on the nasal bridge and other pressure points.
- Secure the mask with the headgear, avoiding a tight fit. Allow enough space to pass two fingers beneath the head straps.
- Increase CPAP to ≥5 cmH_2O.
- Increase pressure support to obtain an exhaled tidal volume ≥7 ml/kg, a respiratory rate ≤25 breaths/min, and patient comfort.
- In hypoxemic patients, increase CPAP in increments of 2 to 3 cmH_2O until FiO_2≤0.6.
- Avoid peak mask pressure above 30 cmH_2O. Allow minimal air leaks if exhaled tidal volume is adequate.
- Set the ventilator alarms and apnea backup parameters.
- Ask the patient to call for needs (repositioning of the mask, pain or discomfort, expectoration) or if complications occur (respiratory difficulties, abdominal distention, nausea, vomiting).
- Monitor with oximetry and adjust ventilator settings following arterial blood gas results.

NPPV Methodology

Because correct implementation and monitoring are critical to the success of NPPV, physicians and hospital respiratory technicians and nurses should develop familiarity with the methodology. Factors vital to the success of NIV include careful patient selection, properly timed intervention, a comfortable, well-fitting interface, patient coaching and encouragement, careful monitoring, and a skilled and motivated team [26]. The methodology adopted at the University of Tennessee, Memphis is shown in Table 2 [27].

Patient Selection

It is critical that the patient be alert and cooperative when initiating NPPV or mask CPAP (Table 3). To initiate NPPV, the patient must be able to voluntarily synchronize respiratory efforts with the ventilator or allow fully controlled ventilation in the intermittent mandatory ventilation (IMV) or assist control ventilation (ACV) mode. However, patients with COPD and CO_2 narcosis are an exception. In our experience and in the experience of others [28] most of these patients will improve mentation within 15–30 min of effective NPPV, and only a minority will require intubation. Although extremely anxious patients may be better served by sedation and ET intubation, a moderate degree of anxiety is frequently overcome once a patient's ventilatory needs are met. During NPPV, patients can achieve a level of control and independence not available while intubated, therefore sedation is infrequently required. When sedation is necessary, we have found intravenous administration of a small dose (2 mg) of morphine to be very effective.

Table 3. Criteria for selecting patients for non-invasive positive pressure ventilation (NPPV)

▌ Alert and cooperative patient[a]
▌ Hemodynamic stability
▌ No need for endotracheal intubation to
  – protect the airways[b]
  – remove excessive secretions
▌ No acute facial trauma
▌ Properly fitted mask

[a] Patients with chronic obstructive pulmonary disease (COPD) and CO_2 narcosis are an exception (see text).
[b] Mental obtundation, impaired swallowing, or active upper gastrointestinal bleeding

NPPV should be avoided in patients with cardiovascular instability (hypotension or life-threatening arrhythmia), in those who require an ET tube to protect the airways (coma, acute abdominal processes, impaired swallowing), and in those who have life-threatening refractory hypoxemia ($PaO_2 < 60$ mmHg on 1.0 FiO_2). Patients with morbid obesity (>200% of ideal body weight) or with unstable angina, or acute myocardial infarction, who are ventilated with NPPV, should be closely monitored by experienced personnel.

Interface

There is no consensus on the optimal interface to use in delivering NPPV [29]. Commercially available mask interfaces include 1) full face masks; 2) nasal masks; 3) nasal pillows or plugs; 4) mouthpieces; and 5) custom-fabricated nasal masks [30]. Full face masks are preferentially used in episodes of acute respiratory failure, while nasal masks are used more often in the chronic setting. Nasal pillows are a useful alternative for patients experiencing skin necrosis of the nasal bridge from other types of masks [31].

Mask CPAP studies have almost exclusively used a facial mask, while nasal and facial masks were used with equal frequency in NPPV studies. The effects of CPAP and PSV delivered by a mask, either alone or in combination, on gas exchange and transdiaphragmatic pressure are shown in Table 1 for patients with obstructive and restrictive lung disease. Nasal masks add less deadspace, cause less claustrophobia (rare occurrence), minimize potential complications if vomiting occurs (rare occurrence), and allow for both expectoration and oral intake without removing the mask. With a nasal mask, patients can vocalize more clearly and can voluntarily discontinue ventilation by opening the mouth. On the other hand, a facial mask is preferable in severe respiratory failure because dyspneic patients are mouth-breathers; mouth breathing bypasses resistances of the nasal passages, and mouth opening during nasal mask ventilation results in air leakage and decreased effectiveness [22, 32, 33]. With nasal masks, an elastic chin strap is often sufficient to control mask leaks, although rarely successful in edentulous patients. Preliminary studies in normal adults suggest that nasal ventilation is of limited effectiveness when nasal resistance exceeds 5 $cmH_2O/l/s$ [34].

Studies comparing the efficacy of the various interfaces used in NPPV are limited. One group has reported a higher success with face mask NPPV compared with their institution's historical ventilation control with nasal mask [35]. Another study that directly compared nasal masks, nasal plugs, and full face masks found that although nasal masks were better tolerated subjectively, full face masks were superior in improving minute ventilation (through an increase in tidal volume) and lowering $PaCO_2$ values [36]. This is supported by previous studies which suggested that improvements in arterial blood gases appear to be slower in those using a nasal mask [5, 22, 37–39] in comparison to those using a face mask [1, 2, 23, 40, 41]. In one study, CPAP via face mask was superior to CPAP via ET tube in improving oxygen saturation [42]. At our institution, face masks are the preferred interface for patients with severe acute respiratory failure and dyspnea. The deadspace volumes of a facial and a nasal mask are 250 ml and 105 ml, respectively [43], while nasal pillows add virtually no deadspace volume [36]. Deadspace volume from the mask and the oropharynx does not appear to affect the effectiveness of ventilation. In mild forms of acute respiratory failure, a nasal mask could be tried first, switching to a facial mask if necessary. A mask with a transparent dome is preferred because it allows visual monitoring of the oral airway for the presence of secretions. The mask should be lightweight to aid in its application and have a soft, pliable, adjustable seal to reduce trauma and leaking [44]. Types of available seals include contoured cushion, air bladder cushion, foam cushion, and double spring. The mask is secured with head straps. Masks have four prongs for attaching head straps. Masks with prongs positioned peripherally allow for a more uniform distribution of pressure on the facial surface. The nasal masks by Respironics have a spacer to fill the space between the patient's forehead and the mask to reduce pressure on the nasal bridge.

Aerophagia during NPPV is unusual when the applied pressure is ≤ 25 cmH$_2$O [45, 46]. Routine placement of a nasogastric tube is therefore not required. Trauma patients, however, frequently have gastric atony and may require nasogastric (NG) tube placement [44]. The mask is connected to the ventilator, similar to an ET tube. To prevent drying of the nasal passages and oropharynx, a humidifier should be connected, but the heater should be turned off because the upper airways that naturally warm inspired gas are not bypassed with NIV.

Comfort

Because patient tolerance is essential to the success of NPPV, a tight, uncomfortable fit should be avoided whenever possible [47, 48]. Even in patients with hypoxemic respiratory failure and receiving mask CPAP alone, a small leak will not cause airway pressure to drop [44, 47, 49]. When securing the mask, we allow enough space to pass two fingers beneath the head straps. Masks with an air cushion fit most facial contours and do not require tight strapping. Small degrees of air leakage are well tolerated if the returned tidal volume is adequate (≥ 7 ml/kg). When necessary, a skin patch [Restore® (Hollister, Libertyville, Ill) or Duoderm® (Bristol-Myers Squibb, Princeton, NJ)] can be used to plug air leaks. Similar to others [33, 50], we have often found that proper fitting of the mask is difficult in edentulous patients and in those with a beard (in the latter, a nasal mask may be more effective). In one report, edentulous patients on NPPV by nasal mask had persistent leaks despite using a chin strap [33]. Placing a NG tube is indicated only for patients developing gastric distention (see below) or to provide access for enteral feeding. In our intensive care unit (ICU), patients are fed by mouth with a liquid diet, while other investigators allow patients on nasal pressure ventilation to eat small meals [38]. Enteral feeding can be provided during the night for patients who do not achieve required caloric intake during the daytime.

Mode of Ventilation

Most NPPV studies used pressure-limited ventilation delivered by a broad range of ventilators. Pressure-limited ventilation improves the efficacy of spontaneous breathing by allowing an optimal synchrony between patient effort and delivered assistance. Inspiration is initiated by the patient's activation of the inspiratory muscles and of the inspiratory glottic abductors, with consequent glottis widening. During PSV, the patient's effort determines volume and duration of inspiration. Gas flow begins after the patient's inspiratory effort reduces pressure in the inspiratory circuit of the ventilator by a predetermined value, usually 1–2 cmH_2O. Pressure-control ventilation (PCV) has a preset inspiratory time and respiratory rate. PCV may ventilate more effectively those patients with low ventilatory drive. In comparison to volume-cycled ventilation, pressure-limited ventilation minimizes peak inspiratory mask pressure and air leakage. Although tidal volume may vary as a function of change in airway resistance and compliance, this variance has been an uncommon problem in our experience. In three comparison studies (patients with hypercapnic acute respiratory failure) with ACV, PSV was equally effective in reducing WOB [51] and improving gas exchange [35, 51] but was better tolerated [35, 51, 52] and associated with fewer complications [35]. During NPPV of stable COPD patients, flow triggering reduces the respiratory effort and intrinsic PEEP (PEEPi) during both PSV and ACV when compared to pressure triggering [53]. No differences were found between 1 and 5 l/min flow triggers [53]. Two reports found nasal ventilation with ACV to be ineffective and time consuming in end-stage obstructive lung disease [32, 54].

Patients may inform the physician as to which mode of ventilation is most effective in ameliorating dyspnea [55]. Portable units have been used frequently in patients with less severe forms of acute respiratory failure. A comparison of several ICU and portable ventilators found that portable units performed as well as the larger ICU ventilators in NPPV [56].

The glottic aperture is influenced by vocal cord angle and represents the main factor regulating effective ventilation in healthy subjects submitted to NPPV. The width of the glottic aperture can be influenced by chemical factors (lower CO_2 levels narrow the glottic width), sleep effects (glottis narrows during sleep with variations in width during different sleep stages), and mechanical factors (see below) [30, 57]. A positive correlation ($r = 0.945$; $p < 0.0001$) exists between vocal cord angle and effective tidal volume reaching the lung [58]. In healthy volunteers, mechanical factors (pressure and flow) can influence glottic behavior during passive (control mode) NPPV. With volumetric respirators, increments in effective ventilation are achieved by increasing flow up to 0.9 l/s and respiratory rate up to 20 breaths per min. Further increases in flow and respiratory rate or increases in delivered tidal volume above 10–15 ml/kg resulted in no change or a reduction in effective ventilation [59]. With passive two-level PPV, effective ventilation was found to be less predictable, especially when intermittent positive airway pressure (IPAP) was kept below 15 cmH_2O [58]. Two-level PPV set in the spontaneous mode may obviate this problem [58].

Mechanical Ventilation

The physiologic effects of NPPV with PSV have been described previously. With NPPV, tidal volume, gas exchange, respiratory rate, and diaphragmatic activity are improved in proportion to the amount of pressure applied [20, 22, 23]. The methodology for NPPV at the University of Tennessee is shown in Table 2. The initial ventilator settings are: CPAP, 0 cmH_2O; and PSV, 10 cmH_2O – the mask is then gently held on the patient's face until the patient is comfortable and in synchrony with the ventilator. Inspired fraction of oxygen (FiO_2) is titrated to achieve an oxygen saturation over 90%. After the mask is secured, CPAP is slowly increased to 3–5 cmH_2O, and PSV is increased to obtain the largest (>5 to 7 ml/kg) exhaled tidal volume, a respiratory rate <25 breaths/min, and patient comfort. These objectives may not be achieved in patients with severe lung disease or with a leaky interface.

In intubated patients with obstructive airway disease, criteria for optimal PSV level have varied [60]. It is important to recognize that excessive PSV levels can cause excessive inflation with consequent patient-ventilator dyssynchrony and activation of expiratory muscles during inspiration [60]. To avoid gastric distention, peak mask pressure should be kept <30 cmH_2O. In one study, patients noticed the best sensation of comfort at a mask CPAP level of 5.3 ± 2.8 cmH_2O [61]. When patients on mechanical ventilation (intubated) are given the option of choosing their tidal volume without mechanical constraints, they frequently opt for a lower tidal volume (7.1 ml/kg, range 3.0–10.4 ml/kg) than conventionally targeted (10–12 ml/kg) [62]. In patients with hypoxemia, CPAP is increased in increments of 2 to 3 cmH_2O until a preselected end point is achieved ($FiO_2 \leq 0.6$ or $PaO_2:FiO_2 \leq 300$) [55, 63]. CO_2 rebreathing can occur during bilevel positive airway pressure (BiPAP) ventilatory assistance using the standard exhalation device (Whisper-Swivel) and can be eliminated with a plateau exhalation device or a nonrebreather valve [64]. Application of expiratory positive airway pressure (EPAP) (>4 cmH_2O) decreases inhaled CO_2 which is eliminated at a level of 8 cmH_2O [64].

Few studies have remarked on patient positioning during NPPV [1, 2]. A recent study in stable hypercapnic COPD patients showed that changing posture position did not significantly influence breathing patterns and respiratory muscle workload during NPPV, suggesting that NPPV may be performed in different positions without any relevant difference in its effectiveness [65]. At our institution we choose to maintain the head of the bed elevated at $\geq45°$ angle at all times during NPPV. Although the original purpose of this intervention was to facilitate manipulation of the mask and to minimize the risk of aspiration in patients without airway protection, we have come to appreciate that, in some patients, NPPV may be more effective (larger delivered tidal volume) in the upright position. In the upright position, increased deployment of inspiratory muscles acting directly on the rib cage and decreased abdominal compliance (gravitationally induced) increase rib cage expansion [66].

Special precautions should be taken when PSV is used with a Puritan-Bennett 7200 ventilator. The breath cycle is terminated when the flow drops below 5 l/min, and a significant leak from the mask can create a 5-s inspiratory pause due to the failure of the ventilator to sense a decrease in flow. If air leakage is not improved, despite manipulations of the mask and application of a skin patch, CPAP first and then applied pressure (or tidal volume) are decreased to reduce peak mask pressure. Portable units, such as Respironics' BiPAP®, Puritan-Bennett's PB-335®, and Healthdyne's Quantum TM PSV, automatically compensate for mask leaks and mouth opening. A pressure and flow sensor in the ventilator monitors system pressure and total system flow. As the system flow fluctuates, the control valve changes position to either let more or less flow out to the patient. This will compensate for changes in flow and the system pressure to maintain the set pressure in the face of leaks.

In most studies, mechanical ventilation was delivered continuously until acute respiratory failure resolved. Intermittent 5- to 15-min periods off NPPV were provided for oral intake or expectoration. Some groups, treating less severe forms of respiratory failure, have delivered NPPV for a few hours a day over extended periods of time [67, 68]. After the initial stabilization period on NPPV (4–6 h), patients with hypercapnic respiratory failure or with hypoxemia on low-level CPAP (<5 cmH$_2$O) can safely remove the mask for 5–15 min, during which time they can talk, drink small amounts of liquid, expectorate, or receive nebulized bronchodilator therapy. Because mask ventilation provides a great degree of flexibility, it can be adjusted to meet a patient's individual needs. In some of our patients with COPD and mild forms of respiratory acidosis, nocturnal ventilation is continued for a few days following resolution of respiratory failure.

Monitoring

Continuous pulse oximetry with an alarm should be provided. Ventilator settings should be adjusted based on results of arterial blood gases obtained within 1 h and, as necessary, at 2- to 6-h intervals. Patients ventilated via an ET tube are heavily sedated and, when indicated, correction of respiratory acidosis can be achieved within the first hour of mechanical ventilation. Patients receiving NPPV or mask CPAP need not be heavily sedated; relief of dyspnea and resolution of signs of respiratory distress are usually achieved soon after adequate positive pressure is provided. Correction of acidosis may be slower with NPPV, depending on the mode of ventilation, amount of applied pressure, and severity of underlying disease. Patients showing improved gas exchange in the first hour of NPPV are more likely to avoid intubation (see below). In our experience, the first 30 to 60 min of NPPV is labor intensive. The bedside presence of a respiratory therapist or nurse familiar with this mode of ventilation is essential for adjusting the mask and the ventilator settings.

In addition to gas exchange response, the following clinical parameters should be monitored: patient's subjective response (dyspnea, comfort, and mental status), patient's objective response (respiratory rate, heart rate, and use of accessory muscle of respiration), and possible complications (abdominal distention, facial pressure necrosis, retention of secretions). The use of the accessory muscles of respiration (respiratory load) [41] and contraction of the transversus abdominis muscle (activated with excessive inflation) [69] can be monitored visually or by palpation. Providing reassurance and adequate explanation to the patient about what to expect is of the utmost importance. Patients are instructed to call the nurse if they have needs or develop complications. Needs include repositioning the mask for comfort or leaks or removing the mask for oral intake or expectoration. Complications include respiratory difficulties, development of abdominal distention, or nausea/vomiting.

Table 4. Criteria to discontinue non-invasive positive pressure ventilation (NPPV)

Inability to tolerate the mask due to discomfort or pain.
Inability to improve gas exchange or dyspnea.
Need for endotracheal intubation to manage secretions or protect the airways.
Hemodynamic instability.
Electrocardiographic instability with evidence of ischemia or significant ventricular arrhythmias.
Failure to improve mental status, within 30 min of initiating non-invasive ventilation, in patients who are lethargic from CO$_2$ retention or agitated from hypoxemia.

In our experience, after the first hour of uncomplicated NPPV, most patients do not require bedside observation; ventilator and oximetry alarms provide warnings for early intervention. In three randomized studies and one prospective control trial, bedside time commitment by nurses and therapists was similar for patients receiving NPPV or conventional treatment [5, 10, 18, 70]. Criteria to discontinue NPPV are shown in Table 4.

Predictors of Success

In patients with hypercapnic acute respiratory failure and receiving NPPV, most studies have found that arterial blood gas response and need for intubation cannot be predicted by the severity of the underlying lung disease (forced expiratory volume in 1 second [FEV1] and arterial blood gases) nor by the arterial blood gas values (PCO_2, pH) obtained before implementing NPPV [2, 37, 39, 67, 71]. Two studies involving 125 patients with COPD and acute respiratory failure found nonresponders to have a higher PCO_2 at initiation of NPPV [2, 37, 39, 67, 71]. In three studies, the underlying cause of acute respiratory failure did not predict the outcome of NPPV [39, 41, 72]. Patients with COPD and pneumonia or congestive heart failure as cause of acute respiratory failure have a higher intubation rate [72, 73]. Three studies [4, 32, 74] found a higher failure rate in COPD patients with higher APACHE II or SAPS scores; however, this finding was not confirmed by others [55, 72].

We found consistently that a reduction in PCO_2 or an increase in pH within 1–2 h of NPPV predicted a sustained improvement in gas exchange [2, 72] and requirement for shorter duration of ventilatory support (mean 26 h of NPPV vs 323 h of mechanical ventilation with endotracheal intubation) [2]. This observation was confirmed by others [5, 71, 74]. In three studies, an inability to improve PCO_2 was related to mask (nasal) leak [32, 33, 75]. This finding suggests that proper selection of the interface leads to higher efficacy of NPPV. Furthermore, we have observed that inability to improve arterial blood gases in hypercapnic patients is in part related to inadequate delivery of inspiratory pressure (12 ± 2 vs 15 ± 4, p=0.016) [72].

In patients with hypoxemic acute respiratory failure, predictors of response to mask CPAP therapy have included degree of hypoxemia at initiation of therapy [47, 76], improvement in gas exchange [77], and respiratory rate shortly after applying CPAP [44, 77]. In one study, however, improvement in PaO_2 after 1 h of NPPV did not predict success [41]. Also, if BiPAP is used as the ventilatory mode in hypoxemic acute respiratory failure, the risk of failure is significantly greater (risk ratio = 2.6, 95% CI = 1.1 to 6.1) than when used in patients with hypercapnic acute respiratory failure [78]. A low $PaCO_2$ may be a factor for failure in patients with cardiogenic pulmonary edema [79].

Weaning

Following improvement in respiratory failure, patients are weaned from mechanical ventilation either by lowering the amount of delivered pressure or by titrating periods off mechanical ventilation to patient tolerance and objective findings, similar to a T-piece weaning trial. At a low level of pressure support (5–8 cmH$_2$O), the patient is disconnected from the ventilator while receiving supplemental oxygen by nasal cannula or face mask. During weaning, NPPV eliminates the 'reintubation factor' associated with premature removal of conventional ventilation, and this may contribute to shorter duration of ventilation.

■ Conclusion

The correct implementation of NPPV by mask has opened new opportunities for the management of acute respiratory failure. It is my hope that the present review provides the reader with useful information for the practical application of NPPV in patients with acute respiratory failure.

References

1. Meduri GU, Conoscenti CC, Menashe P, Nair S (1989) Noninvasive face mask ventilation in patients with acute respiratory failure. Chest 95:865–870
2. Meduri GU, Abou-Shala N, Fox RC, Jones CB, Leeper KV, Wunderink RG (1991) Noninvasive face mask mechanical ventilation in patients with acute hypercapnic respiratory failure. Chest 100:445–454
3. Gregoretti C, Burbi L, Berardino M, et al (1992) Non invasive mask ventilation (NIMV) in trauma and major burn patients. Am Rev Respir Dis 145:A75 (Abst)
4. Antonelli M, Conti G, Rocco M, et al (1998) A comparison of noninvasive positive-pressure ventilation and conventional mechanical ventilation in patients with acute respiratory failure. N Engl J Med 339:429–435
5. Bott J, Carroll MP, Conway JH, et al (1993) Randomised controlled trial of nasal ventilation in acute ventilatory failure due to chronic obstructive airways disease. Lancet 341:1555–1557
6. Ahmed AH, Fenwick L, Angus RM, Peacock AJ (1992) Nasal ventilation vs doxapram in the treatment of type II respiratory failure complicating chronic airflow obstruction. Thorax 1:858 (Abst)
7. Daskalopoulou E, Tsara V, Fekete K, Koutsantas V, Christaki P (1993) Treatment of acute respiratory failure in COPD patients with positive airway pressure via nasal mask (NPPV). Chest 103:271S (Abst)
8. Brochard L, Mancebo J, Wysocki M, et al (1995) Noninvasive ventilation for acute exacerbations of chronic obstructive pulmonary disease. N Engl J Med 333:817–822
9. Martin TJ, Sanders MH, Bierman MI, Hovis JD (1994) Non-invasive application of bi-level positive airway pressure to prevent endotracheal intubation in acute respiratory failure. Crit Care Med 23:A129 (Abst)
10. Kramer N, Meyer TJ, Meharg J, Cece RD, Hill NS (1995) Randomized, prospective trial of noninvasive positive pressure ventilation in acute respiratory failure. Am J Respir Crit Care Med 151:1799–1806
11. Martin TJ, Hovis JD, Costantino JP, et al (2000) A randomized, prospective evaluation of noninvasive ventilation for acute respiratory failure. Am J Respir Crit Care Med 161:807–813
12. Bardi G, Pierotello R, Desideri M, Valdisserri L, Bottai M, Palla A (2000) Nasal ventilation in COPD exacerbations: early and late results of a prospective, controlled study. Eur Respir J 15:98–104
13. Rasanen J, Heikkila J, Downs J, Nikki P, Vaisanen I, Viitanen A (1985) Continuous positive airway pressure by face mask in acute cardiogenic pulmonary edema. Am J Cardiol 55:296–300
14. Bersten AD, Holt AW, Vedig AE, Skowronski GA, Baggoley CJ (1991) Treatment of severe cardiogenic pulmonary edema with continuous positive airway pressure delivered by face mask. N Engl J Med 325:1825–1830
15. Lin M, Yang YF, Chiang HT, Chang MS, Chiang BN, Cheitlin MD (1995) Reappraisal of continuous positive airway pressure therapy in acute cardiogenic pulmonary edema. Short-term results and long-term follow-up. Chest 107:1379–1386

16. Takeda S, Takano T, Ogawa R (1997) The effect of nasal continuous positive airway pressure on plasma endothelin-1 concentrations in patients with severe cardiogenic pulmonary edema. Anesth Analg 84:1091–1096
17. Pang D, Keenan SP, Cook DJ, Sibbald WJ (1998) The effect of positive pressure airway support on mortality and the need for intubation in cardiogenic pulmonary edema: a systematic review. Chest 114:1185–1192
18. Confalonieri M, Potena A, Carbone G, Porta RD, Tolley EA, Meduri GU (1999) Acute respiratory failure in patients with severe community-acquired pneumonia. A prospective randomized evaluation of noninvasive ventilation. Am J Respir Crit Care Med 160:1585–1591
19. Antonelli M, Conti G, Bufi M, et al (2000) Noninvasive ventilation for treatment of acute respiratory failure in patients undergoing solid organ transplantation: a randomized trial. JAMA 283:235–241
20. Appendini L, Patessio A, Zanaboni S, et al (1994) Physiologic effects of positive end-expiratory pressure and mask pressure support during exacerbations of chronic obstructive pulmonary disease. Am J Respir Crit Care Med 149:1069–1076
21. de Lucas P, Tarancon C, Puente L, Rodriguez C, Tatay E, Monturiol JM (1993) Nasal continuous positive airway pressure in patients with COPD in acute respiratory failure. A study of the immediate effects. Chest 104:1694–1697
22. Carrey Z, Gottfried SB, Levy RD (1990) Ventilatory muscle support in respiratory failure with nasal positive pressure ventilation. Chest 97:150–158
23. Brochard L, Isabey D, Piquet J, et al (1990) Reversal of acute exacerbations of chronic obstructive lung disease by inspiratory assistance with a face mask. N Engl J Med 323:1523–1530
24. Ambrosino N, Nava S, Bertone P, Fracchia C, Rampulla C (1992) Physiologic evaluation of pressure support ventilation by nasal mask in patients with stable COPD. Chest 101:385–391
25. Elliott MW, Aquilina R, Green M, Moxham J, Simonds AK (1994) A comparison of different modes of noninvasive ventilatory support: effects on ventilation and inspiratory muscle effort. Anaesthesia 49:279–283
26. Mehta S, Hill NS (1996) Noninvasive ventilation in acute respiratory failure. Respir Care Clin North Am 2:267–292
27. Meduri GU (1996) Noninvasive positive-pressure ventilation in patients with acute respiratory failure. Clin Chest Med 17:513–553
28. Barach AL, Martin J, Eckman L (1937) Positive pressure respiration and its application to the treatment of acute pulmonary edema and respiratory obstruction. Proc Am Soc Clin Invest 16:664–680
29. Meyer TJ, Hill NS (1994) Noninvasive positive pressure ventilation to treat respiratory failure. Ann Intern Med 120:760–770
30. American Thoracic Society (2001) International Consensus Conferences in Intensive Care Medicine: Noninvasive positive pressure ventilation in acute respiratory failure. Am J Respir Crit Care Med 163:283–291
31. Tsuboi T, Ohi M, Kita H, et al (1999) The efficacy of a custom-fabricated nasal mask on gas exchange during nasal intermittent positive pressure ventilation. Eur Respir J 13:152–156
32. Soo Hoo GW, Santiago S, Williams AJ (1994) Nasal mechanical ventilation for hypercapnic respiratory failure in chronic obstructive pulmonary disease: determinants of success and failure. Crit Care Med 22:1253–1261
33. Chiang AA, Lee KC (1993) Use of nasal mask BiPAP in patients with respiratory distress after extubation. Chest 104:135S (Abst)
34. Ohi M, Chin K, Tsuboi T, Fukui M, Kuno K (1994) Effect of nasal resistance on the increase in ventilation during noninvasive ventilation. Am J Respir Crit Care Med 149:A643 (Abst)
35. Vitacca M, Rubini F, Foglio K, Scalvini S, Nava S, Ambrosino N (1993) Non-invasive modalities of positive pressure ventilation improve the outcome of acute exacerbations in COPD patients. Intensive Care Med 19:450–455
36. Navalesi P, Fanfulla F, Frigerio P, Gregoretti C, Nava S (2000) Physiologic evaluation of noninvasive mechanical ventilation delivered with three types of mask in patients with chronic hypercapnic respiratory failure. Crit Care Med 28:1785–1790

37. Elliott MW, Steven MH, Phillips GD, Branthwaite MA (1990) Non-invasive mechanical ventilation for acute respiratory failure. Br Med J 300:358–360
38. Pennock BE, Kaplan PD, Carlin BW, Sabangan JS, Magovern JA (1991) Pressure support ventilation with a simplified ventilatory support system administered with a nasal mask in patients with respiratory failure. Chest 100:1371–1376
39. Benhamou D, Girault C, Faure C, Portier F, Muir JF (1992) Nasal mask ventilation in acute respiratory failure. Experience in elderly patients. Chest 102:912–917
40. Meduri GU, Mauldin GL, Wunderink RG, et al (1994) Causes of fever and pulmonary densities in patients with clinical manifestations of ventilator-associated pneumonia. Chest 106:221–235
41. Wysocki M, Tric L, Wolff MA, Gertner J, Millet H, Herman B (1993) Noninvasive pressure support ventilation in patients with acute respiratory failure. Chest 103:907–913
42. Jousela I (1993) Endotracheal tube versus face mask with and without continuous positive airway pressure (CPAP). Acta Anaesthesiol Scand 37:381–385
43. Criner GJ, Travaline JM, Brennan KJ, Kreimer DT (1994) Efficacy of a new full face mask for noninvasive positive pressure ventilation. Chest 106:1109–1115
44. Branson RD, Hurst JM, DeHaven CB Jr (1985) Mask CPAP: state of the art. Respir Care 30:846–857
45. Linton DM, Potgieter PD (1982) Conservative management of blunt chest trauma. S Afr Med J 61(24):917–919
46. Dodds WJ, Hogan WJ, Lydon SB, Stewart ET, Stef JJ, Arndorfer RC (1975) Quantitation of pharyngeal motor function in normal human subjects. J Appl Physiol 39:692–696
47. Covelli HD, Weled BJ, Beekman JF (1982) Efficacy of continuous positive airway pressure administered by face mask. Chest 81:147–150
48. Pennock BE, Crawshaw L, Kaplan PD (1994) Noninvasive nasal mask ventilation for acute respiratory failure. Institution of a new therapeutic technology for routine use. Chest 105:441–444
49. DeVita MA, Friedman Y, Petrella V (1993) Mask continuous positive airway pressure in AIDS. Crit Care Clin 9:137–151
50. Gregg RW, Friedman BC, Williams JF, McGrath BJ, Zimmerman JE (1990) Continuous positive airway pressure by face mask in Pneumocystis carinii pneumonia. Crit Care Med 18:21–24
51. Girault C, Bonmarchand G, Richard JC, et al (1995) Physiologic assessment of ventilatory mode during non invasive ventilation in acute hypercapnic respiratory failure (AHRF): assist-control (ACV). Am J Respir Crit Care Med 151:A426 (Abst)
52. Richard JC, Molano C, Tengang B, Benhamou D, Cuvellier A, Muir JF (1996) Nasal intermittent positive pressure ventilation vs bilevel pressure ventilation during acute respiratory failure in patients with COPD. Am J Respir Crit Care Med 153:A609 (Abst)
53. Nava S, Bruschi C, Ambrosino N, Paturno V, Confalonieri M (1995) Inspiratory effort during non-invasive mechanical ventilation with flow and pressure triggers in COPD patients. Intensive Care Med 21:S120 (Abst)
54. Chevrolet JC, Jolliet P, Abajo B, Toussi A, Louis M (1991) Nasal positive pressure ventilation in patients with acute respiratory failure. Difficult and time-consuming procedure for nurses. Chest 100:775–782
55. Fernandez R, Blanch L, Valles J, Baigorri F, Artigas A (1993) Pressure support ventilation via face mask in acute respiratory failure in hypercapnic COPD patients. Intensive Care Med 19:456–461
56. Bunburaphong T, Imanaka H, Nishimura M, Hess D, Kacmarek RM (1997) Performance characteristics of bilevel pressure ventilators: a lung model study. Chest 111:1050–1060
57. Jounieaux V, Aubert G, Dury M, Delguste P, Rodenstein DO (1995) Effects of nasal positive-pressure hyperventilation on the glottis in normal awake subjects. J Appl Physiol 79:176–185
58. Parreira VF, Jounieaux V, Aubert G, Dury M, Delguste PE, Rodenstein DO (1996) Nasal two-level positive-pressure ventilation in normal subjects. Effects of the glottis and ventilation. Am J Respir Crit Care Med 153:1616–1623
59. Parreira YV, Jounieaux V, Delguste P, Dury M, Aubert G (1996) Effects of systematic changes in delivered tidal volume, inspiratory flow and respirator frequency on effective

ventilation (VI) during intermittent positive pressure ventilation applied through a nasal mask (nIPPV), in healthy subjects awake and asleep. Am J Respir Crit Care Med 153:A762 (Abst)

60. Jubran A, Van de Graaff WB, Tobin MJ (1995) Variability of patient-ventilator interaction with pressure support ventilation in patients with chronic obstructive pulmonary disease. Am J Respir Crit Care Med 152:129–136

61. Shivaram U, Donath J, Khan FA, Juliano J (1987) Effects of continuous positive airway pressure in acute asthma. Respiration 52:157–162

62. Marantz S, Webster K, Patrick W, Roberts D, Oppenheimer L, Younes M (1992) Respiratory responses to different levels of proportional assist (PAV) in ventilator dependent patients. Am Rev Respir Dis 145:A525 (Abst)

63. Rocker GM, Mackenzie MG, Williams B, Logan PM (1999) Noninvasive positive pressure ventilation: successful outcome in patients with acute lung injury/ARDS. Chest 115:173–177

64. Ferguson GT, Gilmartin M (1995) CO_2 rebreathing during BiPAP ventilatory assistance. Am J Respir Crit Care Med 151:1126–1135

65. Porta R, Vitacca M, Clini E, Ambrosino N (1999) Physiological effects of posture on mask ventilation in awake stable chronic hypercapnic COPD patients. Eur Respir J 14:517–522

66. Druz WS, Sharp JT (1981) Activity of respiratory muscles in upright and recumbent humans. J Appl Physiol 51:1552–1561

67. Leger P, Jennequin J, Gaussorgues P, Robert D (1988) Acute respiratory failure in COPD patient treated with noninvasive intermittent mechanical ventilation (control mode) with nasal mask. Am Rev Respir Dis 137:A63 (Abst)

68. Marino W (1991) Intermittent volume cycled mechanical ventilation via nasal mask in patients with respiratory failure due to COPD. Chest 99:681–684

69. Ninane V, Rypens F, Yernault JC, De Troyer A (1992) Abdominal muscle use during breathing in patients with chronic airflow obstruction. Am Rev Respir Dis 146:16–21

70. Nava S, Bruni M, Evangelisti I, et al (1996) Is non-invasive mechanical ventilation (NIMV) really time-consuming procedure compared to invasive mechanical ventilation (IMV)? Am J Respir Crit Care Med 153:A607 (Abst)

71. Richard JC, Muir JF, Girault C, Benhamou D, Merignac G (1995) Determinants of success of non-invasive positive pressure ventilation for hypercapnic respiratory failure in chronic obstructive pulmonary disease. Am J Respir Crit Care Med 151:A236 (Abst)

72. Meduri GU, Turner RE, Abou-Shala N, Wunderink R, Tolley E (1996) Noninvasive positive pressure ventilation via face mask. First-line intervention in patients with acute hypercapnic and hypoxemic respiratory failure. Chest 109:179–193

73. Soto L, Chernilo S, Gavilán J, Isamit D, Arancibia F, Vargas M (1996) Non invasive mechanical ventilation in COPD patients with acute hypercapnic respiratory failure. Am J Respir Crit Care Med 153:A610 (Abst)

74. Ambrosino N, Foglio K, Rubini F, Clini E, Nava S, Vitacca M (1995) Non-invasive mechanical ventilation in acute respiratory failure due to chronic obstructive pulmonary disease: correlates for success. Thorax 50:755–757

75. Meecham Jones DJ, Paul EA, Grahame-Clarke C, Wedzicha JA (1994) Nasal ventilation in acute exacerbations of chronic obstructive pulmonary disease: effect of ventilator mode on arterial blood gas tensions. Thorax 49:1222–1224

76. Greenbaum DM, Miller JE, Eross B, Snyder JV, Grenvik A, Safar P (1976) Continuous positive airway pressure without tracheal intubation in spontaneously breathing patients. Chest 69:615–620

77. Suter PM, Kobel N (1981) Treatment of acute pulmonary failure by CPAP via face mask: when can intubation be avoided? Klin Wochenschr 59:613–616

78. Alsous F, Amoateng-Adjepong Y, Manthous CA (1999) Noninvasive ventilation: experience at a community teaching hospital. Intensive Care Med 25:458–463

79. Rusterholtz T, Kempf J, Berton C, et al (1995) Efficacy of facial mask pressure support ventilation (FMPSV) during acute cardiogenic pulmonary edema: a descriptive study. Am J Respir Crit Care Med 151:A422 (Abst)

Non-invasive Mechanical Ventilation and Prevention of Pneumonia in Patients with Acute Respiratory Failure

M. Antonelli, G. Mercurio, and M. A. Pennisi

▌ Introduction

Critically ill patients are at high risk of developing nosocomial infections due to their severity of illness, immunosuppression, and prolonged hospitalization. Among nosocomial infections, pneumonia affects from 20 to 30% of intensive care unit (ICU) patients and is the leading cause of death [1]. The use of the endotracheal (ET) tube to deliver ventilatory support is the single most important predisposing factor for developing nosocomial bacterial pneumonia [2]. Fagon et al. [3] have demonstrated that the risk of pneumonia is incremental in ventilated patients and increases by about 1% per day of continuous invasive ventilation.

Nevertheless, patients with acute respiratory failure often require life-supporting mechanical ventilation. The target points of ventilatory support in patients with acute respiratory failure are reduction in the work of breathing (WOB) and alveolar recruitment to increase the functional residual capacity.

Recently, several authors have demonstrated that non-invasive mechanical ventilation (NIV) may represent a valid, complementary, or alternative approach to conventional ventilation with ET tube in selected groups of patients [4–6].

The application of pressure support ventilation (PSV) and positive end-expiratory pressure (PEEP), delivered by a nasal or a full-face mask, seems to be effective in unloading the respiratory muscles and improving gas-exchange by the recruitment of under-ventilated alveoli [7–9]. This approach may have several advantages in terms of prevention of infections, mainly reducing the rate of ET intubation. Factors involved in reducing the rate of ventilator-associated pneumonia (VAP) may include the maintenance of natural barriers provided by the glottis and the upper respiratory tract, the reduction in need of sedation and the shortening of duration of mechanical ventilation.

Patients with acute on chronic respiratory failure are the most likely to benefit from NIV treatment in term of both additive morbidity and mortality [10–16]. However, clinical evidence exists to propose NIV treatment as first line intervention in early hypoxemic acute respiratory failure [17–24]. Randomized and non-randomized studies on the application of NIV in patients with hypoxemic acute respiratory failure have showed promising results, with reduction of complications, including sinusitis and VAP, and shorter duration of ICU stay [24–36].

NIV can be applied at different phases of the acute respiratory failure (Fig. 1):

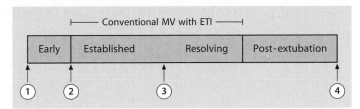

Fig. 1. Timing 1–4, see text, of application of non-invasive ventilation (NIV) (reproduced with permission from G. Umberto Meduri MD, University of Tennessee Health Science Center Memphis, TN). ETI: endotracheal intubation

1) during the early phases to prevent ET intubation;
2) when the respiratory failure is already established as a treatment alternative to ET intubation and
3) during the resolution of acute respiratory failure as a means to wean patients from mechanical ventilation or
4) post-extubation, in order to prevent re-intubation.

In the present chapter, the efficacy of NIV in preventing episodes of pneumonia in patients with acute respiratory failure will be discussed through randomized and non-randomized studies where NIV has been adopted as a modulated approach at different times of acute respiratory failure.

Early NIV: Randomized Trials in Immunocompetent Patients

Several prospective randomized studies have evaluated the usefulness of NIV in avoiding ET intubation and reducing complications related to intubation in patients with hypercapnic and hypoxemic acute respiratory failure.

In a controlled study including 85 patients with chronic obstructive pulmonary disease (COPD), Brochard et al. [16] randomized 43 patients to receive NIV via face mask for at least 6 hours per day and 42 patients to receive standard therapy with oxygen supplementation. The authors found that NIV improved gas-exchange and decreased both the rate of ET intubation and the length of stay in the ICU. There was a trend to reduction of VAP in the NIV group in comparison to patients receiving conventional treatment (5 vs 17%, $p=NS$). In this study, the crude mortality was significantly decreased in patients receiving NIV treatment.

Wysocki et al. [25] compared NIV delivered through a face mask versus conventional therapy in a group of 41 patients with acute respiratory failure. A reduction in ET intubation (36 vs 100%, $p=0.02$), duration of ICU length of stay (13 ± 15 vs 32 ± 30 days, $p=0.04$), and in mortality rate (9 vs 66%, $p=0.06$) was observed only in hypercapnic patients. The authors concluded that NIV may not be effective in all forms of acute respiratory failure not related to COPD, but the incidence of pneumonia and severe sepsis was not reported.

In a randomized, controlled, prospective trial, Wood et al. [27] evaluated the effects of early NIV in 27 patients with hypoxemic acute respiratory failure requiring admission to the emergency department. Sixteen patients (59.3%) were randomly assigned to receive conventional medical therapy plus NIV and 11 patients (40.7%) to receive conventional medical therapy alone. NIV was delivered by a nasal mask with biphasic positive airway pressure (BiPAP) ventilator. The rate of pneumonia was higher in the group receiving conventional medical therapy than in the NIV group (18 vs 0%, $p < 0.05$).

Confalonieri et al. [28] conducted a multicenter, prospective, randomized study comparing standard treatment plus NIV delivered through a face mask to standard treatment alone, in patients with acute respiratory failure caused by severe community-acquired pneumonia. Fifty-six consecutive patients (28 in each arm) were enrolled, and the two groups were similar at study entry. Patients randomized to NIV had a significantly lower rate of ET intubation (21 vs 50%, $p = 0.03$) and a shorter duration of ICU stay (1.8 ± 0.7 vs 6 ± 1.8 days, $p = 0.04$). Among patients with COPD, those randomized to NIV had a lower intensity of nursing care workload ($p = 0.04$) and improved 2-month survival (88.9 vs 37.5%, $p = 0.05$). Timing to ET intubation was similar in both groups, and rate of complications developing during intubation was not increased in patients failing NIV and requiring intubation. Complications associated with conventional mechanical ventilation included two cases of broncho-alveolar lavage (BAL)-proven VAP, one case of otitis and mastoiditis, and one of pneumothorax. All these complications occurred in patients originally randomized to standard treatment.

In a prospective randomized trial, Martin et al. [29] compared non-invasive positive pressure ventilation (NPPV) with usual medical care in the treatment of patients with acute respiratory failure of various origins. Thirty-two patients were randomized to receive NPPV and 29 to receive usual medical care (UMC). NPPV was delivered through a BiPAP system, using initial inspiratory (IPAP) and expiratory (EPAP) positive airway pressure levels of 5 cmH$_2$O. A significantly lower rate of ET intubation was observed in the NPPV group than in the usual medical care group (6.38 intubations vs 21.25 intubations per 100 ICU days; $p = 0.002$). Mortality rates in the ICU were similar for the two treatment groups (2.39 [NPPV group] vs 4.27 deaths [UMC group] per 100 ICU days, $p = 0.21$). Patients with hypoxemic acute respiratory failure in the NPPV group had a significantly lower ET intubation rate than those in the usual medical care group (7.46 intubations vs 22.64 intubations per 100 ICU days, $p = 0.026$); a similar trend was reported also in patients with hypercapnic acute respiratory failure (5.41 intubations [NPPV group] vs 18.52 intubations [UMC group] per 100 ICU days, $p = 0.064$). No infectious complications were evidenced in the two groups.

▌ Randomized Trials in Immunocompromised Patients

Avoiding intubation is a major goal in the treatment of acute respiratory failure in immunosuppressed patients. However, few clinical data are available on the efficacy of NIV in these high risk patients. Two different randomized studies suggest that early NIV application is a therapeutic challenge in patients after transplantation or with immunosuppression of various origins. In a prospective randomized study, Antonelli et al. [30] compared the use of NIV delivered through a face mask with standard treatment using oxygen supplementation to avoid ET intubation, in 40 patients with hypoxemic acute respiratory failure after solid organ transplantation. Twenty patients were randomly assigned to each group and the two groups were similar for baseline characteristics at study entry. All COPD patients were excluded.

Within the first hour of treatment, 14 (70%) of the 20 patients in the NIV group improved their PaO_2/FiO_2 ratio vs five (25%) in the standard treatment group. The improvement of gas-exchange over time was more prolonged in the NIV group than in the standard treatment group (60 vs 25%; p = 0.03). The use of NIV was well tolerated, safe, and associated with a significant reduction in ET intubation (20 vs 70%, p = 0.05) and in severe sepsis and septic shock rates, including VAP (20 vs 50%, p = 0.047). Patients in the NIV group had lower durations of ICU stay (mean [SD] days, 5.5 [3] vs 9 [4], p = 0.03) and lower rates of ICU mortality (20 vs 50%, p = 0.05) than those in the standard treatment group. Hospital mortality did not differ in the two groups.

Hilbert et al. [31] investigated the ability of NIV to prevent ET intubation and serious complications in patients with hematological malignancies, immunosuppression, bone marrow transplantation or human immunodeficiency virus (HIV). Fifty-two patients were enrolled into the study and randomized (26 in each arm) to receive standard treatment with oxygen therapy through a Venturi mask or standard treatment plus intermittent face mask NIV. The authors found that patients in the NIV group required less ET intubation (46 vs 77%, p = 0.03) and had fewer serious complications (50 vs 81%, p = 0.02) than patients in the standard treatment group. The early application of NIV was associated with a decrease in the rate of VAP (12 vs 35%, p = 0.05), and in ICU and hospital mortality (10 vs 18 patients, p = 0.03 and 13 vs 21 patients, p = 0.02, respectively).

These results confirm that the early application of NIV to immunosuppressed patients with hypoxemic acute respiratory failure may be effective in preventing episodes of VAP, by avoiding ET intubation. Moreover, the reduction in additive morbidity may improve patient survival.

∎ NIV as a Means of Treating Established Acute Respiratory Failure: Randomized Trials

Recently, Antonelli et al. [24] conducted a prospective, randomized trial comparing NIV via face mask to ET intubation with conventional ventilation in hypoxemic acute respiratory failure patients who met well defined criteria for mechanical ventilation. Sixty-four consecutive patients were enrolled (32 in each arm) and randomly assigned to each group. The study had a true 'intention to treat' approach and represents the first trial that used NIV as an alternative to conventional mechanical ventilation with ET intubation when the acute respiratory failure is already established. After 1 hour of mechanical ventilation, 20 out of the 32 patients (62%) in the NIV group and 15 of the 32 patients (47%) in the conventional ventilation group improved their ratio of PaO_2 to FiO_2 (PaO_2/FiO_2) (p <0.05). Patients in the conventional ventilation group had more serious complications (66 vs 38%, p = 0.02) and ET intubation-related complications, including pneumonia and sinusitis (31 vs 3%, p = 0.003), than patients in the NIV group. Among patients who failed NIV and required ET intubation, 12 patients (38%) developed serious complications. One of these 12 patients had pneumonia after 6 days of ET intubation. Among survivors, patients in the NIV group had a shorter duration of mechanical ventilation (3 ± 3 vs 6 ± 5 days, p = 0.006) and a shorter stay in the ICU (6.6 ± 5 vs 14 ± 13 days, p = 0.002) than those in the conventional ventilation group.

Factors that may have been involved in shortening the duration of mechanical ventilation in the NIV group included avoidance of sedation, lower rate of VAP, elimination of the extra-work imposed by the ET tube and earlier removal from MV. The authors concluded that NIV is as effective as conventional ventilation in improving gas-exchange in patients with hypoxemic acute respiratory failure and that when ET intubation is avoided the development of VAP is unlikely.

▌ NIV as a Weaning Strategy or to Avoid Re-Intubation: Randomized Trials

The rationale for NIV as a weaning strategy may be related to the ability of NIV to decrease the workload of respiratory muscles, and the development of rapid and shallow breathing associated with unsuccessful weaning from mechanical ventilation.

Nava et al. [12] conducted a prospective randomized controlled study to evaluate the use of non-invasive PSV in the weaning of COPD patients with acute respiratory failure. Fifty patients who had failed a T-piece trial were randomized (25 in each group) to extubation with immediate application of NIV with pressure support or to weaning with ET intubation in pressure support mode. Twenty-two out of the 25 patients (88%) in the NIV group were successfully weaned vs 17 in the invasively ventilated group (68%). None of the patients (0%) in the NIV group developed VAP whereas 7 patients (28%) in the invasive weaning group did (p=0.005). The use of NIV significantly decreased the duration of ICU stay (15±5 vs 24±13 days; p<0.05) and increased the 60-day-survival rate (92 vs 72%, p=0.009).

This study showed that by using NIV as a weaning strategy, the likelihood of weaning success increases, with a decrease in the additive morbidity and the overall mortality.

The effect of NIV during persistent weaning failure was evaluated in another randomized clinical trial [13] including 43 patients who had failed a spontaneous breathing trial for three consecutive days. Thirty-three of these patients had underlying chronic obstructive failure. Patients were randomly assigned to be extubated with NIV or to follow a conventional weaning approach. In this study, the authors found that NIV was effective in facilitating the weaning process, reducing the duration of mechanical ventilation and need for tracheostomy. NIV was associated with a decrease in additive morbidity, including the incidence of VAP, septic shock and multiple organ failure (MOF), and with improvement in the ICU and 90-day cumulative mortality.

▌ NIV: Non-randomized Studies

The ability of NIV to prevent nosocomial pneumonia was also demonstrated in a prospective epidemiological survey on a cohort of 320 consecutive patients with acute respiratory failure on more than 48 hours of mechanical ventilation [32]. The authors reported a lower (p=0.004) rate of VAP in non-invasively supported patients (0.16 per 100 days of NIV) versus those on conventional ventilation (0.85 per 100 days of ET intubation).

Similar results were reported by Nourdine et al. [33] in a prospective study comparing a group of 159 patients with acute respiratory failure of various origins, treated with NIV and 607 patients with ET intubation and mechanical ventilation. The authors described a significantly lower incidence of VAP (4.4 vs 13.2 per 1000 patients/days, p<0.05) and other nosocomial infections in the NIV group in comparison to the conventional ventilation group.

Recently, Girou et al. [34] conducted a matched-case control study that described the application of NIV in everyday clinical practice on 100 patients with acute exacerbation of COPD or hypercapnic cardiogenic pulmonary edema, to evaluate whether the use of NIV was associated with a decreased risk of nosocomial infection and improvement of survival. NIV was delivered in 134 out of 1040 patients. Only 50 of these patients were eligible as cases and treated with NIV for at least two hours. Fifty control patients receiving conventional ventilation with ET intubation were matched for diagnosis, age, simplified acute physiology score II (SAPS II), logistic organ dysfunction (LOD) score and absence of contraindications to NIV treatment.

The 50 patients treated with NIV developed significantly fewer complications (p=0.006) during their ICU stay and received fewer antibiotics for nosocomial infection (8 vs 26%, p=0.01) than controls. Rates of nosocomial infection (18 [NIV group] vs 60% [ET group], p<0.001) and pneumonia (8 [NIV group] vs 22% [ET group]; p=0.04) were significantly decreased when NIV was applied. Interestingly, the authors also observed that the mean duration of ventilation (mean [SD]; 6 [6] vs 10 [12] days, p=0.01), mean duration of ICU stay (9 [7] vs 15 [14] days, p=0.02), and crude mortality (4 vs 26%; p=0.002) were lower in the NIV group than in the ET intubation group.

In a prospective survey among 42 ICUs, Carlucci et al. [35] enrolled 689 patients with acute respiratory failure who required ventilatory support. In 108 of these patients, NIV treatment was delivered through a face mask. Among the 581 patients receiving conventional treatment with ET intubation, 382 were intubated before ICU admission. SAPS II score was significantly higher in patients receiving conventional treatment with ET intubation (mean [SD]; 47 [21] vs 36 [20]; p<0.001) than in patients receiving NIV treatment. Eleven patients (10%) in the NIV group and 72 patients (19%) in the ET intubation group developed nosocomial pneumonia (p=0.03). Overall mortality was significantly decreased in the NIV group (22 vs 41%; p<0.001). The authors concluded that NIV may be successful in selected patients and is associated with a decreased risk of pneumonia and death.

In a prospective multicenter cohort study [36], Antonelli et al. prospectively investigated outcome descriptors for NIV in a population of 354 hypoxemic patients with acute respiratory failure of various origins. The authors found that NIV was successful in 264 (70%) patients whereas 108 (30%) patients failed NIV treatment and required ET intubation. A multivariate analysis identified age >40 years (OR=1.72, 95% CI: 0.92–3.23), SAPS II score ≥35 (OR=1.81, 95% CI: 1.07–3.06), the presence of ARDS or community-acquired pneumonia (OR=3.75, 95% CI: 2.25–6.24), and a $PaO_2:FiO_2 \leq 146$ mmHg after 1 hour of NPPV (OR=2.51, 95% CI: 1.45–4.35), as factors independently associated with NPPV failure. Throughout the study period, patients avoiding ET intubation had shorter duration of mechanical ventilation (median [range], 48 [1–216] vs 24 [1–192] days, p=0.06) and ICU length of stay (median [range], 5 [3–31] vs 9 [1–72] days, p<0.001) than those requiring ET intubation. Successful NIV was associated with a significant decrease in the rate of VAP (0.4 [NIV success] vs 28% [NIV failure], p<0.01), severe sepsis and septic shock (3 [NIV success] vs 65% [NIV failure], p<0.01).

∎ Future Perspectives

During the early phases of hypoxemic acute respiratory failure, if disconnection from mechanical ventilation occurs, patients can rapidly deteriorate gas exchange with potential life threatening consequences. Thus, the improvement of patient-ventilator interface seems crucial to achieve a prolonged application of NIV.

NIV can fail due to: a) conditions related to the disease (inability to correct hypoxia, manage copious secretions, etc.) or b) technical causes (intolerance, skin necrosis).

Attempting to improve tolerance of patients we adopted a transparent Helmet® (Starmed, Mirandola, Italy) (Fig. 2) made in latex-free PVC as an interface during non-invasive PSV. The device allows patients to see, read and speak, and actively interact with the environment.

We conducted a prospective clinical pilot investigation [37], on 33 consecutive non-COPD patients with hypoxemic acute respiratory failure treated by pressure support delivered by helmet and 66 matched controls treated with pressure support delivered by facial mask. Eight patients (33%) in the helmet group and 21 patients (32%) in the facial mask group (p=0.3) failed non-invasive PSV and were intubated. No patients failed non-invasive PSV due to intolerance of the technique in the helmet group in comparison with 8 patients (38%) in the mask group (p=0.047). Complications related to the technique (skin necrosis, gastric distension and eye irritation) were fewer in the helmet group compared to the mask group (no patients vs 14 patients; p=0.002). Four patients (12%) in the helmet group and 10 patients (20%) in the mask group developed nosocomial pneumonia after the study entry (p=0.3).

Interestingly, three of the four pneumonias in the helmet group and six of the 10 nosocomial pneumonia in the mask group developed only after the failure of non-invasive PSV and ET intubation. Helmets allowed the continuous application of non-invasive PSV for a longer period of time (p=0.05). Length of stay in the ICU, intensive care, and hospital mortality were not different in the two groups. We showed that non-invasive PSV by helmet successfully treated hypoxemic acute respiratory failure, with better tolerance and fewer complications than facial mask non-invasive PSV.

• Latex-free transparent PVC secured by 2 arm-pit braces (A) at two hooks (B) of the metallic ring (C) joining helmet with a soft collar (D)
• A seal connection (E) allows the passage of NGT
• Inlet and outlet of the helmet are connected to the inspiratory and expiratory valves of the ventilator through conventional circuits

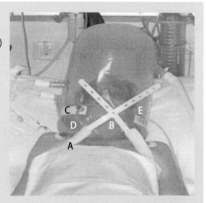

Fig. 2. NIV delivered by Helmet® (Starmed, Mirandola, Italy). NGT: nasogastric tube

If larger studies confirm these preliminary data, the helmet could become another valid therapeutic option to deliver non-invasive PSV to patients with hypoxemic acute respiratory failure.

Conclusion

Randomized and non-randomized clinical studies [17–36] conducted on more than 2000 patients have demonstrated that NIV is really effective in the clinical management of patients with acute respiratory failure.

When NIV is successful, and ET intubation is avoided, the development of nosocomial pneumonia is unlikely (Table 1). Recent studies [24–37] have also reported that NIV treatment may be attempted as a first line intervention for hypoxemic acute respiratory failure with significant reductions in nosocomial infection, including VAP, as well as in antibiotic use, duration in ICU stay, and overall mortality. However, large prospective randomized multicenter trials are needed to obtain a definitive consensus.

Table 1. Randomized studies evaluating the usefulness of early non-invasive ventilation (NIV) as a means of preventing nosocomial pneumonia

Author	Year	N. of pts NIV vs ETI	Episodes of PNEU in CT group (%)	Episodes of PNEU in NIV group (%)	p-value	Mortality in CT group (%)	Mortality in NIV group (%)	p-value
Brochard [16]	1995	43 vs 42	17	5	NS	29	9	0.02
Wysocki [25]	1995	21 vs 20	NR	NR	NR	66	9	NS
Antonelli [24]	1998	32 vs 32	25	3	0.003	47	28	NS
Wood [27]	1998	16 vs 11	18	0	<0.05	0	25	NS
Confalonieri [28]	1999	28 vs 28	7	0	<0.05	88.9*	37.5*	0.05*
Martin [29]	2000	14 vs 11	0	0	NS	34	16	NS
Antonelli [30]	2000	20 vs 20	20	10	0.047	50	20	0.05
Hilbert [31]	2001	26 vs 26	35	12	0.05	69	38	0.03

PNEU = pneumonia; Pts = patients; ETI = endotracheal intubation; CT = conventional treatment; NR = not reported; NS = not significant.
* Refers only to patients with chronic obstructive pulmonary disease

References

1. Torres A, Aznar R, Gatell JM, et al (1990) Incidence, risk and prognosis factors of nosocomial pneumonia in mechanically ventilated patients. Am Rev Respir Dis 142:523–528
2. Meduri GU. (1998) Non invasive ventilation. In: Marini J, Slutsky A (eds) Physiological Basis of Ventilatory Support: A Series on Lung Biology in Health and Disease. Marcel Dekker, New York, pp 921–998
3. Fagon JY, Chastre J, Domart Y, et al (1989) Nosocomial pneumonia in patients receiving continuous mechanical ventilation: prospective analysis of 52 episodes with use of protective specimen brush and quantitative culture techniques. Am Rev Respir Dis 139:877–884
4. Meduri GU, Conoscenti CC, Menashe P, et al (1989) Non invasive face mask ventilation in patients with acute respiratory failure. Chest 95:865–870
5. Benhamou D, Girault C, Faure C, et al (1992) Nasal mask ventilation in acute respiratory failure: experience in elderly patients. Chest 102:912–917
6. Bersten AD, Holt AW, Vedig AE, et al (1991) Treatment of severe cardiogenic pulmonary edema with continuous positive airway pressure delivered by face mask. N Engl J Med 325:1825–1830
7. Duncan AW, Oh TE, Hillman DR (1986) PEEP and CPAP. Anaesth Intensive Care 14:236–250
8. Branson DR (1988) PEEP without endotracheal intubation. Respir Care 33:598–610
9. Amato MB, Barbas CS, Medeiros DM, et al (1998) Effect of a protective-ventilation strategy on mortality in the acute respiratory distress syndrome. N Engl J Med 338 (6):347–354
10. Brochard L, Isabey D, Piquet J, et al (1990) Reversal of acute exacerbations of chronic obstructive lung disease by inspiratory assistance with a face mask. N Engl J Med 323:1523–1530
11. Jubran A, Van de Graaf WB, Tobin MJ (1995) Variability of patient-ventilator interaction with pressure support ventilation in patients with chronic obstructive pulmonary disease. Am J Respir Crit Care Med 152:129–136
12. Nava S, Ambrosino N, Clini E, et al (1998) Non invasive mechanical ventilation in the weaning of patients with respiratory failure due to chronic obstructive pulmonary disease. A randomized, controlled trial. Ann Intern Med 128:721–728
13. Ferrer M, Arancibia F, Esquinas A, et al (2000) Non invasive ventilation for persistent weaning failure. Am J Respir Crit Care Med 161:A262 (Abst)
14. Appendini L, Patessio A, Zanaboni S, et al (1994) Physiologic effects of positive end-expiratory pressure support during exacerbations of chronic obstructive pulmonary disease. Am J Respir Crit Care Med 149:1069–1076
15. Bott J, Carroll MP, Conway JH, et al (1993) Randomized controlled trial of nasal ventilation in acute ventilatory failure due to chronic obstructive airways disease. Lancet 341:1555–1558
16. Brochard L, Mancebo J, Wysocki M, et al (1995) NIV for acute chronic obstructive pulmonary disease. N Engl J Med 333:817–822
17. Meduri GU (1996) Noninvasive positive-pressure ventilation in patients with acute respiratory failure. Clin Chest Med 17:513–553
18. Bersten AD, Holt AW, Vedig AE, et al (1991) Treatment of severe cardiogenic pulmonary edema with continuous positive airway pressure delivered by face mask. N Engl J Med 325:1825–1830
19. Rasanen J, Heikkila J, Downs J, et al (1985) Continuous positive airway pressure by face mask in acute cardiogenic pulmonary edema. Am J Cardiol 55:296–300
20. Lin M, Yang Y, Chiany H, et al (1995) Reappraisal of continuous positive airway pressure therapy in acute cardiogenic pulmonary edema: short-term results and long-term follow-up. Chest 107:1379–1386
21. Masip J, Betbes AJ, Vecilla F, et al (2000) Non-invasive pressure support ventilation versus conventional oxygen therapy in acute cardiogenic pulmonary edema: a randomized trial. Lancet 356:2126–2132
22. Delclaux C, L'Her E, Alberti C, et al (2000) Treatment of acute hypoxemic non hypercapnic respiratory insufficiency with continuous positive airway pressure delivered by a face mask: a randomized controlled trial. JAMA 284:2352–2360

23. Mehta S, Jay GD, Woolard RH, et al (1997) Randomized, prospective trial of bilevel versus continuous positive airway pressure in acute pulmonary edema. Crit Care Med 25:620–628
24. Antonelli M, Conti G, Rocco M, et al (1998) A comparison of noninvasive positive-pressure ventilation and conventional mechanical ventilation in patients with acute respiratory failure. N Engl J Med 339:429–435
25. Wysocki M, Tric L, Wolff MA, et al (1995) Noninvasive pressure support ventilation in patients with acute respiratory failure: A randomized comparison with conventional therapy. Chest 107:761–768
26. Keenan SP, Kernerman PD, Cook DJ, et al (1997) The effect of non invasive positive pressure ventilation on mortality in patients admitted with acute respiratory failure: A meta-analysis. Crit Care Med 25:1685–1692
27. Wood KA, Lewis L, Von Harz B, et al (1998) The use of non invasive pressure support ventilation in the emergency department: Results of a randomized clinical trial. Chest 113:1339–1346
28. Confalonieri M, della Porta R, Potena A, et al (1999) Acute respiratory failure in patients with severe community-acquired pneumonia: a prospective randomized evaluation of non invasive ventilation. Am J Respir Crit Care Med 160:1585–1591
29. Martin TJ, Hovis JD, Costantino JP, et al (2000) A randomized prospective evaluation of non invasive ventilation for acute respiratory failure. Am J Respir Crit Care Med 161:807–813
30. Antonelli M, Conti G, Bufi M, et al (2000) Noninvasive ventilation for treatment of acute respiratory failure in patients undergoing solid organ transplantation. JAMA 283:235–241
31. Hilbert G, Gruson D, Vargas F, et al (2000) Non invasive continuous positive airway pressure in neutropenic patients with acute respiratory failure requiring intensive care unit admission. Crit Care Med 28:3185–3190
32. Guerin C, Girard R, Chemorin C, et al (1997) Facial mask non invasive mechanical ventilation reduces the incidence of nosocomial pneumonia. A prospective epidemiological survey from a single ICU. Intensive Care Med 23:1024–1032
33. Nourdine K, Combes P, Carton MJ, et al (1999) Does NIV reduce the ICU nosocomial infection risk? A prospective clinical survey. Intensive Care Med 25:567–573
34. Girou E, Schortgen F, Delclaux C, et al (2000) Association of non invasive ventilation with nosocomial infections and survival in critically ill patients. JAMA 284:2376–2378
35. Carlucci A, Richard JC, Wysocki M, et al (2001) Non invasive versus conventional mechanical ventilation. An epidemiologic survey. Am J Respir Crit Care Med 163:874–880
36. Antonelli M, Conti G, Moro ML, et al (2001) Predictors of failure of non invasive positive pressure ventilation in patients with acute hypoxemic respiratory failure: a multi-center study. Intensive Care Med 27:1718–1728
37. Antonelli M, Conti G, Pelosi P, et al (2002) A new treatment of acute hypoxemic respiratory failure: Non invasive pressure support ventilation delivered by Helmet. A pilot controlled trial. Crit Care Med (in press)

Infectious Challenges

Evaluation of Non-responding Patients with Ventilator-associated Pneumonia

M. Ferrer, M. Ioanas, and A. Torres

▌ Introduction

Ventilator-associated pneumonia (VAP) is a major challenge in the intensive care unit (ICU), with an incidence varying between 5 and 50% in mechanically ventilated patients [1, 2]. Because of its high mortality rate (around 30%) [3, 4], aggressive evaluation of patients who fail to improve during the first days of treatment is indicated.

Lack of response to empirical antibiotic treatment should be recognized early and an operative strategy to evaluate the causes of failure should be started. The most important questions arising in this situation are:

▌ what is the most appropriate moment to evaluate the response/non-response of VAP to antibiotic treatment and based on which criteria?
▌ what are the possible causes of non-response?
▌ what are the basic investigations to perform in order to detect the alternative causes and to optimize therapy?

▌ Response of Ventilator-Associated Pneumonia to Empirical Antibiotic Treatment: Timing and Criteria for Evaluation

Because of the severity of the disease and the high mortality rate, the evaluation of the response of VAP to empirical antibiotic treatment should be performed early and be based on objective criteria.

Apparently, the most suitable moment for assessment is 72 hours after initial diagnosis. This timing is justified by the study of Montravers et al. [5], who reported that 67% of patients with VAP had sterile secretions, obtained by protected specimen brush (PSB), after 3 days of antibiotic therapy and another 21% had microbial growth below the 10^3 colony-forming units (CFU)/ml threshold. Clinical improvement was associated with bacterial eradication in 96% of cases, while only 44% of patients with persistent growth over the threshold showed a favorable evolution. In addition, complete results of initial microbial investigations are available after 72 hours, allowing the adequacy of empirical treatment to be checked.

The evaluation of the response of VAP to the empirical antibiotic treatment should rely basically on the same criteria used for the initial diagnosis of VAP, namely: presence of fever or hypothermia; leukocytosis or leukopenia; purulent tracheobronchial secretions; and radiographic pulmonary infiltrates. It is known that the diagnosis of VAP based on all these criteria has a good specificity but with the cost of a loss in sensitivity. The most reasonable diagnostic accuracy is provided by the combination of radiographic infiltrates and two of three clinical criteria [6].

An additional benefit for evaluation could be obtained by using the clinical pulmonary infection score (CPIS) [7]. This score includes the traditional parameters (fever, leukocytes, tracheal secretions, oxygenation, radiograph abnormalities). However, because the score also takes into account the culture results of tracheal aspirates, the VAP evaluation may be delayed at least 24 hours. In addition, using the cut-off of 6 points, it appears that a fall below 6, which was compatible with clinical improvement, was observed only after 5 days of antibiotic treatment [8].

Useful tools to improve the accuracy of the follow-up evaluation could be clinical scores such as the lung injury score (LIS), focusing exclusively on lung parameters in ventilated patients (radiographic infiltrates, oxygenation, compliance, positive end-expiratory pressure [PEEP]), and the multiple organ dysfunction score (MODS), allowing concomitant disorders to be monitored also.

In practice, the persistence of fever and/or leukocytosis and/or purulent secretions or the progression of the radiographic infiltrate (increase of the initial opacity, cavitation, pleural effusion), reflect an abnormal evolution of VAP under antibiotic treatment. Additional functional pulmonary parameters, such as oxygenation, compliance, or need of PEEP, must be considered, as well as certain parameters of other organ dysfunction, such as creatinine, bilirubin, thrombocytes, Glasgow coma score, blood pressure, or central venous pressure.

▌ Causes of Non-Response of VAP to Empirical Antibiotic Treatment

The causes of non-response of VAP to the empirical antibiotic treatment are various (Table 1) and can be divided into three categories:
1) causes related to the antibiotic treatment or to the responsible microorganism;
2) infections other than VAP; and
3) non-infectious conditions.

Despite the large numbers of possible causes, few are common in clinical practice, facilitating the diagnostic approach.

Table 1. Causes of non-response of ventilator-associated pneumonia (VAP) to empirical antibiotic treatment. ARDS: acute respiratory distress syndrome; BOOP: bronchiolitis obliterans organizing pneumonia; CMV: cytomegalovirus

Causes related to the antibiotic treatment or to the responsible microorganism	Infections other than VAP	Non-infectious conditions
▌ Inappropriate election/combination of antibiotics	▌ Sinusitis	▌ ARDS
▌ Low dosage/serum level of antibiotics	▌ Vascular catheter-related sepsis	▌ Atelectasis
▌ Resistance to antibiotics (MRSA, P. aeruginosa, Acinetobacter spp, S. maltophilia)	▌ Abdominal sepsis (cholecystitis, pancreatitis, colitis)	▌ BOOP
	▌ Pulmonary abscess	▌ Pulmonary hemorrhage
	▌ Pleural effusion/empyema	▌ Pulmonary embolism
▌ Microorganisms not covered by the empiric antibiotic treatment (Candida spp, Aspergillus spp, CMV, Legionella spp, P. carinii)	▌ Urinary sepsis	▌ Congestive heart failure
		▌ Lung contusion
		▌ Pulmonary edema after lung resection
▌ Superinfection		▌ Drug-related fever

Causes Related to the Antibiotic Treatment or the Etiological Microorganism

The most frequent situation is lack of response due to the persistence of the etiological microorganism. This situation occurs in the following circumstances: inadequate treatment (inappropriate empirical selection of antibiotics, inappropriate dosage, low blood level of antibiotics) or infection caused by microorganisms not covered by the initial therapy (i.e., resistance to antibiotics or infection by unusual organisms).

Initial resistance of the microorganism to antibiotics or inappropriate dosage or combination of antibiotics could result in microbial persistence and lack of clinical resolution. Over the last decade, lung infections caused by strains with multiple resistance to the usual antibiotics, like *Pseudomonas aeruginosa*, *Acinetobacter* spp, and methicillin-resistant *Staphylococcus aureus* (MRSA), have become a common problem in ICUs, being responsible for more than 50% of VAP episodes [2, 9, 10].

The American Thoracic Society recommendation [11] for the treatment of hospital-acquired pneumonia, and other subsequent studies [10], have described a number of risk factors related to infections by multiresistant strains and have made suggestions for optimal empirical antibiotic coverage in these situations. Thus, this approach allows the clinician to safely avoid possible non-response related to antibiotic resistance or inappropriate drug strategy. In fact, several studies [12, 13] support the importance of adequate initial therapy, reporting a statistically significant difference in mortality rate between patients receiving correct antibiotic therapy versus those with inadequate treatment.

Although the persistence of the microorganism can be proved only by a second bacterial investigation, the results of the initial microbial investigation are already available at 72 hours, and treatment should be adjusted accordingly. A second respiratory sampling could reveal a superinfection with another microorganism that is not covered by the initial antibiotic treatment, for example MRSA.

The initial infection, or the superinfection, with MRSA could be a cause of non-response in a significant number of cases, because vancomycin is not usually administered empirically. The fear of developing vancomycin-resistant strains justifies this conservative attitude, but if certain risk factors (i.e., head trauma or low level of consciousness [14] are present, empirical vancomycin is more than appropriate. In addition, the increasing proportion of methicillin-resistant staphylococci in the ICU and the promising new agents against Gram-positive organisms both support the empirical use of vancomycin [15].

Infections with unusual microorganims such as *Aspergillus* spp, *Legionella pneumophila*, *Candida* spp, or *Cytomegalovirus* (CMV) are frequently associated with an immunocompromised condition (solid organ transplant, hematological disorder, prolonged corticosteroid therapy) [16, 17] and must be considered in these particular situations. Rapid techniques of antigen detection may facilitate diagnosis in cases of infection with CMV, *Aspergillus* spp or *L. pneumophila*. Due to its presence in normal flora, infection with *Candida* spp should be considered only in patients with multiple courses of antibiotics and more than 10 days of ICU stay [18], and if no other microorganism is isolated in the respiratory samples.

Infections other than VAP

A concomitant infection in a patient with VAP is not uncommon and can contribute to the persistence of the systemic inflammatory response syndrome (SIRS) and especially to the persistence of fever. In addition, fever in critically ill patients could be related to a variety of non-infectious causes (i.e., myocardial infarction, gastrointestinal bleeding) but in these cases it does not usually exceed 38.9 °C. Therefore, we will focus only on the most frequent nosocomial infections that can occur in an ICU patient.

Nosocomial Sinusitis. Nosocomial sinusitis is commonly associated with nasotracheal intubation and nasogastric tubes but also with head trauma and neurological disorders [19, 20]. It usually occurs after 7 days of nasal intubation, in up to 85% of patients [21, 22]. However, apparently only 20–40% of patients with radiological evidence of maxillary sinusitis have true infectious sinusitis, namely with the presence of pus and positive cultures of the responsible microorganism [21]. Infectious sinusitis seems to be a risk factor for subsequent infections of the lower respiratory tract, supported by a recent study in an animal model [23]. Furthermore, Rouby et al. [21] reported an incidence of nosocomial pneumonia of 67% in patients with infectious nosocomial sinusitis.

The diagnosis of sinusitis is based on computed tomography (CT) scan rather than on the classic x-ray. Microorganisms frequently associated with nosocomial sinusitis in mechanically ventilated patients are *P. aeruginosa*, *Acinetobacter* spp, *Staph. aureus* and anaerobes [19, 20]. Treatment consists of removal of nasal tube, if possible, and maxillary sinus drainage and lavage. Antibiotic treatment is controversial but still recommended.

Vascular Catheter-related Sepsis. Vascular catheter-related sepsis should be considered in patients with positive blood culture and persistent fever. The incidence of catheter-related bacteremia ranges between <1 and 18% [24], depending mainly on the number of days of catheterization (usually more than 2 days), the frequency of manipulation, and the number of ports. The most common microorganisms isolated in blood cultures and in the culture of the catheter tip are the staphylococci, with *Staph. epidermidis* accounting for 50% [25]. Removal of the catheter with reinsertion in a different site is recommended if catheter-related sepsis is suspected.

Abdominal Sepsis. Cholecystitis occurs in 1.5% of critically-ill patients [26] as a result of several non-infectious mechanisms such as gallbladder ischemia, bile stasis, use of PEEP, or parenteral nutrition [27]. Bacterial invasion is just a secondary phenomenon. The diagnosis is particularly difficult in intubated patients and usually occurs when the gallbladder is perforated. Therefore, a persistent fever without evident focus of infection should indicate, among others, a radiological investigation of the gallbladder. Ultrasound and CT scan both provide good diagnostic accuracy. The therapeutic approach in these patients is somewhat controversial. The procedure of choice seems to be percutaneous cholecystectomy and open cholecystectomy is only recommended if this fails [28].

Pancreatitis is sometimes associated with left pleural effusion and has been related also to the development of acute respiratory distress syndrome (ARDS) [29]. Therefore, a new pulmonary infiltrate in patients with a diagnosis of pancreatitis should alert to the possibility of ARDS rather than a pneumonia.

Pseudomembranous colitis caused by *Clostridium difficile* occurs in 20% of all hospitalized patients and about one third of them develop diarrhea [30]. Cephalosporins and clindamycin are usually associated with the development of pseudomembranous colitis [31]. Diagnosis is based on ELISA test for *C. difficile* toxins and/or on CT scan of the abdomen.

Urinary Sepsis. Urinary tract infection (UTI) is a common event in ICU patients, with a reported incidence of 50% of all nosocomial infections. Bacteriuria usually occurs in 30% of catheterized hospitalized patients [32], although this condition does not always imply a real UTI. The differentiation between colonization and infection is not clear, while the bacterial load ($>10^5$ CFU/ml) is similar in both cases. Furthermore, only 3% of these patients develop bacteremia with the same microorganism as isolated in the urine. Therefore, treatment is recommended only if there is ultrasound evidence of stones or urinary tract obstruction.

Pulmonary Abscess. A cavitating image on standard radiograph or CT scan suggests a pulmonary abscess, a condition that prevents good penetration of antibiotics into the lung tissue and can results in the persistence of VAP. In this situation, antibiotic treatment should be revised in order to provide a better coverage for anaerobes and an adequate drainage technique should be considered.

Pleural Effusion/Empyema. Pleural effusion may be associated with VAP [33], contributing to the persistence of clinical and radiological manifestations of pulmonary infection despite adequate antibiotic treatment. A CT scan or ultrasound are often required to reveal pleural effusion in VAP patients. When a significant amount of pleural effusion is present, thoracentesis is mandatory in order to rule out an empyema. Grossly purulent fluid or a pH <7.20 and positive Gram stain and culture are indications for chest tube insertion.

Non-infectious Causes

Different non-infectious conditions can mimic or complicate VAP. The diagnosis is often difficult because these conditions are usually responsible for the lack of resolution of the pulmonary infiltrate and can also be accompanied by fever or other manifestations of SIRS. The most frequent non-infectious situations that should be considered in case of non-response of VAP are listed in Table 1.

ARDS. The distinction between ARDS and VAP is not always easy, especially in post-operative or trauma patients. Fever and leukocytosis can be present in the late phase of ARDS as a consequence of the fibroproliferative changes [34]. Furthermore, these two findings along with the radiographic infiltrate are also criteria to suspect the diagnosis of VAP. On the other hand, pneumonia is one of the main direct lung injuries related to the development of ARDS [29]. However, the presence of a bilateral radiographic infiltrate and severe hypoxemia associated with one of the accepted risk factors for ARDS (i.e., trauma, multiple transfusion, cardiopulmonary bypass, acute pancreatitis) could facilitate the distinction from pneumonia. In addition, a negative or under cut-off microbiologic result usually rules out a respiratory infection in these particular situations.

The relationship between these two conditions is bilateral, some studies reporting an incidence of nosocomial pneumonia varying between 15 [35] and 60% [36] in patients with ARDS. Because critically ill patients usually present with two or more criteria of SIRS [37] and become rapidly colonized with potential pathogenic microorganisms, the diagnosis of pneumonia in ARDS patients should be based on suggestive microbiological findings.

Atelectasis. The mechanical effect of the decubitus and the increased volume of tracheobronchial secretions facilitate the occurrence of atelectasis in ventilated patients. This circumstance could result in a progression of the initial radiological infiltrate. In addition, atelectasis could be associated with fever [38]. Appropriate hydration and physiotherapy may prevent the development of atelectasis in intubated patients.

Bronchiolitis Obliterans Organizing Pneumonia. Bronchiolitis obliterans organizing pneumonia (BOOP) is usually related to specific conditions such as collagen vascular diseases, viral infection, aspiration of gastric contents, lung irradiation, drugs or lung transplant [39]. Clinical presentation may mimic pneumonia and the presence of bilateral radiographic infiltrates is common. Diagnosis is usually delayed but a persistent infiltrate with negative microbial cultures and lack of clinical improvement with antibiotic treatment should alert to this alternative. Although it does not provide diagnostic findings, CT scan investigation can be useful, while open lung biopsy is the last option in mechanically ventilated patients. The administration of corticosteroids usually results in rapid clinical and radiological improvement.

Pulmonary Hemorrhage. Pulmonary hemorrhage is more frequent in patients with hematological disorders or receiving immunosuppressive therapy [40] and should be considered as a differential diagnosis in intubated patients with marked thrombocytopenia. Nevertheless, pulmonary infection in these particular patients could also result in bleeding into the alveolar space [41], so that microbiological investigation of the respiratory sample is mandatory.

Pulmonary Embolism. Pulmonary embolism should be suspected in postoperative patients, patients with prolonged bed-stay or signs of thrombophlebitis. The development of a new pulmonary infiltrate in these patients, associated with a marked deterioration in gas exchange and hemodynamic instability should raise the suspicion of embolism and a supplemental investigation by ventilation-perfusion scintigraphy or pulmonary artery arteriography should be performed.

Congestive Heart Failure. The classical radiographic image of pulmonary edema and high central venous pressure facilitate the diagnosis, but asymmetric patterns of pulmonary edema are not infrequently observed, for example in patients with chronic obstructive pulmonary disease (COPD) or with mitral valve insufficiency. Echocardiography and pulmonary artery catheterization may be helpful in the management of these patients.

Pulmonary Contusion. Probably the most challenging condition in ICU is trauma, because of the frequent presence of SIRS and multiple evident or masked injuries, which make the diagnosis of VAP rather difficult. Thoracic trauma with lung contusion may be followed by infection of the injured pulmonary region with poor radiological improvement and apparent lack of response to antibiotic treatment.

Pulmonary Edema After Pulmonary Resection. Pulmonary edema after pulmonary resection is defined by lung injury after pneumonectomy, lobectomy or bilobectomy [42]. It occurs in approximately 7% of lung resections [43], usually developing 1 to 3 days after surgery [44], and its clinical and pathological manifestations are very similar to ARDS. The diagnosis of pneumonia in the postoperative patient with pulmonary resection is particularly difficult, because fever in the first 48 hours after surgery is a common event and a new pulmonary infiltrate may reflect post-resection lung injury.

Drug-induced Fever. Drug-induced fever is associated with antibiotics, antiarrhythmic drugs, and phenytoin [45]. Although these drugs are frequently administered in the ICU, their role as a cause of fever must be consider only when all possible foci of infection have been ruled out and when blood eosinophilia is present.

▌ Basic Investigations in Non-responding Patients With VAP

The evaluation of the response of VAP to empirical antibiotic treatment should be practical and performed early (Fig. 1). The first approach in cases who fail to improve should be the assessment of the antibiotic treatment based on the microbiological results of the respiratory samples collected on the day of the diagnosis. Therefore, a microbial investigation prior to initiation of the empirical therapy is extremely useful. Although some authors recommend bronchoscopic invasive techniques (PSB, bronchoalveolar lavage [BAL]) [46], the quantitative endotracheal aspirate seems to have similar diagnostic yield [47], is less expensive, and is easier to perform. Complete bacteriological results (Gram stain, cultures, and susceptibility tests) are usually available after 72 hours, facilitating the evaluation of the adequacy of the empirical therapy.

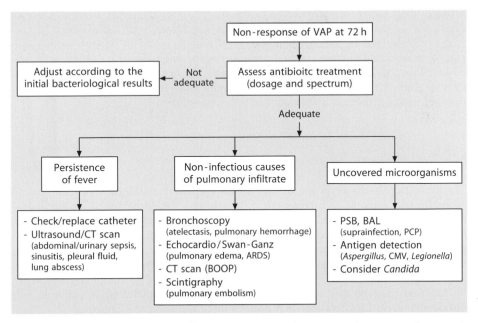

Fig. 1. Basic investigations to be considered in patients with non-responding ventilator associated pneumonia (VAP) after 72 hours of empirical antibiotic treatment. PSB: protected specimen brush; BAL: bronchoalveolar lavage; ARDS: acute respiratory distress syndrome; BOOP: bronchiolitis obliterans organizing pneumonia; CMV: cytomegalovirus; PCP: *Pneumocystis carinii* pneumonia

If the antibiotic treatment is inadequate in terms of spectrum, dosage or serum level, it should be correctly readjusted. If the empirical antibiotic treatment is adequate, the investigation should move on towards the next step and consider: 1) an infection/superinfection due to a microorganism not covered by the initial therapy; and, 2) causes of non-response other than VAP.

In the first case, a new microbial investigation, preferably by invasive methods (i.e., bronchoscopy with PSB and BAL) is recommended. The antigen detection techniques for *Aspergillus* spp, *Legionella*, and CMV are useful, especially in immunocompromised patients (hematological disorders, organ transplants). An infection by *Pneumocystis carinii* should be considered in patients at risk of human immunodeficiency virus (HIV) infection.

Other causes of non-response (infectious or non-infectious) require further investigations, based mainly on the suspicion of the most common alternative diagnosis compatible with the clinical and radiological manifestations (Fig. 1). Fever > 38.9 °C is usually associated with an infection [48], and the investigation must focus on the possible sources of pathogens. If a bacteremia is caused by staphylococci, vascular catheters should be replaced. A thoracic and abdominal ultrasound investigation may reveal a possible pleural effusion or abdominal source of sepsis. A progression of a pulmonary infiltrate under correct antibiotic treatment or a bilateral radiological pattern should mandate the investigation of other alternative causes, especially non-infectious. Because 72 hours is too early to observe any radiological improvement, the persistence of the initial infiltrate should indicate further investigation only if it is accompanied by the persistence of other clinical signs (fever, purulent tracheobronchial secretion or leukocytosis). Fiberoptic bronchoscopy represents the cornerstone for the investigation of the pulmonary infiltrates. Respiratory samples facilitate the diagnosis of bacterial, viral and fungal infections as well as of other non-infectious conditions such as alveolar hemorrhage or atelectasis by mucus plugging. A CT scan is useful in patients with suspicion of pulmonary abscess, pleural effusion, nosocomial sinusitis, pseudomembranous colitis and BOOP. When pulmonary embolism is suspected, ventilation-perfusion scintigraphy is required. Echocardiography and pulmonary artery catheterization are useful if there is a suspicion of pulmonary edema.

▌ Conclusion

The evaluation of the response of VAP to the empirical antibiotic treatment should be performed early, at 72 hours from diagnosis and should be based on the assessment of the initial criteria of diagnosis and on certain additional scores of organ function (LIS, MODS). Lack of response to the antibiotic treatment must be suspected in the following circumstances: persistence of fever, purulent tracheal secretions, leukocytosis; progression of the radiographic pulmonary infiltrate; lack of improvement or further impairment of gas exchange. Other parameters of organ dysfunction must be assessed (i.e., creatinine, bilirubin, platelets) in order to rule out concomitant disorders that may contribute to the failure to improve.

The first approach in case of non-response consists of revising the antibiotic treatment based on the initial bacteriological results and adjusting the combination and dosage, if necessary. Some microorganisms that are not covered by the empirical treatment (MRSA, fungi, *Legionella* spp, CMV) must be consider when risk factors are present (i.e., head trauma for MRSA, immunocompromised condition for fungi and viruses). Other frequent causes of fever in critically ill patients could be concomitant to VAP, like catheter-related sepsis, sinusitis or urinary infection. The radiographic pulmonary infiltrate in critically ill patients could be related to ARDS, atelectasis, BOOP, pulmonary embolism or pulmonary edema after lung resection. Fiberoptic bronchoscopy with respiratory sampling (PSB, BAL), ultrasound, CT scan, echocardiography and pulmonary scintigraphy are the basic investigations recommended when a condition other than VAP is suspected to be responsible for the lack of improvement of the patient with VAP.

References

1. Celis R, Torres A, Gatell JM, Almela M, Rodriguez-Roisin R, Aqusti-Vidal A (1988) Nosocomial pneumonia: A multivariate analysis of risk and prognosis. Chest 93:318–324
2. Fagon JY, Chastre J, Domart Y, et al (1989) Nosocomial pneumonia in patients receiving continuous mechanical ventilation. Prospective analysis of 52 episodes with use of a protected specimen brush and quantitative culture techniques. Am Rev Respir Dis 139:877–884
3. Fagon JY, Chastre J, Hance AJ, Montravers P, Novara A, Gibert C (1993) Nosocomial pneumonia in ventilated patients: A cohort study evaluating attributable mortality and hospital stay. Am J Med 94:281–288
4. Leu HS, Kaiser DL, Mori M, Woolson RF, Wenzel RP (1989) Hospital-acquired pneumonia. Attributable mortality and morbidity. Am J Epidemiol 129:1258–1267
5. Montravers P, Fagon JY, Chastre J, et al (1993) Follow-up protected specimen brushes to assess treatment in nosocomial pneumonia. Am Rev Respir Dis 147:38–44
6. Fabregas N, Ewig S, Torres A, et al (1999) Clinical diagnosis of ventilator associated pneumonia revisited: comparative validation using immediate postmortem lung biopsies. Thorax 54:867–873
7. Pugin J, Auckenthaler R, Mili N, Janssens JP, Lew PD, Suter PM (1991) Diagnosis of ventilator associated pneumonia by bacteriologic analysis of bronchoscopic and non-bronchoscopic "blind" bronchoalveolar lavage fluid. Am Rev Respir Dis 143:1121–1129
8. Garrad ChS, A Court ChD (1995) The diagnosis of pneumonia in the critically ill. Chest 108:17s–25s
9. Torres A, Aznar R, Gatell JM, et al (1990) Incidence, risk, and prognosis factors of nosocomial pneumonia in mechanically ventilated patients. Am Rev Respir Dis 142:523–528
10. Trouillet JL, Chastre J, Vuagnat A, et al (1998) Ventilator-associated pneumonia caused by potentially drug-resistant bacteria. Am Rev Respir Dis 157:531–539
11. American Thoracic Society (1996) Hospital-acquired pneumonia in adults: Diagnosis, assessment, initial therapy, and prevention: A consensus statement. Am J Respir Crit Care Med 153:1711–1725
12. Kollef MH, Ward S (1998) The influence of mini-BAL cultures on patient outcomes: implications for the antibiotic management of ventilator-associated pneumonia. Chest 113:412–420
13. Nava S, Ambrosino N, Bruschi C, Confalonieri M, Rampulla C (1997) Physiological effects of flow and pressure triggering during non-invasive mechanical ventilation in patients with chronic obstructive pulmonary disease. Thorax 52:249–254
14. Rello J, Ausina V, Castella J, Net A, Prats G (1992) Nosocomial respiratory tract infections in multiple trauma patients. Influence of level of consciousness with implications for therapy. Chest 102:525–529
15. Ravindra M, Niederman MS (2000) Adequate empirical therapy minimizes the impact of diagnostic methods in patients with ventilator-associated pneumonia. Crit Care Med 28:3092–3093
16. Singh N (2000) Infection in solid organ transplant recipient. Curr Opin Infect Dis 13:343–347
17. Donnelly JP (2000) Infection in the neutropenic and haematopoietic stem cell transplant recipient. Curr Opin Infect Dis 13:337–342

18. Petri MG, König J, Moecke HP, et al (1997) Epidemiology of invasive mycosis in ICU patients: a prospective multicenter study in 435 non-neutropenic patients. Intensive Care Med 23:317–325
19. Bert F, Lambert-Zechovsky N (1996) Sinusitis in mechanically ventilated patients and its role in the pathogenesis of nosocomial pneumonia. Eur J Clin Microbiol Infect Dis 15:533–544
20. Le Moal G, Lemerre D, Grollier G, Desmont C, Klossek JM, Robert R (1999) Nosocomial sinusitis with isolation of anaerobic bacteria in ICU. Intensive Care Med 25:1066–1071
21. Rouby JJ, Laurent P, Gosnach M, et al (1994) Risk factors and clinical relevance of nosocomial maxillary sinisitis in the critically ill. Am J Respir Crit Care Med 150:776–783
22. Holzapfel L, Chastang C, Demingeon G, Bohe J, Piralla B, Coupry A (1999) Randomized study assessing the systematic search for maxillary sinusitis in nasotracheal mechanically ventilated patients. Am J Respir Crit Care Med 159:695–701
23. Berglof A, Norlander T, Feinstein R, Otori N, Stierna P, Sandstedt K (2000) Association of bronchopneumonia with sinusitis due to Bordetella bronchiseptica in an experimental rabbit model. Am J Rhinol 14:125–130
24. Elliott TSJ (1997) Catheter-associated infections: new developments in prevention. Current Topics in Intensive Care 4:182–205
25. Elliott TSJ (1993) Line-associated bacteraemias. Commun Dis Rep CDR Rev 3:R91–R96
26. Orlando R, Gleason E, Drezner AD (1983) Acute acalculous cholecystitis in the critically ill patient. Am J Surg 145:472–476
27. Barie PS, Fischer E (1995) Acute acalculous cholecystitis. J Am Coll Surg 180:232–244
28. Kiviniemi H, Makela JT, Autio R, et al (1998) Percutaneous cholecystostomy in acute cholecystitis in high risk patients: an analysis of 69 cases. Int Surg 83:299–302
29. Ware LB, Matthay MA (2000) The acute respiratory distress syndrome. N Engl J Med 342:1334–1349
30. Lai KK, Melvin ZS, Menard MJ, Kotilainen MR, Baker S (1997) *Clostridium difficile*-associated diarrhea: epidemiology, risk factors and infection control. Infect Control Hosp Epidemiol 18:628–632
31. Pear SM, Williamson TH, Bettin KM, Gerding DN, Galgiani JN (1994) Decrease in nosocomial *Clostridium difficile*-associated diarrhea by restricting clindamycin use. Ann Intern Med 120:272–277
32. Paradisi F, Corti G, Mangani V (1998) Urosepsis in the critical care unit. Crit Care Clin 114:165–180
33. Winer-Muram HT, Rubin SA, Ellis JV, et al (1993) Pneumonia and ARDS in patients receiving mechanical ventilation: diagnostic accuracy of chest radiography. Chest 188:479–485
34. Meduri GU, Belenchia JM, Estes RJ, Wunderink RG, el Torky M, Leeper KV Jr (1991) Proliferative phase of ARDS. Clinical findings and effects of corticosteroids. Chest 100:943–952
35. Sutherland KR, Steinberg PS, Maunder RJ, Millberg JA, Allen DL, Hudson LD (1995) Pulmonary infection during the acute respiratory distress syndrome. Am J Respir Crit Care Med 152:550–556
36. Delclaux C, Roupie E, Blot F, Brochard L, Lemaire F, Brun-Buisson C (1997) Lower respiratory tract colonization and infection during severe acute respiratory distress syndrome. Am J Respir Crit Care Med 156:1092–1098
37. Brun-Buisson C (2000) The epidemiology of the systemic inflammatory response. Intensive Care Med 26 (suppl 1):S64–S74
38. Engoren M (1995) Lack of association between atelectasis and fever. Chest 107:81–84
39. Wright L, King TE (1997) Cryptogenic organizing pneumonia (Idiopathic bronchilitis obliterans organizing pneumonia): An update. Clin Pulm Med 4:152–158
40. Xaubet A, Torres A, Marco F, Puig-De la Bellacasa J, Faus R, Aqusti-Vidal A (1989) Pulmonary infiltrates in immunocompromised patients. Diagnostic value of telescoping plugged catheter and bronchoalveolar lavage. Chest 95:130–135
41. Kahn FW, Jones JH (1988) Analysis of bronchoalveolar lavage specimens from immunocompromised patients with a protocol applicable in the microbiology laboratory. J Clin Microbiol 26:1150–1155
42. Jordan S, Mitchell, Quinlan GJ, Goldstraw P, Evans TW (2000) The pathogenesis of lung injury following pulmonary resection. Eur Respir J 15:790–799

43. Waller DA, Gebitekin C, Saunders NR, Walker DR (1993) Non-cardiogenic pulmonary edema complicating lung resection. Ann Thorac Surg 55:140–143
44. Turnage WS, Lunn JJ (1993) Postpneumonectomy pulmonary edema. A retrospective analysis of associated variables. Chest 103:1646–1650
45. Wunderink RG (1995) Ventilator-associated pneumonia: failure to response to antibiotic therapy. Clin Chest Med 16:173–193
46. Fagon JY, Chastre J, Wolff M (2000) Invasive and non-invasive strategies for management of suspected ventilator-associated pneumonia. Ann Intern Med 132:612–630
47. Sanchez-Nieto JM, Torres A, Garcia-Cordoba F, et al (1998) Impact of invasive and noninvasive quantitative culture sampling on outcome of ventilator-associated pneumonia: a pilot study. Am J Respir Crit Care Med 157:371–376
48. Cunha BA (1998) Fever in the critical care unit. Crit Care Clin 14:1–14

The Prevention of Invasive *Candida* Infection in Critically Ill Surgical Patients

S. L. Sylvester and P. Lipsett

▍ Introduction

Over the past three decades, the significant morbidity and mortality associated with candidemia and invasive candidiasis have been well established. Technological and scientific advancement has led to an increase in the incidence of serious *Candida* infections. With the introduction of the azoles and more recently with the development of the echinocandin class of antifungals, our ability to treat these infections has improved; however, our ability to diagnose these infections in a timely fashion remains limited, and patient outcomes remain poor. Antifungal prophylaxis has emerged as a method to attempt to decrease the occurrence of these serious infections in selected high-risk patient populations. The role of antifungal prophylaxis is well established in bone marrow transplant recipients [1, 2]. In this chapter, we will review the role of antifungal prophylaxis in the surgical patient, with particular attention to the prevention of candidemia and invasive candidiasis in surgical intensive care unit (ICU) patients and abdominal organ transplant recipients.

▍ Epidemiology of *Candida* Infections in Surgical Patients

The incidence of *Candida* bloodstream infections has increased markedly over the past three decades, due, in part, to factors such as parenteral hyperalimentation, the use of broad-spectrum antibiotics and intravascular catheters [3]. National Nosocomial Infection Survey (NNIS) data published almost a decade ago indicated that the nosocomial fungal infection rate for surgical wounds increased from 1.0 infection/10,000 discharges to 3.1 infections/10,000 discharges between 1980 and 1990 [4]. The rate of nosocomial fungemia rose from 1.0/10,000 discharges to 4.9/10,000 discharges, and the proportion of nosocomial bloodstream infections due to fungi increased from 5.4% in 1980 to 9.9% in 1990 [4]. More recent data from the NNIS (1989–1998) indicated that *C. albicans* was the seventh most common pathogen causing nosocomial infection in an ICU setting, and accounted for 4.9% of bloodstream infections, and 4.8% of surgical site infections, in the ICU [5].

Surgical patients in particular have been shown to have a high incidence of fungal infection [4]. Blumberg and colleagues in the National Epidemiology of Mycosis Survey (NEMIS), identified 42 candidal bloodstream infections (CBSI) among 4276 patients admitted to six surgical ICUs between 1993 and 1995 [6], yielding an incidence rate of 9.8 CBSIs/1000 admissions. In this study, *Candida* species caused 9.2% of all bloodstream infections diagnosed in the surgical ICUs, and more than half of these were non-*albicans* [6].

Among surgical patients, solid organ transplant recipients, and in particular liver, pancreas and small bowel transplant patients, appear to have a greater risk of developing invasive fungal infections. Incidences of invasive *Candida* infection in liver transplant patients vary from 1.3–15% among those receiving antifungal prophylaxis [7–9], to 23% in patients not receiving prophylaxis [10]. Among pancreas transplant recipients the incidence of invasive fungal infection has been estimated to be approximately 9% [11], and among small bowel transplant recipients the incidence has been estimated to be as high as 59% [12].

▌ Risk Factors for Invasive *Candida* Infection

The determination of risk factors associated with invasive candidiasis in the surgical patient is complicated by the variety of definitions of invasive candidiasis in the literature and the heterogeneity of study populations. In studies evaluating risk factors associated with candidiasis, invasive disease has generally been defined by the isolation of *Candida* from cultures of abscess material or normally sterile body tissues, and/or the presence of invasive organisms consistent with *Candida* on histological examination of body tissues, in the presence of signs of infection. Recognizing the variations in definitions and patients, risk factors associated in multivariate analyses with invasive candidiasis are shown in Table 1.

Risk factors associated with invasive fungal disease in organ transplant patients are somewhat different than those identified for heterogeneous surgical patient populations (Table 2). Risk factors for invasive fungal infection in other solid organ transplant populations are not as well defined. In a study of post-transplant intraabdominal fungal infections in pancreas transplant recipients, those with older donors, those whose transplants were drained into bowel as compared to those drained via the bladder, those receiving living, related donor organs and those undergoing pancreas and renal transplantation (as compared to pancreas alone) were at higher risk of infection [11].

Table 1. Risk factors associated with invasive *Candida* infection in critically ill surgical patients

Risk Factor	Point Estimate*	95% Confidence Interval	Reference
▌ Surgery (any)	8.7	1.2–63.5	17
▌ Central venous catheter	8.1	1.1–59.6	17
▌ Triple lumen catheter	5.1	1.5–16.8	17
▌ *Candida* colonization	4.01 (OR)	2.16–7.45	18
	10.64	1.43–78.74	20
▌ Hyperalimentation	3.8	1.9–7.6	17
	NS	NS	19
▌ Hemodialysis	2.6	1.2–5.6	17
▌ Anti-anaerobic agents	2.2	1.1–4.6	17
▌ Severity of illness[a]	1.03 (OR)	1.01–1.05	18
	1.02	1.01–1.04	20

*Values represent relative risk, except where indicated. OR=odds ratio. NS=not specified.
[a] Severity of illness measured by APACHE II score [18] and by APACHE III score [20]

Table 2. Risk factors associated with risk of invasive *Candida* infection in liver transplant recipients

Risk Factor	Point Estimate*	95% Confidence Interval	Reference
▌Hyperglycemia within 2 weeks of candidemia	16.15 (OR)	2.77–94.07	11
▌Exposure to >3 antibiotics	11.15 (OR)	2.04–61.02	11
▌Cytomegalovirus infection	3.4	1.1–10.2	13
	8.5	3.3–21.7	22
▌Choledochojejunostomy anastomosis	4.9	1.8–13.8	13
▌United Organ Sharing classification 1 (life support in intensive care)	3.5	1.7–7.0	14
▌Repeated transplantation	3.7	2.0–6.8	14
	3.2	1.5–6.5	22
▌Abdominal or thoracic reoperation	2.5	1.6–3.8	22
▌Fungal colonization[a]	2.3	1.2–4.3	14
▌Transfusion of cellular blood products	2.2	2.1–4.4	13
▌Creatinine >3 mg/dl	1.4	1.2–1.6	22
▌Operation time ≥11 h	1.2	1.1–1.4	22

*Values represent relative risk, except where indicated. OR=odds ratio.
[a] In [13] and [22], fungal colonization

▌High Mortality Associated with Serious *Candida* Infections

Despite advances in diagnostic technologies and therapy, patients with fungemia continue to do poorly, with an attributable mortality of 38% [13]. Although mortality rates remain high, improvements in outcome have occurred. McNeil and colleagues analyzed data from the National Center of Health Statistics to determine trends in mortality associated with invasive fungal disease in the United States between 1980 and 1997 [14]. The overall mortality rate associated with invasive mycoses increased over the study period; the mortality rate associated with candidiasis occurring in non-human immunodeficiency virus (HIV)-infected individuals increased steadily to a peak of greater than 60% in 1989, but since 1989 has decreased by 50% [14], perhaps reflecting enhanced awareness of the possibility of occult infection in high-risk patients and a lower threshold to treat empirically before culture or biopsy results are available.

▌Challenges in the Diagnosis of Invasive *Candida* Infection

The lack of highly sensitive and specific diagnostic techniques accounts in part for the poor outcome associated with invasive *Candida* infection. Despite the increasing frequency with which *Candida* species have been isolated from blood cultures in recent years the diagnosis of invasive candidiasis remains problematic [15], and the sensitivity of current blood culture technology for diagnosis of disseminated disease is unclear [16]. Sensitivities of 61–82% have been reported for blood cultures in neutropenic patients with invasive candidiasis proven by tissue biopsy

[17, 18]. It has been estimated that only 15–40% of cases of invasive candidiasis are diagnosed early enough for the initiation of appropriate therapy [19].

A number of new diagnostic techniques, including serological, antigen and DNA-based assays, have been under evaluation for use in the diagnosis of candidemia and invasive *Candida* infection but are not yet well developed enough for routine use [20, 21]. A recent study of nested polymerase chain reaction (PCR) for the diagnosis of fungal disease in febrile, neutropenic patients yielded promising results, but a comparative, controlled evaluation of this strategy remains to be performed [22]. Evaluation of serological and antigen assays in a study of non-neutropenic ICU patients yielded sensitivities of 50–100%, and sensitivities of only 26–73% [23]. The diagnosis of invasive *Candida* infection therefore continues to be based on the accumulation of a multitude of data, including patient risk profile, clinical status, and the results of traditional blood cultures and histological examination of tissues.

Antifungal Prophylaxis in the Critically Ill Surgical Patient

The use of antifungal prophylaxis has not been routinely advocated for critically ill, non-neutropenic patients in the ICU [24]. Recently published practice guidelines discuss antifungal prophylaxis in HIV-infected, neutropenic and solid-organ transplant patients but not in the critically ill ICU patient who does not fit into one of these categories [25].

The possible benefits of antifungal prophylaxis were recognized in the surgical literature as early as the 1970s. In 1975, Evans published the results of an uncontrolled, comparative study in 137 patients undergoing open-heart surgery [26]. Oral and fecal swabs were done on admission and post-operatively to determine the incidence of *Candida* colonization. The risk of *Candida* colonization and sepsis was compared in the 87 patients receiving standard treatment and the 50 patients receiving preoperative prophylaxis with oral and vaginal nystatin plus oral amphotericin B. He found that patients who received prophylaxis were less likely to become colonized with *Candida* during the study; no cases of *Candida* sepsis occurred, and so effects on infection rates were not determined [26].

The first randomized, double blind, placebo-controlled trial of systemic antifungal prophylaxis in critically ill surgical patients was published by Slotman and Burchard in 1987 [27]. Patients admitted to the surgical ICU with three or more of 16 identified risk factors were eligible. Patients were excluded if they had liver disease. Enrolled patients were randomized to receive ketoconazole 200 mg enterally per day, or placebo. Of 74 subjects enrolled, 17 were found to be colonized with yeast on study entry, and so were not evaluated. Of the remaining 57 patients, 27 received ketoconazole and 30 received placebo. Patients received the study treatment for 21 days, or until discharge from the surgical ICU. Invasive fungal disease was defined as a positive fungal culture obtained from blood, the peritoneum, deep tissue, or burn wound. The investigators found that ketoconazole was associated both with a lower incidence of yeast colonization and with a lower risk of invasive *Candida* infection [27]. Infection developed in none of the patients receiving prophylaxis and in 17% of the patients receiving placebo ($p < 0.01$). Mortality was not significantly different in the two groups, but length of hospital stay and median surgical ICU patient charges were lower for those receiving ketoconazole (6 days versus 12.5 days, $p < 0.01$; $4800 versus $10 000, $p < 0.01$) [27].

Limitations of this study include the heterogeneity of the study population and the choice of prophylactic agent. It is possible that the benefits of antifungal prophylaxis were realized in a single subset of the study population – those undergoing abdominal surgery, for example. In addition, ketoconazole is not reliably absorbed and has a multitude of drug interactions and toxicities that make it a poor choice for a prophylactic agent in a critically ill patient on numerous other medications and with multisystem disease.

In a second trial performed by Savino and colleagues between 1990 and 1991, 292 patients were randomized to one of four arms: no therapy, oral clotrimazole, oral ketoconazole, and oral nystatin [28]. Patients admitted to the surgical ICU for more than 48 hours were eligible. Those who were pregnant, on antifungals within two weeks of the study, with evidence of systemic fungal infection or colonization at the time of the study, or who were burn patients or transplant patients were excluded. *Candida* infection was broadly defined as a positive blood or peritoneal culture, or positive cultures from three or more sites. Because the study was underpowered, no significant differences among the treatment arms were detected. Fungal sepsis was diagnosed in only 3% of patients on no prophylaxis, 1% of patients on clotrimazole, 2% of patients on ketoconazole and 7% of patients on nystatin [28]. In addition, the authors included fungal colonization (three or more sites) as a diagnostic criterion for fungal infection, making the definition of infection in this study problematic.

The advent of a new generation of azole antifungals, most notably fluconazole, brought new promise to investigators looking for a way to reduce the occurrence of invasive fungal disease in critically ill patients. Garbino and colleagues [29] randomized 220 patients who were receiving selective digestive decontamination (SDD) and mechanical ventilation in the medical or surgical ICU to receive either fluconazole 100 mg intravenously per day or placebo. Of 204 evaluable patients, 103 received fluconazole and 101 placebo. No patients receiving fluconazole prophylaxis developed serious *Candida* infection, whereas six patients in the placebo group developed infection [29]. Limitations of this study again include its lack of power to detect a significant difference in rates of infection, as well as the absence of a clear definition of *Candida* infection.

The two most recent studies in the literature demonstrate that prophylaxis can be efficacious when administered to a highly select group of surgical patients. Eggimann et al. [30] conducted a randomized, double blind, placebo-controlled trial of intravenous fluconazole prophylaxis administered to surgical patients with recurrent gastrointestinal perforations or anastomotic leakages. Patients were excluded if they had a documented or probable fungal infection at the time of the study, or if they had received systemic antifungals in the two weeks prior to the study. Patients with significant hepatic dysfunction were also excluded, as were those on dialysis and those felt likely to die within 72 hours. *Candida* infection was defined in this study as follows: intraabdominal candidiasis (abscess with pure or mixed growth of *Candida*, or signs of peritonitis with isolation of *Candida* from peritoneal fluid at laparotomy or from drains); candidemia (one or more positive blood cultures); urinary tract infection ($>10^5$ *Candida* colonies per ml of urine, plus pyuria and symptoms of infection); or evidence of infection with *Candida* isolated from a tissue biopsy [30].

The infection rate in this small study was strikingly high: 35% of patients receiving placebo developed infection, as compared to 9% in the group receiving intravenous fluconazole at a dose of 400 mg per day ($p=0.06$) [30]. The relative risk of

Candida infection associated with fluconazole prophylaxis was 0.25 (95% CI 0.06–1.06). All infections but one were cases of peritonitis. If only intraabdominal infection was considered, the differences between fluconazole and placebo achieved statistical significance (relative risk 0.12, 95% CI 0.02–0.93) [30]. One potential concern here is the definition of *Candida* peritonitis used; positive cultures obtained from abdominal drains were accepted as evidence of infection, and this may have artificially elevated the incidence of infection observed. Nonetheless, this small study suggests a beneficial effect of prophylaxis in the highest-risk patient population.

In the most recently published study by Pelz et al., 260 patients with an expected surgical ICU stay of three or more days were randomized to receive fluconazole 400 mg enterally per day or placebo [31]. Patients under the age of 18, pregnant patients, those who had received antifungals within seven days of the study, and those expected to die within 24 hours were excluded. *Candida* infection was defined in this study as definite, presumed or suspected. Definite infection meant histologic evidence of yeast invasion on tissue biopsy or at autopsy, or microbiologic evidence of infection in two separate, closed, normally sterile sites, except for urine or sputum. Presumed infection was defined as a positive blood culture by venipuncture; a positive culture from a single, closed, normally sterile site, excluding cultures from peritoneal drains or biliary catheters; an intradermal catheter tip culture with more than 15 colonies of growth; a deep surgical site infection; or a urinary tract infection (two positive urine cultures obtained by straight catheterization, or before and after removal of an indwelling catheter). Suspected infection was defined as the administration of empiric antifungal therapy by the treating clinician, in the presence of signs of end-organ dysfunction and fungal colonization [31].

Of the 260 patients in the initial intent-to-treat analysis, 11 of 130 patients receiving fluconazole and 20 of 130 receiving placebo developed *Candida* infections. In an intent-to-treat analysis the absolute reduction in risk of fungal infection was 7%. In analyses excluding patients with fungal urinary tract infections or central venous catheter infections, fluconazole prophylaxis was associated with a decreased risk of infection that was statistically significant. In a time-to-event analysis the protective effect of fluconazole was also statistically significant ($p = 0.01$, log-rank test). A Cox proportional hazards regression analysis yielded an overall adjusted risk reduction of 55% in the fluconazole group as compared to the placebo group (relative risk 0.45, 95% confidence interval 0.21–0.98). Mortality was not significantly different in the two treatment groups [31].

The major limitations of this study are: that this is a single center report with patients that may be at greater risk than the general surgical ICU population; that enrollment criteria were based on estimated length of stay at a tertiary care center; and that not all of the infection definitions (for example, the inclusion of urinary tract infections) would be generally accepted as indicative of invasive disease. However, the definitions were strict, based on microbiological evidence, and did not include fungal colonization of drains or other body sites.

Despite their individual shortcomings, these studies demonstrate that antifungal prophylaxis may be appropriate for selected high-risk patient populations in the surgical ICU. One of the major challenges to be met in future studies is the development of a reliable method to identify these patients.

▌ Antifungal Prophylaxis in Liver, Pancreas and Small Bowel Transplantation

Several studies evaluating the efficacy of antifungal prophylaxis in liver transplant recipients have been published. At least three of these studies were randomized, and two were double blind, placebo-controlled trials. Tollemar et al. [32] evaluated 86 consecutive liver transplant patients in a multicenter study between 1990 and 1992; subjects were randomized to receive liposomal amphotericin B 1 mg/kg/d intravenously, or placebo. Proven fungal infection was defined as a positive culture from blood, sterile body site, or deep organ biopsy, in the setting of fever and leukocytosis. Suspected fungal infection was defined as fever of unknown etiology plus positive fungal serology or antigen testing, in the absence of culture or histological evidence of fungal disease [32]. In patients receiving antifungal prophylaxis, no proven infections and two suspected infections occurred, while in patients receiving placebo six proven infections (five *Candida* and one *Aspergillus*) and three suspected infections occurred (p < 0.05) [32].

A second study compared oral fluconazole 100 mg daily to oral nystatin suspension every six hours [8]. Patients were eligible for the trial if they were over eight years of age and if they had had their transplant within the preceding 24 hours. Patients were excluded for renal insufficiency, receipt of antifungals within one week of study entry, preexisting fungal infection, retransplantation and azole allergy. Of 143 eligible patients, 76 were randomized to receive fluconazole and 67 to receive nystatin during the first 28 days following transplantation. Invasive *Candida* infection was defined as evidence of *Candida* infection in blood, tissues, or bloody fluids plus organ-specific symptoms [8]. Invasive infection developed in 1.3% of patients on fluconazole and in 6% of patients on nystatin (p = 0.12). Overall mortality also was not significantly different in the two arms [8].

Winston et al. [10] conducted the most recent study of antifungal prophylaxis in liver transplant recipients between 1992 and 1993. Of the 236 patients in this trial randomized to receive fluconazole 400 mg per day or placebo, 30 developed proven fungal infection. Proven infection was defined as presence of fungus in blood, lung tissue or secretions, sinuses, the peritoneal cavity or other organs, in addition to sign and symptoms of infection not explained by other pathogens [10]. Of the 30 patients with proven fungal infection, 24 had received placebo (23% of all patients receiving placebo) and 6 had received fluconazole (6% of all patients receiving fluconazole). This difference was statistically significant [10]. However, the rate of invasive infection in the placebo group was quite high compared to rates seen in other studies, bringing into question the rigor of the event definition and the possible contribution of other factors to the high infection rate.

For recipients of pancreas and small bowel transplants, the rates of fungal infection appear to be high; however, few data exist regarding the efficacy of prophylaxis in these populations. Benedetti et al. [11] conducted a retrospective analysis of 445 patients who underwent pancreas transplantation. Recipients who received prophylaxis with fluconazole 400 mg per day for one week following transplantation had a somewhat lower rate (although not statistically significant) of intraabdominal fungal infection than those who did not receive prophylaxis (6% versus 10%) [11].

Another observational study described the incidence of surgical complications following 580 pancreas transplants occurring during two periods: 1985–1994 and 1994–1997. Subjects undergoing transplantation in the second period received fluconazole prophylaxis, whereas those in the first period did not. Half of the intraabdominal infections occurring in these patients were polymicrobial. Fungal pathogens were implicated in 34% of polymicrobial infections in the first period, but in only two transplant recipients with polymicrobial intraabdominal infection in the second period [33].

These studies suggest, as do the studies of antifungal prophylaxis in critically ill surgical patients, that prophylaxis strategies should be carefully applied to select groups of patients, and not broadly to all surgical ICU patients, or to all those undergoing abdominal organ transplantation. Based on the risk factors discussed above, Singh [34] has recently suggested that anti-*Candida* prophylaxis be considered for liver transplant patients who are undergoing reoperation, who have longer operations, renal failure, or who require multiple blood transfusions. Furthermore, she has suggested that pancreas transplant patients be considered for anti-*Candida* prophylaxis if their transplanted organ is drained into the bowel, if the pancreas transplant has occurred following renal transplant, if retransplantation is performed, if there is post-reperfusion pancreatitis, or if there is renal failure requiring dialysis [34].

▌ The Impact of Antifungal Prophylaxis on the Emergence of Resistance

The most significant drawback to routine antifungal prophylaxis of surgical patients is the development of resistance to available agents among *Candida* species. Studies in oncology patient populations and in hospitalized patient populations have demonstrated the emergence of drug resistance among *Candida* species and a shift in species distribution patterns to those that are inherently more resistant to drugs such as fluconazole.

In a retrospective analysis of patients who had undergone bone marrow transplant or treatment for leukemia at the Johns Hopkins Hospital in 1989 and 1990, those patients who received fluconazole prophylaxis had a seven-fold greater frequency of infection with *C. krusei*, which is inherently resistant to azole antifungals (8.3 versus 1.2%, $p=0.002$) [35]. Furthermore, colonization with *C. krusei* was found in 40.5% of those who received fluconazole prophylaxis, as compared to 16.7% of those who did not ($p<0.0001$) [35].

A second study performed at Johns Hopkins revealed that leukemia and bone marrow transplant patients who received fluconazole were more likely to develop bloodstream infections with *C. glabrata* than those who did not receive fluconazole [36]. Seventy-five percent of candidemias occurring in patients who received fluconazole were due to *C. glabrata*, whereas only 1% of candidemias occurring in patients who did not receive fluconazole were due to *C. glabrata* [36].

Other studies have shown that although prolonged fluconazole prophylaxis has been shown to improve mortality in allogeneic bone marrow transplant patients [37], it may also lead to the emergence of more resistant *Candida* species. Marr et al. [38] collected mouth washings from patients before, during, and bone marrow transplant during the period 1994–1997. They found that *C. albicans* was the most common species isolated from patients prior to transplantation and fluconazole exposure, whereas species such as *C. glabrata* and *C. krusei*, which are tolerant or resistant to fluconazole, were most commonly isolated after transplant and exposure to fluconazole [38]. Although a causal connection between fluconazole exposure and the emergence of resistant species could not be established from this study, the data are suggestive [38].

In hospitalized patients, some investigators have observed similar trends. Nguyen et al. conducted a prospective, observational study of 427 candidemic patients in a tertiary care medical center between 1990 and 1994, and found that non-*albicans* species accounted for more than half of all candidemias in the second half of the study period [39].

Over a period of increasing azole use at the University of Iowa, Berrouane et al. showed that the proportion of fungal infections caused by *C. glabrata* increased from zero in 1987–88 to approximately 30% in 1993–94, while the proportion of infections caused by *C. albicans* decreased from 49% in 1987–88 to 23% in 1993–94 [40].

By contrast, Pelz et al. found that over the year's duration of their fluconazole prophylaxis trial in critically ill surgical patients [31], fluconazole minimum inhibitory concentrations (MICs) of infecting *Candida* isolates did not increase significantly. There was no association between the use of fluconazole and fluconazole MIC and there was no shift toward non-*albicans* species [31]. However, MIC testing was performed only on the small number of infecting isolates, rather than on infecting and colonizing isolates, and the assessment of resistance and species distribution was performed only over the duration of the clinical trial.

Winston and colleagues [10] also found no increases in colonization with species such as *C. krusei* or *C. glabrata* associated with fluconazole use over the 10 weeks of their trial, but it is difficult to know the significance of such a finding, given the short period of observation.

Results of a larger surveillance study [41] have indicated that the majority of *Candida* bloodstream infections in the United States continue to be due to *C. albicans*, and the majority of *C. albicans* isolates remain susceptible to fluconazole. Pfaller and colleagues [41] reported the results of an analysis of 1579 *Candida* bloodstream isolates from over 50 medical centers in the United States during the period from 1992–1998. Fifty-two percent of these were *C. albicans*, consistent with results of earlier multicenter studies [41]. In addition, the fluconazole MIC_{90} was observed to remain stable over the period of the study. The proportion of candidemias due to *C. glabrata*, however, did appear to increase; this organism was the second most common *Candida* species causing bloodstream infection during the period 1995–1998 [41].

The emergence of *C. glabrata*, which is often fluconazole-resistant, as a prominent fungal pathogen in the ICU setting should be a consideration when planning antifungal prophylaxis strategies for critically ill patients. Fluconazole has been an attractive choice for prophylaxis because it can be administered enterally or intravenously, and because it has a favorable safety profile. Amphotericin B deoxycholate, while effective against most *Candida* species, is too toxic to use as routine prophylaxis, particularly in patients with multi-organ system dysfunction; its lipid formulations, while better tolerated, are only available for intravenous administration and may be prohibitively expensive. New azole antifungals such as voriconazole have been shown to be active *in vitro* against fluconazole-resistant strains of *C. albicans*, *C. glabrata* and *C. krusei* [42], but their role in the prophylaxis and treatment of *Candida* infection has yet to be established. Caspofungin, an echinocandin, is the first of this new class of antifungal agents that inhibit the synthesis of (1,3)-β-D-glucan, and is currently indicated for the treatment of refractory invasive aspergillosis. In a recently published study, caspofungin compared favorably to amphotericin B for the treatment of esophageal candidiasis in HIV-infected patients [43]; like voriconazole, however, its role in the prophylaxis and treatment of invasive *Candida* infection is not yet clear. While these newer agents appear to have favorable safety profiles, only further clinical experience will determine their promise as prophylactic agents.

▌ Conclusion

Invasive *Candida* infections are highly morbid and often fatal, particularly in critically ill patients and organ transplant recipients who often have multiple comorbid diseases. While techniques for early diagnosis are lacking, the early administration of antifungal agents to patients at high risk for developing invasive *Candida* infection has emerged as a viable strategy by which to improve outcomes. Surgical patients in recent years have been found to have particularly high rates of *Candida* infection, and a few carefully conducted studies have shown the potential benefit of antifungal prophylaxis in selected high-risk patients in the surgical ICU and certain abdominal organ transplant recipients.

In some circumstances, the favorable results of these studies are extrapolated to patient populations who are not necessarily comparable to those in the trials, and antifungal prophylaxis may be administered to such patients in the absence of data suggesting a clinical benefit. In addition to evaluating new diagnostic modalities, future studies need to better define guidelines for deciding which patients will benefit from prophylaxis; to establish effective prophylaxis regimens for various high risk patient populations; to determine the long-term impact of antifungal prophylaxis on the ecology of *Candida* species in various patient populations; and to determine the role of the newer antifungal agents in the prevention of these infections.

References

1. Goodman JL, Winston DJ, Greenfield RA, et al (1992) A controlled trial of fluconazole to prevent fungal infections after bone marrow transplantation. N Engl J Med 326:845–851
2. Slavin MA, Osborne B, Adams R, et al (1995) Efficacy and safety of fluconazole prophylaxis for fungal infections after bone marrow transplantation: a prospective, randomized, double-blind study. J Infect Dis 171:1545–1552
3. Fraser VJ, Jones M, Dunkel J, Storfer S, Medoff G, Dunagan WC (1992) Candidemia in a tertiary care hospital: epidemiology, risk factors, and predictors of mortality. Clin Infect Dis 15:414–421
4. Beck-Sague CM, Jarvis W, and the National Nosocomial Infections Surveillance System (1993) Secular trends in the epidemiology of nosocomial fungal infections in the United States, 1980–1990. J Infect Dis 167:1247–1251
5. Fridkin SK, Gaynes RP (1999) Antimicrobial resistance in intensive care units. Clin Chest Med 20:303–316
6. Blumberg HM, Jarvis WR, Soucie JM, et al (2001) Risk factors for candidal bloodstream infections in surgical intensive care unit patients: the NEMIS prospective multicenter study. Clin Infect Dis 33:177–186
7. Nieto-Rodriguez JA, Kusne S, Manez R, et al (1996) Factors associated with the development of candidemia and candidemia-related death among liver transplant recipients. Ann Surg 223:70–76
8. Lumbreras C, Cuervas-Mons V, Jara P (1996) Randomized trial of fluconazole versus nystatin for the prophylaxis of Candida infection following liver transplantation. J Infect Dis 174:583–588
9. Hadley S, Samore MH, Lewis WD, Jenkins RL, Karchmer AW, Hammer SM (1995) Major infectious complications after orthotopic liver transplantation and comparison of outcomes in patients receiving cyclosporine or FK506 as primary immunosuppression. Transplantation 59:851–859
10. Winston DJ, Pakrasi A, Busuttil RW (1999) Prophylactic fluconazole in liver transplant recipients: a randomized, double-blind, placebo-controlled trial. Ann Intern Med 131:729–737

11. Benedetti E, Gruessner AC, Troppmann C, et al (1996) Intra-abdominal fungal infections after pancreatic transplantation: incidence, treatment, and outcome. J Am Coll Surg 183:307–316
12. Kusne S, Furukawa H, Abu-Elmagd K, et al (1996) Infectious complications after small bowel transplantation in adults: an update. Transplant Proc 28:2761–2762
13. Wey SB, Mori M, Pfaller MA, Woolson RF, Wenzel RP (1988) Hospital-acquired candidemia: the attributable mortality and excess length of stay. Arch Intern Med 148:2642–2645
14. McNeil MM, Nash SL, Hajjeh RA, et al (2001) Trends in mortality due to invasive mycotic diseases in the United States, 1980–1997. Clin Infect Dis 33:1692–1696
15. Pfaller MA (1992) Laboratory aids in the diagnosis of invasive candidiasis. Mycopathologia 120:65–72
16. Richardson MD, Kokki MH (1999) New perspectives in the diagnosis of systemic fungal infections. Ann Med 31:327–335
17. Ness MJ, Vaughan WP, Woods GL (1989) Candida antigen latex test for detection of invasive candidiasis in immunocompromised patients. J Infect Dis 159:495–502
18. Walsh TJ, Hathorn JW, Sobel JD, et al (1991) Detection of circulating Candida enolase by immunoassay in patients with cancer and invasive candidiasis. N Engl J Med 324:1026–1031
19. Edwards JE (2000) Candida species. In: Mandell GL, Bennett JE, Dolin R (eds) Principles and Practice of Infectious Diseases. Churchill Livingstone, New York, pp 2656–2673
20. Jones JM (1990) Laboratory diagnosis of invasive candidiasis. Clin Micro Rev 3:32–45
21. Rex JH, Sobel JD (2001) Prophylactic antifungal therapy in the intensive care unit. Clin Infect Dis 32:1191–2000
22. Lin MT, Lu HC, Chen WL (2001) Improving efficacy of antifungal therapy by polymerase chain reaction-based strategy among febrile patients with neutropenia and cancer. Clin Infect Dis 33:1621–1627
23. Petri MG, Konig J, Moecke HP, et al (1997) Epidemiology of invasive mycosis in ICU patients: a prospective multicenter study in 435 non-neutropenic patients. Intensive Care Med 23:317–325
24. Edwards JE, Bodey GP, Bowden RA, et al (1997) International Conference for the development of a consensus on the management and prevention of severe candidal infections. Clin Infect Dis 25:43–59
25. Rex JH, Walsh TJ, Sobel JD, et al (2000) Practice guidelines for the treatment of candidiasis. Clin Infect Dis 30:662–678
26. Evans EGV (1975) The incidence of pathogenic yeast among open-heart surgery patients – the value of prophylaxis. J Thoracic Cardiovasc Surg 70:466–470
27. Slotman GJ, Burchard KW (1987) Ketoconazole prevents Candida sepsis in critically ill surgical patients. Arch Surg 122:147–151
28. Savino JA, Agarwal N, Wry P, Policastro A, Cerabona T, Austria L (1994) Routine prophylactic antifungal agents (clotrimazole, ketoconazole, and nystatin) in nontransplant/nonburned critically ill surgical and trauma patients. J Trauma 36:20–26
29. Garbino J, Lew D, Romand J-A, Auckenthaler R, Suter P, Pittet D (1997) Fluconazole prevents severe Candida spp infections in high-risk critically ill patients: a randomized, double-blind, placebo-controlled study. In: Program and Abstracts of the 37th Interscience Conference on Antimicrobial Agents and Chemotherapy. ASM Press, Herndon, pp LM-23b
30. Eggimann P, Francioli P, Bille J, et al (1999) Fluconazole prophylaxis prevents intra-abdominal candidiasis in high-risk surgical patients. Crit Care Med 27:1066–1072
31. Pelz RK, Hendrix CW, Swoboda SM, et al (2001) Double-blind placebo-controlled trial of fluconazole to prevent candidal infections in critically ill surgical patients. Ann Surg 233:542–548
32. Tollemar J, Hockerstedt K, Ericzon B-G, Jalanko H, Ringden O (1995) Liposomal amphotericin B prevents invasive fungal infections in liver transplant recipients: a randomized, placebo-controlled study. Transplantation 59:45–50
33. Humar A, Kandaswamy R, Granger D, Gruessner RW, Gruessner AC, Sutherland DER (2000) Decreased surgical risks of pancreas transplantation in the modern era. Ann Surg 231:269–275

34. Singh N (2000) Antifungal prophylaxis for solid organ transplant recipients: seeing clarity amidst controversy. Clin Infect Dis 31:545–553
35. Wingard JR, Merz WG, Rinaldi MG, Johnson TR, Karp JE, Saral R (1991) Increase in Candida krusei infection among patients with bone marrow transplantation and neutropenia treated prophylactically with fluconazole. N Engl J Med 325:1274–1277
36. Wingard JR, Merz WG, Rinaldi MG, Miller CB, Karp JE, Saral R (1993) Association of Torulopsis glabrata infections with fluconazole prophylaxis in neutropenic bone marrow transplant patients. Antimicrob Agents Chemother 37:1847–1849
37. Marr KA, Seidel K, Slavin MA, et al (2000) Prolonged fluconazole prophylaxis is associated with persistent protection against candidiasis-related death in allogeneic marrow transplant recipients: long-term follow-up of a randomized, placebo-controlled trial. Blood 96:2055–2061
38. Marr KA, Seidel K, White TC, Bowden RA (2000) Candidemia in allogeneic blood and marrow transplant recipients: evolution of risk factors after the adoption of prophylactic fluconazole. J Infect Dis 181:309–316
39. Nguyen MH, Peacock JE, Morris AJ, et al (1996) The changing face of candidemia: emergence of non-Candida albicans species and antifungal resistance. Am J Med 1900:617–623
40. Berrouane YF, Herwaldt LA, Pfaller MA (1999) Trends in antifungal use and epidemiology of nosocomial yeast infections in a university hospital. J Clin Microbiol 37:531–537.
41. Pfaller MA, Messer SA, Hollis RJ, et al (1999) Trends in species distribution and susceptibility to fluconazole among blood stream isolates of Candida species in the United States. Diagn Microbiol Infect Dis 33:217–222
42. Nguyen MH, Yu CY (1998) Voriconazole against fluconazole-susceptible and resistant Candida isolates: in-vitro efficacy compared to that of itraconazole and ketoconazole. J Antimicrob Chemother 42:253–256
43. Villanueva A, Arathoon EG, Gotuzzo E, Berman RS, DiNubile MJ, Sable CA (2001) A randomized double-blind study of caspofungin versus amphotericin for the treatment of candidal esophagitis. Clin Infect Dis 33:1529–1535

Bacterial CpG DNA in Septic Shock

E. Wiel, G. Lebuffe, and B. Vallet

▌ Introduction

Septic shock develops when specific microbial components gain access to the circulation and are recognized by the immune system, generating exaggerated mediator and cytokine production. The main microbial components responsible for this recognition are lipopolysaccharide (LPS) in Gram-negative bacteria, or peptidoglycan and teichoic acid in Gram-positive bacteria. Microbial compounds display molecular pattern recognition receptors (PRR) – such as LPS receptors (Toll-like receptor [TLR]4 and CD14) which are expressed constitutively on innate immune system cells (macrophages and dendritics cells) [1].

Bacterial DNA, by the presence of unmethylated sequences, is able to activate innate immune defenses [2]. In contrast, methylation of these sequences containing cytosine poly-guanine dinucleotides, called CpG motifs, abolishes this immune stimulatory effect [3–5]. In the vertebrate genome, CpG dinucleotides are suppressed and constitute only 25% of the level expected from random base utilization [6]. Whereas C5 methylation is common in eukaryote cells, it is uncommon in bacterial DNA [3]. These structural differences of CpG motifs in bacterial DNA – sensed as 'danger codes' – have been adopted by vertebrate immune cells to recognize pathogens [1, 7, 8]. In other terms, CpG motifs represent a type of PRR to detect early evidence of microbial invasion resulting in the activation of protective defense mechanisms. Furthermore, vertebrate immune systems have evolved a specific receptor termed TLR9, by which bacterial DNA and self-DNA can be differentiated [9]. The TLR family is a phylogenetically conserved mediator of innate immunity known to play an essential role in microbial recognition [1].

However, the sole recognition of CpG DNA does not seem to be sufficient to stimulate the immune system against bacteria. Because bacteria live outside human cells shielding their DNA from detection, CpG DNA recognition does not seem to evolve as a general defense strategy against bacteria. Thus, the CD14 pathway is more involved in detection of endotoxins and defense against extracellular Gram-negative bacteria. CpG DNA triggers protective defenses against intracellular pathogens replicating inside host cells (intracellular bacteria, viruses and retroviruses) [10]. The effectiveness of immune defense by CpG is inferred from the fact that DNA viruses have very low CpG content, with a little as 6% of the CpGs predicted based on random base utilization, indicating an evolutionary adaptation to replication in eukaryotic hosts [6, 8].

Similar to LPS, bacterial DNA induces acute inflammatory responses. The immunostimulatory effects of bacterial DNA can be mimicked by synthetic oligodeoxynucleotides (ODN) containing the proper CpG-DNA motif [11]. These ODN have been used as vaccine adjuvants and as immunotherapeutics for treatment of cancer and allergic diseases [12, 13]. Thus, CpG-ODN may represent potent agents for the treatment of sepsis-associated immunoparalysis [14].

This chapter is divided into 2 parts: first the recent advances in the CpG-induced and LPS signaling pathways, and second the specific CpG-mediated effects in different type of cells.

Molecular Mechanisms of Action of CpG DNA

Cell-surface Receptors

The adaptive immune system responds to a pathogen, only after it has been recognized by the innate immune system which has specific receptors for recognition of microbial pathogen allowing to signal the presence of infection. This signal then controls the activation of the adaptive immune system [15].

Recent data demonstrate that CpG DNA and LPS are recognized by a family of vertebrate PRR called TLR [1]. These receptors are transmembrane proteins and play a major role in the induction of immune and inflammatory responses. They contain extracellular leucine-rich repeats and a cytoplasmic Toll/interleukin (IL)-1R (TIR) homology domain. TLR4 was the first human TLR identified being also known to activate the nuclear factor-κB (NF-κB) signaling pathway. Recently, in a mouse model, TLR4 has been identified as the receptor for LPS [16]. However, TLR4 does not seem to be the sole protein involved in LPS recognition. LPS also interacts with a serum protein (LBP) – LPS-binding protein – transferring LPS to CD14 which is a receptor present on macrophages and B-cells that are anchored to the cell surface [17]. Another protein named MD-2 is required for TLR4-mediated recognition of LPS [18]. Therefore, LPS recognition requires the CD14, TLR4 and MD-2 complex [15].

In parallel, it was recently demonstrated that the cellular response to bacterial CpG DNA is mediated by TLR9 [9]. In this study, Hemmi et al. [9] found a transmembrane segment in the TLR9 gene suggesting that TLR9 is inserted into the membrane, but not present in the cytoplasm. Their confocal data showed that tagged myeloid differentiation marker 88 (MyD88) – an adapter molecule involved in the signaling through the IL-1R and TLR families and essential for the responses to CpG DNA – colocalizes with tagged CpG DNA in endosomal structures, but not on the cell membrane. This contrasts with LPS which colocalizes with MyD88 at the cell membrane. Together, these results suggest that signaling is triggered by LPS at the cell membrane, whereas CpG DNA initiates signaling after translocation to endosomes.

Cellular Uptake

In principle, mechanisms mediating cellular uptake of CpG DNA might include receptor-mediated endocytosis, adsorptive endocytosis, pinocytosis, and phagocytosis [10]. The cellular uptake is energy- and temperature-dependent and saturable [19]. CpG are non-sequence specific translocated into endosomes [3, 20]. This intracellular location appears within the first minutes after uptake.

Endosomal Acidification

In this endosomal compartment, DNA becomes progressively acidified and digested by nucleases [21, 22]. Only a small fraction of CpG DNA leaves the endosomes by a non-sequence specific way and reaches the nucleus [23]. It has been shown that acidification is essential for CpG DNA release from the endosomes to the cytoplasm, based on the observation that reagents such as chloroquine or bafilomycin A act as potent inhibitors of immune activation by CpG DNA by interfering with endosomal acidification [5, 22].

▌ Signal Transduction Pathways Activated by CpG DNA

CpG DNA activates several signaling pathways and mediates different cellular activation and cytokine release [24]. The main signaling pathways include production of reactive oxygen species (ROS) [25], NF-κB activation [22, 26, 27], and mitogen-activated protein kinase (MAPK) [5, 28] in B cells and monocytic cells line in both humans and mice.

ROS and Nitric Oxide (NO) Production

Recently, CpG DNA has been shown to induce cellular injury by a free radical mechanism [25]. Production of ROS may be of importance in the CpG signaling pathways, rather than a byproduct of activation, leading to NF-κB activation because antioxidants, which block the ROS production, block the stimulatory effects of CpG DNA. ROS are implicated in signal transduction through the B cell antigen receptor and CD40, resulting in either stimulation or apoptosis [29]. Depending on the type, concentration, and intracellular localization of ROS, their biological effects result in either cell activation or apoptosis. For example, excessive intracellular ROS are linked to apoptosis. ROS induced by CpG alter the cell redox balance and may result in activation of redox-sensitive transcription factors (NF-κB, p53, SP-1 and activating protein (AP)-1).

CpG DNA have been shown to produce NO only after priming macrophages with interferon (IFN-)γ which increases expression of the inducible NO synthase (iNOS) gene [29]. NO production is, thus, not a direct consequence of CpG DNA administration, in contrast with LPS.

MAPK Pathways and Transcription Factor Activation

The MAPK superfamily is a group of serine/threonine-specific kinases that can be activated by many different extracellular stimuli such as cytokines and environmental stress [30]. In vertebrates, there are three major MAPK pathways organized as sequentially working modules, sensing and integrating incoming signals from different sources, and transducing them into specific gene expression: the extracellular receptor kinase or Erk pathway, the p38 MAPK pathway, and the c-Jun N-terminal kinase or Jnk pathway. The two last pathways are activated by CpG DNA in B cells and macrophages within 7 minutes after their administration [4, 5], whereas the Erk pathway is induced by CpG DNA in macrophages but not in B cells [28].

Activation of the Jnk pathway leads to the phosphorylation of the AP-1 [5, 28]. The target transcription factor of the p38 MAPK pathway, is the activating factor-2

(ATF-2) [5, 28]. This phosphorylation increases binding to DNA and enhances transcriptional activity in B cells and macrophages exposed to CpG DNA [5, 28].

Transcription Factor Activation and the NF-κB Pathway

Several previous studies have reported that bacterial DNA and synthetic ODN containing CpG motifs are inducers of NF-κB in macrophages [26]. NF-κB is bound to its inhibitory subunit, I-κB, in the cytoplasm toward activation. I-κB inhibits both NF-κB translocation and DNA binding in the nucleus. Phosphorylation and degradation of I-κB allows translocation of NF-κB to the nucleus [31]. This activation is initiated by cellular stress and results in induction of CpG DNA induced tumor necrosis factor (TNF)-α, iNOS, and IL-12. The signaling pathway between IL-1 receptor and NF-κB activation is allowed by the proteins TNF-receptor-associated factor 6 (TRAF-6), IL-1-receptor-associated kinase (IRAK) and MyD88 [32]. In contrast with LPS for which signaling is triggered at the cell membrane, CpG DNA initiates signaling after translocation to endosomes. All NF-κB inducers can be blocked by antioxidants [33], suggesting that ROS play a major role in NF-κB activation. However, it was found that NF-κB activation does not involve ROS as second messengers [34] although the redox state of certain signaling molecules upstream of the NF-κB should be important in allowing activation. In conclusion, the NF-κB pathway seems to be a general mechanism through which CpG DNA transduces its signal via ROS activation.

Gene and Cytokine Induction by DNA

Nuclear gene transcription is induced within 30 minutes after CpG DNA administration [35]. CpG DNA increases mRNA levels for several genes, regulating the cellular cycle or apoptosis (c-*myc*, bcl-X_L, *myn*, and bcl-2 [29]) and mRNA levels for several transcription factors, such as egr-1, ets-2, C/enhancing binding protein (EBP)-β and -δ, and c-Jun [36]. This leads to mRNA translation and the induction of others genes. mRNA for IL-1, IL-6, IL-10, IL-18, IFN-α/β, IFN-γ, macrophage inflammatory protein (MIP)-1β, and monocyte chemoattractant protein (MCP)-1 are also increased in CpG-treated leukocytes within 30 minutes after CpG stimulation [29]. In macrophages and dendritic cells, CpG DNA is also a strong inducer of IL-12 expression. IL-12 is known to induce IFN-γ in natural killer (NK) cells and to promote T-helper-1 (Th1)-type immunity [37]. This Th1-like cytokine profile is dominated by IL-12, IL-18 and IFN-γ which appear as the faster DNA response [37]. IL-18 cooperates with IL-12 in the promotion of IFN-γ production and the development of Th1-type immunity, the level of IL-12 being controlled by IL-10 produced by B cells stimulated by CpG DNA. However, IL-10 acts as a counter-regulating agent for limiting CpG-induced toxicity [29] while Th2-like cytokines such as IL-4 and IL-5 are not induced by CpG DNA [38]. In spleen cells exposed to CpG DNA, TNF-α is released resulting, as observed with IL-12, in IFN-γ production. Apart from its important role in the normal inflammatory response, TNF-α is responsible for the induction of the systemic inflammatory-response syndrome (SIRS) in mice sensitized to the effects of TNF-α [27].

Cellular Mechanisms of Action of CpG DNA

All the stimulation pathways described above are involved in mediating CpG DNA effects in monocytic cells and B cells in both mice and humans. However, some CpG DNA-induced effects are different according to the type of cells stimulated.

Monocyte-macrophage and Dendritic Cell Activation

CpG DNA can directly activate these antigen-presenting cells resulting in cytokine production such as TNF-a (with a peak of TNF-a mRNA at 1 hour after DNA exposure) [27, 37, 39, 40], IL-1, IL-6, and IL-12 via Th1-like responses [41], and in increased expression of cell surface class-II major histocompatability complex (MHC) and the costimulatory molecules B7-1 and B7-2 [12, 37]. Stimulation of macrophages by CpG DNA leads to IL-12 production, this leading further to NK cell-induced IFN-γ production. This creates a sort of self-amplifying loop resulting in an enhancement of the macrophage response to DNA with an increase of compounds such as TNF-a, NO and IL-12 itself. *In vivo*, this loop has to be kept under control to avoid the development of toxic shock. IL-10 plays an important role in this loop control where it inhibits CpG DNA-induced IL-12 release in macrophage. IL-10 keeps the response to foreign DNA under control. CpG DNA has been shown to induce slower differentiative responses in the maturation of antigen-presenting cell function [37]. Furthermore, CpG DNA-treated cells produce more IL-12 and less IL-6 and TNF-a than LPS-treated cells.

In human monocytes, CpG DNA induces the release of TNF-a and IL-6 and the expression of intercellular adhesion molecule 1 (ICAM-1) [42]. However, the magnitude is less important and the kinetics are much slower than after LPS exposure. TNF-a and IL-6 are produced only 18 to 24 hours after CpG DNA stimulation compared to the 4 hours after LPS stimulation [42]. However, the comparison of CpG DNA and LPS stimulation between mouse and human is difficult. In the mouse, macrophages are mature (peritoneal or bone-marrow-derived macrophages) while human circulating monocytes are immature. The studies showing IL-18, IFN-a and -β mRNA macrophage production in response to DNA were obtained from human macrophages purified from peripheral mononuclear cells.

Human dendritic cells are activated by CpG DNA resulting in an increase in costimulatory molecules associated with much faster kinetics than that observed within macrophages. Therefore, these cells appear to be the most effective inducers of allogenic T cell proliferative responses [12].

B Cell Activation

CpG DNA is the most potent single B cell mitogen. It can drive more than 95% of B cells into the cell cycle [3]. Low concentrations of CpG DNA synergize for B cell activation through the B cell antigen receptor (BCR). B cell proliferation increases at least tenfold more [3]. B cells proliferate in a polyclonal T cell independent manner [3]. This activation leads to secretion of IL-6, IL-10, and immunoglobulin such as IgM in an IL-6-dependent manner [25]. Thus, the synergistic costimulation of B cells by CpG DNA and the BCR provides a mechanism for crosstalk between PRR of the innate immune system and the antigen-specific features of the adaptive system. This synergy provides a mechanism for the preferential activation of B cells.

These are specific for bacterial antigens in an area of infection in which CpG DNA is present. Opposite to LPS, IFN-γ synergizes with CpG DNA in B cell activation promoting stronger CpG-induced effects [10]. CpG DNA can also increase the expression of B cell class-II MHC molecules, and costimulatory molecules B7-1 and B7-2 [3]. This suggests that CpG DNA might directly enhance by itself the antigen-presenting function of B cells.

In experimental models, CpG DNA has been implicated in preventing B cell apoptosis produced through the Fas-mediated pathway [43], and in cultured primary B cells [25]. Indeed, CpG DNA was found to rescue from apoptosis a murine immature B cell line WEHI-231 that normally undergoes apoptosis in response to BCR cross-linking [10]. The phenomenon requires the induction of NF-κB [22, 35]. In this WEHI-231 model, the anti-apoptotic activity is observed to persist when CpG DNA is added as late as 8 hours after BCR ligation [29].

In humans, B cell responses to CpG DNA appear to be very similar to those of murine B cells. However, the optimal ODN motifs for stimulation are different:

5' TCCATGA<u>CG</u>TTCCTGA<u>CG</u>TT 3' activates only mouse;

5' <u>TCGTCG</u>;TTTTGT<u>CG</u>TTTTGT<u>CG</u>TT 3' activates human and mouse cells.

T Cell Activation

Klinman et al. [38] found first that CpG DNA directly stimulates cytokine production in T cells, but this study was performed on partially purified T cells. Direct CpG DNA activation on T cells was not found in further studies [44, 45]. It seems that CpG DNA induces in adherent cells type-I IFN production with the consequence of T cell activation by CD 69 and B7-2 expression. However, their proliferative responses to ligation of the T cell receptor in response to type-1 IFN production by antigen-presenting cells are reduced [45]. Also, purified T cells have been shown to have synergistic proliferative responses to CpG DNA, which promote antigen-specific T cell responses [46]. However, no study has been performed *in vivo* to assess the inhibitory and stimulatory effects of CpG DNA on T cell activation.

NK Cell Activation

Tokunaga et al. [2] were the first to show that bacterial DNA could activate NK cells resulting in their lytic activity with IFN-γ production. The effect of CpG DNA on NK cell activation seems to be indirect. Antibodies neutralizing IL-12, TNF-α, and type-I IFN, which are cytokines produced by adhering cells, block this NK activation [36]. Therefore, it is assumed that NK cells could be costimulated by the combination of CpG DNA and specific activating cytokines, as with T cells [36].

▌ Comparison of CpG DNA and LPS Responses

CpG DNA shares many similarities with LPS for monocyte cytokine production, but there are many differences in the signaling pathways. In experimental models, these agents are both mitogenic for mouse B cells, and increase monocyte production of TNF-α, IL-6 and other cytokines. CpG DNA induces expression of iNOS only after priming with IFN-γ [47] whereas this priming is not required for LPS to induce iNOS. LPS action differs from CpG DNA action in relation to its cytokine secretion kinetics.

To differentiate the signaling pathway activated by CpG from that activated by LPS, an LPS non-responder mice model has been developed. These mice, termed C3H/HeJ, retain normal responses to CpG DNA [27, 36]. The principle difference is the presence of an LPS receptor molecule – TLR4 – which is not necessary for the CpG DNA-mediated effect [48]. Furthermore, LPS-induced activation is not inhibited by chloroquine and bafilomycin A, which are molecules interfering with endosomal acidification. Even though the recognition structures for LPS and CpG DNA may be distinct, the signaling in response to LPS and CpG DNA converges toward the activation of MAPK [5, 28], and activation of transcription factors such as NF-κB, AP-1, C/EBP-β, C/EBP-δ and ets-2 [37]. Finally, the signaling pathways triggered by CpG DNA are remarkably similar to those triggered by LPS.

LPS leads to toxic shock by cytokine production released by macrophages. Although CpG DNA by itself is non toxic, demonstration of its toxic effects requires sensitizing mice with D-galactosamine which is a liver specific inhibitor sensitizing liver to TNF-α-mediated apoptosis. A single dose of CpG DNA alone is not responsible for toxic shock, by contrast with LPS [49]. But two doses of CpG DNA given within 1 week can cause a sepsis-like condition. This effect can result from a priming effect of cytokines by the first dose. A synergy between CpG DNA and LPS on cytokine production *in vitro* and *in vivo* has been reported [49]. In a mouse model, Cowdery et al. [36] found that CpG DNA given 4 hours before a sublethal dose of LPS was responsible for a very high mortality associated with an increase of TNF-α production. The author concluded that this effect might be the consequence of IFN-γ production. We demonstrated that CpG acts as a sensitizing agent for LPS [49]. A sublethal dose of CpG injected 1 hour before a sublethal dose of LPS was responsible for an increase in TNF-α serum level associated with a 100% mortality. This sensitizing effect was inhibited by administration of a specific TNF-α transcription inhibitor (pentoxifylline). We suggested that this sensitizing effect was in relation to mRNA neosynthesis [49]. In human monocytes, CpG DNA and LPS also synergize in the induction of IL-6 [42]. This toxicity difference between LPS and CpG DNA when given separately could be important for the therapeutic application of CpG DNA.

▮ Is there a Role for CpG DNA Activation for Immunostimulation in Sepsis?

Unmethylated CpG sequences have demonstrated utility as vaccine adjuvants for antigen presenting cell (such as macrophage) stimulation, and as immunological treatment for cancer and allergic diseases such as asthma. However, their immunostimulant role in natural infection is difficult to assess. Pisetsky et al. [50], suggested that DNA detection is important in viral infections, because viruses do not contain the necessary range of lipid and sugar molecules allowing identification of bacteria and pathogens in the innate immune system. LPS present in bacteria is more stimulant than DNA and has a quantitatively greater effect on the immune system than foreign DNA. But, detection of this foreign DNA is of importance in synergizing with activating molecules and in detection of bacterial strains that have avoided other ways of surveillance [37]. Recently, Weighardt et al. [14] suggested that CpG DNA acts as a protective agent by increasing resistance in acute polymicrobial infection and so enhances effector cell response of innate immunity. These authors suggested that CpG DNA could act as a potent agent for the treatment of sepsis-associated immunoparalysis.

▌ Conclusion

It is well known that bacterial DNA is recognized by immune cells through its unmethylated CpG motifs. Both the innate and acquired immune systems are involved in CpG sequence detection: innate by monocytes and macrophages, and acquired via B cell activation. CpG DNA and LPS share many similarities in term of signaling pathway. However, the main difference lies in the time course of cytokine expression which is delayed for CpG DNA compared to LPS. The greatest advance in the understanding of the mechanism of action of CpG DNA has been the identification of its species-specific receptor TLR9 which is the first step of activation of its molecular signaling pathways.

CpG DNA can induce toxic effects but this requires high doses that are inconsistent with any rationale for therapeutic effect. However, CpG DNA emerges as a non-toxic vaccine adjuvant in multiple disease categories and the preclinical studies seem to be promising. The place of CpG DNA treatment in human sepsis remains to be explored, although a recent study [14] proposes that CpG DNA could represent a potent agent for the treatment of sepsis-associated immunoparalysis.

References

1. Medzhitov R, Janeway CA Jr (1997) Innate immunity: the virtues of a nonclonal system recognition. Cell 91:295–298
2. Tokunaga T, Yamamoto H, Shimada S, et al (1984) Antitumor activity of deoxyribonucleic acid fraction from *Mycobacterium bovis* BCG. I. Isolation, physicochemical characterization, and antitumor activity. J Natl Cancer Inst 72:955–962
3. Krieg AK, Yi A-K, Matson S, et al (1995) CpG motifs in bacterial DNA trigger direct B-cell activation. Nature 374:546–549
4. Krieg AM, Wu T, Weeratna R, et al (1998) Sequence motifs in adenoviral DNA block immune activation by stimulatory CpG motifs. Proc Natl Acad Sci USA 95:12631–12636
5. Häcker H, Mischak H, Miethke T, et al (1998) CpG-DNA-specific activation of antigen-presenting cells requires stress kinase activity and is preceded by non-specific endocytosis and endosomal maturation. EMBO J 17:6230–6240
6. Karlin S, Doerfler W, Cardon LR (1994) Why is CpG suppressed in the genomes of virtually all small eukaryotic viruses but not in those of large eukaryotic viruses? J Virol 68:2889–2897
7. Krieg AM, Yi AK, Schorr J, Davis HL (1998) The role of CpG dinucleotides in DNA vaccines. Trends Microbiol 6:23–27
8. Krieg AM (1996) An innate immune defense mechanism based on the recognition of CpG motifs in microbial DNA. J Lab Clin Med 128:128–133
9. Hemmi H, Takeuchi O, Kawai T, et al (2000) A toll-like receptor recognizes bacterial DNA. Nature 408:740–745
10. Krieg AM, Hartmann G, Yi AK (2000) Mechanism of action of CpG DNA. Curr Top Microbiol Immunol 247:1–21
11. Yamamoto S, Yamamoto T, Shimada S, et al (1992) DNA from bacteria, but not from vertebrates, induces interferons, activates natural killer cells and inhibits tumor growth. Microbiol Immunol 36:983–997
12. Krieg AM (2001) Immune effects and mechanisms of action of CpG motifs. Vaccine 19:618–622
13. Krieg AM (2001) From bugs to drugs: therapeutic immunomodulation with oligodeoxynucleotides containing CpG sequences from bacterial DNA. Antisense Nucleic Acid Drug Dev 11:181–188
14. Weighardt H, Feterowski C, Veit M, Rump M, Wagner H, Holzmann B (2000) Increased resistance against acute polymicrobial sepsis in mice challenged with immunostimulatory CpG oligodeoxynucleotides is related to an enhanced innate effector cell response. J Immunol 165:4537–4543

15. Medzhitov R, Janeway C Jr (2000) Innate immunity. N Engl J Med 343:338–344
16. Hoshino K, Takeuchi O, Kawai T, et al (1999) Cutting edge: Toll-like receptor 4 (TLR4)-deficient mice are hyporesponsive to lipopolysaccharide: evidence for TLR4 as the Lps gene product. J Immunol 162:3749–3752
17. Wright SD, Ramos RA, Tobias PS, Ulevitch RJ, Mathison JC (1990) CD14, a receptor for complexes of lipopolysaccharide (LPS) and LPS binding protein. Science 249:1431–1433
18. Shimazu R, Akashi S, Ogata H, et al (1999) MD-2, a molecule that confers lipopolysaccharide responsiveness on Toll-like receptor 4. J Exp Med 189:1777–1782
19. Beltinger C, Saragovi HU, Smith RM, et al (1995) Binding, uptake, and intracellular trafficking of phosphothioate-modified oligodeoxynucleotides. J Clin Invest 95:1814–1823
20. Hanss B, Stein CA, Klotman PE (1998) Cellular uptake and biodistribution of oligodeoxynucleotides. In: Stein CA, Krieg AM (eds) Applied Oligonucleotide Technology. John Wiley and Sons, Inc, New York, pp 431–448
21. Bennett RM, Gabor GT, Merritt MM (1985) DNA binding to human leukocytes. Evidence for a receptor-mediated association, internalization, and degradation of DNA. J Clin Invest 76:2182–2190
22. Yi AK, Tuetken R, Redford T, Kirsch J, Krieg AM (1998) CpG motifs in bacterial DNA activates leukocytes through the pH-dependent generation of reactive oxygen species. J Immunol 160:4755–4761
23. Zhao Q, Matson S, Herrera CJ, et al (1993) Comparison of cellular binding and uptake of antisense phosphodiester, phosphorothioate, and mixed phosphorothioate and methylphosphonate oligonucleotides. Antisense Res Dev 3:53–66
24. Häcker H (2000) Signal transduction pathways activated by CpG-DNA. Curr Top Microbiol Immunol 247:77–92
25. Yi AK, Klinman DM, Martin TL, Matson S, Krieg AM (1996) Rapid immune activation by CpG motifs in bacterial DNA: systemic induction of IL-6 transcription through an anti-oxidant-sensitive pathway. J Immunol 157:5394–5402
26. Stacey KJ, Sweet MJ, Hume DA (1996) Macrophages ingest and are activated by bacterial DNA. J Immunol 157:2116–2122
27. Sparwasser T, Miethke T, Lipford G, et al (1997) Macrophages sense pathogens via DNA motifs: induction of tumor necrosis factor-a-mediated shock. Eur J Immunol 27:1671–1679
28. Yi AK, Krieg AM (1998) Rapid induction of mitogen activated protein kinases by immune stimulatory CpG DNA. J Immunol 161:4493–4497
29. Krieg AM (2000) Signal transduction induced by immunostimulatory CpG DNA. Springer Semin Immunopathol 22:97–105
30. Lewis TS, Shapiro PS, Ahn NG (1998) Signal transduction through MAP kinases cascades. Adv Cancer Res 74:49–139
31. Baldwin As Jr (1996) The NF-κB and I-κB proteins: New discoveries and insights. Annu Rev Immunol 14:649–681
32. Wesche H, Henzel WJ, Shillinglaw W, Li S, Cao Z (1997) MyD88: an adapter that recruits IRAK to the IL-1 receptor complex. Immunity 7:837–847
33. Baeuerle PA, Henkel T (1994) Function and activation of NF-κB in the immune system. Annu Rev Immunol 12 :141–179
34. Brennan P, O'Neil L (1995) Effects of oxidants and antioxydants on NF-κB activation in three different cell lines: evidence against a universal hypothesis involving oxygen radicals. Biochem Biophys Acta 1260 :1670–1675
35. Yi AK, Chang M, Peckham DW, Krieg AM, Ashman RF (1998) CpG oligodeoxynucleotides rescue mature spleen B cells from spontaneous apoptosis and promote cell cycle reentry. J Immunol 160:4755–4761
36. Cowdery JS, Chace JH, Yi AK, Krieg AM (1996) Bacterial DNA induces NK cells to produce interferon-γ in vivo and increases the toxicity of lipopolysaccharides. J Immunol 156:4570–4575
37. Stacey KJ, Sester DP, Sweet MJ, Hume DA (2000) Macrophage activation by immunostimulatory DNA. Curr Top Microbiol Immunol 247:41–58
38. Klinman D, Yi AK, Beaucage SL, Conover J, Krieg AM (1996) CpG motifs expressed by bacterial DNA rapidly induce lymphocytes to secrete IL-6, IL-12 and IFNγ. Proc Natl Acad Sci USA 93:2879–2883

39. Lipford GB, Sparwasser T, Bauer M, et al (1997) Immunostimulatory DNA: sequence-dependent production of potentially harmful or useful cytokines. Eur J Immunol 27:3420–3426

40. Sparwasser T, Miethke T, Lipford G, et al (1997) Bacterial DNA causes septic shock. Nature 386:336–337

41. Jakob T, Walker PS, Krieg AM, Udey MC, Vogel JC (1998) Activation of cutaneous dendritic cells by CpG-containing oligodeoxynucleotides: A role for dendritic cells in the augmentation of Th1 responses by immunostimulatory DNA. J Immunol 161:3042–3049

42. Hartmann G, Krieg AM (1999) CpG DNA and LPS induce distinct patterns of activation in human monocytes. Gene Therapy 6:893–903

43. Wang Z, Karras JG, Colarusso TP, Foote LC, Rothstein TL (1997) Unmethylated CpG motifs protect murine B lymphocytes against Fas-mediated apoptosis. Cell Immunol 180:162–167

44. Lipford GB, Bauer M, Blank C, Reiter R, Wagner H, Heeg K (1997) CpG-containing synthetic oligonucleotides promote B and cytotoxic T cell responses to protein antigen: a new class of vaccine adjuvants. Eur J Immunol 27:2340–2344

45. Sun S, Zhang X, Tough DF, Sprent J (1998) Type I interferon-mediated stimulation of T cells by CpG DNA. J Exp Med 188:2335–2342

46. Bendigs S, Salzer U, Lipford GB, Wagner H, Heeg K (1999) CpG-oligodeoxynucleotides costimulate primary T cells in the absence of APC. Eur J Immunol 29:1209–1218

47. Sweet MJ, Stacey KJ, Kakuda DK, Markovich D, Hume DA (1998) IFN-γ primes macrophage responses to bacterial DNA. J Interferon Cytokines Res 18:263–271

48. Poltorak A, He X, Smirnova I, et al (1998) Defective LPS signaling in C3H/HeJ and C57BL/10ScCr mice: mutations in Tlr4 gene. Science 282:2085–2088

49. Wiel E, Ban E, Lund N, Riveau G, Vallet B (2001) CpG motifs are sensitizing agents for LPS in toxic shock model. Intensive Care Med 27 (suppl 2):S233 (Abst)

50. Pisetsky DS (1996) The immunologic properties of DNA. J Immunol 156:421–423

Antibiotics by Continuous Infusion: Time for Re-evaluation?

D. L. A. Wyncoll, R. Bowry, and L. J. Giles

▌ Introduction

Severe sepsis and septic shock account for 15–20% of intensive care unit (ICU) admissions and when associated with multi-organ dysfunction there is a 55% mortality [1]. Surgical evacuation of any focus of infection should be undertaken where possible, however, the mainstay of treatment is antibiotic therapy. In recent years there have been considerable advances in the support of these patients with emphasis being placed on early, adequate volume resuscitation [2], administration of stress-dose corticosteroids [3], immunonutrition [4], and, more recently, manipulation of coagulation pathways [5]. However, the way in which antibiotics are administered has remained largely unchanged since the 1940s. At a time when many standard therapies are being re-evaluated we should ask the question 'Are we using antibiotics to their greatest potential?'

A significant clinical problem in the ICU today is the increased prevalence of highly resistant organisms. The development of resistance is undoubtedly a multifactorial problem, but inappropriate and over use of antimicrobials may be a key factor. In fact, very few patients pass through the ICU without being exposed to antibiotics at some point, whether for prophylaxis or treatment. The development of new classes of antimicrobials is likely to be only a temporary solution and other mechanisms must be found to deal with this problem. The use of surveillance programs, and rotational, restrictive prescribing policies has been recommended [6]. Another valuable strategy may be administration of high dose, short course antibiotics.

▌ How is Antibiotic Dose Related to Antimicrobial Effect?

Antibiotic dosing regimens were originally determined from data relating to *in vitro* antimicrobial activity and an appreciation of the pharmacokinetic characteristics of the drug concerned. This information combined with clinical experience led to intermittent bolus dosing. These schedules were rarely validated and yet have been used for several decades [7]. This approach should be challenged based on improved understanding of the pharmacodynamics of these drugs in the critically ill.

To achieve the most efficient killing of bacteria, both the pharmacokinetic and pharmacodynamic properties of the antibiotic must provide the rationale for dosing. These include the post-antibiotic effect (PAE), exponential versus stationary growth phase, glycocalyx and biofilms, synergism, time-kill kinetics, and protein binding.

In vitro experiments with inoculate of bacteria are used to find the minimum inhibitory concentration (MIC) of antibiotic required to inhibit growth. These experiments rely on maintaining a steady concentration of antibiotic, yet the information gained can be unpredictable. The MIC for an antibiotic will vary depending upon the size of the inoculums and the type of medium used, as well as for different bacteria. Although it is possible to get an idea of the MIC required, it is only accurate to ±one 2-fold dilution [8]. The bactericidal effect of β-lactams is closely related to the time during which serum concentration is above the MIC ($T>$MIC) [9] and maximum killing is seen when $T>$MIC is at least 60–70% of the dosage interval [10].

Antibiotics may exert antimicrobial effects even after the tissue level has fallen below the MIC. This is known as the PAE. PAE can be used as justification for intermittent bolus dosing, but it is both antibiotic and bacteria specific and so its relevance in the critically ill patient remains uncertain. For example, β-lactams exhibit a PAE that ranges from 4 for Gram-positive organisms to undetectable for Gram-negative organisms, whereas aminoglycosides have significant PAEs for Gram-negative organisms. Furthermore, PAE studies are performed by exposing bacteria to a one-time dose of antibiotic. Whether PAE remains constant after multiple doses is unresolved [11]. Tissue concentrations vary widely in critically ill patients due to abnormalities in drug clearance, protein binding and drug interactions. For antibiotics that require a prolonged time above MIC, one approach is to achieve the therapeutic level rapidly with a generous loading dose and ensure that the dosing interval is short enough to maintain high tissue levels.

Unnecessarily high peaks may be produced, significant antibiotic may be wasted, and repeated administrations are time consuming for nursing staff. Conversely, a simpler way of achieving this goal is to administer antimicrobials by continuous infusion. The pharmacodynamic rationale for dosing the key classes of antimicrobial has been recently reviewed [12] and is summarized in Table 1.

Table 1. Pharmacodynamic rationale for dosing the key classes of antimicrobial agents

Antimicrobial class	Rationale for dosing
Penicillins	$T>$MIC & PAE
Cephalosporins	$T>$MIC & PAE
Carbapenems	$T>$MIC & PAE
Quinolones	AUC/MIC & peak MIC
Glycopeptides	$T>$MIC & AUC/MIC
Aminoglycosides	AUC/MIC & peak MIC
Macrolides	? peak MIC
Metronidazole	?

AUC: area under the concentration time curve; MIC: minimum inhibitory concentration; PAE: post-antibiotic effect; T: serum concentration

▌ Pharmacokinetics of Infusions

Continuous infusions are already frequently used in the ICU setting with most drugs initially given in small boluses until the desired clinical effect occurs. This initial rapid titration is effectively giving a loading dose. When the appropriate clinical effect is achieved, an infusion is started to maintain serum concentrations and consequently prolong the effect. Using the two equations below an appropriate loading dose (Eqn. 1) and infusion rate (Eqn 2) may be calculated if a target concentration, volume of distribution, and clearance are known.

Loading dose = Concentration desired × volume of distribution   (Eqn 1)

Infusion Rate = Concentration desired × clearance   (Eqn 2)

Volume and clearance values quoted in the literature have usually been determined in healthy volunteers and will vary considerably from the true values in critically ill patients. Volume of distribution may be affected by hypoalbuminemia, change in binding affinity, and fluid status. Clearance will be altered by changes in protein binding, liver or renal dysfunction, and the use of extracorporeal techniques. Values should be sought from published pharmacokinetic studies carried out in critically ill patients.

▌ What is the Evidence Supporting the Use of Continuous Infusion in Critically Ill Patients?

Over the past couple of decades there have been many case reports and small series of patients treated with continuous infusions of antibiotics. The earliest reports were with 'second generation' cephalosporins. Most of the more recent data comparing continuous infusion with intermittent bolus dosing of antibiotics has been carried out with ceftazidime, meropenem and vancomycin; three antibiotics commonly used in the ICU.

Ceftazidime, when given at the recommended 2 g 8-hourly, produces very erratic plasma concentrations with troughs well below the MIC. Young et al. [13] investigated 10 patients who were being treated for *Pseudomonas aeruginosa* infections with conventional intermittent dosing. On day 1, plasma ceftazidime concentrations were less than the MIC in three patients and in nine, concentrations were less than the recommended 4–5×MIC. The results were not better by day 3. This dosing regimen may result in treatment failure and potentially encourage the emergence of resistant bacteria. The same group has also demonstrated that when a loading dose of ceftazidime is used followed by a continuous infection, no patient had levels less than the target 4–5×MIC for *P. aeruginosa* after eight hours [14]. Once again they confirmed that 80% of patients receiving intermittent bolus dosing had trough levels that were below the ideal plasma concentration.

Meropenem, a carbapenem, has a bactericidal effect with efficacy predominantly related to $T > MIC$. Carbapenems differ however from other β-lactams in that they also exhibit concentration-dependent killing, which suggests some benefit from attaining high peak concentrations [15]. Nevertheless, in a fifteen patient crossover study, Thalhammer et al. [16] demonstrated that it was possible to maintain appropriate tissue levels via either continuous infusion or intermittent bolus. More interestingly, however, the continuous infusion regimen (3 g/24 h) achieved adequate bactericidal serum levels using only 50% of the drug required for intermittent administration (2 g every 8 h).

For the glycopeptide vancomycin $T > MIC$ is again the pharmacodynamic variable best related to outcome. Unlike β-lactams which are relatively safe given in high doses, vancomycin exhibits toxic effects at high concentrations; specifically ototoxicity is recognized when concentrations exceed 40 mg/l. Logically, the safest method to administer vancomycin would be to infuse a slow loading dose avoiding high peak levels, and then a continuous infusion to maintain a steady plasma level. It has been known for some years that intermittent dosing of vancomycin risks treatment failure since it may take several days to achieve adequate tissue levels. A study using intermittent vancomycin prior to cardiac surgery showed that adequate bone levels were only achieved after 48 hour's administration [17]. This may have clinical relevance to the treatment of *Staphylococcal* osteomyelitis. Additionally, there are further data which demonstrate that vancomycin, using standard intermittent dosing, has very poor penetration into pulmonary tissue with $T > MIC$ often less than 20% [18, 19]. Interestingly, detection of vancomycin in pulmonary tissue correlated with serum concentration exceeding 20 mg/l. This has direct clinical importance in treating patients with methicillin-resistant Staphylococcus aureus (MRSA) where MICs are considerably higher than for sensitive *Staphylococci* and, moreover, the requirement for $8-10 \times MIC$ has been recommended by some authors [20]. These factors could account for the slow response and 20–30% failure rate in treating certain MRSA infections [21].

One of the first comparative studies of conventional dosing vancomycin and continuous infusion was performed by James and colleagues [22]. In a ten patient crossover study they showed that continuous infusion produced more stable plasma concentrations than intermittent bolus, and that $T > MIC$ was achieved for the duration of treatment only with continuous infusion. With reasonable certainty, we can suppose that continuous infusion would result in a reduced risk of toxicity, and a reduced risk of under dosing and treatment failure.

▌ Is there Improved Outcome for Antibiotic Infusions?

At present the largest study evaluating whether continuous infusion has an outcome advantage over intermittent bolus is from Paris [23]. One hundred and nineteen patients with severe hospital-acquired MRSA were randomized to receive continuous or intermittent infusion of vancomycin. Microbiological and clinical outcomes, and safety were similar, however, the daily dose given over 10 days was lower with continuous infusion resulting in a 23% lower 10-day treatment cost (p < 0.0001). The largest study using ceftazidime by continuous infusion involved only 35 patients [24]. Not surprisingly, clinical efficacy was judged to be similar and adverse events and length of stay did not differ among the two groups. Again costs associated with continuous infusion were significantly lower ($627 versus $1007, p < 0.001). Further larger studies are now required to evaluate clinical outcomes comparing the two routes.

▌ Therapeutic Drug Monitoring

Therapeutic drug monitoring (TDM) has always been important in the ICU to reduce the toxic effects of therapy. Antibiotics such as vancomycin, particularly when used in combination with an aminoglycoside, can exhibit significant toxicity. For many years, it was thought necessary to measure peak and trough vancomycin concentrations to determine the appropriate dose and dosing interval, with the consequent expense of monitoring and interpreting levels. It has been demonstrated that toxic peak levels are unlikely to be generated, as long as trough concentrations do not exceed 15 mg/l, and therefore need not to be monitored routinely [25]. Unfortunately this approach risks trough levels below MIC and potentially risks under treating patients with severe infection. A significant advantage with continuous infusion is that only a single daily level need be measured to target a chosen concentration range well above MIC (e.g., for vancomycin 15–25 mg/l). Moreover, this level can be taken at the most convenient time of day and batched with other assays resulting in further cost savings.

One final advantage that may arise from maintaining adequate levels of antibiotics from the onset of treatment could well be an opportunity to reduce the length of the antibiotic course. More than fifty years ago, it was known that the total dose required to cure infection was significantly less if the drug was administered in multiple doses at frequent intervals [26]. A short, sharp and effective course of antibiotics, which has adequately penetrated the relevant body tissues, is likely to produce a greater clinical effect than an approach where antibotics are given intermittently with levels subsequently dropping significantly below MIC. Although the suggestion that continuous infusion might allow shorter courses of antimicrobials is theoretical and requires further study, it is not a novel concept. Table 2 outlines the established and potential advantages and disadvantages of continuous infusions of antibiotics.

Table 2. Arguments for and against administering β-lactam and glycopeptide antibiotics by continuous infusion

Arguments 'for'	Arguments 'against'
▌ **Established**	▌ **Established**
– Cheaper	– Limited outcome data
– Less risk of under dosing	– More infusion lines/pumps required
– Less risk of toxicity	– Lag time to achieve steady state after change
– Single daily level tested at most convenient time of day	in infusion rate
– Serum samples may be assayed as a single batch	
▌ **Theoretical**	▌ **Theoretical**
– Shorter duration of treatment	– Concern over stability of drugs in the syringe
– Less nursing time	– Limited data on compatibility with other infusions

What about Drug Stability?

Most dissolved antimicrobials are stable for at least 24 hours [10]. The manufacturers of meropenem suggest that when reconstituted in isotonic saline stability cannot be guaranteed for longer than 8 hours at room temperature. Ceftazidime has been more extensively studied and remains stable for 24 hours if kept at temperatures less than 25 °C. Nevertheless, incompatibility with several commonly used drugs, including propofol and midazolam, has been noted [27]. Vancomycin has been used by continuous infusion and remains stable for 24 hours after dilution.

Protocol for Vancomycin by Continuous Infusion

Vancomycin has been given by continuous infusion in our ICU since 1997. We describe here our protocol, which includes dosing guidance for patients with renal dysfunction and those requiring renal support.

All patients receive a weight-related loading dose of either 1 g (weight <65 kg) or 1.5 g (weight >65 kg) given over 1 hour to ensure rapid attainment of target concentrations. This is especially important for patients with significant renal impairment who will have a prolonged vancomycin half-life and would otherwise take several days to achieve the steady state serum concentrations. A continuous intravenous infusion is started immediately after the loading, at a dose based on an estimate of the patient's renal function (Table 3).

A serum vancomycin level is measured every day at 06.00 h using a Syvia EMIT assay. The daily dose and hence infusion rate is then adjusted according to the level

Table 3. Starting daily dose for vancomycin by continuous infusion

	Estimated creatinine clearance (ml/min)	Starting daily vancomycin dose	Starting infusion rate (mg/hr)
▌ Normal renal function	>50	2000 mg	83
▌ Mild impairment	20–50	1500 mg	63
▌ Moderate impairment	10–20	1000 mg	42
▌ Severe impairment	<10	500 mg	21
▌ CVVH		1000 mg	42

CVVH: Continuous veno-venous hemofiltration at flow rate of 2–2.5 l/h

Table 4. Daily dose adjustment for vancomycin by continuous infusion

Vancomycin level	Dosage change required
<15 mg/l	Increase the daily dose by 500 mg
15–25 mg/l	No change
>25 mg/l	Decrease the daily dose by 500 mg[a]
>30 mg/l	Stop infusion for 6 h and re-check level

[a] If the patient is receiving 500 mg/day, the dose is decreased to 250 mg/day

Table 5. Vancomycin compatibility information

Compatibility at a vancomycin concentration of 10 mg/l	Compatibility at a vancomycin concentration of 5 mg/l
▌ Propofol	▌ Morphine
▌ Fluconazole	▌ Midazolam
	▌ Cisatracurium
	▌ Amiodarone
	▌ Labetalol

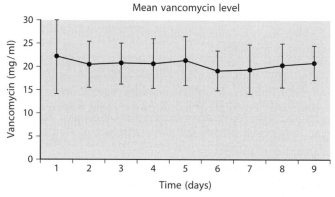

Fig. 1. Plasma concentrations achieved using protocol in Tables 3 and 4

(Table 4). If treatment with vancomycin is started within 6 h of the usual 6.00 h level, the first level is taken on the following morning.

Vancomycin is infused at a concentration of 10 mg/l when given via a central line. Whenever possible a separate lumen is used for the vancomycin infusion otherwise it shares a lumen based on the available compatibility information [28] (Table 5).

We have experience using this protocol for at least 300 treatment episodes and preliminary data (Fig. 1) suggest that it is safe and effective at achieving concentrations within our chosen target range.

▌ Conclusion

Antibiotics administered to critically ill patients are still routinely dosed using schedules that were determined in healthy volunteers. Antibiotics that have a time-related antimicrobial effect are still being used in a way that produces trough concentrations below the MIC several days into a treatment course in critically ill patients. Giving antimicrobials by continuous infusion can effectively eliminate the risk of this occurrence. Theoretical benefits of antibiotic infusions requiring further investigation include greater efficacy, reduction in drug expenditure, and the possibility of shorter courses resulting in less risk of the emergence of resistant bacteria.

References

1. Brun-Buisson C, Doyon F, Carlet J, et al (1995) Incidence, risk factors, and outcome of severe sepsis and septic shock in adults. A multicenter prospective study in intensive care units. French ICU Group for Severe Sepsis. JAMA 274:968–974
2. Rivers E, Nguyen B, Havstad S, et al (2001) Early goal directed therapy in the treatment of severe sepsis and septic shock. N Engl J Med 345:1368–1377
3. Bollaert P-E, Charpentier C, Levy B, et al (1998) Reversal of late septic shock with supraphysiological doses of hydrocortisone. Crit Care Med 26:645–650
4. Wyncoll D, Beale R (2001) Immunologically enhanced enteral nutrition: current status. Curr Opin Crit Care 7:128–132
5. Bernard GR, Vincent JL, Laterre PF, et al (2001) Efficacy and safety of recombinant human activated protein C for severe sepsis. N Engl J Med 344:699–709
6. de Man P, Verhoeven B, Verbrugh H, Vos M, van den Anker J (2000) An antibiotic policy to prevent emergence of resistant bacilli. Lancet 355:973–978
7. Carbón C (1992) Single-dose antibiotic therapy: what has the past taught us? J Clin Pharmacol 32:686–691
8. Rotschafer JC, Zabinski RA, Walker KJ, Vance-Bryan K (1992) Pharmacotherapy and pharmacodynamics in the management of bacterial infection. J Clin Pharmacol 32:1083–1088
9. Drusano GL (1988) Role of pharmacokinetics in the outcome of infections. Antimicrob Agents Chemother 32:289–297
10. Craig WA (1995) Antibiotic selection factors and description of a hospital-based outpatient antibiotic therapy program in the USA. Eur J Clin Microbiol Infect Dis 14:636–642
11. MacGowan AP, Bowker KE (1998) Continuous infusion of β-lactam antibiotics. Clin Pharmacokinet 35:391–402
12. MacGowan AP, Bowker KE (1997) Pharmacodynamics of antimicrobial agents and rationale for their dosing. J Chemotherapy 9:64–73
13. Young RJ, Lipman J, Gin T, Gomersall CD, Joynt GM, Oh TE (1997) Intermittent bolus dosing of ceftazidime in critically ill patients. J Antimicrob Chemother 40:269–273
14. Lipman J, Gomersall CD, Gin T, Joynt GM, Young RJ (1999) Continuous infusion ceftazidime in intensive care: a randomised controlled trial. J Antimicrob Chemother 43:309–311
15. Gould IM (1997) Pharmacodynamics and the relationship between in vitro and in vivo activity of antimicrobial agents. J Chemother 9:73–83
16. Thalhammer F, Traunmüller F, Menyawi IE, et al (1999) Continuous infusion versus intermittent administration of meropenem in critically ill patients. J Antimicrob Chemother 43:523–527
17. Massias L, Dubois C, de Lentdecker P, et al (1992) Penetration of vancomycin in uninfected sternal bone. Antimicrob Agents Chemother 36:2539–2541
18. Cruciani M, Gatti G, Lazzarini L, et al (1996) Penetration of vancomycin into human lung tissue. J Antimicrob Chemother 38:865–869
19. Georges H, Leroy O, Alfandari S, et al (1997) Pulmonary disposition of vancomycin in critically ill patients. Eur J Clin Microbiol Infect Dis 16:385–388
20. Ellner PD, Neu HC (1981) The inhibitory quotient. A method for interpreting minimum inhibitory concentration data. JAMA 246:1575–1578
21. Levine DP, Fromm BS, Reddy BR (1991) Slow response to vancomycin or vancomycin plus rifampin in methicillin-resistant Staphylococcus aureus endocarditis. Ann Intern Med 115:674–680
22. James JK, Palmer SM, Levine DP, Rybak MJ (1966) Comparison of conventional dosing versus continuous-infusion vancomycin therapy for patients with suspected or documented gram-positive infections. Antimicrob Agents Chemother 40:696–700
23. Wysocki M, Delatour F, Faurisson F, et al (2001) Continuous versus intermittent infusion of vancomycin in severe Staphylococcal infections: prospective multicenter randomised study. Antimicrob Agents Chemother 45:2460–2467
24. NcNabb JJ, Nightingale CH, Quintiliani R, Nicolau DP (2001) Cost-effectiveness of ceftazidime by continuous infusion versus intermittent infusion for nosocomial pneumonia. Pharmacotherapy 21:549–555
25. Saunders NJ (1994) Why monitor peak vancomycin concentrations. Lancet 344:1748–1750

26. Eagle HR, Fleischman R, Musselman (1950) Effect of schedule of administration on the therapeutic efficacy of penicillin: importance of the aggregate time penicillin remains at effectively bactericidal levels. Am J Med 9:280–299
27. Servaais H, Tulkens PM (2001) Stability and compatibility of ceftazidime administered by continuous infusion to intensive care patients. Antimicrob Agents Chemother 45:2643–2647
28. Trissel LA (1998) Handbook on Injectable Drugs, 10th ed. American Society of Health System Pharmacists, Bethesda

Extended Spectrum Beta-lactamases in Gram-negative Sepsis

D. L. Paterson

▌ Introduction

Escherichia coli, Klebsiella pneumoniae, and other enteric Gram-negative bacilli are commonly associated with sepsis. Bacteremia caused by such organisms may arise from infections of the urinary tract, the gastrointestinal tract and peritoneal cavity, the lungs, and less commonly from central venous lines and wounds. In many hospitals, at least one third of *E. coli* strains and greater than 95% of *K. pneumoniae* strains are resistant to ampicillin. This resistance is usually mediated in *E. coli* by a plasmid mediated *β*-lactamase known as TEM-1 and in *K. pneumoniae* by a chromosomally encoded *β*-lactamase known as SHV-1 (TEM refers to Temoneira, a patient from Athens, Greece, from whom a urinary tract isolate of *E. coli* bearing the TEM-1 *β*-lactamase was first isolated in the 1960s. SHV refers to sulfhydryl variable, in reference to the interaction of SHV-1 with p-chloromercuribenzoate). Both TEM-1 and SHV-1 can mediate resistance to ampicillin and first generation cephalosporins, but not to the third generation cephalosporins.

In 1983, a cefotaxime resistant *Klebsiella* isolate was described which produced a *β*-lactamase with an ability to hydrolyze the third generation cephalosporins [1]. The gene encoding this *β*-lactamase had a mutation of a single nucelotide compared to the gene encoding SHV-1. Other *β*-lactamases were soon discovered which were closely related to TEM-1, but which had the ability to confer resistance to the third generation cephalosporins [2, 3]. Since these new *β*-lactamases had an extended spectrum of activity compared to their parent enzymes, they were termed the extended-spectrum *β*-lactamases (ESBLs).

It should be noted that the chromosomally encoded AmpC type *β*-lactamases, commonly produced by organisms such as *Pseudomonas aeruginosa* and *Enterobacter cloacae,* are not referred to as ESBLs, even though they can hydrolyze third generation cephalosporins. Structurally and functionally, such *β*-lactamases are different from the true ESBLs. The ESBLs and the AmpC type *β*-lactamases can be differentiated by their susceptibility to *β*-lactamase inhibitors (for example, clavulanic acid) and their ability to inactivate the cephamycins (such as cefoxitin and cefotetan). The ESBLs are inhibited by clavulanic acid, but are not able to inactivate the cephamycins. AmpC type *β*-lactamases are not inhibited by clavulanic acid and are able to inactivate the cephamycins.

▌ Epidemiology

Geographic Variation

There is considerable geographic diversity in the epidemiology of ESBL producing organisms. However, almost universally *Klebsiellae* are the most likely organisms to produce ESBLs. *Klebsiellae* isolated from patients in intensive care units (ICUs) are more likely to produce ESBLs than organisms from other wards of the hospital. Community-acquired infections with ESBL producing organisms are distinctly uncommon.

How frequent are ESBL producing organisms in ICUs? In a large survey performed in 1997 and 1998 in 24 ICUs in Western and Southern Europe, 25% of *Klebsiellae* possessed ESBLs [4]. A similar survey was performed by the same researchers in 1994; the overall proportion of *Klebsiellae* which possessed ESBLs did not differ significantly between the two time periods, but the percentage of ICUs that recorded ESBL producing *Klebsiellae* rose significantly from 74 to >90% [4, 5]. Another large study from more than 100 European ICUs, found that the prevalence of ESBLs in *Klebsiellae* ranged from as low as 3% in Sweden to as high as 34% in Portugal [6]. A third study, which included both ICU and non-ICU isolates from 25 European hospitals, found that 21% of *K. pneumoniae* isolates had reduced susceptibility to ceftazidime (indicative of ESBL production) [7]. In Turkey, a survey of *Klebsiella* from ICUs from 8 hospitals showed that 58% of 193 isolates harbored ESBLs [8].

In a survey of nearly 400 ICUs in North America, resistance rates of *Klebsiella* to third generation cephalosporins increased from 3.6 to 14.4% between 1990 and 1993. However, National Nosocomial Infection Surveillance (NNIS) figures for the 2nd half of 1999 reveal that only 6.5% of 4,294 *K. pneumoniae* isolates from 125 ICUs were resistant to third generation cephalosporins [9]. In contrast, ESBLs have been found in 30–60% of Klebsiella from ICUs in Brazil, Colombia and Venezuela [10, 11]. Rates of ESBL production by *K. pneumoniae* have been as low as 5% in Japan [12–15] and 20–50% elsewhere in Asia.

Risk Factors for Colonization and Infection with ESBL Producers

Prior use of third generation cephalosporins is a very important risk factor for acquisition of an ESBL-producing organism [16–19]. Approximately one third of patients colonized or infected with an ESBL-producing strain have had recent previous exposure to third generation cephalosporins. Furthermore, a tight correlation has existed between ceftazidime use in individual wards within a hospital and prevalence of ceftazidime resistant strains in those wards [20]. In a survey of 15 different hospitals, an association existed between cephalosporin and aztreonam usage at each hospital and the isolation rate of ESBL-producing organisms at each hospital [21].

How might patients acquire ESBL-producing organisms in the absence of antibiotic selection from third generation cephalosporins? Patients at high risk for developing colonization or infection with ESBL-producing organisms are usually seriously ill patients with prolonged duration of hospital stay and in whom invasive medical devices are present (urinary catheters, endotracheal tubes, central venous lines) for a prolonged duration (usually at least 10 days). Individual studies have found a variety of other risk factors including administration of total parenteral nutrition [22], recent surgey, hemodialysis [23], presence of nasogastric tubes [16], gastrostomy or jejunostomy tubes [17, 24] and arterial lines [22, 25, 26], decubitus ulcers [24] and poor nutritional status [25].

Molecular epidemiologic studies have shown that in most ICUs, multiple patients are colonized with genotypically identical strains, indicating patient to patient spread. The hands of healthcare workers are presumably the vector. Common environmental sources of infection are rarely found. Like other organisms colonizing the gastrointestinal tract, ESBL producing *K. pneumoniae* or *E. coli* also colonize the skin of hospitalized patients. Contact with the skin of colonized patients by healthcare workers with suboptimal hand hygiene may then occur. It is important to recognize that many patients have asymptomatic colonization with ESBL producing organisms without signs of overt infection. These patients represent an important reservoir of organisms. For every patient with clinically significant infection with an ESBL-producing organism, at least one other patient exists in the same unit with gastrointestinal tract colonization with an ESBL-producer [26]. In some hyperendemic ICUs and transplants units, 30–70% of patients have gastrointestinal tract colonization with ESBL-producers at any one time [22, 27, 28].

▌ Treatment Options for ESBL-producing Organisms

ESBL-producing organisms are usually resistant to at least one third generation cephalosporin plus first generation cephalosporins and antipseudomonal penicillins. Unfortunately many ESBL-producing organisms actually produce multiple β-lactamses – this may overwhelm the effects of β-lactamase inhibition provided by agents such as tazobactam or clavulanic acid. Indeed, in the previously mentioned study of isolates from 35 ICUs in Europe, 63% of ESBL-producing Klebsiellae were resistant to piperacillin/tazobactam [4].

The plasmids which carry the genes encoding ESBLs often carry genes encoding resistance to aminoglycosides and trimethoprim/sulfamethoxazole. Most frequently gentamicin and tobramycin are inactive, with amikacin remaining susceptible. There is a strong association between quinolone resistance and ESBL production [4, 29, 30]. Presumably patients at high risk of developing colonization with an ESBL-producer may also have a high likelihood of receipt of a quinolone, with subsequent selection of chromosomal gene mutations. There has been only one report of plasmid-mediated quinolone resistance in a ceftazidime resistant *K. pneumoniae* isolate [31].

Curiously, approximately 40% of ESBL-producing isolates tested 'susceptible' to at least one of the third generation cephalosporins [32]. The reason for this apparent susceptibility to some cephalosporins is the result of varying degrees of hydrolysis of cephalosporins by different β-lactamases and enhanced penetration through the bacterial outer membrane of some cephalosporins compared to others. Usually the third generation cephalosporin minimum inhibitory concentrations (MICs) of seemingly 'susceptible' ESBL-producing strains are 2–8 µg/ml – this is several fold less susceptible than the MICs for the same antibiotics seen in non-ESBL producing strains of the same organism (0.03–0.25 µg/ml).

It should also be noted that the MICs of cephalosporins rise as the inoculum of ESBL-producing organisms increases [32–34]. Many times, this MIC rises into the frankly resistant range [35]. Animal studies have demonstrated that the 'inoculum effect' may be clinically relevant. In animal models of infection, failure of cephalosporin therapy has been demonstrated despite levels of antibiotics in serum far exceeding the MIC of the antibiotic when tested at the conventional inoculum of 10^5 CFU/ml [34, 36].

In previously published clinical reports in humans, more than 50% of patients treated with a cephalosporin against seemingly susceptible, but ESBL-producing, organisms experienced failure of therapy [32]. Cefepime and piperacillin/tazobactam also suffer from the 'inoculum effect'; unexplained clinical failure has also been observed when treatment has been given for infections due to apparently susceptible organisms [32, 37].

In vitro, the cephamycins (for example, cefoxitin and cefotetan) have consistently good activity against ESBL-producing organisms. This arises from their stability to hydrolysis by ESBLs. However, there are just two published reports of the use of cephamycins in the treatment of ESBL-producers [38, 39]. In one of these reports, selection of porin resistant mutants occurred during therapy, resulting in cefoxitin resistance and relapse of infection. In addition, combined cephamycin and carbapenem resistance in *K. pneumoniae* has been observed in the setting of widespread cephamycin use in response to an outbreak of infection with ESBL-producing organisms. Therefore, cephamycins may not be suitable as first-line therapy for ESBL producing organisms, despite their good *in vitro* activity.

Like the cephamycins, the carbapenems (imipenem, meropenem, ertapenem) are stable to the hydrolytic effects of ESBLs. In most studies, close to 100% of ESBL-producing isolates are found to be susceptible to carbapenems. Additionally there is increasingly extensive clinical experience with carbapenems for ESBL-producers [32, 40, 41]. There is no evidence that combination therapy with a carbapenem and antibiotics of other classes is superior to use of a carbapenem alone.

Unfortunately, case reports have recently emerged documenting carbapenem resistance in organisms such as *K. pneumoniae*. Such isolates have been resistant to virtually all antibiotics which are currently available. Much scientific attention has been devoted to antibiotic resistance in Gram-positive cocci such as *Staphylococcus aureus* and *Enterococcus faecium*. However, two new antibiotics active against such organisms have recently become available and more will become available in the near future. Unfortunately there are no such new antibiotics active against multiply resistant Gram-negative bacilli. This underscores the importance of prevention of spread of multiply resistant organisms such as ESBL-producers.

▌ Prevention

Changes in antibiotic policy may play a role in reducing occurrence of ESBL-producing organisms. Restriction of use of third generation cephalosporins as empiric workhorse antibiotics is important. However, a number of authors have shown that ceftazidime restriction alone is insufficient to control continued infections with ESBL-producing organisms [42–44]. Rahal et al. [44] were forced to withdraw cephalosporins as an entire class from their hospital in order to exact control over endemic ESBL-producers. Use of β-lactam/β-lactamase inhibitor combinations as empiric therapy, rather than cephalosporins, may facilitate control of ESBL-producers [20, 45, 46]. The mechanism by which these drugs may reduce infections with ESBL-producers is not certain, although the β-lactamase inhibitors themselves are partially active against ESBLs. Cycling of various antibiotic classes through ICUs may also prove to be useful in controlling development of resistance in Gram-negative bacilli.

Classical infection control interventions should also be instituted when outbreaks of ESBL-producing organisms occur. A comprehensive infection control intervention would include:

1) performance of rectal swabs to delineate patients colonized (but not infected) with ESBL-producers;
2) evaluation for the presence of a common environmental source of infection;
3) a campaign to improve hand hygiene;
4) introduction of contact isolation for those patients found to be colonized or infected [46]. Contact isolation implies use of gloves and gowns when contacting the patient. Several studies have documented that this practice alone can lead to reduction in horizontal spread of ESBL-producing organisms. However, compliance with these precautions needs to be high in order to maximize the effectiveness of these precautions. Furthermore, it is recommended that patients who have gastrointestinal tract colonization as well as those with frank infection undergo contact isolation.

Selective digestive decontamination (SDD) has been considered as a means of reducing transmission of ESBL-producing organisms. SDD with polymyxin, neomycin and nalidixic acid [48], colistin and tobramycin or norfloxacin [47] have been used to interrupt outbreaks of infection with ESBL-producing infections that had not been completely controlled using traditional infection control measures. Erythromycin based therapies have not been effective [49, 50].

▌ Conclusion

ESBL-production by organisms such as *K. pneumoniae* or *E. coli* can be a significant problem in ICUs. ESBL-producing organisms are usually multiresistant. Third generation cephalosporins, cefepime, ticarcillin/clavulanate and piperacillin/tazobactam should be avoided in treatment of serious infections with ESBL-producing organisms even in the presence of apparent susceptibility. Quinolones are the therapy of choice for urinary infections due to ESBL-producers (Table 1). Carbapenems (imipenem, meropenem, ertapenem) are the agents of choice for serious infections due to ESBL-producers (Table 1). ESBL-producing organisms are a prominent example of the need for new antibiotics active against common Gram-negative bacilli.

Table 1. Treatment options for infections due to extended-spectrum β-lactamase (ESBL) producing organisms

	First-choice	Second-choice
▌ Urinary tract infection	Quinolone	Amoxycillin/clavulanate
▌ Ventilator-associated pneumonia	Carbapenem (imipenem or meropenem)	Quinolone
▌ Bacteremia	Carbapenem (imipenem or meropenem)	Quinolone
▌ Intra-abdominal infection	Carbapenem (imipenem, ertapenem or meropenem)	Quinolone
▌ Post-neurosurgical meningitis	Meropenem	? Cefepime (in very high dose)

References

1. Knothe H, Shah P, Krcmery V, Antal M, Mitsuhashi S (1983) Transferable resistance to ce-
    fotaxime, cefoxitin, cefamandole and cefuroxime in clinical isolates of *Klebsiella pneumo-
    niae* and *Serratia marcescens*. Infection 11:315–317
2. Brun-Buisson C, Legrand P, Arlet G, Jarlier V, Paul G, Philippon A (1987) Transferable en-
    zymatic resistance to third-generation cephalosporins during nosocomial outbreak of mul-
    tiresistant *Klebsiella pneumoniae*. Lancet ii:302–306
3. Sirot D, Sirot J, Labia R, et al (1987) Transferable resistance to third-generation cephalo-
    sporins in clinical isolates of *Klebsiella pneumoniae*: identification of CTX-1, a novel beta-
    lactamase. J Antimicrob Chemother 20:323–334
4. Babini GS, Livermore DM (2000) Antimicrobial resistance amongst *Klebsiella* spp. collected
    from intensive care units in Southern and Western Europe in 1997–1998. J Antimicrob
    Chemother 45:183–189
5. Livermore DM, Yuan M (1996) Antibiotic resistance and production of extended-spectrum
    beta-lactamases amongst *Klebsiella* spp. from intensive care units in Europe. J Antimicrob
    Chemother 38:409–424
6. Hanberger H, Garcia-Rodriguez JA, Gobernado M, Goossens H, Nilsson LE, Struelens MJ
    (1999) Antibiotic susceptibility among aerobic Gram-negative bacilli in intensive care units
    in 5 European countries. JAMA 281:67–71
7. Fluit AC, Jones ME, Schmitz FJ, Acar J, Gupta R, Verhoef J (2000) Antimicrobial suscept-
    ibility and frequency of occurrence of clinical blood isolates in Europe from the SENTRY
    antimicrobial surveillance program, 1997 and 1998. Clin Infect Dis 30:454–460
8. Gunseren F, Mamikoglu L, Ozturk S, et al (1999). A surveillance study of antimicrobial re-
    sistance of gram-negative bacteria isolated from intensive care units in eight hospitals in
    Turkey. J Antimicrob Chemother 43:373–378
9. NNIS (1999) Semiannual Report. http://www.cdc.gov/ncidod/hip/NNIS/dec99sar.pdf
10. Pfaller MA, Jones RN, Doern GV (1999) Multicenter evaluation of the antimicrobial activity
    for six broad-spectrum beta-lactams in Venezuela: comparison of data from 1997 and 1998
    using the Etest method. Diagn Microbiol Infect Dis 35:153–158
11. Pfaller MA, Jones RN, Doern GV, Salazar JC (1999) Multicenter evaluation of antimicrobial
    resistance to six broad-spectrum beta-lactams in Colombia: comparison of data from 1997
    and 1998 using the Etest method. Diagn Microbiol Infect Dis 35:235–241
12. Lewis MT, Biedenbach DJ, Jones RN (1999) In vitro evaluation of broad-spectrum beta-lac-
    tams tested in medical centers in Korea: role of fourth-generation cephalosporins. Diagn
    Microbiol Infect Dis 35:317–323
13. Lewis MT, Biedenbach DJ, Jones RN (1999) In vitro evaluation of cefepime and other
    broad-spectrum beta-lactams against bacteria from Indonesian medical centers. Diagn Mi-
    crobiol Infect Dis 35:285–290
14. Lewis MT, Yamaguchi K, Biedenbach DJ, Jones RN (1999) In vitro evaluation of cefepime
    and other broad-spectrum beta-lactams in 22 medical centers in Japan: a phase II trial
    comparing two annual organism samples. Diagn Microbiol Infect Dis 35:307–315
15. Yamaguchi K, Mathai D, Biedenbach DJ, Lewis MT, Gales AC, Jones RN (1999) Evaluation
    of the in vitro activity of six broad-spectrum beta-lactam antimicrobial agents tested
    against over 2000 clinical isolates from 22 medical centers in Japan. Japan Antimicrobial
    Resistance Study Group. Diagn Microbial Infect Dis 34:123–134
16. Asensio A, Oliver A, Gonzalez-Diego P, et al (2000) Outbreak of a multiresistant *Klebsiella
    pneumoniae* strain in an intensive care unit: antibiotic use as risk factor for colonization
    and infection. Clin Infect Dis 30:55–60
17. Schiappa DA, Hayden MK, Matushek MG, et al (1996) Ceftazidime-resistant *Klebsiella
    pneumoniae* and *Escherichia coli* bloodstream infection: a case-control and molecular epi-
    demiologic investigation. J Infect Dis 174:529–536
18. Lautenbach E, Patel JB, Bilker WB, Edelstein PH, Fishman NO (2001) Extended-spectrum
    beta-lactamase producing *Escherichia coli* and *Klebsiella pneumoniae*: risk factors for infec-
    tion and impact of resistance on outcome. Clin Infect Dis 32:1162–1171
19. Ariffin H, Navaratnam P, Mohamed M, et al (2000) Ceftazidime-resistant *Klebsiella pneu-
    moniae* bloodstream infection in children with febrile neutropenia. Int J Infect Dis 4:21–25

20. Rice LB, Eckstein EC, DeVente J, Shlaes DM (1996) Ceftazidime-resistant *Klebsiella pneumoniae* isolates recovered at the Cleveland Department of Veterans Affairs Medical Center. Clin Infect Dis 23:118–124

21. Saurina G, Quale JM, Manikal VM, Oydna E, Landman D (2000) Antimicrobial resistance in Enterobacteriaceae in Brooklyn, NY: epidemiology and relation to antibiotic usage patterns. J Antimicrob Chemother 45:895–898

22. Pena C, Pujol M, Ricart A, et al (1997) Risk factors for faecal carriage of *Klebsiella pneumoniae* producing extended-spectrum beta-lactamase (ESBL-KP) in the intensive care unit. J Hosp Infect 35:9–16

23. D'Agata E, Venkataraman L, DeGirolami P, Weigel L, Samore M, Tenover F (1998) The molecular and clinical epidemiology of enterobacteriaceae-producing extended-spectrum beta-lactamase in a tertiary care hospital. J Infect 36:279–285

24. Wiener J, Quinn JP, Bradford PA, et al (1999) Multiple antibiotic-resistant *Klebsiella* and *Escherichia coli* in nursing homes. JAMA 281:517–523

25. Mangeney N, Niel P, Paul G, et al (2000) A 5-year epidemiological study of extended-spectrum beta-lactamase producing *Klebsiella pneumoniae* isolates in a medium- and long-stay neurological unit. J Appl Microbiol 88:504–511

26. Lucet JC, Chevret S, Decre D, et al (1996) Outbreak of multiply resistant *Enterobacteriaceae* in an intensive care unit: epidemiology and risk factors for acquisition. Clin Infect Dis 22:430–436

27. Green M, Barbadora K (1998) Recovery of ceftazidime-resistant *Klebsiella pneumoniae* from pediatric liver and intestinal transplant recipients. Pediatr Transplant 2:224–230

28. Soulier A, Barbut F, Ollivier JM, Petit JC, Lienart A (1995) Decreased transmission of *Enterobacteriaceae* with extended-spectrum beta-lactamases in an intensive care unit by nursing reorganization. J Hosp Infect 31:89–97

29. Paterson DL, Mulazimoglu L, Casellas JM, et al (2000) Epidemiology of ciprofloxacin resistance and its relationship to extended-spectrum beta-lactamase production in *Klebsiella pneumoniae* isolates causing bacteremia. Clin Infect Dis 30:473–478

30. Brisse S, Milatovic D, Fluit AC, Verhoef J, Schmitz FJ (2000) Epidemiology of quinolone resistance of *Klebsiella pneumoniae* and *Klebsiella oxytoca* in Europe. Eur J Clin Microbiol Infect Dis 19:64–68

31. Martinez-Martinez L, Pascual A, Hernandez-Alles S, et al (1999) Roles of beta-lactamases and porins in activities of carbapenems and cephalosporins against *Klebsiella pneumoniae*. Antimicrob Agents Chemother 43:1669–1673

32. Paterson DL, Ko WC, Von Gottberg A, et al (2001) Outcome of cephalosporin treatment for serious infections due to apparently susceptible organisms producing extended-spectrum beta-lactamases: implications for the clinical microbiology laboratory. J Clin Microbiol 39:2206–2212

33. Medeiros AA, Crellin J (1997) Comparative susceptibility of clinical isolates producing extended spectrum beta-lactamases to ceftibuten: effect of large inocula. Pediatr Infect Dis 16 (3 Suppl):S49–S55

34. Rice LB, Yao JD, Klimm K, Eliopoulos GM, Moellering RC Jr (1991) Efficacy of different beta-lactams against an extended-spectrum beta-lactamase-producing *Klebsiella pneumoniae* strain in the rat intra-abdominal abscess model. Antimicrob Agents Chemother 35:1243–1244

35. Thauvin-Eliopoulos C, Tripodi MF, Moellering RC Jr, Eliopoulos GM (1997) Efficacies of piperacillin-tazobactam and cefepime in rats with experimental intra-abdominal abscesses due to an extended-spectrum beta-lactamase producing strain of *Klebsiella pneumoniae*. Antimicrob Agents Chemother 41:1053–1057

36. Fantin B, Pangon B, Potel G, et al (1990) Activity of sulbactam in combination with ceftriaxone in vitro and in experimental endocarditis caused by *Escherichia coli* producing SHV-2-like beta-lactamase. Antimicrob Agents Chemother 34:581–586

37. Paterson DL, Singh N, Gayowski T, Marino IR (1999) Fatal infection due to extended-spectrum beta-lactamase-producing *Escherichia coli*: implications for antibiotic choice for spontaneous bacterial peritonitis. Clin Infect Dis 28:683–684

38. Siu LK, Lu PL, Hseuh PR, et al (1999) Bacteremia due to extended-spectrum beta-lactamase-producing *Escherichia coli* and *Klebsiella pneumoniae* in a pediatric oncology ward:

clinical features and identification of different plasmids carrying both SHV-5 and TEM-1 genes. J Clin Microbiol 37:4020–4027

39. Pangon B, Bizet C, Bure A, et al (1989) In vivo selection of a cephamycin-resistant, porin deficient mutant of *Klebsiella pneumoniae* producing a TEM-3 beta-lactamase. J Infect Dis 159:1005–1006

40. Wong-Beringer A (2001) Therapeutic challenges associated with extended-spectrum, beta-lactamase-producing *Escherichia coli* and *Klebsiella pneumoniae*. Pharmacotherapy 21:583–592

41. Meyer KS, Urban C, Eagan JA, Berger BJ, Rahal JJ (1993) Nosocomial outbreak of *Klebsiella pneumoniae* resistant to late generation cephalosporins. Ann Intern Med 119:353–358

42. Rice LB, Willey SH, Papanicolaou GA, et al (1990) Outbreak of ceftazidime resistance caused by extended-spectrum beta-lactamases at a Massachusetts chronic-care facility. Antimicrob Agents Chemother 34:2193–2199

43. Szabo D, Filetoth Z, Szentandrassy J, et al (1999) Molecular epidemiology of a cluster of cases due to *Klebsiella pneumoniae* producing SHV-5 extended-spectrum beta-lactamase in the premature intensive care unit of a Hungarian hospital. J Clin Microbiol 37:4167–4169

44. Rahal JJ, Urban C, Horn D (1998) Class restriction of cephalosporin use to control total cephalosporin resistance in nosocomial *Klebsiella*. JAMA 280:1233–1237

45. Piroth L, Aube H, Doise JM, Vincent-Martin M (1998) Spread of extended-spectrum beta-lactamase-producing *Klebsiella pneumoniae*: are beta-lactamase inhibitors of therapeutic value? Clin Infect Dis 27:76–80

46. Patterson JE, Hardin TC, Kelly CA, Garcia RC, Jorgensen JH (2000) Association of antibiotic utilization measures and control of multiple drug resistance in *Klebsiella pneumoniae*. Infect Control Hosp Epidemiol 21:455–458

47. Paterson DL, Singh N, Rihs JD, Squier C, Rihs BL, Muder RR (2001) Control of an outbreak of infection due to extended-spectrum beta-lactamase-producing *Escherichia coli* in a liver transplantation unit. Clin Infect Dis 33:126–128

48. Brun-Buisson C, Legrand P, Rauss A, et al (1989) Intestinal decontamination for control of nosocomial multiresistant Gram-negative bacilli. Ann Intern Med 110:873–881

49. De Champs CL, Guelon DP, Garnier RM, et al (1993) Selective digestive decontamination by erythromycin-base in a polyvalent intensive care unit. Intensive Care Med 19:191–196

50. Decre D, Gachot B, Lucet JC, et al (1998) Clinical and bacteriologic epidemiology of extended-spectrum beta-lactamase-producing strains of *Klebsiella pneumoniae* in a medical intensive care unit. Clin Infect Dis 27:834–844

Fluid Therapy

Towards Safer Central Venous Access

D. W. M. Jones and A. Bodenham

Introduction

Central venous access is ubiquitous, with some 200,000 UK procedures annually. Success is marred by significant numbers of early (1–10%) and later complications. The frequency of such complications has been highlighted by the medical and lay press in the USA and UK, with demands for systematic approaches for their reduction [1].

There are many aspects to consider in the practice of safe central venous access, in this chapter we will review two facets:

- The use of ultrasound to guide successful first pass central venous cannulation without damage to collateral structures.
- The optimum site for the tip of the central venous catheter.

Ultrasound Guidance for Central Venous Access

Background

The indications, techniques and complications of central venous access are well documented [2–4]. There are increasing numbers of medico-legal cases resulting from such mishaps and many conscious patients suffer unnecessarily whilst clinicians struggle with repeated painful attempts at access, often under inadequate local anesthesia [5].

The majority of central venous access procedures are performed utilizing surface markings alone. However obscured or pathologically altered anatomy can make procedures difficult. Multiple attempts and inexperienced operators have been shown to be associated with increased risk of complications during central venous access [3, 4].

A key question is whether the wider use of ultrasound to visualize anatomy and guide interventions would improve overall success and reduce complication rates of such procedures in both adults and children. There is increasing evidence that this is so, particularly in the higher risk/difficult case.

Ultrasound may be perceived to be difficult to learn, time consuming, and of little assistance to experienced operators [6]. Diagnostic and interventional ultrasound techniques have long been in the domain of non-radiologists e.g., cardiology, and obstetrics and gynecology. North American trauma surgeons have developed practice in the use of ultrasound for imaging in abdominal trauma, echocardiography, and pleural drainage. From this experience, there is evidence to suggest that clinicians from outside radiology can rapidly become proficient in limited areas of ultrasound practice [7, 8].

What Equipment is Available?

The range and capability of ultrasound machines has increased enormously in recent years. In common with other technological devices the image quality and diversity of functions is very dependent on price. However, smaller, cheaper, good quality, portable ultrasound imaging equipment is now available from a number of manufacturers. This equipment ranges from small devices designed specifically for a particular purpose (e.g., vascular access) and costing $8–12000 to more sophisticated general purpose machines ($15–25000 upwards) that offer better image quality and many of the features of radiology department scanners. These machines provide B mode 2-dimensional real time images, generally utilizing 2.5–10 MHz probes. More sophisticated Doppler functions are not usually a feature on this size of machine.

There are other inexpensive Doppler ultrasound devices specifically designed to aid vascular access. These provide an auditory signal rather than a visual display and are used to distinguish between arterial and venous pulsations each of which produces a characteristic signal. Such devices utilize either relatively expensive disposable probes that lie within the seeking needle, or a reusable Doppler probe and disposable extras that encircle the seeking needle [9].

Practicalities of Using Ultrasound

With B mode ultrasound, structures can be visualized in transverse and longitudinal section to allow the user to build up a three-dimensional image. Anatomy may be visualized prior to procedures but should ideally be imaged real-time during the procedure. In general, scanning in longitudinal section will allow easier visualization of needles, as repeated segments of the needle are shown to build up an image. However, the relationship of the needle path to target and adjacent structures is often better seen in transverse section. Tissue distortion produced with repeated movements of the needle or acoustic shadows will give a guide to needle direction in the absence of direct visualization. The visualization of needles can be improved by incorporating a roughened surface to improve scatter of ultrasound. Many ultrasound probes incorporate either fixed or detachable guides to facilitate the accurate insertion of needles.

Applied Vascular Anatomy

Larger central and peripheral arteries and veins are easily visualized with high-resolution ultrasound in adults and children [10]. Arteries are round in cross-section, pulsatile and are not easily compressible with pressure applied through the ultrasound probe. Veins are more irregular in cross-section, easily compressible, vary in size with respiration, the valsalva maneuver and head-down tilt. The variability of vessel anatomy in the neck has been documented [11, 12]. Traditional anatomical descriptions of femoral vascular anatomy have been challenged, showing that the femoral artery overlies the vein much higher than generally realized [13]. The presence of the clavicle limits ultrasound access to the subclavian vessels. However it may be used to image and guide axillary vessel puncture more laterally. This may have an advantage in reducing risk of pleural or arterial puncture, and also lessen the risk of 'pinch off' to catheters between clavicle, first rib, and the ligamentous complex between them [14].

How Does Ultrasound Help?

Ultrasound imaging indicates the presence, patency, position, and direction of vessels in the neck, axilla, antecubital fossa, femoral triangle and other sites. Vessels can be visualized in the presence of hematoma, morbid obesity, or other abnormalities, and valves and thrombus can be seen so enabling the choice of optimum site for access. A site can be chosen to avoid veins overlying arteries, which is a common feature, or worse when the artery lies over the vein. The actual cannulation procedure can be visualized to ensure centralized needle placement and maximize first pass needle placement, which has been shown to reduce the rate of complications [15]. This may be particularly useful in the high risk/difficult patient with, for instance, coagulopathy [16], or in the teaching situation [6]. Using ultrasound it is possible to check for malposition of central venous catheters (catheter lies in the neck veins, or opposite subclavian vein) prior to X-ray or for successful passage of long venous catheters passed from the antecubital fossa into the subclavian vein [17]. Unfortunately, overlying ribs and aerated lung prevent tip position in the chest being assessed with transthoracic techniques.

What is the Evidence to Support the Use of Ultrasound in Vascular Access?

Surface landmark guided venous access is a procedure with high success rates when performed in optimal circumstances and some clinicians have questioned the role of ultrasound in this area [18]. Other authors have specifically noted the usefulness of ultrasound in difficult cases [5, 15, 16, 19]. A 1996 meta-analysis reviewed eight randomized, prospective studies [20]. It concluded that ultrasound improved success rate, reduced the number of passes, and decreased complications. A recent pediatric study reinforced these findings [21].

Equivocal ultrasound studies during vascular access have tended to focus on uncomplicated patients, using Doppler-only equipment, which provides no image [22, 23] or two-dimensional ultrasound to mark the vessel site on the skin prior to subsequent blind attempts at catheterization. Other authors have noted the usefulness of ultrasound in patients in the emergency room [24, 25] or when femoral arterial pulsation cannot be felt during resuscitation.

There have been a number of studies supporting the use of ultrasound in relation to vascular access for dialysis patients [19]. These patients represent a difficult population due to multiple previous cannulations with vein thrombosis, the need to insert stiff large-bore dual lumen catheters, the inability to tolerate a head-down position, the presence of platelet dysfunction and anticoagulation; scenarios common in many critically ill patients.

A possible list of indications for using ultrasound is shown in Table 1.

Limitations of Ultrasound for Vascular Access

A major limitation of ultrasound is that the presence of a patent vein does not guarantee free passage of the catheter into the great veins or right atrium. Narrowing and obstruction of the great veins is more common than generally realized, usually secondary to long-term vascular access for parenteral nutrition/chemotherapy, or to tumor invasion/compression. The characteristic venous chest collaterals, which bypass the obstruction, take time to develop and may not be visible in the large or obese patient.

Table 1. When to consider using ultrasound to aid successful central venous access

▌ Lack of operator experience or in a teaching setting
(particularly if accompanied by one of the indications below)
▌ Previous difficulties during catheterization
(e.g., failure to gain access; >3 punctures at one site; 2 sites attempted)
▌ Previous complication
(e.g., arterial puncture, pneumothorax)
▌ Limited access sites
(e.g., other catheters *in situ*; pacemaker *in situ*; catheters recently removed; burns, local surgery, infection)
▌ Surface landmarks difficult to identify/utilize
(e.g., obesity, local swelling, scars, previous surgery)
▌ Pediatric cannulation
(less than 2 years old, less than 10 kg, congenital heart disease)
▌ Deranged hemostasis
(congenital or acquired)
▌ Supine position not tolerated by patient
(e.g., short of breath, raised intracranial pressure)
▌ Others
(e.g., suspected vascular abnormality, hypovolemia, left-sided cannulation)

▌ The Optimum Position of the Central Venous Catheter Tip

The devastating effects of central venous catheter-induced tamponade have been highlighted by the American Food and Drugs Administration (FDA), and equipment manufacturers warn of the requirement for catheter tips to lie outside the heart in their package inserts [26]. The awareness of physicians regarding this problem has been reported to be low [27].

Although cardiac perforation and subsequent tamponade can be minimized by keeping catheter tips outside the heart, having the tip outside does not guarantee freedom from other potentially life-threatening complications.

We shall first review the possible sequels of poorly placed central venous catheter tips, and then discuss where the optimal site(s) should be.

Arrhythmias

These are common, but partial withdrawal of the guide wire or catheter usually solves the problem [28].

Perforation

Cardiac tamponade from perforation of the right ventricle, right atrium (RA) or superior vena cava (SVC) was the most common fatal complication of central venous cannulation among approximately 3500 cases in the ASA Closed Claims Project [26]. Approximately 90% of perforations occur from catheter tips located in the right atrium or right ventricle, with only 10% occurring from catheters in the superior vena cava. Peripherally inserted central venous catheters pose an increased risk due to the intracardiac migration of the tip during arm abduction.

Most cases of perforation occur in the first week following insertion [27]. Chest pain, nausea, dyspnea, cyanosis, tachycardia, hypotension, engorged neck veins and pulsus paradoxus may occur hours before decompensation. The correct clinical diagnosis is rarely made and cardiac arrest usually ensues, with significant mortality.

Central vein perforation has also been widely reported resulting in complications such as pleural effusion, pneumothorax, hydrothorax, hemothorax, pneumo- or hydromediastinum and pericardial tamponade [29, 30]. Clinically, visceral type chest pain on drug infusion, and a curved appearance of the distal part of the catheter on chest radiograph, are both strongly suggestive of impending vessel perforation [31]. The effects of central vessel perforation are less dramatic than for cardiac perforation but there is an appreciable mortality [32]. A bewildering range of other complications has also been described [33].

The mechanism for perforation in both cardiac and central vessels is probably due to physical trauma or chemical erosion from infusates. *In vitro* studies have demonstrated that the risk of perforation increases as the catheter becomes more perpendicular to the vessel wall [34].

Other factors implicated in vessel perforation include: trauma due to guide wire or dilator insertion, left sided line insertion (due to the fact that the left brachiocephalic vein drains almost perpendicularly into the superior vena cava) [29, 30], and stiffer catheters (related to material used and multiple lumens) [34]. Fluid infused under pressure through multi-lumen catheters, adherent thrombosis between catheter and vessel wall, and excessive catheter tip movement, are also likely to be prominent risks for vessel perforation.

Subcutaneous Extravasation

This usually occurs via proximal side holes of multi-lumen catheters not inserted to an adequate depth [35]. This is particularly relevant in the pediatric population where the distance from the catheter entry site to the right atrium may be less than 5 cm, so that a high catheter tip position may result in the proximal side hole being in an extravascular position.

Thrombosis

Although usually asymptomatic or causing catheter blockage, catheter related thrombus formation may result in fatal complications such as superior vena caval obstruction or septic thrombophlebitis. Thrombus formation is extremely common in patients with central venous catheters with rates estimated at between 25 and 70% [36]. The incidences of pulmonary embolic phenomena resulting from this have been suggested to be as high as 60%, even with short-term catheterization [36, 37], with mortality as high as 12% [37].

Evidence is emerging which shows a relationship between catheter tip placement high in the superior vena cava (or above) and thrombosis formation [38]. Thrombosis occurs where there are signs of repeated trauma to the vascular endothelium from the catheter tip. The morbidity and mortality that result from a high lying catheter tip, which causes thrombus formation, may therefore quantitatively exceed that related to perforation.

Catheter-related Sepsis (and its Link with Thrombosis)

With a direct mortality rate of up to 25% [39], catheter-related sepsis is probably the most significant problem regarding central venous catheterization; its relationship with thrombus has been established [36]. From this it is easy to see that the combination of sepsis and thrombosis may produce devastating consequences.

▌ Guidance for Correct Positioning of the Catheter Tip

Clinical

Catheters placed via the subclavian or brachial route are more likely to lie outside the superior vena cava or right atrium than those via the internal jugular route. In adults, an audit of subclavian catheter insertion has shown that when inserted to a depth of 15 cm, over half were positioned too far centrally radiographically [35], and position improved with a tailored technique. Detection of arrhythmia is not a reliable indicator and the catheter may move with guide wire withdrawal. Easy aspiration through all ports should be confirmed before use, to rule out vessel wall abutment or extravascular placement.

Chest Radiography

This is still the standard method of identifying the site of the catheter tip. Various criteria have been suggested to ensure the safe extra-pericardial position of the tip, none of which has gained universal acceptance.

Suggested landmarks for catheter tip position are:
▪ Posterior-anterior X-ray (erect): no lower than 2 cm inferior to a line drawn between the lower borders of the clavicles [40].
▪ Anterior-posterior X-ray (supine): no lower than the level of the carina [41].

The carina is more reliable for anterior-posterior films due to its central position and close proximity to the superior vena cava thus limiting any parallax effect [41].

Real Time Electrocardiography

The intra-atrial position is identified by a change in p wave morphology and the catheter then withdrawn into the superior vena cava by 2–3 cm or until the original p wave reappears. Success rates of greater than 80% have been claimed [42]; however catheter malpositioning, e.g., looping or pre-existing myocardial electrocardiographic abnormalities may undermine this technique.

Transesophageal Echocardiography (TEE)

At the present time, the vast majority of patients receiving central venous catheters will not have a TEE examination. However, in patients who do, it may be used to verify guide-wire placement in the right atrium hence confirming venous cannulation and position of the catheter tip [43]. TEE allows two dimensional real time imaging to give more accurate visualization and positioning of the catheter within the superior vena cava/right atrium.

Others

Transthoracic ultrasound has limited uses (see above). Venography, computed to-mography, or magnetic resonance studies may be useful in difficult cases where catheter re-insertion may be undesirable.

▌ Suitable Positions for the Catheter Tip

Intracardiac positioning of a catheter tip does pose the risk of tamponade and is thus the focus of current guidelines. However, given the other possible sequels, we should not blindly accept a potentially more unsatisfactory extracardiac position. Each site for catheter tip position has its own problems, and route of insertion is an important factor. Using a schematic diagram we will demonstrate what we feel to be suitable sites for catheter tip position [44] (Fig. 1).

▌ Zone 1. Mid-point of innominate vein: Suitable position for catheter tip following insertion via left internal jugular or subclavian vein [30].

▌ Zone 2. Upper superior vena cava: Suitable position for catheter tip following insertion via right internal jugular vein [29, 32].

▌ Zone 3. Lower superior vena cava/upper right atrium: Provided that the tip does not abut the atrial wall end on, enter the coronary sinus or pass through the tricuspid valve, we believe that this is a suitable position for a catheter tip from any upper body access point [31, 38, 45]

From the femoral route there are no good data to identify the optimum tip site, it would therefore seem sensible to ensure the catheter is in the inferior vena cava, with tip parallel to its walls, and in an infradiaphragmatic position.

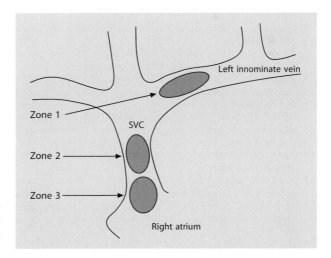

Fig. 1. Schematic diagram of optimum catheter tip position (see text for explanation of zones). SVC: superior vena cava

▌ Conclusion

Several factors have been linked with an improved chance of successful central venous cannulation, including increased operator experience, right-sided cannulation, Seldinger wire techniques, and cannulating anesthetized patients. An increasing number of studies support the use of ultrasound to facilitate safe central venous access in adults and children, particularly in the more difficult cases, and for teaching. It is likely that, in the future, such techniques will become a standard and routine part of central venous access [6].

When considering the question of the catheter tip position, all have their potential problems. Each case must be judged individually based upon patient factors, indication for the catheter, type of catheter, duration of placement, and route of insertion. Unfortunately there is a lack of good evidence upon which to base our practice. The risks of possible cardiac perforation with low superior vena cava/right atrium placement must be balanced against risks of thrombosis/infection from less central placement.

References

1. Alberti KGMM (2001) Medical errors: a common problem. It is time to get serious about them. Br Med J 322:501–502
2. Gualtieri E, Deppe SA, Sipperly ME, Thompson DR (1995) Subclavian venous catheterization: Greater success rate for less experienced operators using ultrasound guidance. Crit Care Med 23:692–697
3. Mansfield PF, Hohn DC, Fornage BD, Gregurich MA, Ota DM (1994) Complications and failures of subclavian-vein catheterisation. N Engl J Med 331:1735–738
4. Sznajder JI, Zveibil FR, Bitterman H, Weiner P, Bursztein S (1986) Central vein catheterisation. Failure and complication rates by three percutaneous approaches. Arch Intern Med 146:259–261
5. Hatfield A, Bodenham A (1999) Portable ultrasound for difficult central venous access. Br J Anaesth 82 822–826
6. Scott DHT (1999) In the country of the blind, the one-eyed man is king. Br J Anaesth 82:820–821
7. Smith RS, Kern SJ, Fry WR, Helmer SD (1998) Institutional learning curve of surgeon-performed trauma ultrasound. Arch Surg 133:530–536
8. Buzzas GR, Kern SJ, Smith RS, Harrison PB, Helmer SD, Reed JA (1998) A comparison of sonographic examinations for trauma performed by surgeons and radiologists. J Trauma 44:604–608
9. Gilbert TB, Seneff MG, Becker RB (1995) Facilitation of internal jugular venous cannulation using an audio-guided doppler ultrasound vascular access device. Results from a prospective dual center, randomized crossover clinical study. Crit Care Med 23:60–65
10. Denys BG, Uretsky BF (1991) Anatomical variations of the internal jugular vein. Crit Care Med 19:1516–1519
11. Sulek CA, Gravenstein N, Blackshear RH, Weiss L (1996) Head rotation during internal jugular vein cannulation and the risk of carotid artery puncture. Anesth Analg 82:125–128
12. Troianos CA, Kuwik RJ, Pasqual JR, Lim AJ, Odasso DP (1996) Internal jugular vein and carotid artery anatomic relation as determined by ultrasonography. Anaesthesiology 85:43–48
13. Hughes P, Scott C, Bodenham A (2000) Ultrasonography of femoral vessels, implications for vascular access. Anaesthesia 55:1199–1202
14. Aitken DR, Minton JP (1984) The Pinch-off sign: A warning of impending problems with permanent subclavian catheters. Am J Surg 148:633–636
15. Troianos CA, Jobes DR, Ellison N (1991) Ultrasound-guided cannulation of the internal jugular vein. A prospective, randomized study. Anesth Analg 72:823–826

16. Gallieni M, Cozzolino M (1995) Uncomplicated central vein catheterisation of high-risk patients with real time ultrasound guidance. Int J Artif Organs 18:117–121
17. Skolnick ML (1994) The role of sonography in the placement and management of jugular and subclavian central venous catheters. Am J Roentegenol 163:291–295
18. Muhm M, Waltl B, Sunder-Plassman G, Apsner R (1998) Is ultrasound guided cannulation of the internal jugular vein really superior to landmark techniques? Nephrol Dial Transplant 13:522–523
19. Forauer AR, Glockner JF (2000) Importance of US findings in planning jugular vein hemodialysis catheter placements. J Vasc Interv Radiol 11:233–238
20. Randolph AG, Cook DJ, Gonzales CA, Pribble CG (1996) Ultrasound guidance for placement of central venous catheters: A meta-analysis of the literature. Crit Care Med 24:2053–2058
21. Verghese ST, Mcgill WA, Patel, et al (1999) Ultrasound guided internal jugular venous cannulation in infants; a prospective comparison with the traditional palpation method. Anaesthesiology 91:71–77
22. Lefrant JY, Cuvillon P, Benezet JF, et al (1998) Pulsed Doppler ultrasonography guidance for catheterization of the subclavian vein: a randomized study. Anesthesiology 88:1195–201
23. Vucevic M, Tehan B, Gamlin F, Berridge JC, Boylan M (1994) The SMART needle. A new Doppler ultrasound-guided vascular access needle. Anaesthesia 49:889–891
24. Hrics P, Wilber S, Blanda MP, Gallo U (1998) Ultrasound-assisted internal jugular vein catheterization in the ED. Am J Emerg Med 16:401–403
25. Hilty WM, Hudson PA, Levitt MA, Hall JB (1997) Real-time ultrasound-guided femoral vein catheterization during cardiopulmonary resuscitation. Ann Emerg Med 29:331–336
26. Bowdle TA (1996) Central line complications from the ASA Closed Claims Project. Am Soc Anesthesiol Newsletter 60:22
27. Collier PE, Goodman GB (1995) Cardiac tamponade caused by central venous catheter perforation of the heart: a preventable complication. J Am Coll Surg 181:459–463
28. Royster RL, Johnston WE, Gravelee GP (1985) Arrythmias during venous cannulation prior to pulmonary artery catheterisation. Anesth Analg 64:1214–1216
29. Tocino IM, Watanabe A (1986) Impending catheter perforation of superior vena cava: radiographic recognition. Am J Roentgenol 146:487–490
30. Dailey RH (1988) Late vascular perforations by CVP catheter tips. J Emerg Med 6:137–140
31. Passaro ME, Steiger E, Curtas S, Seidner DL (1994) Long-term Silastic catheters and chest pain. J Parenter Enteral Nutr 18:240–242
32. Duntley P, Siever J, Korwes ML, Harpel K, Heffner JE (1992) Vascular erosion by central venous catheters. Chest 101:1633–1638
33. Latto IP (2000) Complications following internal jugular cannulation In: Latto IP, Ng WS, Jones PL, Jenkins BJ (eds) Percutaneous Central Venous and Arterial Catheterisation, 3rd edn. WB Saunders, Philadelphia, pp 184–190
34. Gravenstein N, Blackshear RH (1991) In vitro evaluation of relative perforating potential of central venous catheters: comparison of materials, selected models, number of lumens, and angles of incidence to simulated membrane. J Clin Monit 7:1–6
35. Chalkiadis GA, Gouke CR (1998) Depth of central venous catheter insertion in adults: an audit and assessment of a technique to improve tip position. Anaesth Intensive Care 26:61–66
36. Timsit JF, Farkas JC, Boyer JM, et al (1998) Central vein catheter-related thrombosis in intensive care patients: incidence, risk factors and relationship with catheter-related sepsis. Chest 114:207–213
37. Dollery CM, Sullivan ID, Bauralind O, Bull C, Milla PJ (1994) Thrombosis and embolism in long-term central venous access for parenteral nutrition. Lancet 344:1043–1045
38. Stanislav GV, Fitzgibbons RJ, Bailey RT, Mailliard JA, Johnson S, Feole JB (1987) Reliability of implantable central venous access devices in patients with cancer. Arch Surg 122:1280–1283
39. Pittet D (1994) Nosocomial bloodstream infections in the critically ill. JAMA 272:1819–1820
40. Greenall MJ, Blewitt RW, McMahon MJ (1975) Cardiac tamponade and central venous catheters. Br Med J 2:595–597

41. Schuster M, Nave H, Piepenbrock, Pabst R, Panning B (2000) The carina as a landmark in central venous catheter placement. Br J Anaesth 85:192–194
42. Parigi GB (1997) Accurate placement of central venous catheters in pediatric patients using endocavity electrocardiography: reassessment of a personal technique. J Pediatr Surg 32:1226–1228
43. D'Souza MG, Schwartz AJ, Scwarzenberger JC (2001) Safe central venous access and trans-esophageal echocardiography. J Cardio Vasc Anesth 15:275–276
44. Fletcher SJ, Bodenham AR (2000) Safe placement of central venous catheters. Where should the tip of the catheter lie? Br J Anaesth 85:188–191
45. Taber SW, Bergamimi TM (1997) Long-term venous access: indications and choice of site and catheter. Semin Vasc Surg 10:130–134

Strong Ions, Acid-base, and Crystalloid Design

T. J. Morgan and B. Venkatesh

▌ Introduction

It is now generally accepted that whenever large volumes of saline are administered intravenously, metabolic acidosis can result [1–3]. Examples of at risk situations include acute normovolemic hemodilution, cardiopulmonary bypass, hypovolemic and septic shock, multitrauma, burns, liver transplantation, diabetic ketoacidosis and hyperosmolar non-ketotic coma. The conventional explanation is that there is simple dilution of extracellular bicarbonate (HCO_3^-) by large volumes of non-HCO_3^- containing fluid [4–7]. However, Stewart's physical-chemical approach to acid-base analysis provides a different perspective. In this chapter, we will see how Stewart's concepts might assist in the design of crystalloid solutions with predetermined acid-base effects. We will begin by reviewing some important principles of acid-base analysis with an emphasis on the physical-chemical approach.

▌ Acid-base Analysis: Fundamental Principles

Usually, the first step in the laboratory evaluation of arterial acid-base status is to measure the arterial $PaCO_2$ and pH. The $PaCO_2$/pH relationship then allows us to distinguish respiratory from metabolic (non-respiratory) acid-base perturbations, traditionally using offsets in bicarbonate concentration ($[HCO_3^-]$) (the Boston school) [8, 9] or standard base excess (the Copenhagen school) [10–12]. In acute respiratory acid-base disturbances, $PaCO_2$ is abnormal but its relationship to pH is normal (Fig. 1). Here there is no $[HCO_3^-]$ offset, and standard base excess lies in the normal range. If the $PaCO_2$/pH relationship is shifted to the left, there is a metabolic acidosis, in which case $[HCO_3^-]$ and standard base excess are low. If the $PaCO_2$/pH relationship is shifted to the right, there is a metabolic alkalosis (Fig. 1), and $[HCO_3^-]$ and standard base excess are elevated.

▌ The Physical Chemical Approach [13–15]

The Stewart approach looks at acid-base analysis from a different perspective. Here $[HCO_3^-]$ and pH are both seen as dependent variables determined by three independent variables. These are PCO_2, strong ion difference ($[SID]$), and the total concentration of non-volatile weak acid buffer ($[A_{TOT}]$). A_{TOT} consists primarily of protein histidine residues. In plasma, A_{TOT} is largely albumin (with a small contribution

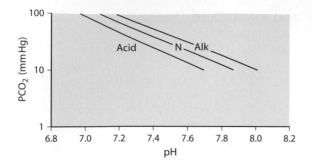

Fig. 1. PaCO$_2$/pH relationships. Illustrated are the normal relationship (N) and examples of metabolic acidosis (Acid) and metabolic alkalosis (Alk)

from inorganic phosphate). In whole blood the predominant contributor to A$_{TOT}$ is hemoglobin. The [SID] concept is based on the observation that certain ions such as Na$^+$, K$^+$, Cl$^-$ and lactate remain essentially fully ionized under all physiologic acid-base conditions, and do not bind to other molecules such as albumin. They are therefore termed 'strong ions': [SID]=[strong cations] – [strong anions]. In normal plasma, [SID] is approximately 40 mEq/l. [SID] in whole blood is harder to quantify, but can be derived using expressions for intra-erythrocytic buffering and plasma/erythrocyte distribution equations [16, 17].

In the Stewart analysis, as in all other 'schools' of acid-base analysis, respiratory acid-base disturbances arise because of primary alterations in PaCO$_2$. What is different about the physical-chemical approach is the contention that metabolic acid-base derangements can be caused only by alterations in one or both of [SID] and [A$_{TOT}$]. To improve our understanding of this idea, we now need to explore the concept of 'buffer base'.

∎ The 'Buffer Base' Concept

To preserve electrical neutrality, the 'space' left by the surfeit of strong cations is filled passively by weak anions (i.e., anions that can bind protons to form their parent molecules in the physiological pH range) (Fig. 2). These are the buffer base anions, and consist of two basic types – the anions of non-volatile weak acids (the A$^-$ component of A$_{TOT}$ where [A$_{TOT}$]=[HA]+[A$^-$]), and the weak anion HCO$_3^-$. Buffer base is, therefore, ([A$^-$]+[HCO$_3^-$]), and is numerically the same as [SID]. [A$^-$] is also numerically the same as the anion gap, provided no other unmeasured anions

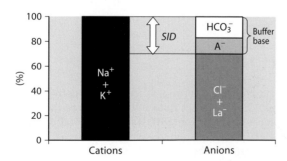

Fig. 2. Illustration of the mirror image relationship between strong ion difference ([SID]) and the buffer base anions. The total concentration of buffer base anions ([A$^-$]+[HCO$_3^-$]) is determined by [SID] in order to maintain electroneutrality. La$^-$ is the lactate anion

are present. Protons generated in biological fluids are buffered exclusively by either or both of these anions in the following manner:

$$H^+ + A^- \leftrightarrow HA \tag{1}$$

$$H^+ + HCO_3^- \leftrightarrow H_2CO_3 \leftrightarrow CO_2 + H_2O \tag{2}$$

It is certainly true that [SID] is the independent variable which defines, controls and is numerically identical to the buffer base anion concentration [12]. However, in the final analysis it is buffer base which determines metabolic acid-base status, despite its being the dependent variable. As we will see, buffer base also plays an important buffering role in respiratory acid-base alterations.

▌ Metabolic Acid-base Disturbances and Buffer Base

We have stated that metabolic acid-base disturbances are due to alterations in either [SID] or [A_{TOT}]. [SID] reductions occur when strong anions such as lactate or beta-hydroxybutyrate appear in the plasma unaccompanied by strong cations (thus causing a raised anion gap acidosis), or when [Cl$^-$] and [Na$^+$] simply move closer together (causing a normal anion gap acidosis). An isolated reduction in [SID] by either mechanism reduces the total buffer base concentration, with both [HCO$_3^-$] and [A$^-$] participating in the buffering process. Since PCO$_2$ also remains constant, the fall in [HCO$_3^-$] shifts the fundamental PCO$_2$/pH relationship to the left (via the Henderson-Hasselbalch equation), creating a metabolic acidosis (Fig. 1).

The effect of [A_{TOT}] is more complicated. Studies performed *in vitro* confirm that isolated [A_{TOT}] elevations cause a metabolic acidosis, and reductions cause a metabolic alkalosis [18]. The mechanism can be thought of as follows: An isolated increase in [A_{TOT}] increases the A$^-$ component of buffer base. However, the total buffer base concentration ([A$^-$]+[HCO$_3^-$]) cannot alter, since it is constrained by [SID]. As a result [HCO$_3^-$] is reduced by an equal amount. Since PCO$_2$ remains unchanged, this shifts the PCO$_2$/pH relationship to the left and creates a metabolic acidosis (Fig. 1). In similar manner, an isolated fall in [A_{TOT}] creates a metabolic alkalosis.

The situation *in vivo* is probably different, in that alterations in [A_{TOT}] take days rather than hours to appear (in the absence of hemodilution), and seem to stimulate compensatory changes in [SID] via alterations in [Cl$^-$] [19]. Under these circumstances [A_{TOT}] is better thought of as setting the normal range for [SID] rather than causing primary metabolic acid-base disturbances. However, during crystalloid fluid loading the [SID] changes accompanying dilutional [A_{TOT}] reductions are governed solely by the [SID] of the diluting crystalloid. As a result, appropriate [SID] compensation for acute A_{TOT} dilution can only occur if the diluent crystalloid [SID] is calibrated for this purpose.

Thus, in summary, isolated decreases in [SID] or uncompensated increases in [A_{TOT}] cause a metabolic acidosis, whereas increases in [SID] or decreases in A_{TOT} cause a metabolic alkalosis. All such disturbances are mediated by alterations in the components of buffer base. The metabolic effects of chronic *in vivo* [A_{TOT}] reductions are probably compensated by reduced [SID].

▌ Respiratory Acid-base Disturbances and Buffer Base

In respiratory acid-base disturbances, A^- alone participates in the buffering process, since protons generated by changes in PCO_2 cannot be buffered by the system in which they are produced. Total buffer base concentration is fixed as always by [SID], so that any alteration in $[HCO_3^-]$ is mirrored by an equal and opposite alteration in $[A^-]$. Thus, as changes in PCO_2 cause HCO_3^- (and H^+) to be generated or consumed, the total concentration of buffer base does not change, merely the ratio of $[HCO_3^-]$ to $[A^-]$. In respiratory acidosis, $[HCO_3^-]$ increases and $[A^-]$ decreases by the same amount, and the converse applies in respiratory alkalosis.

Hence, it can be seen that the buffer base anions are vital determinants of the acid-base status of biological fluids, even though in the Stewart analysis they are dependent variables. Knowledge of how [SID], $[A_{TOT}]$ and $PaCO_2$ interact with buffer base anions improves our understanding of the Stewart approach, and how physical chemical principles can improve our understanding of crystalloid acid-base effects.

▌ Interpreting Crystalloid-induced Acid-base Effects

Using this model, crystalloid infusions can have two separate effects on metabolic (non-respiratory) acid-base balance. There will always be a tendency to reduce $[A_{TOT}]$ by simple dilution, since crystalloid solutions by definition contain no hemoglobin or albumin. Such $[A_{TOT}]$ reductions must produce a metabolic alkalosis as we have discussed [18]. However, there is a simultaneous effect on [SID], the specifics of which depend on the [SID] of the crystalloid fluid [20]. If the [SID] of the diluting crystalloid is lower than that of the extracellular space, there will be a tendency to reduce extracellular [SID] and thus buffer base, creating a co-existent metabolic acidosis. Conversely, fluids with high [SID] (such as sodium bicarbonate solutions) increase extracellular [SID] and, therefore, buffer base concentrations, superimposing a further metabolic alkalosis on that of A_{TOT} dilution. With any large volume crystalloid infusion, the final acid-base outcome is thus a summation of the effects of altered extracellular [SID] and the metabolic alkalosis of reduced $[A_{TOT}]$.

All NaCl solutions have a zero [SID], since Na^+ and Cl^- are present in equimolar concentrations. This is also true of dextrose in saline solutions. The [SID] of water, dextrose solutions and mannitol is also zero, since no strong ions are present in these fluids. Infusion of large volumes of this group of fluids will thus have a tendency to reduce extracellular [SID], pushing acid-base balance in the direction of a metabolic acidosis [21, 22]. Importantly, although this type of acidosis is commonly hyperchloremic, the same phenomenon can occur with a reduction in chloride concentrations depending on the fluid infused [23]. Either way the anion gap will not be elevated. In fact, as A_{TOT} is diluted the anion gap will be reduced (since the anion gap is really $[A^-]$, provided no other unmeasured anions are present).

Determining the 'Neutral' Crystalloid [SID]

For a crystalloid not to produce acid-base disturbances during large volume infusion, some [SID] reduction must be necessary to offset the metabolic alkalosis of A_{TOT} dilution, but the two processes should balance exactly. However, theoretical determination of the crystalloid [SID] required to create this balance is difficult. This is because infused strong ions are distributed amongst plasma, erythrocytes and interstitial fluid in complex ways governed by Gibbs-Donnan equilibria, and the laws of electroneutrality and of chemical equilibrium. In contrast, A_{TOT} (especially hemoglobin) is concentrated primarily in the intravascular space and remains so during crystalloid infusions.

We recently performed an *in vitro* experiment to gain a more exact picture of the relationship between crystalloid [SID] and its acid-base effects [24]. We found that there was a linear relationship between crystalloid [SID] and the rate of change (slope) of base excess as hemoglobin concentration fell during hemodilution of normal blood. If this relationship also holds true *in vivo*, the [SID] of any given crystalloid might perform as a simple descriptor of its potential acid-base effects. From our *in vitro* data, a crystalloid [SID] of 24 mEq/l exactly balances the metabolic alkalosis of A_{TOT} dilution [24].

An [SID] of 24 mEq/l is very similar to the effective *in vivo* [SID] of Hartmann's solution (Table 1), assuming that all contained lactate is metabolized on infusion. Dr Alexis Hartmann himself considered his modification of Ringer's injection to be alkalinizing rather than neutral in its effects. In fact his intention was to create a solution less severely alkalinizing than sodium bicarbonate solutions [25] by adding lactate in its slowly metabolized racemic form to Ringer's solution [26]. Most of the resultant metabolic delay in his original preparation was due to the *d*-lactate component of the racemic mixture.

Of interest, for some years, preparations of Hartmann's solution used in Australia have contained only the *l*-lactate form (personal communication, Bill Houghton, Baxter, Australia). This isomer should disappear quite rapidly after infusion by the process of oxidation or by undergoing gluconeogenesis. Although our *in vitro* data indicate that once the exogenous lactate is metabolized, Hartmann's solution should be neither alkalinizing nor acidifying (i.e., it should be neutral in its effects), confirmatory *in vivo* experimentation is required.

Does Infusion-Related Metabolic Acidosis Really Matter?

There have been calls for a simple resuscitation crystalloid which does not cause acid-base disturbances [27]. However, whether an infusion-related metabolic acidosis is likely to cause harm remains uncertain. There is even a theoretical potential benefit – a reduction in hemoglobin-oxygen affinity due to the Bohr effect, which increases tissue oxygen availability [28]. However, this affinity shift is rapidly corrected by a pH-induced fall in 2,3-diphosphoglycerate (2,3-DPG) levels [29].

The detrimental effects of acidosis are mediated via reduced pH within the cell, a milieu with its own specific buffering mechanisms [30]. Severe acidemia reduces myocardial contractility and can stimulate tachy- and bradydysrhythmias, systemic arteriolar dilatation, venoconstriction, and pulmonary vasoconstriction. There is an increased respiratory drive combined with depressed diaphragmatic function, and there are other adverse effects on brain, liver, and the musculoskeletal system [30].

However, most significant adverse responses occur only in acidemia of a severity seldom seen after crystalloid infusions. Furthermore, intracellular pH is much more resistant to metabolic than respiratory acidosis.

At this time it, therefore, remains to be determined whether fluids with neutral acid-base effects produce better results in terms of tissue oxygenation, organ function or survival.

Nevertheless, the onset of an infusion-related metabolic acidosis introduces a risk of incorrect diagnoses such as unresolved ketoacidosis or persistent tissue dysoxia. In the face of persisting metabolic acidosis despite resuscitation, clinicians may overlook the fact that the anion gap or concentrations of beta-hydroxybutyrate or lactate are inconsistent with these diagnoses. Inappropriate and perhaps harmful therapies such as further aggressive insulin therapy or fluid loading might then follow.

▍ Altering Crystalloid [SID]: Practical Considerations

To increase the [SID] of fluids such as saline above zero it is necessary to replace some Cl^- ions (strong anions) with weak anions such as HCO_3^-. HCO_3^- in solution equilibrates with dissolved carbon dioxide (CO_2), a highly diffusible gas. Such solutions must be stored in glass and infused promptly to prevent CO_2 loss. Because HCO_3^- ions are unstable, commercially produced balanced salt solutions are manufactured with organic acid anions (lactate, acetate, or gluconate) as stable surrogates for HCO_3^- (Table 1). Although these anions are actually strong ions with pKa values of approximately 3.5, they are metabolized *in vivo* following infusion. Provided their metabolic clearance is rapid, the effective *in vivo* [SID] of these solutions can be calculated as though the contained organic anions are weak ions (Table 1). Of note, in all [SID] determinations we take the view of Schlichtig and colleagues that Ca^{++} and Mg^{++} are not strong ions, since they bind reversibly to albumin in a pH dependent manner [17]. This is contrary to the more widely held opinion that they are strong ions [14].

Available evidence indicates that fluid replacement using balanced salt solutions can reduce the incidence of infusion related metabolic acidosis [2, 31]. In fact some

Table 1. Three balanced salt solutions (electrolyte concentrations in mmol/l)

	Hartmann's [a]	Plasmalyte [a]	Plasmalyte-R [a]
▍ Sodium	129	140	140
▍ Chloride	109	98	103
▍ Potassium	5	5	10
▍ Calcium	2		5
▍ Magnesium		1.5	3
▍ Lactate	29		8
▍ Acetate		27	47
▍ Gluconate		23	
▍ Effective [SID] [b]	25	47	47

[a] Baxter, Australia; [b] mEq/l

balanced salt solutions are likely to cause metabolic alkalosis on large volume equilibration with the extracellular space, because of a high effective [SID]. For example, the effective [SID] of Plasmalyte (Baxter, Sydney, Australia) is 47 mEq/l, assuming complete metabolism of the contained acetate and gluconate anions (Table 1). Data on its acid–base effects are limited, but if Plasmalyte is used to prime cardio-pulmonary bypass circuits, arterial base excess becomes elevated by the end of bypass [32].

■ Conclusion

By applying Stewart's physical–chemical principles of acid-base it should be possible to design crystalloids with specific acid-base effects on large volume infusion. Our *in vitro* evidence suggests that a crystalloid [SID] of 24 mEq/l has neutral effects on acid-base balance in patients without pre-existing acid-base disturbances. Confirmation by *in vivo* experimentation is required. Either way, it remains to be established that infusion-related metabolic acidosis causes significant harm.

References

1. Scheingraber S, Rehm M, Sehmisch C, Finsterer U (1999) Rapid saline infusion produces hyperchloremic acidosis in patients undergoing gynecologic surgery. Anesthesiology 90:1265–1270
2. McFarlane C, Lee A (1994) A comparison of Plasmalyte 148 and 0.9% saline for intra-operative fluid replacement. Anaesthesia 49:779–781
3. Prough DS, Bidani A (1999) Hyperchloremic metabolic acidosis is a predictable consequence of intraoperative infusion of 0.9% saline. Anesthesiology 90:1247–1249
4. Mathes DD, Morell RC, Rohr MS (1997) Dilutional acidosis: Is it a real clinical entity? Anesthesiology 86:501–503
5. Goodkin DA, Raja RM, Saven A (1990) Dilutional acidosis. South Med J 83:354–355
6. Garella S, Chang BS, Kahn SI (1975) Dilutional acidosis and contraction alkalosis: Review of a concept. Kidney Int 8:279–283
7. Prough DS (2000) Acidosis associated with perioperative saline administration. Dilution or delusion? Anesthesiology 93:1167–1169
8. Schwartz WB, Relman AS (1963) A critique of the parameters used in the evaluation of acid-base disorders. N Engl J Med 268:1382–1388
9. Narins RB, Emmett M (1980) Simple and mixed acid-base disorders: A practical approach. Medicine 59:161–187
10. Siggaard-Andersen O, Engel K (1960) A micro method for determination of pH, carbon dioxide tension, base excess and standard bicarbonate in capillary blood. Scand J Clin Lab Invest 12:172–176
11. Astrup P, Jorgensen K, Siggaard-Andersen O, et al (1960) Acid-base metabolism: New approach. Lancet 1:1035–1039
12. Siggaard-Andersen O, Fogh-Andersen N (1995) Base excess or buffer base (strong ion difference) as measure of a non-respiratory acid-base disturbance. Acta Anesth Scand Suppl 107:123–128
13. Stewart PA (1981) How to understand acid-base. In: Stewart PA (ed) A Quantitative Acid-base Primer for Biology and Medicine. Elsevier, New York, pp 1–286
14. Stewart PA (1983) Modern quantitative acid-base chemistry. Can J Physiol Pharmacol 61:1444–1461
15. Story DA, Liskaser F, Bellomo R (2000) Saline infusion, acidosis and the Stewart approach. Anesthesiology 92:624
16. Schlichtig R (1997) [Base excess] vs [strong ion difference]: Which is more helpful? Adv Exp Med Biol 411:91–95

17. Schlichtig R, Grogono AW, Severinghaus JW (1998) Current status of acid-base quantitation in physiology and medicine. Anesthesiol Clin North Am 16:211–233
18. Rossing TH, Maffeo N, Fencl V (1986) Acid-base effects of altering plasma protein concentration in human blood in vitro. J Appl Physiol 61:2260–2265
19. Wilkes P (1998) Hypoproteinemia, strong-ion difference, and acid-base status in critically ill patients. J Appl Physiol 84:1740–1748
20. LeBlanc M, Kellum J (1998) Biochemical and biophysical principles of hydrogen ion regulation. In: Ronco C, Bellomo R (eds) Critical Care Nephrology. Kluwer Academic Publishers, Dordrecht, pp 261–277
21. Miller LR, Waters JH (1997) Mechanism of hyperchloremic nonanion gap acidosis. Anesthesiology 87:1009–1010
22. Storey DA (1999) Intravenous fluid administration and controversies in acid-base. Crit Care Resuscitation 1:151–156
23. Makoff DL, da Silva JA, Rosenbaum BJ, Levy SE, Maxwell MH (1970) Hypertonic expansion: acid-base and electrolyte changes. Am J Physiol 218:1201–1207
24. Morgan TJ, Venkatesh B, Hall J (2002) Crystalloid strong ion difference determines metabolic acid-base change during in vitro hemodilution. Crit Care Med (in press)
25. White SA, Goldhill DR (1997) Is Hartmann's the solution? Anaesthesia 52:422–427
26. Hartmann AF, Senn MJ (1932) Studies in the metabolism of sodium r-lactate. 1. Response of normal human subjects to the intravenous injection of sodium r-lactate. J Clin Invest 11:337–344
27. Dorje P, Adhikary G, Tempe DK (2000) Avoiding iatrogenic hyperchloremic acidosis – call for a new crystalloid fluid. Anesthesiology 92:625–626
28. Morgan TJ (1999) The significance of the P50. In: Vincent JL (ed) Yearbook of Intensive Care and Emergency Medicine. Springer-Verlag, Heidelberg pp 433–447
29. Morgan TJ, Koch D, Morris D, Clague A, Purdie DM (2001) Red cell 2,3-diphosphoglycerate concentrations are reduced in critical illness without net effect on in vivo P50. Anaesth Intensive Care 29:479–483
30. Forrest DM, Walley KR, Russell JA (1998) Impact of acid-base disorders on individual organ systems In: Ronco C, Bellomo R (eds) Critical Care Nephrology. Kluwer Academic Publishers, Dordrecht, pp 313–326
31. Traverso LW, Lee WP, Langford MJ (1986) Fluid resuscitation after an otherwise fatal hemorrhage: 1. Crystalloids solutions. J Trauma 26:168–175
32. Liskaser FJ, Bellomo R, Hayhoe M, et al (2000) Role of pump prime in the etiology and pathogenesis of cardiopulmonary bypass-associated acidosis. Anesthesiology 93:1170–1173

Reactive Oxygen Species as Mediators of Organ Dysfunction: Potential Benefits of Resuscitation with Ringer's Ethyl Pyruvate Solution

M. P. Fink

▌ Introduction

Reactive oxygen species (ROS) are reactive, partially reduced derivatives of molecular oxygen (O_2). Important ROS in biological systems include superoxide radical anion ($O_2^{-\bullet}$), hydrogen peroxide (H_2O_2), hydroxyl radical ($OH^\bullet$), and peroxynitrite ($ONOO^-$). Other related nitrogen-containing moieties, such as nitroso-peroxocarboxylate ($ONOOCO_2^-$) and nitrogen dioxide ($NO_2^\bullet$), may also be significant [1, 2]. Most cell types are capable of generating ROS under certain conditions. However, the major sources of these reactive molecules are phagocytic cells, especially macrophages, Kupffer cells, and polymorphonuclear neutrophils (PMN), endothelial cells, and various epithelial cell types, including enterocytes, hepatocytes, alveolar epithelial cells, and renal tubular epithelial cells.

A variety of enzymatic and non-enzymatic process can generate ROS in mammalian cells. Among the most important sources are the reactions catalyzed by the enzymes nicotinamide adenine dinucleotide phosphate (NADPH) oxidase and xanthine oxidase (XO).

NADPH oxidase catalyzes the one-electron reduction of molecular oxygen to form $O_2^{-\bullet}$ using NADPH as an electron donor. NADPH oxidase is an enzyme complex that is assembled following activation of phagocytes by microbes or microbial products, such as lipopolysaccharide (LPS) or various pro-inflammatory mediators. In resting cells, the components of NADPH oxidase are present in the cytosol and the membranes of various intracellular organelles. When the cell is activated, the components are assembled on a membrane-bound vesicle, which then fuses with the plasma membrane, resulting in the release of $O_2^{-\bullet}$ outward into the extracellular milieu and inward into the phagocytic vesicle. The reaction catalyzed by NADPH oxidase is critical for the formation of ROS in macrophages and PMN. NADPH oxidase, however, is present in other cell types as well, including vascular smooth muscle cells [3] and endothelial cells [4]. Some data suggest that the endothelial form of NADPH oxidase is structurally distinct from the form of the enzyme present in PMN [5], whereas other findings indicate that the form of NADPH oxidase present in endothelial cells is identical to the one in leukocytes [6, 7].

Xanthine oxidase (XO) catalyzes the oxidation of xanthine (or hypoxanthine) by molecular oxygen to form uric acid and $O_2^{-\bullet}$. An enzyme related to XO, namely xanthine dehydrogenase (XDH), utilizes reduced nicotinamide adenine dinucleotide (NADH) as a cofactor, and coverts xanthine (or hypoxanthine) to uric acid without forming ROS. It has been postulated that XDH is converted to XO during episodes of tissue ischemia [8, 9], although the importance of this phenomenon has been disputed [10]. Since the liver and the gut are rich sources of XO, and the lung receives the venous drainage from these organs, some investigators have proposed that pulmonary injury following hepatosplanchnic ischemia and reperfusion or hemorrhagic shock is caused, at least in part, by the release of XO + XDH into the circulation [11–13]. This notion is supported, in part, by a recent study showing that XO binds to the endothelium with high affinity [14].

The reactions catalyzed by both NADPH oxidase and XO produce $O_2^{-\bullet}$ as the predominant ROS. $O_2^{-\bullet}$ while only moderately reactive can be converted to other more reactive moieties by a series of additional reactions. Superoxide dismutase (SOD) catalyzes the conversion (dismutation) of two moles of $O_2^{-\bullet}$ to form one mole each of O_2 and H_2O_2. Because H_2O_2 can diffuse over long distances and penetrate cytoplasmic and organellar membranes, this compound can be quite toxic to cells. In addition, in the presence of free ionized iron or copper in a low oxidation state (i.e., Fe^{2+} or Cu^+, respectively), H_2O_2 can be converted further to the extremely reactive species, $OH^\bullet$ according to this non-enzymatic reaction:

$$H_2O_2 + Fe^{2+} \rightarrow OH^\bullet + OH^- + Fe^{3+}.$$

The lower oxidation state of the transition metal cation can then be regenerated by the action of any number of reducing agents within the cellular milieu (e.g., ascorbic acid) [15], and the cycle repeated. In phagocytic cells containing the enzyme, myeloperoxidase, H_2O_2 also can react with chloride to form hypochlorous acid.

Strictly speaking, nitric oxide (NO) is not itself an ROS. NO is synthesized in biological systems from the amino acid, L-arginine, in a complex five-electron redox reaction that requires molecular oxygen and a number of other co-factors. This reaction is catalyzed by a family of enzymes called NO synthase (NOS). If L-arginine availability is limiting, NOS can generate $O_2^{-\bullet}$ [16–18]. NO reacts rapidly and non-enzymatically with $O_2^{-\bullet}$ to form $ONOO^-$.

In addition to the reactions listed above, another important source of ROS production is the mitochondrion, the subcellular organelle that carries out the tricarboxylic acid (TCA) cycle and the coupled oxidative metabolism of pyruvate and phosphorylation of adenosine diphosphate (ADP) to generate adenosine triphosphate (ATP). Even under normal conditions, electrons can 'leak' from the mitochondrial electron transport chain, leading to the partial reduction of O_2 and, hence, the formation of $O_2^{-\bullet}$. Production of $O_2^{-\bullet}$ via this process is increased during cellular hypoxia or after oxidant-mediated mitochondrial damage [19, 20]. Interestingly, hyperglycemia also can promote $O_2^{-\bullet}$ production by mitochondria [21].

The oxidizing agents that are produced via these reactions can interact with numerous cellular constituents including proteins, DNA, and lipids. One of the results of oxidative stress can include the inactivation of key enzymes involved in intermediary metabolism. For example, the glycolytic enzyme, glyceraldehyde-3-phosphate dehydrogenase (GAPDH), can be inactivated by oxidation of key sulfhydryl residues by H_2O_2 [22] or S-nitrosylation and subsequent ADP-ribosylation induced by NO [23]. ROS, such as H_2O_2, can also inactivate a number of phosphatases, and thereby dramatically alter signaling mediated by various intracellular kinase cascades [24]. H_2O_2-, $OH^\bullet$, or $ONOO^-$-mediated oxidative stress can lead to single-strand breaks in nuclear DNA, an event that can trigger activation of the enzyme, poly(ADP-ribose) polymerase (PARP), leading to depletion of cellular stores of NAD and 'cytopathic hypoxia' on this basis [25]. Oxidants also can alter key structural proteins. Thus, H_2O_2 can oxidize sulfhydryl groups in actin (particularly, the one at Cys-374), impairing the interaction of the protein's subunits and its binding with various other proteins [26].

▌ Effects of ROS on Activation of NF-κB and Other Intracellular Signaling Pathways

ROS have been implicated in the activation or modulation of a number of important intracellular signaling pathways, most notably those dependent upon the transcription factor, nuclear factor-kappa B (NF-κB), a *trans*-acting protein that is important in regulating the expression of iNOS, cyclo-oxygenase II (COX-2) and numerous cytokines, such as tumor necrosis factor (TNF) [27–29]. Delineating the role of oxidant stress in the activation of NF-κB, however, has been far from straightforward.

The transcriptionally active form of NF-κB is a homo- or heterodimer made up of various proteins belonging to the NF-κB family. These proteins include p50, RelA, c-Rel, p52 and RelB [30]. In resting cells, however, these homo- or heterodimeric forms of NF-κB exist in the cytoplasm in an inactive form due to binding by a third inhibitory protein, called IκB [30]. Upon stimulation of the cell by a pro-inflammatory trigger (e.g., TNF, interleukin [IL]-1 or LPS), IκB is phosphorylated on two key serine residues (Ser^{32} and Ser^{36}), which targets the molecule for ubiquination and subsequent proteosomal degradation. Phosphorylation of IκB is thought be mediated by various IκB kinases (IKKs) [31]. Phosphorylation and degradation of IκB permits translocation of the transcriptionally active (dimeric) form of NF-κB into the nucleus and subsequent binding of the transcription factor to *cis*-acting elements in the promoter regions of various NF-κB-responsive genes.

Although the upstream events that lead to IKK activation are unclear (and probably differ depending on the inciting pro-inflammatory stimulus), it has been proposed that ROS are important in this process. Several lines of evidence support this view. First, numerous studies have shown that providing an exogenous source of ROS (e.g., by adding H_2O_2 to the medium for cultured cells) can trigger activation of NF-κB [28, 29, 32]. Second, stimulating cells with various pro-inflammatory substances (e. g., TNF) leads to endogenous production of ROS [33]. Third, various compounds with known anti-oxidant activity, such as N-acetylcysteine (NAC) and pyrolidine dithiocarbamate (PDTC) have been shown to block activation of NF-κB in cultured cells, not only by exogenous ROS but also by other pro-inflammatory stimuli [33, 34]. Fourth, certain ROS scavengers, such as PDTC and dimethylthiourea (DMTU), have been shown to block NF-κB activation *in vivo* as well [35, 36]. Fifth, cytokine-stimulated activation of NF-κB tends to be exaggerated when cells are pretreated with an agent, such as buthionine sulfoximine (BSO) that depletes intracellular levels of glutathione (GSH), an important endogenous ROS scavenger [37].

The mechanisms whereby ROS lead to activation of NF-κB are not completely understood. Recently, Schoonbroodt et al. [28] provided evidence that H_2O_2-induced NF-κB activation in a lymphocytic cell line (EL4) is not mediated by phosphorylation of the Ser^{32} and Ser^{36} residues on IκB, but rather as a result of phosphorylation of a key tyrosine residue (Tyr^{42}) or serine and threoninine residues in a C-terminal portion of the molecule called the PEST domain. These H_2O_2-induced phosphorylation events apparently are not mediated by activation of IKKs, but might involve activation of other kinases. One candidate for this role is casein kinase II, because an inhibitor of this enzyme (5,6-dichloro-1-beta-D-ribofuranosyl-benzimidazole) blocks NF-κB activation initiated by oxidant stress [28]. Recently, however, Livolsi et al. [29] presented convincing data suggesting that H_2O_2-induced phosphorylation of Tyr^{42} on IκB is mediated as a result of activation of the tyrosine kinases, p56(lck) and ZAP-70.

Despite the preceding information, other findings suggest that the role of ROS as initiators of the NF-κB signaling pathway is probably not universal, but rather dependent on the pro-inflammatory stimulus and the cell type in question. For example, in an elegant series of studies using primary and immortalized cultures of human endothelial cells, Bowie and colleagues [30] showed that activation of NF-κB by H_2O_2 was demonstrable only in transformed cells. Furthermore, incubation of ECV304 (transformed endothelial) cells with either TNF or IL-1-failed to stimulate formation of H_2O_2 [30]. Additionally, incubation of ECV304 cells with NAC blocked activation of NF-κB induced by exogenous H_2O_2, but failed to block activation of NF-κB induced by TNF or IL-1 [30].

Recently, Jaspers et al. [31] showed that exposing primary normal human bronchial epithelial cells to H_2O_2 resulted in increased IKK activity and phosphorylation and ubiquitination of IκB. However, degradation of IκB was not enhanced by H_2O_2, nor was nuclear binding of NF-κB enhanced by exposure of the cells to H_2O_2 [31]. Indeed, in this system, H_2O_2-mediated oxidant stress inhibited TNF-stimulated IκB degradation and NF-κB nuclear binding [31]. Thus, these data support the view that the formation of ROS might actually *inhibit* activation of NF-κB. This view is supported by a recent study by Keffer et al. [38], showing that TNF-mediated NF-κB activation in endothelial cells is impaired if GSH levels are depleted by exposing the cells to BSO.

From the preceding, it is apparent that NF-κB activation is not universally driven by an ROS-mediated process. Nevertheless, PDTC and other related thiocarbamates are almost uniformly effective as inhibitors of NF-κB activation. Although these compounds are known to be ROS scavengers, their pharmacological effects relative to NF-κB activation are probably not related to ROS scavenging. Thus, Bowie et al. [30] presented data in support of the idea that PDTC blocks NF-κB activation by chelating free iron in the cytosol. Subsequently, Brennan and O'Neill [39] showed that PDTC blocks nuclear binding of NF-κB by promoting oxidation of a critical thiol group, possible on the p50 subunit of the transcription factor. Apparently, PDTC can function as an antioxidant at low concentrations (0–25 µM), but acts as a pro-oxidant at higher concentrations [40].

In addition to NF-κB, ROS have been implicated in activating other signaling pathways. For example, activation of activator protein (AP)-1, another important transcription factor involved in regulation of the inflammatory response, is also at least partially redox-dependent, possibly because of H_2O_2-mediated activation of the upstream mitogen activated protein kinases, Erk1/2 [41, 42], or the signaling molecule, apurinic/apyrimidinic endonuclease [1, 43].

▋ Blocking the Effects of ROS Animal Models of Critical Illness

There is an extensive body of evidence showing that acute respiratory distress syndrome (ARDS) can be prevented or ameliorated in numerous different animal models by timely pharmacological intervention with agents that either block the synthesis of ROS or scavenge these reactive molecules once they have been formed. For example, one of the most extensively studied animal models of ARDS is the ovine paradigm, wherein adult sheep are infused with LPS to induce a transient syndrome characterized by pulmonary hypertension, widening of the alveolar-arterial PO_2 gradient, and increased transudation of protein-rich fluid into the pulmonary lymphatic system. Using this model, Bernard et al. [44] showed that treatment with NAC ameliorated the development of LPS-induced pulmonary injury. Using a similar ovine model, Seekamp et al. [45] and Milligan et al. [46] subsequently showed that infusion of catalase, an enzyme that catalyzes the conversion of H_2O_2 to water and O_2, prevented both biochemical evidence of oxidant stress and the development of acute lung injury (ALI) following the injection of endotoxin [45]. More recently, Amari et al. [47] showed that recombinant human SOD ameliorated TNF-induced ALI in sheep.

Infusing pigs with LPS also induces a sepsis-like state characterized by arterial hypotension and severe ALI. Using this model, Gonzalez et al. showed that LPS-induced lung injury was significantly ameliorated when anesthetized pigs were pretreated or even post-treated with EUK-8, a salen-manganese derivative that 'mimics' the activities of both SOD and catalase and hence scavenges $O_2^{\bullet}$ and H_2O_2 [48, 49].Using a similar model, Olson et al. [50] showed that other antioxidants, such as the $OH^{\bullet}$ scavenger, dimethylthiourea (DMTU), and catalase [51], ameliorated LPS-induced lung injury in swine.

Various ROS scavengers have been shown to ameliorate multiple organ dysfunction, blunt pro-inflammatory cytokine release, and/or improve survival in various animal models of sepsis or endotoxemia. For example, the cell-permeable SOD mimic, 4-hydroxy-2,2,6,6-tetramethylpiperidine-N-oxyl (tempol), has been shown to ameliorate renal and hepatocellular dysfunction in rats challenged with LPS [52] or lipoteichoic acid and peptidoglycan (components of the cell wall of Gram-positive bacteria) [53]. Administration of the $OH^{\bullet}$ scavenger, dimethyl sulfoxide, has been shown to blunt NF-κB activation and TNF release and ameliorate hepatocellular injury in galactosamine-sensitized mice challenged with LPS [54]. Another ROS scavenger, phenyl-N-tert-butyl nitrone (PBN) has been shown to decrease the release of TNF and IL-6 and improve survival in mice injected with LPS [55].

▌ Pyruvate and Ethyl Pyruvate

The three-carbon carboxylic acid, pyruvic acid, is a vital compound in the intermediary metabolism of glucose as well as a number of aliphatic amino acids. The reaction of pyruvate with co-enzyme A to form acetyl-coA is the rate-limiting step in the oxidative metabolism of glucose via the tricarboxylic acid (TCA) cycle. Although the importance of pyruvate as a metabolic fuel is beyond question, it is also likely that pyruvate functions as an endogenous ROS scavenger.

In 1904, Holleman [56] reported that pyruvate and related a-keto acids with the general structure, R–CO–COOH, reduce H_2O_2 non-enzymatically in a reaction that yields carbon dioxide and water. In the case of pyruvic acid, this oxidative decarboxylation reaction can be written as follows:

$$CH_3COCOO^- + H_2O_2 \rightarrow CH_3COO^- + H_2O + CO_2 .$$

Subsequent studies have verified that this reaction is rapid and stoichiometric [57, 58]. In addition to scavenging H_2O_2, pyruvate is also capable of scavenging $OH^{\bullet}$ [59].

Many years ago, biologists recognized that the addition of various a-keto acids, especially pyruvate but also oxalacetate, and a-ketoglutarate (AKG), facilitates the growth of cells in vitro [60]. Prompted in part by this observation, O'Donnell-Tormey and colleagues [61] carried out a series of investigations, leading to the proposal that cells actively secrete pyruvate into the extracellular milieu as a defense against ROS-mediated injury. In this study, the authors reported that the presence of pyruvate, oxalacetate, and AKG in the growth medium could protect cells from death induced by exposure to exogenous H_2O_2 [61]. Similar findings were reported roughly contemporaneously by Andrae et al. [62]. A subsequent study by Salahudeen et al. [63] further extended this line of investigation. These authors reported that intravenous infusion of sodium pyruvate protects rats from renal parenchymal injury induced by injecting H_2O_2 into the renal artery. After the publication of this paper, a number of other investigators reported that treatment with pyruvate could protect animals from the deleterious effects of a variety of conditions thought to be mediated by ROS, including myocardial ischemia/reperfusion [59, 64–67], intestinal ischemia/reperfusion [68], and hemorrhagic shock/resuscitation [69].

Despite these promising observations, the usefulness of pyruvate as a therapeutic agent is hampered by the compound's poor stability in solution [70, 71]. Aqueous solutions of pyruvate spontaneously undergo an aldol-like condensation reaction to form 2-hydroxy-2-methyl-4-ketoglutarate, also known as parapyruvate [70, 72, 73]. This compound can undergo spontaneous cyclization and dehydration to form the enolic lactone form or nonenzymatic reduction to form 2,4-dihydroxy-2-methylglutarate, which has been shown to be a mitochondrial poison [73].

Prompted by these considerations, we sought to develop a more stable analog of pyruvate for use as a component of an intravenous fluid for administration under conditions that are likely to be associated with the formation of ROS. Basic principles of organic chemistry suggest that ethyl pyruvate should be more stable in solution than the parent a-ketoacid. Indeed, preliminary studies suggest that this prediction holds true (A. Ajami, personal communication).

An additional potential benefit of using ethyl pyruvate rather than the parent acid as a therapeutic agent may relate to the relative lipophilicities of the two compounds. Pyruvate is transported across the plasma membrane by a family of proton-linked monocarboxylate transporters (MCTs) [74]. Pyruvate is also transported by a similar mechanism into mitochondria [75, 76]. Being more lipophilic than the parent acid, ethyl pyruvate should enter cells and cross into mitochondria more readily than pyruvate. Published studies using a related compound, methyl pyruvate, support this view [77]. It is also possible that pyruvate esters exert biochemical effects that are distinct from those caused by pyruvate itself [78]. For example, recently reported data suggest that methyl pyruvate (or some downstream metabolite of this compound) is capable of inhibiting K^+_{ATP} channels in pancreatic islet cells [78]. Whatever the biochemical basis, ethyl pyruvate has been shown to be more potent than the parent acid as an inhibitor of ROS-mediated toxicity in cultured cells [79].

Despite the potential advantages of ethyl pyruvate, this compound has not been extensively evaluated as a therapeutic agent. One reason for the paucity of prior work with ethyl pyruvate may relate to its poor solubility in pure water (0.25% wt/vol; 22 mM). Sims et al. [80], however, discovered that the use of a balanced, calcium-containing salt solution (analogous to Ringer's lactate solution) markedly increases the solubility of ethyl pyruvate to 1.5% (wt/vol) or 130 mM. The basis for the increased solubility of ethyl pyruvate in a Ringer's-type solution is thought to be stabilization of the enolate form of ethyl pyruvate by Ca^{2+} (Fig. 1) [80].

A formulation of ethyl pyruvate in a Ringer's type balanced salt solution – Ringer's ethyl pyruvate solution (REPS) – has been evaluated in two published studies.

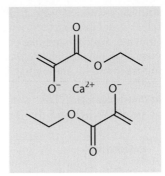

Fig. 1. Proposed mechanism for stabilization of the enolate form of ethyl pyruvate by ionized calcium. Stabilization of the enolate form of the ethyl pyruvate by calcium ion markedly increases the solubility of the ester in an aqueous solvent. (From [80] with permission)

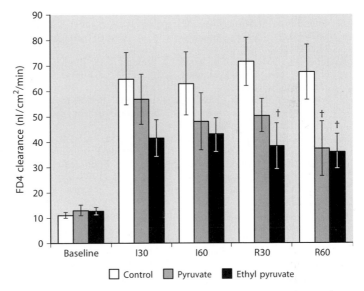

Fig. 2. Effect of treatment with Ringer's pyruvate or Ringer's ethyl pyruvate solution on intestinal mucosal permeability to fluorescein-labeled dextran with an average molecular weight of 4,000 Da (FD4) in rats subjected to mesenteric ischemia and reperfusion. The time points depicted along the abscissa are baseline (prior to the onset of ischemia), I30 and I60 (after 30 and 60 min of ischemia, respectively), R30 and R60 (after 30 and 60 min of reperfusion, respectively). Permeability was assessed using an everted gut sac method. Results are expressed as mean clearances ± SE. Higher values indicate greater permeability. Clearance of FD4 increased significantly in all three groups studied following the onset of ischemia and remained significantly elevated relative to baseline through the final measurements at R60. † indicates $p < 0.05$ versus the time-matched value in the control group (treated with LR). (From [80] with permission)

In the first, Sims et al. [80] showed that pre- and post-treatment of rats subjected to mesenteric ischemia/reperfusion tended to preserve normal intestinal mucosal histology, and also significantly ameliorated the development of gut mucosal hyperpermeability following reperfusion (Fig. 2). Subsequently, Tawadrous et al. [81] showed that resuscitating rats with REPS instead of Ringer's lactate solution resulted in improved survival, decreased intestinal mucosal damage, and amelioration of lipid peroxidation, a marker of ROS-mediated stress, in liver and gut. In other studies, treatment with REPS has been shown to improve survival and block TNF release in mice injected with LPS and to decrease TNF production by RAW 264.7 (murine macrophage-like) cells in culture [82]. Collectively, these data support the view that ethyl pyruvate warrants further evaluation as a therapeutic agent for the management of hemorrhagic shock, ARDS, sepsis and other similar conditions.

Acknowledgement. This work was supported by grants from the National Institutes of Health (NIH) and the Defense Advance Research Projects Agency (DARPA).

References

1. Radi R, Peluffo G, Alvarez MN, Naviliat M, Cayota A (2001) Unraveling peroxynitrite formation in biological systems. Free Rad Biol Med 30:463–488
2. Wink DA, Mitchell JB (1998) Chemical biology of nitric oxide: insights into regulatory, cytotoxic, and cytoprotective mechanisms of nitric oxide. Free Rad Biol Med 25:434–456
3. Griendling KK, Minieri CA, Ollerenshaw JD, Alexander RW (1994) Angiotensin I stimulates NADH and NADPH oxidase activity in cultured vascular smooth muscle cells. Circ Res 74:1141–1148
4. Jones SA, O'Donnell VB, Wood JD, Broughton JP, Hughes EJ, Jones OT (1996) Expression of phagocyte NADPH oxidase components in human endothelial cells. Am J Physiol 271:H1626–H1634
5. Souza HP, Laurindo FRM, Ziegelstein RC, Berlowitz CO, Zweier JL (2001) Vascular NAD(P)H oxidase is distinct from the phagocytic enzyme and modulates vascular reactivity control. Am J Physiol 280:H658–H667
6. Meyer JW, Holland JA, Ziegler LM, Chang MM, Beebe G, Schmitt ME (1999) Identification of a functional leukocyte-type NADPH oxidase in human endothelial cells: a potential atherogenic source of reactive oxygen species. Endothelium 7:11–22
7. Bayraktutan U, Draper N, Lang D, Shah AM (1998) Expression of functional neutrophil-type NADPH oxidase in cultured rat coronary microvascular endothelial cells. Cardiovasc Res 38:256–262
8. Parks DA, Granger DN (1986) Xanthine oxidase: biochemistry, distribution and physiology. Acta Physiol Scand Suppl 548:87–99
9. Parks DA, Williams TK, Beckman JS (1988) Conversion of xanthine dehydrogenase to oxidase in ischemic rat intestine: a reevaluation. Am J Physiol 254:G768–G774
10. Jaseschke H, Smith CV, Mitchell JR (1988) Reactive oxygen species during ischemia-reflow injury in isolated perfused rat liver. J Clin Invest 81:1240–1246
11. Yokoyama Y, Beckman JS, Beckman TK, et al (1990) Circulating xanthine oxidase: potential mediator of ischemic injury. Am J Physiol 258:G564–G570
12. Tan S, Yokoyama Y, Dickens E, Cash TG, Freeman BA, Parks DA (1993) Xanthine oxidase activity in the circulation of rats following hemorrhagic shock. Free Rad Biol Med 15:407–414
13. Terada LS, Dormish JJ, Shanley PF, Leff JA, Anderson BO, Repine JE (1992) Circulating xanthine oxidase mediates lung neutrophil sequestration after intestinal ischemia-reperfusion. Am J Physiol 263:L394–L401
14. Houston M, Estevez A, Chumley P, et al (1999) Binding of xanthine oxidase to vascular endothelium. Kinetic characterization and oxidative impairment of nitric oxide-dependent signaling. J Biol Chem 274:4985–4994
15. Higson FK, Kohen R, Chevion M (1988) Iron enhancement of ascorbate toxicity. Free Rad Res Commun 5:107–115
16. Xia Y, Roman LJ, Masters BS, Zweier JL (1998) Inducible nitric-oxide synthase generates superoxide from the reductase domain. J Biol Chem 273:22635–22639
17. Pou S, Pou WS, Bredt DS, Snyder SH, Rosen GM (1992) Generation of superoxide by purified brain nitric oxide synthase. J Biol Chem 267:24173–24176
18. Xia Y, Tsai AL, Berka V, Zweier JL (1998) Superoxide generation from endothelial nitric-oxide synthase. A Ca^{2+}/calmodulin-dependent and tetrahydrobiopterin regulatory process. J Biol Chem 273:25804–25808

19. Dawson TL, Gores GJ, Nieminen AL, Herman B, Lemasters JJ (1993) Mitochondria as a source of reactive oxygen species during reductive stress in rat hepatocytes. Am J Physiol 264:C961–C967

20. Du G, Mouithys-Mickalad A, Sluse FE (1988) Generation of superoxide anion by mitochondria and impairment of their functions during anoxia and reoxygenation in vitro. Free Rad Biol Med 25:1066–1074

21. Du XL, Edelstein D, Rossetti L, et al (2000) Hyperglycemia-induced mitochondrial superoxide overproduction activates the hexosamine pathway and induces plasminogen activator inhibitor-1 expression by increasing Sp1 glycosylation. Proc Natl Acad Sci USA 97:12222–12226

22. Janero DR, Hreniuk D, Sharif HM (1994) Hydroperoxide-induced oxidative stress impairs heart muscle cell carbohydrate metabolism. Am J Physiol 266:C179–C188

23. Mohr S, Stamler JS, Brune B (1996) Posttranslational modification of glyceraldehyde-3-phosphate dehydrogenase by S-nitrosylation and subsequent NADH attachment. J Biol Chem 271:4209–4214

24. Mahadev K, Zilbering A, Zhu L, Goldstein BJ (2001) Insulin-stimulated hydrogen peroxide reversibly inhibits protein-tyrosine phosphatase 1b in vivo and enhances the early insulin action cascade. J Biol Chem 276:21938–21942

25. Fink MP (2001) Cytopathic hypoxia: mitochondrial dysfunction as a mechanism contributing to organ dysfunction in sepsis. Crit Care Clin North Am 17:219–237

26. Dalledonne I, Milzani A, Colombo R (1995) H_2O_2-treated actin: assembly and polymer interactions with cross-linking proteins. Biophys J 69:2710–2719

27. Verhasselt V, Berghe WV, Vanderheyde N, Willems F, Haegeman G, Goldman M (1999) N-acetyl-L-cysteine inhibits primary human T cell responses at the dendritic cell level: association with NF-κB inhibition. J Immunol 162:2569–2574

28. Schoonbroodt S, Ferreira V, Best-Belpomme M, et al (2000) Crucial role of the amino-terminal tyrosine residue 42 and the carboxyl-terminal PEST domain of Iκ κB in NF-B activation by oxidative stress. J Immunol 164:4292–4300

29. Livolsi A, Busuttil V, Imbert V, Abraham RT, Peyron J-F (2001) Tyrosine phosphorylation-dependent activation of NF-κB: Requirement for p56 LCK and ZAP-70 protein tyrosine kinases. Eur J Biochem 268:1508–1515

30. Bowie AG, Moynagh PN, O'Neill LAJ (1997) Lipid peroxidation is involved in the activation of NF-κB by tumor necrosis factor but not interleukin-1 in the human endothelial cell line ECV304. J Biol Chem 272:25941–25950

31. Jaspers I, Zhang W, Fraser A, Samet JM, Reed W (2001) Hydrogen peroxide has opposing effects on IKK activity and Iκ Bα breakdown in airway epithelial cells. Am J Respir Cell Mol Biol 24:769–777

32. Rahman I, Mulier B, Gilmour PS, et al (2001) Oxidant-mediated lung epithelial cell tolerance: the role of intracellular glutathione and nuclear factor-kappaB. Biochem Pharmacol 62:787–794

33. Schreck R, Meier B, Mannel DN, Droge W, Baeuerle PA (1992) Dithiocarbamates as potent inhibitors of nuclear factor kappa B activation in intact cells. J Exp Med 175:1181–1194

34. Oka S, Kamata H, Kamata K, Yagisawa H, Hirata H (2000) N-acetylcysteine suppresses TNF-induced NF-kappaB activation through inhibition of IkappaB kinases. FEBS Lett 472:196–202

35. Sprong RC, Aarsman CJ, van Oirschot JF, van Asbeck BS (1997) Dimethylthiourea protects rats against gram-negative sepsis and decreases tumor necrosis factor and nuclear factor kappaB activity. J Lab Clin Med 129:470–481

36. Liu SF, Ye X, Malik AB (1999) Inhibition of NF-kappaB activation by pyrrolidine dithiocarbamate prevents in vivo expression of proinflammatory genes. Circulation 100:1330–1337

37. Sen CK, Khanna S, Reznick AZ, Roy S, Packer L (1997) Glutathione regulation of tumor necrosis factor-alpha-induced NF-kappa B activation in skeletal muscle-derived L6 cells. Biochem Biophys Res Comm 237:645–649

38. Keffer J, Rahman A, Anwar KN, Malik AB (2001) Decreased oxidant buffering impairs NF-kappaB activation and ICAM-1 transcription in endothelial cells. Shock 15:11–15

39. Brennan P, O'Neill LAJ (1996) 2-mercaptoethanol restores the ability of nuclear factor B (NF-B) to bind DNA in nuclear extracts from interleukin 1-treated cells incubated with pyrollidine dithiocarbamate (PDTC). Biochem J 320:975–981

40. Moellering D, McAndrew J, Jo H, Darley-Usmar VM (1999) Effects of pyrrolidine dithiocarbamate on endothelial cells: protection against oxidative stress. Free Rad Biol Med 26:1138–1145

41. Ranganathan AC, Nelson KK, Rodriguez AM, et al (2001) Manganese superoxide dismutase signals matrix metalloproteinase expression via H_2O_2-dependent ERK1/2 activation. J Biol Chem 276:14264–14270

42. Lakshminarayanan V, Drab-Weiss EA, Roebuck KA (1998) H_2O_2 and tumor necrosis factor-alpha induce differential binding of the redox-responsive transcription factors AP-1 and NF-kappaB to the interleukin-8 promoter in endothelial and epithelial cells. J Biol Chem 273:32670–32678

43. Ramana CV, Boldogh I, Izumi T, Mitra S (2001) Activation of apurinic/apyrmidinic endonuclease in human cells by reactive oxygen species and its correlation with their adaptive response to genotoxicity of free radicals. Proc Natl Acad Sci USA 95:5061–5066

44. Bernard GR, Lucht WD, Niedermeyer ME, Snapper JR, Ogletree ML, Brigham KL (1984) Effect of N-acetylcysteine on the pulmonary response to endotoxin in the awake sheep and upon in vitro granulocyte function. J Clin Invest 73:1772–1784

45. Seekamp A, Lalonde C, Deguang Z, Demling R (1988) Catalase prevents prostanoid release and lung lipid peroxidation after endotoxemia in sheep. J Appl Physiol 65:1210–1216

46. Milligan SA, Hoeffel JM, Goldstein IM, Flick MR (1988) Effect of catalase on endotoxin-induced acute lung injury in unanesthetized sheep. Am Rev Respir Dis 137:420–428

47. Amari T, Kubo K, Kobayashi T, Sekiguchi M (1993) Effects of recombinant human superoxide dismutase on tumor necrosis factor-induced lung injury in awake sheep. J Appl Physiol 74:2641–2648

48. Gonzalez PK, Zhuang J, Doctorow SR, et al (1995) EUK-8, a synthetic superoxide dismutase and catalase mimetic, ameliorates acute lung injury in endotoxemic swine. J Pharmacol Exp Ther 275:798–806

49. Gonzalez PK, Zhuang J, Doctorow SR, et al (1995) Delayed treatment with EUK-8, a novel synthetic superoxide dismutase (SOD) and catalase (CAT) mimetic, ameliorates acute lung injury in endotoxemic pigs. Surg Forum 46:72–73

50. Olson NC, Anderson DL, Grizzle MK (1987) Dimethylthiourea attenuates endotoxin-induced acute respiratory failure in pigs. J Appl Physiol 63:2426–2432

51. Olson NC, Grizzle MK, Anderson DL (1987) Effect of polyethylene glycol-superoxide dismutase and catalase on endotoxemia in pigs. J Appl Physiol 63:1526–1532

52. Leach M, Frank S, Olbrich A, Pfeilschifter J, Thiemermann C (1998) Decline in the expression of copper/zinc superoxide dismutase in the kidney of rats with endotoxic shock: effects of the superoxide anion radical scavenger, tempol, on organ injury. Br J Pharmacol 125:817–825

53. Zacharowski K, Olbrich A, Cuzzocrea S, Foster SJ, Thiemermann C (2000) Membrane-permeable radical scavenger, tempol, reduces multiple organ injury in a rodent model of Gram-positive shock. Crit Care Med 28:1953–1961

54. Essani NA, Fisher MA, Jaeschke H (1997) Inhibition of NF-κB activation by dimethyl sulfoxide correlates with suppression of TNF-α formation, reduced ICAM-1 gene transcription, and protection against endotoxin-induced liver injury. Shock 7:90–96

55. Pogrebniak HW, Merino MJ, Hahn MJ, Mitchell JB, Pass HI (1992) Spin trap salvage from endotoxemia: the role of cytokine down regulation. Surgery 112:130–139

56. Holleman MAF (1904) Notice sur l'action de l'eau oxygénée sur les acétoniques et sur le dicétones 1.2. Recl Trav Chim Pays-bas Belg 23:169–171

57. Bunton CA (1949) Oxidation of α-diketones and α-keto-acids by hydrogen peroxide. Nature 163:144

58. Melzer E, Schmidt H (1988) Carbon isotope effects on the decarboxylation of carboxylic acids. Biochem J 252:913–915

59. Dobsak P, Courdertot-Masuyer C, Zeller M, et al (1999) Antioxidative properties of pyruvate and protection of the ischemic rat heart during cardioplegia. J Cardiovasc Pharmacol 34:651–659

60. Neuman RE, McCoy TA (1958) Growth-promoting properties of pyruvate, oxalacetate, and α-ketoglutarate for isolated Walker carcinosarcoma 256 cells. Proc Soc Exp Biol Med 98:303–307

61. O'Donnell-Tormey J, Nathan CF, Lanks K, DeBois CJ, de la Harpe J (1987) Secretion of pyruvate. An antioxidant defense of mammalian cells. J Exp Med 165:500–514

62. Andrae U, Singh J, Ziegler-Skylakakis K (1985) Pyruvate and related α-ketoacids protect mammalian cells in culture against hydrogen peroxide-induced cytotoxicity. Toxicol Lett 28:93–98

63. Salahudeen AK, Clark EC, Nath KA (1991) Hydrogen peroxide-induced renal injury. A protective role for pyruvate in vitro and in vivo. J Clin Invest 88:1886–1893

64. Bunger R, Mallet RT, Hartman DA (1989) Pyruvate-enhanced phosphorylation potential and inotropism in normoxic and postischemic isolated working heart. Near-complete prevention of reperfusion contractile failure. Eur J Biochem 180:221–233

65. Deboer LWV, Bekx PA, Han L, Steinke L (1993) Pyruvate enhances recovery of hearts after ischemia and reperfusion by preventing free radical generation. Am J Physiol 265:H1571–H1576

66. Park TW, Chun YS, Kim MS, Park YC, Kwak SJ, Park SC (1998) Metabolic modulation of cellular redox potential can improve cardiac recovery from ischemia-reperfusion injury. Int J Cardiol 65:139–147

67. Crestanello JA, Lingle DM, Millili J, Whitman GJ (2001) Pyruvate improves myocardial tolerance to reperfusion injury by acting as an antioxidant: a chemiluminescence study. Surgery 124:92–99

68. Cicalese L, Lee K, Schraut W, Watkins S, Borle A, Stanko R (1999) Pyruvate prevents ischemia-reperfusion mucosal injury of rat small intestine. Am J Surg 171:97–100

69. Mongan PD, Fontana JL, Chen R, Bunger R (1999) Intravenous pyruvate prolongs survival during hemorrhagic shock in swine. Am J Physiol 277:H2253–H2263

70. von Korff RW (1964) Pyruvate-C^{14}, purity and stability. Anal Biochem 8:171–178

71. Montgomery CM, Webb JL (1956) Metabolic studies on heart mitochondria. II. The inhibitory action of parapyruvate on the tricarboxylic acid cycle. J Biol Chem 221:359–368

72. Margolis SA, Coxon B (1986) Identification and quantitation of the impurities in sodium pyruvate. Anal Biochem 58:2504–2510

73. Willems JL, de Kort AFM, Vree TB, Trijbels JMF, Veerkamp JH, Monnens LAH (1978) Nonenzymatic conversion of pyruvate in aqueous solution to 2,4-dihydroxy-2-methylglutaric acid. FEBS Lett 86:42–44

74. Halestrap AP, Price NT (1999) The proton-linked monocarboxylate transporter (MCT) family: structure, function and regulation. Biochem J 343:281–299

75. Halestrap AP (1975) The mitochondrial pyruvate carrier. Kinetics and specificity for substrates and inhibitors. Biochem J 148:85–96

76. Brooks GA, Brown MA, Butz CE, Sicurello JP, Dubouchaud H (1999) Cardiac and skeletal muscle mitochondria have a monocarboxylate transporter MCT1. J Appl Physiol 87:1713–1718

77. Mertz RJ, Worley JFI, Spencer B, Johnson JJ, Dukes ID (1996) Activation of stimulus-secretion coupling in pancreatic β-cells by specific products of glucose metabolism. J Biol Chem 271:4838–4845

78. Lembert N, Joos HC, Idahl L-Å, Ammon HPT, Wahl MA (2001) Methyl pyruvate initiates membrane depolarization and insulin release by metabolic factors other than ATP. Biochem J 354:345–350

79. Varma SD, Devamanoharan PS, Ali AH (1998) Prevention of intracellular oxidative stress to lens by pyruvate and its ester. Free Rad Res 28:131–135

80. Sims CA, Wattanasirichaigoon S, Menconi MJ, Ajami AM, Fink MP (2001) Ringer's ethyl pyruvate solution ameliorates ischemia/reperfusion-induced intestinal mucosal injury in rats. Crit Care Med 29:1513–1518

81. Tawadrous ZS, Delude RL, Fink MP (2002) Resuscitation from hemorrhagic shock with Ringer's ethyl pyruvate solution improves survival and ameliorates intestinal mucosal hyperpermeability in rats. Shock (in press)

82. Ulloa L, Ochani M, Fink MP, Tracey KJ (2001) Ethyl pyruvate prevents endotoxin lethality. Shock 15 (Suppl):118 (Abst)

The Immunological Effects of Hypertonic Saline

S. B. Rizoli, O. D. Rotstein, and W. J. Sibbald

▌ Introduction

Sporadic reports on the use of high salt crystalloid solutions, or hypertonic saline, date back to the beginning of the 20th century. Hypertonic solutions were most often used to correct electrolyte abnormalities, but also to induce peripheral vasodilatation and to transiently increase blood pressure [1]. De Felippe et al. [2] reported the first clinical study with hypertonic saline solution in 1980. This Brazilian study reported that small volumes of hypertonic saline administered to 12 trauma patients *in extremis* of hemorrhagic shock resulted in a remarkable increase in blood pressure, with nine patients leaving the hospital alive. Curiously, during the following 10 years, a large number of studies and considerable effort focused on trying to understand how hypertonic saline increased blood pressure instead of focusing on why nine out of 12 patients who should have died, survived.

▌ Focusing on Hemodynamics

It is easy to understand why the remarkable hemodynamic effects of hypertonic saline solutions have shadowed other possible effects. A single bolus of 250 ml of 7.5% NaCl (usually combined with 6% dextran 70) causes plasma volume to expand 8 to 10 times more than with a similar infusion of isotonic saline. This happens because water is osmotically shifted from the extravascular compartment. For a patient in hemorrhagic shock, this volume expansion can normalize blood pressure for hours [1]. Hypertonic saline causes no significant change in blood pressure in normovolemic individuals.

Hypertonic saline augments cardiac output by increasing venous return, by exerting direct inotropic and chronotropic effects on the heart, and by reducing afterload. Afterload reduction is the consequence of vasodilatation of both pulmonary and systemic circulations [1]. The combination of an augmented cardiac output and capillary dilatation causes an improvement in microcirculation and organ perfusion [3]. Overall, hypertonic saline resuscitation results in lower fluid requirements, including blood transfusion, less whole body edema, and normalization of laboratorial parameters such as pH, base excess, lactate levels and improved pulmonary function [1].

Following the first clinical report, hypertonic saline resuscitation has been examined in over 1500 trauma patients in hemorrhagic shock, mostly in North America [1, 4]. In all studies, hypertonic saline was found to be extremely safe. The hypothesis behind these studies was that an improvement in hemodynamics would increase survival. While two meta-analyses of the randomized controlled trials demonstrated a better survival with hypertonic saline versus isotonic crystalloid resuscitation, evidence of bias in the primary studies makes these results doubtful [4, 5]. An historic paper, unrelated to hypertonic saline, raised theoretical concerns about normalizing blood pressure prior to surgical hemostasis [6]. Because hypertonic saline had been explored primarily as a therapy to improve blood pressure, enthusiasm for hypertonic saline resuscitation for hemorrhagic shock became tempered and was almost completely abandoned.

▌ Expanding the Focus

A renewed interest in hypertonic saline has occurred recently when the focus moved from hemodynamics to immunomodulation. In the 1990s, many investigators demonstrated that variations in cell volume under hypertonic conditions profoundly influenced cellular function, including cellular metabolism and gene expression [7]. In fact, cell volume is an essential element of the cellular machinery and regulates cell performance and adaptation to a changing environment.

Based on these concepts, Rizoli and colleagues initiated a series of studies to investigate the cellular effects of hypertonic saline resuscitation. In a rodent model of hemorrhagic shock complicated by acute lung injury (ALI), hypertonic saline reduced lung tissue damage, capillary leak and neutrophil accumulation in the lungs [8]. Neutrophils have long been implicated in the pathogenesis of acute respiratory distress syndrome (ARDS). In this model, a transient elevation of serum osmolarity protected the lungs from damage by preventing neutrophil margination in the pulmonary vessels and subsequent migration into the alveoli. The mechanisms responsible for the reduced accumulation of neutrophils in the lungs with hypertonic saline included major changes in surface adhesion molecules in both neutrophils and vascular endothelium [8]. The finding that hypertonicity had no effect on chemokine production by alveolar macrophages suggested that only cells directly exposed to hypertonicity were affected.

The hypertonic effect on neutrophils was the determinant factor in reducing both neutrophil accumulation and lung damage. This fact was demonstrated by an experiment where isolated neutrophils treated *ex vivo* with hypertonicity and returned to the models' circulation failed to accumulate in the lungs. In contrast to neutrophils treated *ex vivo* with isotonic solution, hypertonicity markedly reduced lung injury [8].

The experimental observation that hypertonic saline resuscitation reduces lung injury is supported by clinical trials. A 1991 randomized clinical trial in trauma patients with hemorrhagic shock, reported that hypertonic saline resuscitation was associated with a lower incidence of ARDS and pneumonia [9]. Other trials also reported significantly less lung morbidity with hypertonic saline [10, 11]. These studies showed less respiratory dysfunction (ARDS), a decreased need of mechanical ventilation and a shorter intensive care unit (ICU) stay with hypertonic saline. Walker et al. [12] recently undertook a clinical study in which ischemic limbs were perfused with a hypertonic hyperoncotic solution after surgical embolectomy. While local effects of hypertonic saline were undetermined (it did not reduce the amputation rate in these patients), the systemic effects were remarkable. Hypertonicity reduced distant organ dysfunction (renal, cardiac) and mortality. Even though only the ischemic limb was perfused with hypertonic saline, systemic neutrophil activation was significantly reduced [12].

▊ Understanding the Immunological Effects of Hypertonic Saline

A well-characterized homeostatic response follows an insult such as trauma or infection [13]. When homeostasis cannot be restored, the inflammatory response that follows is known as systemic inflammatory response syndrome or SIRS. Neutrophil and endothelial activation, increased capillary leak and maldistribution of blood flow characterize this early inflammatory phase. SIRS often results in multiple organ dysfunction. A later excessive compensatory response to SIRS may lead to a state of immunosuppression. Impaired lymphocyte and macrophage function, anergy and increased susceptibility to infections characterize this immunosuppression phase.

Hypertonic Saline Reduces Early Inflammation

As mentioned earlier, hypertonicity abolishes the neutrophil mediated inflammatory response and attenuates tissue injury and organ dysfunction [8]. In SIRS, neutrophil mediated organ damage involves a complex sequence of events and mediators. Initially, naïve circulating neutrophils roll over the vascular endothelium through the binding of their surface adhesion molecule L-selectin to its endothelial ligand. During rolling, neutrophils become activated and upregulate surface expression of another class of adhesion molecules, the β_2 integrins CD11b/CD18, which mediate the firm adhesion to the endothelium [14]. Neutrophils then leave the vascular space and migrate into tissues. Once activated, neutrophils are capable of producing tissue injury by generating reactive oxygen species (ROS) and releasing the contents of their granules.

This entire process is disabled by hypertonicity. We, and others, have found that a transient increase in serum osmolarity causes extensive shedding of L-selectin from the neutrophil surface and prevents the surface upregulation of CD11b/CD18 [8, 15–17]. Under hypertonic conditions, neutrophils do not roll nor adhere to the vascular endothelium [8, 9]. The absence of neutrophil-endothelial adhesive interaction is compounded by the fact that hypertonicity also prevents upregulation of endothelial adhesion molecules, such as E-selectin, P-selectin, intercellular adhesion molecule (ICAM)-1 and vascular cell adhesion molecule (VCAM) [8, 19, 20]. Even under static conditions, when neutrophils are placed on top of activated endothelium and stimulated with chemotactic agents, they neither attach nor migrate across the endothelium [8]. Hypertonicity renders neutrophils non-functional, unable to be activated, to migrate, to form ROS or to release granule contents [8, 16, 21, 22].

All these characteristics are explained by the fact that in a hypertonic environment neutrophils shrink and are incapable of increasing their volume back to normal. In addition, hypertonicity induces the formation of a submembranous ring of filamentous actin [16]. This ring prevents granules from reaching and fusing with the plasma membrane and releasing their contents (Fig. 1). It acts as a physical barrier both to granule exocytosis and shape changing [16]. Since neutrophil activation requires major shape and volume changes [21], they remain non-functional for as long as they are in a hypertonic environment. This effect is however transi-

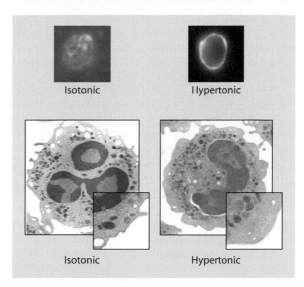

Fig. 1. Distribution of filamentous actin (F-actin) in human neutrophils under isotonic and hypertonic conditions. *Top pictures*: hypertonicity induced the formation of a thick actin ring under the entire surface of the plasma membrane. Neutrophils were stained for F-actin and visualized by fluorescent microscopy. *Bottom pictures*: after neutrophils were visualized by electron microscopy under isotonic and hypertonic conditions. The actin ring was not stained and appears as a thick and homogenous empty area, separating granules and organelles away from the plasma membrane. Enclosed insets show details of the submembranous area (from [16] with permission).

ent, and most functions are fully regained once the neutrophils are returned to an isotonic environment [23].

Having neutrophils temporarily disabled is desirable and potentially beneficial during the initial overwhelming inflammatory response and might account for the reduced incidence of organ dysfunction. Yet, there is also evidence suggesting that hypertonicity affects the state of impaired immunity and suppressed cytokine release that follows SIRS, often ending in sepsis and death.

Hypertonic Saline Restores late Immunosuppression and Reduces Sepsis

While hypertonic saline exerts inhibitory effects on neutrophils, it has opposite effects on macrophages and lymphocytes. In 1994, Junger and colleagues demonstrated that hypertonicity enhances cellular immune function [24]. Hypertonic saline markedly increased both T-cell proliferation and function, with a 300% increase in monocyte tumor necrosis factor (TNF) production and improvement in delayed type hypersensitivity skin reaction [24]. In subsequent studies, the same group demonstrated, both *in vivo* and *in vitro*, that hypertonic saline reverts post-trauma cellular immunosuppression. Hypertonic saline enhanced T-cell function as measured by a three-fold increase in interleukin (IL)-2 expression, restored T-cell function even in the presence of suppressive factors such as prostaglandin E_2 (PGE_2), IL-4, IL-10 and transforming growth factor(TGF)-β_1 [25, 26]. Hypertonic saline resuscitation also restored splenocyte function and reduced production and/or release of suppressive factors such as IL-4 and PGE_2 [27].

The many complementary effects of hypertonicity can also be observed in a recent study by Oreopoulos et al. [28]. Using peritoneal macrophages, Oreopoulos and colleaques demonstrated that hypertonic saline inhibited production of pro-inflammatory cytokines, such as TNF, while enhancing the expression of anti-inflammatory cytokines such as IL-10 [28].

The strongest argument that hypertonic saline reverses immunosuppression and subsequent sepsis is seen in a study by Coimbra et al. [29]. In a mouse model of hemorrhage and sepsis (cecal ligation and puncture), hypertonic saline resuscitation improved survival, improved infection containment, and minimized distant organ injury, including lung and liver [29].

In addition to restoring cellular immunocompetence, other mechanisms can also explain the benefits of hypertonic saline on sepsis. Hypoperfusion of the gut mucosa with subsequent impairment of the epithelial barrier predisposes to bacterial translocation, triggering or aggravating a septic state. In this scenario, a rapid restoration of intravascular volume and cardiac output (hallmarks of hypertonic saline resuscitation), are conceptually valuable. However, even more important might be the ability of hypertonic saline to improve microvascular blood flow. Hypertonic saline reduces shock-induced endothelial and red blood cell swelling, preventing leukocyte or red blood cell (RBC) plugging and restores flow and surface for tissue oxygen exchange in the microcirculation [30, 31]. Besides intravascular expansion, hypertonic saline induces prostacyclin (PGI_2) production from endothelial cells, which leads to capillary vasodilatation and reduction of platelet aggregation [3].

While causing vasodilatation, hypertonic saline has also been reported to reduce capillary leak. Hypertonic saline reduces fluid and protein extravasation from the intravascular space, even under direct challenge with endotoxin [32]. Furthermore, hypertonic saline also reduces translocation of bacteria [33] and increases oxygen extraction [34]. Finally, using a porcine model of endotoxin shock, a recent study demonstrated that hypertonic saline improved portal and gut mucosal blood flow with a significant improvement in survival [30]. Hypertonicity induced changes in microcirculation may also account for the reduction in organ dysfunction.

▮ Hypertonic Saline Reduces Organ Dysfunction

Lung Dysfunction

Most of the evidence for the protective effect of hypertonic saline on the lung comes from experimental studies. Yet, clinical evidence can be gathered from some human trials as presented earlier in this chapter. Most experimental studies focused on post hemorrhagic shock lung injury [8]; Shields et al. [35] however, reported on severe pancreatitis. In a rodent model of L-arginine induced pancreatitis, hypertonic saline resuscitation reduced both local (pancreatic) and distant organ injury, in this case, the lungs [35]. Shields also found a marked reduction in neutrophil sequestration in the lungs.

The overall evidence suggests that hypertonic saline protects the lung from inflammatory damage by attenuating neutrophil-mediated injury.

Liver Dysfunction

In experimental models of ischemia/reperfusion, hypertonic saline resuscitation reduced neutrophil accumulation in the liver and decreased biochemical and histological evidence of liver damage [19].

Brain Dysfunction

According to a recent meta-analysis by Wade et al. [36], patients with severe head injury and hypotension are twice as likely to survive if resuscitated with hypertonic saline rather than isotonic crystalloids. The improved survival may relate solely to the hemodynamic and osmotic effects of hypertonic saline resuscitation. Hypertonic saline rapidly corrects hypotension, improves cerebral perfusion pressure and cerebral blood flow, and reduces brain edema and intracranial pressure [37]. However, other known effects of hypertonic saline may also account for limiting secondary pathological events and improving both survival and outcome [37]. Hypertonicity normalizes and stabilizes membrane resting potential, increases blood flow to the choroid plexus and reduces the inflammatory response to trauma by reducing neutrophil adhesion to the microvasculature and attenuating pial vasodilatation [18]. A study currently under way in Australia is investigating the effect of hypertonic saline resuscitation on the neurological outcome of head injury patients (D.J. Cooper, personal notification).

Spinal Cord Dysfunction

In experimental models, Tuma et al. [38] and Sumas et al. [39] reported that hypertonic saline resuscitation both preserves spinal cord function and expedites recovery after injury. Although the studies propose that improvement in local spinal cord flow was responsible for these effects, other vasodilators such as nitroprusside did not have any protective effect in these models. This suggests that other factors related to hypertonic saline might be responsible for the reported benefits.

Organ Death

Cell death by apoptosis has been implicated in organ dysfunction following trauma and sepsis. Deb et al. [40] described that standard resuscitation of hemorrhagic shock with Ringer's solution resulted in a significant increase in apoptosis of both liver and small bowel. Hypertonic saline resuscitation, however, protected both organs from apoptosis [40].

Hypertonicity has also been reported to protect other cells from apoptosis, potentially preventing progression to organ dysfunction including renal medullary epithelial cells [41] and thymic lymphocytes [42]. Interestingly hypertonic saline protects organs from apoptosis but accelerates apoptosis of neutrophils that cause organ damage [15].

▌ Conclusion

Hypertonic saline exerts many potentially beneficial effects. The hemodynamic effects were extensively characterized during the 1980s. A small infusion of hypertonic saline rapidly shifts fluid into the intravascular space, expands plasma volume, increases cardiac output and transiently normalizes blood pressure and organ perfusion.

Hypertonic saline also has immunological properties. Hypertonic saline minimizes excessive SIRS response to trauma and shock, mostly by abolishing neutrophil-mediated inflammation and tissue damage. Furthermore, hypertonic saline reverses the subsequent immune suppression by enhancing lymphocyte and macrophage function. The conclusion is that hypertonic saline has the potential to reduce both organ dysfunction and susceptibility to infection, fascinating possibilities to a simple, safe and inexpensive therapy that unfortunately still lacks well designed clinical trials.

References

1. Rocha e Silva M (1998) Hypertonic saline resuscitation. Medicina (B Aires) 58:393–402
2. de Felippe J, Timoner J, Velasco IT, Lopes OU, Rocha E, Silva M Jr (1980) Treatment of refractory hypovolaemic shock by 7.5% sodium chloride injections. Lancet 2:1002–1004
3. Arbabi S, Garcia I, Bauer G, Maier RV (1999) Hypertonic saline induces prostacyclin production via extracellular signal-regulated kinase (ERK) activation. J Surg Res 83:141–146
4. Wade CE, Grady JJ, Kramer GC, Younes RN, Gehlsen K, Holcroft JW (1997) Individual patient cohort analysis of the efficacy of hypertonic saline/dextran in patients with traumatic brain injury and hypotension. J Trauma 42:S61–S65
5. Schierhout G, Roberts I (1998) Fluid resuscitation with colloid or crystalloid solutions in critically ill patients: a systematic review of randomised trials. Br Med J 316:961–964
6. Bickell WH, Wall MJJ, Pepe PE, et al (1994) Immediate versus delayed fluid resuscitation for hypotensive patients with penetrating torso injuries. N Engl J Med 331:1105–1109
7. Lang F, Busch GL, Ritter M, et al (1998) Functional significance of cell volume regulatory mechanisms. Physiol Rev 78:247–306
8. Rizoli SB, Kapus A, Fan J, Li YH, Marshall JC, Rotstein OD (1998) Immunomodulatory effects of hypertonic resuscitation on the development of lung inflammation following hemorrhagic shock. J Immunol 161:6288–6296
9. Mattox KL, Maningas PA, Moore EE (1991) Prehospital hypertonic saline/dextran infusion for post-traumatic hypotension: the USA multicenter trial. Ann Surg 213:482–491
10. Holcroft JW, Vassar MJ, Turner JE, Derlet RW, Kramer GC (1987) 3% NaCl and 7.5% NaCl/dextran 70 in the resuscitation of severely injured patients. Ann Surg 206:279–288
11. Simma B, Burger R, Falk M, Sacher P, Fanconi S (1998) A prospective, randomized, and controlled study of fluid management in children with severe head injury: lactated Ringer's solution versus hypertonic saline. Crit Care Med 26:1265–1270
12. Walker PM, Romaschin AD, Davis S, Piovesan J (1999) Lower limb ischemia: phase 1 results of salvage perfusion. J Surg Res 84:193–198
13. Bone RC (1996) Immunologic dissonance: a continuing evolution in our understanding of the systemic inflammatory response syndrome (SIRS) and the multiple organ dysfunction syndrome (MODS). Ann Intern Med 125:680–687
14. Aplin AE, Howe A, Alahari SK, Juliano RL (1998) Signal transduction and signal modulation by cell adhesion receptors: the role of integrins, cadherins, immunoglobulin-cell adhesion molecules, and selectins. Pharmacol Rev 50:197–263
15. Rizoli SB, Rotstein OD, Kapus A (1999) Cell volume-dependent regulation of L-selectin shedding in neutrophils. A role for p38 mitogen-activated protein kinase. J Biol Chem 274:22072–22080
16. Rizoli SB, Rotstein OD, Parodo J, Phillips MJ, Kapus A (2000) Hypertonic inhibition of exocytosis in neutrophils: central role for osmotic actin skeleton remodeling. Am J Physiol 279:C619–C633
17. Thiel M, Buessecker F, Eberhardt K, et al (2001) Effects of hypertonic saline on expression of human polymorphonuclear leukocyte adhesion molecules. J Leukoc Biol 70:261–273
18. Hartl R, Medary MB, Ruge M, Arfors KE, Ghahremani F, Ghajar J (1997) Hypertonic/hyperoncotic saline attenuates microcirculatory disturbances after traumatic brain injury. J Trauma 42:S41–S47

19. Oreopoulos GD, Hamilton J, Rizoli SB, et al (2000) In vivo and in vitro modulation of intercellular adhesion molecule (ICAM)-1 expression by hypertonicity. Shock 14:409–414
20. Alam HB, Sun L, Ruff P, Austin B, Burris D, Rhee P (1994) E- and P-selectin expression depends on the resuscitation fluid used in hemorrhaged rats. J Surg Res 2000 94:145–152
21. Worthen GS, Henson PM, Rosengren S, Downey GP, Hyde DM (1994) Neutrophils increase volume during migration in vivo and in vitro. Am J Respir Cell Mol Biol 10:1–7
22. Junger WG, Hoyt DB, Davis RE, et al (1998) Hypertonicity regulates the function of human neutrophils by modulating chemoattractant receptor signaling and activating mitogen-activated protein kinase p38. J Clin Invest 101:2768–2779
23. Rizoli SB, Kapus A, Parodo J, Fan J, Rotstein OD (1999) Hypertonic immunomodulation is reversible and accompanied by changes in CD11b expression. J Surg Res 83:130–135
24. Junger WG, Liu FC, Loomis WH, Hoyt DB (1994) Hypertonic saline enhances cellular immune function. Circ Shock 42:190–196
25. Junger WG, Coimbra R, Liu FC, et al (1997) Hypertonic saline resuscitation: a tool to modulate immune function in trauma patients? Shock 8:235–241
26. Loomis WH, Namiki S, Hoyt DB, Junger WG (2001) Hypertonicity rescues T cells from suppression by trauma-induced anti-inflammatory mediators. Am J Physiol 281:C840–848
27. Coimbra R, Junger WG, Hoyt DB, Liu FC, Loomis WH, Evers MF (1996) Hypertonic saline resuscitation restores hemorrhage-induced immunosuppression by decreasing prostaglandin E2 and interleukin-4 production. J Surg Res 64:203–209
28. Oreopoulos GD, Bradwell S, Lu Z, et al (2001) Synergistic induction of IL-10 by hypertonic saline solution and lipopolysaccharides in murine peritoneal macrophages. Surgery 130: 157–165
29. Coimbra R, Hoyt DB, Junger WG, et al (1997) Hypertonic saline resuscitation decreases susceptibility to sepsis after hemorrhagic shock. J Trauma 42:602–606
30. Oi Y, Aneman A, Svensson M, Ewert S, Dahlqvist M, Haljamae H (2000) Hypertonic saline-dextran improves intestinal perfusion and survival in porcine endotoxin shock. Crit Care Med 28:2843–2850
31. Mazzoni MC, Borgstrom P, Intaglietta M, Arfors KE (1990) Capillary narrowing in hemorrhagic shock is rectified by hyperosmotic saline-dextran reinfusion. Circ Shock 31:407–418
32. de CH, Matos JA, Bouskela E, Svensjo E (1999) Vascular permeability increase and plasma volume loss induced by endotoxin was attenuated by hypertonic saline with or without dextran. Shock 12:75–80
33. Assalia A, Bitterman H, Hirsh TM, Krausz MM (2001) Influence of hypertonic saline on bacterial translocation in controlled hemorrhagic shock. Shock 15:307–311
34. Maciel F, Mook M, Zhang H, Vincent JL (1998) Comparison of hypertonic with isotonic saline hydroxyethyl starch solution on oxygen extraction capabilities during endotoxic shock. Shock 9:33–39
35. Shields CJ, Winter DC, Sookhai S, Ryan L, Kirwan WO, Redmond HP (2000) Hypertonic saline attenuates end-organ damage in an experimental model of acute pancreatitis. Br J Surg 87:1336–1340
36. Wade CE, Kramer GC, Grady JJ, Fabian TC, Younes RN (1997) Efficacy of hypertonic 7.5% saline and 6% dextran-70 in treating trauma: a meta-analysis of controlled clinical studies. Surgery 122:609–616
37. Qureshi AI, Suarez JI (2000) Use of hypertonic saline solutions in treatment of cerebral edema and intracranial hypertension. Crit Care Med 28:3301–3313
38. Tuma RF, Vasthare US, Arfors KE, Young WF (1997) Hypertonic saline administration attenuates spinal cord injury. J Trauma 42:S54–S60
39. Sumas ME, Legos JJ, Nathan D, Lamperti AA, Tuma RF, Young WF (2001) Tonicity of resuscitative fluids influences outcome after spinal cord injury. Neurosurgery 48:167–172
40. Deb S, Martin B, Sun L, et al (1999) Resuscitation with lactated Ringer's solution in rats with hemorrhagic shock induces immediate apoptosis. J Trauma 46:582–588
41. Dmitrieva N, Kultz D, Michea L, Ferraris J, Burg M (2000) Protection of renal inner medullary epithelial cells from apoptosis by hypertonic stress-induced p53 activation. J Biol Chem 275:18243–18247
42. Luo X, Huang Z, Xiao G, Tang A, Deng Y (1998) Protection of hypertonic saline/mannitol to thymic cell apoptosis induced by endotoxin (LPS) in mice. Hunan Yi Ke Da Xue Xue Bao 23:14–16

Does Albumin Infusion Affect Survival?
Review of Meta-analytic Findings

M. M. Wilkes and R. J. Navickis

▊ Introduction

Since its introduction more than 50 years ago, albumin has been in widespread use for the fluid management of acutely ill patients. In the US, the licensed indications for albumin include hypovolemia/shock, burns, hypoalbuminemia/hypoproteinemia, surgery, trauma, cardiopulmonary bypass (CPB), adult respiratory distress syndrome (ARDS), hemodialysis, acute nephrosis, hyperbilirubinemia, acute liver failure, ascites, and sequestration of protein rich fluids in acute peritonitis, pancreatitis, mediastinitis, and extensive cellulitis.

Although the effectiveness of albumin in improving clinical outcomes has been a subject of controversy and its economic impact has prompted concerns, the safety of albumin was long judged "so high that it rarely warrants discussion" [1]. However, a 1998 meta-analysis of randomized trials by the Cochrane Injuries Group Albumin Reviewers for the first time seriously called the safety of albumin into question [2]. In that meta-analysis, mortality was significantly higher overall in albumin recipients than in patients receiving crystalloid, no albumin, or lower-dose albumin. However, this observation of excess albumin-associated mortality could not be confirmed in a larger more recent meta-analysis of Wilkes and Navickis [3].

Clinicians are now faced with the need to reconcile the disparate findings of the two meta-analyses and weigh their implications for clinical practice. In this chapter, we compare and contrast the meta-analyses, endeavor to account for their differences and offer conclusions regarding their validity.

▊ The Cochrane Meta-Analysis and its Impact

The Cochrane meta-analysis addressed three categories of clinical indications: hypovolemia from surgery or trauma; burns; and hypoalbuminemia. There was no significant effect of albumin on survival in trials of hypovolemia from surgery or trauma. However, among trials of burns and hypoalbuminemia mortality was significantly higher in albumin recipients. The pooled mortality for all three categories of indications was significantly increased by albumin therapy. Although this meta-analysis has been updated [4], no further trials with mortality data were included, and the results remain unchanged. Based on their results, the Cochrane Group advocated restricting albumin usage to randomized trials and "urgently" reviewing the safety of albumin [2].

The Cochrane meta-analysis provoked immediate and intense criticism. Commentators called attention to an array of flaws that cast doubt on the validity of the meta-analysis, including omission of relevant trials, heterogeneity of included trials, inadequate assessment of trial methodological quality, and absence of plausible pathophysiological mechanisms to explain a deleterious effect of albumin [5, 6]. Evidence external to the meta-analysis also failed to support the conclusion that albumin therapy is harmful. In a randomized trial of patients with spontaneous bacterial peritonitis, albumin administration significantly improved survival and ameliorated renal impairment [7].

Also inconsistent with the Cochrane results was the excellent long-term safety record of albumin. This record has been further enhanced by the recent report of a large-scale pharmacovigilance study focusing on spontaneously reported, serious adverse events and encompassing 100 million albumin doses distributed worldwide during 1990–1997 [8]. No deaths were judged "probably" attributable to albumin, and the incidence of fatal serious adverse events "possibly" related to albumin was 5.24 per 100 million doses. Thus, fatal adverse events in albumin recipients were very rare.

Notwithstanding the doubts as to its validity, the Cochrane meta-analysis prompted a decline in albumin usage. This impact likely reflected, at least in part, the absence of evidence that rectifying any of the perceived flaws in the meta-analysis would have altered its conclusions. With the appearance of the meta-analysis by Wilkes and Navickis [3] such evidence now exists.

▍ A More Comprehensive Meta-Analysis and a Different Conclusion

Wilkes and Navickis [3] included all the trials of the Cochrane meta-analysis, as well as additional trials. Therefore, the Cochrane trials constituted a subset of those in the Wilkes and Navickis meta-analysis. Some trials included in both meta-analyses involved zero deaths in both groups, and in such cases relative risk of death cannot be calculated. Only trials with at least one death can contribute to pooled estimates of relative risk, and we will restrict our discussion to such trials.

The meta-analysis of Wilkes and Navickis [3] encompassed six categories of clinical indications: surgery or trauma; burns; hypoalbuminemia; high-risk neonates; ascites; and other indications. In this meta-analysis there was no significant overall effect of albumin therapy on survival either across all indications or in any individual category of indications. However, mortality was substantially and consistently lower among trials of higher methodological quality, as indicated for instance by a relative risk for death of 0.73 with a 95% confidence interval (CI) of 0.48–1.12 in blinded trials and 0.94 (CI, 0.77–1.14) in larger trials. Relative risk < 1 signifies lower mortality in albumin recipients. Relative risk was also < 1 in all six subsets of trials sharing two or more attributes indicative of higher quality (blinding, larger size, a mortality endpoint, absence of crossover). It is well established that trial quality can alter the conclusions of meta-analyses. In one meta-analysis, for example, an apparent benefit of low-molecular weight heparin did not persist when the analysis was restricted to blinded trials [9].

Even without trial quality taken into account, the difference in pooled relative risk estimates between the two meta-analyses was striking. The pooled overall relative mortality risk reported by the Cochrane Group (1.68; CI, 1.26–2.23) was 51% higher than that of Wilkes and Navickis (1.11; CI, 0.95–1.28). Furthermore, there was minimal overlap in the confidence intervals, and as shown in Fig. 1 the difference in relative risk estimates was statistically significant.

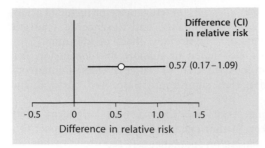

Fig. 1. Difference in pooled overall relative risk estimates of the Cochrane Group [2] and Wilkes and Navickis [3]. The confidence interval (CI) for the difference was calculated by bootstrapping with bias correction. The difference was statistically significant as indicated by the absence of zero from the CI

Nonetheless, trial quality *should* be taken into account [10]. Detailed sensitivity analyses reported by Wilkes and Navickis [3] revealed consistent bias favoring control among lower quality trials. This bias is reflected in the pooled relative risk estimate of 1.11 from their meta-analysis. In the absence of bias, a relative risk >1 might suggest a trend toward harm, but such an interpretation would clearly be unsound when the presence of bias has been demonstrated.

▌ Why the Conflicting Results?

In methodology there were many similarities between the two meta-analyses (Table 1). Both involved the same types of included trials, control groups, data sources, endpoint, effect size measure, and statistical model. Search methods were similar, and no language restrictions were applied. However, the inclusion criteria of the Cochrane meta-analysis [2] were more restrictive, and several exclusion rules were imposed. Wilkes and Navickis [3], by contrast, adopted a broad 'all comers' approach and did not exclude any trials.

Differing trial selection criteria could clearly have contributed to the disparate results. The adoption of particular trial selection rules is a recognized potential source of bias in meta-analysis. For instance, in a meta-analysis of cholesterol lowering after myocardial infarction [11], the seven included trials revealed a trend toward improved survival; whereas, 11 excluded trials indicated significant harm [12]. One missed trial also pointed toward harm. Thus, biased inclusion criteria and selective identification of supportive studies appear to have distorted the results of that meta-analysis [12].

Similar biases were also at work in the Cochrane meta-analysis. As shown in Table 2, there were 18 trials [7, 13–18, 22, 23, 25–33] included by Wilkes and Navickis [3] that were absent from the Cochrane meta-analysis [2]. Of these, the Cochrane Group specifically excluded four trials and missed at least two trials fulfilling the selection criteria of their meta-analysis. The four excluded trials accounted for 38% of all patients determined to be eligible by the Cochrane Group. Both the excluded trials and the missed trials suggested a survival benefit due to albumin therapy; whereas, the included trials indicated harm (Fig. 2). Importantly, the included trials accounted for only 36% of the total meta-analytic weight, primarily because the median size of the excluded and missed trials (130 patients per trial) was greater by more than 3.5 fold than that of the included trials (36 patients per trial). Thus, based on these observations the conclusions of the Cochrane meta-analysis rested

Table 1. Comparative attributes of the two meta-analyses [2, 3]

Attribute	Meta-Analysis	
	Cochrane Group [2]	Wilkes and Navickis [3]
Type of trials included	Randomized	Randomized
Control group	Crystalloid, no albumin or lower-dose albumin	Crystalloid, no albumin or lower-dose albumin
Data sources	Published and unpublished	Published and unpublished
Language restrictions	None	None
Search methods	Bibliographic database searches; hand searching; contacts with investigators and albumin suppliers; and perusal of reference lists	Bibliographic database searches; full-text Internet searches; hand searching; contacts with investigators and albumin suppliers; and perusal of reference lists
Endpoint	All-cause mortality based on intention to treat	All-cause mortality based on intention to treat
Effect size measure	Relative risk	Relative risk
Statistical model	Fixed effects	Fixed effects
Clinical indications	Hypovolemia due to surgery or trauma; burns; or hypoalbuminemia	"All comers"
Exclusion criteria	Preoperative volume loading; hemodilution; or albumin administration during paracentesis	None
Quality assessment	Allocation concealment	Allocation concealment; blinding; mortality endpoint; crossover; and trial size
Funding source	Britain's National Health Service, which bears the cost for albumin therapy in the UK	Plasma Protein Therapeutics Association, which represents albumin suppliers, and the American Red Cross, which supplies albumin
Type of funding	Support for the infrastructure of the Cochrane Injuries Group	Unrestricted grant
Role of funding source	Undisclosed	No participation in either the design, conduct, interpretation and analysis of the study or the review and approval of the manuscript

on a biased and relatively small sample from the total weight of relevant evidence that the Cochrane Group either explicitly considered or clearly failed to identify.

Varying underlying risk within the patient population can also contribute to differences in effect size estimates by meta-analysis. In neither meta-analysis were studies selected on the basis of "critical illness," a term for which there exists as yet no consensus definition. The population included by Wilkes and Navickis [3] appears to have been more "critically ill" as judged by a control group mortality rate of 17% compared with 10% in the Cochrane meta-analysis.

Table 2. Trials with one or more deaths included by Wilkes and Navickis [3] but not the Cochrane Group [2]

Trial	Basis for Absence from the Cochrane Meta-Analysis
Wilkinson and Sherlock [13]	Hypovolemia due to ascites rather than surgery or trauma
Bland et al. [14]	Missed
Recinos et al. [15]	Missed
Hallowell et al. [16]	Either missed or excluded on unspecified grounds, possibly hemodilution
Virgilio et al. [17]	Hypovolemia due to ARDS rather than surgery or trauma
Metildi et al. [18]	Specifically excluded, because it involved both non-trauma and trauma patients [a]
Bodenhamer et al. [22]	Either missed or excluded on unspecified grounds
Grundmann and Heistermann [23]	Specifically excluded, because it involved "different criteria for albumin supplementation" [4] [b]
Grundmann and von Lehndorff [25]	Specifically excluded, because both the intervention and control groups received albumin [4] [c]
Ginès et al. [26]	Hypovolemia due to ascites rather than surgery or trauma; paracentesis
Marelli et al. [27]	Either missed or excluded on unspecified grounds
Adam et al. [28]	Either missed or excluded on unspecified grounds
Goslinga et al. [29]	Specifically excluded, because the intervention was directed at hemodilution rather than volume replacement [4] [d]
London et al. [30]	Either missed or excluded on unspecified grounds
Gentilini et al. [31]	Hypovolemia due to ascites rather than surgery or trauma
Oca et al. [32]	Mortality data available subsequent to update of Cochrane meta-analysis [4]
Sort et al. [8]	Hypovolemia due to ascites rather than surgery or trauma
Lennihan et al. [33]	Either missed or excluded on unspecified grounds

[a] Three trials involving neither surgery nor trauma [19–21] were, however, included in the hypovolemia from surgery or trauma category.

[b] A burns trial with higher mortality in the albumin group [24] was nevertheless included, even though albumin was administered by different criteria, viz, for the albumin group whether serum albumin fell below 25–35 g/l or for the control group below 15–20 g/l.

[c] According to the explicit inclusion criteria of the meta-analysis, however, trials "that compared different levels of albumin supplementation were also included" [2]. Also, the included burns trial of Greenhalgh et al. [24] involved low vs high albumin administration.

[d] In the published report of this trial the investigators indicated that the therapeutic intervention entailed both "viscosity reduction and optimization of the circulatory volume" [29].

▌ Which Results were more Reliable?

By virtue of its far greater comprehensiveness and the higher quality of included trials, the Wilkes and Navickis meta-analysis arguably provided a more reliable estimate of mortality risk associated with albumin therapy. These authors identified 42 randomized trials with at least one death, versus 24 such trials in the Cochrane meta-analysis (Fig. 3a), and the total number of patients in the 42 trials (2958) was 2.5 fold greater than the 1204 patient total for the Cochrane trials (Fig. 3b).

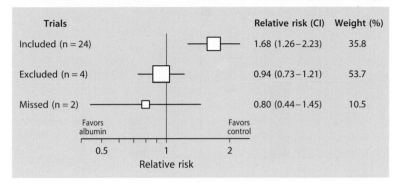

Fig. 2. Relative mortality risk in trials with one or more deaths included, excluded and missed by the Cochrane Group

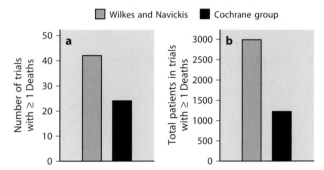

Fig. 3. a Number of trials with one or more deaths in the two meta-analyses and **b** total numbers of patients in those trials

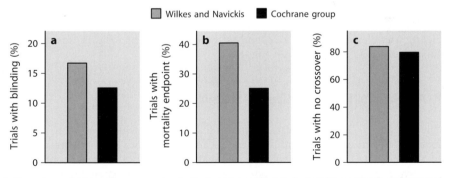

Fig. 4. Percentages of trials with one or more deaths involving **a** blinding, **b** mortality as a study endpoint and **c** no crossover

The percentages of trials with blinding (Fig. 4a) and mortality as a study endpoint (Fig. 4b) were substantially higher in the Wilkes and Navickis meta-analysis [3], and the percentage of trials without crossover was modestly greater (Fig. 4c). Additionally, the size of the trials included by Wilkes and Navickis was much larger. For the 42 trials with deaths in their meta-analysis, the median number of pa-

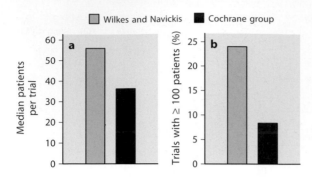

Fig. 5. a Median numbers of patients per trial for trials with one or more deaths and **b** percentages of such trials with 100 or more patients

tients per trial was 56 (range, 16–300) vs 36 (range, 17–219) for the 24 Cochrane trials (Fig. 5a). The percentage of trials with 100 or more patients included by Wilkes and Navickis (24%) exceeded that of the Cochrane Group (8%) by 3 fold (Fig. 5b).

Limitations of the Meta-Analyses

Both meta-analyses were subject to several limitations. Due to the low event rate in broad populations of acutely ill patients, mortality is an inherently insensitive endpoint. Although statistical heterogeneity was not detected, the included trials of both meta-analyses involved widely differing clinical indications, fluid management regimens, and patient populations. Albumin dosages varied and were frequently poorly described, and the infusion of blood products that contain albumin in many studies further compounds the complexity of ascertaining administered dose. Many of the currently available trials were small and low in quality. In light of these uncertainties it is perhaps more reasonable to view meta-analyses of such broad design and clinical heterogeneity as helpful in generating hypotheses rather than in guiding fluid management practice. Nonetheless, the Cochrane meta-analysis clearly *did* alter clinical practice, and to the extent that its validity was questionable this impact may not have been salutary.

Are Harmful Effects of Albumin Plausible?

The Cochrane Group suggested two mechanisms by which albumin could exert harmful effects: anticoagulant activity that might promote hemorrhage, and leakage of albumin into the extravascular spaces that might induce edema. In a recent comparative review, however, no report was identified of increased bleeding tendency related to albumin infusion [34]. Rather, albumin is "generally considered not to influence blood coagulation" [34]. Of all deaths possibly related to albumin exposure in the recent large-scale pharmacovigilance study [8], none was attributed to a hemorrhagic complication. Indeed in certain indications such as CPB surgery the ability of albumin to coat the fluid pathway surface, diminish fibrinogen binding sites, reduce platelet granule release, and preserve the functional and morphologic integrity of platelets is viewed as a major advantage [35], since acquired transient platelet dysfunction is a major cause of excessive postoperative bleeding in these patients. In a randomized trial, an albumin-containing CPB priming solution was judged superior to priming solutions of either crystalloid, hydroxyethyl starch or gelatin in preserving platelet function [36]. Furthermore, in a recent meta-analysis of randomized trials comparing albumin with hydroxyethyl starch of either high or medium molecular weight, postoperative bleeding in CPB patients was significantly lower in albumin recipients [37].

Although promotion of interstitial fluid accumulation by colloids in states of increased vascular permeability such as sepsis has often been speculated, prompting concerns, particularly of pulmonary edema, empirical support for this concept is lacking. For instance, according to guidelines for hemodynamic support of adult patients with sepsis issued by the Society of Critical Care Medicine, "a number of studies, including a variety of models of increased microvascular permeability as well as clinical studies in patients with septic shock and the acute respiratory distress syndrome, have not found evidence of increased lung water or compromised lung function with the administration of colloids" [38].

Conversely, there are a variety of mechanisms whereby albumin therapy might bestow benefit. Albumin exerts 75–80% of the normal colloid osmotic pressure and thus plays a pivotal role in maintaining fluid balance. Additionally, albumin possesses a wide array of nononcotic properties that may help preserve physiological homeostasis, including antioxidant and free radical-scavenging activity as well as binding affinity for lipids, drugs, toxic substances and other ligands [39]. For instance, albumin is the only currently identified plasma factor that specifically inhibits endothelial cell apoptosis at physiological concentrations [40] as well as a major serum survival factor for renal tubular cells and macrophages [41]. During CPB albumin prevents erythrocyte crenation and may thus improve microcirculatory performance [42].

The importance of the physiological roles played by albumin is suggested by the pervasive increase in risk of poor clinical outcomes associated with reduced serum albumin levels. Hypoalbuminemia is a potent, dose-dependent independent risk factor for mortality and morbidity in acutely ill patients [43], suggesting that albumin exerts a direct protective effect in averting these unfavorable outcomes.

▌ Beyond Mortality: Assessing the Clinical Utility of Albumin

Albumin therapy is administered for the purpose of deriving clinical benefit, and lack of excess mortality is of course insufficient justification *per se* for such therapy. While one randomized trial did demonstrate a survival advantage due to albumin therapy [7], most studies to date have been inadequately powered to assess mortality. Accordingly, it is appropriate to consider other clinically relevant endpoints such as morbidity and length of stay when appraising the clinical utility of albumin. For example, in 11 of the trials included by Wilkes and Navickis [3] no between-group survival difference could be detected; however, significant differences did exist in complications or length of stay. In all 11 trials, those differences favored albumin. Thus, albumin therapy reduced: the incidences of acute complications among adults without inhalational injury [14], respiratory dysfunction, escharotomy and ileus [44], hypotension associated with spinal anesthesia for cesarean section [45], pulmonary edema [18], septicemia, pneumonia and total complications [46]; hyponatremia and renal impairment [25], oliguria [19], moderate or severe ovarian hyperstimulation syndrome [47]; the severity of intestinal edema [48]; the frequency of reoperations [22]; and the length of hospital stay [30]. These observations suggest that, at least in particular clinical settings, albumin may confer significant benefit. Of course, the totality of evidence should be considered, and in certain indications such as hypoalbuminemia, some trials have failed to detect benefit, although these results may have reflected lower albumin dosages.

Perhaps the most frequent objection to albumin therapy is its cost. However, thus far this issue has been considered seldom in light of the overall pharmacoeconomic impact of albumin, including not just its acquisition cost, but also the savings attributable to reduced complications and length of stay in some clinical settings [49]. For instance, albumin may reduce overall costs of care by minimizing bleeding in CPB patients [50] and shortening hospital stay in ascites patients [30].

▌ Conclusion

Although albumin therapy has been the subject of numerous clinical trials, many of the trials have been small in size and deficient in quality. Consequently, much uncertainty remains as to the clinical utility of albumin in particular indications. Newer, higher quality trials such as the pending large-scale randomized trial being conducted by the Australian and New Zealand Intensive Care Society Clinical Trials Group, as well as other currently ongoing trials, should further elucidate the value of albumin infusion.

The Cochrane meta-analysis [2] prompted a curtailment of albumin usage because of a possible adverse impact on survival. The more comprehensive and reliable meta-analysis of Wilkes and Navickis [3] reveals no overall effect of albumin on mortality. However, results in higher quality trials suggest a possible survival benefit of albumin therapy. Hence, currently available evidence does not provide a sound basis for withholding albumin therapy because of safety concerns.

References

1. Tullis JL (1977) Albumin. 1. Background and use. JAMA 237:355–360
2. Cochrane Injuries Group Albumin Reviewers (1998) Human albumin administration in critically ill patients: systematic review of randomised controlled trials. Br Med J 317:235–240
3. Wilkes MM, Navickis RJ (2001) Patient survival after human albumin administration: a meta-analysis of randomized, controlled trials. Ann Intern Med 135:149–164
4. The Albumin Reviewers, Alderson P, Bunn F, et al (2000) Human albumin solution for resuscitation and volume expansion in critically ill patients. Cochrane Database Syst Rev CD 001208
5. Erstad BL (1999) Concerns with defining appropriate uses of albumin by meta-analysis. Am J Health Syst Pharm 56:1451–1454
6. Webb AR (2000) The appropriate role of colloids in managing fluid imbalance: a critical review of recent meta-analytic findings. Crit Care 4 (suppl 2):S26–S32
7. Sort P, Navasa M, Arroyo V, et al (1999) Effect of intravenous albumin on renal impairment and mortality in patients with cirrhosis and spontaneous bacterial peritonitis. N Engl J Med 341:403–409
8. von Hoegen I, Waller C (2001) Safety of human albumin based on spontaneously reported serious adverse events. Crit Care Med 29:994–996
9. Juni P, Witschi A, Bloch R, Egger M (1999) The hazards of scoring the quality of clinical trials for meta-analysis. JAMA 282:1054–1060

10. Moher D, Pham B, Jones A, et al (1998) Does quality of reports of randomised trials affect estimates of intervention efficacy reported in meta-analyses? Lancet 352:609–613
11. Rossouw JE, Lewis B, Rifkind BM (1990) The value of lowering cholesterol after myocardial infarction. N Engl J Med 323:1112–1119
12. Egger M, Dickersin K, Davey Smith G (2001) Problems and limitations in conducting systematic reviews. In: Egger M, Davey Smith G, Altman DG (eds) Systematic Reviews in Health Care: Meta-Analysis in Context, 2nd edn. BMJ Publishing Group, London, pp 43–68
13. Wilkinson P, Sherlock S (1962) The effect of repeated albumin infusions in patients with cirrhosis. Lancet 2:1125–1129
14. Bland RD, Clarke TL, Harden LB, et al (1973) Early albumin infusion to infants at risk for respiratory distress. Arch Dis Child 48:800–805
15. Recinos PR, Hartford CA, Ziffren SE (1975) Fluid resuscitation of burn patients comparing a crystalloid with a colloid containing solution: a prospective study. J Iowa Med Soc 65:426–432
16. Hallowell P, Bland JH, Dalton BC, et al (1978) The effect of hemodilution with albumin or Ringer's lactate on water balance and blood use in open-heart surgery. Ann Thorac Surg 25:22–29
17. Virgilio RW, Metildi LA, Peters RM, Shackford SR (1979) Colloid vs crystalloid volume resuscitation of patients with severe pulmonary insufficiency. Surg Forum 30:166–168
18. Metildi LA, Shackford SR, Virgilio RW, Peters RM (1984) Crystalloid versus colloid in fluid resuscitation of patients with severe pulmonary insufficiency. Surg Gynecol Obstet 158:207–212
19. Rackow EC, Falk JL, Fein IA, et al (1983) Fluid resuscitation in circulatory shock: a comparison of the cardiorespiratory effects of albumin, hetastarch, and saline solutions in patients with hypovolemic and septic shock. Crit Care Med 11:839–850
20. Pockaj BA, Yang JC, Lotze MT, et al (1994) A prospective randomized trial evaluating colloid versus crystalloid resuscitation in the treatment of the vascular leak syndrome associated with interleukin-2 therapy. J Immunother 15:22–28
21. So KW, Fok TF, Ng PC, Wong WW, Cheung KL (1997) Randomised controlled trial of colloid or crystalloid in hypotensive preterm infants. Arch Dis Child Fetal Neonatal Ed 76:F43–46
22. Bodenhamer RM, Johnson RG, Randolph JD, et al (1985) The effect of adding mannitol or albumin to a crystalloid cardioplegic solution: a prospective, randomized clinical study. Ann Thorac Surg 40:374-379
23. Grundmann R, Heistermann S (1985) Postoperative albumin infusion therapy based on colloid osmotic pressure. A prospectively randomized trial. Arch Surg 120:911–915
24. Greenhalgh DG, Housinger TA, Kagan RJ, et al (1995) Maintenance of serum albumin levels in pediatric burn patients: a prospective, randomized trial. J Trauma 39:67–73
25. Grundmann R, von Lehndorff C (1986) Zur Indikation der postoperativen Humalbumintherapie auf der Intensivstation – eine prospektiv randomisierte Studie. Langenbecks Arch Chir 367:235–246
26. Ginès P, Tító L, Arroyo V, et al (1988) Randomized comparative study of therapeutic paracentesis with and without intravenous albumin in cirrhosis. Gastroenterology 94:1493–1502
27. Marelli D, Paul A, Samson R, Edgell D, Angood P, Chiu RC (1989) Does the addition of albumin to the prime solution in cardiopulmonary bypass affect clinical outcome? A prospective randomized study. J Thorac Cardiovasc Surg 98:751–756
28. Adam R, Astarcioglu I, Castaing D, Bismuth H (1991) Ringer's lactate vs serum albumin as a flush solution for UW preserved liver grafts: results of a prospective randomized study. Transplant Proc 23:2374–2375
29. Goslinga H, Eijzenbach V, Heuvelmans JH, et al (1992) Custom-tailored hemodilution with albumin and crystalloids in acute ischemic stroke. Stroke 23:181–188
30. London MJ, Franks M, Verrier ED, Merrick SH, Levin J, Mangano DT (1992) The safety and efficacy of ten percent pentastarch as a cardiopulmonary bypass priming solution. A randomized clinical trial. J Thorac Cardiovasc Surg 104:284–296
31. Gentilini P, Casini-Raggi V, Di Fiore G, et al (1999) Albumin improves the response to diuretics in patients with cirrhosis and ascites: results of a randomized, controlled trial. J Hepatol 30:639–645

32. Oca MJ, Nelson M, Donn SM (1999) Randomized trial of normal saline (NS) versus 5% albumin (ALB) for the treatment of neonatal hypotension. Pediatr Res 45:1265 (Abst)
33. Lennihan L, Mayer SA, Fink ME, et al (2000) Effect of hypervolemic therapy on cerebral blood flow after subarachnoid hemorrhage: a randomized controlled trial. Stroke 31:383–391
34. de Jonge E, Levi M (2001) Effects of different plasma substitutes on blood coagulation: a comparative review. Crit Care Med 29:1261–1267.
35. Addonizio VP, Macarak J, Nicolaou KC, Edmunds LH, Colman RW (1979) Effects of prostacyclin and albumin on platelet loss during in vitro simulation of extracorporeal circulation. Blood 53:1033–1042
36. Boldt J, Zickmann B, Ballesteros BM, Stertmann F, Hempelmann G (1992) Influence of five different priming solutions on platelet function in patients undergoing cardiac surgery. Anesth Analg 74:219–225
37. Wilkes MM, Navickis RJ, Sibbald WJ (2001) Albumin versus hydroxyethyl starch in cardiopulmonary bypass surgery: a meta-analysis of postoperative bleeding. Ann Thorac Surg 72:527–534
38. Task Force of the American College of Critical Care Medicine, Society of Critical Care Medicine (1999) Practice parameters for hemodynamic support of sepsis in adult patients in sepsis. Crit Care Med 27:639–660
39. Emerson TE (1989) Unique features of albumin: a brief review. Crit Care Med 17:690–694
40. Zoellner H, Jing Yun H, Lovery M, et al (1999) Inhibition of microvascular endothelial apoptosis in tissue explants by serum albumin. Microvasc Res 57:162–173
41. Iglesias J, Abernethy VE, Wang Z, Lieberthal W, Koh JS, Levine JS (1999) Albumin is a major serum survival factor for renal tubular cells and macrophages through scavenging of ROS. Am J Physiol 277:F711–722
42. Kamada T, McMillan DE, Sternlieb JJ, Bjork VO, Otsuji S (1988) Albumin prevents erythrocyte crenation in patients undergoing extracorporeal circulation. Scand J Thorac Cardiovasc Surg 22:155–158
43. Gibbs J, Cull W, Henderson W, Daley J, Hur K, Khuri SF (1999) Preoperative serum albumin level as a predictor of operative mortality and morbidity: results from the National VA Surgical Risk Study. Arch Surg 134:36–42
44. Jelenko C, Williams JB, Wheeler ML, et al (1979) Studies in shock and resuscitation I: Use of a hypertonic, albumin-containing, fluid demand regimen (HALFD) in resuscitation. Crit Care Med 7:157–167
45. Mathru M, Rao TL, Kartha RK, Shanmugham M, Jacobs HK (1980) Intravenous albumin administration for prevention of spinal hypotension during cesarean section. Anesth Analg 59:655–658
46. Brown RO, Bradley JE, Bekemeyer WB, Luther RW (1988) Effect of albumin supplementation during parenteral nutrition on hospital morbidity. Crit Care Med 16:1177–1182
47. Isik AZ, Gokmen O, Zeyneloglu HB, Kara S, Keles G, Gulekli B (1996) Intravenous albumin prevents moderate-severe ovarian hyperstimulation in in vitro fertilization patients: a prospective, randomized and controlled study. Eur J Obstet Gynecol Reprod Biol 70:179–183
48. Prien T, Backhaus N, Pelster F, Pircher W, Bünte H, Lawin P (1990) Effect of intraoperative fluid administration and colloid osmotic pressure on the formation of intestinal edema during gastrointestinal surgery. J Clin Anesth 2:317–323
49. Vincent JL (2000) Fluid management: the pharmacoeconomic dimension. Crit Care 4 (suppl 2):S33–35
50. Herwaldt LA, Swartzendruber SK, Edmond MB, et al (1998) The epidemiology of hemorrhage related to cardiothoracic operations. Infect Control Hosp Epidemiol 19:9–16

Metabolic Support

Lipids in Parenteral Nutrition:
Benefits in Critically Ill Patients?

I. Kelbel, P. L. Radermacher, and H. Suger-Wiedeck

▍ Introduction

Currently, total parenteral nutrition (TPN) is used for nutritional support in a wide variety of patients when the enteral route cannot be used. Over the past 30 years, long-chain triglycerides (LCT) derived from soybean or safflower oil have been the source of lipid emulsions for parenteral nutrition. Traditionally, lipid emulsions are included in parenteral nutrition regimes both as part of energy supply and as a source of essential fatty acids. It has become obvious during the last two decades that the amount and type of long-chain fatty acids consumed in the diet can profoundly influence biological responses. Therefore, efforts to further develop and optimize lipid emulsions have focused on replacing part of the LCT by medium-chain triglycerides (MCT). As a result, the physical MCT/LCT mixture is a well proven concept in TPN regimes. Mixed triglyceride molecules obtained by interesterifying MCT and LCT – so called structured triglycerides – are the latest result of this chain of development.

Another concept to reduce the content of LCT is based on the idea of mixing soybean oil with olive oil, the latter being rich in the monounsaturated oleic acid. A more promising step in the evolution of lipid emulsions can be seen in adding fish oil to lipid emulsions in order to combine parenteral nutrition with an anti-inflammatory intervention.

Biochemistry of Lipids

The length and the degree of saturation of the incorporated fatty acids largely determine the physical properties of triglycerides. Under current classification, different groups of fatty acids are defined by their degree of saturation:
▍ Saturated fatty acids (SFA; fatty acids with no double bond),
▍ mono-unsaturated fatty acids (one double bond on position 9; ω-9)
▍ poly-unsaturated fatty acids (PUFA).

SFAs are mainly used for energy supply. Long chain fatty acids of this family are even integral parts of membrane structures. The mono-unsaturated fatty acids, as well as their derivatives, can be synthesized by the organism itself. When the mono-unsaturated fatty acids are not acting as energy donors they are incorporated in triacylglycerides and phospholipids. The PUFA contain two or more double bonds. Based on the position of the first double bond ω-3, ω-6 and ω-9 groups can be identified when the first double bonds are between C3 and C4, C6 and C7, and C9 and C10, respectively. Common dietary fatty acids of the ω-6 series are linoleic acid (18:2 ω-6) and arachidonic acid (20:4 ω-6) and those of the ω-3 series are α-linolenic acid (18:3 ω-3), eicosapentaenoic acid (EPA, 20:5 ω-3) and docosahexaenoic acid (DHA, 22:6 ω-3). These fatty acids have important structural and functional roles and ideally should not be utilized for energy purposes.

▌ Fat as an Essential Component of Nutrition

The human body is unable to synthesize linoleic acid or α-linolenic acid, the main components of the ω-3 and ω-6 series of PUFA. Essential fatty acid deficiency can develop in patients who receive fat-free parenteral nutrition for longer than two weeks. This deficiency is clinically characterized by hepatomegaly, thrombocytopenia, impaired wound healing, hair loss, and dry, desquamated skin. In trauma patients the concentration of linoleic acid in blood decreases severely, especially when fat-free parenteral nutrition is administrated to the patient. There is also agreement about the need for α-linolenic acid as an essential part of nutrition. Thus, Holman et al. [1] first reported a case of a fat-fed child, who exhibited episodes of neuropathy. When TPN was changed to a soybean oil-preparation, the neuropathy disappeared.

In an adequate TPN, 10 g of linoleic acid and 1.2 g of α-linolenic acid, respectively, will prevent essential fatty acid deficiency. In critically ill patients, however, the demand on linoleic acid can rise up to 50 g per day.

▌ Fat as an Energy Source

Intensive care patients with sepsis and trauma are characterized by hypermetabolism, insulin resistance with hyperglycemia and marked catabolism. If requirement for muscle protein continues unabated, protein breakdown will result in severe depletion of vital proteins. Thus, the main goal of nutrition in critically ill patients must be the improvement in protein economy, avoiding muscle protein breakdown for the purpose of energy supply. The administration of lipids alone, however, has minimal, or no, effect on nitrogen metabolism. By contrast, in association with amino acids, lipid emulsions induce significant improvements in net nitrogen balance [2], although some of these effects can also be attributed to the glycerol-containing lipid emulsion.

Intravenous fat emulsions are usually added to the TPN regime as they provide a concentrated source of calories (9 kcal/g) with a relatively low osmotic load. Lipid application offers diversification of energy input with reduced effects of excessive glucose supply. Carbohydrate overfeeding is associated with significant side effects such as excessive CO_2-production and increased adrenergic activation, indicating the need for a non-carbohydrate energy source. Glucose-based TPN has been shown to cause adverse effects related to glucose storage, particularly as fat. This might account for the extensive lipid deposition reported both in liver and adipose tissue. It is conceivable that lipid administration could prevent such hepatic steatosis [3].

The lipid component of most emulsions for parenteral nutrition consists of LCT, which have proven to be both an effective and a reliable source of energy and of essential fatty acids. Lipids should account for 20 to 30% of the total caloric input. The maximum lipid elimination capacity is about 3.8 g/kg/day. At this rate, excessive hepatic uptake of lipids would lead to steatosis.

For parenteral nutrition, commercial fat emulsions with 10 or 20% triglycerides are available. The use of the 20% fat emulsions seems to be more appropriate because of a reduced triglyceride/phospholipid ratio [4]. However, the use of high levels of LCT has been implicated as the cause of impaired host defense and increased infectious complications [5–7], which in turn has emphasized the need for alternatives.

Lipid Emulsions Containing MCT/LCT

MCT might be preferable for patients in stress due to their higher need for energy. Because of their smaller molecular size and greater solubility, MCT offer a more rapid clearance from the circulation than LCT. In contrast to LCT they are not stored as body fat and are oxidized more rapidly. Furthermore, they are independent of carnitine acyltransferase and are promptly transferred into mitochondria for β-oxidation. Compared to pure LCT emulsions, MCT have an increased rate of oxidation [8]. MCT induce the synthesis of ketone bodies in the liver to a greater extent than LCT [9], thus offering an additional source of energy for the gut and central nervous system.

MCT are better substrates for hepatocytes, induce less fat deposition, and have a lower ability to acquire and transport cholesteryl ester and, therefore, induce fewer alterations in bile composition. The above qualities may be responsible for protective effects on liver function [10]. Prolonged administration of LCT leads to immunosuppressive effects, in terms of a reduction in lymphokine-activated killer cell activity [6] and impairment of neutrophil bactericidal [7] and RES (reticuloendothelial system) function [11], which could be virtually avoided by the administration of MCT/LCT emulsions. In addition, pure LCT emulsions are known to reduce oxygen tension (PaO_2) and increase both the pulmonary venous admixture (Qva/Qt) and the mean pulmonary artery pressure (PAP) [12]. These effects are probably due to the production of arachidonic acid and increased production of prostaglandin (PG)I_2 and thromboxane (TX)A_2. Sepsis appears to aggravate this metabolic cascade. Radermacher et al. [13] investigated the pulmonary vascular and gas exchange effects of a fat emulsion containing MCT in patients with sepsis syndrome receiving TPN. These authors demonstrated that LCT/MCT 1:1 emulsions did not increase the formation of TXA_2 and PGI_2 and did not cause any significant alterations in pulmonary hemodynamics and gas exchange. Finally, Suchner et al. [14] concluded from their studies in patients with acute respiratory distress syndrome (ARDS), that a changing balance of PGI_2 and TXA_2 modulates gas exchange, presumably via interference with hypoxic pulmonary vasoconstriction [14].

Therefore, and probably by minimizing the amount of ω-6 fatty acid disposal for arachidonic acid metabolism to produce proinflammatory eicosanoids, LCT/MCT emulsions appear to be particularly beneficial for patients with ARDS.

Lipid Emulsions containing Structured Triglyceride

Hydrolysis of a mixture of LCT and MCT followed by random reesterification on the same glycerol backbone gives a structured triglyceride as endproduct (Fig. 1). Structured triglycerides may be less toxic and have a lower tendency to promote acidosis compared to physical mixtures of MCT and LCT, because these tri-

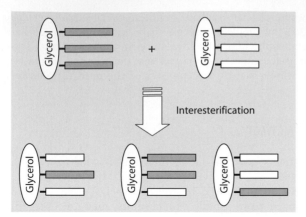

Fig. 1. Grey columns present long-chain fatty acids (LCFA), white indicate medium-chain fatty acids (MCFA). By interesterification between medium-chain triglycerides (MCT) and long-chain triglycerides (LCT) a number of different new molecules are formed comprising one to two LCFA and two to one MCFA per molecule, respectively

glycerides seem to interact with each other during plasma and tissue elimination. Sandström et al. [15] demonstrated that intravenous administration of structured triglyceride versus pure LCT emulsions was associated with increased whole body fat oxidation in stressed postoperative patients. Structured triglyceride has been shown to improve nitrogen balance in human studies [16, 17] when compared to LCT emulsions and a physical mixture of MCT/LCT. However, Chambrier et al. [18] did not find a significant difference in nitrogen balance between patients receiving either structured triglyceride or a physical MCT/LCT mixture for TPN after abdominal surgery.

In conclusion, although it has been shown, both in healthy volunteers and in postoperative patients, that structured triglyceride is a save and well tolerated lipid emulsion, further studies are obligatory to investigate potential benefits of structured triglyceride compared to the conventional LCT or LCT/MCT emulsions in clinical settings.

▍ Lipid containing Olive Oil

Long-term TPN with soybean oil-based lipid emulsions may be associated with increased lipid oxidation and decreased vitamin E nutritional status. Patients undergoing major surgery are exposed to metabolic stress situations together with an increased synthesis of radicals and other highly reactive compounds, i.e., in the situation of ischemic reperfusion injury. Supplementation with antioxidants such as vitamin E was shown to reduce the production of free radicals and lipid peroxidation products and to decrease cell damage, indicating a benefit on the clinical outcome of these patients [18, 19].

Consequently, the recently developed olive oil-based lipid emulsion contains the more biologically active a-tocopherol. From their animal studies, Dutot et al. [20] obtained evidence that olive oil emulsions are a better source of antioxidants and should contribute to decreased peroxidation. Gracia de Lorenzo and colleagues [21], however, found no differences between olive/soy bean oil lipid emulsions and a physical mixture of MCT and LCT on the nutritional status in burned patients. A controversial statement was made by Arborati et al. [22], who concluded that reduction of the PUFA and simultaneous substitution with MCT constitutes the best approach to the reduction in susceptibility of lipid emulsions to peroxidative modification.

In contrast to linoleic acid-rich lipid emulsions, known to decrease cell-mediated immunity, oleic acid-rich emulsions do not affect lymphocyte proliferation and interleukin (IL)-2 production by cultured cells [23]. In rats fed with a diet rich in oleic acid, greater lymphocyte activation was measured compared to rats fed with a soybean oil emulsion [24]. These results indicate that olive oil may offer an immunological alternative to soybean oil for nutrition.

Therefore, further studies on the potential advantages of lipid emulsions containing olive oil compared to MCT/LCT are necessary.

▌ Fish Oil as a Modulator of Biochemical Functions

Eicosanoids

The lipid requirement of all mammals is met by their dietary intake or by the *de novo* synthesis of fatty acids. The ω-3 and ω-6 PUFAs are essential fatty acids that cannot be synthesized by mammals and, therefore, must be obtained from dietary sources. The precursor of the ω-6 is linoleic acid, a major component of plant oils such as corn, sunflower, soybean and safflower oils primarily in the form of α-linolenic acid. The precursor of the ω-3 family of PUFAs is α-linolenic acid found in green plant tissue and some plant oils. Marine fish oils have a considerably higher content of the ω-3 fatty acids, mostly in the form of EPA and DHA. The epidemiological studies of Bang and Dyberg [25] showed that Innuit, consuming mainly fish oil, have a lower rate of coronary disease and cancer, asthma, psoriasis and diabetes compared to a matched population of Danes. These findings point towards anti-thrombotic and anti-inflammatory properties of EPA, the major ω-3 fatty acid in fish oil. The biochemical basis for the proposed beneficial effects may be the inhibitory action of ω-3 fatty acids on the cyclooxygenase pathway. When ω-3 fatty acids are included in the diet, EPA competes with arachidonic acid (the main fatty acid of the ω-6 family) at the cyclooxygenase and the 5-lipoxygenase levels. This circumstance causes modulation of the products of diene prostanoids (e.g., PGE_2, PGI_2, TXA_2) and of tretaene leukotrienes (i.e., leukotriene C_4) derived from arachidonic acid in favor of the corresponding triene prostanoids (i.e., PGE_3, PGI_3, TXA_3) and pentaene leukotriene (LTC_5) derived from EPA (Fig. 2). Examination of the EPA/AA ratio in several cells, i.e., erythrocytes, neutrophils, platelets, endothelial cells, monocytes, and brain and liver cells, demonstrated that ω-3 FA are preferentially incorporated into membranes. This results in an enhanced release of EPA-derived products with an attenuated spectrum of biological activity than products derived from arachidonic acid [26]. Compared to arachidonic acid, the derivatives of EPA have less-proinflammatory and chemotactic characteristics.

To profit from this knowledge, ω-3 fatty acid-enriched lipid infusions have been used to combine parenteral nutrition with an anti-inflammatory intervention, by shifting the arachidonic acid/EPA ratio towards predominance of the latter lipid precursor [27]. Consequently, attempts have been made to use fish oil (ω-3 FA) in the treatment of numerous diseases.

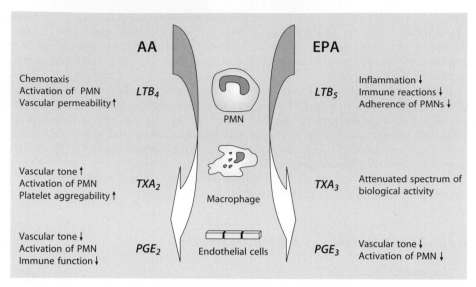

Fig. 2. Influence of arachidonic acid (AA) and eicosapentaenoic acid (EPA) on immune function. LT: leukotriene; TX: thromboxane; PG: prostaglandin; PMN: polymorphonuclear leukocyte. (From [37] with permission)

Immune system

The results of several studies on dietary supplementation with ω-3 FA have shown a favorable influence of fish oil nutrition on pathophysiological responses to endotoxin, and important effects on eicosanoid and cytokine biology [28]. The modulation of cytokine biology may occur by changing the substrate availability for lipid-derived mediators and altering membrane fluidity by the modified fatty acid composition of the cell membrane [29]. Membrane fluidity influences the binding of cytokines and cytokine-induced agonists to the receptors and may alter G-protein activity, thereby changing adenylate kinase, phospholipase A_2 and phospholipase C activity. The incorporation of ω-3 FA into cell phospholipids also alter the production of non-eicosanoid secondary messengers such as PAF (platelet activating factor), phosphatidic acid, diacylglycerol, and ceramide [30]. Indeed, inflammatory symptoms of rheumatoid arthritis, psoriasis, Crohn's disease and ulcerative colitis are ameliorated by fish oil preparations whether or not directly related to cytokine production (IL-1α, IL-1β, IL-6, tumor necrosis factor [TNF]-α and -β) in response to inflammatory stimulation [31]. In addition, intravenous application of a 10% lipid emulsion rich in fish oil significantly improved survival from endotoxemia in guinea pigs compared with infusion of a 10% (v/v) safflower oil (enriched in ω-6 fatty acids) emulsion [32]. These clinical effects could be explained as follows: Dietary fish oil leads to a decreased production of proinflammatory substances like LTB$_4$ and PAF, released by the action of cytokines. Since ω-3 fatty acids lead to a reduced production of PGE$_2$, they might act as a PGE$_2$ antagonist and thus enhance production of Th1-type cytokines (IL-2 and interferon [IFN]-γ) and T-lymphocyte proliferation and decrease production of Th2-type cytokines (IL-4, IL-10) and TGF-β (transforming growth factor). Th1-type cytokines are important in promoting the activity of macrophages, natural killer cells, and cytotoxic lymphocytes and therefore are relevant for host defense against bacteria, viruses, and fungi [33]. If these effects indeed occur, the ω-3 FA would be a useful therapeutic agent in systemic inflammatory response syndrome (SIRS) and sepsis.

ω-3 fatty acids may also modulate regional blood flow and possibly prevent intestinal ischemia. In an endotoxin rat model, fish oil administration abolished the endotoxin-induced decrease of splanchnic blood flow and ameliorated the bacterial defense of the splanchnic region [34]. The lower content of viable bacteria in the gut of fish oil treated rats was interpreted as a result of an improved killing of translocated bacteria rather than a reduction of translocation.

Considering clinical and experimental evidence that dietary intake of ω-3 FA may influence the immune function of the RES and circulating phagocytes [35], we investigated whether or not blood clearance and organ distribution of systemically applied *E. coli* might be improved after infusion of lipid emulsions enriched with ω-3 FA compared with clinically used ω-6 FA emulsions [36]. ω-6 FA infusion produced a significant delay in blood clearance compared to saline and ω-3 FA treatment (Fig. 3). The diminished systemic bacterial elimination after ω-6 FA was accompanied by increased numbers of viable bacteria in lung (Fig. 4) and spleen. Moreover, Cukier et al. [37] demonstrated that four days of lipid infusion with ω-3 FA emulsions improved phagocytotic activity of alveolar macrophages in comparison to placebo and soybean oil application. A series of functional alterations induced by diets enriched with ω-3 FA might contribute to the described effects, i.e., an increased production of cytokines [38], improved cell-mediated immunity [39] and opsonization index [40], as well as an increase in antigen-induced lymphocyte generation [40]. In animal experiments, Ertel et al. [41] observed increased cytokine production (IL-1, IL-2), reduced PGE_2 release from macrophages, and an improvement in both the capacity of antigen presentation and splenocyte proliferation following hemorrhagic shock in those animals which had been fed ω-3 FA instead of ω-6 FA. Finally, a recently published animal study [42] demonstrated that in

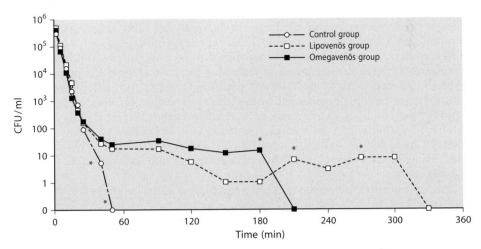

Fig. 3. Time course of bacterial elimination from blood after injection of *E. coli* (1.3×10^8 colony-forming units, CFU) in rabbits pretreated with a fish oil (Omegavenös group), a soybean oil (Lipovenös group) emulsion (1.5 g/kg/d for 3 days), or the equivalent volume of 0.9% saline (control group). *=p < 0.05 versus all other groups. (From [37] with permission)

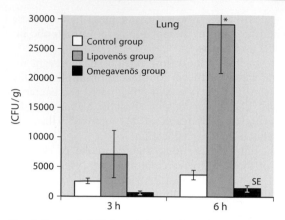

Fig. 4. Counts of viable bacteria in lung homogenates taken 3 hours and 6 hours after injection of *E. coli* in rabbits pretreated with a fish oil (Omegavenös group), a soybean oil (Lipovenös group) emulsion (1.5 g/kg/d for 3 days), or the equivalent volume of 0.9% saline (control group). *=p<0.01 versus all other groups. (From [37] with permission)

Sprague-Dawley rats infused with a 1:1 fish oil-soybean oil mix following the onset of sepsis, mortality was significantly decreased compared to saline infused rats. Fish oil lowered PGE$_2$ production, totally prevented sepsis-induced suppression of splenocyte proliferation and IL-2 production as well as TGF-β production. Synthesis of IL-10 by splenocytes was significantly reduced after fish oil feeding compared with saline or soybean oil infusion. In conclusion, fish oil prevents the production of the immunosuppressive cytokine TGF-β and maintains the Th-1 response during sepsis [43].

In contrast to this, in autoimmune disease [43], ω-3 FA are known to promote the synthesis of TGF-β. The reason for this cannot be discerned from the results of this study [44], but they provide evidence that fish oil can alter the responses to different types of immunology challenges in different ways, and, at least partly, acts to restore the balance between Th1- and Th2-type responses.

Nevertheless, it must be taken into account that the response to an inflammatory stimulus is biphasic: Persistent and uncontrolled secretion of pro-inflammatory cytokines (TNF-α, IL-1, IL-6, and IL-8) has been implicated in the pathophysiology of SIRS [44] and multiple organ dysfunction [45]. In response to this pro-inflammatory reaction, the body also mounts an anti-inflammatory response [46]. IL-4, IL-10 and IL-11 participate in this compensatory anti-inflammatory response syndrome (CARS) by, for example, inhibiting T- and B-lymphocyte activity [47]. If CARS is sufficiently severe, it will manifest as anergy and increased susceptibility to infection.

The key components of early sepsis are regarded as suitable targets for therapeutical interventions with fish oil emulsions, whereas it remains to be elucidated whether ω-3 FA can have beneficial effects in late chronic sepsis with anti-inflammatory features.

Pulmonary Functions

In the early phase of SIRS and sepsis, overwhelming activation of humoral and cellular mediator systems can alter vascular resistance and cause capillary leakage – the major pathophysiological event during the development of ARDS. ω-6 FA are released from lipid pools of cellular membranes during inflammation and are metabolized to pro-inflammatory prostaglandins and leukotrienes, which are essentially involved in the pathogenesis of pulmonary lesions after shock, trauma and sepsis by changing vascular tone and disturbing epithelial and endothelial barrier function in the microcirculation of the lung and other organs. We investigated the efficacy of short-term ω-3 FA supplementation with respect to the inflammatory pulmonary vascular reaction in isolated perfused rabbit lungs [48, 49]. A rapid increase in free fatty acids (EPA and DHA) in plasma and lung tissue could be observed in the ω-3 FA infused lung (Figs. 5, 6). In this study, a synthetic calcium ionophor, A 23187, was used as a stimulus for ionized calcium-influx by forming artificial pores in the cell membranes resembling the effects of pore-forming bacterial toxins. In ω-3 FA treated lungs, a shift in A 23187-stimulated leukotriene synthesis from LTC_4 to LTC_5 (Fig 7), as well as reduced TXA_2 biosynthesis was observed. These findings paralleled the observations of an effectively attenuated pressure increase (Fig. 8a) and weight gain (Fig. 8b) as well as reduced pulmonary capillary filtration [50]. Taking into account that TXA_2 is known to be the predominant mediator of the arachidonic acid-induced pressure response, surpassing the vasodilator properties of the simultaneously liberated prostacyclin, this assumption might explain the reduced vascular reaction brought about by pre-treatment with fish oil. The reduced pulmonary capillary filtration and edema formation may be due to the decreased LTC_4 production and shift to LTC_5 during and after dietary supplemention with fish oil.

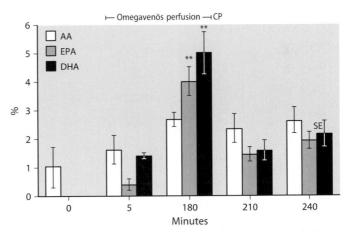

Fig. 5. Time course of detection of arachidonic acid (AA, *reverse-hatched bars*), eicosapentaenoic acid (EPA, *open bars*), and docosahexaenoic acid (DHA, *dotted bars*) in the perfusate lipids of isolated, recirculation-perfused rabbit lungs. Perfusate was collected during and after fish oil emulsion supplementation. Values at 210 and 240 minutes were obtained after elimination of circulating lipids by exchanging the perfusion fluid (CP). The quantities of AA, EPA, and DHA were expressed as a percentage of the total amount of free fatty acids. Data are presented as mean ±SEM from six lungs. **p<0.001 vs. corresponding baseline values (0 min), as well as vs. values after 5 minutes of lipid infusion. (From [49] with permission)

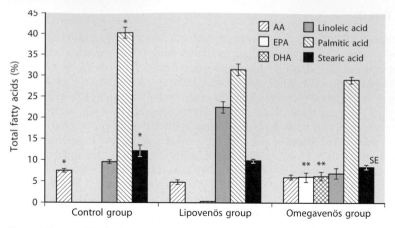

Fig. 6. Influence of lipid infusion on fatty acid content of lung tissue. Lung tissue samples were collected from rabbit lungs following treatment with saline (control group), soybean oil preparation (Lipovenös group), or fish oil emulsion (Omegavenös group).* $p < 0.05$, ** $p < 0.001$ vs. all other groups. Data are expressed as mean ± SEM. AA: arachidonic acid; EPA: eicosapentaenoic acid; DHA: docosahexaenoic acid. (From [49] with permission)

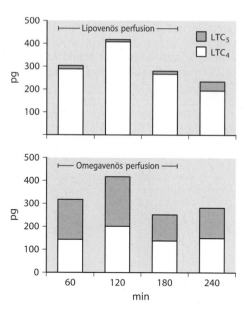

Fig. 7. Leukotriene (LT) C_4 (*open bars*) and leukotriene C_5 (*dotted bars*) generation in isolated rabbit lungs perfused with either 10% fish oil emulsion (*bottom*) or 10% soybean oil preparation (*top*). Samples were taken 30 minutes after activation of the lungs by calcium-ionophore A 23187 (10^{-8} M). Values at 60, 120, and 180 minutes represent leukotriene synthesis in the presence of either soybean oil preparation or fish oil emulsion in the perfusion fluid, whereas the value at 240 minutes was obtained after the infusion had been stopped. (From [49] with permission)

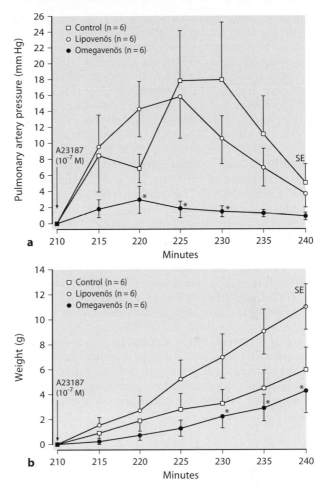

Fig. 8. a Increase in pulmonary arterial pressure and **b** weight changes (as an indicator of extravascular lung water after calcium ionophore A 23187 (10^{-7} M) application following a preceding 3-hour perfusion period with saline (*open squares*), 10% soybean oil preparation (*open circles*), or 10% fish oil emulsion (*solid circles*) in an experimental rabbit lung model. Data are mean ± SEM, *$p < 0.05$ vs. corresponding values in the soybean oil preparation group. (From [49] with permission)

In view of the pivotal role of lipid mediators in mediating inflammatory reactions after shock, trauma and sepsis, these studies may suggest that short-term ω-3 FA supplementation could be an additional, acute, anti-inflammatory therapeutic approach in patients with inflammatory disorders.

▌ Conclusion

In clinical practice, lipids are a suitable energy source whenever TPN is indicated. Withholding lipid emulsions from parenteral nutrition dependent patients is not free from risk as carbohydrate overfeeding and the symptoms of essential fatty acid deficiency with impaired wound healing and hepatic steatosis must be avoided, especially in critically ill patients. Isolated organ failure *per se* is not a contraindication for parenteral application of lipid emulsions [50], but it should be used with care in cases of impaired tissue blood flow and peripheral oxygen deficiency.

Lipid emulsions derived from soybean oil with a high PUFA content and an insufficient amount of the antioxidant α-tocopherol may cause impaired host defense and increased infectious complications. Increasing PUFA intake mounts oxidative stress, which, if not counterbalanced by antioxidants, can cause lipid peroxidation and tissue damage. Therefore, physical mixtures of MCT and LCT may be an optimal fatty acid composition of lipid emulsions for parenteral nutrition of critically ill patients. This emulsion carries the positive qualities of a higher oxidative rate, the preservation of liver function, and the maintenance of immune and RES function. Finally, MCT/LCT emulsions seem not to interfere with pulmonary hemodynamics and gas exchange.

To improve these attributes of lipid emulsions a variety of new emulsions based on structured triglycerides, olive oil, or fish oil have been developed. An important common characteristic of these emulsions is the reduction of the high PUFA load of soybean oil. These new emulsions have been shown to be safe and well tolerated, but further studies are necessary to investigate potential advantages compared to LCT/MCT emulsions in clinical settings.

A promising emulsion in the development of lipid emulsions seems to be fish oil. Although the published studies have only investigated in part the broad spectrum of biological effects induced by ω-3 FA, the results suggest that ω-3 FA, apart from nutritional aspects, may be a useful approach in critically ill patients. In view of the current data, it can be concluded that the infusion of EPA-enriched lipid emulsions is capable of inducing important modulation on eicosanoid and cytokine biology and beneficially influencing the pathophysiological response to inflammation.

References

1. Holman R, Johnson S, Hatch T (1982) A case of human linolenic acid deficiency involving neurological abnormalities. Am J Clin Nutr 35:617–623
2. Radermacher P, Grote H, Herbertz L, Reinauer H (1982) Effect of lipid infusions on triglyceride and protein metabolism. Infusionther Klin Ernahr 9:279–85
3. Nussbaum M, Li S, Bower R, McFadden D, Dayal R, Fischer J (1992) Addition of lipid to total parenteral nutrition prevents hepatic steatosis in rats by lowering the portal venous insulin/glucagon ratio. J Parenter Enteral Nutr 16:106–109
4. Roulet M, Wiesel P, Chapuis G, Carpentier Y (1993) Effects of intravenously infused egg phospholipids on lipid and lipoprotein metabolism in postoperative trauma. J Parenter Enteral Nutr 17:107–112
5. Fisher GW, Hunter KW, Wilson SR, Mease D (1980) Diminished bacterial defense with Intralipid. Lancet ii:819–820
6. Sedman PC, Somers SS, Ramsden CW, Brennan TG, Guillou PJ (1991) Effects of different lipid emulsions on lymphocyte function during total parenteral nutrition. Br J Surg 78:1396–1399
7. Waitzberg DL, Bellinati-Pires R, Salgado MM, et al (1997) Effect of total parenteral nutrition with different lipid emulsions on human monocyte and neutrophil functions. Nutrition 13:128–132
8. Adolph M, Hailer S, Eckart J (1995) Serum phospholipid fatty acids in severely injured patients on total parenteral nutrition with medium chain/long chain triglyceride emulsions. Ann Nutr Metab 39:251–260

9. Jansing P, Reinauer H (1978) Human catabolism of medium and long chain triglycerides after intravenous infusion. Infusionsther Klin Ernähr 5:26–32
10. Carpentier YA, Dubois DY, Siderova VS, Richelle M (1994) Exogenous lipids and hepatic function. In: Kinney JM, Tucker HN (eds) Organ Metabolism and Nutrition. Raven Press, New York, pp 349–367
11. Sobrado J, Moldawer LL, Pomposelli JJ, Mascioli EA (1985) Lipid emulsions and reticuloendothelial system function in healthy and burned guinea pigs. Am J Clin Nutr 42:855–863
12. Smyrniotis VE, Kostopanagiotou GG, Arkadopoulos NF, et al (2001) Long-chain versus medium-chain lipids in acute pancreatitis complicated by acute respiratory distress syndrome: effects on pulmonary hemodynamics and gas exchange. Clin Nutr 20:139–143
13. Radermacher P, Santak B, Strobach H, Schrör K, Tarnow J (1992) Fat emulsions containing medium chain triglycerides in patients with sepsis syndrome: Effects on pulmonary hemodynamics and gas exchange. Intensive Care Med 18:231–234
14. Suchner U, Katz DP, Furst P, et al (2001) Effects of intravenous fat emulsions on lung function in patients with acute respiratory distress syndrome or sepsis. Crit Care Med 29:1569–1574
15. Sandström R, Hyltander A, Körner U, Lundholm K (1995) Structured triglycerides were well tolerated and induced increased whole body fat oxidation compared with long-chain triglycerides in postoperative patients. J Parenter Enteral Nutr 19:381–386
16. Lindgren BF, Ruokonen E, Magnusson-Borg K, Takala J (2001) Nitrogen sparing effect of structured triglycerides containing both medium- and long-chain fatty acids in critically ill patients; a double blind randomised controlled trial. Clin Nutr 20:43–48
17. Kruimel JW, Naber TH, van der Vliet JA, Carneheim C, Katan MB, Jansen JB (2001) Parenteral structured triglyceride emulsion improves nitrogen balance and is cleared faster from the blood in moderately catabolic patients. J Parenter Enteral Nutr 25:237–244
18. Rabl H, Ratschek M, Khoschsorur G, et al (1997) Limitation of intestinal reperfusion injury in the rat by vitamin treatment. Med Sci Res 25:315–318
19. Linseisen J, Hoffmann J, Lienhard S, Jauch KW, Wolfram G (2000) Antioxidant status of surgical patients receiving TPN with an ω-3-fatty acid-containing lipid emulsion supplemented with α-tocopherol. Clin Nutr 19:177–184
20. Dutot G, Melin C (1991) Assessment of lipid peroxidation during lipid infusion: influence of fatty acid composition of fat emulsion. Clin Nutr 10 (Suppl 2):50 (Abst)
21. Gracia de Lorenzo A, Denia R, Martinez Ratero S, et al (2000) Randomised, double-blinded study in severely burned patients under short term total parenteral nutrition (TPN) with a new olive-oil based lipid emulsion vs. MCT/LCT lipid emulsion. Clin Nutr 19 (Suppl 1):177 (Abst)
22. Arborati M, Ninio E, Chapman MJ, Sultan F (1997) Comparison of lipoperoxide content and lipoperoxidability in parenteral fat emulsions with different triglyceride content. Clin Nutr 16 (Suppl 2):O18 (Abst)
23. Granato D, Blum S, Rössle C, Le Boucher J, Malnoe A, Dutot G (2000) Effects of parenteral lipid emulsions with different fatty acid composition on immune cell functions *in vitro*. J Parenter Enteral Nutr 24:113–118
24. Moussa M, Boucher LE, Garcia J, et al (2000) In vivo effects of olive oil-based lipid emulsion on lymphocyte activation in rats. Clin Nutr 19:49–54
25. Dyerberg J, Bang HO, Hjorne N (1975) Fatty acid composition of the plasma lipids in Greenland eskimos. Am J Clin Nutr 28:958–966
26. Weber PC, Fischer S, von Schacky C, et al (1986) Dietary omega-3 polyunsaturated fatty acids and eiosanoid formation in man. In: Simopoulos AP, Kifer RR, Martin RE (eds) Health Effects of Polyunsaturated Acids in Seafoods. Academic Press, Orlando, pp: 49–60
27. Weber PC (1989) Clinical studies on the effect of n-3 fatty acids on cells and eicosanoids in cardiovascular system. J Intern Med 225:61–68
28. Fürst P (1998) Old and new substrates in clinical nutrition. J Nutr 128:789–796
29. Grimble RF (1998) Dietary lipids and the inflammatory response. Proc Nutr Soc 57:535–542
30. Ross JA, Moses AGW Fearon KCH (1999) The anti-catabolic effects of n-3 fatty acids. Curr Opin Clin Nutr Met Care 2:219–226

31. Caughey GE, Mantzioris E, Gibson RA, Cleland LG, James MJ (1996) The effect on human tumor necrosis factor alpha and interleukin 1 beta production of diets enriched in n-3 fatty acids from vegetable oil or fish oil. Am J Clin Nutr 63:116–122
32. Mascioli EA, Leader L, Flores E, Trimbo S, Bistrian B, Blackburn G (1988) Enhanced survival to endotoxin in guinea pigs fed iv fish oil emulsion. Lipids 23:623–625
33. Mossman TR, Sad S (1996) The expanding universe of T-cell subsets: Th1, Th2 and more. Immunol Today 17:138–146
34. Pscheidl E, Schywalsky M, Tschaikowski K, Böke-Pröls T (2000) Fish oil supplemented parenteral diets normalize splanchnic blood flow and improve killing of translocated bacteria in a low-dose endotoxin rat model. Crit Care Med 28:1489–1496
35. Fritsche KL, Shahabazian LM, Feng C, Berg JN (1997) Dietary fish oil reduces survival and impairs bacterial clearance in C3H/Hen mice challenged with Listeria monocytogenes. Clin Sci (Lond) 92:95–101
36. Kelbel I, Koch T, Prechtl A, et al (1999) Effects of parenteral application of fish oil versus soy oil emulsion on bacterial clearance functions. Infusionsther Transfusionsmed 26:226–232
37. Cukier C, Waitzberg DL, Logullo AF, et al (1999) Lipid and lipid-free total parenteral nutrition: differential effects on macrophage phagocytosis in rats. Nutrition 15:885–889
38. Watanabe S, Hayashi H, Onozaki K, Okuyama H (1991) Effect of dietary alpha-linolenate/linoleate balance on lipopolysaccharide-induced tumor necrosis factor production in mouse macrophages. Life Sci 28:2013–2020
39. Alexander JW, Saito H, Trocki O, Ogle CK (1986) The importance of lipid type in the diet after burn injury. Ann Surg 204:1–8
40. Cerra FB, Alden PA, Negro F, et al (1988) Sepsis and exogenous lipid modulation. J Parenter Enteral Nutr 12 (6 Suppl):63S–68S
41. Ertel W, Morrison MH, Ayala A, Chaudry IH (1993) Modulation of macrophage membrane phospholipids by n-3 polyunsaturated fatty acids increases interleukin-1 release and prevents suppression of cellular immunity following hemorrhagic shock. Arch Surg 128:15–21
42. Lanza-Jacoby S, Flynn JT, Miller S (2001) Parenteral supplementation with fish oil emulsion prolongs survival and improves lymphocyte function during sepsis. Nutrition 17:112–116
43. Fernades G, Bysani C, Venkatramen JT, Tomar V, Zhao W (1994) Increased TGF-β and decreased oncogene expression by ω-3 fatty acids in the spleen delays onset of autoimmune disease in B/W mice. J Immunol 152:5979–5987
44. Shayevitz JR, Miller C, Johnson KJ, Rodriguez JL (1995) Multiple organ dysfunction syndrom: end organ and systemic inflammatory response in a mouse model of nonseptic origin. Shock 4:389–396
45. Pinsky MR, Vincent JL, Deviere J, Alegre M, Kahn RJ, Dupont E (1993) Serum cytokine levels in human septic shock; Relation to multiple-system organ failure and mortality. Chest 103:565–575
46. Bone RC (1996) Sir Isaac Newton, sepsis, SIRS, and CARS. Crit Care Med 24:1125–1128
47. Abraham E (1991) Physiological stress and cellular ischemia: Relationship to immunosuppression and susceptibility to infection. Crit Care Med 19:613–618
48. Breil I, Koch T, Heller A, et al (1996) Alteration of n-3 fatty acid composition in lung tissue after short-term infusion of fish oil emulsion attenuates inflammatory vascular reaction. Crit Care Med 24:1893–1902
49. Koch T, Heller A, Breil I, van Ackern K, Neuhof H (1995) Alterations of pulmonary capillary filtration and leukotriene-synthesis, due to infusion of a lipid emulsion enriched with omega-3 fatty acids. Clin Intensive Care 6:112–120
50. Druml W, Fischer M, Ratheiser K (1998) Use of intravenous lipids in critically ill patients with sepsis without and with hepatic failure. J Parenter Enteral Nutr 22:217–223

Early Enteral Nutrition in the Intensive Care Unit

F. M. P. van Haren and J. G. van der Hoeven

▌ Introduction

Nutritional support for critically ill patients independently influences outcome and should be considered an integral component of critical care. Decisive factors are route of feeding, timing, composition, and amount of different nutrients delivered. A recent survey among European intensivists showed that the preferred modality was enteral nutrition, instituted before the 48th hour after admission [1].

This chapter focuses on the role of early administration of enteral nutrition in the intensive care unit (ICU). Arbitrarily we define enteral nutrition within 6 hours of admission to the ICU as immediate, within 24 hours as early, and after 24 hours as late. We will discuss the pathophysiological concepts of early enteral nutrition and review available clinical studies.

▌ Concepts behind Early Initiation of Enteral Feeding

Failure of the gut barrier function after injury may result in increased bacterial and endotoxin translocation as has been shown in both animal and human studies [2, 3]. According to the so-called gut hypothesis this causes or contributes to the development of multiple organ failure (MOF). An increase in intestinal permeability has been shown in patients with severe injuries and burns, ischemia-reperfusion, after cardiac surgery, and in those receiving only parenteral nutrition [4, 5–12]. Recently, a lot of work has been done trying to understand the link between gut barrier failure and lung injury. Mesenteric lymph appears to be the route by which gut-derived toxic factors exit the gut to induce lung injury, through up-regulation of microvascular adhesion molecules [13–16]. This hypothesis is supported by the fact that this phenomenon can be prevented by mesenteric lymph duct ligation [16, 17].

The beneficial effects of early administration of enteral nutrition are probably mediated through preservation of the gut barrier function and attenuation of the hypermetabolic stress response. This concept is based on animal experiments performed in the mid-1980s. Following major thermal injury in guinea pigs, immediate enteral feeding was associated with a decrease in hypermetabolism and suppression of the catabolic hormones glucagon, cortisol, and norepinephrine [18]. Resting energy expenditure measured 2 weeks after the injury was lower in the early feeding group. Atrophy of the short bowel was more severe in the delayed enteral feeding group. A decade after this experiment, the link with bacterial translocation was made. Delayed enteral feeding led to an increase in bacterial translocation that was associated with an increase in serum cortisol and hypermetabolism [19]. A delay of more than 6 hours following the injury diminished the positive effect of early enteral feeding, suggesting that feeding should be instituted immediately [20].

In human studies, early enteral nutrition has also been shown to decrease intestinal permeability [4, 6, 8, 12, 21]. For example, in one study, 28 multiple injury patients who had recovered from shock within 6 hours where randomized in two groups [22]. The first group received immediate intragastric tube feeding a median of 4.4 hours after ICU admission; the second group received total parenteral nutrition (TPN) within 6 hours, followed by enteral feeding a median of 36.6 hours after admission. Intestinal permeability was measured on days 2 and 4 using a lactose/mannitol (L/M) clearance assay. On postinjury day 4, the L/M ratio was significantly higher in the second group suggesting that immediate enteral nutrition protects against an increase in intestinal permeability induced by multiple injury.

There are some difficulties interpreting this and other studies. The use of differential sugar absorption tests as a measure for intestinal permeability has several limitations. First, intestinal permeability measured with these methods does not represent (immunological) gut barrier function and cannot easily be extrapolated to bacterial and endotoxin translocation. Second, reported values for healthy subjects vary considerably and interpretation of values obtained in the ICU population is even more difficult. Differential sugar absorption using mannitol after red blood cell transfusion is unreliable since bank blood contains mannitol. Tests that use sucrose (to assess gastroduodenal permeability) as well as cellobiose are influenced by renal function (endogenous creatinine clearance); in contrast, mannitol is not [23].

Direct measurement of endotoxin concentration in sera bypasses the above-mentioned problems. In a study comparing enteral with parenteral nutrition 1 week before until 2 weeks after thoracic esophagectomy, patients who received enteral feeding had significantly lower endotoxin concentrations in sera [24]. Moreover, the TPN group had significantly higher serum interleukin (IL)-6 and IL-10 concentrations, suggesting that the reduced inflammatory responses were related to the inhibition of the development of postoperative immunosuppression. In another study in multiple trauma patients, early enteral nutrition seemed to stabilize the immunosuppression of polytraumatized patients in an earlier phase via consolidation of lymphocyte counts and of T (CD3$^+$)- and T-helper (CD4$^+$) cells [25]. This implies that immunological phenomena may also contribute to the effects of early enteral nutrition. Lack of enteral nutrition induces endothelial activation, which may change the response to injury or infection, probably by increasing neutrophil accumulation in the small intestine and expression of intestinal intercellular adhesion molecule (ICAM)-1 and P-selectin [26]. Furthermore, enteral feeding may decrease distant organ inflammation by reducing gut apoptotic activity [27]. Finally, IgA-dependent upper respiratory tract immunity is influenced by the route of nutrition [28]. Both decreased IgA production due to gut-associated lymphoid tissue (GALT) atrophy and impaired mucosal transport occur when enteral feeding is not provided [29]. These changes are likely to be cytokine mediated [27, 30, 31].

In conclusion, many studies support the theory that loss of mechanical and immunological gut barrier function is induced by injury or illness, leading to distant organ injury. Early initiation of enteral nutrition seems to prevent or attenuate this problem, in part by cytokine-mediated inhibition of post-injury immunosuppression.

▌ Clinical Studies

The question now is whether the observed effects of early enteral nutrition contribute to favorable, clinically relevant endpoints. For example, one would expect a decrease in the number or severity of infections due to inhibition of post-injury immunosuppression. Many studies have been conducted addressing to this question, using different patient categories and different feeding strategies. The endpoints can be divided into metabolic parameters, immunological parameters, morbidity (incidence of stress ulceration and ileus, rate of infections, severity of MOF), length of stay, cost effectiveness, and mortality.

Surgical Patients

The first controlled study in humans comparing early versus delayed enteral nutrition was conducted in seriously burned patients (average burn size of 38%). Patients who received enteral feeding within 4.4 ± 0.5 hours postburn had fewer positive blood cultures and significantly shortened hospital stays compared to the group with delayed feeding (57.7 ± 2.6 hours postburn) [32]. Other trials showed a decrease in postburn hypermetabolism and endotoxin translocation [33, 34]. In a retrospective study of severely burned patients, mortality was significantly lower in patients who accepted early intragastric nutrition (mean 11.5 h postburn) [35]. Early enteral nutrition is also effective in preventing stress ulceration in burn patients [36]. Intestinal permeability and gut-derived endotoxemia due to burns is decreased by early enteral nutrition [37].

Many studies have been conducted in patients who underwent major abdominal surgery including liver transplantation and pancreaticoduodenectomy. An important conclusion is that early enteral nutrition is safe and well tolerated in this group, even in the light of recent intestinal anastomoses. Withholding enteral nutrition following surgery because bowel sounds are absent is therefore considered obsolete. Animal experiments showed that early enteral feeding promotes gastrointestinal anastomotic healing. Early intragastic feeding following colon anastomosis increased colonic anastomotic bursting pressure by preservation of structural collagen, enhancing the ability of the gut to hold sutures [38]. Positioning the feeding tube either distal or proximal of the (gastric) anastomosis is equally safe [39]. In a very interesting prospective, randomized trial in 43 patients with nontraumatic intestinal perforation and peritonitis, the study group underwent a feeding jejunostomy and received enteral feeding from 12 hours after laparotomy. Early enteral nutrition proved not only to be safe and feasible but also resulted in a decrease in septic morbidity and an improvement in nutritional parameters [40]. However, even late institution of jejunal feeding in patients with secondary peritonitis or severe pancreatitis improves outcome [41].

The other effects of early enteral nutrition following major abdominal surgery can be summarized as follows. Early initiation of enteral feeding led to a decrease in postoperative complications such as infections [42–46], a decrease in length of hospital stay [43, 44, 46–51] and an improvement in nutritional and immunological status [52]. No effects on mortality were noticed [45, 53–57]. The implementation of an early postoperative enteral feeding protocol, in which patients were fed via a jejunal feeding tube within 12 hours after bowel resection, was cost-effective [58].

Multiple trauma patients also benefit from early enteral nutrition, as was shown in a meta-analysis of the earlier studies [59]. Duodenal tube feeding immediately after injury is feasible in severely injured patients (mean Injury Severity Score [ISS] 40.3) [60]. This strategy results in a decrease in the number and severity of septic complications [61], and in a less severe form of MOF [22]. One prospective randomized controlled study of 38 patients showed an increase in survival rate, a lower complication rate, as well as a decrease in length of ICU stay and earlier weaning from the ventilator [62].

Whether early enteral nutrition is beneficial in neurotrauma patients remains unclear. The Cochrane group performed an analysis of the available randomized controlled trials [63]. The trials suggest that early feeding may be associated with a trend towards better outcomes in terms of survival and disability, but further trials are required.

Non-surgical Patients

In septic patients, early enteral nutrition is well tolerated [64]. Although early enteral nutrition is recommended by experts [65], there are no definite data to support early administration of enteral nutrition in this group of patients.

This is not true for severe acute pancreatitis. Although long considered to be an indication for TPN, prospective randomized trials showed the opposite. Early enteral nutrition via a jejunal feeding tube is safe, cost-effective and leads to a decrease in toxic and hypermetabolic stress responses without worsening the pancreatitis [66–69]. Early enteral nutrition also may prevent bacterial translocation from the gut, which is thought to be responsible for secondary infection of necrotic pancreatic tissue [67, 70].

In conclusion, in adult surgical patients, the early introduction of enteral feeding is safe, well tolerated and cost-effective. It is associated with a reduction in complications and possibly a shorter hospital stay (level II evidence); early enteral nutrition is recommended in critically ill surgical and trauma patients (grade B recommendation), and in severe acute pancreatitis. Early enteral nutrition can also be considered in other critically ill patient populations (grade C recommendation) [71, 72].

▌ Contraindications and Complications

In general, enteral nutrition is contraindicated in gastrointestinal perforation, obstruction, proven bowel ischemia, or toxic megacolon. Obviously these situations prompt for a surgical solution. As has been shown, enteral nutrition can be safely initiated immediately after (gastrointestinal) surgery.

Most experts will agree that severe hemodynamic instability is a contraindication to enteral nutrition, based on the idea that feeding the hypoperfused gut might result in (worsening of) ischemia, or in a steal phenomenon impairing oxygen transport to other (vital) organs. The problem is how to define hemodynamic instability. Is it safe to initiate enteral nutrition when a patient has stable hemodynamics or should one wait until normal hemodynamics have been regained? And what about the use of inotropic agents and vasopressors?

Recently, a prospective study was undertaken to assess the hemodynamic and metabolic adaptations to enteral nutrition in patients with circulatory compromise [73]. Nine patients requiring hemodynamic support by dobutamine and/or norepinephrine received postpyloric enteral nutrition one day after cardiac surgery. Enteral nutrition increased cardiac index and splanchnic blood flow compared to baseline (fasted) condition, and nutrients were utilized. This small study suggests that early enteral nutrition may be appropriate, even in patients requiring inotropes. However, in ICU patients receiving nasogastric tube feeding, the use of catecholamines is associated with high gastric aspirate volumes [74]. It seems reasonable to state that once a patient is properly volume resuscitated, enteral nutrition can be initiated even in the presence of inotropic support. One should switch from intragastric to postpyloric tube feeding when, in the light of using catecholamines, gastric aspirate volume is high despite the use of prokinetic agents.

Nonocclusive bowel necrosis and intestinal obstruction have been reported as serious complications of enteral feeding [75–77]. An early useful clinical indicator to recognize these rare complications has not been identified. Clinical findings resemble systemic inflammatory response syndrome (SIRS).

The complex association of ventilator-associated pneumonia (VAP) and enteral feeding is beyond the scope of this chapter.

▌ Practical Considerations

Introduction of a simple feeding algorithm such as shown in Fig. 1 is cost-effective [58] and improves nutritional parameters as well as outcome. The flowchart shown is just an example and should be adapted to the local situation. However, every algorithm should emphasize the initiation of enteral nutrition within 6 hours after admission to the ICU provided a hemodynamic stable condition and in the absence of contraindications. As gastric emptying often is impaired in critically ill patients [74, 78], measures should be undertaken to reduce upper digestive intolerance to enteral feeding. Surgeons should consider routine insertion of jejunal feeding tubes (needle catheter jejunostomy placement) in patients undergoing major abdominal surgery, anticipating prolonged tube feeding [79]. In other patients, a gastric challenge should be undertaken with measurement of gastric aspirate volume [80]. A gastric aspirate volume of 150 ml after 6 hours is considered to be safe; more than 150 ml at least twice is an indication for the use of prokinetic agents. Recently, a more aggressive approach allowing gastric aspirate volumes to be more than 250 ml along with the mandatory use of prokinetic agents appeared to be safe and effective as well [80]. No evidence-based recommendations can be made on which prokinetic agent is to be preferred. Cisapride, metoclopramide, and erythromycin are all effective in promoting gastric emptying in critically ill patients [81–84]. Postpyloric feeding should be considered in cases of intragastric intolerance despite prokinetic agents. Different techniques for postpyloric placement of feeding tubes have been described. Endoscopic placement is the most reliable [85–87]. Other techniques involve sonographic or fluoroscopic guiding [88]. Blind techniques can be facilitated by the use of erythromycin and position of the patient [89], or by the use of weighted feeding tubes [90].

Finally, adding parenteral to enteral nutrition has no clinically relevant effect on outcome [91].

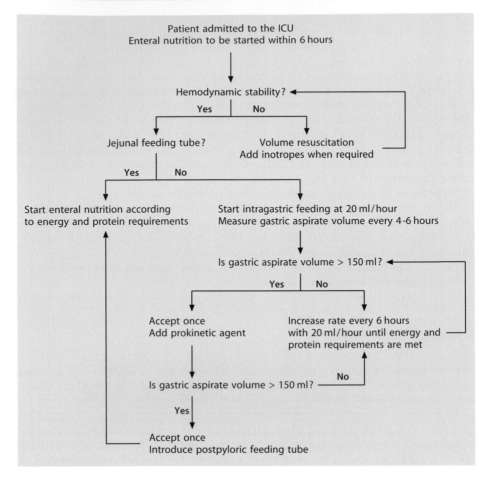

Fig. 1. Suggested flowchart for early initiation of enteral nutrition

▌ Conclusion

Early enteral nutrition in critically ill patients is safe and feasible, resulting in a decrease in morbidity and in a shorter hospital length of stay, especially in surgical patients. Improvement of the (immunological) gut barrier function, resulting in cytokine-mediated inhibition of post-injury immunosuppression is considered to be an important mechanism. Implementation of a simple feeding algorithm is both cost-effective and very useful to achieve early initiation of enteral nutrition in critically ill patients.

As Baskin stated almost a decade ago, the old adagio "if the gut works, use it" should be replaced by "use it, or lose it" [92].

References

1. Preiser JC, Berre J, Carpentier Y, et al (1999) Management of nutrition in European intensive care units: results of a questionnaire. Working Group on Metabolism and Nutrition of the European Society of Intensive Care Medicine. Intensive Care Med 25:95–101
2. Brathwaite CE, Ross SE, Nagele R, Mure AJ, O'Malley KF, Garcia-Perez FA (1993) Bacterial translocation occurs in humans after traumatic injury: evidence using immunofluorescence. J Trauma 34:586–589
3. Landow L, Andersen LW (1994) Splanchnic ischaemia and its role in multiple organ failure. Acta Anaesthesiol Scand 38:626–639
4. Pape HC, Dwenger A, Regel G, et al (1994) Increased gut permeability after multiple trauma. Br J Surg 81:850–852
5. Roumen RM, van d V Wevers RA, Goris RJ (1993) Intestinal permeability is increased after major vascular surgery. J Vasc Surg 17:734–737
6. Roumen RM, Hendriks T, Wevers RA, Goris JA (1993) Intestinal permeability after severe trauma and hemorrhagic shock is increased without relation to septic complications. Arch Surg 128:453–457
7. LeVoyer T, Cioffi WGJ, Pratt L, et al (1992) Alterations in intestinal permeability after thermal injury. Arch Surg 127:26–29
8. Harris CE, Griffiths RD, Freestone N, Billington D, Atherton ST, Macmillan RR (1992) Intestinal permeability in the critically ill. Intensive Care Med 18:38–41
9. Sinclair DG, Haslam PL, Quinlan GJ, Pepper JR, Evans TW (1995) The effect of cardiopulmonary bypass on intestinal and pulmonary endothelial permeability. Chest 108:718–724
10. Deitch EA (1990) Intestinal permeability is increased in burn patients shortly after injury. Surgery 107:411–416
11. van der Hulst RR, von Meyenfeldt MF, van Kreel BK, et al (1998) Gut permeability, intestinal morphology, and nutritional depletion. Nutrition 14:1–6
12. Hadfield RJ, Sinclair DG, Houldsworth PE, Evans TW (1995) Effects of enteral and parenteral nutrition on gut mucosal permeability in the critically ill. Am J Respir Crit Care Med 152:1545–1548
13. Adams CAJ, Magnotti LJ, Xu DZ, Lu Q, Deitch EA (2000) Acute lung injury after hemorrhagic shock is dependent on gut injury and sex. Am Surg 66:905–912
14. Magnotti LJ, Upperman JS, Xu DZ, Lu Q, Deitch EA (1998) Gut-derived mesenteric lymph but not portal blood increases endothelial cell permeability and promotes lung injury after hemorrhagic shock. Ann Surg 228:518–527
15. Magnotti LJ, Xu DZ, Lu Q, Deitch EA (1999) Gut-derived mesenteric lymph: a link between burn and lung injury. Arch Surg 134:1333–1340
16. Adams CAJ, Sambol JT, Xu DZ, Lu Q, Granger DN, Deitch EA (2001) Hemorrhagic shock induced up-regulation of P-selectin expression is mediated by factors in mesenteric lymph and blunted by mesenteric lymph duct interruption. J Trauma 51:625–631
17. Sambol JT, Xu DZ, Adams CA, Magnotti LJ, Deitch EA (2000) Mesenteric lymph duct ligation provides long term protection against hemorrhagic shock-induced lung injury. Shock 14:416–419
18. Mochizuki H, Trocki O, Dominioni L, Brackett KA, Joffe SN, Alexander JW (1984) Mechanism of prevention of postburn hypermetabolism and catabolism by early enteral feeding. Ann Surg 200:297–310
19. Gianotti L, Nelson JL, Alexander JW, Chalk CL, Pyles T (1994) Post injury hypermetabolic response and magnitude of translocation: prevention by early enteral nutrition. Nutrition 10:225–231
20. Gianotti L, Alexander JW, Nelson JL, Fukushima R, Pyles T, Chalk CL (1994) Role of early enteral feeding and acute starvation on postburn bacterial translocation and host defense: prospective, randomized trials. Crit Care Med 22:265–272
21. Langkamp-Henken B, Donovan TB, Pate LM, Maull CD, Kudsk KA (1995) Increased intestinal permeability following blunt and penetrating trauma. Crit Care Med 23:660–664
22. Kompan L, Kremzar B, Gadzijev E, Prosek M (1999) Effects of early enteral nutrition on intestinal permeability and the development of multiple organ failure after multiple injury. Intensive Care Med 25:157–161

23. Oudemans-van Straaten HM, Van der Voort PHJ, Hoek FJ, Bosman RJ, Van der Spoel JI, Zandstra DF (2002) Pitfalls in gastrointestinal permeability measurement in ICU patients with multiple organ failure using differential sugar absorption. Intensive Care Med (In Press)

24. Takagi K, Yamamori H, Toyoda Y, Nakajima N, Tashiro T (2000) Modulating effects of the feeding route on stress response and endotoxin translocation in severely stressed patients receiving thoracic esophagectomy. Nutrition 16:355–360

25. Engel JM, Menges T, Neuhauser C, Schaefer B, Hempelmann G (1997) [Effects of various feeding regimens in multiple trauma patients on septic complications and immune parameters]. Anasthesiol Intensivmed Notfallmed Schmerzther 32:234–239

26. Fukatsu K, Lundberg AH, Hanna MK, et al (2000) Increased expression of intestinal P-selectin and pulmonary E-selectin during intravenous total parenteral nutrition. Arch Surg 135:1177–1182

27. Alscher KT, Phang PT, McDonald TE, Walley KR (2001) Enteral feeding decreases gut apoptosis, permeability, and lung inflammation during murine endotoxemia. Am J Physiol 281:G569–G576

28. Kudsk KA, Li J, Renegar KB (1996) Loss of upper respiratory tract immunity with parenteral feeding. Ann Surg 223:629–635

29. Renegar KB, Kudsk KA, Dewitt RC, Wu Y, King BK (2001) Impairment of mucosal immunity by parenteral nutrition: depressed nasotracheal influenza-specific secretory IgA levels and transport in parenterally fed mice. Ann Surg 233:134–138

30. Wu Y, Kudsk KA, Dewitt RC, Tolley EA, Li J (1999) Route and type of nutrition influence IgA-mediating intestinal cytokines. Ann Surg 229:662–667

31. Fukatsu K, Kudsk KA, Zarzaur BL, Wu Y, Hanna MK, Dewitt RC (2001) TPN decreases IL-4 and IL-10 mRNA expression in lipopolysaccharide stimulated intestinal lamina propria cells but glutamine supplementation preserves the expression. Shock 15:318–322

32. Chiarelli A, Enzi G, Casadei A, Baggio B, Valerio A, Mazzoleni F (1990) Very early nutrition supplementation in burned patients. Am J Clin Nutr 51:1035–1039

33. Wang S, Li A (1997) [A clinical study of early enteral feeding to protect the gut function in burned patients]. Chung Hua Cheng Hsing Shao Shang Wai Ko Tsa Chih 13:267–271

34. Wang S, You Z (1997) [Clinical study of the effect of early enteral feeding on reducing hypermetabolism after severe burns]. Chung Hua Wai Ko Tsa Chih 35:44–47

35. Raff T, Hartmann B, Germann G (1997) Early intragastric feeding of seriously burned and long-term ventilated patients: a review of 55 patients. Burns 23:19–25

36. Raff T, Germann G, Hartmann B (1997) The value of early enteral nutrition in the prophylaxis of stress ulceration in the severely burned patient. Burns 23:313–318

37. Peng YZ, Yuan ZQ, Xiao GX (2001) Effects of early enteral feeding on the prevention of enterogenic infection in severely burned patients. Burns 27:145–149

38. Kiyama T, Efron DT, Tantry U, Barbul A (1999) Effect of nutritional route on colonic anastomotic healing in the rat. J Gastrointest Surg 3:441–446

39. Velez JP, Lince LF, Restrepo JI (1997) Early enteral nutrition in gastrointestinal surgery: a pilot study. Nutrition 13:442–445

40. Singh G, Ram RP, Khanna SK (1998) Early postoperative enteral feeding in patients with nontraumatic intestinal perforation and peritonitis. J Am Coll Surg 187:142–146

41. Pupelis G, Selga G, Austrums E, Kaminski A (2001) Jejunal feeding, even when instituted late, improves outcomes in patients with severe pancreatitis and peritonitis. Nutrition 17:91–94

42. Beier-Holgersen R, Boesby S (1996) Influence of postoperative enteral nutrition on postsurgical infections. Gut 39:833–835

43. Braga M, Vignali A, Gianotti L, Cestari A, Profili M, Carlo VD (1996) Immune and nutritional effects of early enteral nutrition after major abdominal operations. Eur J Surg 162:105–112

44. Braga M, Vignali A, Gianotti L, Cestari A, Profili M, Di CV (1995) Benefits of early postoperative enteral feeding in cancer patients. Infusionsther Transfusionsmed 22:280–284

45. Hasse JM, Blue LS, Liepa GU, et al (1995) Early enteral nutrition support in patients undergoing liver transplantation. J Parenter Enteral Nutr 19:437–443

46. Bozzetti F, Braga M, Gianotti L, Gavazzi C, Mariani L (2001) Postoperative enteral versus parenteral nutrition in malnourished patients with gastrointestinal cancer: a randomised multicentre trial. Lancet 358:1487–1492
47. Schilder JM, Hurteau JA, Look KY, et al (1997) A prospective controlled trial of early postoperative oral intake following major abdominal gynecologic surgery. Gynecol Oncol 67:235–240
48. Reissman P, Teoh TA, Cohen SM, Weiss EG, Nogueras JJ, Wexner SD (1995) Is early oral feeding safe after elective colorectal surgery? A prospective randomized trial. Ann Surg 222:73–77
49. Choi J, O'Connell TX (1996) Safe and effective early postoperative feeding and hospital discharge after open colon resection. Am Surg 62:853–856
50. Stewart BT, Woods RJ, Collopy BT, Fink RJ, Mackay JR, Keck JO (1998) Early feeding after elective open colorectal resections: a prospective randomized trial. Aust NZJ Surg 68:125–128
51. Detry R, Ciccarelli O, Komlan A, Claeys N (1999) Early feeding after colorectal surgery. Preliminary results. Acta Chir Belg 99:292–294
52. Hochwald SN, Harrison LE, Heslin MJ, Burt ME, Brennan MF (1997) Early postoperative enteral feeding improves whole body protein kinetics in upper gastrointestinal cancer patients. Am J Surg 174:325–330
53. Heslin MJ, Latkany L, Leung D, et al (1997) A prospective, randomized trial of early enteral feeding after resection of upper gastrointestinal malignancy. Ann Surg 226:567–577
54. Harrison LE, Hochwald SN, Heslin MJ, Berman R, Burt M, Brennan MF (1997) Early postoperative enteral nutrition improves peripheral protein kinetics in upper gastrointestinal cancer patients undergoing complete resection: a randomized trial. J Parenter Enteral Nutr 21:202–207
55. Carr CS, Ling KD, Boulos P, Singer M (1996) Randomised trial of safety and efficacy of immediate postoperative enteral feeding in patients undergoing gastrointestinal resection. Br Med J 312:869–871
56. Shirabe K, Matsumata T, Shimada M, et al (1997) A comparison of parenteral hyperalimentation and early enteral feeding regarding systemic immunity after major hepatic resection – the results of a randomized prospective study. Hepatogastroenterology 44:205–209
57. Wicks C, Somasundaram S, Bjarnason I, et al (1994) Comparison of enteral feeding and total parenteral nutrition after liver transplantation. Lancet 344:837–840
58. Hedberg AM, Lairson DR, Aday LA, et al (1999) Economic implications of an early postoperative enteral feeding protocol. J Am Diet Assoc 99:802–807
59. Moore FA, Feliciano DV, Andrassy RJ, et al (1992) Early enteral feeding, compared with parenteral, reduces postoperative septic complications. The results of a meta-analysis. Ann Surg 216:172–183
60. Bastian L, Weimann A, Regel G, Trautwein C, Tscherne H (1996) [Feasibility and complications in early enteral nutrition of severely injured polytrauma patients via duodenal tubes.] Unfallchirurg 99:642–649
61. Moore EE, Moore FA (1991) Immediate enteral nutrition following multisystem trauma: a decade perspective. J Am Coll Nutr 10:633–648
62. Chuntrasakul C, Siltharm S, Chinswangwatanakul V, Pongprasobchai T, Chockvivatanavanit S, Bunnak A (1996) Early nutritional support in severe traumatic patients. J Med Assoc Thai 79:21–26
63. Yanagawa T, Bunn F, Roberts I, Wentz R, Pierro A (2000) Nutritional support for head-injured patients. Cochrane Database Syst Rev 2:CD001530
64. Bower RH, Cerra FB, Bershadsky B, et al (1995) Early enteral administration of a formula (Impact) supplemented with arginine, nucleotides, and fish oil in intensive care unit patients: results of a multicenter, prospective, randomized, clinical trial. Crit Care Med 23:436–449
65. Vincent JL, Preiser JC (1999) Management of the critically ill patient with severe sepsis. J Chemother 11:524–529
66. McClave SA, Greene LM, Snider HL, et al (1997) Comparison of the safety of early enteral vs parenteral nutrition in mild acute pancreatitis. J Parenter Enteral Nutr 21:14–20

67. Kalfarentzos F, Kehagias J, Mead N, Kokkinis K, Gogos CA (1997) Enteral nutrition is superior to parenteral nutrition in severe acute pancreatitis: results of a randomized prospective trial. Br J Surg 84:1665–1669
68. Nakad A, Piessevaux H, Marot JC, et al (1998) Is early enteral nutrition in acute pancreatitis dangerous? About 20 patients fed by an endoscopically placed nasogastrojejunal tube. Pancreas 17:187–193
69. Windsor AC, Kanwar S, Li AG, et al (1998) Compared with parenteral nutrition, enteral feeding attenuates the acute phase response and improves disease severity in acute pancreatitis. Gut 42:431–435
70. Lehocky P, Sarr MG (2000) Early enteral feeding in severe acute pancreatitis: can it prevent secondary pancreatic (super) infection? Dig Surg 17:571–577
71. Heyland DK (1998) Nutritional support in the critically ill patient. A critical review of the evidence. Crit Care Clin 14:423–440
72. Heyland DK (2000) Enteral and parenteral nutrition in the seriously ill, hospitalized patient: a critical review of the evidence. J Nutr Health Aging 4:31–41
73. Revelly JP, Tappy L, Berger MM, Gersbach P, Cayeux C, Chiolero R (2001) Early metabolic and splanchnic responses to enteral nutrition in postoperative cardiac surgery patients with circulatory compromise. Intensive Care Med 27:540–547
74. Mentec H, Dupont H, Bocchetti M, Cani P, Ponche F, Bleichner G (2001) Upper digestive intolerance during enteral nutrition in critically ill patients: frequency, risk factors, and complications. Crit Care Med 29:1955–1961
75. Marvin RG, McKinley BA, McQuiggan M, Cocanour CS, Moore FA (2000) Nonocclusive bowel necrosis occurring in critically ill trauma patients receiving enteral nutrition manifests no reliable clinical signs for early detection. Am J Surg 179:7–12
76. Frey C, Takala J, Krahenbuhl L (2001) Non-occlusive small bowel necrosis during gastric tube feeding: a case report. Intensive Care Med 27:1422–1425
77. Scaife CL, Saffle JR, Morris SE (1999) Intestinal obstruction secondary to enteral feedings in burn trauma patients. J Trauma 47:859–863
78. Heyland DK, Tougas G, King D, Cook DJ (1996) Impaired gastric emptying in mechanically ventilated, critically ill patients. Intensive Care Med 22:1339–1344
79. Biffi R, Lotti M, Cenciarelli S, et al (2000) Complications and long-term outcome of 80 oncology patients undergoing needle catheter jejunostomy placement for early postoperative enteral feeding. Clin Nutr 19:277–279
80. Pinilla JC, Samphire J, Arnold C, Liu L, Thiessen B (2001) Comparison of gastrointestinal tolerance to two enteral feeding protocols in critically ill patients: a prospective, randomized controlled trial. J Parenter Enteral Nutr 25:81–86
81. Spapen HD, Duinslaeger L, Diltoer M, Gillet R, Bossuyt A, Huyghens LP (1995) Gastric emptying in critically ill patients is accelerated by adding cisapride to a standard enteral feeding protocol: results of a prospective, randomized, controlled trial. Crit Care Med 23:481–485
82. Jooste CA, Mustoe J, Collee G (1999) Metoclopramide improves gastric motility in critically ill patients. Intensive Care Med 25:464–468
83. Boivin MA, Levy H (2001) Gastric feeding with erythromycin is equivalent to transpyloric feeding in the critically ill. Crit Care Med 29:1916–1919
84. MacLaren R, Kuhl DA, Gervasio JM, et al (2000) Sequential single doses of cisapride, erythromycin, and metoclopramide in critically ill patients intolerant to enteral nutrition: a randomized, placebo-controlled, crossover study. Crit Care Med 28:438–444
85. Dranoff JA, Angood PJ, Topazian M (1999) Transnasal endoscopy for enteral feeding tube placement in critically ill patients. Am J Gastroenterol 94:2902–2904
86. Ott L, Annis K, Hatton J, McClain M, Young B (1999) Postpyloric enteral feeding costs for patients with severe head injury: blind placement, endoscopy, and PEG/J versus TPN. J Neurotrauma 16:233–242
87. Reed RL, Eachempati SR, Russell MK, Fahkry C (1998) Endoscopic placement of jejunal feeding catheters in critically ill patients by a "push" technique. J Trauma 45:388–393
88. Hernandez-Socorro CR, Marin J, Ruiz-Santana S, Santana L, Manzano JL (1996) Bedside sonographic-guided versus blind nasoenteric feeding tube placement in critically ill patients. Crit Care Med 24:1690–1694

89. Komenaka IK, Giffard K, Miller J, Schein M (2000) Erythromycin and position facilitated placement of postpyloric feeding tubes in burned patients. Dig Surg 17:578–580
90. Ugo PJ, Mohler PA, Wilson GL (1992) Bedside postpyloric placement of weighted feeding tubes. Nutr Clin Pract 7:284–287
91. Bauer P, Charpentier C, Bouchet C, Nace L, Raffy F, Gaconnet N (2000) Parenteral with enteral nutrition in the critically ill. Intensive Care Med 26:893–900
92. Baskin WN (1992) Advances in enteral nutrition techniques. Am J Gastroenterol 87:1547–1553

Relative Adrenal Insufficiency Syndrome

J.J.M. Ligtenberg and J.G. Zijlstra

▮ Introduction

Several recent studies have given rise to optimism concerning steroid treatment in septic shock. 'Physiological' doses of steroids have been shown to reduce time to shock reversal and may even be able to decrease mortality [1–3]. Assuming that forthcoming studies will confirm these results, steroid treatment will go through a revival [4]. The term: 'relative adrenal insufficiency syndrome' has already become established and – as mortality from severe sepsis is still more than 40% despite advances in critical care – expectations for therapeutic consequences are high.

The current definition of the so-called relative adrenal insufficiency syndrome is rapid clinical and hemodynamic improvement of catecholamine-dependent patients after substitution with 300 mg (or less) hydrocortisone per day, which also seems the best available clue to its diagnosis until now. Another definition mentions a 'blunted' response of cortisol to the rapid corticotropin test [5, 6]. As a matter of fact, several questions remain: how accurate are our actual diagnostic tools, and, second, what is the evidence that the cause of this 'adreno-cortical insufficiency syndrome' is really situated in the adrenal cortex?

▮ Accuracy of the Current Tools for Diagnosis of the 'Relative Adrenal Insufficiency Syndrome'

We need tools to diagnose this syndrome, because it has important therapeutic consequences. Probably derived from the diagnostic approach to *absolute* adrenal insufficiency, much effort has been put into the determination of basal and corticotropin-stimulated blood cortisol concentrations, electrolyte disturbances, and changes in eosinophilic cell counts in critically ill patients [6, 7, 12–14]. In the next paragraphs we discuss how precise these various parameters are in diagnosing 'relative adrenal insufficiency' in intensive care unit (ICU) patients.

Cortisol

In general, as has been extensively shown, critically ill patients appear to have high normal to raised plasma cortisol concentrations (Fig. 1). In a prospective study in 40 septic shock patients (Fig. 1 a), the cortisol level was measured over the 72 hours following the onset of shock. Cortisol levels on admission were elevated (mean value 1015 nmol/l); basal cortisol levels did not differ significantly between survivors (858 nmol/l) and non-survivors (1073 nmol/l). Cortisol in survivors did not rise,

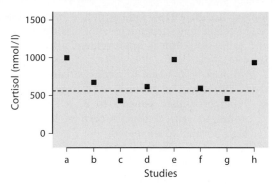

Fig. 1. Each point represents the mean serum cortisol level found in one of 8 different studies (**a–h**) in a total of 616 intensive care patients. **a** 40 medical ICU patients with septic shock [7]; **b** 54 post-operative patients after ruptured aortic aneurysm [8]; **c** 20 patients on a multidisciplinary ICU surviving septic shock [9]; **d** 32 patients with septic shock [12]; **e** 70 intensive care patients [10]; **f** 159 intensive care patients, >7 days ICU-stay [11]; **g** 52 surgical ICU patients [13]; **h** 189 septic shock patients [6]; *Dotted line*: maximum (unstimulated) serum cortisol level in healthy persons [37]

whereas an increase to 1840 nmol/l was found in non-survivors after 72 hours. Cortisol response to the ACTH test did not differ between survivors and non-survivors [7]. In 54 post-operative patients with a rupture of the abdominal aorta, a moderately increased morning cortisol (within 24 hr after admission) was found; cortisol was lower – though within 'normal' limits – in patients who had received etomidate during surgery (Fig. 1b) [8]. In 20 relatively young patients (out of 33) surviving hyperdynamic septic shock, basal cortisol levels were slightly increased (Fig. 1c) [9]. In 159 patients who stayed in the ICU for at least 7 days cortisol levels were elevated (Fig. 1f); non-survivors again showed higher values than survivors: 780 vs 540 nmol/l [11]. In 52 surgical ICU patients random cortisol levels were found to be in the high-normal range (Fig. 1g) [13]. In 189 patients mean cortisol level at the onset of septic shock was 940 mmol/l; overall mortality in this study was 59% (Fig. 1h). Non-survivors once more had significantly higher cortisol levels than survivors: 1076 vs 772 nmol/l. In this study [6], the patients with the poorest prognosis (mortality rate 82%) showed a basal cortisol >940 nmol/l and a corticotropin stimulated cortisol rise of <250 nmol/l. Oppert et al. found that hydrocortisone treatment in septic shock patients resulted in faster weaning from catecholamine-infusion in the group with 'inadequate' endogenous cortisol production (defined as a baseline level of <1000 nmol/l and a 'blunted' response to ACTH) than in patients with higher basal and stimulated cortisol levels, despite the same plasma cortisol levels reached during hydrocortisone therapy (between 1310–3587 nmol/l!) [15].

The prevalence of *absolute* adrenal insufficiency in ICU patients turns out to be low: 2–3% [16]; e.g., in the above-mentioned study of Bouachour et al. only one out of 40 septic patients fulfilled the criteria for absolute adrenal insufficiency [7].

The incidence of *relative* adrenal insufficiency in critically ill patients is unknown and is strongly dependent on the population studied, the test methods and the definition used [17]. For instance, Barquist et al. [18] measured cortisol levels in more than 1000 surgical ICU admissions and proposed defining 'relative' adrenal insufficiency as a basal cortisol level of <410 nmol/l and a synacthen-stimulated cortisol level stayed below 690 nmol/l. Based on these criteria, 0.7% of their patients had relative adrenal insufficiency, with an increase to 6% in those with prolonged ICU stay [18]. Others define the syndrome of relative adrenal insufficiency as catecholamine-dependent shock without other curable causes of hypertension and with fast clinical improvement after 'supraphysiological' doses of hydrocortisone [5].

Although – as usual in intensive care based research – the reviewed studies include a case-mix of patients, we can nevertheless conclude that:

▌ Hypercortisolism appears to be a normal physiological response to acute and prolonged critical illness: cortisol levels in intensive care patients usually are 'high normal' to increased.
▌ Recent studies demonstrate a relation between mortality rate and cortisol concentration; non-survivors tend to have higher cortisol levels.
▌ The prevalence of *absolute* adrenal insufficiency in critically ill patients is fairly low.
▌ There seems to be no consensus concerning 'reference values' for baseline and stimulated cortisol concentrations in ICU patients.

Do these findings help us in diagnosing patients with the relative adrenal insufficiency syndrome, and thus in selecting patients who will benefit from steroid treatment? Unfortunately, the answer must be 'no'. The data we have gathered demonstrate increased cortisol levels in critically ill patients, but are not suitable for sorting out patients who will or will not respond to steroid treatment. The same goes for the prognostic classification based on the cortisol concentration; again these data do not help us to diagnose 'relative adrenal insufficiency syndrome' or to select patients in whom steroid therapy could be withheld. Furthermore, the prognostic data derived from corticotropin stimulation tests are useful for research purposes, but are insignificant in diagnosing relative adrenal insufficiency syndrome [19]. Reference values of the ACTH stimulation test – determined under standardized circumstances [20, 21] – cannot be applied to the population under stress in the ICU [22]. Additionally, the usually high unstimulated cortisol levels are associated with a relatively small increment in cortisol, without a clear association between basal and stimulated levels [7, 8]. This 'blunted' response may be found:

▌ because the hypothalamic-pituitary-adrenal axis is already maximally stimulated;
▌ because pituitary glucocorticoid feedback might be altered;
▌ because the adrenal glands are already (maximally) stimulated by the increased secretion of peptides with corticotropin-releasing hormone (CRH)-like activity (e.g., cytokines) [23]; or have been damaged by adrenal hemorrhage, which is not uncommon in e.g., meningococcal septic shock [24].

Summarizing, on the basis of the available data, we cannot find sound evidence supporting the use of cortisol concentrations or a 'blunted' response as diagnostic tools for relative adrenal insufficiency syndrome nor are they helpful in selecting septic shock patients in whom steroid therapy can be withheld.

Electrolyte Disturbances

Probably analogous to the diagnosis of absolute adrenal insufficiency, the recommendation has been made to look into electrolyte disturbances (hyponatremia, hyperkalemia) as indicators of relative adrenal insufficiency [16]. As we pointed out in the preceding section, critically ill patients show high-normal to increased cortisol levels, thus indicating that the adrenal cortex is working – perhaps relatively –

well. It is difficult to imagine why this would cause electrolyte disorders comparable to those found in *absolute* adrenal insufficiency. Apart from that, assessment of serum electrolyte concentrations in patients treated in the ICU is complicated because of treatment related factors such as infusion of various volume-expanding solutions in variable volumes, routine potassium supplementation and treatment with diuretics.

A relationship between cortisol levels and serum calcium values, which has been described in *absolute* adrenal insufficiency, could not be demonstrated in 52 patients on a surgical ICU: mean $\pm$ SD cortisol 464 $\pm$ 292, mean (corrected) calcium 2.00 $\pm$ 0.29 mmol/l: Pearson correlation 0.025, p = 0.8 [13].

In conclusion, serum electrolyte determinations for this purpose are not very practical in ICU practice [25].

Eosinophilia

A rise in the number of circulating eosinophilic cells has been described as an indicator for adrenocortical dysfunction [26]. DiPiro et al. [27] performed blood eosinophil counts in 100 patients admitted to a trauma ICU and found a significant rise in patients with (severe) sepsis: 1225/µl vs 446/µl. Hormone determinations were not carried out in this study. Beishuizen et al. [28] studied 612 severely ill ICU patients by daily measuring the percentage of eosinophils. In 40 patients with eosinophilic cell counts >3%, a low-dose (1 µg) synacthen stimulation test was performed: ten patients responded abnormally (in this case 'abnormal' was defined as: cortisol levels <550 nmol/l and an increase of <150 nmol/l, both after stimulation). Treatment with steroids resulted in rapid hemodynamic improvement in seven patients. Patients with normal and abnormal synacthen stimulation tests did not differ significantly in % eosinophilic cells: 5.1 vs 5.8. The investigators state that relative eosinophilia should be thought of as a warning sign of insufficient adrenocortical function. However, eosinophilia was used as an inclusion criterion to enter the study, so we do not know what proportion of the remaining patients, who did not show eosinophilia, could have benefited from glucocorticoid administration [29].

The idea that a rise in eosinophilic cells and an abnormal response to synacthen point to relative adrenal insufficiency again is an extrapolation of the diagnostic approach to *absolute* adrenal insufficiency, which – adding up the evidence discussed up to now – seems to be a completely different syndrome.

▌ Is the Cause of this 'Adreno-cortical Insufficiency Syndrome' Situated in the Adrenal Cortex?

On theoretical grounds, one would expect relative hypofunction of the adrenal cortex in *prolonged* critical illness, to be caused either by 'exhaustion' of the adrenal cortex or by a decreased secretory activity of the anterior pituitary gland, resulting in reduced neuroendocrine stimulation [30].

Yet, as we mentioned in the preceding sections, both in acute and prolonged critical illness, cortisol levels have consistently been found to be increased and adrenal stimulation tests with synthetic ACTH may give all sorts of results. Since we do not have reference values for this test in critically ill patients, we could just as well consider the limited or so-called 'blunted' cortisol response as a functional adaptation of the adrenal cortex instead of a pathological condition.

The data we have reviewed give rise to an intriguing question: why should one consider an organ (the adrenal cortex) insufficient when it has been proven to function adequately, given normal to increased 'product' (cortisol) levels?

Evidence is certainly accumulating that treatment of critically ill septic shock patients with this 'product' (hydrocortisone) has beneficial effects: it reduces time to shock reversal and may be able to decrease mortality [1–3]. So, we have to look for other explanations why this treatment works [31]. Hypotheses focus on two areas: a) hemodynamic effects and b) effects on cell activation and subsequent cytokine release. Corticosteroids can modulate blood pressure, in part in close relation with the adrenergic system. They are able to attenuate the down regulation of adrenergic receptors, which has been found in sepsis, and can be induced by the prolonged use of catecholamines – resulting in an increase in the number of receptors [32]. Steroids have a positive effect on myocardial contractility and can exert vasoconstrictive effects by increasing the number of α_1-adrenoreceptors and β-adrenoreceptors and by stimulating the function of these receptors [33].

Hypercortisolism can also be effective as a defense mechanism against the cascade of cell activation and subsequent cytokine release involved in the systemic inflammatory response, which has been described to be a universal reaction of the body during stress [34]. In patients with septic shock (or acute respiratory distress syndrome [ARDS]), prolonged treatment with glucocorticoids is associated with a significant reduction in proinflammatory cytokines and an increase in interleukin (IL)-4 and IL-10 [35], which may increase cortisol receptor binding affinity [36], thus positively influencing blood pressure.

▌ Conclusion

There certainly is an evolving place for 'supplementation' doses of steroids in catecholamine-dependent septic shock patients. In this chapter, we have built up a line of reasoning to demonstrate that the adrenal cortex functions very well in septic shock and that there must be other explanations why steroid supplementation therapy works. We suggest replacing the confusing term 'relative adrenal insufficiency syndrome' as soon as we know more about its pathophysiology.

References

1. Briegel J, Forst H, Haller M, Schelling G, et al (1999) Stress doses of hydrocortisone reverse hyperdynamic septic shock: a prospective, randomized, double-blind, single-center study. Crit Care Med 27:723–732
2. Bollaert PE, Charpentier C, Levy B, Debouverie M, Audibert G, Larcan A (1998) Reversal of late septic shock with supraphysiologic doses of hydrocortisone. Crit Care Med. 26:645–650
3. Chawla K, Kupfer Y, Goldman I, Tessler S (1999) Hydrocortisone reverses refractory septic shock. Crit Care Med 27:A33 (Abst)
4. Spijkstra JJ, Girbes AR (2000) The continuing story of corticosteroids in the treatment of septic shock. Intensive Care Med 26:496–500
5. Bollaert PE (2000) Stress doses of glucocorticoids in catecholamine dependency: a new therapy for a new syndrome? Intensive Care Med 26:3–5

6. Annane D, Sebille V, Troche G, Raphael JC, Gajdos P, Bellissant E (2000) A 3-level prognostic classification in septic shock based on cortisol levels and cortisol response to corticotropin. JAMA 283:1038–1045
7. Bouachour G, Tirot P, Gouello JP, Mathieu E, Vincent JF, Alquier P (1995) Adrenocortical function during septic shock. Intensive Care Med 21:57–62
8. Braams R, Koppeschaar HP, van de Pavoordt HD, van Vroonhoven TJ (1998) Adrenocortical function in patients with ruptured aneurysm of the abdominal aorta. Intensive Care Med 24:124–127
9. Briegel J, Schelling G, Haller M, Mraz W, Forst H, Peter K (1996) A comparison of the adrenocortical response during septic shock and after complete recovery. Intensive Care Med 22:894–899
10. Jurney TH, Cockrell JL Jr., Lindberg JS, Lamiell JM, Wade CE (1987) Spectrum of serum cortisol response to ACTH in ICU patients. Correlation with degree of illness and mortality. Chest 92:292–295
11. Span LF, Hermus AR, Bartelink AK, et al (1992) Adrenocortical function: an indicator of severity of disease and survival in chronic critically ill patients. Intensive Care Med 18:93–96
12. Rothwell PM, Udwadia ZF, Lawler PG (1991) Cortisol response to corticotropin and survival in septic shock. Lancet 337:582–583
13. Ligtenberg JJM, Pieters RC, Nijsten MWN, Delwig H (2001) No correlation between serum calcium and serum cortisol in critically ill patients. Am J Respir Crit Care Med 163:D41 (Abst)
14. Beishuizen A, Vermes I, Hylkema BS, Haanen C (1999) Relative eosinophilia and functional adrenal insufficiency in critically ill patients. Lancet 353:1675–1676
15. Oppert M, Reinicke A, Graf KJ, Barckow D, Frei U, Eckardt KU (1999) Plasma cortisol levels before and during 'low-dose' hydrocortison therapy and their relationship to hemodynamic improvement in patients with septic shock. Intensive Care Med 26:1747–1755
16. Lamberts SW, Bruining HA, de Jong FH (1997) Corticosteroid therapy in severe illness. N Engl J Med 337:1285–1292
17. Van den Berghe, de Zegher F, Veldhuis JD, et al (1997) Thyrotrophin and prolactin release in prolonged critical illness: dynamics of spontaneous secretion and effects of growth hormonesecretagogues. Clin Endocrinol 47:599–612
18. Barquist E, Kirton O (1997) Adrenal insufficiency in the surgical intensive care unit patient. J Trauma 42:27–31
19. Ligtenberg JJM, Nieboer P, Beentjes JA, van der Werf TS, Tulleken JE, Zijlstra JG (2000) A new therapy for a new syndrome. Intensive Care Med 26:1013–1014
20. Bos Kuil MJ, Endert E, Fliers E, Prummel MF, Romijn JA, Wiersinga WM (1998) Establishment of reference values for endocrine tests. I: Cushing's syndrome. Neth J Med 53:153–163
21. Dickstein G, Shechner C, Nicholson WE, et al (1991) Adrenocorticotropin stimulation test: effects of basal cortisol level, time of day, and suggested new sensitive low dose test. J Clin Endocrinol Metab 72:773–778
22. Streeten DH (1999) What test for hypothalamic-pituitary-adrenocortical insufficiency? Lancet 354:179–180
23. Reincke M, Allolio B, Wurth G, Winkelmann W (1993) The hypothalamic-pituitary-adrenal axis in critical illness: response to dexamethasone and corticotropin-releasing hormone. J Clin Endocrinol Metab 77:151–156
24. Ligtenberg JJM, Zijlstra JG, Girbes AR (2000) Noradrenaline in meningococcal septic shock. Intensive Care Med 26:1588–1589
25. Ligtenberg JJM, Girbes AR, Beentjes JA, Tulleken JE, Der Werf TS, Zijlstra JG (2001) Hormones in the critically ill patient: to intervene or not to intervene? Intensive Care Med 27:1567–1577
26. Thorn GW, Forsham PH, Prunty FTG, Hills AG (2001) A test for adrenal cortical insufficiency. JAMA 137:1005–1009
27. DiPiro JT, Howdieshell TR, Hamilton RG, Mansberger AR Jr (1998) Immunoglobulin E and eosinophil counts are increased after sepsis in trauma patients. Crit Care Med 26:465–469

28. Beishuizen A, Vermes I (1999) Relative eosinophilia (Thorn test) as a bioassay to judge the clinical relevance of cortisol values during severe stress. J Clin Endocrinol Metab 84:3400
29. Ligtenberg JJ, van der Werf TS, Tulleken JE, Beentjes JA, Zijlstra JG (1999) Diagnosis of relative adrenal insufficiency in critically ill patients. Lancet 354:774–775
30. Van den Berghe, de Zegher F, Baxter RC et al (1998) Neuroendocrinology of prolonged critical illness: effects of exogenous thyrotropin-releasing hormone and its combination with growth hormone secretagogues. J Clin Endocrinol Metab 83:309–319
31. Annane D (2001) Corticosteroids for septic shock. Crit Care Med 29:S117-S120
32. Saito T, Takanashi M, Gallagher E, et al (1995) Corticosteroid effect on early beta-adrenergic down-regulation during circulatory shock: hemodynamic study and beta-adrenergic receptor assay. Intensive Care Med 21:204–210
33. Walker BR, Williams BC (1992) Corticosteroids and vascular tone: mapping the messenger maze. Clin Sci (Colch) 82:597–605
34. Bone RC, Grodzin CJ, Balk RA (1997) Sepsis: a new hypothesis for pathogenesis of the disease process. Chest 112:235–243
35. Meduri GU, Headley AS, Golden E, et al (1998) Effect of prolonged methylprednisolone therapy in unresolving acute respiratory distress syndrome: a randomized controlled trial. JAMA 280:159–165
36. Kam JC, Szefler SJ, Surs W, Sher ER, Leung DY (1993) Combination IL-2 and IL-4 reduces glucocorticoid receptor-binding affinity and T cell response to glucocorticoids. J Immunol 151:3460–3466
37. Williams GH, Dluhy RG (1998) Endocrinology and metabolism. In: Fauci AS, Braunswald E, Isselbacher KJ (eds) Harrison's Principles of Internal Medicine (Single Volume). McGraw Hill, New York, pp 2040–2041

Metabolic Effects of Adrenergic Drugs

E. Ensinger and K. Träger

Introduction

Vasoactive drugs are widely used in intensive care medicine to restore hemody-namic stability. Therapy can be led by blood pressure and cardiac output, but it can also be extended to regional hemodynamic and integrative parameters such as gastric tonometry or systemic regional oxygen extraction. The drugs used for this purpose are mainly catecholamines or synthetic sympathomimetic drugs. These drugs not only mediate hemodynamic actions, but they also have metabolic effects. They act on receptors that are targets of the sympathetic nervous system. The ob-jective in the use of all these compounds is to improve hemodynamic and meta-bolic performance in order to avoid a deficit in ATP production and to maintain homeostasis.

This chapter will focus on the metabolic effects of the endogenous catechola-mines and vasoactive drugs with emphasis on compounds acting on adrenoceptors.

The Autonomic Nervous System

The autonomic nervous system serves as an integrative system for the control and maintenance of all non- or semi-voluntary functions of the body. The hypothala-mus and the nucleus of the solitary tract are regarded as the principal loci of the autonomic nervous system including regulation of the cardiovascular system, respi-ration, water balance, metabolism with control of metabolic rate, food uptake, star-vation and body temperature, reproductive functions, and in part the control of immune defense [1, 2].

The sympathetic nervous system consists of the preganglionic fibers originating from the spinal cord, and the postganglionic fibers originating from the paraver-tebral ganglia. The neurotransmitter of all preganglionic autonomic fibers is acetyl-choline acting on the muscarinic receptor. The second sympathetic neuron releases norepinephrine with the exception of the adrenal medulla where primarily epi-nephrine is released. The sympathetic nervous system with the associated adrenal medulla is not essential to life in a controlled environment. However, it enables us to live in areas with adverse climatic conditions, it has major functions during physical exercise, stress, aggression, and trauma. The sympathetic nervous system is continuously active. The degree of activity varies from moment to moment and from organ to organ. However, it can also react as a unit, as seen in the fight and/or flight reaction.

Table 1. Specificity at adrenoceptor subtypes

a_1	epinephrine $\geq$ norepinephrine $\gg$ isoproterenol
a_2	epinephrine $\geq$ norepinephrine $\gg$ isoproterenol
β_1	isoproterenol $>$ epinephrine $=$ norepinephrine
β_2	isoproterenol $>$ epinephrine $\gg$ norepinephrine
β_3	isoproterenol $=$ norepinephrine $>$ epinephrine

▌ The Endogenous Catecholamines

The releative potencies of epinephrine and norepinephrine at the different adrenoceptor subtypes are listed in Table 1. Epinephrine originates almost exclusively from the adrenal medulla and serves as a hormone. It is a full agonist at the β_1-, β_2-, a_1- and a_2-adrenoceptors. Norepinephrine is the neurotransmitter in the second sympathetic neuron and in the central nervous system (CNS). The potency of norepinephrine in comparison to epinephrine is equal at the β_1-adrenoceptor and it is equal or less potent at both a-adrenoceptor subtypes [1]. Norepinephrine is 10 to 50-fold less potent at the β_2-adrenoceptor than epinephrine [3]. Norepinephrine is more effective at the β_3-adrenoceptor that is resistant to blockade by propranolol [1].

Dopamine is a central neurotransmitter, which is of particular importance in the control of movement. At low doses it acts on the D_1- and D_2-receptor subtypes. Outside the CNS, activation of the D_1-receptor causes renal vasodilation; activation of the D_2-receptor decreases action potential-evoked norepinephrine release by a presynaptic mechanism and interferes with the release of some pituitary hormones. Dopamine stimulates the release of growth hormone and suppresses the release of thyroid stimulating hormone (TSH) and prolactin [4]. A decrease in prolactin release can suppress immune function [5]. At somewhat higher concentrations, dopamine acts on β_1- and a_1-adrenoceptors both directly and as an indirect sympathomimetic agent. There are no reports of major actions on a_2- and β_2-adrenoceptors.

▌ The Synthetic Adrenergic Activating Drugs:
Isoproterenol, Fenoterol, Phenylephrine, Dobutamine, and Dopexamine

The relative potencies of the synthetic adrenergic drugs at the adrenoceptor subtypes are given in Table 2. Isoproterenol is a non-selective β-adrenoceptor agonist. Fenoterol is a selective β_2-adrenoceptor agonist. Phenylephrine acts selectively on a_1-adrenoceptors [1]. The two newer adrenergic agents, dobutamine and dopexamine, have a more complex profile. Dobutamine is a racemic mixture. It is devoid of a_2-agonist activity. The (–) isomer is a partial a_1-adrenoceptor agonist reaching 60% of the maximal effect of phenylephrine. In contrast, the (+) isomer is an a_1-adrenoceptor antagonist, which can block the effects of the (–) isomer or of the endogenous catecholamines [6]. The (+) isomer is seven to ten times more potent at the β_1-adrenoceptor [6] and about 18-fold more potent at the β_2-adrenoceptor [7] than the (–) isomer. The dose to reach half of the maximal effect is two fold higher for the β_2-effect than for the β_1-effect [7]. Furthermore, these receptor interactions were obtained in isolated tissues from different species. There are no conclusive studies of dobutamine dose (plasma concentration) effect in man for selective adrenoceptor activity.

Table 2. Catecholamines and receptors

	a_1	a_2	β_1	β_2	DA_1	DA_2	indirect
Dopamine	1	0	1	0	1	1	+++[d]
(+) Dobutamine	0[a]	0	1[b, c]	1[b, c]	0	0	0
(−) Dobutamine	0.6	0	0.7[c]	0.7[c]	0	0	0
(+/−) Dobutamine	0.6	0	1	?	0	0	0
Dopexamine	0	0	++	+	0.3	0.16	+++[d]
Fenoterol	0	0	+	+++	0	0	0

indirect: indirect sympathomimetic action

[a] a_1-adrenoceptor antagonist

[b] For (+) dobutamine the concentration of the half maximal response is 30-fold higher for the β_2-effect as for the β_1-effect

[c] For (−) dobutamine the concentration of the half maximal effect for the β_1-effect is 9.5-fold higher, and for the β_2-effect 18-fold higher than (+) dobutamine, respectively

[d] The contribution of the indirect sympathomimetric effect of dopamine and dopexamine to the total drug effect is not known. The indirect sympathomimetric effect for vasopressor action by a-adrenoceptor-stimulation is not important whereas β-adrenoceptor mediated chronotropic and inotropic effects of dopamine are mediated by direct receptor stimulation and indirectly released norepinephrine

In clinical use, (+,−)-dobutamine appears to be a selective β_1-adrencoceptor agonist. It is not known whether the sometimes-observed hypotension in critically ill patients is related to the a_1-antagonist activity of the (+) isomer. A contribution to this effect by β_2-adrenoceptor activation is discussed, though unlikely since no increase in cAMP production by dobutamine was observed in human lymphocytes [8]. Dobutamine has no indirect sympathomimetic activity.

Dopexamine is an agonist at the D_1- and D_2-receptors with an activity of 1/3 and 1/6, respectively when compared to dopamine. Dopexamine is a full β_2-adrenoceptor agonist. However, the activity of dopexamine is only 1/300 compared with isoproterenol at a molar level [9]. The clinical importance of the β_2-action is questioned since MacGregor et al. [8] found no cAMP production by dopexamine in human lymphocytes. Dopexamine possesses an indirect sympathomimetic action by inhibiting neuronal norepinephrine reuptake [10], resulting in an increase in the norepinephrine plasma concentration. This release of endogenous norepinephrine contributes to the effect of dopexamine.

▌ Metabolic Effects

The actions of adrenoceptor activation can be investigated by either using an agonist or by administration of an antagonist in a state with an increased endogenous agonist release. Systematic studies on the metabolic effects of adrenergic drugs in healthy volunteers were mainly conducted using agonists. In patients, studies on the metabolic action of vasoactive compounds are rare with the exception of the investigation of oxygen consumption and carbohydrate metabolism. However, a few studies in which antagonists were administered have led to some conclusions regarding the consequences of the activated endogenous sympatho-adrenergic system.

Table 3. Metabolic effects mediated by adrenoceptor-subtypes

	α_1	α_2	β_1	β_2	β_3
Metabolic rate	0	0	+++	+++	+++
Glucose production	+[a]	0	0	(+)[a]	?
Gluconeogenesis	0	0	0	+++[b]	0
Glycogenolysis	+++	0	0	0	0
Lactate concentration	0	0	0	+++[b]	0
Insulin concentration	0	−[c]		+[c]	0
Lipolysis	0	0	+++	?	+++
Proteolysis	0	0	0	−	?

[a] Only a combined stimulation of α and β_2-adrenoceptor stimulation results in a maximal stimulation of glucose production since insulin release is suppressed

[b] An increase in gluconeogenesis is critically dependent on an increase in precursor supply, such as lactate, alanine and glycerol

[c] The suppression of insulin release by α-adrenoceptors overrides the stimulation of insulin release by β_2-adrenoceptors

Administration of catecholamines has an impact on metabolic rate, carbohydrate, fat and protein metabolism in healthy volunteers. In Table 3, the metabolic actions of adrenergic drugs are related to the different adrenoceptor subtypes. Catecholamines also can affect the release of certain hormones and interfere with the immune system. Both of these actions do not play a major role in the volunteer studies. In patients after trauma or with sepsis the interaction between the hemodynamic system, metabolism, hormone release, and the immune system becomes very complex as a general activation of the immune system with release of cytokines and the expression of genes makes the underlying situation completely different from that of healthy volunteers. Furthermore, the immune system and the sympathetic nervous system interact [1, 2, 11, 12].

▌ Resting Metabolic Rate

The sympatho-adrenergic system is involved in thermogenesis. Activation of all β-adrenoceptor subtypes increases resting metabolic rate and hence oxygen consumption in humans, while α-adrenoceptor agonists are without effect [13]. However, the contribution of the β_3-adenoceptor subtype in humans has not been well investigated. The mechanism leading to the increase in resting metabolic rate is not completely understood. Uncoupling of mitochondrial oxidative phosphorylation in brown adipose tissue and skeletal muscle by a β-adrenoceptor mediated effect contributes to the thermogenic effect of catecholamines [14, 15]. This increase in metabolic rate is related to an increase in free fatty acid availability [16].

Gluconeogenesis is an energy consuming process and an increase in Cori-cycle activity may also contribute to the increase in metabolic rate [17]. Gylcolysis from glucose to pyruvate produces two mol of ATP per mol glucose. The synthesis of one mol glucose from lactate consumes six to seven mol of ATP. Hepatic gluconeogenesis may contribute up to 50% of hepatic oxygen consumption [18]. Epinephrine causes a considerable increase in oxygen consumption [19], that is sustained over time [20].

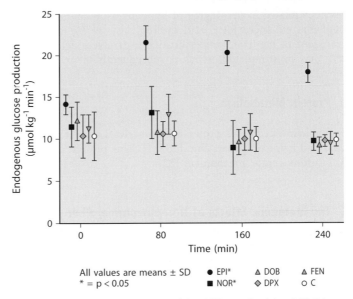

Fig. 1. Effects of adrenergic agonists on glucose production. EPI epinephrine, NOR norepinephrine, DOB dobuta-mine, DPX dopexamine, FEN fenoterol, C control. Means ± standard deviation are given. * p < 0.05 drug versus control, two way analysis of variance

▌ Carbohydrate Metabolism

Epinephrine causes hyperglycemia and hyperlactatemia [21]. The plasma concentration of insulin remains low since insulin release is suppressed despite the elevated glucose plasma concentration by an α-adrenergic effect [22].

Hyperglycemia results from an increase in glucose production and a decrease in peripheral insulin-dependent glucose uptake [23]. The increase in glucose production is caused by an increase in hepatic glycogenolysis which is caused by α_1-adrenoceptor activation and an increase in gluconeogenesis which is related to β_2-adrenoceptor activation in dogs [24]. Species differences are obvious. However, Kawai et al. [25] found that canine and human liver plasma membranes have a similar adrenoceptor distribution with α_1- and β_2-adrenoceptors predominating, suggesting that these mechanisms are active in humans as well.

In skeletal muscle, epinephrine enhances glycogenolysis and glycolysis resulting in an increase in peripheral lactate and alanine release. This increase in alanine release is not related to an enhanced protein breakdown [26]. Both, lactate and alanine serve as substrates for hepatic gluconeogenesis. Thus epinephrine causes an increase in Cori-cycle- and glucose-alanine-cycle activity [26–29]. In Figure 1 the effect of some adrenergic agonists on glucose production is shown.

▌ Fat Metabolism

Epinephrine increases lipolysis as shown by an increase in the rate of appearance by palmitic acid [30]. The increase in the plasma concentration of free fatty acids may be transient or lasting [20], depending on the adrenergic agonist used and perhaps related to the degree of hyperglycemia and subsequent insulin release. Epinephrine enhances fatty acid cycling, i.e., release of fatty acids from adipocytes, transport to the liver, reesterification to triglyceride, and hepatic release of lipoprotein may be stimulated, which is subsequently taken up in adipocytes [17].

▌ Protein Metabolism

Epinephrine decreases proteolysis in skeletal muscle as shown by a decrease in leucine and ketoisocaproate flux [26, 31]. This protein preserving effect is mediated by a β_2-adrenoceptor mechanism [32].

▌ The Metabolic Effects of Norepinephrine, Phenylephrine, Fenoterol, Dobutamine, and Dopexamine in Volunteers

Norepinephrine increases oxygen consumption to a lesser extent than epinephrine [19]. There is only a slight transient increase in glucose production [19] which is most likely only due to glycogenolysis and not to gluconeogenesis [24]. The plasma lactate concentration remains in the physiologic range. Norepinephrine induces a persistent increase in plasma fatty acid concentration [20]. It has no effect on protein metabolism. The α_1-agonist, phenylephrine, induces neither calorigenic nor other metabolic effects in volunteers [33].

The preferential β_2-agonist, fenoterol, has similar effects on oxygen consumption and metabolism as epinephrine with the exception that the plasma insulin concentration increases and the rise in plasma glucose concentration is only 20% of that found with epinephrine [33]. The lack of an increase in glucose production may be due to the elevated plasma insulin concentration. The increase in the plasma lactate concentration may lead to an increase in hepatic gluconeogenesis. The decrease in proteolysis as shown by a decrease in leucine flux may be due to a direct β_2-adrenoceptor effect and/or to the increase in the plasma insulin concentration.

Dobutamine causes an increase in oxygen consumption and plasma fatty acid concentration, like epinephrine. It does not affect glucose or insulin plasma concentration [33]. However, it decreases the rate of production of glucose. The decreased leucine flux suggests a decrease in skeletal muscle proteolysis.

Dopexamine also increases oxygen consumption and plasma fatty acid concentration. There is only a minor enhancement in carbohydrate metabolism at infusion rates above 2–3 µg/kg min [34]. No increase in glucose production is observed. Like dobutamine, dopexamine decreases skeletal muscle proteolysis.

▌ Are the Metabolic Actions of Adrenergic Drugs Important for the Critically Ill?

Sepsis and trauma result in a 10–30% increase in metabolic rate. Patients with severe burn injury and septic complications can have an increase in metabolic rate of up to 100% [35]. But, even patients with a minor increase in metabolic rate suffer from protein catabolism and a loss of lean body mass, since in contrast to fasting and starvation there is an increase in skeletal muscle protein breakdown. Hyperglycemia and an elevated glucose production are present in patients with sepsis or trauma paralleled by an increase in splanchnic oxygen uptake [36, 37]. Gluconeogenesis from lactate and alanine is markedly enhanced. Hyperglycemia and the enhanced gluconeogenesis are not sensitive to insulin. Similarly, lipolysis is increased [38] and also not sensitive to insulin, resulting in fatty acid cycling [17] and hepatic steatosis [39].

The counterregulatory hormones (epinephrine, glucagon, cortisol) are thought to mediate this metabolic reaction in trauma or sepsis. Bessey et al. [40] showed that only a combined infusion of epinephrine, cortisol, and glucagon, mimicked in part the response seen after mild to moderate injury, while epinephrine alone did not evoke that response. Additionally, cytokines play a pivotal role in the metabolic response. Fong et al. [41] investigated the effect of a six hour infusion of epinephrine followed by a six hour infusion of epinephrine and cortisol on volunteers during parenteral nutrition. They found the typical response outlined above with an increase in metabolic rate by approximately 30%, hyperglycemia, and hyperlactatemia and a decrease in leg amino acid outflow suggesting a decrease in proteolysis by epinephrine, which was reversed by the addition of cortisol [41]. The same group later on investigated the effect of a bolus of endotoxin during the subsequent six hours [42]. Metabolic rate was increased by 40% and hyperglycemia was similar to in the study cited above. The leg amino acid outflow resembled that obtained by infusion of the combination of epinephrine and cortisol. However, values for cortisol and plasma epinephrine concentrations were far lower in the endotoxin study than in the study with cortisol and epinephrine infusion, suggesting that these hormones were not solely responsible for the metabolic effects after endotoxin administration.

Studies in Patients with Adrenergic Agonists

The short-term effect of dobutamine on glucose production was investigated in patients with septic shock and after coronary artery bypass surgery. The patients with septic shock required norepinephrine to maintain a mean arterial pressure (MAP) of more than 70 mmHg. Dobutamine was added to obtain a 20% increase in cardiac output. Despite an increase in oxygen delivery (DO_2), oxygen consumption (VO_2) did not increase. Dobutamine decreased glucose production in these patients who had an elevated baseline rate of production of glucose [43].

After coronary artery bypass-grafting, dobutamine was infused at a dosage to increase cardiac output by at least 25%. This goal was achieved at an infusion rate of 6 µg/kg min. Dobutamine increased systemic and splanchnic blood flow. Whole body VO_2 increased by 10% while splanchnic VO_2 did not change. There was a decrease in glucose production over time in both the dobutamine and the control group. These patients had a glucose production which was slightly less than in normal post-absorptive volunteers. No changes in interorgan lactate or amino acid transportation rates were observed [44]. In both patient populations, dobutamine had a similar effect as seen in volunteers except that the increase in VO_2 in the coronary artery bypass surgery group was only half of that found in volunteers [33].

Dopexamine was investigated in patients with septic shock, requiring norepinephrine in order to maintain MAP above 60 mmHg. Dopexamine was infused to increase cardiac output by 18 to 35%. The infusion rate of dopexamine was one to four µ/kg min. Despite an increase in DO_2, VO_2 did not increase. The median lactate/pyruvate ratio in these patients was 14, and thus slightly above the normal value of 10 showing that some patients might have had an oxygen limited ATP-production. Glucose production, splanchnic lactate and alanine balance and the lactate/pyruvate ratio were not changed [45], also a similar finding to that in volunteers.

The effect of phenylephrine on splanchnic VO_2 and glucose production was investigated in patients with septic shock requiring norepinephrine administration [46]. A switch from norepinephrine to phenylephrine titrated to obtain a similar MAP (phenylephrine infusion rate: median 3.2 mg/kg min, range 1.08 to 9.62 µg/kg min) did not change cardiac output or systemic or splanchnic VO_2. Splanchnic blood flow, DO_2, glucose production and splanchnic lactate uptake decreased during phenylephrine infusion. Switching back to norepinephrine again, restored the values of all variables except the glucose production which remained suppressed. Glucose production was not correlated with splanchnic VO_2. The author does not have an explanation for these results in terms of metabolic action mediated by adrenoceptors.

▌ Studies in Patients with Hypermetabolism and β-adrenoceptor Blockade

Wolfe et al. [17] showed that in patients with severe burns, substrate cycling of glucose and fatty acids is increased. All patients had an increased plasma concentration of the counter-regulatory hormones and an increased rate of appearance of glucose and fatty acids. Infusion of propranolol decreased the fatty acid cycling but not that of glucose, suggesting that in hypermetabolic patients the increase in lipolysis is enhanced by a β-adrenergic mechanism. The increase in metabolic rate brought about by catecholamines is related to the uncoupling of the respiration chain and to an increase in lipolysis (see above). In a very recent study, the same group showed that in children with severe burns, propranolol at a dosage to decrease heart rate by 20% resulted in a 20% decrease in metabolic rate as compared to baseline over a 14 day period. Furthermore, the loss of lean body mass was 1% as compared to 9% in the control group. While skeletal muscle proteolysis was not affected by propranolol, skeletal muscle protein synthesis was enhanced in the propranolol group suggesting that a β-adrenergic mechanism is involved in the suppression of muscle protein synthesis [47]. There might also be a link between the decrease in metabolic rate and protein wasting since catecholamines are at least in part responsible for the hypermetabolism seen after burn injury [48], and metabolic rate is one of the determinants of protein loss in burn patients [49].

▌ Conclusion

In volunteers, catecholamines have clearly defined metabolic effects besides their impact on the hemodynamic system. Activation of the sympatho-adrenergic system leads to the stand by or provision of maximal physical exercise. In injury or sepsis, the sympatho-adrenergic system leads to a hypermetabolic and hypercatabolic state. The studies on metabolic actions of vasoactive drugs are rather limited, mainly to metabolic rate and glucose metabolism. In studies on septic patients, the adrenergic agonists dobutamine and dopexamine did not induce a major increase in metabolic rate and there was either no change or a decrease in glucose production. Hence, from these studies, no adverse effects of dobutamine or dopexamine can be derived. However, studies with β-adrenoceptor antagonists suggest that the increase in metabolic rate, that in part is mediated by adrenoceptor stimulation by endogenous epinephrine and norepinephrine, results in an increase in protein wasting.

References

1. Lefkowitz RJ, Hofman BB, Taylor P (1996) Neurotransmission. In: Hardman JG, Limbird LE (eds) The Pharmacological Basis of Therapeutics, 9th edn., McGraw-Hill, New York, pp 105–139
2. Elenkov IJ, Wilder RL, Chrousos GP, Vizi ES (2000) The sympathetic nerve–an integrative interface between two supersystems: the brain and the immune system. Pharmacol Rev 52:595–638
3. Lands AM, Arnold A, McAuliff JP, Luduena FP, Brown TG (1967) Differentiation of receptor systems activated by sympathomimetic amines. Nature 214:597–598
4. Tuomisto J Männistö P (1985) Neurotransmitter regulation of anterior pituitary hormones. Pharmacol Rev 37:249–332
5. Chikanza IC (1999) Prolactin and neuroimmunomodulation: in vitro and in vivo observations. Ann N Y Acad Sci 876:119–130
6. Ruffolo RR, Spradlin TA, Pollock GD, Waddell JE, Murphy PJ (1981) Alpha and beta adrenergic effects of the stereoisomers of dobutamine. J Pharmacol Exp Ther 219:447–452
7. Ruffolo RR Yaden EL (1983) Vascular effects of the stereoisomers of dobutamine. J Pharmacol Exp Ther 224:46–50
8. MacGregor DA, Prielipp RC, Butterworth JF, James RL, Royster RL (1996) Relative efficacy and potency of beta-adrenoceptor agonists for generating cAMP in human lymphocytes. Chest 109:194–200
9. Brown RA, Dixon J, Farmer JB, et al (1985) Dopexamine: a novel agonist at peripheral dopamine receptors and β 2-adrenoceptors. Br J Pharmacol 85:599–608
10. Brown RA, Farmer JB, Hall JC, Humphries RG, O'Connor SE, Smith GW (1985) The effects of dopexamine on the cardiovascular system of the dog. Br J Pharmacol 85:609–619
11. De Luigi A, Terreni L, Sironi M, De Simoni MG (1998) The sympathetic nervous system tonically inhibits peripheral interleukin–1betaand interleukin–6 induction by central lipopolysaccharide. Neuroscience 83:1245–1250
12. Farmer P Pugin J (2000) beta-adrenergic agonists exert their "anti-inflammatory" effects in monocytic cells through the IkappaB/NF-kappaB pathway. Am J Physiol 279:L675–L682
13. Blaak EE, Saris WH, van Baak MA (1993) Adrenoceptor subtypes mediating catecholamine-induced thermogenesis in man. Int J Obes Relat Metab Disord 17 (suppl 3):S78-S81
14. Nagase I, Yoshida T, Saito M (2001) Up-regulation of uncoupling proteins by β-adrenergic stimulation in L6 myotubes. FEBS Lett 494:175–180
15. Nedergaard J, Golozoubova V, Matthias A, Asadi A, Jacobsson A, Cannon B (2001) UCP1: the only protein able to mediate adaptive non-shivering thermogenesis and metabolic inefficiency. Biochim Biophys Acta 1504:82–106
16. Schiffelers SL, Brouwer EM, Saris WH, van Baak MA (1998) Inhibition of lipolysis reduces beta1-adrenoceptor-mediated thermogenesis in man. Metabolism 47:1462–1467
17. Wolfe RR, Herndon DN, Jahoor F, Miyoshi H, Wolfe M (1987) Effect of severe burn injury on substrate cycling by glucose and fatty acids. N Engl J Med 317:403–408
18. Jungas RL, Halperin ML, Brosnan JT (1992) Quantitative analysis of amino acid oxidation and related gluconeogenesis in humans. Physiol Rev 72:419–448
19. Ensinger H, Weichel T, Lindner KH, Grünert A, Ahnefeld FW, Grunert A (1993) Effects of norepinephrine, epinephrine, and dopamine infusions on oxygen consumption in volunteers. Crit Care Med 21:1502–1508
20. Ensinger H, Weichel T, Lindner KH, Grunert A, Georgieff M (1995) Are the effects of noradrenaline, adrenaline and dopamine infusions on vo2 and metabolism transient? Intensive Care Med 21:50–56

21. Cryer PE (1993) Adrenaline: a physiological metabolic regulatory hormone in humans? Int J Obes Relat Metab Disord 17 (suppl 3):S43–S46
22. Porte D (1967) A receptor mechanism for the inhibition of insulin release by epinephrine in man. J Clin Invest 46:86–94
23. Nonogaki K (2000) New insights into sympathetic regulation of glucose and fat metabolism. Diabetologia 43:533–549
24. Chu CA, Sindelar DK, Igawa K, et al (2000) The direct effects of catecholamines on hepatic glucose production occur via alpha(1)- and beta(2)-receptors in the dog. Am J Physiol 279:E463–E473
25. Kawai Y, Powell A, Arinze IJ (1986) Adrenergic receptors in human liver plasma membranes: predominance of beta 2- and alpha 1-receptor subtypes. J Clin Endocrinol Metab 62:827–832
26. Ensinger H, Träger K, Geisser W, et al (1994) Glucose and urea production and leucine, ketoisocaproate and alanine fluxes at supraphysiological plasma adrenaline concentrations in volunteers. Intensive Care Med 20:113–118
27. Kusaka M, Ui M (1977) Activation of the Cori cycle by epinephrine. Am J Physiol 232:E145–E155
28. Sacca L, Vigorito C, Cicala M, Corso G, Sherwin RS (1983) Role of gluconeogenesis in epinephrine-stimulated hepatic glucose production in humans. Am J Physiol 245:E294–E302
29. Cherrington AD, Fuchs H, Stevenson RW, Williams PE, Alberti KGMM, Steiner KE (1984) Effect of epinephrine on glycogenolysis and gluconeogenesis in conscious overnight-fasted dogs. Am J Physiol 247:E137–E144
30. Galster AD, Clutter WE, Cryer PE, Collins JA, Bier DM (1981) Epinephrine plasma thresholds for lipolytic effects in man. J Clin Invest 67:1729–1738
31. Matthews DE, Pesola G, Campbell RG (1990) Effect of epinephrine on amino acid and energy metabolism in humans. Am J Physiol 258:E948–E956
32. Navegantes LC, Resano NM, Migliorini RH, Kettelhut IC (2000) Role of adrenoceptors and cAMP on the catecholamine-induced inhibition of proteolysis in rat skeletal muscle. Am J Physiol 279:E663–E668
33. Erb JM, Ensinger H, Gaissmaier S, Weichel T, Schricker T, Georgieff M (1995) Oxygen uptake and metabolic changes during infusion of dobutamine in comparison to fenoterol and phenylephrine in volunteers. Clin Intensive Care 6:159–165
34. Geisser W, Trager K, Hahn A, Georgieff M, Ensinger H (1997) Metabolic and calorigenic effects of dopexamine in healthy volunteers. Crit Care Med 25:1332–1337
35. Kinney JM Elwyn DH (1983) Protein metabolism and injury. Ann Rev Nutr 3:433–466
36. Dahn MS, Lange P, Lobdell K, Hans B, Jacobs LA, Mitchell RA (1987) Splanchnic and total body oxygen consumption differences in septic and injured patients. Surgery 101:69–80
37. Wilmore DW, Goodwin CW, Aulick LH, Powanda MC, Mason AD, Pruitt BA (1980) Effect of injury and infection on visceral metabolism and circulation. Ann Surg 192:491–504
38. Miles JM (1993) Lipid fuel metabolism in health and disease. Curr Opin Gen Surg 78–84
39. Feingold KR, Grunfeld C (1987) Tumor necrosis factor-alpha stimulates hepatic lipogenesis in the rat in vivo. J Clin Invest 80:184–190
40. Bessey PQ, Watters JM, Aoki TT, Wilmore DW (1984) Combined hormonal infusion simulates the metabolic response to injury. Ann Surg 200:264–280
41. Fong YM, Albert JD, Tracey K, et al (1991) The influence of substrate background on the acute metabolic response to epinephrine and cortisol. J Trauma 31:1467–1476
42. Fong Y, Marano MA, Moldawer LL, et al (1990) The acute splanchnic and peripheral tissue metabolic response to endotoxin in humans. J Clin Invest 85:1896–1904
43. Reinelt H, Radermacher P, Fischer G, et al (1997) Effects of a dobutamine-induced increase in splanchnic blood flow on hepatic metabolic activity in patients with septic shock. Anesthesiology 86:818–824
44. Ensinger H, Rantala A, Vogt J, Georgieff M, Takala J (1999) Effect of dobutamine on splanchnic carbohydrate metabolism and amino acid balance after cardiac surgery. Anesthesiology 91:1587–1595
45. Kiefer P, Tugtekin I, Wiedeck H, et al (2001) Effect of dopexamine on hepatic metabolic activity in patients with septic shock. Shock 15:427–431

46. Reinelt H, Radermacher P, Kiefer P, et al (1999) Impact of exogenous beta-adrenergic receptor stimulation on hepatosplanchnic oxygen kinetics and metabolic activity in septic shock. Crit Care Med 27:325–331
47. Herndon DN, Hart DW, Wolf SE, Chinkes DL, Wolfe RR (2001) Reversal of catabolism by beta-blockade after severe burns. N Engl J Med 345:1223–1229
48. Wilmore DW, Long JM, Mason AD, Skreen RW, Pruitt BA (1974) Catecholamines: mediator of the hypermetabolic response to thermal injury. Ann Surg 180:653–668
49. Hart DW, Wolf SE, Chinkes DL, et al (2000) Determinants of skeletal muscle catabolism after severe burn. Ann Surg 232:455–465

Acidemia: Good, Bad or Inconsequential?

J. A. Kellum, M. Song, and S. Subramanian

Introduction

Despite significant advances in the understanding of cellular physiology and acid-base chemistry, and despite progress in the treatment of acid-base disorders, a central clinical question remains unanswered: Is acidemia harmful? To address this question we will consider both theory and evidence. Acid-base theory is important because it impacts greatly on the interpretation of the limited clinical, epidemiologic, and experimental evidence. It is also important because most clinicians fail to understand or apply basic physical-chemical principles. This said, let us first review the basics of acid-base chemistry.

Acid-base Physiology and Physical Chemistry

At the clinical level, acid-base physiology is really the study of blood pH. While intracellular acid-base balance is, no doubt, of great interest, it varies widely between cell types [1] and cannot be measured clinically (note gastric tonometry does not measure pHi [2]). Thus, we are confined to evaluating acid-base balance in the blood. As such, it is important to appreciate that the determinants of blood pH are the physical chemical determinants of hydrogen ion concentration in aqueous solutions where water dissociation (into H^+ and OH^-) is a critical factor [3, 4]. Governed by the principles of electrical neutrality and conservation of mass, H^+ concentration is determined by three independent variables: CO_2, the weak acids and the strong ions. Importantly, the Henderson-Hasselbalch equation defines equilibrium for only one of these variables (i.e., CO_2). While the system as a whole can be accurately *described* using only one equation, the *determinants* of blood pH include all three [3, 4]. The key point here is that pH (really H^+ concentration) is not an independent variable and neither is bicarbonate ion (for a complete discussion of this topic, the reader is referred to a number of recent reviews [4–6]. Thus, it is impossible to separate the effects of pH *per se* from the effects of the independent variables controlling it. Indeed, changes in blood pH due to alterations in CO_2 vs those secondary to metabolic causes often appear to produce very different clinical effects.

Nonetheless, there are good reasons to believe that changes in H^+ concentration itself are associated with important biological effects. First, H^+ ions have very high charge densities and thus very large electric fields. In the plasma, four to five fold changes in H^+ concentration are possible within the physiologic range, and even greater variability can exist inside cells [1]. Thus, enormous changes in electric field strength are possible and likely have important effects on nearby cellular structures. Second, the strengths of hydrogen bonds, ubiquitous in biologic systems, are very sensitive to local H^+ concentration. Third, enzyme activities are profoundly influenced by local pH and finally, H^+ concentration affects the rates of biochemical reactions in which it is involved.

Clinical Evidence

Whether acidemia itself causes clinical effects, or whether these effects are caused by the variables producing the acidosis, is uncertain. Some insight can be gained by comparing the effects associated with respiratory vs metabolic acidosis (Table 1). Undoubtedly, some of the differences in effect between respiratory and metabolic acidosis are due to differences in the diffusibility of CO_2 compared to strong ions. CO_2 can move rather quickly into the cells and across the blood-brain barrier, whereas strong ions such as lactate and chloride (Cl^-), must be actively transported

Table 1. Clinical effects associated with acidosis

	Metabolic	Respiratory
Cardiovascular		
decreased inotropy*	+	
conduction defects	+	
arterial vasodilatation	+	++
venous vasoconstriction	+	
pulmonary vasoconstriction	+	++
Oxygen Delivery		
decreased oxy-Hb binding	+	+
decreased 2,3 DPG (late)	+	+
Neuromuscular		
respiratory depression	+	++
decreased sensorium	+	++
increased intracranial pressure		+
Metabolism		
bone demineralization	+	
catecholamine, stimulation*	+/++	+/++
insulin resistance	+	
decreased oxygen utilization	+	
Gastrointestinal/Hepatic		
nausea/vomiting	+	
decreased protein synthesis	+	
Electrolytes		
hyperkalemia	+	
hypercalcemia	+	
hyperuricemia	+	

+/++ Denote relative effects between respiratory and metabolic acidosis. *The effect seen with acidosis may be variable depending on the state of endogenous catecholamine release and exogenous catecholamine use.

or move through channels. As ionized species, their movement alters local charge and has electrical consequences that are not easily overcome. Thus, when metabolic acidosis is exogenous (e.g., HCl infusion) or regional (e.g., lactate from an exercising muscle) its effects will not be rapidly or evenly distributed across all cells in the body. However, it is not yet known whether the clinical consequences associated with acidosis are related to the intracellular acid-base status or that of the extracellular fluid.

A quick examination of Table 1 will reveal that most of the clinical effects associated with acidosis are undesirable – but not all. Healthy, conditioned, exercising subjects routinely experience severe metabolic (lactic) acidosis without apparent sequel [7]. And recently, some authors have suggested the possibly beneficial effects of acidosis in patients. In conditions of unresuscitated shock, acidosis decreases cellular function, conserving metabolic substrate, and decreasing oxygen utilization [8]. The effects of acidosis on the shape of the oxyhemoglobin dissociation curve may also be beneficial in some circumstances. Correcting acidosis in such conditions may be quite harmful [9] and even when harm cannot be proved, there is little or no evidence of benefit [10]. However, as we will discuss later, cautioning against the correction of metabolic acidosis with sodium bicarbonate is very different from allowing acidosis to occur in the first place.

One place where we allow acidosis to occur is in the ventilator management of acute lung injury (ALI), a practice commonly referred to as 'permissive hypercapnia'. Arterial PCO_2 is determined by the balance between production by cellular respiration and elimination by alveolar ventilation. Arterial PCO_2 is adjusted by the respiratory center in response to altered arterial pH produced by metabolic acidosis or alkalosis in predictable ways. While it is desirable to maintain a normal PCO_2 of 40 mmHg, in certain instances one has to accept higher levels of CO_2 tension as a consequence of concomitant therapeutic interventions. While this strategy may be useful in some patients with ALI, it is not clear whether it is necessary to achieve the desired levels of airway pressure recently shown to improve outcome in such patients [11]. Furthermore, some authors have postulated that high CO_2 levels in themselves may be protective [12]. This hypothesis is based on the yet unproven, but potentially beneficial, effects of hypercarbia including arterial vasodilatation and improved PO_2. However, a rise in PCO_2 and the resulting intracellular acidosis, may contribute to increased catecholamine synthesis, increased intracranial and pulmonary artery pressures, and a variety of other effects (Table 1) that are potentially deleterious. The arterial PO_2 may actually fall owing to a decrease in alveolar PO_2. If an improvement in oxygenation is seen with this strategy, it might instead be explained by improvements in ventilation perfusion matching and minimization of ventilator induced lung injury. The improvements in hemodynamics can also be related to these factors. Although CO_2 is a vasodilator in local vascular beds, hypercarbia has not been convincingly shown to either induce systemic vasodilatation or improve cardiac output. Thus, CO_2 may be considered a potentially useful but dangerous drug.

▎ Epidemiological Evidence

There is little question that, regardless of whether or not there is a true cause-effect relationship, acidosis is a powerful marker of poor prognosis in critically ill patients. Again there does seem to be a difference between patients with respiratory

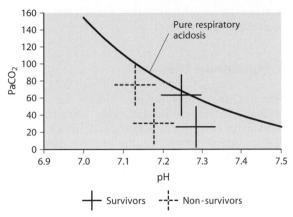

Fig. 1. Relationship between acidosis and mortality in two different populations. Shown are ranges of blood gas data for survivors and non-survivors with either permissive hypercapnia (upper pair) or lactic acidosis (lower pair). In both series, non-survivors were more acidemic than survivors. Furthermore, in both series, the mean values for non-survivors were further from the line of pure respiratory acidosis. (Figure adapted from [11] and [24])

and metabolic acidosis (Fig. 1) and this might temper concerns over the dangers of hypercarbia. However, in all cases, the lower the pH, the higher the mortality. Interestingly, in both groups, non-survivors had blood gases that were further separated from the line of pure respiratory acidosis. In other words, non-survivors had more *metabolic* acidosis.

In the ICU, metabolic acidosis is usually due to either elevated lactate or another strong ion such as Cl^- (commonly seen during resuscitation with saline). While factors such as hypoperfusion and hypoxia will play important roles in generation of lactic acidosis in ischemic states, current evidence does not support a prominent role for anaerobiosis as a mechanism for acidosis in patients. Indeed, increased aerobic metabolism and decreased lactate utilization appear to be much more important mechanisms in resuscitated states [13].

The effect of Cl^- administration on the development of metabolic acidosis has been known for many years. Recently, there has been renewed interest in this area in light of better understanding of the mechanisms responsible for this effect. It has now been shown in animal models of sepsis and in patients undergoing surgery that saline causes metabolic acidosis not by 'diluting' bicarbonate (HCO_3^-), but rather by its Cl^- content [14–18]. From a physical-chemical prospective this is completely expected. HCO_3^- is a dependent variable and its reduction *per se* cannot be the cause of the acidosis. Instead, Cl^- administration decreases the strong ion difference (SID, an independent variable) and produces an increase in water dissociation and hence H^+ concentration. The reason this occurs with saline administration is that, although saline contains equal amounts of both Na^+ and Cl^-, the plasma does not. When large amounts of salt are added, the Cl^- concentration increases much more than the sodium concentration. For example, 0.9% ('normal') saline contains 154 mEq/l of Na^+ and Cl^-. Administration of large volumes of this fluid will have a proportionally greater effect on total body Cl^- than on total body Na^+. Of note, it is the total body concentrations of these strong ions that must be considered and although the true volume of distribution of Cl^- is less, like Na^+, the effective volume of distribution (after some time of equilibration) is equal to total body water [14].

▌ Experimental Evidence

However, these data do not address the clinical significance of hyperchloremic acidosis. To answer this question, controlled studies are needed. Such studies are difficult in critically ill humans with shock but are easier to do in elective surgery and in animal models. Neither of these fully simulates human shock and resuscitation, but we may never have data that directly address this population. In one recent study, elective surgery patients were loaded with two fluid regimens [19]. One was composed of 0.9% saline and hydroxyethyl starch in saline (Hespan®); the other was composed of lactated Ringers and hydroxyethyl starch in a balanced electrolyte solution (Hextend®). The primary outcome measures included acidosis and morbidity. Hyperchloremic acidosis occurred exclusively in the saline/Hespan® group and morbidity was significantly higher in this group as well. Morbid events were primarily those attributable to the acidosis (abdominal pain and nausea). In our studies using a rat model of septic shock induced by endotoxin infusion, we compared fluid resuscitation with saline to Hextend® in terms of acidosis and survival time [20]. Our results demonstrate a significant improvement in survival time with Hextend® (567 ± 140 min) vs saline (391 ± 151 min), $p < 0.0001$. Overall survival (at 12 hrs) was 20% with Hextend®, vs 0% with saline, $p = 0.05$. After resuscitation with Hextend®, arterial standard base excess and plasma apparent strong ion difference (SID) were both significantly higher (-12.1 ± 5.7 vs -19.3 ± 5.2, $p < 0.001$ and 30.3 ± 2.9 vs 23.0 ± 6.2, $p < 0.0001$, respectively) compared to saline. Furthermore, survival time was inversely correlated with the change in plasma Cl^-, $R^2 = 0.4$, $p < 0.01$.

Short-term survival in experimental septic shock is likely a function of hemodynamics. As shown in Table 1, metabolic acidosis is associated with reductions in arterial blood pressure and myocardial contractility. Recent work suggests that the hypotension associated with acidosis is in part mediated by release of nitric oxide (NO). Pedoto et al. [21] have evaluated the consequences of acid infusion on NO, blood pressure and lung injury in rats. Their results suggest that moderate acidosis causes increases in NO, hypotension, and lung inflammation and they were the first to report a direct effect of persistent acidosis on NO production and lung injury. These results have profound implications on the role of acidosis on NO production and lung injury during sepsis. We have preliminarily demonstrated this effect of acidosis not only in septic animals [22] but also in cultured macrophages stimulated with endotoxin [23]. Therefore, a plausible link has been established between acidosis and mortality in sepsis.

▌ Conclusion

Is acidemia good, bad, or inconsequential? The answer is likely yes, all three. In healthy exercising humans, brief periods of even severe acidosis are probably inconsequential. In unresuscitated states, acidosis may provide some benefit to the organism. Even in fully resuscitated states, treating metabolic acidosis with sodium bicarbonate is of unproven benefit. However, metabolic acidosis may be avoided or at least reduced by avoiding hyperchloremic solutions commonly used in resuscitation (e.g., saline) in favor of balanced solutions (e.g., Hextend®). The benefit of this approach is also unproven but the clinical, epidemiological, and experimental evidence to date suggest that benefit is likely. Whether, hypercarbia is safer than hyperchloremia as a source of acidosis is still unknown.

References

1. Magder S (2002) A "post-Copernican" analysis of intracellular pH. In: Gullo, A (ed) Anaesthesia, Pain, Intensive Care and Emergency Medicine. Springer, Milan, pp 589–609
2. Kellum JA, Rico P, Garuba AK, Pinsky MR (2000) Accuracy of mucosal pH and mucosal-arterial carbon dioxide tension for detecting mesenteric hypoperfusion in acute canine endotoxemia. Crit Care Med 28:462–466
3. Stewart P (1983) Modern quantitative acid-base chemistry. Can J Physiol Pharmacol 61: 1444–1461
4. Kellum JA (2000) Determinants of blood pH in health and disease. Crit Care 4:6–14
5. Kellum JA (2000) Diagnosis and treatment of acid-base disorders. In: Grenvik A, Ayres SM, Holbrook PR, Shoemaker WC (eds) Textbook of Critical Care. WB Saunders, Philadelphia, pp 839–853
6. Leblanc M, Kellum JA (1998) Biochemical and biophysical principles of hydrogen ion regulation. In: Ronco C, Bellomo R (eds) Critical Care Nephrology. Kluwer, Dordrecht, pp 261–277
7. Lindinger MI, Heigenhauser GJF, McKelvie RS, Jones NL (2001) Blood ion regulation during repeated maximal exercise and recovery in humans. Am J Physiol 262:R126–R136
8. Schurr A, Payne RS, Miller JJ, Rigor BM (1997) Brain lactate, not glucose, fuels recovery of synaptic function from hypoxia upon reoxygenation: an in vitro study. Brain Res 744:105–111
9. Laffey JG, Engelberts D, Kavanagh BP (2000) Injurious effects of hypocapnic alkalosis in the isolated lung. Am J Respir Crit Care Med 162:399–405
10. Forsythe SM, Schmidt GA (2000) Sodium bicarbonate for the treatment of lactic acidosis. Chest 117:260–267
11. Hickling KG, Walsh TJ, Henderson SJ, Jackson R (1994) Low mortality rate in adult respiratory distress syndrome using low volume pressure limited ventilation with permissive hypercapnia: a prospective study. Crit Care Med 22:1568–1578
12. Laffey JG, Kavanagh BP (1999) Carbon dioxide and the critically ill-too little of a good thing? Lancet 354:1283–1286
13. Gore DC, Jahoor F (1996) Lactic acidosis during sepsis is related to increased pyruvate Production, not deficits in oxygen availability. Ann Surg 224:97–102
14. Kellum JA, Bellomo R, Kramer DJ, Pinsky MR (1998) Etiology of metabolic acidosis during saline resuscitation in endotoxemia. Shock 9:364–368
15. Scheingraber S, Rehm M, Sehmisch C, Finsterer U (1999) Rapid saline infusion produces hyperchloremic acidosis in patients undergoing gynecologic surgery. Anesthesiology 90:1265–1270
16. Rehm M, Orth V, Scheingraber S, et al. (2000) Acid-base changes caused by 5% albumin versus 6% hydroxyethyl starch solution in patients undergoing acute normovolemic hemodilution: A randomized prospective study. Anesthesiology 93:1174–1183
17. Waters JH, Miller LR, Clack S, Kim JV (1999) Cause of metabolic acidosis in prolonged surgery. Crit Care Med 27:2142–2146
18. Waters JH, Bernstein CA (2000) Dilutional acidosis following hetastarch or albumin in healthy volunteers. Anesthesiology 93:1184–1187
19. Wilkes NJ, Woolf R, Mutch M, et al (2001) The effects of balanced versus saline-based hetastarch and crystalloid solutions on acid-base and electrolyte status and gastric mucosal perfusion in elderly surgical patients. Anesth Analg 93:811–816
20. Kellum JA (2002) Fluid resuscitation and hyperchloremic acidosis in experimental sepsis: Improved survival and acid-base balance with a synthetic colloid in a balanced electrolyte solution compared to saline. Crit Care Med (in Press)

21. Pedoto A, Caruso JE, Nandi J (1999) Acidosis stimulates nitric oxide production and lung damage in rats. Am J Respir Crit Care Med 159:397–402
22. Kellum JA, Song M, Schmigel J, Venkataraman R (2002) Effects of hyperchloremic acidosis on hemodynamics and circulating inflammatory molecules in experimental sepsis. Crit Care Med (Abst, in press)
23. Kellum JA, Song M (2002) Effects of acidosis on LPS-mediated production of inflammatory cytokine and nitric oxide in RAW macrophages. Am J Respir Crit Care Med (Abst, in press)
24. Stacpoole PW, Lorenz AC, Thomas RG, Harman EM (1998) Dichloroacetate in the treatment of lactic acidosis. Ann Intern Med 108:58–63

Cardiorespiratory Monitoring

Monitoring Left Heart Performance in the Critically Ill

J. Poelaert, C. Roosens, and P. Segers

▌ Introduction

Pre-existing ventricular dysfunction in the critically ill patient significantly determines outcome. The importance of this feature has been demonstrated both in septic and in perioperative non-cardiac surgical patients [1, 2]. When admitted to the ICU, patients with extensive hemodynamic deterioration, either due to distributive shock, cardiogenic shock or posttraumatic hypovolemia, should be examined rapidly to correctly assess the main determinants of cardiovascular function. Table 1 summarizes intrinsic and extrinsic determinants governing ventricular function. Rapid decision making will have a major impact on further therapeutic strategies [3, 4]. In this respect, it is of paramount importance to estimate accurately both changing loading conditions and cardiac function. Traditional measures, such as stroke volume, cardiac output, and ejection fraction have proven their validity in

Table 1. Determinants of ventricular function

Extrinsic
- ▌ Neurotransmitters: autonomic
- ▌ Metabolic components
  - Locally produced metabolites
  - pH, O_2, CO_2
- ▌ Endocrine function
  - Catecholamines
  - Mineralocorticoids
- ▌ Coordination of contraction
  - Presence and timing of atrial systole
  - Mode of ventricular excitation

Intrinsic (Frank-Starling mechanism)
- ▌ Contractility
- ▌ End-diastolic fiber length (preload)
  - Filling
  - Duration of diastole (heart rate)
  - Ventricular compliance, distensibility
  - – Pericardial constraint
  - – Coronary vascular tree
- ▌ Arterial elastance, aortic impedance (afterload)
- ▌ Heart rate

clinical practice, although caution is warranted because of their strong load dependency. The load dependency precludes the use of ejection fraction as a parameter in patients with either disturbed preload or afterload. Left ventricular (LV) ejection fraction does not show any prognostic value with respect to outcome prediction in patients with normal systolic LV function in septic shock [5]. With the advent of more powerful and more specific technology, a different framework for evaluating LV performance must be proposed.

There are at least three mechanisms regulating contractile strength of the heart: sympathetic and vagal nervous system, the Frank-Starling mechanism, and the force-frequency relationship [6]. The altered sensitivity to β-adrenergic agents, linked to a decreased receptor density [7], and the changed response to the force-frequency relationship [8] have been described extensively in cardiac failure patients. Current, albeit advanced, monitoring permits a separate and independent determination of all three features determining the Frank-Starling mechanism, namely preload, afterload, and contractility. The importance of estimating the contractile capability of a ventricle is exemplified in a patient with ischemic heart failure. The contractile ability of the ventricle will not be comparable with the contractile capability present in a patient with aortic stenosis; ventricular function in this setting is characterized by an increased myocardial end-systolic wall stress. The balance between all three parameters will only be restored when either coronary perfusion is optimized or aortic valve replacement has been performed. Over the last decades, several investigators have proposed various physical entities to describe contractility, independent of preload and afterload. Although two-dimensional, and Doppler, echocardiography may suggest defective contractile function of a ventricle, their interpretation is hampered by interference of loading conditions. The secret of future hemodynamic monitoring is to combine several technologies, which merge different approaches to the same problem, in order to investigate the hemodynamic impairment rapidly and meticulously. In addition, it is evident that the monitoring technique of choice should not solely take into account the parameter to be monitored at that particular time, but also other, potentially present, dysfunctions, e.g., concomitant right ventricular (RV) failure [9, 10], valvular dysfunction [11, 13].

To comply with this approach, echocardiography must be integrated in a concept of pressure monitoring and other monitoring techniques, significantly augmenting key information about hemodynamic assessment. This chapter will focus on the assessment of cardiac performance, which should be the basis of each hemodynamic assessment, incorporating accurate and quick assessment of contractility and loading conditions by combined use of different hemodynamic monitors.

▌ Pressure and Preload

There is straightforward evidence that preload influences cardiac performance. In order to optimize ventricular performance, preload must be adjusted to the appropriate level, also in failing hearts [14]. Although preload is defined as the end-diastolic fiber length, traditionally pressures have been utilized to assess preload.

Pressure and LV Area

Central venous pressure (CVP) has always been the hallmark of filling pressure; as it is a simple, cheap, and relatively safe mode of continuous monitoring of the filling status, it has been rehabilitated recently [15, 16]. Nevertheless, in specific clinical situations, such as patients with acute respiratory failure, CVP monitoring will not allow adequate preload estimation and transesophageal echocardiography (TEE) and Doppler may be more useful [17]. In contrast, in changing loading conditions, it has been shown several times that both pulmonary artery diastolic pressure (PADP) and pulmonary artery occlusion pressure (PAOP) are poor guides to estimate LV preload, in particular when ventilatory adjustments frequently alter intrathoracic pressures. In cardiac surgical patients with normal LV function, and also in septic patients, two-dimensional echocardiography provides a better index of LV preload than conventional hemodynamic monitoring [18–21]. The correlation of LV preload with PAOP or PADP is inexistent and does not reflect changes in LV size [22]. Data from these investigators showed that TEE provides useful information about endpoints for intravenous fluid administration as defined by maximum cardiac output and LV stroke work, whereas PAOP did not show any significant relationship to changes in cardiac output and LV stroke work [22].

At the short axis level (with the two papillary muscles of the LV in the transverse plane), certain signs are typical to identify a low filling status: kissing walls [23], small LV end-diastolic area (LVEDA) indexed for body surface, although it appears difficult to define a threshold value for LVEDA [21].

Nevertheless, the problem still exists in patients with severely decreased LV systolic function or when valvular dysfunction is present [24], where LVEDA can be a measure of preload only if a fluid challenge is administered to find maximum cardiac output. In patients suffering from distributive shock, several techniques have been utilized to assess optimal preload. Respiratory variations of the arterial pressure waveform have been shown to be a reasonable indicator of LV preload [25–27]. Significant correlation was found between LVEDA and systolic pressure variation during acute preload augmentation [28]. A delta down of 5 mmHg or more during inspiration represents a low filling status in sepsis induced hypotension [27]. Interference of pulmonary compliance could preclude use in patients with altered lung or/and chest wall compliance [28]. Whether afterload may interfere with respiratory systolic pressure variation remains controversial: extreme vasodilatory septic shock could interact with the magnitude of the systolic pressure variation for a particular decrease in stroke volume.

Indirectly estimating filling pressures, TEE could offer relevant information in this respect. In particular, visualization of the pulmonary venous flow revealed high correlation with filling pressures [29, 30]. Several authors showed close correlations between pulmonary venous Doppler indices and left sided filling pressures [31–35]. When the duration of the atrial pulmonary venous Doppler flow wave exceeds the duration of the transmitral flow wave, good evidence of a LV end-diastolic pressure (LVEDP) above 15 mmHg is provided [36]. In addition, indirect estimation of LVEDP has been shown recently to present bedside and quick information about the filling status of the left heart [37]. The deceleration time of the diastolic wave (expressed in ms) is more accurate than PAOP in estimating left atrial pressure (LAP) in cardiac surgical patients. These investigators found a correlation ($r = -0.92$) between deceleration time of the D wave and LAP in the entire group of patients (Fig. 1), according to the formula:

$$LAP = 53.236 - [0.302 - decT] + [0.000484(decT)^2]$$

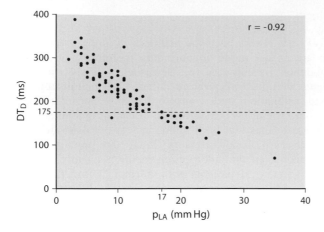

Fig. 1. The relationship between pulmonary venous deceleration time (DT) and PAOP (see text for details). (From [37] with permission)

Intrathoracic Blood Volume

Both intrathoracic blood volume and extravascular lung water are increasingly utilized for extended hemodynamic monitoring with a low grade of invasiveness [38–40]. Using the indocyanine green (ICG) dye dilution technique, Hinder et al. showed that changes in LVEDA and intrathoracic blood volume correlated closely (r=0.87) [41]. Both intrathoracic blood volume and global end-diastolic blood volume are reliable indicators of myocardial preload in critically ill patients [42]. Besides information about preload, this device also routinely offers cardiac output as a parameter, based on the area under the arterial pressure tracing [43]. The morphology of the arterial pressure tracing is, however, often disturbed or crushed, necessitating frequent calibration to allow correct cardiac output measurements to be made. Other determinants of ventricular function such as afterload and contractility cannot, or can at best only indirectly, be assessed by dye dilution (Table 2).

Right Ventricular End-diastolic Volume (RVEDV)

Another more recent advance in the monitoring of cardiac preload, is the development of a RV ejection fraction, volumetric thermodilution, pulmonary artery catheter for the calculation of right end-diastolic volume [44]. Cardiac index (CI) corre-

Table 2. Comparison of various bedside hemodynamic monitoring techniques, to demonstrate their ability to assess separately various hemodynamic parameters.

Parameter	Pulmonary artery catheter	Doppler-TEE	Double dye dilution technique
Preload	(+)	+	+
Afterload	(+)	+	(+)
Contractility	–	+	–
Cardiac output	+	+	+
Diastolic function	–	+	–

TEE, transesophageal echocardiography

lates significantly better with RVEDV index than with PAOP at different levels of positive end-expiratory pressure (PEEP) [44]. RV volume measurements are independent of zero pressure references and unlike intrathoracic filling pressures, not confounded by higher levels of PEEP. The correct place of this tool in the framework of hemodynamic monitoring has yet to be determined.

Contractility

Cardiac dysfunction is a commonly encountered disorder in critical care medicine. The correct assessment of contractility is a pertinent question with respect to multiple critical situations in the ICU, from evaluation for potential donorship in brain-dead patients due to extensive traumatic brain injury or massive central nervous system damage [45], to patients without a history of cardiac disease, with sepsis or septic shock with regard to evaluating the myocardial depressant effects of e.g., tumor necrosis factor (TNF)-α [46, 47].

Cardiac dysfunction is mainly governed by pump failure of one or both ventricles. The pump function provides hydraulic energy to maintain the circulation. In this respect both pressure production and flow generation encompass the capacity of the heart to compensate for the energy dissolution into the vasculature. Ventricular performance is, hence, governed, in physiological terms, by pressure and flow. Traditional measures such as ejection fraction or maximum rate of change of LV pressure (dP/dt_{max}) are governed by load dependency [48]. A more complete evaluation of ventricular performance ideally includes relatively load-insensitive measures of systolic pump properties in a beat-to-beat fashion, and the assessment of inotropic state and cardiac reserve.

Pressure-volume Loops

From the pressure-volume framework, the end-systolic pressure-volume relationship [49–52], preload-recruitable stroke work [50, 53], dP/dtmax–end-diastolic volume relationship [54, 55] and the ejection fraction-afterload stress correlation [56] can each be obtained with echocardiography in conjunction with pressure measurements, measuring a pump function variable corrected for a loading parameter. This correction permits higher specificity, although not complete, to changes of contractile state.

The slope of the end-systolic pressure-volume relationship is referred to as end-systolic elastance (Ees) [49, 51]. In a well-controlled animal investigation, comparing preload-recruitable stroke work, maximum dP/dt – end-diastolic volume relation and the end-systolic pressure-volume relation, it is clear that the first, provides the most stable data; the volume-axis intercept is the least sensitive to enhanced contractile state or increased afterload indices [57] and, thus, preload-recruitable stroke work has advantages over the other techniques to monitor LV performance. In contrast, dP/dt_{max} – end-diastolic LV volume is the least reproducible but most sensitive index of contractility alterations.

Utilizing echocardiographic automated border detection, LVEDA changes can be linked with invasive LV or arterial pressure [58], to calculate nearly on-line Ees (Fig. 2). This methodology permits independent quantification of changes of ventricular performance and vascular load in both well-controlled animal [51] and hu-

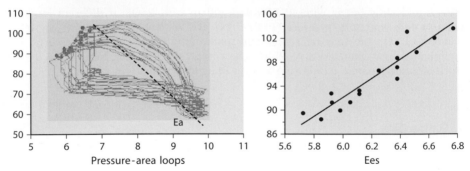

Fig. 2. Pressure-area loops can be obtained by combining digitized arterial pressure tracings and a preload parameter (e.g., LVEDA), measured with echocardiography (left panel). Connecting the end-systolic points of the different loops, resulting from changed preloading conditions, provides end-systolic elastance, Ees (dashed line on the left panel). Arterial elastance (Ea) is determined graphically as the relationship between the end-diastolic and the end-systolic points

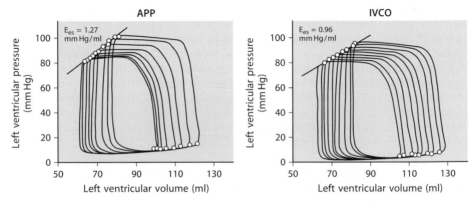

Fig. 3. Example of a series of pressure-volume loops in an animal model, obtained with progressive inferior caval vein occlusion (right panel: IVCO), and generated with airway pressure plateau (left panel: APP). (From [64] with permission)

man studies [59, 60]. Ees, however, may be quite variable with respect to different levels of preload, stroke volume, or coronary perfusion pressure. In addition, a linear approximation may not always be appropriate [61] and the arterial loading conditions may shift the relation [62]. Moreover, in order to obtain a complete data set (i.e., end-diastolic points in the pressure-volume loop), invasive instrumentation of the LV is needed, in conjunction with simultaneous pressure and volume measurements in order to obtain end-diastolic indices. Finally, technical difficulties compromise the clinical determination of Ees in the critically ill at the bedside [63]. Therefore, it can be speculated that this technique, although apparently useful in stable cardiac surgical patients, will never be used in patients in whom fluid shifts could lead to disastrous hemodynamic instability (e.g., severely hypovolemic posttraumatic, septic shock patients). Some authors [64], however, described a striking similarity in the LV pressure-volume relationship during a well-controlled and limited positive airway pressure plateau of a clinically relevant duration and magnitude, and during controlled preload reduction by transient balloon occlusion of the intrathoracic caval vein to rapidly alter LV preload by occlusion of blood flow (Fig. 3). The big advantage of this method is the use of physiological ranges of variations of preload with a routine technique of mechanical ventilation, besides the minimal invasiveness and the reproducibility of the technique, without need to implement transmural LV pressures [65].

Single Beat Techniques

Several investigators have suggested single beat techniques to estimate LV performance [66–68].

Experimental. On the basis of contraction-relaxation coupling and relative load, and with an intraventricular high fidelity pressure catheter in place, LV contractile function can be assessed in one single beat, independent of LV dimension measurements [66, 69]. A coupling of the alteration of cardiac systolic load and the response to LV contraction and relaxation was shown [70]. Preserved or increased relaxation rate suggests conserved LV function. Each retarded relaxation during increased preload would be indicative of impaired LV function [71]. Nevertheless, considerable drawbacks to this method should be considered. First, the invasiveness is significant with the use of an intraventricular high fidelity pressure catheter. Second, the RV plays the role of a preload buffer, making the technique dependent on RV function and afterload. Finally, this technique tests contraction and relaxation characteristics close to each other, although a break up of these parameters should be made; recently, caffeine has been proposed for this purpose as it permits the fragmentation of contraction and relaxation into two separate entities [72].

Clinical. In the search for more clinically useful and load insensitive methods to determine LV contractile function, Tan [73] suggested that the cardiac pumping performance is better estimated by utilizing a pressure-*flow* index, such as total hydraulic power output. The concept is based on work of previous studies [74]. Myocardial performance is strongly linked with myocardial force, velocity and fiber length. Hence, the ejection rate of change of power also must be related to these variables. The ejection rate of change of ventricular power measured at peak tension describes in an uncomplicated manner the contractile characteristics of muscle fibers. Improvement of cardiac pumping reserve and optimalization of regional blood flow should be considered, rather than optimalization of cardiac output. Therapeutic trials to improve cardiac exercise capacity should be gauged against the ability to augment cardiac reserve [75]. As cardiac failure is most often brought back to pump failure, the function of the heart is to provide hydraulic energy to the systemic circulation. The instantaneous product of pressure and flow is the ventricular rate of performing work, i.e., hydraulic power [76]. Maximal ventricular power is an ejection phase index at a time point of maximal flow through the open aortic valve and at the time point of maximum aortic pressure. Recent developments in pressure, echocardiographic flow, and dimension techniques allow the relatively non-invasive determination of this descriptor of ventricular performance. The combined use of TEE continuous-wave Doppler in the LV outflow tract [77] and aortic pressure recording, permits the calculation of this power parameter in clinical conditions [67]. Correction for preload (LVEDA or LV length), preload-adjusted maximal-power, provides insight in alterations of contractility.

Total hydraulic power can be described as the continuous product of pressure and flow and is not significantly influenced by afterload [78]. Also, maximal ventricular power (product of maximal pressure and maximal flow) corrected for the square of the LVEDV, provides a good measure for contractile function of that ventricle, although more sensitive to afterload alterations [79]. Following the Frank-Starling mechanism, both peak flow and ejection pressure vary directly with preload. This preload influence is parabolic in nature and can be virtually completely abolished by correction of maximal power by the square of end-diastolic volume [76], or a regional echocardiographic surrogate (LVEDA or length) [67, 78, 80], diminishing the influence of preload significantly. Hence, a considerable advantage is the non-invasive potential of the technique [67]. LV power variables calculated from invasive and non-invasive techniques were closely related [78, 81]. In an experimental setting, the preload adjustment appeared to be less dependent on Emax [79], resulting in a correction factor of 2.17–2.20 (preload adjusted total power: $PWR/EDV^{2.2}$). Clinical trials supporting the improved accuracy are, however, not yet available.

Determination of Ventricular Performance

Ees/Ea

The ratio of ventricular Ees to arterial elastance (Ea) is one of the most direct indexes of ventricular-arterial coupling and reflects both ventricular and energetic performance. Again, the shortcomings commented on in the previous section suggest that the relationship between Ees and Ea will be disturbed, hampering its routine clinical use. Recently, a single beat framework was proposed to estimate Ees/Ea from ventricular and aortic pressures [68]. Approximation of the waveform of the ventricular time-varying elastance curve was performed with a line for the isovolumic phase and another for the ejection phase (Fig. 2). The ratio Ees/Ea is dependent on the slope ratio of these two straight lines, aortic pressure and systolic time intervals (pre-ejection and ejection period). Incorporation of the slope ratio (k) into the estimation of Ees/Ea permits determination of Ees/Ea from ventricular and aortic pressure:

$$Ees/Ea = Pad/Pes\ (1 + k \times ET/PEP) - 1$$

with Pad is the LV pressure at onset of ejection; Pes the end-systolic pressure; ET the ejection period; PEP the pre-ejection period. In this setup, the authors still claim the use of ventricular and aortic pressures, which are far more invasive than what is used in daily routine practice [68]. Nevertheless, the authors bring the intriguing relationship of Ees and Ea back to a simple ratio of pressures and PEP and ET, two easy obtainable Doppler echocardiographic parameters.

MPI

Another Doppler derived index of myocardial performance (MPI) has been described by Tei [82]. This Doppler index, void from any necessity to link with pressure data, incorporates both systolic and diastolic indices of ventricular performance and is independent of ventricular geometric dimensions. It is defined as the sum of the isovolumetric contraction and relaxation time, corrected for the ejection time [83]:

$$MPI = (ICT + IRT)/ET$$

where ET is the ejection time, ICT the isovolumetric contraction time, and IRT the isovolumetric relaxation time.

The great advantage of this index is the simplicity with which MPI can be obtained: the time interval between two transmitral flow patterns must be diminished by the ejection time period, and be corrected for that same time period (Fig. 4).

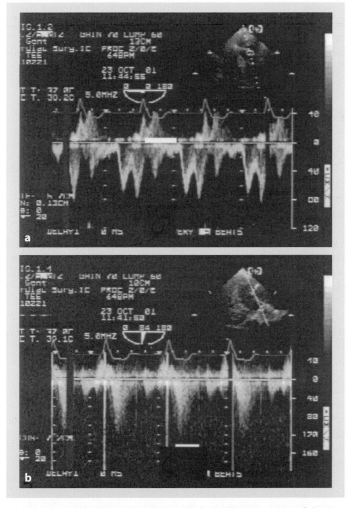

Fig. 4. Definition of myocardial performance index (MPI). The upper panel shows the measurement of the time between the end of the atrial contraction and the start of filling. The lower panel demonstrates the measurement of the ejection time interval. ET, ejection time; ICT, isovolumic contraction index; IRT, isovolumic relaxation time; MPI, myocardial performance index

The different time intervals show their own and relative dependency to heart rate, afterload and contractility changes:

▌ isovolumetric contraction time: dependent on heart rate [84];

▌ isovolumetric relaxation time: is related to +dP/dt and τ [83];

▌ ejection time: dependent on heart rate [85, 86] and relies strongly on +dP/dt [85].

Overall, MPI appears to be independent of heart rate [87], but load independency is still under debate with some contradictory reports [83, 88–90]. Tei et al. showed both a close relationship between MPI and the load dependent +dP/dt and between MPI and τ [83].

MPI has already been utilized to assess global LV [82–84, 88] and RV [89, 91] function, and in the estimation of prognosis of various diseases [83]. Also in children <1 year old with double outlet right ventricle, operated on for bicavopulmonary shunt, MPI fell significantly, suggesting an improvement in (systemic) ventricular function [90]. Recently, clinical trials using MPI in critically ill patients have been reported [92].

▌ Diastolic Performance of the Left Ventricle

The clinical picture of diastolic dysfunction is presented by a retardation in filling of the LV. Congestive heart failure is characterized by diastolic dysfunction, which presents itself before systolic dysfunction becomes overt [93, 94]. Also, diastolic dysfunction is an early marker of myocardial ischemia [93]. Considerable advances have been made in the on-line and bedside echocardiographic evaluation of diastolic dysfunction of the cardiac compromised patient [30].

The analysis of transmitral flow pattern has provided information about filling and abnormal diastolic function. The early transmitral flow wave velocity (E) is strongly dependent on loading conditions. In particular in patients with a LV fractional area contraction above 50%, it is clear that a E/A <1 is seldom linked with impaired relaxation and should be interpreted primarily as a low filling state (often aggravated by 'overmedication' with diuretics). In addition, important alterations in transmitral filling patterns may vary significantly within the same patient. A dynamic test is a more appealing technique to differentiate within and between patients with diastolic dysfunction with respect to assessment of systolic cardiac performance (see above [95]). This technique is, however not always appropriate and sometimes dangerous. Indices of pulmonary venous Doppler patterns have been proposed as an adjunct to differentiate the type of diastolic dysfunction, albeit both are sensitive to loading conditions and depend on compliance of both left atrium and LV, and elevated left atrial filling pressures. Several authors have proposed, therefore, some supplementary measurements to assess more accurately the presence of diastolic dysfunction.

A preload independent, non-invasive index of relaxation has been proposed utilizing tissue velocities. Tissue Doppler velocities may be shown either by color M-mode [96–98], tissue Doppler imaging (TDI) [99, 100], or two-dimensional mode [101]. Whereas Doppler ultrasound has been traditionally utilized to measure flow velocities of red blood cells, TDI allows measurement of velocities of myocardial tissue (typically low velocities, high intensity Doppler signals) at certain points.

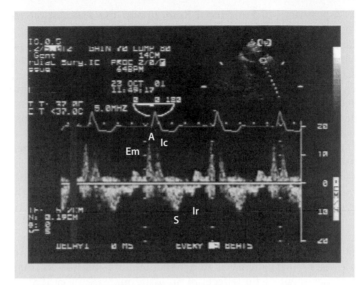

Fig. 5. Tissue Doppler imaging, here obtained at the lateral wall of the mitral annulus, gives insight into both systolic and diastolic characteristics of the left ventricle. A: atrial contraction filling wave; Em: early diastolic filling wave; Ic: isovolumetric contraction time; Ir: isovolumetric relaxation time; S: systolic flow wave

TDI, which has a high reproducibility rate [102, 103], has several advantages. First, determination of isovolumic relaxation and contraction time is much more simple to assess. Second, unlike mitral inflow Doppler, where fusion of the different flow waves is seen during tachycardia, TDI remains useful with respect to assessment of diastolic function in this condition [104]. Third, peak systolic myocardial velocity, which is part of the TDI transmitral pattern (Fig. 5), correlates well with non-invasively estimated LV peak dP/dt [105]. Finally, the ratio between the transmitral early filling wave and TDI early wave can be used to estimate PCWP [106, 107]. Utilizing TDI in conjunction with routine Doppler parameters may hold a promising future in the non-invasive hemodynamic assessment of critically ill patients with a view to discriminating preload problems, systolic, and diastolic dysfunction (Table 3).

Table 3. Diagnosis of diastolic dysfunction following the respective stage, as determined by Doppler-TEE, utilizing both transmitral flow parameters, pulmonary vein Doppler and tissue Doppler techniques.

	E/A	Dect E (ms)	S/D	Ar (m/s)	Em (m/s)
Normal	>1	160–240	≥1	<0.35	>0.08
Delayed relaxation	<1	>240	≥1	<0.35	<0.08
Pseudonormal filling	1–2	160–240	<1	≥0.35	<0.08
Restrictive filling	>2	<160	<1	≥0.35	<0.08

Ar, reverse flow velocity at the level of a pulmonary vein, owing to atrial contraction; DT, deceleration time; E/A, ratio of early to late filling wave velocity; Em, early flow velocity obtained with spectral Doppler tissue imaging; IVRT, isovolumetric relaxation time; S/D, ratio of systolic to diastolic Doppler flow velocity in a pulmonary vein

▌ Assessment of Functional Reserve and the Association with Outcome

Ejection fraction does not reflect contractility, due to its load dependency [108]. Nevertheless, this parameter has been incorporated in several preoperative cardiac scoring indices [109–111]. In contrast, several other contractility indices, such as ejection rate of change of power [74] and the relation of end-systolic stress to the velocity of shortening [112–114], have been related with estimation of prognosis and outcome [115]. Peak rate of change of power was defined as the difference between maximal cardiac power at peak dobutamine dosage and at baseline value [116, 117]. Cardiac peak power had a predicted mortality rate with a 100% sensitivity, 56% specificity and 64% positive predictive value in NYHA III and IV patients [118]. Cardiac failure patients with a cardiac peak power reserve of <1.5 W/ml were shown to have a ±90% mortality [117]. The strength of this index, however, has not yet been evaluated in a critically ill subset of patients.

Using the relatively load-insensitive concepts of pressure-volume relations with automated echocardiographic measures of RV cross-sectional area, it was shown that patients in NYHA functional class IV who showed an increase in RV contractile reserve with increases in dobutamine infusion had an improved outcome [119].

Assessment of the effects of an acute increase in cardiac preload permits a dynamic determination of LV functional reserve. This allowed identification of a subset of patients, who responded to an acute increase of preload with a decrease in stroke volume and dP/dtmax, a delayed myocardial relaxation and a marked increase in the LVEDP [95].

Regional indices have also been utilized to estimate contractile reserve [120]. In this context, strain and rate of strain have been forwarded. In general terms, strain means tissue deformation as a function of applied force (stress) [101]. Strain rate is the temporal derivative of strain and is a measure of the rate of deformation. A negative strain rate means that the tissue segment becomes shorter or thinner. A positive strain rate exemplifies a wall segment that becomes longer or thicker [101]. In patients with stunned myocardium, inotropic stimulation could characterize the regional contractile function using the maximal systolic strain rate. The result is a decrease in regional systolic strain with a concomitant augmentation of postsystolic thickening [120]. Nevertheless, load dependency accounts in part for the observed changes in contractility [121], potentially limiting the value of quantitative strain-rate measurements at the moment.

▌ Conclusion

Echocardiography, in conjunction with other hemodynamic monitoring techniques, in particular the arterial waveform, plays a key role in the separate determination of preload, afterload, and contractility of both the right and left ventricle. This information gives the clinician a mighty weapon to improve the efficiency of management and therapy for the critically ill patient: less invasiveness, less transportation, and independent information of both global and regional function. Further studies are necessary to obtain data regarding the value of combining different hemodynamic monitoring techniques with respect to improving care of the critically ill and refining quality of life.

References

1. Vallet B, Chopin C, Curtis S, et al (1993) Prognostic value of the dobutamine test in patients with sepsis syndrome and normal lactate values: a prospective, multicenter study. Crit Care Med 21:1868–1875
2. Mangano D, Browner W, Hollenberg M, London M, Tubau J, Tateo I (1990) Association of perioperative myocardial ischemia with cardiac morbidity and mortality in men undergoing noncardiac surgery. N Engl J Med 323:1781–1788
3. Bergquist BD, Bellows WH, Leung JM (1996) Transesophageal echocardiography in myocardial revascularisation: II. Influence on intraoperative decision making. Anesth Analg 82:1139–1145
4. Poelaert JI, Trouerbach J, De Buyzere M, Everaert J, Colardyn FA (1995) Evaluation of transesophageal echocardiography as a diagnostic and therapeutic aid in a critical care setting. Chest 107:774–779
5. Jardin F, Fourme T, Page B, et al (1999) Persistent preload defect in severe sepsis despite fluid loading. A longitudinal echocardiographic study in patients with septic shock. Chest 116:1354–1359
6. Braunwald E (1997) Mechanisms of cardiac contraction and relaxation. In: Braunwald E (ed) Heart disease. A Textbook of Cardiovascular Medicine. W.B. Saunders, Philadelphia, pp 360–393
7. Ogletree-Hughes ML, Stull LB, Sweet WE, Smedira NG, McCarthy PM, Moravec CS (2001) Mechanical unloading restores beta-adrenergic responsiveness and reverses receptor downregulation in the failing human heart. Circulation 104:881–886
8. Mulieri L, Hasenfuss G, Ittleman F, et al (1992) Altered myocardial force-frequency relation in human heart failure. Circulation 85:1743–1750
9. Goldstein J, Tweddell J, Barzilai B, Yagi Y, Jaffe A, Cox J (1992) Importance of left ventricular function and systolic ventricular interaction to the right ventricular performance during acute right heart ischemia. J Am Coll Cardiol 19:704–711
10. Marcus J, Noordegraaf A, Roeleveld R, et al (2001) Impaired left ventricular filling due to right ventricular pressure overload in primary pulmonary hypertension. Chest 119:1761–1765
11. Berger M, Haimowitz A, Van Tosh A, Berdoff R, Goldberg E (1985) Quantitative assessment of pulmonary hypertension in patients with tricuspid regurgitation using continuous wave Doppler ultrasound. J Am Coll Cardiol 6:359–365
12. Bajzer C, Stewart W, Cosgrove D, Azzam S, Arheart K, Klein A (1998) Tricuspid valve surgery and intraoperative echocardiography. J Am Coll Cardiol 32:1023–1031
13. Pathi V, Jones B, Davidson K (1996) Mitral valve disruption following blunt trauma: case report and review of the literature. Eur J Cardiothorac Surg 10:806–808
14. Holubarsch C, Ruf T, Goldstein D, et al (1996) Existence of the Frank-Starling mechanism in the failing human heart. Investigations on the organ, tissue and sarcomere levels. Circulation 94:683–689
15. Mark J (1991) Central venous pressure monitoring: clinical insights beyond the numbers. J Cardiothorac Vasc Anesth 5:163–173
16. Magder S (1998) More respect for the CVP. Intensive Care Med 24:651–653
17. Soliman D, Maslow A, Bokesch P, et al (1998) Transoesophageal echocardiography during scoliosis repair: comparison with CVP monitoring. Can J Anaesth 45:925–932
18. Hansen RM, Viquerat CE, Matthay MA, et al (1986) Poor correlation between pulmonary arterial wedge pressure and left end-diastolic volume after coronary artery bypass graft surgery. Anesthesiology 64:764–770
19. Thys D, Hillel Z, Goldman M, Mindich B, Kaplan J (1987) A comparison of hemodynamic indices derived by invasive monitoring and two-dimensional echocardiography. Anesthesiology 67:630–634
20. Jardin F, Valier B, Beauchet A, Dubourg O, Bourdarias J (1994) Invasive monitoring combined with two-dimensional echocardiographic study in septic shock. Intensive Care Med 20:550–554
21. Tousignant C, Walsh F, Mazer C (2000) The use of transesophageal echocardiography for preload assessment in critically ill patients. Anesth Analg 90:351–355

22. Swenson JD, Harkin C, Pace NL, Astle K, Bailey P (1996) Transesophageal echocardiography: An objective tool in determining maximum ventricular response to intravenous fluid therapy. Anesth Analg 83:1149–1153
23. Leung JM, Levine EH (1994) Left ventricular end-systolic cavity obliteration as an estimate of intraoperative hypovolemia. Anesthesiology 81:1102–1109
24. Mirsky I, Corin WJ, Murakami T, Grimm J, Hess OM, Kraeyenbuehl HP (1988) Correction for preload in assessment of myocardial contractility in aortic and mitral valve disease. Circulation 87:68–80
25. Perel A, Pizov R, Cotev S (1987) Systolic blood pressure variation is a sensitive indicator of hypovolaemia in ventilated dogs subjected to graded hemorrhage. Anesthesiology 67:498–502
26. Coriat P, Vrillon M, Perel A, et al (1994) A comparison of systolic blood pressure variations and echocardiographic estimates of end-diastolic left ventricular size in patients after aortic surgery. Anesth Analg 78:46–53
27. Tavernier B, Makhotine O, Lebuffe G, Dupont J, Scherpereel P (1998) Systolic pressure variation as a guide to fluid therapy in patients with sepsis-induced hypotension. Anesthesiology 89:1313–1321
28. Tournadre JP, Allacouchiche B, Cayrel V, Mathion L, Chassard D (2000) Estimation of cardiac preload changes by systolic pressure variation in pigs undergoing pneumoperitoneum. Acta Anaesthesiol Scand 44:231–235
29. Keren G, Sherez J, Megidish R, Levitt B, Laniado S (1985) Pulmonary venous flow pattern – its relationship to cardiac dynamics. Circulation 71:1105–1112
30. Appleton C, Hatle L, Popp R (1988) Relation of transmitral flow velocity patterns to left ventricular diastolic function: new insights from a combined hemodynamic and Doppler echocardiographic study. J Am Coll Cardiol 12:426–440
31. Kuecherer H, Muhiudeen I, Kusumoto F, et al (1990) Estimation of mean left atrial pressure from transesophageal pulsed Doppler echocardiography of pulmonary venous flow. Circulation 82:1127–1139
32. Rossvoll O, Hatle L (1993) Pulmonary venous flow velocities recorded by transthoracic Doppler ultrasound: relation to left ventricular diastolic pressures. J Am Coll Cardiol 21:1687–1696
33. Hoit B, Shao Y, Gabel M, Walsh R (1992) Influence of loading conditions and contractile state on pulmonary venous flow. Validation of Doppler velocimetry. Circulation 86:651–659
34. Hofmann T, Keck A, van Ingen G, Simic O, Ostermeyer J, Meinertz T (1995) Simultaneous measurement of pulmonary venous flow by intravascular catheter Doppler velocimetry and transesophageal Doppler echocardiography: relation to left atrial pressure and left atrial and left ventricular function. J Am Coll Cardiol 26:239–249
35. Yamamuro A, Yoshida K, Hozumi T, et al (1999) Noninvasive evaluation of pulmonary wedge pressure in patients with acute myocardial infarction by deceleration time of pulmonary venous flow velocity iin diastole. J Am Coll Cardiol 34:90–94
36. Appleton C, Galloway J, Gonzalez M, Gaballa M, Basnight M (1993) Estimation of left ventricular filling pressures using two-dimensional and Doppler echocardiography in adult patients with cardiac disease. Additional value of analyzing left atrial size, left atrial ejection fraction and the difference in duration of pulmonary venous and mitral flow velocity at atrial contraction. J Am Coll Cardiol 22:1972–1982
37. Kinnaird T, Thompson C, Munt B (2001) The deceleration time of pulmonary venous diastolic flow is more accurate than the pulmonary artery occlusion pressure predicting left atrial pressure. J Am Coll Cardiol 37:2025–2030
38. Hoeft A, Schorn B, Weyland A, et al (1994) Bedside assessment of intravascular volume status in patients undergoing coronary bypass surgery. Anesthesiology 81:76–86
39. Goedje O, Thiel C, Lamm P, et al (1999) Less invasive, continuous hemodynamic monitoring during minimally invasive coronary surgery. Ann Thorac Surg 68:1532–1536
40. Sakka S, Rühl C, Pfeiffer U, et al (2000) Assessment of cardiac preload and extravascular lung water by single transpulmonary thermodilution. Intensive Care Med 26:180–187
41. Hinder F, Poelaert J, Schmidt C, et al (1998) Assessment of cardiovascular volume status by transoesophageal echocardiography and dye dilution during cardiac surgery. Eur J Anaesth 15:633–640

42. Goedje O, Seebauer T, Peyerl M, Pfeiffer U, Reichart B (2000) Hemodynamic monitoring by double-indicator dilution technique in patients after orthotopic heart transplantation. Chest 118:775–781

43. Wesseling K, Jansen J, Settels J, Schreuder J (1993) Computation of aortic flow from pressure in humans using a nonlinear, three-element model. J Appl Physiol 74:2566–2573

44. Cheatham M, Nelson L, Chang M, Safcsak K (1998) Right ventricular end-diastolic volume index as a predictor of preload status in patients on positive end-expiratory pressure. Crit Care Med 26:1801–1805

45. Shivalkar B, Van Loon J, Wieland W, et al (1993) Variable effects of explosive or gradual increase of intracranial pressure on myocardial structure and function. Circulation 87:230–239

46. Goddard C, Allard M, Hogg J, Walley K (1996) Myocardial morphometric changes related to decreased contractility after endotoxin. Am J Physiol 270:H1446-H1452

47. Murray D, Freeman G (1996) Tumor necrosis factor-alpha induces a biphasic effect on myocardial contractility in conscious dogs. Circ Res 78:154–160

48. Kass DA, Maughan WL, Guo ZM, Kono A, Sunagawa K, Sagawa K (1987) Comparative influence of load versus inotropic states on indexes of ventricular contractility: experimetntal and theoretical analysis based on pressure-volume relationships. Circulation 76:1422–1436

49. Sagawa K (1981) The end-systolic pressure-volume relation of the ventricle: definition, modification, and clinical use. Circulation 63:1223–1227

50. Pagel P, Kampine J, Schmeling W, Warltier D (1990) Comparison of end-systolic pressure-length relations and preload recruitable stroke work as indices of myocardial contractility in the conscious and anesthetized, chronically instrumented dog. Anesthesiology 73:278–290

51. Kass D, Grayson R, Marino P (1990) Pressure-volume analysis as a method for quantifying simultaneous drug (amrinone) effects on arterial load and contractile state in vivo. J Am Coll Cardiol 16:726–732

52. Gorcsan J, Gasior T, Mandarino W, Deneault L, Hattler B, Pinsky M (1994) Assessment of the intermediate effects of cardiopulmonary bypass on left ventricular performance by on-line pressure-area relations. Circulation 89:180–190

53. Glower DD, Spratt JA, Snow ND, et al (1985) Linearity of the Frank-Starling relationship in the intact heart: the concept of preload recuitable stroke work. Circulation 71:994–1009

54. Broka S, Eucher P, Jamart J, et al (1999) Doppler-derived left ventricular rate of pressure rise determination in presence of severe acute mitral regurgitation in pigs. J Am Soc Echocardiogr 12:827–833

55. Rhodes J, Udelson J, Marx G, et al (1993) A new noninvasive method for the estimation of peak dP/dt. Circulation 88:2693–2699

56. Greim C, Roewer N, Meissner C, Bause H, Schulte am Esch J (1995) Estimation of acute left ventricular afterload alterations. A transesophageal echocardiographic evaluation. Anaesthesist 44:108–115

57. Little W, Cheng C, Mamma M, Igarashi Y, Vinten-Johansen J, Johnston W (1989) Comparison of measures of left ventricular performance derived from pressure-volume loops in conscious dogs. Circulation 80:1378–1387

58. Gorcsan J III, Denault A, Gasior TA, et al (1994) Rapid estimation of left ventricular contractility from end-systolic relations by echocardiographic automated border detection and femoral arterial pressure. Anesthesiology 81:553–562

59. De Hert SG, Rodrigus IE, Haenen LR, De Mulder PA, Gillebert TC (1996) Recovery of systolic and diastolic left ventricular function early after cardiopulmonary bypass. Anesthesiology 85:1063–1075

60. Declerck C, Hillel Z, Shih H, Kuroda M, Connery C, Thys D (1998) A comparison of left ventricular performance indices measured by transesophageal echocardiography with automated border detection. Anesthesiology 89:341–349

61. Kass D, Beyar R, Lankford E, Heard M, Maughan W, Sagawa K (1989) Influence of contractile state on curvilinearity of in situ end-systolic pressure-volume relation. Circulation 79:167–178

62. Baan J, Van Der Velde E (1988) Sensitivity of left ventricular end-systolic pressure-volume relation to type of loading intervention in dogs. Circ Res 62:1247–1258

63. Poortmans G, Schüpfer G, Roosens C, Poelaert J (2000) Transesophageal echocardiographic evaluation of left ventricular function. J Cardiothorac Vasc Anesth 14:588–598
64. Haney M, Johansson G, Häggmark S, Biber B (2001) Heart-lung interactions during positive pressure ventilation: left ventricular pressure-volume momentary response to airway pressure elevation. Acta Anaesthesiol Scand 45:702–709
65. Haney M, Johansson G, Häggmark S, Biber B (2001) Analysis of left ventricular systolic function during elevated external cardiac pressure: an examination of measured transmural left ventricular pressure during pressure-volume analysis. Acta Anaesthesiol Scand 45:868–874
66. Leite-Moreira A, Gillebert T (1994) Nonuniform course of left ventricular pressure fall and its regulation by load and contractile state. Circulation 90:2481–2491
67. Schmidt C, Roosens C, Struys M, et al (1999) Contractility in humans after coronary artery surgery. Echocardiographic assessment with preload-adjusted maximal power. Anesthesiology 91:58–70
68. Hayashi K, Shigemi K, Shishido T, Sugimachi M, Sunagawa K (2000) Single-beat estimation of ventricular end-systolic elastance-effective arterial elastance as an index of ventricular mechanoenergetic performance. Anesthesiology 92:1769–1776
69. Gillebert TC, Leite-Moreira AF, De Hert SG (1997) Relaxation-systolic pressure relation. A load dependent assessment of left ventricular contractility. Circulation 95:745–752
70. Ishizaka S, Asanoi H, Wada O, Kameyama T, Inoue H (1995) Loading sequence plays an important role in enhanced laod sensitivity of left ventricular relaxation in conscious dogs with tachycardia-induced cardiomyopathy. Circulation 92:3560–3567
71. Gillebert T, Leite-Moreira A, De Hert S (1997) The hemodynamic manifestation of normal myocardial relaxation. A framework for experimental and clinical evaluation. Acta Cardiologica 52:223–246
72. Leite-Moreira A, Correia-Pinto J, Gillebert T (1999) Load dependence of left ventricular contraction and relaxation. Effects of caffeine. Basic Res Cardiol 94:284–293
73. Tan L (1991) Evaluation of cardiac dysfunction, cardiac reserve and inotropic response. Postgrad Med J 67:S10–S20
74. Stein P, Sabbah H (1976) Rate of change of ventricular power: An indicator of ventricular performance during ejection. Am Heart J 91:219–227
75. Yi KD, Downey HF, Bian X, Fu M, Mallet RT (2000) Dobutamine enhances both contractile function and energy reserves in hypoperfused canine right ventricle. Am J Physiol 279:H2975–H2985
76. Kass DA, Beyar R (1991) Evaluation of contractile state by maximal ventricular power divided by the square of end-diastolic volume. Circulation 84:1698–1708
77. Katz WE, Gasior TA, Quinlan JJ, Gorcsan III J (1993) Transgastric continuous-wave Doppler to determine cardiac output. Am J Cardiol 71:853–857
78. Mandarino W, Pinsky M, Gorcsan J (1998) Assessment of left ventricular contractile state by preload-adjusted maximal power using echocardiographic automated border detection. J Am Coll Cardiol 31:861–868
79. Segers P, Carlier S, Westerhof B, Poelaert J, Verdonck P (2001) Significance du pouvoir hydraulique du VG: étude d'un modèle mathématique. J Cardiologie 13:3–11
80. Pagel PS, Nijhawan N, Warltier DC (1993) Quantitation of volatile anesthetic-induced depression of myocardial contractility using a single beat index derived from maximal ventricular power. J Cardiothor Vasc Anesth 7:688–695
81. Kelly R, Fitchett D (1992) Noninvasive determination of aortic input impedance and external left ventricular power output: a validation and repeatability study of a new technique. J Am Coll Cardiol 20:952–963
82. Tei C (1995) New non-invasive index for combined systolic and diastolic ventricular function. J Cardiol 26:396–404
83. Tei C, Nishimura R, JB S, Tajik A (1997) Noninvasive Doppler-derived myocardial performance index: correlation with simultaneous measurements of cardiac catheterisation measurements. J Am Soc Echocardiogr 10:169–178
84. Tei C, Dujardin K, Hodge D, Kyle R, Tajik A, Seward J (1996) Doppler index combining systolic and diastolic myocardial performance: clinical value in cardiac amyloidosis. J Am Coll Cardiol 27:658–664

85. Weissler A, Harris W, Schoenfeld C (1968) Systolic time intervals in heart failure in man. Circulation 37:149–159
86. Kyriakidis M, Antonopoulos A, Georgiakodis F, et al (1994) Systolic time intervals after phenylephrine administration for early stratification of patients after acute myocardial infarction. Am J Cardiol 73:6–10
87. Poulsen S, Nielsen J, Andersen H (2000) The influence of heart rate on the Doppler-derived myocardial performance index. J Am Soc Echocardiogr 13:379–84
88. Moller J, Poulsen S, Egstrup K (1999) Effect of preload alterations on a new Doppler echocardiographic index of combined systolic and diastolic performance. J Am Soc Echocardiogr 12:1065–1072
89. Eidem B, O'Leary P, Tei C, Seward J (2000) Usefulness of the myocardial performance index for assessing right ventricular function in congenital heart disease. Am J Cardiol 86:654–658
90. Williams R, Ritter S, Tani L, Pagotto L, Minich L (2000) Quantitative assessment of ventricular function in children with single ventricles using Doppler myocardial performance index. Am J Cardiol 86:1106–1110
91. Eidem B, Tei C, O'Leary P, Cetta F, Seward J (1998) Nongeometric quantitative assessment of right and left ventricular function: Myocardial Performance Index in normal children and patients with Ebstein Anomaly. J Soc Echocardiogr 11:849–856
92. Schmidt C, Berendes E (2001) Myocardial performance before and after sympathectomy. Anesthesiology 96:(Abst)
93. Grossman W (1991) Diastolic dysfunction in congestive heart failure. N Engl J Med 325:1557–1564
94. Pagel P, Grossman W, Haering J, Warltier D (1993) Left ventricular diastolic function in the normal and diseased heart: persepctives for the anesthesiologist (first of two parts). Anesthesiology 79:836–854
95. De Hert S, Vander Linden P, Ten Broecke P, De Mulder P, Rodrigus I, Adriaensen H (2000) Assessment of length-dependent regulation of myocardial function in coronary surgery patients using transmitral flow velocity patterns. Anesthesiology 93:374–381
96. Sutherland G, Stewart M, Groundstroem K, et al (1994) Color Doppler myocardial imaging: a new technique for the assessment of myocardial function. J Am Soc Echocardiogr 7:441–458
97. Takatsuji H, Mikami T, Urasawa K, et al (1996) A new approach for evaluation of left ventricular diastolic function: spatial and temporal analysis of left ventricular filling flow propagation by color M-mode Doppler echocardiography. J Am Coll Cardiol 27:365–371
98. Sohn DW, Chai IH, Lee DJ, et al (1997) Assessment of mitral annulus velocity by Doppler tissue imaging in the evaluation of left ventricular diastolic function. J Am Coll Cardiol 30:474–480
99. Oki T, Tabata T, Yamada H, et al (1997) Clinical application of pulsed Doppler tissue imaging for assessing abnormal left ventricular relaxation. Am J Cardiol 79:921–928
100. Oki T, Tabata T, Mishiro Y, et al (1999) Pulsed tissue Doppler imaging of left ventricular systolic and diastolic wall motion velocities to evaluate differences between long and short axes in heatly subjects. J Am Soc Echocardiogr 12:308–313
101. Heimdal A, Stoylen A, Torp H (1998) Real-time strain rate imaging of the left ventricle by ultrasound. J Am Soc Echocardiogr 11:1013–1019
102. Sohn DW, Kim YJ, Chun HG, Park YB, Choi YC (1999) Evaluation of left ventricular diastolic function when mitral E and A waves are completely fused: role of assessing mitral annulus velocity. J Am Soc Echocardiogr 12:203–208
103. Sohn DW, Kim YL, Lee MM, Park YB, Choi YS, Lee YW (2000) Differentiation between reversible and irreversible restrictive left ventricular filling pattern with the use of mitral annulus velocity. J Am Soc Echocardiogr 13:891–895
104. Sohn DW, Choi YJ, Oh BH, Lee MM, Lee YW (1999) Estimation of left ventricular end-diastolic pressure with the difference in pulmonary venous and mitral A durations is limited when mitral E and A waves are overlapped. J Am Soc Echocardiogr 12:106–112
105. Bach D (1996) Quantitative Doppler tissue imaging as a correlated of left ventricular contractility. Int J Cardiac Imag 12:191–195

106. Nagueh S, Middleton K, Kopelen H, Zoghibi W, Quinones M (1997) Doppler tissue imaging: a noninvasive technique for evaluation of left ventricular relaxation and estimation of filling pressures. J Am Coll Cardiol 30:1527–1533
107. Nagueh S, Mikati I, Kopelen H, Middleton K, Quinonens M, Zoghbi W (1998) Doppler estimation of left ventricular filling pressure in sinus tachycardia. A new application of tissue Doppler imaging. Circulation 98:1644–1650
108. Robotham J, Takata M, Berman M, Harasawa Y (1991) Ejection fraction revisited. Anesthesiology 74:172–183
109. Tuman K, McCarthy R, Pharm D, March R, Najafi H, Ivankovich A (1992) Morbidity and duration of ICU stay after cardiac surgery: A model for preoperative risk assessment. Chest 102:36–44
110. Tu J, Jaglal S, Naylor D (1995) Multicenter validation of a risk index for mortality, intensive care unit stay, and overall hospital length of stay after cardiac surgery. Circulation 91:677–684
111. Higgins T (1998) Quantifying risk and assessing outcome in cardiac surgery. J Cardiothorac Vasc Anesth 12:330–340
112. Gault J, Ross J, Braunwald E (1968) Contractile state of the left ventricle in man. Circ Res 22:451–463
113. Borow KM, Neumann A, Marcus RH, Sarelli P, Lang RM (1992) Effects of simultaneous alterations in preload and afterload measurements of left ventricular contractility in patients with dilated cardiomyopathy: comparisons of ejection phase, isovolumetric and end-systolic force-velocity indexes. J Am Coll Cardiol 20:787–795
114. Jin XY, Pepper JR, Gibson DG (1996) Effects of incoordination on left ventricular force-velocity relation in aortic stenosis. Heart 76:695–501
115. Sharir T, Feldman MD, Haber H, et al (1994) Ventricular systolic assessment in patients with dilated cardiomyopathy by preload-adjusted maximal power. Validation and noninvasive application. Circulation 89:2045–2053
116. Marmor A, Raphael T, Marmor M, Blondheim D (1996) Evaluation of contractile reserve by dobutamine echocardiography: noninvasive estimation of the severity of heart failure. Am Heart J 132:1196–1201
117. Marmor A, Schneeweiss A (1997) Prognostic value of noninvasively obtained left ventricular contractile reserve in patients with severe heart failure. J Am Coll Cardiol 29:422–428
118. Avramides D, Perakis A, Voudris V, Gezerlis P (2000) Noninvasive assessment of left ventricular systolic function by stress-shortening relation, rate of change of power, preload-adjusted maximal power, and ejection force in idiopathic dilated cardiomyopathy: prognostic implications. J Am Soc Echocardiogr 13:87–95
119. Gorcsan J, Murali S, Counihan PJ, Mandarino WA, Kormos RL (1996) Right ventricular performance and contractile reserve in patients with severe heart failure. Circulation 94:3190–3197
120. Jamal F, Strotmann J, Weidemann F, et al (2001) Noninvasive quantification of the contractile reserve of stunned myocardium by ultrasonic strain rate and strain. Circulation 104:1059–1065
121. Seeberger M, Cahalan M, Rouine-Rapp K, et al (1997) Acute hypovolemia may cause segmental wall motion abnormalities in the absence of myocardial ischemia. Anesth Analg 85:1252–1257

Functional Hemodynamic Monitoring:
Applied Physiology at the Bedside

M. R. Pinsky

▌ Introduction

The goal of cardiovascular therapy is to create a physiological condition wherein blood flow and oxygen delivery to the tissues is adequate to meet the metabolic demands of the tissues without inducing untoward cardiorespiratory complications. Cardiovascular insufficiency is often referred to as circulatory shock and is often the primary manifestation of critical illness. In most clinical conditions associated with circulatory shock, the primary concerns and therapeutic options relate to three functional performance-based questions:

▌ Will blood flow to the body increase (or decrease) if the patient's intravascular volume is increased (or decreased), and if so, by how much?

▌ Is any decreased in arterial pressure due to loss of vascular tone or merely due to inadequate blood flow?

▌ Is the heart capable of maintaining an effective blood flow with an acceptable perfusion pressure without going into failure?

▌ The Problem

The immediate questions asks by doctors are functional and physiological in their language but practical and concrete in their application. Presently, highly invasive hemodynamic monitoring is needed to define the specific hemodynamic profiles seen in these complex and heterogeneous conditions. Regrettably, data from one large retrospective clinical trial failed to document any benefit of pulmonary arterial catheterization on outcome [1]. Furthermore, data from numerous clinical trials have documented repeatedly that neither right atrial pressure (RAP) or pulmonary artery occlusion pressure (PAOP) predict well the subsequent response of the subject to an intravascular fluid challenge [2]. In addition, measures of absolute left ventricular (LV) volumes are only slightly better at predicting preload-responsiveness. Clearly, subjects with small LV end-diastolic volumes (LVEDV) can have a limited response to a volume challenge if their filling is limited either by tamponade, cor pulmonale or diastolic stiffening. Finally, ventilation and ventilatory therapies, such as the use of positive end-expiratory pressure (PEEP), often complicate this analysis by dissociating filling pressures from measured intrathoracic vascular pressure because of both increasing intrathoracic pressure and cardiac compression by lung expansion [3]. However, ventilation, by phasically altering RAP, also serves as a sine wave forcing function on venous return and can be used to define cardiovascular performance. Several groups have applied this concept to assess preload-responsiveness. The importance of these applications to bedside monitoring is finally being understood.

Unfortunately, present diagnostic and treatment protocols lack generalized acceptance and do not directly address the three fundamental questions asked above. Furthermore, existing complex and poorly validated monitoring systems of hemodynamic profile analysis belie the simple fact that most treatments for hemodynamically unstable patients can be resolved by answering these three specific questions. Thus, the stage is set for a more functional method of assessing cardiovascular performance using hemodynamic monitoring.

▌ Functional Measures of 'Preload Responsiveness'

Since RAP is the backpressure to venous return, if RAP decreases during spontaneous inspiration, then venous return will transiently increase, increasing cardiac output. If, however, the right ventricle (RV) is unable to dilate further, then RAP will not decrease during inspiration even though intrathoracic pressure decreases. At the extreme, spontaneous inspiration-associated increases in RAP reflect severe RV failure and are referred to as Kussmaul's sign. Magder et al. [4] used the fall in RAP to predict which patients would increase their cardiac output in response to a defined fluid challenge. These authors found that if RAP decreased by >2 mmHg during a spontaneous breath then cardiac output increased in 16 or 19 patients in response to 250–500 ml bolus saline infusion. If RAP did not decrease, then cardiac output increased in only one of 14 patients. These data are important because they focus on both RV function and spontaneous ventilation, two areas of study with markedly few clinical trials. These workers recently documented that this approach can also be used to predict subsequent changes in cardiac output in response to increasing levels of PEEP in mechanically ventilated subjects [5]. However, these studies rely on RV performance as the signal transducer for blood flow. Though appealing on physiological grounds, this approach does not address the issue of LV performance, which would need to be assessed separately.

Other studies have focused on the effects of positive-pressure ventilation on LV output. Positive-pressure ventilation induces phasic changes in LV stroke volume though similar cyclic changes in venous return. The magnitude of these changes in stroke volume are a function of the size of the tidal breath, the subsequent increase in intrathoracic pressure and the extent that changes in LV output are determined by changes in LV filling pressure. Beat-to-beat changes in LV stroke volume can be easily monitored as beat-to-beat changes in arterial pulse pressure variation (PPV), since the only other determinants of pulse pressure, arterial resistance and compliance, cannot change enough to alter pulse pressure during a single breath. Based on this logic, Perel et al. [6, 7] examined the systolic pressure variation (SPV) induced by a defined positive-pressure breath in animals made hypovolemic and in heart failure and in humans, demonstrating that the SPV, as specifically the decrease in systolic pressure from an apneic baseline, referred to as Δdown, identified hemorrhage and was minimized by fluid resuscitation. Tavernier et al. [8] validated these findings. The concept of SPV assumes that all the changes in systolic pressure can be explained by parallel changes in LV stroke volume. Unfortunately, Denault et al. [9] could not demonstrate any relation between LV stroke volume, estimated by transesophageal echocardiographic (TEE) analysis, and SPV, suggesting that factors other than LV stroke volume contribute to SPV. Michard et al. [10, 11] reasoned that arterial PPV rather than SPV would more accurately reflect changes in LV stroke volume because arterial PPV is not influenced by the intrathoracic pressure-induced changes in both systolic and diastolic arterial pressure. These authors compared SPV with PPV as predictors of the subsequent increase in cardiac output in response to fluid loading in septic ventilator-dependent patients. Their data convincingly demonstrated that both PPV and SPV of ≥15% were far superior to measures of either RAP or PAOP in predicting an increase in cardiac output response to volume loading. Furthermore, the greater the PPV or SPV, the greater was the increase in cardiac output. However, PPV claimed a slight, though significant, advantage over SPV in terms of greater precision and less bias. Since PPV attempts to monitor LV stroke volume changes, it was not surprising that Feissel et al. [12] demonstrated that aortic flow variation, as measured by transesophageal 2-D echocardiography pulsed Doppler of the aortic outflow tract, followed a similar response to PPV in response to fluid loading. The flow variation data are very important because flow is the primary variable from which SPV and arterial PPV derive their validity. Though less invasive than arterial pressure monitoring, echocardiographic analysis is far from ideal as a hemodynamic monitoring tool: It requires the continuous presence of an experienced operator; echocardiography requires using expensive and often scare equipment; and finally, measures of aortic root flow variation cannot be made on-line or continuously over prolonged periods of time. Still, recent, minimally invasive, esophageal pulsed Doppler techniques have been developed that continuously measure descending aortic flow on a beat-to-beat basis. To the extent that descending aortic flow varies proportionally with aortic outflow, then these measures of descending aortic flow accurately access stroke volume variation (SVV).

▌ Applying Functional Measures to Practical Questions: Is the Cardiovascular System 'Preload Responsive'?

Meaning, "If blood flow back to the heart, referred to as venous return, is changed, will cardiac output also change in the same direction and by how much?". The manner by which one increases or decreases venous return will be a function of the specific clinical or pathological intervention. For example, bleeding induces loss of blood volume while the use of artificial ventilation to support a patient in respiratory distress will impede venous return reducing the amount of blood returning to the heart in a fashion similar to hemorrhage. It would be highly advantageous to be able to accurately predict ahead of time if cardiac output will decrease by the application of PEEP or increase if a patient's blood volume is increased by transfusion of fluids or blood. And, it would be even more important if this monitoring system could continually monitor the dynamic response to the treatment so as to allow the accurate delivery of potentially dangerous therapies, such as intravascular fluid loading or artificial ventilation.

Measuring either the PPV change or SVV during positive-pressure breathing allows us to accurately predict if this patient will increase cardiac output in response to fluid loading or decrease cardiac output in response to increasing artificial ventilation support [11–13]. In patients with acute respiratory distress syndrome (ARDS) requiring artificial ventilation, the degree of PPV during a breath was quantitatively related to the subsequent decrease in cardiac output in response to the addition of increasing amounts of airway pressure [11]. Furthermore, we

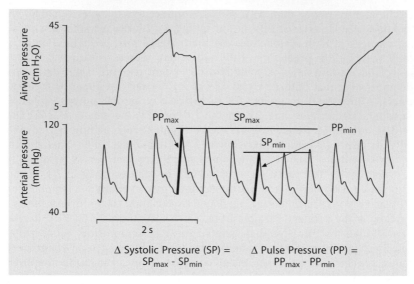

Fig. 1. Strip chart recording of airway pressure and arterial pressure for a subject during positive pressure venti-lation, illustrating the technique of calculating both systolic pressure variation (ΔSP) and pulse pressure varia-tion (ΔPP)

showed that in critically ill patients with severe sepsis, PPV predicted the amount of increase of the cardiac output in response to intravascular fluid loading [12]. Arterial pulse pressure is the difference between the systolic arterial pressure and diastolic arterial pressure (Fig. 1). For example, if a patient's blood pressure were 120/80 then their pulse pressure would be 120 minus 80, or 40 mmHg. During breathing, the actual pulse pressure will vary slightly. If PPV >15% of the baseline pulse pressure (e.g., 6 mmHg for a mean pulse pressure of 40 mmHg) for a normal tidal breath (<6 ml/kg), then that patient will increase their cardiac output in re-sponse to intravascular volume challenges. Furthermore, this PPV changes inversely as cardiac output changes. Thus, PPV will decrease as cardiac output increases with intravascular fluid loading. Since the primary determinant of arterial pulse pressure is the phasic aortic flow generated by the heart's contraction with each heart beat, aortic flow variation can also be used to determine preload-responsiveness and the subsequent change in cardiac output in response to a treatment [12]. Thus, either PPV or SVV can be used to assess preload-responsiveness. This simple fact allows one to answer the question "If I were to increase venous return, will cardiac output increase and by how much?".

The Science. The heart pumps blood into the arteries to deliver blood to the body. The heart does this by phasically ejecting its stroke volume into the arterial circuit under an increasing pressure. This results in the usual arterial pulse pressure and phasic aortic flow. Ventilation causes a dynamic change in the rate of venous return during the breath. Because the pressure inside the chest decreases with sponta-neous inspiration and increases with artificial ventilation inspiration, a dynamic and cyclic variation in venous return is induced [13, 14]. The greater the degree to which the heart's stroke volume is dependent of this venous return, the greater the

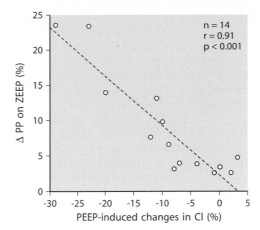

Fig. 2. Relation between 10 cm H$_2$0 PEEP-induced changes in cardiac index and initial pulse pressure variation (ΔPP) prior to the addition of PEEP. (From [10] with permission)

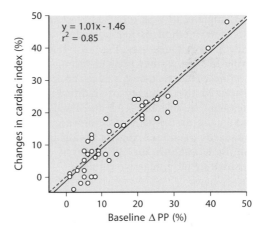

Fig. 3. Relation between change in cardiac index and initial pulse pressure variation (PP) in septic patients given an intravenous bolus of 500 ml hydroxyethyl starch (HES). (From [11] with permission)

change in stroke volume over the breath. Arterial PPV analysis assumes that the phasic effects of either spontaneous inspiration or positive-pressure (artificial) inspiration cause venous return to vary in a cyclic fashion throughout the breath. The major assumption of the PPV technique is that changes in the downstream pressure for venous return (usually assumed to be RAP also referred to as central venous pressure [CVP]) will reduce the pressure gradient for venous return, and that this reduction in venous return will reduce LV filling. This implies that the entire cardiac circuitry in the chest, from the RV and pulmonary circulation to the LV will transpose all the variation in venous flow rate. If this were not the case, as will occur in patients with selective RV failure, tamponade or LV failure, then no change in pulse pressure can occur [15]. Importantly, these are just the conditions in which intravascular fluid loading may cause serious and often fatal complications. A potential limitation of the pulse-pressure responsiveness index, is that it was validated under conditions in which the percent change in pulse pressure during ventilation was >15%. The size of the breath should also influence the magnitude of the change in venous return as well as pulmonary venous blood flow [16]. Thus, if small breaths are given by artificial ventilation, then the maximal PPV will also decrease, although the directional change in pulse pressure will still be accurate.

Using this approach Michard et al. [10] showed that the arterial PPV predicted the subsequent decrease in cardiac output in patients with acute lung injury (ALI) who were given increasing amounts of positive airway pressure at end-expiration, referred to as PEEP, a maneuver often associated with a decrease in cardiac output. The greater the baseline PPV (ΔPP), the greater the subsequent decrease in cardiac index (CI) (Fig. 2). Note that not all patients had a decrease in cardiac index, but that the PPV predicted the degree of CI decrease. These authors also showed that in patients with severe septic shock, the ΔPP predicted the subsequent increase in cardiac output in response to intravascular fluid loading (Fig. 3), a maneuver usually associated with an increase in cardiac index [11]. Note that although intravascular volume loading tended to increase CI, as it should, some patients had no increase in CI and the degree to which CI increased was predictable from the PPV. Finally, as CI increased in these critically ill patients, their degree of PPV decreased, such that changes in PPV could be used to monitor the effect of intravascular volume loading on flow.

Using the PPV as a bedside test, we then documented the test characteristics of this new method of hemodynamic assessment relative to other novel, and established, techniques (see Fig. 1 of following chapter, p. 554). Others had proposed using SPV to predict preload-responsiveness so we also compared pulse pressure to systolic pressure using a receiver-operator characteristic (ROC) analysis. We also examined the accuracy of traditional measures of preload-responsiveness, namely measures of absolute RAP and PAOP. Both these techniques have a long history of use in the assessment of cardiovascular insufficiency and both are considered the standards of monitoring for assessing preload-responsiveness. As can be seen from our ROC analysis the PPV analysis was superior to all others with minimal false positive or false negative results.

▌ Functional Measures of Arterial Tone

Critically ill patients often have a low blood pressure or systemic hypotension. The relationship between arterial pressure and regional blood flow is both non-linear and different among vascular beds. Thus, a change in arterial pressure may induce blood flow redistribution and/or frank ischemia in specific vascular beds [17]. Normally, baroreceptors on the carotid body vary arterial tone to keep cerebral perfusion pressure constant. If cardiac output were to increase, then arterial tone would decrease to maintain cerebral perfusion pressure (CPP) constant. Similarly, hypoperfusion seen early in hypovolemic shock induces peripheral vasoconstriction, tending to maintain arterial pressure constant. Thus, under all conditions, arterial hypotension connotes cardiovascular dysfunction, whereas normotension does not insure a lack of cardiovascular dysfunction. Accordingly, arterial pressure and vasomotor tone can be evaluated in two steps: first determining the actual perfusion pressure, and second determining arterial tone.

Hypotension for any reason causes a decrease in brain, heart, gut and kidney blood flow. If sustained, hypotension results in end-organ failure and death. However, even if cardiac output is supranormal, if systemic hypotension co-exists, then blood flow regulation and pressure-dependent flow to all organs may still be impaired. Primary loss of vasomotor tone is a hallmark of septic shock, hypoglycemia, hypoxemia, and adrenocortical insufficiency. Thus, independent of knowing if a patient will increase their cardiac output in response to volume loading, knowing the level of vasomotor tone and its change in response to changes in cardiac output and vasoactive therapy is relevant in deciding on specific therapies and their titration.

To assess arterial tone it is necessary to know the relation between changes in blood flow and changes in blood pressure, not absolute pressure and flow values. Here, the same measures of arterial pulse pressure and aortic flow variation during a positive-pressure breath can be used to characterize arterial tone. Importantly, one needs to examine the proportional changes in each, rather than their specific values. The ratio of PPV to SVV defines arterial tone and allows for the continual tracking of vascular tone as either treatment or time evolve.

The Science. The cause of the pulse pressure in the first place is the interaction of the ejected LV stroke volume with the arterial impedance circuit. As the blood is rapidly ejected it causes the arterial pressure to rise. The degree to which arterial pressure rises generating the arterial pulse pressure is a function of both LV stroke volume and arterial tone [18]. Increasing LV stroke volume, all else being equal, increases arterial pulse pressure by a proportional amount. Thus, if LV stroke volume were to increase 20% from one beat to the next, arterial pulse pressure would also increase by 20%. The slope of the change in arterial pulse pressure to stroke volume describes the tone of the arterial circuit at that time and is referred to as arterial elastance (Ea) (Fig. 4). If arterial tone were to increase, then for the same stroke volume the arterial pulse pressure would be greater and the ratio of the pulse pressure to stroke volume would increase proportionally along a series of varying LV stroke volumes. As can be seen, increasing tone increases the 'slope' of the pressure to flow relation but does not alter its primary relationship. Thus, by measuring the ratio if arterial pulse pressure to aortic flow as both vary, one can derive an accurate measure of arterial tone or Ea.

The primary limitation to the bedside application of Ea analysis is not its scientific validity. Physiologists have used this analysis to assess arterial tone for over 20 years. However, its bedside use was previously impractical because of the inherent difficulty in measuring LV stroke volume at the bedside from beat-to-beat. Prior to

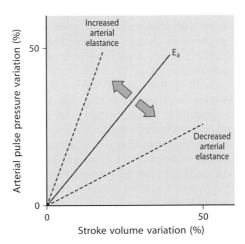

Fig. 4. Effect of changes in arterial vasomotor tone on the relation between arterial pulse pressure and stroke volume

the advent of esophageal pulsed Doppler and robust arterial pulse contour techniques, the routine measure of LV stroke volume on a beat-to-beat basis over prolonged time intervals was not realistic. Although TEE measures of aortic outflow tract flow, using pulsed Doppler techniques, are accurate and have been applied in this manner [12], they are limited to specific centers with the expertise and equipment and also cannot be used continually over prolonged intervals to assess changes in LV stroke volume.

Now we have a unique advantage in the field of hemodynamic monitoring, because of the introduction of novel, and hopefully accurate, estimates of LV stroke volume on a beat-to-beat basis using both esophageal pulsed Doppler from a small indwelling esophageal probe or via the arterial pulse contour technique using mathematical modeling to derive LV stroke volume from arterial pressure profiles over a single cardiac cycle [19]. Importantly, the PPV response to positive-pressure ventilation lends itself to arterial tone analysis as well. Since LV stroke volume will vary slightly during the ventilatory cycle, owing to changes in preload, noting the ratio of PPV to SVV as a percent of baseline will define Ea. This concept is just now being studied, but appears to be as robust as the measures of beat-to-beat changes in LV stroke volume define. One can easily imagine a diagnostic and treatment protocol algorithm incorporating this measure as is described below.

▌ Functional Measures of Ventricular Performance

Absolute cardiac output and blood pressure, by themselves do not tell one much about cardiac pump performance. Furthermore, in a subject with an artificially reduced LVEDV, LV performance is proportionally reduced even if under greater filling volumes it is normal. This preload-dependent cardiac performance is another way of describing the Frank-Starling relationship (Fig. 5). Thus, measures of LV performance, as an independent measure of cardiovascular function, cannot be made until the subject is no longer preload responsive. Importantly, cardiac output is a very poor measure of ventricular performance, as cardiac output is often elevated in acute myocardial infarctions and during the post-resuscitated septic state, although clear impairment of cardiac contractility is seen [20, 21]. Both cardiac output and arterial pressure are often elevated in acute ventricular failure associated with myocardial infarction [20]. In severe septic shock, cardiac output is often elevated despite profound impairment in contractility [21]. The poor LV contractile reserve associated with sepsis is 'unmasked' by increasing arterial tone, thereby impeding LV ejection, reducing cardiac output and potentially inducing acute LV failure. Measuring stroke work, rather than stroke volume, in the Frank-Starling relation minimizes this weakness of using the Frank-Starling relationship to assess LV contractility, but does not eliminate it (Fig. 6). Still, knowing the degree of contractile reserve is important is assessing a subject's response to subsequent stress (weaning from mechanical ventilation, surgery), the ability of the patient to sustain an adequate cardiac output once the work load it has to perform is markedly increased by treatments that increase arterial pressure and LV afterload, and in following the subject's response to treatments aimed at improving contractility (coronary vasodilation during ischemia, dobutamine infusion). The best measures of contractility are those that are not affected by changes in either cardiac size just prior to contraction, referred to as end-diastole, or the pressure and mus-

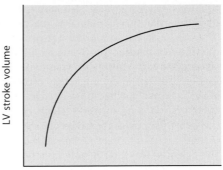

Fig. 5. The Frank-Starling relationship: The relation between preload (LV end-diastolic volume) and the ejection phase index LV stroke volume

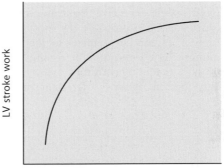

Fig. 6. The Frank-Starling relationship: The relation between preload (LV end-diastolic volume) and the ejection phase index LV stroke work. This is the same concept as shown in Figure 6, except now both pressure and flow are included into the ejection phase index

cle tension needed to develop the ejection pressure during contraction, referred to as afterload. Measures used by cardiac physiologists to measure cardiac contractility include complex derived measures such as LV end-systolic elastance (the slope of the LV end-systolic pressure-volume relation), preload-recruitable stroke work, and preload-adjusted maximal cardiac power. Although accurate, the use of these parameters in the routine monitoring and management of critically ill patients is impractical. Importantly, however, one can derive the same qualitative data from analyzing the instantaneous relationship between LV ejection and developed pressure. The product of flow and pressure is power. Thus, the product of peak aortic flow – arterial pressure or stroke volume and arterial pulse pressure are excellent measures of maximal cardiac power. Measures of cardiac power can be made from instantaneous stroke volume and arterial pressure data. This method of analysis of heart function, like all measures of heart pump function, is limited by not knowing the actual LV preload, which is the primary factor other than contractility that determines cardiac power.

However, the assessment of maximal cardiac power can be done along a reductionism line as follows: Is apneic cardiac power below a certain minimal level? If yes, is the subject preload-responsive (arterial PPV)? If the subject is preload-responsive, then volume resuscitation should be given prior to ascertaining if cardiac failure is a contributing factor in the cardiovascular state. If the subject is no longer preload responsive and still has a reduced cardiac power, then one assumes impaired cardiac performance is the primary cause of lack of preload-responsiveness. The cause of this impaired performance is not defined by this analysis. Equal reductions in cardiac performance could occur by tamponade, cor pulmonale, massive pulmonary embolism, traumatic ventricular septal defect (VSD), acute myocardial infarction, and congestive cardiomyopathy, to name just a few. In summary, since maximal cardiac power varies directly with preload, only when the cardiovascular system is no longer preload-responsive will a low cardiac power clear identify the heart as a primary cause of circulatory shock and critical illness.

The Science. The heart's only function is to take what blood it receives under a low filling pressure and transfer it to the arterial system under a higher pressure. The amount of stroke volume the heart ejects for a given heart beat is determined by three factors: the amount of blood in the heart prior to contractions (called preload), the contractile state of the heart (contractility), and the resistance of the arterial vessels to receive the stroke volume (called afterload). Preload, or pre-ejection heart volume is probably the most important single factor determining stroke volume. This concept returns to the first issue raised by the above hemodynamic monitoring questions: Will cardiac output increase if preload increases, and if so, by how much? The relation between LVEDV, or preload and LV stroke volume is described in Figure 5. Increasing preload increases stroke volume. For any level of

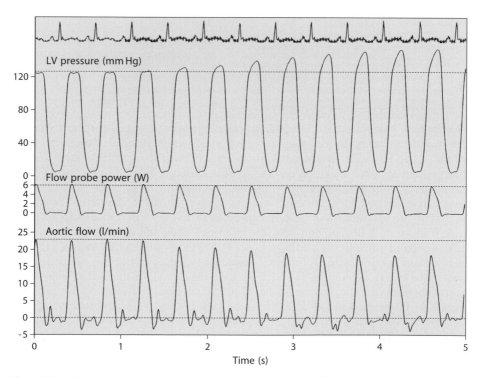

Fig. 7. Effect of partial aortic occlusion on cardiac power in a canine model. Note that as left ventricular (LV) pressure increases, aortic flow decreases, but cardiac power remains constant. (From [22] with permission)

preload, however, stroke volume will decrease if the ejection pressure increases because the work the heart has to do to ejects its blood increases. Cardiac work during ejection if measured as stroke work (the product of the stroke volume and the pressure generated) and when expressed relative to preload, also describes the Frank-Starling relationship (Fig. 6). Since stroke volume may vary with changing ejection pressures, a patient with a poorly functioning heart may still have a good stroke volume if they also have a low blood pressure. However, their stroke work, which it the product of stroke volume and blood pressure will be reduced. These points are illustrated in Figures 7 and 8 from recent animal studies [22]. These data show that the product of flow and pressure remains constant during transient partial aortic occlusion (Fig. 7), but is markedly increased (or decreased) by inotropic (negative inotropic) therapy (Fig. 8).

Importantly, LV stroke work will also be reduced under conditions where LV preload is also low. Thus, in a subject with low preload, a low stroke work may reflect inadequate heart filling rather than impaired contractility. If, however, the initial step in resuscitation is bringing the subject to hemodynamic stability by fluid resuscitation, then once preload-responsiveness is lost in a hemodynamically unstable patient, measures of cardiac performance will have purchase. If a subject is not preload-responsive and has a low cardiac stroke work, then a primary cause of any hemodynamic instability centers with the heart. The reason for heart failure is on the intrathoracic contents. Many critical clinical conditions have both a decreased LV preload and a decreased ability to fill the heart with intravascular vol-

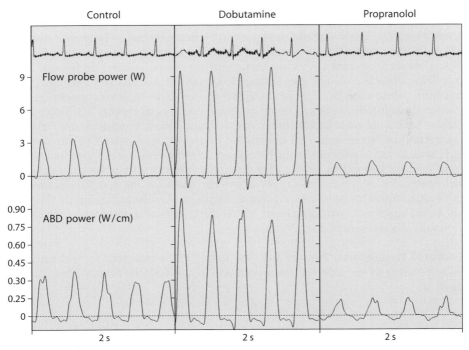

Fig. 8. Effect of changing cardiac contractility on measured cardiac power in a canine model. Note that dobutamine (5 mg/kg/min) increases cardiac power, whereas propranolol (5 mg IV) decreases it. (From [22] with permission)

ume replacement. Examples include acute RV failure, mitral stenosis and cardiac tamponade. All these conditions have many specific causes but still are not pre-load-responsive and need specific cardiac treatments. Thus, any hemodynamically unstable subject in whom preload-responsiveness is no longer present and who also has a reduced stroke work has a primary cardiac cause of their dysfunction. Accordingly, both diagnostic efforts and treatments must be focused on improving cardiac performance.

The numeric value for the lower limit of stroke work below which impaired cardiac performance is said to be present will be a function of the method by which aortic flow or stroke volume are measured. If stroke volume is calculated from the pulse contour method and estimates of absolute stroke work index (ratio of stroke work to body surface area) are given, then a stroke work index < 1625 mmHg/ml/m^2 would be considered low. However, if descending aortic flow were used to derive stroke volume, then a relative stroke work index would need to be defined specific for each measuring device. Although not presently defined, as part of the usual output of these pulsed Doppler monitors, the calculation would be easy.

▌ Simple Measures of Cardiovascular Performance

Arterial Pressure. An essential component to this analysis is the accurate measure of central arterial pressure waveform. This information allows for the definition of hypotension and also to analyze the PPV.

Aortic Flow. The other essential component of this analysis is LV stroke volume, either absolute or relative. Importantly since relative stroke volume and its changes over a breath are central to this analysis, there are several monitoring systems commercially available that may give acceptable signals for this analysis. However, none has been validated to be accurate on a beat-to-beat basis as stroke volume rapidly varies. Assuming that such validation occurs, then these techniques will become valuable monitoring tools for functional hemodynamic monitoring analyses. Descending aorta flow can be measured directly by transesophageal pulse Doppler technology; several such devices are available. However, stroke volume can also be inferred from the arterial pressure profile by a technique referred to as pulse contour analysis. Potentially, either of these types of system allow for the accurate measure of the beat-to-beat change in stroke volume. Although the descending aortic flow signal is not equal to LV stroke volume, its variation in flow from beat-to-beat closely approximates the variation in LV output.

Calculated Variables from Pressure and Flow Data. PPV is measured form the arterial pulse pressure as the difference between systolic and diastolic arterial pressure, defined as:

$$(PP_{max} - PP_{min})/[(PP_{max} - PP_{min})/2]$$

a) Aortic flow variation as an estimate of SVV is measured from the transesophageal pulsed Doppler recording of stroke distance (SD) measured in cm, defined as:

$$(SD_{max} - SD_{min})/[(SD_{max} - SD_{min})/2] .$$

For the pulse contour method, derived stroke volume measures are used to calculate SVV.

b) Arterial elastance (Ea) is defined as the ratio of PPV to arterial flow variation (AFV).

c) Maximal cardiac power is defined as the maximal value for the product of paired pulse pressure and stroke distance data during a breath (usually occurring at end-expiration) while the operating stroke work of the patient is defined as the product of the calculated stroke volume and mean arterial pressure (MAP).

▌ A Simplified Treatment Algorithm

Although many specific treatment algorithms may be constructed form this model, the basic structure follows. The treatment algorithm is divided into two sequential treatment arms and one contingent treatment arm based on MAP, PPV and SVV data. The algorithm is put into operation only if the patient develops signs and symptoms of cardiovascular compromise because preload-responsiveness is also a characteristic of normal stable subjects.

Criteria for the diagnosis of hemodynamic instability are readily available and may include:

a) MAP <60 mmHg, or a decrease in MAP of >20 mmHg in a previously hypertensive patient and one of the two (b and c below).

b) Evidence of end-organ hypoperfusion: a decrease in urine output to <20 ml/hr, confusion, new onset tachycardia, lactic acidosis, ileus.

c) Symptoms of increased sympathetic tone: agitation, confusion, restlessness.

If hemodynamic instability were present one would proceed with the treatment algorithm.

1. Measures of MAP and PPV during positive pressure breathing (A/C, IMV ≥10/min, or pressure support [PS] ≥15 cmH$_2$O; with a tidal volume of 10 ml/kg and a frequency between 10 and 20 with a 30% inspiratory time). Alternatively, measure aortic flow variation during a positive pressure breath.

   a) If PPV >12% then give a bolus infusion of 500 ml fluid (the choice of specific fluid is probably more a matter of religion than science) over 15 minutes and reassess.

   b) Repeat these bolus infusions of 500 ml fluid every 15 minutes until PPV becomes <12%, then stop fluid boluses.

   c) If MAP remains >60 mmHg after the initial fluid bolus then start norepinephrine protocol as described in step 3 below.

2. Measure aortic flow or estimated LV stroke volume as described above. Calculate the PPV to SVV ratio (Ea*).

   a) If MAP is <60 mmHg and Ea >1.2 then the subject has increased arterial tone and fluid resuscitation alone should rapidly increase MAP and vasopressor should be withheld during after this initial fluid bolus.

   b) If MAP is <60 mmHg and Ea is <0.8 then the patient should be simultaneously started on a vasopressor infusion titrated to increase MAP to >60 mmHg, since increasing cardiac output in response to fluid loading alone may not induce as much of an increase in arterial pressure.

   c) If MAP is <60 mmHg and Ea is <1.2 but >0.8 initial vasopressor therapy may be given to maintain MAP >60 mmHg at the discretion of the physician.

   d) Vasopressor therapy would include the infusion of norepinephrine at 0.02–0.05 μg/kg/min and titrate upward every 15 minutes in 0.02 to 0.05 μg/kg/min increments until MAP is >60 mmHg. When Ea becomes >2 further increases in vasopressor infusion rate should be stopped until the next fluid bolus is given, assuming the PPV remains >12%.

3) Once the PVV or SVV becomes <12%, if vasopressor therapy is still required measure both maximal cardiac power and stroke work.

   a) If either is less than normal value then cardiac performance is also impaired and attention should shift to including assessment of cardiac performance. A reasonable initial approach would be to start an infusion of dobutamine 5–10 μg/mg/min and reassess in 15 minutes, since most cardiac impairment has a component of depressed contractility.

   b) If hemodynamic insufficiency persists, the assessment of cardiac function directly by use of a balloon floatation pulmonary artery catheter and/or echocardiographic study is indicated with treatment following diagnosis. Using this approach, a pulmonary artery catheters would not be inserted early during resuscitation but would be used when specific diagnostic information related to cardiac performance was needed.

Perspective. The above management protocol is merely an example of how this simplified approach can be easily applied to the management of any critically ill patient. Several comments about ignored hemodynamic measures and ancillary clinical conditions also need to be made. The measures and treatments described above occur independent of measures of cardiac output, arterial oxygenation, mixed venous oxygen saturation (SvO_2), tonometric ΔPCO_2 and other ancillary monitoring techniques. Many physicians would argue that these 'ignored' variables are equally as important, if not more so, than MAP and stroke volume. Recall, that MAP is an absolute determinant of organ perfusion independent of cardiac output. However, the PPV and SVV calculations are made not to define adequacy but to determine preload-responsiveness, arterial tone and cardiac power.

   Clearly, both cardiac output and arterial oxygenation are essential aspects of cardiovascular performance and primary determinants of survival. However, cardiac output is linked to cardiac function by stroke volume and heart rate. Thus, as long as heart rate remains in the normal range (e.g., 60–100 beats/min) this algorithm accounts for CI. Importantly, arterial oxygenation may be impaired by fluid resuscitation in patients with ALI or severe LV failure. Although some impact of arterial desaturation may limit overall fluid management of the hemodynamically unstable patient, the prudent physician would still treat a hypotensive, hypodynamic patient who is also preload-responsive with intravascular volume expansion. If this patient became increasingly more hypoxemic, artificial ventilation and PEEP therapy would also be used. Controversy exists as to the optimal fluid management goals in the critically ill patient and whether or not to add an inotrope to keep pulmonary vascular pressures low while maintaining cardiac output at some minimal levels. Importantly, this protocol approach would allow investigators to explore different treatment goals in a controlled and easily managed fashion.

▌ Conclusion

Cardiovascular insufficiency is a complex process with several adaptive and maladaptive forces intertwined. By dissecting out preload-responsiveness from arterial perfusion pressure and arterial tone, as well as from cardiac performance, the physician should be able to diagnose and treat multiple aspects of cardiovascular performance simultaneously and base don an easily articulated logic. The stage is now set to study specific treatment algorithms for efficacy and long-term outcome based on these strong physiological principals.

Acknowledgements. This work was supported in part by a grant from the Laerdal Foundation and the NIH (NRSA 4-T32 HL07820-01A5).

References

1. Connors AF Jr, Speroff T, Dawson NV, et al (1996) The effectiveness of right heart catheterization in the initial care of critically ill patients. SUPPORT Investigators. JAMA 276:889–997

2. Lichtwarck-Aschoff M, Zeravik J, Pfeiffer UJ (1992) Intrathoracic blood volume accurately reflects circulatory volume status in critically ill patients with mechanical ventilation. Intensive Care Med 18:137–138

3. Pinsky MR, Vincent JL, DeSmet JM (1991) Estimating left ventricular filling pressure during positive end-expiratory pressure in humans. Am Rev Respir Dis 143:25–31

4. Magder S, Georgiadis G, Cheong T (1992) Respiratory variations in right atrial pressure predict the response to fluid challenge. J Crit Care 7:76–85

5. Magder S, Lagonidis D, Erice F (2001) The use of respiratory variations in right atrial pressure to predict the cardiac output response to PEEP. J Crit Care 16:108–114

6. Perel A, Pizov R, Cotev S (1987) Systolic blood pressure variation is a sensitive indicator of hypovolemia in ventilated dogs subjected to graded hemorrhage. Anesthesiology 67:498–502

7. Szold A, Pizov R, Segal E, Perel A (1989) The effect of tidal volume and intravascular volume state on systolic pressure variation in ventilated dogs. Intensive Care Med 15:368–371

8. Tavernier B, Makhotine O, Lebuffe G, Dupont J, Scherpereel P (1998) Systolic pressure variation as a guide to fluid therapy in patients with sepsis-induced hypotension. Anesthesiology 89:1313–1321

9. Denault AY, Gasior TA, Gorcsan J, Mandarino WA, Deneault LG, Pinsky MR (1999) Determinants of aortic pressure variation during positive-pressure ventilation in man. Chest 116:176–186

10. Michard F, Chemla D, Richard C, et al (1999) Clinical use of respiratory changes in arterial pulse pressure to monitor the hemodynamic effects of PEEP. Am J Respir Crit Care Med 159:935–939

11. Michard F, Boussat S, Chemla D, et al (2000) Relation between respiratory changes in arterial pulse pressure and fluid responsiveness in septic patients with acute circulatory failure. Am J Respir Crit Care Med 162:134–138

12. Feissel M, Michard F, Mangin I, Ruyer O, Faller JP, Teboul JL (2001) Respiratory changes in aortic blood velocity as an indicator of fluid responsiveness in ventilated patients with septic shock. Chest 119:867–873

13. Pinsky MR (1984) Determinants of pulmonary artery flow variation during respiration. J Appl Physiol 56:1237–1245

14. Pinsky MR (1984) Instantaneous venous return curves in an intact canine preparation. J Appl Physiol 56:765–771

15. Sharpey-Schaffer EP (1955) Effects of Valsalva maneuver on the normal and failing circulation. Br Med J 1:693–699

16. Brower R, Wise RA, Hassapoyannes C, Bromberger-Barnea B, Permutt S (1985) Effect of lung inflation on lung blood volume and pulmonary venous flow. J Appl Physiol 58:954–963

17. Schlichtig R, Kramer D, Pinsky MR (1991) Flow redistribution during progressive hemorrhage is a determinant of critical O_2 delivery. J Appl Physiol 70:169–178

18. Sunagawa K, Maughn WL, Burkhoff, Sagawa K (1983) Left ventricular interaction with arterial load studied in the isolated canine ventricle. Am J Physiol 245:H773–H785

19. Wesseling K, Wit Bd, Weber J, Smith NT (1983) A simple device for the continuous measurement of cardiac output. Adv Cardiovasc Physiol 5:16–52

20. Sagawa K, Suga H, Shoukas AA, Bakalar KM (1977) End-systolic pressure-volume ratio: A new index of contractility. Am J Cardiol 40:748–756

21. Cariou A, Monchi M, Laurent I, et al (2001) Noninvasive estimation of left ventricular elastance during sepsis. Am J Respir Crit Care Med 163:A135 (Abst)

22. Mandarino W, Gorcsan J, Pinsky MR (1998) Assessment of left ventricular contractile state by preload-adjusted maximal power using echocardiographic automated border detection. J Am Coll Cardiol 31:861–868

Detection of Fluid Responsiveness

F. Michard and J. L. Teboul

▌ Introduction

Volume expansion is frequently used in critically ill patients to improve hemodynamics. However, in studies designed to examine fluid responsiveness, only around 50% of critically ill patients have been shown to respond to volume expansion by a significant increase in stroke volume or cardiac output [1]. This finding emphasizes the need for predictive factors of fluid responsiveness to avoid ineffective or even deleterious effects of volume expansion (increase of extravascular lung water potentially resulting in worsening in gas exchange and longer ventilation time) in non-responder patients, in whom inotropic and/or vasopressor support should preferentially be used to improve hemodynamics. Clinical examination has been shown to be of minimal value in detecting inadequate cardiac preload and fluid responsiveness [2–5]. Therefore, many parameters derived from pulmonary artery catheterization, arterial pressure wave form analysis, echocardiography-Doppler and the PiCCO system have been proposed to help the caregiver in the decision making process concerning volume expansion.

▌ Pulmonary Artery Catheter

Right Atrial and Pulmonary Artery Occlusion Pressures

It has been suggested that a beneficial hemodynamic effect of volume expansion cannot be expected in critically ill patients with a central venous pressure (CVP) [6] or a pulmonary artery occlusion pressure (PAOP) [7] greater than 12 mmHg. In this regard, right atrial pressure (RAP) or PAOP have been reported to be lower in responder, than in non-responder, patients in a few studies [8–10]. Moreover, a significant relationship between the increase in stroke volume in response to volume expansion and the baseline RAP ($r^2 = 0.20$) or the baseline PAOP ($r^2 = 0.33$) has also been reported by Wagner et al. [9], suggesting that the lower RAP or PAOP before volume expansion, the greater the increase in stroke volume in response to fluid infusion. However, although statistically significant, these relationships were weak because a given value of RAP or of PAOP could not be used to discriminate responders and non-responders before fluid was given [9]. Moreover, in many other clinical studies, no difference between responder and non-responder patients was observed with regard to the baseline value of RAP [11–13] and of PAOP [8, 11–15] and no relationship was reported between cardiac filling pressures before volume expansion and the hemodynamic response to volume expansion (Fig. 1). One study

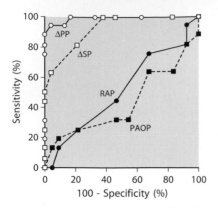

Fig. 1. ROC curves comparing the ability of the respiratory changes in pulse pressure (ΔPP), the respiratory changes in systolic pressure (ΔSP), right atrial pressure (RAP) and pulmonary artery occlusion pressure (PAOP) to discriminate responder (cardiac index increase > 15%) and non-responder patients to volume expansion. The area under the ROC curves for RAP and PAOP indicates that measuring these parameters to detect fluid responsiveness is no better than chance. The area under the ROC curve for ΔPP is greater (p < 0.01) than for ΔSP, indicating that ΔPP is a better indicator of fluid responsiveness than SP. (From [13] with permission)

[16] even reported a significantly higher value of PAOP in responder than in non-responder patients (14±7 vs 7±2 mmHg, p < 0.01) and fluid infusion has been shown to significantly increase cardiac output in critically ill patients with central venous pressures greater than 15 mmHg [17].

Inspiratory Decrease in Right Atrial Pressure

Assuming that respiratory changes in pleural pressure induce greater changes in RAP when the right ventricle is highly compliant than when it is poorly compliant, Magder et al. [18, 19] investigated whether the inspiratory decrease in RAP could be used to predict fluid responsiveness. In patients with spontaneous breathing activity, two studies demonstrated that a positive response to volume expansion was very likely in patients with an inspiratory decrease in RAP < 1 mmHg, while it was unlikely if the inspiratory decrease in RAP was < 1 mmHg.

Right Ventricular End-Diastolic Volume (RVEDV)

The RVEDV can be evaluated at the bedside by fast response pulmonary artery catheters. Two studies of Diebel et al. [14, 16] reported a lower value of RVEDV index in responder than in non-responder patients and suggested that a beneficial hemodynamic effect of volume expansion was likely when the RVEDV index was below 90 ml/m^2 and very unlikely when the RVEDV index was greater than 138 ml/m^2. However, when the RVEDV index ranged between 90 and 138 ml/m^2, no cutoff value could be proposed to discriminate responder and non-responder patients. In four other studies [8, 9, 11, 12], no significant difference was observed between responders and non-responders with regard to the baseline RVEDV index.

❚ Arterial Pressure Wave Form Analysis

Respiratory Changes in Pulse Pressure

Analysis of the respiratory changes in left ventricular (LV) stroke volume recently has been proposed to predict fluid responsiveness. Indeed, the respiratory changes in LV stroke volume reflect the sensitivity of the heart to changes in preload induced by mechanical ventilation. Therefore, they also reflect the sensitivity of the heart to changes in preload induced by volume expansion [1]. Because the arterial pulse pressure (systolic minus diastolic pressure) is directly proportional to LV stroke volume [20], the respiratory changes in LV stroke volume have been shown reflected by changes in peripheral pulse pressure [21]. Accordingly, the respiratory changes in pulse pressure (ΔPP) have been recently proposed as a predictor of fluid responsiveness. In patients mechanically ventilated with a positive end-expiratory pressure (PEEP) for an acute lung injury (ALI), we observed a very tight relationship between ΔPP before volume expansion, and the percent increase in cardiac output in response to fluid infusion [22]. In sedated and mechanically ventilated patients with acute circulatory failure related to sepsis, we demonstrated that ΔPP was significantly greater (24 ± 9 vs $7\pm3\%$, $p<0.001$) in responders than in non-responders, and that a ΔPP threshold value of 13% allowed discrimination between responder and non responder patients with a positive predictive value of 94% and a negative predictive value of 96% [13] (Fig. 1). Moreover, in this study [13], the value of ΔPP before fluid administration was closely correlated ($r^2=0.85$, $p<0.001$) with the volume expansion-induced changes in cardiac output, such that the higher the ΔPP at baseline, the greater was the increase in cardiac output in response to fluid infusion.

Expiratory Decrease in Systolic Pressure

The analysis of the respiratory changes in systolic pressure has also been proposed to detect fluid responsiveness [23]. However, because the systolic pressure depends on diastolic pressure (systolic pressure = diastolic pressure + pulse pressure) and because the diastolic pressure may increase during mechanical insufflation (due to the rise in aortic extramural pressure), significant changes in systolic pressure can be observed independent of changes in pulse pressure and hence in stroke volume [24, 25]. In other words, significant changes in systolic pressure over a single respiratory cycle can be observed in some patients unsensitive to changes in preload induced by mechanical insufflation, and hence non-responders to a fluid challenge (Fig. 2). In this regard, the respiratory changes in systolic presssure have been shown to be less accurate that changes in pulse pressure to discriminate responders and non-responders before fluid infusion [13] (Fig. 1). Therefore, in order to use the systolic pressure variation as an indicator of fluid responsiveness, it has been proposed to perform an end-expiratory pause to discriminate the inspiratory increase in systolic pressure (not necessarily due to an increase in stroke volume) and the expiratory decrease in systolic pressure (Δdown), which in contrast necessarily reflects a change in stroke volume [26]. In sedated and mechanically ventilated patients with sepsis-induced hypotension, one study [15] demonstrated that the Δdown was significantly greater (11 ± 4 vs 4 ± 2 mmHg, $p=0.0001$) in responders than in non-responders, and that a Δdown threshold value of 5 mmHg was able to discriminate responders and non-responders with a positive predictive value

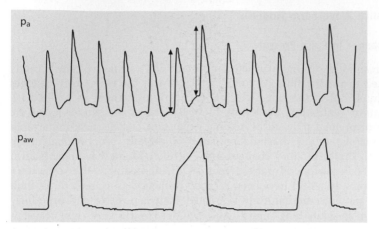

Fig. 2. Simultaneous recordings of arterial pressure (Pa) and airway pressure (Paw) curves in an illustrative patient with large respiratory changes in systolic pressure but small changes in pulse pressure (systolic minus diastolic pressure, dotted arrow). The small pulse pressure variation reflects the fact that left ventricular stroke volume varies only a little over the respiratory cycle. This patient was a non-responder to fluid infusion

of 95% and a negative predictive value of 93%. This study [15] also reported a significant relationship ($r^2 = 0.58$, p = 0.001) between the baseline value of Δdown and the percent increase in stroke volume in response to volume expansion.

▌ Echocardiography-Doppler

Left Ventricular End-diastolic Area (LVEDA)

The LVEDA can be evaluated at the bedside by transthoracic or transesophageal echocardiography (TEE) using the short axis view of the LV. The LVEDA has been shown to reflect more accurately the LV preload when compared with PAOP [27]. The LVEDA was found to be significantly lower in responders than in non-responders in two clinical studies [10, 15] and a significant relationship between the baseline LVEDA index and the changes in stroke volume induced by volume expansion has been reported by Tavernier et al. [15] in patients with sepsis-induced hypotension. However, using receiver operating (ROC) curve analysis, the same authors [15] also demonstrated the minimal value of a given LVEDA index value to discriminate responders and non-responders before fluid was given. Moreover, in the study of Tousignant et al. [10] including medical-surgical ICU patients, considerable overlap of baseline individual values of LVEDA was also observed between responders and non-responders supporting the interpretation that a specific LVEDA value cannot reliably predict fluid responsiveness in an individual patient. More recently, in patients with septic shock, we did not observe any difference between the mean baseline value of LVEDA index in responders and non-responders nor any relationship between the baseline value of LVEDA index and the percent change in cardiac index in response to volume expansion [28].

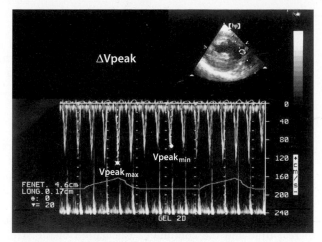

Fig. 3. Recording of aortic blood flow in one illustrative patient. Beat-to-beat measurement of aortic peak velocity (Vpeak) allows the determinantion of maximal (Vpeak$_{max}$) and minimal (Vpeak$_{min}$) values of Vpeak over a single respiratory cycle. The respiratory changes in Vpeak (ΔVpeak) are calculated as the difference between Vpeak$_{max}$ and Vpeak$_{min}$, divided by the mean of the two values, and expressed as a percentage

Respiratory Changes in Aortic Blood Velocity

The Doppler imaging of aortic blood flow can be used to assess non-invasively the respiratory changes in aortic blood velocity and has recently been proposed to detect fluid responsiveness (Fig. 3). Indeed, in sedated and mechanically ventilated patients with septic shock, we demonstrated that the respiratory changes in peak velocity of aortic blood flow (ΔVpeak) were significantly greater (20±6 vs 10±3%, p<0.01) in responder than in non-responder patients and that a ΔVpeak threshold value of 12% allowed discrimination between responder and non-responder patients with a positive predictive value of 91% and a negative predictive value of 100% [28]. Moreover, a positive and tight linear correlation (r^2=0.83, p<0.001) was also found between the ΔVpeak before volume expansion and the volume expansion-induced changes in cardiac output [28].

Respiratory Changes in Vena Caval Diameter

Using TEE-Doppler, Vieillard-Baron et al. [29] recently compared the magnitude of the inspiratory collapse of the superior vena cava to the magnitude of the respiratory changes in RV stroke volume. They found that a marked inspiratory collapse of the superior vena cava was associated with a major inspiratory drop in RV outflow. Therefore, this finding suggests that the inspiratory collapse of the superior vena cava could be a predictor of fluid responsiveness. Using abdominal echography, Feissel et al. (unpublished data) recently studied the relationship between the respiratory changes in inferior vena caval diameter and fluid responsiveness. They found that the higher the magnitude of the respiratory changes in inferior vena caval diameter, the greater was the increase in cardiac output in response to fluid infusion.

▌ PiCCO Monitoring

In patients instrumented with a central venous line and a femoral arterial catheter, the PiCCO monitor (PULSION Medical Systems, Munich, Germany) allows the assessment of hemodynamic parameters derived from two different techniques: pulse contour analysis and transpulmonary thermodilution.

Pulse Contour Analysis

Pulse contour analysis is based on the physiological relationship between stroke volume and the area (A) under the systolic portion of the aortic pressure curve: stroke volume = A×cal., where cal. is a calibration factor obtained by an independent technique of stroke volume measurement [30]. On the PiCCO device, the pulse contour analysis is calibrated by the transpulmonary thermodilution technique [31]. Pulse contour analysis allows the beat-to-beat measurement of stroke volume in real time and the continuous calculation of the stroke volume variation (SVV), which is defined as the percentage change in stroke volume over a floating period of 30 seconds [32]. The close correlation between SVV and arterial pressure variations was shown recently in patients after cardiac surgery [33]. Assuming that the main determinant of SVV is the respiratory variation in stroke volume, Berkenstadt et al. [32] recently demonstrated the value of SVV to predict fluid responsiveness in the operating room. In this study, small fluid challenges of 100 ml of 6% hydroxyethylstarch were performed in patients undergoing brain surgery and a positive response to fluid infusion was defined by an increase in stroke volume of at least 5% [32]. Using ROC analysis, Berkenstadt et al. [32] demonstrated that the SVV cut off value of 9.5% could be used to discriminate responders and non-responders to fluid infusion with a sensitivity of 79% and a specificity of 93% [32] (Fig. 4). The usefulness of SVV to detect and predict volume responsiveness has also been demonstrated in a recent study including cardio-surgical patients [34]. In addition, pulse contour analysis provides continuous measurement of cardiac output with a delay of just a few seconds. Thus, time consuming diagnostic interventions or wait-

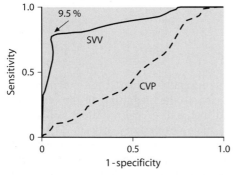

Fig. 4. ROC curves comparing the ability of the stroke volume variation (SVV) and the central venous pressure (CVP) to discriminate responder (stroke volume increase > 5%) and non-responder patients to volume expansion. The SVV is evaluated by the pulse contour analysis (PiCCO monitor, PULSION Medical Systems, Munich, Germany). A SVV value equal to or more than 9.5% predicts positive fluid responsiveness with a sensitivity of 79% and a specificity of 93%. (From [32] with permission)

ing for the delayed stabilization of so-called continuous cardiac output measurements with right heart catheters are no longer required [31].

Transpulmonary Thermodilution

The measurement of cardiac output by the transpulmonary thermodilution technique has been validated against the pulmonary artery thermodilution [31, 35], and the Fick, methods [36]. On the PiCCO device, the transpulmonary thermodilution technique allows not only the calibration of the pulse contour analysis (see above) but also the evaluation of the global end-diastolic volume (GEDV) and the extravascular lung water (EVLW) [37]. The changes in global end-diastolic volume have been shown to be better correlated with the changes in cardiac output than the changes in RAP or PAOP [38, 39], suggesting that the GEDV is a better indicator of preload than cardiac filling pressures. The cardiac function index (CFI), which is calculated as the ratio of cardiac output to GEDV, has been proposed as an indicator of cardiac performance [40]. Because the slope of the relationship between ventricular preload and stroke volume depends on ventricular contractility, assessing ventricular preload alone is not sufficient to predict fluid responsiveness. Indeed, a given change in ventricular preload results in a greater change in stroke volume in case of normal ventricular function than in case of ventricular dysfunction. Therefore, the simultaneous assessment of cardiac preload and cardiac performance may be particularly useful to guide fluid therapy [41]. Indeed, in sepsis-induced low flow states, a positive response to volume expansion has been shown to be very unlikely in patients with a low CFI and very likely in the others (Fig. 5) [41].

▍ Overview

Cardiac filling pressures are used by a majority of ICU physicians to decide to give fluid [42] and several recommendations support their use to guide fluid therapy in critically ill patients [43–45]. However, all clinical studies have emphasized the

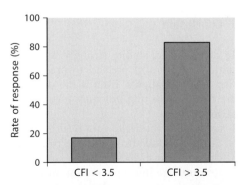

Fig. 5. Rate of response to volume expansion (defined as a cardiac output increase >15%) in sepsis-induced low flow states according to the pre-infusion value of the cardiac function index (CFI). The CFI is calculated as the ratio of cardiac output to global end-diastolic volume, which are evaluated by the transpulmonary thermodilution technique

minimal value of cardiac filling pressures in detecting fluid responsiveness. The RVEDV index evaluated by thermodilution and the LVEDA index evaluated by echocardiography have also been shown to be of little value in predicting the effects of volume expansion on cardiac output. Several reasons could be advanced to explain these findings. First, these parameters are not always accurate indicators of ventricular preload because of erroneous readings of pressure tracings [46], discrepancy between measured and transmural pressures [47], ventricular compliance alterations [48], tricuspid regurgitation [49], poor relationship between LVEDA and LVEDV [50]. Second, the physiological values of these parameters vary widely from one patient to another. For example, hypovolemic patient may have a 'normal' LVEDA in case of dilated cardiopathy or a 'normal' PAOP in case of hypertrophic cardiopathy! Third, considering only one ventricle (i.e., right or left ventricular preload) may be misleading to detect fluid responsiveness since both ventricles have to operate on the ascending portion of the preload/stroke volume relationship to turn the volume expansion-induced increase in RV preload into a significant increase in LV output [1]. Finally, as mentioned above, the slope of the relationship between ventricular preload and stroke volume depends on ventricular contractility. Therefore, a given change in ventricular preload results in a greater change in stroke volume in case of normal ventricular function than in ventricular dysfunction. In this regard, it is not so surprising that bedside indicators of preload are not accurate predictors of fluid responsiveness in intensive care unit (ICU) patients in whom ventricular contractility is frequently altered.

In contrast, dynamic parameters (ΔRAP, ΔPP, Δdown, ΔVpeak, SVV), testing the sensitivity of the heart to changes in pleural pressure, have been shown to accurately discriminate between responders and non-responders before fluid was given. However, it must be noted that:

▌ analysis of the respiratory changes in LV stroke volume (ΔPP, Δdown, ΔVpeak and SVV) is not possible in patients with cardiac arrhythmias because the beat-to-beat changes in LV stroke volume do not reflect anymore the effects of mechanical insufflation on stroke volume;

▌ these parameters have been validated in deeply sedated patients. Whether they also predict fluid responsiveness in non-sedated, spontaneously breathing patients, remains to be determined.

▌ Conclusion

To date, clinical studies strongly support the use of dynamic parameters rather than static indicators of preload to predict the hemodynamic effects of volume expansion in ICU patients. Even if the detection of fluid responsiveness is very useful in the decision making process concerning volume expansion in such patients, it must be noted that:

▌ since both ventricles of a healthy subject are operating on the ascending portion of the preload/stroke volume relationship, the fluid responsiveness is physiological and hence does not necessarily require fluid infusion but it may be helpful to minimize inotropic and/or vasopressor support;

▌ in shock states, the decision of volume expansion has to be balanced with the potential risk of worsening gas exchange in patients with pulmonary edema (EVLW measurement by transpulmonary thermodilution may be useful in identifying such patients);

▌ the use of a vasoactive agent appears to be more logical than fluid infusion to correct a hypotensive state when cardiac output is high (even if a significant increase in cardiac output can be predicted). Therefore, the decision of volume expansion should be based on the measurement of several parameters, which emphasizes the value of techniques allowing the simultaneous assessment of cardiac preload, cardiac output and fluid responsiveness. Such measurements are provided by the transpulmonary thermodilution technique and, in real time and continuously, by online pulse contour analysis.

References

1. Michard F, Teboul JL (2000) Using heart-lung interactions to assess fluid responsiveness during mechanical ventilation. Crit Care 4:282–289
2. Connoars AF, McCaffee DR, Gray RA (1983) Evaluation of right heart catheterization in the critically ill patient without acute myocardial infarction. N Engl J Med 308:263–267
3. Shippy CR, Appel PL, Shoemaker WC (1984) Reliability of clinical monitoring to assess blood volume in critically ill patients. Crit Care Med 12:107–112
4. McGee S, Abernethy WB 3rd, Simel DL (1999) Is this patient hypovolemic? JAMA 281:1022–1029
5. Michard F, Ruscio L, Teboul JL (2001) Clinical prediction of fluid responsiveness in acute circulatory failure related to sepsis. Intensive Care Med 27:1238
6. Magder S (1998) More respect for the CVP. Intensive Care Med 24:651–653
7. Packman MI, Rackow EC (1983) Optimum left heart filling pressure during fluid resuscitation of patients with hypovolemic and septic shock. Crit Care Med 11:165–169
8. Schneider AJ, Teule GJJ, Groeneveld ABJ, et al (1988) Biventricular performance during volume loading in patients with early septic shock, with emphasis on the right ventricle: a combined hemodynamic and radionuclide study. Am Heart J 116:103–112
9. Wagner JG, Leatherman JW (1998) Right ventricular end-diastolic volume as a predictor of the hemodynamic response to a fluid challenge. Chest 113:1048–1054
10. Tousignant CP, Walsh F, Mazer CD (2000) The use of transesophageal echocardiography for preload assessment in critically ill patients. Anesth Analg 90:351–355
11. Calvin JE, Driedger AA, Sibbald WJ (1981) The hemodynamic effect of rapid fluid infusion in critically ill patients. Surgery 90:61–76
12. Reuse C, Vincent JL, Pinsky MR (1990) Measurements of right ventricular volumes during fluid challenge. Chest 98:1450–1454
13. Michard F, Boussat S, Chemla D, et al (2000) Relation between respiratory changes in arterial pulse pressure and fluid responsiveness in septic patients with acute circulatory failure. Am J Respir Crit Care Med 162:134–138
14. Diebel L, Wilson RF, Heins J, et al (1994) End-diastolic volume versus pulmonary artery wedge pressure in evaluating cardiac preload in trauma patients. J Trauma 37:950–955
15. Tavernier B, Makhotine O, Lebuffe G, et al (1998) Systolic pressure variation as a guide to fluid therapy in patients with sepsis-induced hypotension. Anesthesiology 89:1313–1321
16. Diebel LN, Wilson RF, Tagett MG, et al (1992) End-diastolic volume. A better indicator of preload in the critically ill. Arch Surg 127:817–822
17. Baek S-E, Makabali GG, Bryan-Brown CW, et al (1975) Plasma expansion in surgical patients with high central venous pressure (CVP); the relationship of blood volume to hematocrit, CVP, pulmonary wedge pressure, and cardiorespiratory changes. Surgery 78:304–315
18. Magder S, Georgiadis G, Cheong T (1992) Respiratory variations in right atrial pressure predict the response to fluid challenge. J Crit Care 7:76–85
19. Magder S, Lagonidis D (1999) Effectiveness of albumin versus normal saline as a test of volume responsiveness in post-cardiac surgery patients. J Crit Care 14:164–171
20. Chemla D, Hébert JL, Coirault C, et al (1998) Total arterial compliance estimated by the stroke volume-to-aortic pulse pressure ratio in humans. Am J Physiol 274:H500–H505
21. Jardin F, Farcot JC, Gueret P, Prost JF, Ozier Y, Bourdarias JP (1983) Cyclic changes in arterial pulse during respiratory support. Circulation 68:266–274

22. Michard F, Chemla D, Richard C, et al (1999) Clinical use of respiratory changes in arterial pulse pressure to monitor the hemodynamic effects of PEEP. Am J Respir Crit Care Med 159:935–939
23. Michard F, Teboul JL (2000) Respiratory changes in arterial pressure in mechanically ventilated patients. In: Vincent JL (ed) Yearbook of Intensive Care and Emergency Medicine. Springer, Heidelberg, pp 696–704
24. Robotham JL, Cherry D, Mitzner W, et al (1983) A re-evaluation of the hemodynamic consequences of intermittent positive pressure ventilation. Crit Care Med 11:783–793
25. Denault YD, Gasior TA, Gorcsan III J, et al (1999) Determinants of aortic pressure variation during positive-pressure ventilation in man. Chest 116:176–186
26. Perel A, Pizov R, Cotev S (1987) Systolic blood pressure variation is a sensitive indicator of hypovolemia in ventilated dogs subjected to graded hemorrhage. Anesthesiology 67:498–502
27. Thys DM, Hillel Z, Goldman ME, et al (1987) A comparison of hemodynamic indices derived by invasive monitoring and two-dimensional echocardiography. Anesthesiology 67:630–634
28. Feissel M, Michard F, Mangin I, et al (2001) Respiratory changes in aortic blood velocity as an indicator of fluid responsiveness in ventilated patients with septic shock. Chest 119:867–873
29. Vieillard-Baron A, Augarde R, Prin S, et al (2001) Influence of superior vena caval zone condition on cyclic change in right ventricular outflow during respiratory support. Anesthesiology 95:1083–1088
30. Wesseling KH, deWit B, Weber JAP, et al (1983) A simple device for the continuous measurement of cardiac output. Adv Cardiovasc Physiol 5:16–52
31. Goedje O, Hoeke K, Lichtwarck-Aschoff M, et al (1999) Continuous cardiac output by femoral arterial thermodilution calibrated pulse contour analysis: comparison with pulmonary arterial thermodilution. Crit Care Med 27:2407–2412
32. Berkenstadt H, Margalit N, Hadani M, et al (2001) Stroke volume variation as a predictor of fluid responsiveness in patients undergoing brain surgery. Anesth Analg 92:984–989
33. Reuter DA, Kirchner A, Felbinger TW, et al (2002) Optimising fluid therapy in mechanically ventilated patients after cardiac surgery by on-line monitoring of left ventricular stroke volume variations: a comparison to aortic systolic pressure variations. Br J Anaesth (in press)
34. Reuter DA, Felbinger TW, Schmidt C, et al (2002) Stroke volume variations for assessment of cardiac responsiveness to volume loading in mechanically ventilated patients after cardiac surgery. Intensive Care Med (in press)
35. Sakka SG, Reinhart K, Meier-Hellmann A (1999) Comparison of pulmonary artery and arterial thermodilution cardiac output in critically ill patients. Intensive Care Med 25:843–846
36. Tibby SM, Hatherill M, Marsh MJ, et al (1997) Clinical validation of cardiac output measurements using femoral artery thermodilution with direct Fick in ventilated children and infants. Intensive Care Med 23:987–991
37. Sakka SG, Ruhl CC, Pfeiffer UJ, et al (2000) Assessment of cardiac preload and extravascular lung water by single transpulmonary thermodilution. Intensive Care Med 26:180–187
38. Gödje O, Peyerl M, Seebauer T, et al (1998) Central venous pressure, pulmonary capillary wedge pressure and intrathoracic blood volume as preload indicators in cardiac surgery patients. Eur J Cardiothorac Surg 13:533–540
39. Goedje O, Seebauer T, Peyerl M, et al (2000) Hemodynamic monitoring by double-indicator dilution technique in patients after orthotopic heart transplantation. Chest 118:775–781
40. Wisner-Euteneir AJ, Lichtwarck-Aschoff M, Zimmermann G, et al (1994) Evaluation of the cardiac function index as a new bedside indicator of cardiac performance. Intensive Care Med 20:S21 (Abst)
41. Michard F and Teboul JL (2001) Usefulness of transpulmonary thermodilution to predict fluid responsiveness in humans with septic shock. Intensive Care Med 27:S148 (Abst)
42. Boldt J, Lenz M, Kumle B, Papsdorf M (1998) Volume replacement strategies on intensive care units: results from a postal survey. Intensive Care Med 24:147–151

43. Société de réanimation de langue française (1997) Quels sont les critères diagnostiques d'une hypovolémie nécessitant un remplissage vasculaire? Réanim Urg 6:347–360
44. Vincent JL (2001) Hemodynamic support in septic shock. Intensive Care Med 27:S80–S92
45. Task Force of the American College of Critical Care Medicine, Society of Critical Care Medicine (1999) Practice parameters for hemodynamic support in adult patients in sepsis. Crit Care Med 27:639–660
46. Iberti TJ, Fischer EP, Leibowitz AB, et al (1990) A multicenter study of physician's knowledge of the pulmonary artery catheter. JAMA 264:2928–2932
47. Teboul JL, Pinsky MR, Mercat A, et al (2000) Estimating cardiac filling pressure in mechanically ventilated patients with hyperinflation. Crit Care Med 28:3631–3636
48. Raper R, Sibbald WJ (1986) Misled by the wedge? The Swan-Ganz catheter and left ventricular preload. Chest 89:427–434
49. Hoeper MM, Tongers J, Leppert A, et al (2001) Evaluation of right ventricular ejection fraction thermodilution catheter and MRI in patients with pulmonary hypertension. Chest 120:502–507
50. Urbanowicz JH, Shaaban MJ, Cohen NH, et al (1990) Comparison of transesophageal echocardiographic and scintigraphic estimates of left ventricular end-diastolic volume index and ejection fraction in patients following coronary artery bypass grafting. Anesthesiology 72:607–612s

Volumetric Capnography in the Non-intubated Critically Ill Patient

F. Verschuren, F. Thys, and G. Liistro

▮ Introduction

Direct application of physiopathology at the bedside represents an enthusiastic challenge for the clinician. CO_2 kinetics has been the focus of attention of several laboratories in the past, but the clinical implications did not always follow the enthusiasm of the physiologists, principally because of technical limitations and artefacts. With the recent development of analytic devices, acquisition systems and microcomputers, it is now possible to obtain quick and reliable information that in the past required patiently recorded data. Moreover, if these new methods are characterized by their non-invasiveness, and if they can help the diagnostic and therapeutic process while limiting the recourse to invasive or expensive procedures, then it is worth reassessing them in the clinical setting.

Volumetric capnography, also known as the single breath test for CO_2 (SBT-CO_2) displaying an expirogram (the three terms will be used indifferently in the text), seems to possess these characteristics. Fletcher and colleagues extensively described volumetric capnography in 1981, as the plot of the expired CO_2 concentration against the expired volume [1, 2]. This method has been considered more accurate than time-based capnography in determining the dead space volumes, i.e., the lung regions that do not participate in gas exchange. Emergency departments are confronted daily with pathologies affecting the dead space volumes, such as pulmonary embolism, obstructive lung diseases, or heart failure. This chapter will focus on the way volumetric capnography can help the clinician in diagnosing, excluding or differentiating these diseases, especially in non-intubated critically ill patients.

▮ Deadspace Measurement: Evolution of the Concept [2, 3]

Bohr introduced in 1891 the concept of deadspace (VD) as the part of the tidal volume (VT) that does not participate in gas exchange:

$$VD/VT = 1 - (FeCO_2/F_ACO_2) \qquad \text{(Eqn 1)}$$

where $FeCO_2$ is the mixed expired CO_2 collected in a bag, and F_ACO_2 the fraction of CO_2 in the alveolar gas. Bohr was thus the first to express the deadspace as a CO_2 ratio, i.e., the ratio of the fraction of CO_2 in the alveolar gas to the fraction of CO_2 in the expired gas. In 1938, Enghoff substituted the arterial PCO_2 ($PaCO_2$) for F_ACO_2:

$$VD_{phys}/VT = 1 - (FeCO_2/PaCO_2) \qquad \text{(Eqn 2)}$$

VD_{phys} is called physiologic deadspace because the formula takes into account the physiologic ventilation and perfusion of the lungs, $PaCO_2$ being considered as an ideal F_ACO_2 in a lung with a perfect V/Q ratio.

The concept of airway deadspace, i.e., the volume of the conductive airways, was best described and measured by Fowler (1948). There is no equation to calculate its value, but a graphic representation may be obtained by a single breath test for N_2, a precursor of the $SBT\text{-}CO_2$. The airway deadspace (VD_{aw}) is preferred to the term of anatomical deadspace, since its volume may vary in the same patient. This deadspace may be considered as the volume of the conducting airways above an interface between the alveolar and the airway gas. VD_{aw} depends on the patient's height, posture, tidal volume, and also on the inspiratory flow (a high inspiratory flow increases VD_{aw} by external traction on the airways and by the down movement of the interface), and finally on the respiratory rate (a low frequency makes the interface move up by increasing the diffusion time).

The alveolar deadspace (VD_{alv}) is defined as the lung volumes that are ventilated but not perfused, in other words the deadspace of all causes distal to the airway deadspace:

$$VD = VD_{aw} + VD_{alv} \tag{Eqn 3}$$

In 1967, Severinghaus described VD_{alv} as a ratio between $PaCO_2$ and $EtCO_2$, which was the first easy to calculate method, requiring a blood gas analysis and a CO_2 measurement:

$$VD_{alv}/VT_{alv} = 1 - (EtCO_2/PaCO_2) \tag{Eqn 4}$$

which is the alveolar deadspace fraction corresponding to the efficacy of the alveolar gas exchanges.

The single breath test for CO_2 ($SBT\text{-}CO_2$), also known as volumetric capnography, is a summary of the formulas listed above, since it takes into account in a single graph the measurement of the VD_{aw} according to Fowler's method and the $PaCO_2$ value for determination of the VD_{phys} and VD_{alv}.

$SBT\text{-}CO_2$ represents the plot of expired CO_2 against volume during a single expiration. The tracing may be divided into three phases (Fig. 1).

Phase 1 represents CO_2-free gas from the airway deadspace; phase 2 is the S-shaped transition phase between airway and alveolar gas; phase 3 is the alveolar plateau, representing CO_2-rich gas from the alveoli. The sum of phases 2 and 3 represents the effective VT capable of eliminating CO_2. We will see further in the text factors influencing the slope of this phase 3.

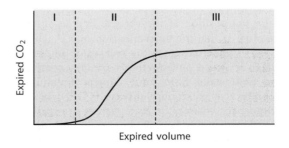

Fig. 1. Single breath test for CO_2 ($SBT\text{-}CO_2$) or CO_2 expirogram: the three phases of the fractional exhaled CO_2 vs exhaled volume

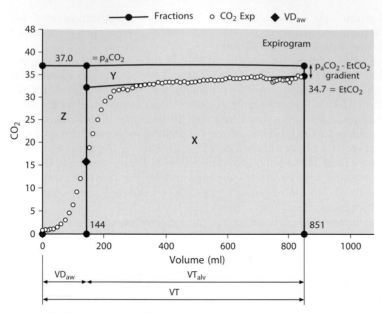

Fig. 2. SBT-CO_2 and its subdivisions in order to calculate surfaces representing volumes of CO_2. *Area X:* tidal elimination of CO_2, which is the effective part of VT; *Area Y:* alveolar deadspace (VD_{alv}); *Area Z:* airway deadspace (VD_{alv}) modified from the Fowler's method

This tracing was modified by Fowler (1948) and Nunn (1977) in order to determine surfaces that represent the three deadspace volumes. A vertical line divides phase 2 in two triangles p and q of equal area, and the $PaCO_2$, that represents the ideal alveolar fraction of CO_2 in equilibrium with the arterial blood, is plotted on a horizontal line (Fig. 2).

These areas can be used to express various deadspace fractions:

$$VD_{phys}/VT = Y + Z/X + Y + Z$$

$$VD_{alv}/VT_{alv} = Y/X + Y$$

which represents the percentage of the alveolar volume occupied by alveolar deadspace per breath.

$$VD_{aw}/VT = Z/X + Y + Z$$

Factors Affecting Alveolar Deadspace. The value of VD_{alv} as expressed by the surface Y is limited by the slope of the phase 3, the gradient between $EtCO_2$ and $PaCO_2$ and the position of the vertical line separating VD_{aw} from VT (see Fig. 2). A first finding is that the determination of VD_{alv} by calculating the gradient $PaCO_2$-$EtCO_2$ (eq. 4) underestimates the real VD_{alv} since the surface Y frequently presents a triangular shape. Both methods are only comparable if phase 3 has no slope. In order to understand how some clinical situations like pulmonary embolism, chronic obstructive pulmonary disease (COPD) or heart failure may modify the alveolar deadspace volumes, it is important to explain the influence of ventilation-perfusion (V/Q) mismatch, venous admixture and other ventilatory parameters, on the slope of the phase 3 and on the $PaCO_2$-$EtCO_2$ gradient.

1. Alveolar dead-space may be due to spatial V/Q mismatching. In this case, unperfused alveoli (high V/Q ratios), unable to eliminate CO_2, are emptying synchronously with normal alveoli during expiration, diluting the CO_2 concentration of the expired gas and causing wasted ventilation. In the clinical setting, this situation is best encountered with pulmonary embolism and right cardiac failure. This synchronous emptying of alveoli from well- and underperfused lung regions, with subsequent dilution of the CO_2 concentration in the expired gas, is expressed by an almost horizontal phase 3 of the SBT-CO_2 curve, which does not reach the PaCO$_2$value. The shape of the area Y is rectangular.

2. Another cause of alveolar deadspace is due to asynchronous emptying of alveoli. In this case, alveoli with low V/Q ratios, containing a relative high CO_2 concentration, empty relatively late. This situation is seen with COPD patients where some lung regions have an increased time constant (the product of resistance and compliance); these areas with low V/Q ratios are filling late in inspiration, and are emptying late in expiration. Since these well-perfused lung regions contain a high CO_2 concentration at the end of expiration because of a longer diffusion time, they participate actively in the CO_2 elimination, but later in the expiration phase. This asynchronous emptying of alveoli from well- and underventilated lung regions is expressed by a sloping phase 3 in the SBT-CO_2 curve. The shape of the area Y is therefore triangular.

3. Time also influences the VD$_{alv}$: a low respiratory rate decreases VD$_{alv}$ because of a better gas mixing and gas distribution within and between the lung units. On the other hand, a rapid respiratory rate increases the VD$_{alv}$ by incomplete diffusion of the CO_2 between the blood and the alveoli.

4. Perfusion of unventilated lung compartments constitutes venous admixture, which contributes to overestimate the VD$_{alv}$ by raising the arterial PCO$_2$, with subsequent increase in the Pa-EtCO$_2$ gradient. This phenomenon seems to play a lesser role in the etiology of VD$_{alv}$. The clinical situations responsible for venous admixture include atelectasis, pneumonia, pulmonary edema acute respiratory distress syndrome (ARDS).

Since the slope of phase 3 of the SBT-CO_2 is of utmost importance in differentiating pulmonary embolism from other pulmonary disease, it has been shown by Eriksson et al. [4] that the extrapolation of phase 3, fit to a logarithmic curve, reaches the PaCO$_2$ value at an equivalent exhaled volume of 15% predicted total lung capacity (TLC, based on patient sex and size) in normal and COPD patients, but fails to reach its value in case of pulmonary embolism (Fig. 3). The term FD$_{late}$ is defined as the late deadspace fraction:

$$FD_{late} = 1 - (FCO_{2\,15\%TLC}/PaCO_2) \qquad \text{(Eqn 5)}$$

where F$_{15\%TLC}$ is the fractional CO_2 value at an exhaled volume of 15% of the TLC. This F$_{15\%TLC}$ may be regarded as a CO_2 value at a forced expiration where time is no longer a limiting factor for the diffusion of CO_2 between the pulmonary blood and the alveoli.

In conclusion, the expirogram generated from a computerized synchronization of flow and CO_2 measurements can bring new information to the clinician concerning alveolar, airway or late deadspace fractions. Can volumetric capnography (expirogram) bring more information than the time-plot CO_2 measurement (capnogram)? To answer this question, we have to remember that the shapes of the curves are different between the two techniques: the alveolar plateau of the capnogram has

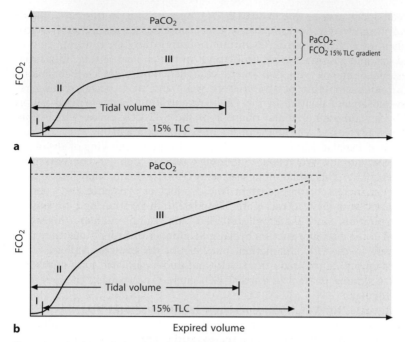

Fig. 3. Late deadspace fraction (FD$_{late}$) values for patient with pulmonary embolism (PE) (**a**) and with chronic obstructive pulmonary disease (COPD) (**b**). TLC: total lung capacity

a shallower slope in comparison with the phase 3 of the expirogram because most of the volume has been exhaled during the early part of the alveolar plateau. Consequently, the last 15% of the expired gas, the richest in CO_2 content, occupies half of the capnogram but a small part of the expirogram. Since the slope of the alveolar plateau is an important factor to differentiate pulmonary embolus from emphysema, the expirogram has a theoretical advantage over the capnogram in separating the two diseases.

Applications of the Deadspace Measurement for Pulmonary Embolism

Pulmonary embolism remains a challenging diagnosis [5]. Several reasons have motivated clinicians to explore the role of capnography as a simple, non-invasive, rapid and bedside method in the diagnostic work-up of pulmonary embolism:

- the limitations in the availability of some complementary testing in small hospitals;
- the time-consuming use of expensive and sometimes inappropriate radiological or nuclear imaging;
- the current trend towards non-invasive procedures attempting to decrease the need for pulmonary angiography;
- the mandatory use of a coherent integration of clinical and paraclinical data in the diagnostic work-up;
- the possibility of unmasking asymptomatic cases of pulmonary embolism [6].

The physiology of gas exchange during pulmonary embolism must be developed first in order to understand why and in which way CO_2 measurements may reflect the VD_{alv} created by a pulmonary embolism.

Physiology of Gas Exchange during Pulmonary Embolism (with Focus on the CO_2)

CO_2 is produced in the tissues by aerobic and anaerobic metabolism, transported in the blood to the lung and then eliminated by ventilation. A pulmonary embolus is first characterized by pulmonary obstruction, responsible for an increased VD_{alv}, which creates hyperoxic and hypocarbic alveolae unable to participate in the CO_2 elimination process (high V/Q ratio) [7]. This phenomenon explains the gradient between the arterial and alveolar CO_2. The next step should be marked by hypercapnia with respiratory acidosis, but on the contrary, hyperventilation with hypocapnia is the most frequent finding during pulmonary embolism. This phenomenon, even if only partially understood, is centrally mediated by chemoreceptors, and explains why the wasted ventilation will be compensated by an increased tidal volume and/or respiratory rate. Consequently, it seems reasonable to assert that an increased alveolar deadspace, measured by whatever capnographic technique, will characterize the beginning of a moderate to large pulmonary embolism in a patient free of previous cardiopulmonary disease. Moreover, a low cardiac output from circulatory shock in case of massive pulmonary embolism emphasizes the alveolar deadspace value (relatively increased V/Q ratio), and reduces the pulmonary CO_2 transport so that CO_2 progressively accumulates in the blood (increased $PaCO_2$ with increased $Pa-EtCO_2$ gradient). Nevertheless, the presence of an easily measurable increased deadspace volume must be evaluated in the light of the physiopathologic knowledge of V/Q ratio distribution during pulmonary embolism. Venous admixture (i.e., the perfusion of unventilated lung units) and deadspace are two parallel phenomena during pulmonary embolism, leading most frequently to hypoxemia and hypocapnia. Experimental data by Delcroix et al. [8] with an inert gas method showed that a small size marble embolus (mimicking a peripheral embolism) resulted more in venous admixture than in deadspace [8]. Even if segmental pulmonary embolism is less frequent than central pulmonary embolism, it is therefore difficult to assert that deadspace determination with a capnographic method will be sensitive enough in case of peripheral lung embolism. On the other hand, several clinical adaptations appear in the course of a pulmonary embolism, limiting the importance of the VD_{alv} volume by redistributing the ventilation to well-perfused lung regions: pulmonary infarction, atelectasis in the occluded segment, the hypocarbic bronchoconstrictive reflex, local edema are all circumstances reducing the value of capnography as a screening test for pulmonary embolism [10].

Review of the Literature

About 15 human clinical studies have been reported in the literature concerning the use of CO_2 measurement in the clinical suspicion of pulmonary embolism. Results are listed in Table 1. All these studies differ in terms of the population's origin (in- or outpatients), patient status (spontaneously breathing or mechanically ventilated), reference tests for pulmonary embolism diagnosis, deadspace calculation, type of capnograph used, combination of CO_2 measurement with other diagnostic tools (D-dimers, spirometry), time of performance (from 1959 to 2001), type and objectives of the study (CO_2 as a screening test versus diagnostic test or therapeutic use). These differences may explain to some extent the lack of sufficient validation and power of the deadspace measurement as a diagnostic tool in pulmonary embolism.

In 1959, Robin et al. [9] were the first authors to suggest "a physiological approach to the diagnosis of pulmonary embolism" by measuring the arterial to end-tidal CO_2 gradient as a percentage of the ventilated but not perfused lung. In this small series of 35 subjects, eight patients with probably very severe pulmonary embolism (four diagnoses made by post-mortem examination) had a gradient higher than 4 mmHg in comparison with a mean difference of 1.8 mmHg in normal subjects. The authors concluded that a normal gradient could rule out large vascular occlusions. They also pointed out the limitations of their promising procedure: the technical measurement difficulties for low VT or high respiratory rates, the lack of diagnostic performance in case of small pulmonary embolism, the physiological absence of VD_{alv} when a pulmonary infarction occurs. Finally, they considered the test as unsuitable in patients with emphysema, because both conditions are associated with a similar increase in the CO_2 gradient.

In 1966, Nutter and Massumi [10] emphasized, with the greatest accuracy, the pitfalls and sources of error when using the a-A CO_2 gradient as assessment of the VD_{alv} in the clinical suspicion of pulmonary embolism. Their analyses were carried out in four groups of patients: 29 control healthy subjects, 14 COPD patients, 20 subjects with documented pulmonary embolism and 15 cases of pulmonary artery balloon occlusion. In the discussion, the authors pointed out the necessity for the physician to be fully aware of the relatively high incidence of false positive and negative results of the gradient.

In 1973, Vereerstraeten et al. [11], a Belgian team, investigated the correlation between deadspace determination (Severinghaus's formula) and lung scintigraphy in 312 patients suspected of having pulmonary embolism. After 91 capnographs were eliminated because of inadequate alveolar plateau phase, these authors showed that an increased gradient (>5 mmHg or >15%) was found in 59% of the proven pulmonary emboli (sensitivity 59%). Even if there was a significant correlation between the vascular defects measured by lung scan and calculated from the alveolo-arterial gradient of PCO_2, the lung scan appeared to have a greater sensitivity (89%), especially for small pulmonary emboli. They also demonstrated the lack of relation between the vascular defect and the duration of the symptoms of the disease. As in the two previous studies, they finally concluded that deadspace calculation, as well as the lung scintigraphy, were useful mainly in patients suspected of pulmonary embolism without other cardio-pulmonary disorder.

Comparable results with similar deadspace measurements were found in the study of Hatle and Rokseth in 1974 [12]. An a-A CO_2 gradient above 5 mmHg was observed in 24 of 25 patients with moderate or massive pulmonary embolism, but in only 7 of 17 with small pulmonary embolism confirmed by angiogram or autopsy. These authors pointed out the role of a maximal expiration in order to correct the false-positive gradients in patients with COPD, left ventricular failure, pneumonia or shock. For instance, they noted a normalization of the gradient in 19 of 21 COPD patients after a forced exhalation. Nevertheless, the use of maximal end-expired CO_2 value instead of end-tidal CO_2 for VD_{alv} determination has three disadvantages: it is dependent on patient cooperation, it suppresses the steady-state condition, and it is difficult to perform in severely ill patients.

In conclusion, all these problems with the measurement of VD_{alv} according to the a-A CO_2 gradient can explain why this test was abandoned and considered as

an 'orphan' test for more than ten years [13]. Three phenomena explain the resurrection of the test in the late 1980s:
1) the use of volumetric capnography according to the publications of Fletcher et al;
2) the combination of the CO_2 measurement with other diagnostic tools to better differentiate pulmonary embolism from other cardio-respiratory diseases;
3) the association with D-dimer assays in order to exclude pulmonary embolism.

In 1986, Burki [14] assessed the combination of the VD_{phys} measurement and spirography in 110 inpatients suspected of having pulmonary embolism. The deadspace value, which was not readily performed at the bedside, was calculated according to Enghoff's modification of Bohr's technique (mean expired CO_2 collected during 3 min in a Douglas bag). Even if diagnostic certainty was made in only 45 of the 110 patients, the study showed that none of the 16 patients with definitively proved pulmonary embolism had a VD/VT value less than 40%, which is a surprising and optimistic finding (sensitivity 100%). Moreover, the absence of pulmonary embolism was associated in 29 patients with either a normal VD/VT gradient <40% or an increased gradient combined with a pathological spirogram, this test allowing to discriminate better the two main causes of an elevated CO_2 gradient.

In an effort to improve the specificity of the deadspace measurement without modifying the stable respiratory status of the patient, three authors have investigated the use of volumetric capnography with focus on the late deadspace fraction (FD_{late}). As explained before (see Fig. 3), the extrapolation of the phase 3 of the SBT-CO_2 curve reaches the $PaCO_2$ value at an expired volume corresponding to 15% of the predicted TLC, except in cases of pulmonary embolism because of a uniform mixing of the gas throughout expiration. Eriksson et al. [4] showed that a FD_{late} cut-off of 12% correlated significantly with the angiographic findings in 38 patients with suspected pulmonary embolism. Moreover, volumetric capnography with FD_{late} appeared to be superior to measurements of the traditional a-A PCO_2 gradient and the VD/VT gradient in differentiating patients with pulmonary embolism from those with normal, obstructive or restrictive lung function; these two methods, the a-A PCO_2 gradient and the VD/VT gradient, showing a substantial overlap between the study groups. Nine years later, Olsson et al. validated the same technique in comparison with lung scintigraphy in a larger number of 223 in- and outpatients [15]. Even if the diagnostic standard reference for the diagnosis of pulmonary embolism was subject to criticism, and if patients with an intermediate probability lung scan were excluded from analysis, the authors showed that the FD_{late} cut-off of 12% suggested by Eriksson et al. [4] allowed a diagnosis of pulmonary embolism with a sensitivity of 85% and a specificity of 93%. In their conclusion, the authors [15] suggested starting anticoagulation when a very high FD_{late} was associated with a high clinical probability of pulmonary embolism, and to limit further investigation for a very low FD_{late} in combination with a low clinical probability. Finally, a study by Anderson et al. [16] explored the use of SBT-CO_2 with FD_{late} in a small group of 12 surgical patients including 10 mechanically ventilated subjects, and four patients with ARDS. The authors pointed out the promising role of this non-invasive bedside screening test for pulmonary embolism in a subset of critically ill patients difficult to transport. In conclusion, these three series showed that volumetric capnography coupled with FD_{late} measurement might provide more accurate information than the a-A CO_2 gradient in terms of sensitivity and specificity, especially by separating obstructive lung diseases from pulmonary embolism without modifying the steady state pattern of the patient.

The most recent publications on deadspace measurement as an adjunctive tool in the clinical evaluation of pulmonary embolism have used capnography in combination with D-dimer assays in order to increase the sensitivity. Kline has been the most prolific author in this area. In a first study in 1997 [17], he showed that the combination of a normal Latex D-dimer <500 ng/ml and a normal VD/VT was 100% sensitive (95% IC = 88–100%) in ruling out pulmonary embolism in 170 ambulatory patients, suggesting that this association could eliminate the need for additional procedure in selected low-risk patients. The authors calculated the alveolar deadspace with a derived Severinghaus's method using the maximal end-tidal CO_2, instead of the end-tidal CO_2, in order to improve the specificity of the test (65%) by separating pulmonary embolism from other obstructive lung diseases. Later research by Kline and Arunachlam [18] did not use any D-dimer assay, but shared the selection of the patients (outpatients) with the previous study. In this study [18], the authors originally analyzed the area under the time-based capnogram waveform as a screening test for pulmonary embolism. In a group of 139 outpatients, they showed that a cut-off of 50 mmHg/sec separated 19 positive pulmonary embolism from 120 negative pulmonary embolism with 100% sensitivity (95% CI = 82–100%) and 53% specificity (95% CI = 44–62%). The area under the waveform was determined with an electronic digitizing tablet. Even if original, the technique used may be criticized because time-based capnographic curves cannot give any volume information, so that calculation of an area under the waveform has no physiological support. For instance, a prolonged expiration may falsely increase the surface, and stress hyperventilation may falsely decrease it. In 1999, Johaning et al. [19] assessed the combination of VD_{alv} and D-dimers in the evaluation of 21 mechanically ventilated patients with suspected pulmonary embolism, a population known to be difficult to investigate and transport. This study suggested that a change in deadspace from a baseline value (in 11 patients) was a potential key to non-invasively diagnosing pulmonary embolism.

In 1999, Patel and Kline [20] made substantial progress in the clinical application of gas exchange and ventilatory control physiology during pulmoanry embolism. They collected volumetric capnograms on 53 outpatients, in whom pulmonary angiography confirmed pulmonary embolism in 30 and ruled out the diagnosis in 23. The capnograms were obtained at the bedside using a commercially available machine (CO_2SMO plus, Novametrix, Wallingford) connected to a portable computer. A software program used 17 variables as input parameters recorded from time-based capnograms, flow, and volume information, in order to determine an output probability of pulmonary embolism according to a neural network analysis. A previous test model on 12 patients had shown that six of the seventeen variables were significantly weighted: end-tidal CO_2, slope of the phase 3 of the volumetric capnography, peak expiratory flow, total minute ventilation, alveolar ventilation, and inspiratory time – all these parameters expressing the increased VD_{alv} and the centrally mediated hyperventilation in pulmonary embolism. No arterial blood gas collection was necessary. Applying this derived neural network model, the authors detected a pulomonary embolism with a sensitivity of 100% (95% CI = 89 to 100%) and a specificity of 48% (95% CI = 27 to 69%). In their conclusion, the authors promoted the use of such a rapid and non-invasive prototype, capable of using computer technology in order to apply the physiopathology of pulmonary embolism at the bedside of a patient, and of reducing dependence on expensive and time-consuming imaging examinations.

The next study by Kline et al. [21] evaluated the VD_{alv} as a predictor of severity of pulmonary embolism. The authors showed a relatively good correlation between VD_{alv}/VT_{alv} and the percentage perfusion defect on lung scintigraphy (regression coefficient $r^2 = 0.41$), and with the pulmonary artery pressures (regression coefficient $r^2 = 0.59$) in 53 patients, including 33 with pulmonary embolism. Since elevated pulmonary arterial pressures precede right ventricular ischemia and left ventricular dysfunction, both responsible for hemodynamically unstable pulmonary embolism, the authors postulated that a very high $VD_{alv}/VT_{alv} > 60\%$ should be a reason to consider thrombolysis. This finding must be considered in the light of the current debate concerning the usefulness of thrombolytic treatment in cases of pulmonary embolism with right heart dysfunction but normal blood pressure [22]. Future investigations should determine whether the correction of a large VD_{alv} by thrombolysis would bring some prognostic benefit.

The next two studies are similar in the way they evaluated the combination of deadspace measurement with D-dimer assays in excluding pulmonary embolism with the best accuracy. In the first multicenter study by Kline et al. [23], the combination of a normal whole blood D-dimer value with a normal $FD_{alv} < 20\%$ (calculated from volume-based capnographic data) could exclude pulmonary embolism with a 98.4% sensitivity (95% CI $= 91.6$–100%), the posttest probability decreasing to less than 1% (which is similar to the long-term prevalence of pulmonary embolism when using current diagnostic strategies). Such a normal combination was observed in 164 of 380 enrolled patients (43%), avoiding the recourse to vascular imaging in this subset of patients regardless of the pretest clinical probability. This interesting figure could be compared to the smaller percentage of patients (21%) in whom vascular imaging could be obviated when a low clinical probability was associated with a normal D-dimer value without taking capnographic data into account. Interestingly, the VD_{alv} measurement as a sole screening test showed a disappointing sensitivity of 67%, confirming that pulmonary embolism is not always associated with a measurable increase in deadspace in a stable ambulatory population. In the study by Rodger et al. [24], the association of VD_{alv} measurement (either measured with a-A PCO_2 gradient or with volumetric capnography) and D-dimers (latex or whole-blood assays) showed similar results in terms of sensitivity and specificity on a series of 246 in- and outpatients suspected of pulmonary embolism. The proportion of patients who could be excluded without additional testing represented 28% of the population. In conclusion, both studies showed that a substantial percentage (respectively 43 and 28%) of the patients (626 in total) could be safely managed without additional time and cost-consuming tests and without considering the pretest clinical probability. Nevertheless, these encouraging results must be compared with the diagnostic performances of much more sensitive ELISA D-dimer assays that have been recently validated as screening tests for the exclusion of pulmonary embolism with a sensitivity of 99.5% (95% CI 92–100%) and with a similar exclusion proportion of 31% of the patients [25]. Consequently, the benefit of associating agglutination D-dimer tests and FD_{alv} measurements in order to better rule out pulmonary embolism (sensitivity 97.8%) is similar to the performance of a rapid ELISA D-dimer alone. Moreover, Wells and co-workers [26] showed recently on 930 outpatients that the association of a well scored clinical probability with a whole-blood agglutination D-dimer assay could safely rule out pulmonary embolism without further imaging in 47% of the enrolled population.

In conclusion, the disimilarity in the study population, as shown in Table 1, may explain why volumetric capnography remains difficult to place in the diagnostic ar-

Table 1. Results of studies using capnography as screening tool for pulmonary embolism (PE)

	Type of study	Diagnostic reference[a]	Deadspace measurement	Additional diagnostic tool	Patient's origin and status	Patients	Prevalence of PE	Sensitivity	Specificity
Robin et al [9]	observational	autopsy in 5 patients	$PaCO_2$-$EtCO_2$ gradient	no	in and out	35	31%	69%	–
Vereerstraeten et al [11]	prospective	level 3	$PaCO_2$-$EtCO_2$ gradient	no	in and out	312	30%	59%	–
Nutter and Massumi [10]	experimental comparative	PE arteriographically documented	$PaCO_2$-$EtCO_2$ gradient	no	in	66	30%	75%	–
Hatle and Rokseth [12]		level 1	$PaCO_2$-$EtCO_2$ gradient	maximal expiration	in	114	37%	–	–
Burki [14]	prospective	level 2	Enghoff	spirography	in	110	31%	100%	94%
Erikkson et al [4]	experimental comparative	level 2	SBT-CO_2+FD_{late}	no	in	130	7%	–	–
Olsson et al [15]	prospective	level 3	SBT-CO_2+FD_{late}	no	in and out	223	9%	85%	93%
Anderson et al [16]	prospective	level 1	SBT-CO_2+FD_{late}	no	in + mech. vent.	12	42%	100%	89%
Kline et al [17]	prospective	level 2	$PaCO_2$-$EtCO_2$ gradient + deep expiration	D-dimers	out	170	15%	100% (88–100%)	65% (52–73%)
Kline and Arunachlam [18]	prospective	level 2	CO_2 waveform area	no	out	139	14%	100% (82–100%)	53% (44–62%)
Johanning et al [19]	prospective	level 3	$PaCO_2$-$EtCO_2$ gradient	D-dimers	in + mech. vent.	21	33%	–	–
Patel et al [20]	prospective	level 1	SBT-CO_2	no	out	53	57%	100% (89–100%)	48% (27–69%)
Kline et al [21]	prospective	partially level 1	SBT-CO_2	no	in and out	53	62%	–	0
Kline et al [23]	prospective and multicenter	level 2	SBT-CO_2	D-dimers	out	380	16.8%	98.4% (91.6–100%)	51% (46–57%)
Rodger et al [24]	prospective	level 2	$PaCO_2$-$EtCO_2$ gradient and SBT-CO_2	D-dimers	in and out	246	20%	97.8% (88.5–99.9%)	38%

[a] diagnostic references: level 1: angiography or autopsy as reference standard; level 2: appropriate combination of clinical suspicion, V/Q scan results, ultrasonography of the lower extremities, and pulmonary angiography, together with clinical follow-up; level 3: V/Q scan as reference standard or incomplete combination of diagnostic tests. in: in-patient; out: out-patient

senal of pulmonary embolism. Nevertheless, if we take into account the two series by Kline and Rodger totalizing 626 patients suspected of having pulmonary embolism [23, 24], we see the outstanding sensitivity of the association between normal capnography and normal D-dimer assays in excluding pulmonary embolism without additional testing. Respectively, 43 and 28% of the population could be safely managed in this way, which is much better than the 14% having a normal/near normal lung scan in the PIOPED (prospective investigation of pulmonary embolism diagnosis) study [27]. Since D-dimer assays have relative low specificities, a study evaluating the non-invasive management of patients with positively D-dimer values when the clinical probability is low and when volumetric capnography shows normal VD_{alv} values, would be of great interest.

Capnography to Monitor Thrombolytic Therapy in Acute Pulmonary Embolism

The use of a pulmonary catheter, serial cardiac echographies, or a second lung scintigraphy, is usually mandatory in the evaluation thrombolytic efficacy after a massive pulmonary embolism. Two small series have recently shown that the time-based capnogram could easily be used as sensitive non-invasive monitoring of thrombolytic efficacy in mechanically ventilated patients [28, 29]. Moreover, recurrence of pulmonary embolism was detected by sudden reduction in $EtCO_2$ in two patients. We have found a similar performance of volumetric capnography in confirming a significant decrease in the VD_{alv}, 40 min after starting the thrombolytic infusion in one spontaneously breathing patient with a massive pulmonary embolism (Fig. 4; F. Verschuren unpublished data).

Capnography as a Diagnostic Aid for Pulmonary Embolism in COPD Patients

There is no ideal test to diagnose pulmonary embolism in a COPD patient, especially when the patient is hospitalized. A normal D-dimer value, an unusual arterial hypocapnia, or a diagnostic lung scintigraphy, constitute interesting signs but are seldom encountered. The spiral CT needs to be fully validated in this indication.

COPD patients are traditionally divided into 'pink puffers' with predominant high V/Q lung units, and 'blue bloaters' with low V/Q lung units due to the ob-

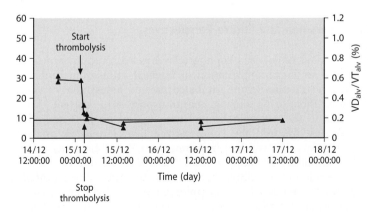

Fig. 4. Evolution of VD_{alv}/VT_{alv} during thrombolysis for massive pulmonary embolism

structed airways. Most COPD patients have a combination of both processes, resulting in shunting as well as deadspace effects. A prolonged breath will attenuate the increased (a-Et) CO_2 gradient due to the high V/Q lung units by the slow exhalation of poorly ventilated but rich in CO_2 alveoli, so that the final gradient must be canceled. Chopin et al. [30] showed that this gradient between the arterial PCO_2 and the maximum expired PCO_2 was not canceled when a COPD patient presented with a pulmonary embolism. A gradient ratio <5% could rule out pulmonary embolism in a study population of 44 mechanically ventilated patients with a sensitivity of 100% and a specificity of 65%. Even though a similar performance with a gradient ratio of 7% was encountered in another French study of 178 patients, the French Society of Reanimation does not recommend its use since capnographic technology is not widely known and is not sufficiently validated in this indication.

▌ Volumetric Capnography as a Non-invasive Measure of Cardiac Output

The continued debate about pulmonary artery catheter morbidity has led to an increased interest for non-invasive methods for cardiac output monitoring. Amongst these, the partial rebreathing method has been validated and commercialized by Novametrix Medical System (NICO System) [31]. This technique determines the pulmonary blood flow by comparing the changes in CO_2 elimination (Δ VCO_2) and the changes in the alveolar CO_2 blood content between a baseline and a rebreathing period. This interesting method is beyond the scope of this chapter, because it requires an adapted ventilation circuit and is not adaptable for spontaneously breathing patients.

However, Arnold et al. [32] investigated the use of volumetric capnography in the prediction of cardiac output in healthy and lung-injured sheep. They speculated that the slope of phase 2, which represents the transition from airway deadspace to alveolar gas, was the most sensitive indicator of pulmonary inefficiency produced by decreases in pulmonary blood flow. The decrease in the slope of phase 2 seemed to be a more powerful predictor of decreased cardiac output than the increase in VD_{alv} (surface Y of the expirogram). More studies are required to confirm such results in humans.

▌ Conclusion and Future Perspectives

Traditional time-based capnography has acquired undeniable indications in several clinical settings: confirmation of tracheal intubation, continuous monitoring of alveolar ventilation in the intubated patient, assessment of cardiopulmonary resuscitation, monitoring during the transport of a patient. Volumetric capnography, thanks to the determination of the slope of phase 3, the adjunct of the late deadspace fraction and the computerized neural network analysis of CO_2 and spirometric data, has resulted in promising new applications and a better knowledge of the pulmonary physiopathology. The role of volumetric capnography in the diagnosis of pulmonary embolism, thrombolytic efficacy in pulmonary embolism, the differential diagnosis between pulmonary embolism and COPD, or the non-invasive evaluation of cardiac output, has been discussed in this chapter. To our knowledge, no other application of volumetric capnography has been investigated in the non-intubated patient. On the other hand, promising clinical application in the intensive care setting and during anesthesia must be cited: first, volumetric capnography has been used to predict successful extubation in infants and children [33]. Secondly, parameters from the expirogram curve (VCO_2, mean alveolar volume, VD/VT) have been implemented in commercially available capnograms to aid the physician in the weaning procedure. Thirdly, Breen et al. showed that the effect of the addition of PEEP on the alveolar deadspace was better displayed by the expirogram than the capnogram [34]. Finally, acute lung injury has been shown to create a steeper slope of phase 3, so that the slope determination may be useful for the early detection of ARDS. Future directions should analyze if volumetric capnography, with its accurate metabolic, hemodynamic, and pulmonary information, may improve the clinical care of the patient and the knowledge of the physiopathological processes.

Acknowledgements. The authors thank Mr. Coffeng and Mr. Sweeney from Datex-Ohmeda-Finland, and Mr. Schmidt, Mr. Buschman and Mr. Morias from Meda-Belgium, for their intellectual and technical support in the development of expirogram curves.

References

1. Fletcher R, Jonson B, Cumming G, Brew J (1981) The concept of deadspace with special reference to the single breath test for carbon dioxide. Br J Anaesth 53:77–78
2. Fletcher R (1985) Deadspace, invasive and non-invasive. Br J Anaesth 57:245–249
3. West JB (1995) Respiratory Physiology: the Essentials, 4th ed. Lippincott, Williams & Wilkins, Philadelphia
4. Eriksson L, Wollmer P, Olsson CG, et al (1989) Diagnosis of pulmonary embolism based upon alveolar dead space analysis. Chest 96:357–362
5. Douketis JD, Kearon C, Bates S, Duku EK, Ginsberg JS (1998) Risk of fatal pulmonary embolism in patients with treated venous thromboembolism. JAMA 279:458–462
6. Ryu JH, Olson EJ, Pellikka PA (1998) Clinical recognition of pulmonary embolism: problem of unrecognized and asymptomatic cases. Mayo Clin Proc 73:873–879
7. Elliott CG (1992) Pulmonary physiology during pulmonary embolism. Chest 101 (Suppl 4): 163S–171S
8. Delcroix M, Melot C, Vachiery JL, et al (1990) Effects of embolus size on hemodynamics and gas exchange in canine embolic pulmonary hypertension. J Appl Physiol 69:2254–2261
9. Robin ED, Julian DG, Travis DM, Crump CH (1959) A physiological approach to the diagnosis of acute pulmonary embolism. N Engl J Med 19:586–591
10. Nutter DO, Massumi RA (1966) The arterial-alveolar carbon dioxide tension gradient in diagnosis of pulmonary embolus. Dis Chest 50:380–387
11. Vereerstraeten J, Schoutens A, Tombroff M, De Koster (1973) Value of measurement of alveolo-arterial gradient of PCO_2 compared to pulmonary scan in diagnosis of thromboembolic pulmonary disease. Thorax 28:306–312
12. Hatle L, Rokseth R (1974) The arterial to end-expiratory carbon dioxide tension gradient in acute pulmonary embolism and other cardiopulmonary diseases. Chest 66:352–357
13. Colp C, Stein M (2001) Re-emergence of an "orphan" test for pulmonary embolism. Chest 120:115–119
14. Burki NK (1986) The dead space to tidal volume ratio in the diagnosis of pulmonary embolism. Am Rev Respir Dis 133:679–685
15. Olsson K, Jonson B, Olsson CG, Wollmer P (1998) Diagnosis of pulmonary embolism by measurement of alveolar dead space. J Intern Med 244:199–207
16. Anderson JT, Owings JT, Goodnight JE (1999) Bedside noninvasive detection of acute pulmonary embolism in critically ill surgical patients. Arch Surg 134:869–874

17. Kline JA, Meek S, Boudrow D, Warner D, Colucciello S (1997) Use of the alveolar dead space fraction (Vd/Vt) and plasma D-dimers to exclude acute pulmonary embolism in ambulatory patients. Acad Emerg Med 4:856–863

18. Kline JA, Arunachlam M (1998) Preliminary study of the capnogram waveform area to screen for pulmonary embolism. Ann Emerg Med 32:289–296

19. Johanning JM, Veverka TJ, Bays RA, Tong GK, Schmiege SK (1999) Evaluation of suspected pulmonary embolism utilizing end-tidal CO_2 and D-dimer. Am J Surg 178:98–102

20. Patel MM, Rayburn DB, Browning JA, Kline JA (1999) Neural network analysis of the volumetric capnogram to detect pulmonary embolism. Chest 116:1325–1332

21. Kline JA, Kubin AK, Patel MM, Easton EJ, Seupal RA (2000) Alveolar dead space as a predictor of severity of pulmonary embolism. Acad Emerg Med 7:611–617

22. Hamel E, Pacouret G, Vincentelli D, et al (2001) Thrombolysis or heparin therapy in massive pulmonary embolism with right ventricular dilation: results from a 128-patient monocenter registry. Chest 120:6–8

23. Kline JA, Israel EG, Michelson EA, O'Neil BJ, Plewa MC, Portelli DC (2001) Diagnostic accuracy of a bedside D-dimer assay and alveolar dead-space measurement for rapid exclusion of pulmonary embolism: a multicenter study. JAMA 285:761–768

24. Rodger MA, Jones G, Rasuli P, et al (2001) Steady-state end-tidal alveolar dead space fraction and D-dimer: bedside tests to exclude pulmonary embolism. Chest 120:115–119

25. Perrier A, Desmarais S, Miron MJ, et al (1999) Non-invasive diagnosis of venous thromboembolism in outpatients. Lancet 353:190–195

26. Wells PS, Anderson DR, Rodger M, et al (2001) Excluding pulmonary embolism at the bedside without diagnostic imaging: management of patients with suspected pulmonary embolism presenting to the emergency department by using a simple clinical model and d-dimer. Ann Intern Med 135:98–107

27. The PIOPED investigators (1990) Value of the ventilation/perfusion scan in acute pulmonary embolism. Results of the prospective investigation of pulmonary embolism diagnosis (PIOPED). JAMA 263:2753–2759

28. Thys F, Elamly A, Marion E, et al (2001) PaCO(2)/ETCO(2) gradient: early indicator of thrombolysis efficacy in a massive pulmonary embolism. Resuscitation 49:105–108

29. Wiegand UK, Kurowski V, Giannitsis E, Katus HA, Djonlagic H (2000) Effectiveness of end-tidal carbon dioxide tension for monitoring thrombolytic therapy in acute pulmonary embolism. Crit Care Med 28:3588–3592

30. Chopin C, Fesard P, Mangalaboyi J, et al (1990) Use of capnography in diagnosis of pulmonary embolism during acute respiratory failure of chronic obstructive pulmonary disease. Crit Care Med 18:353–357

31. Jaffe MB (1999) Partial CO_2 rebreathing cardiac output- operating principles of the NICO system. J Clin Monit 15:387–401

32. Arnold JH, Stenz RI, Thompson JE, Arnold LW (1996) Noninvasive determination of cardiac output using single breath CO_2 analysis. Crit Care Med 24:1701–1705

33. Hubble CL, Gentile MA, Tripp DS, Craig DM, Meliones JN, Cheifetz IM (2000) Deadspace to tidal volume ratio predicts successful extubation in infants and children. Crit Care Med 28:2034–2040

34. Breen PH, Mazumdar B, Skinner SC (1996) Comparison of end-tidal PCO_2 and average alveolar expired PCO_2 during positive end-expiratory pressure. Anesth Analg 82:368–373

Assessment of Lung Function in Mechanically Ventilated Patients

J. H. T. Bates

▊ Introduction

Lung function is often compromised in respiratory failure. Therefore, the management of mechanically ventilated patients is facilitated by knowing the mechanical properties of the patient's lungs. Monitoring mechanical lung function regularly may help in the diagnosis of adverse events such as onset of pulmonary edema or blockage of the endotracheal tube. Ventilator-induced lung injury (VILI), due to over-stretch of the pulmonary tissues, may be minimized if the relationships between volume, flow and pressure in the lungs are understood and ventilatory parameters are chosen accordingly.

Assessment of lung mechanics in a mechanically ventilated patient is an exercise in what an engineer would call system identification, or inverse modeling. This begins with the application of some suitable input to the system under study, together with a measurement of the resultant output. The input and output are then related to each other in terms of a mathematical model encapsulating the important functional components of the system. The parameters of the model, which are evaluated by matching the model's behavior to that of the system, are taken as measures of corresponding quantities within the system itself. The mechanically ventilated patient is well suited to this kind of investigation because the ventilator, by its very action, provides a mechanical perturbation to the lungs that serves as a convenient input. In principle, we are at liberty to choose the flow ($\dot{V}$), volume (V) or pressure (P) provided by the ventilator as the input, but the convention is to consider $\dot{V}$ as the input. The P associated with this $\dot{V}$ is taken as the output. P is determined by $\dot{V}$ and the mechanical properties of the system being ventilated. Determining these properties requires a mathematical model.

The mathematical model should encapsulate the physiology of the lung, as it is manifest in the dynamic relationships between $\dot{V}$ and P. The particular model appropriate in any particular situation depends on the nature of the input $\dot{V}$ used to perturb the system. In general, if $\dot{V}$ is a simple signal, such as a sinewave of modest amplitude, the model required to relate $\dot{V}$ to P will also be simple. Conversely, if $\dot{V}$ contains many different frequency components, or has a large amplitude, the appropriate model will also likely be more complicated. Consequently, our understanding of lung mechanics is equivalent to an understanding of the mathematical model upon which it is based.

The simplest model of lung mechanics that is physiologically reasonable can be visualized as an elastic compartment served by a flow-resistive conduit. The equation relating $\dot{V}$, V, and P in this model is

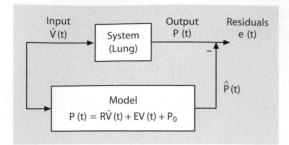

Fig. 1. The system identification paradigm applied to the assessment of lung function. The system under study (the lung) is probed with a time-varying input ($\dot{V}$), giving rise to a correspondingly time-varying output (P). The same input is applied to a model whose parameters (R, E and P_0) are adjusted to make the output from the model ($\hat{P}$) match the measured output as closely as possible. This is equivalent to requiring that the residuals ($e=P-\hat{P}$) be as small as possible

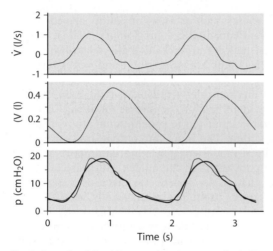

Fig. 2. Example of fit of Eq. 1 to data from a mechanically ventilated patient. The top two panels show two breaths of flow and volume measured at the entrance to the endotracheal tube. The lower panel shows transpulmonary pressure measured at the same site (thin line) together with the best fit provided by the model (thick line). The best fit was determined by multiple linear regression to be

$$Ptp(t) = 7.4\dot{V}(t) + 21.5\,V(t) + 8.6$$

corresponding to a value for R=7.4 cm $H_2O\cdot$s/ml and a value for E=21.5 cmH_2O/l

$$P(t) = R\dot{V}(t) + EV(t) + P_0 \qquad\qquad (Eqn\ 1)$$

where if P is transpulmonary pressure (the difference between airway opening and esophageal pressures) then R is pulmonary resistance and E is pulmonary elastance. P_0 accounts for any positive end-expiratory pressure (PEEP) that might be present. This model describes $\dot{V}$–P data accurately when most of the power in $\dot{V}$ is at a single frequency and its amplitude is not too large. This is generally the case during normal tidal ventilation. Of course, the lung is much more complicated than this simple model, so there are no values for R and E that will make the right-hand side of Eqn 1 match the left-hand side exactly. However, it is possible to find values for R and E that match the two sides of the equation as closely as possible (Fig. 1). This used to be achieved, prior to the widespread use of digital computers, by the electrical subtraction method of Mead and Whittenberger [1]. Now, however, R and E are conveniently evaluated by multiple linear regression (Fig. 2).

■ Methods Based on the Single-compartment Linear Model

The single-compartment linear model and the parameters it provides (R and E) underly most investigations of lung mechanics in mechanically ventilated patients [e.g., 2–4]. The physiological interpretations of R and E appear to be obvious – R is the flow resistance of the airways and E is the stiffness of the lung tissues. However, invasive studies with alveolar capsules in animals [5, 6] have shown that this is incorrect in the case of R, which is composed of both airway resistance (Raw) plus tissue resistance (Rt). R depends markedly on the frequency of ventilation because, while Raw is independent of frequency, Rt decreases asymptotically toward zero as frequency increases.

Frequency dependence of R and E is not something that the single-compartment linear model is able to account for. Other mechanical phenomena, such as a dependence of R upon $\dot{V}$ or a dependence of E upon V, are also beyond the scope of this simple model. The question, therefore, is how the single-compartment linear model should be extended to more accurately represent the mechanical properties of a real lung. There are a number of possibilities.

■ Methods Based on Single-compartment Non-linear Models

The single-compartment linear model is readily extended to include non-linearities of both R and E. If airflow in the lungs is turbulent, the resistance of the airways is not a constant, but is described to a high degree of accuracy by:

$$Raw = K_1\dot{V} + K_2\dot{V}|\dot{V}| \tag{Eqn 2}$$

as first described by Rohrer nearly a century ago [7]. This effect can be incorporated easily into Eqn 1 to yield

$$P(t) = K_1\dot{V}(t) + K_2\dot{V}(t)|\dot{V}(t)| + EV(t) + P_0 \tag{Eqn 3}$$

where $|\dot{V}|$ denotes the absolute value of $\dot{V}$ (necessary to make sure that the sign of the second term in Eqn 3 is correct for both inspiration and expiration). The four parameters K_1, K_2, E and P_0 can again be evaluated by multiple linear regression from records of P, $\dot{V}$ and V. However, just because there is reason to believe there might be turbulent flow in the airways sometimes does not mean one should automatically invoke Eqn 3 over Eqn 1. The real issue is whether the data (i.e., P, $\dot{V}$ and V) support the added complication of the nonlinear model. If the fit to P(t) is not improved significantly by using the more complicated model, or if any of the parameters of the more complicated model do not make physical sense (such as a negative value for E), then one should revert to the simpler model. Nevertheless, non-linearities in resistance have been observed in ventilated patients. For example, the resistance of an endotracheal tube obeys Eqn 2 [8], which has been shown to cause non-linear behavior in patients with acute respiratory distress syndrome (ARDS) [9].

Another non-linear possibility is a volume-dependent elastance, such as:

$$E = E_1 V + E_2 V^2 \qquad \text{(Eqn 4)}$$

which again can be incorporated readily into Eqn 1 to give:

$$P(t) = R\dot{V}(t) + E_1 V(t) + E_2 V^2(t) + P_0 \qquad \text{(Eqn 5)}$$

Bersten [10] has shown that this equation gives a significantly improved fit to data from ventilated patients, and that the parameter E_2 is sensitive to the degree of hyperinflation. The reason is presumably that the lung tissues are not linearly elastic over the vital capacity range, but rather become progressively stiffer as total lung capacity is approached. This is evidenced by the downward concavity of the quasi-static pressure-volume (PV) curve [11]. If a significant fraction of the lung collapses, the remaining open lung may be driven up to the curvilinear portion of its PV curve during normal mechanical ventilation with the concomitant appearance of nonlinear elastic behavior as described by Eqn 5. The important point to note with this model is that the elastic parameters E_1 and E_2 do not mean anything in particular individually. Rather, they are to be considered together as defining a curvilinear dynamic PV curve.

The quasi-static P-V curve is also interpreted in terms of a model – one with a single non-linearly elastic compartment (the presence of an airway is irrelevant in this case because $\dot{V}$ is zero). The elastic properties of this compartment are frequently interpreted, for deflation, in terms of the equation proposed by Salazer and Knowles [11]:

$$V = A - Be^{-Kp} \qquad \text{(Eqn 6)}$$

where A, B and K are parameters. K has been interpreted as a kind of generalized shape factor [12] and varies predictably with diseases, such as emphysema and fibrosis, that affect parenchymal compliance. However, K is merely an empirical quantity and does not relate to any particular structure in the tissues.

Equation 6 only applies above functional residual capacity (FRC). Below FRC in normal lungs, airway closure begins to occur, causing the P-V curve to assume an upward concavity. In an injured lung, significant closure may occur well above FRC. The entire P-V curve is thus sigmoidal and can be described mathematically [13]. The two points on the curve where the rates of change of slope are greatest define the so-called upper and lower inflection points. These have been used to delineate the lung volumes at which overdistension of the tissues (the upper inflection) and airway closure (the lower inflection) start to occur. However, this simple interpretation has been challenged recently [14] on the grounds that the shape of the P-V curve represents a balance between the nonlinear elastic properties of the lung tissues and ongoing recruitment and derecruitment of lung units throughout the entire vital capacity range.

■ Methods Based on Linear Multi-compartment Models

Making sense of the frequency dependence of R and E requires a different kind of model, one that contains more than one mechanical degree of freedom. There are several physiologically plausible possibilities, and sorting them out has been one of the major sagas in the history of respiratory mechanics. In 1956, Otis et al. [15] realized that a model consisting of two elastic compartments connected in parallel (Fig. 3) would have an R and E that varied with frequency provided that the time constants (τ) of the two compartments were different (the τ of a compartment is the ratio of resistance to elastance for that compartment). These authors showed that such a model could account for the main frequency-dependent features of lung compliance that had been observed. Some time later, Mead [16] showed that equivalent behavior could be obtained, in principle, if the two compartments were connected in series (Fig. 3). Prior to both these studies, however, Mount [17] proposed a model for the lung in which a single alveolar compartment was surrounded by viscoelastic tissue. This tissue was not purely elastic, but rather had a viscous component that allowed it to exhibit stress adaptation following sudden volume changes that mimicked observations in real lungs. The viscoelastic model, shown in Fig. 3, features an airway resistance (R_1) together with a double spring and dashpot assembly known as a Kelvin body (R_2, E_1 and E_2) that describes the tissues.

These three models are all described by the same differential equation [18]:

$$P(t) = A\dot{P}(t) + BV(t) + C\dot{V}(t) + D\ddot{V}(t) + E \qquad (Eqn\ 7)$$

where the parameters A, B, C, D and E are derivable (and *vice versa*) from the parameters of each of the models shown in Fig. 3. It is not possible to decide which of the three models is the best in any particular situation from measurements of P and $\dot{V}$ made at the airway opening [18]. Resolving the issue requires additional experimental information. This has been achieved in animals using the alveolar capsule technique to measure alveolar pressure at several sites simultaneously, and has shown that the viscoelastic model is the most appropriate for describing a normal lung [19]. However, this technique has also shown that the lung becomes markedly heterogeneous under pathological conditions [20, 21], so some combination of all three models is likely necessary in the diseased patient.

A number of investigators [22, 23] have invoked the viscoelastic model in ventilated patients to explain data obtained using the constant-flow interrupter method. This technique involves inflating the lungs with a constant inspiratory $\dot{V}$ and then suddenly interrupting $\dot{V}$ at the end of inspiration while P just distal to the point of

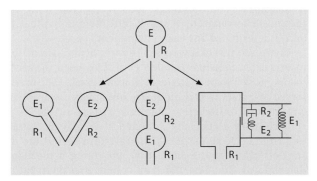

Fig. 3. The single-compartment linear model (*top*) and its three two-compartment extensions: the parallel two-compartment model (*lower left*), the series two-compartment model (*lower middle*) and the viscoelastic model (*lower right*)

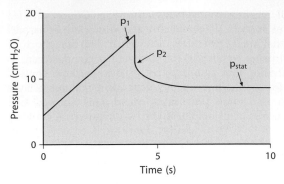

Fig. 4. Transpulmonary pressure (stylized) versus time during a constant flow inspiration terminated in a sudden interruption of flow. The initial rapid change in pressure (P_1–P_2) reflects airways resistance, while the subsequent slower change from P_2 to the final static pressure (P_{stat}) reflects stress adaptation in the tissues plus any gas redistribution that will occur if the lungs are mechanically heterogeneous

interruption is measured. A stylized P tracing is given in Fig. 4, showing the sudden drop at the instant of interruption followed by a subsequent slower decay. The magnitude of the sudden drop is divided by $\dot{V}$ to give Raw. The subsequent drop in P divided by $\dot{V}$ gives the resistance of the tissues in the viscoelastic model [24]. However, a patient with lung disease is likely to have significant regional heterogeneities of lung function. Such heterogeneities are not accounted for by the viscoelastic model. Nevertheless, the viscoelastic interpretation can still be used to characterize lung mechanical function empirically.

A more general approach to the multi-compartment behavior of the lung is provided by a quantity known as input impedance, Zin, which is really nothing more than a description of how R and E vary with frequency over some range. Zin can be obtained, in principle, by oscillating the lungs with flow at a particular frequency, calculating R and E via Eqn 1, moving on to another frequency, and so on until the desired frequency range has been covered. However, it is more usual, and much more convenient, to use the so-called forced oscillation technique [25]. Here, a complex $\dot{V}$ signal containing many different frequencies is applied to the airway opening with an oscillator of some kind (e.g., loudspeaker, piston pump), while P is measured. Computational techniques employing the fast Fourier transform are then used to separate $\dot{V}$ and P into their individual frequency components, and R and E determined for each component.

There are not many recent reports of the use of the forced oscillation technique in ventilated patients. Beraldo et al. [26] used the technique in a tetraplegic patient to diagnose tracheal stenosis. Kaczka et al. [27] used an elegant adaptation of the forced oscillation technique to investigate lung mechanics in ventilated patients with chronic obstructive pulmonary disease (COPD). These authors ventilated their subjects with a specially designed $\dot{V}$ waveform containing a spectrum of frequencies from 0.156 to 8.1 Hz. This waveform served the dual purpose of ventilating the subjects while at the same time providing a mechanical perturbation suitable for determining Zin. The Zin they obtained in their patients were consistent with heterogeneous narrowing of peripheral airways.

The calculation of Zin is based on the assumption that the lung is a linear dynamic system. This means that it behaves like a single-compartment linear model

(Eqn 1) at each frequency, even though the values of R and E may not be the same at all frequencies. Consequently, interpreting Zin globally requires a model of the lung that allows for R and E to be frequency dependent. The models shown in Fig. 3 are possible candidates. However, the lung is far more complicated than this, so future developments may include the use of models with multiple compartments. At an even more complicated level, one might envisage models that are both multi-compartment and nonlinear, although it will be a severe challenge to obtain data of the quality and dynamic range necessary to support such models uniquely.

▌ Conclusion

The quantitative assessment of lung mechanics is always based on some model idealization of the real system. Most investigations invoke the single-compartment linear model that yields estimates of so-called lung resistance (R) and lung elastance (E). These parameters account for the overall behavior of the lung, but must be interpreted with care. This applies especially to R which contains contributions from both airways and tissue resistance. The single-compartment linear model may be extended in various ways to make it more realistic. One way is to make it non-linear by allowing R to depend on $\dot{V}$ and E to depend on V. Another approach is to give the model more degrees of freedom, either by including more than one alveolar compartment or by allowing the tissues to be viscoelastic rather than purely elastic. These models predict that R and E will depend on frequency, as has been observed in both healthy and diseased lungs. The measurement of Zin by the forced oscillation technique allows R and E to be determined over some frequency range, and may be interpreted in terms of these more complicated models.

References

1. Mead J, Whittenberger JL (1953) Physical properties of human lungs measured during spontaneous respiration. J Appl Physiol 5:779–796
2. Peslin R, Felicio da Silva J, Chabot F, Duvivier C (1992) Respiratory mechanics studied by multiple linear regression in unsedated ventilated patients. Eur Respir J 5:871–878
3. Dechman GS, Chartrand DA, Ruiz-Neto RP, Bates JHT (1995) The effect of changing end-expiratory pressure on respiratory system mechanics in open- and closed-chested anesthetized, paralyzed patients. Anesth Analg 81:279–286
4. Fahy BG, Barnas GM, Nagle SE, Flowers JL, Njoku MJ, Agarwal M (1996) Effects of Trendelenburg and reverse Trendelenburg postures on lung and chest wall mechanics. J Clin Anesth 8:236–244
5. Fredberg JJ, Keefe DH, Glass GM, Castile RG, Franz ID (1984) Alveolar pressure nonhomogeneity during small-amplitude high-frequency oscillation. J Appl Physiol 57:788–800
6. Hantos Z, Daroczy B, Suki B, Nagy S, Fredberg JJ (1992) Input impedance and peripheral inhomogeneity of dog lungs. J Appl Physiol 72:168–178
7. Otis AB (1986) History of respiratory mechanics. In: Cherniack NS (ed) Handbook of Physiology. The Respiratory System, vol III. Am Physiol Soc, Bethesda, pp 1–12
8. Fabry B, Guttman J, Eberhard L, Wolff G (1994) Automatic compensation of endotracheal tube resistance in spontaneously breathing patients. Technol Health Care 1:281–291
9. Guttman J, Eberhard L, Fabry B, et al (1995) Time constant/volume relationship of passive expiration in mechanically ventilated ARDS patients. Eur Respir J 8:114–120
10. Bersten AD (1998) Measurement of overinflation by multiple linear regression analysis in patients with acute lung injury. Eur Respir J 12:526–532
11. Salazar E, Knowles JH (1964) An analysis of pressure-volume characteristics of the lungs. J Appl Physiol 19:97–104

12. Colebatch HJH, Ng CKY, Nikov N (1979) Use of an exponential function for elastic recoil. J Appl Physiol 46:387–393
13. Harris RS, Hess DR, Venegas JG (2000) An objective analysis of the pressure-volume curve in the acute respiratory distress syndrome. Am J Respir Crit Care Med 161:432–439
14. Hickling K (1998) The pressure-volume curve is greatly modified by recruitment. Am J Respir Crit Care Med 158:194–202
15. Otis AB, McKerrow CB, Bartlett RA, et al (1956) Mechanical factors in distribution of pulmonary ventilation. J Appl Physiol 8:427–443
16. Mead J (1969) Contribution of compliance of airways to frequency-dependent behavior of lungs. J Appl Physiol 26:670–673
17. Mount LE (1955) The ventilation flow-resistance and compliance of rat lungs. J Physiol (Lond) 127:157–167
18. Similowski T, Bates JHT (1991) Two-compartment modelling of respiratory system mechanics at low frequencies: gas redistribution or tissue rheology? Eur Respir J 4:353–358
19. Bates JHT, Ludwig MS, Sly PD, Brown K, Martin JG, Fredberg JJ (1988) Interrupter resistance elucidated by alveolar pressure measurement in open-chest normal dogs. J Appl Physiol 65:408–414
20. Fredberg JJ, Ingram RH, Castile RG, Glass GM, Drazen JM (1985) Nonhomogeneity of lung response to inhaled histamine assessed with alveolar capsules. J Appl Physiol 58:1914–1922
21. Ludwig MS, Romero PV, Sly PD, Fredberg JJ, Bates JHT (1990) Interpretation of interrupter resistance after histamine-induced constriction in the dog. J Appl Physiol 68:1651–1656
22. Rossi A, Gottfried SB, Higgs BD, Zocchi L, Grassino A, Milic-Emili J (1985) Respiratory mechanics in mechanically ventilated patients with respiratory failure. J Appl Physiol 58:1849–1858
23. D'Angelo E, Tavola M, Milic-Emili J (2000) Volume and time dependence of respiratory system mechanics in normal anaesthetized paralysed humans. Eur Respir J 16:665–672
24. Bates JHT, Rossi A, Milic-Emili J (1985) Analysis of the behavior of the respiratory system with constant inspiratory flow. J Appl Physiol 58:1840–1848
25. Peslin R, Fredberg JJ (1986) Oscillation mechanics of the respiratory system. In: Cherniack NS (ed) Handbook of Physiology, The Respiratory System, vol III. Am Physiol Soc, Bethesda, pp 145–177
26. Beraldo PS, Mateus SR, Arujo LM, Horan TA (2000) Forced oscillation technique to detect and monitor tracheal stenosis in a tetraplegic patient. Spinal Cord 38:445–447
27. Kaczka D, Ingenito EP, Body SC, et al (2001) Inspiratory lung impedance in COPD: effects of PEEP and immediate impact of lung volume reduction surgery. J Appl Physiol 90:1833–1841

Tissue Lactate Concentrations in Critical Illness

B. Venkatesh and T. J. Morgan

▌ Introduction

Perturbations in oxygen delivery to, and consumption by, the tissues are common in critical illness resulting in impaired tissue metabolism. This in turn can result in biochemical changes, which if uncorrected may progress to cell death. Lactic acidosis is a signal of tissue distress associated with altered tissue perfusion and cell metabolism [1, 2]. This is evidenced by the demonstration of high lactate concentrations in the setting of shock and circulatory failure, irrespective of the aetiology [3]. There are also data to show that elevated blood lactate concentrations in critical illness portend a poor prognosis [4–8]. Not surprisingly, arterial plasma lactate measurements have become commonplace in intensive care. However, a number of caveats need to be applied when interpreting plasma lactate concentrations. Certain clinical situations might reduce the sensitivity of plasma lactate concentrations as an indicator of dysoxia (oxygen limited cytochrome turnover) [9]. This might result if regional production of lactate in ischemic tissues was diluted by venous effluent from well perfused tissues or if the liver, kidney and possibly the muscle tissue acted as efficient 'sinks' for the lactate and prevented significant elevations in the plasma [10–12]. Conversely, an elevation in plasma lactate concentration might not always signify dysoxia, thus reducing its specificity. Hyperlactatemia without dysoxia might result from aerobic glycolysis during sepsis, liver failure, altered pyruvate dehydrogenase activity, hyperventilation, elevated catecholamine concentrations and in the presence of certain drugs and toxins [13–15].

It, therefore, stands to reason that lactate production by individual organs may be a more reliable index of anaerobic metabolism than arterial lactate concentrations.

Whilst individual organ production of lactate can be calculated from its blood flow and the arterio-venous (A-V) lactate concentration difference; in practice this is difficult and not routinely applicable at the bedside. With refinement in technology, it is now possible to measure lactate concentrations in the tissues. In this chapter we will:

▌ review the basic physiology of lactate production and clearance by various tissues in health and in shock;

▌ discuss the various methods of monitoring tissue lactate concentrations;

▌ critically examine the evidence on tissue lactate measurements in critical illness;

▌ explore some of the pitfalls in the interpretation of tissue lactate as an indicator of dysoxia; and

▌ deliberate on its future role in intensive care practice and research.

Table 1. Important milestones in the evolution of knowledge on lactic acidosis

1886	Gaglio established the presence of lactate in mammalian blood [73]
1918	Cannon described the association between tissue perfusion and acidosis [74]
1922	A practical technique for lactate analysis described by Clausen [75]
1961	Huckabee's original classification of lactic acidosis proposed [76]
1976	Reclassification of lactic acidosis by Cohen and Woods [77]
1980s	Lactate measurement commonplace in ICU management

Some of the important milestones in the evolution of our knowledge of lactic acidosis are summarized in Table 1.

❙ Lactate Production and Clearance in Health

The estimated daily lactate production in a 70 kg individual is about 1400 mmol. All of this lactate is derived from pyruvate through glycolysis. The chemical reaction is catalyzed by the enzyme lactate dehydrogenase (LDH).

$$\text{Pyruvate} + \text{NADH} + \text{H}^+ \xleftarrow{\text{LDH}} \text{Lactate} + \text{NAD} \qquad \text{(Eqn 1)}$$

Rearranging this equation gives the determinants of lactate production.

$$\text{Lactate} = K_{eq} \times [\text{pyruvate}] \times \text{H}^+ \times \frac{\text{NADH}}{\text{NAD}} \qquad \text{(Eqn 2)}$$

$$\frac{\text{Lactate}}{\text{Pyruvate}} = \frac{K \times [\text{H}^+ \times \text{NADH}]}{\text{NAD}} = \frac{10}{1} \qquad \text{(Eqn 3)}$$

Lactate is the anion of lactic acid (a strong acid with a pKa of 3.8) [16]. Pyruvic acid, the precursor of lactic acid is also a strong acid. As it is present in such small concentrations (approximately a tenth of lactate concentration), it does not contribute in any significant fashion to the development of metabolic acidosis.

Lactate is a metabolic dead-end in that it can only be produced or utilized via pyruvate. The bulk of the lactate is metabolized through the Cori cycle largely by the liver, kidney, and the myocardium and under certain conditions (when blood lactate concentration exceeds 4 mM/l) the skeletal muscle becomes a net consumer of lactate.

The daily individual organ production and uptake of lactate is summarized in Table 2 [17–20].

During pregnancy, the placenta is a source of aerobic generation of lactate with a net transfer to both mother and fetus. The lactate concentration in the cord vein blood is 7% higher than in the arterial blood. The uterine vein has a 3% higher concentration of lactate as compared to the uterine artery [21].

Once produced, the transport of lactate across cell membranes involves one of three pathways: a) free diffusion of undissociated acid, b) exchange for another anion such as Cl^- or HCO_3^-; and c) H^+ linked carrier mechanism, which is pH dependent (the most important of the three mechanisms) [22]. The H^+ linked carrier mechanism is catalyzed by a specific monocarboxylate/proton co-transporter (MCT).

Table 2. Individual organ production and uptake of lactate

Lactate production		Lactate utilization	
Skin	350	Liver	720
Red Blood Cell	300	Kidney	380
Brain	235	Heart	80
Muscle	218	Others	100
Mucosa	115		
White blood cell, platelet	70		

(Values are in mMol/24 hours/70 Kg man)

Kinetics of Lactate Production in Shock

Data have been published on the maximal catalytic capacities of the enzymes involved in the glycolytic and gluconeogenetic pathways in various tissues *in vitro* [20]. Inspection of the data reveals that the glycolytic capacities of muscle, heart, and brain are significantly greater than their gluconeogenetic capacities whilst the reverse is true of the liver and the kidney. Since enzymatic machinery determines substrate flow, the logical conclusion is that during a hypoxic insult, muscle, heart, and brain would be the significant producers of lactate (muscle being the principal source owing to its greatest glycolytic capacity).

Support for this theoretical concept comes from data published by Daniel et al. [23]. Cardiac tamponade was induced in animals to achieve a preset mean arterial pressure (MAP) for varying durations. At the end of the study period, the solid and the hollow organs and the skeletal muscle were biopsied and the tissue lactate concentrations assayed. The primary source of lactate was identified as skeletal muscle, which is consistent with data derived from the enzymatic catalytic capacities in skeletal muscle. Recently, similar conclusions have been arrived at in animal models of hemorrhagic shock [24]. Muscles from shocked rats produced twice as much lactate compared to those from sham rats.

What are the Mechanisms of Lactate Production in Shock?

In animal models of shock, the demonstration of a remarkable level of congruity between reductions in tissue perfusion and elevation of lactate concentrations led to the hypothesis that tissue hypoxia was the predominant source of lactate. However, several lines of evidence suggest that hyperlactatemia may result from adrenaline induced aerobic glycolysis even in the absence of tissue hypoxia [25]. Epinephrine accelerates aerobic glycolysis and lactate production, which is coupled to Na^+, K^+-ATPase activity. In animal studies of hemorrhage, adrenergic blockade prior to the induction of shock blunted the rise in lactate concentrations [26–30]. Epinephrine infusions in critical illness have been known to increase plasma lactate concentrations even in the absence of hypoxia. The plasma epinephrine concentrations encountered in health and in critical illness and the threshold for lactate elevations in arterial blood are summarized in Table 3 [31–34].

Catecholamine mediated plasma lactate elevation appears to originate from skeletal muscle [25]. Although catecholamines are reported to decrease splanchnic

Table 3. Plasma concentrations of epinephrine in physiological and pathological states

Setting	Plasma (pg/ml)
▌ Health (at rest)	50
▌ Threshold for lactate elevation	150–300
▌ Epinephrine infusion*	100–200
▌ Exercise	1500
▌ Severe shock	4000
▌ Post shock	500

* The plasma concentration would be dose dependent

blood flow and intramucosal pH, and elevate plasma lactate concentrations [35, 36], the small bowel does not appear to be the primary source of lactate during catecholamine infusions [37].

▌ Lactate Measurement in the Tissues/Body Fluids

Lactate concentrations are measured using the lactate oxidase technique [38, 39]. The principle behind the technique is the oxidation of lactate in the presence of oxygen to hydrogen peroxide which is detected amperometrically. This technique has found commercial application in most blood gas analyzers [40, 41]. The limitation of the lactate electrode is the dependence on molecular oxygen as an electronic mediator [38]. Low PO_2 values may lead to a substantial decrease in the sensitivity of the sensor to detect lactate when placed directly in a hypoxic environment. However, improvements in the technology are thought to have overcome this 'oxygen dependence' phenomenon.

Sampling of tissue fluid is possible by using microdialysis techniques. This technique enables prolonged measurements of extracellular fluid metabolites. The method uses an internally perfused, semipermeable membrane probe, which allows water soluble substances such as lactate, glucose, amino acids, and electrolytes to be collected for analysis outside the tissue of interest. Normal saline is used as the perfusate. This technique has been put to use in neuro-critical care and shows promise as a potential monitoring tool [42–44]. The main limitation of this method is its intermittent nature.

Recently, continuous intravascular and tissue lactate measuring technologies have been described which incorporate either an electrochemical [45–47] or a fiberoptic system [48]. These probes have been evaluated in both animals and in humans. The performance characteristics of these probes include a broad range of measurement (0–20 mmol), rapid response time (60–120 s), and stable shelf life [47].

Substances Interfering with the Lactate Assay

Substances known to interfere with lactate assays have been identified. These include glycolate, which interferes with the lactate oxidase assay resulting in artifactual elevations in lactate concentrations [40, 41]. Toxic concentrations of isoniazid, acetaminophen and thiocyanate also cause artificial elevations of L-lactate concentrations measured by some blood gas analyzers [40].

Tissue Lactate: Review of Published Data in Critical Illness

There is a paucity of data in the critical care literature concerning tissue lactate measurements. Although site specific measurements can be performed depending on the clinical scenario, e.g., brain PO_2 and lactate as an indicator of cerebral perfusion in neurotrauma [49], what would be desirable is the ability to measure tissue lactate concentration at one site most representative of whole body well being. Based on theoretical considerations and experimental data, muscle would be the obvious choice. Muscle lactate concentrations reflect circulating catecholamines (a marker of stress response) and therefore an elevated muscle lactate would be a marker of tissue distress. Although it is a non-specific signal, it should prompt the search for the cause of the ongoing stress response. However, human data are lacking in this area. What we have is a plethora of isolated studies examining individual organ lactate kinetics in critical illness. To this end, a number of tissue sites has been examined including lung, urine, brain, myocardium, skeletal muscle, and the hepatosplanchnic bed. Considering each in turn:

Lung Lactate

The human lung is capable of generating lactate in normal health [50] and this production is known to increase in disease states such as tuberculosis and malignancy [51]. Recent studies have demonstrated elevated lung lactate production in acute lung injury (ALI) and acute respiratory distress syndrome (ARDS) [52, 53]. Increases in lung lactate production were in direct proportion to the severity of lung injury, A-a gradient and venous admixture and did not appear to be related to hypoxia. The magnitude of the lactate flux across the lung was of the order of 0.4 mmol/l [52]. The lactate is thought to be generated by activated neutrophils in the lung. The above data have potential clinical ramifications. It is likely that there may be a greater release of lactate in sepsis-related ALI and this may explain some of the hyperlactatemia of sepsis. Also, lung lactate flux could be used to monitor severity of lung injury. As an extrapolation, it is tempting to suggest that resolution of raised lung lactate concentrations might signal recovery from ALI and ARDS although this hypothesis has not been tested.

Urinary Lactate

The kidney plays a crucial role in lactate homeostasis through gluconeogenesis and by regulating lactate concentrations in the body fluids. The kidney effectively reabsorbs all of the filtered lactate up to plasma concentrations of 6 to 10 mM/l [19]. Thus lactate does not appear in the urine until these concentrations in plasma are exceeded as long as there is preservation of renal blood flow.

Lactate concentrations in the urine (expressed as urinary lactate/creatinine ratio) have been demonstrated to reflect the severity of perinatal asphyxia in animal models [54] and in infants with perinatal asphyxia [55]. In a study of 40 infants, the ratio of lactate to creatinine in the urine in the first 6 hours after birth was significantly higher (17 ± 27) in those infants who subsequently developed hypoxic ischemic encephalopathy as compared to infants with perinatal asphyxia who did not develop neurological complications (0.19 ± 0.12) and normal newborns (0.09 ± 0.02) [55]. A ratio of 0.64 or higher within 6 hours after birth had a sensitivity and specificity of 94% and 100%, respectively. The two groups with asphyxia did not differ significantly with respect to APGAR scores, arterial pH and base deficit values. The source of lactate may be multifactorial; global circulatory hypoxia or renal injury from marked vasoconstriction resulting in local production of lactate, or skeletal muscle generation of lactate from the sympathetic discharge induced by asphyxia. The appearance of urinary lactate in the group with the poor prognosis would suggest direct renal injury from asphyxia rather than global circulatory failure-induced lactic aciduria as the arterial parameters were similar in both groups.

The results from this study offer an opportunity to identify early, and in a relatively simple way, infants with asphyxia who are most likely to have subsequent brain injury. This clinical study demonstrates the utility of measuring tissue lactate concentrations as a predictor of outcome. The study also adds to the growing list of publications that underscore the limitations of global circulatory parameters as markers of tissue injury.

Hepatosplanchnic Lactate

The liver plays a pivotal role in lactate metabolism. Approximately 50% of the lactate generated daily is metabolized in the liver through gluconeogenesis. Hepatic lactate uptake is a saturable process with a reduction in fractional liver extraction with increasing lactate influx [56]. With impaired hepatic perfusion, both reduced perfusion and impaired hepatic lactate clearance may contribute to the development of systemic hyperlactatemia. The relative contributions of hepatic lactate production versus impaired clearance are difficult to quantify. A number of aspects of hepatosplanchnic lactate kinetics require further clarification. The relationship between intestinal ischemia and systemic hyperlactatemia is not linear. This is because liver perfusion is protected to a certain extent by the hepatic arterial buffer response (an increase in hepatic arterial blood flow when there is a reduction in portal blood flow) [57]. Consequently, hepatic uptake of lactate blunts the rise in lactate generated by the intestines. Also there are conflicting data on whether lactate is released from the hepatosplanchnic bed during sepsis [58, 59]. Whilst lactate measurements across the hepatic bed have provided further insight into lactate physiology and pathophysiology, clinical outcome data are still lacking.

Brain Lactate

Using microdialysis techniques, it has been possible to demonstrate that brain extracellular fluid (ECF) lactate concentrations might be a marker of ischemia and secondary brain injury [60]. A good correlation was also demonstrated between ECF lactate, lactate/pyruvate (L/P) ratios and physiological deterioration. Increased lactate and decreased glucose, indicating accelerated anaerobic glycolysis, commonly occurred with cerebral ischemia or hypoxia and were associated with a poor outcome [61].

As microdialysis is an invasive monitoring tool, we have examined the feasibility of studying cerebrospinal fluid (CSF) lactate concentrations in patients with neurotrauma who have a ventricular drain in place. Many patients with severe head in-

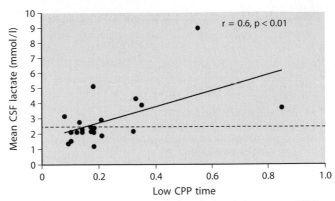

Fig. 1. Cerebrospinal fluid (CSF) lactate versus cerebral hypoperfusion (low cerebral perfusion pressure [CPP])

jury have a ventricular drain inserted for monitoring intracranial pressure (ICP) and intermittent CSF drainage as required. CSF sampling can be performed at regular intervals without additional invasiveness. In a study of 21 head injured patients, we have demonstrated a good correlation between raised levels of CSF lactate and a reduction in cerebral perfusion (Fig. 1) (Venkatesh et al., unpublished data). CSF lactate concentrations correlated inversely with outcome.

Preliminary data indicate that measurement of lactate in brain ECF or in the CSF has the potential to become a monitoring tool in patients at risk of cerebral hypoperfusion. Furthermore, it might be possible to titrate therapies aimed at reducing cerebral metabolism such as induced hypothermia and pentobarbital coma [62] using brain tissue lactate as an end point.

Myocardial Lactate

Lactate is a respiratory fuel for the myocardium under aerobic conditions and is transported from the interstitium into the myocardium for oxidation. During ischemia, lactate is transported out of the cells with protons to maintain glycolysis. This transport is achieved with the aid of MCT [63].

At the present time, myocardial lactate measurements have found greater application in research than in clinical medicine. Myocardial lactate measurements enable us to recognize one of the important endogenous protective mechanisms in myocardial ischemia, i.e., myocardial hibernation, and to distinguish myocardial hibernation from stunning. In both these processes, the ability to respond to an inotropic challenge is preserved, but in myocardial hibernation, the recruitment of an inotropic reserve occurs at the expense of lactate generation [64]. The importance of recognizing this phenomenon is that its presence extends the time frame for a reperfusion intervention. The evolution of ischemic preconditioning, another cardioprotective mechanism, is characterized by an attenuation of glycolysis and lactate in the myocardium [64]. The measurement of myocardial lactate concentrations offers a means of monitoring this phenomenon. Myocardial lactate used as a marker of myocardial injury can be used as an endpoint by which the protective effect of new cardioplegia solutions can be evaluated and new mechanisms of induction of hibernation can be tested [65]. At the present time, direct measurement of myocardial tissue lactate production remains a research tool.

Skeletal Muscle

As mentioned before, muscle lactate measures the global stress response. They might also be useful at the local level in the recognition of muscle fatigue. Although lactate on its own does not cause fatigue [66], the associated intracellular acidosis leads to inhibition of myocytic glycolysis, thus limiting ATP production. As a result there is a failure of the contractile machinery [67]. Measurement of skeletal muscle ECF lactate concentrations may give sufficient indirect information about intracellular concentrations to enable the diagnosis of muscle fatigue. Continuous measurements of diaphragmatic lactate might thus become a useful monitor in slow to wean patients [68].

▌ Is Tissue Lactate a Reliable Indicator of Tissue Dysoxia?

There is uniform agreement and there are plenty of data to show that in acute total body hypoxia, tissue and arterial lactate concentrations become elevated. Consequently, the notion that elevated lactate is specific for tissue dysoxia is deep rooted in the minds of most clinicians. However this is not the case. To illustrate why this is so, we need to explore some concepts of hypoxia and dysoxia. There are three thresholds of cellular hypoxia [9]. The first threshold is reached when ATP supply and demand are matched by metabolic adaptation despite a decrease in oxygen tension within the cell. The second threshold is when ATP supply can be maintained only by supplementary production from glycolysis. The third threshold is when glycolysis produces insufficient ATP to maintain cell function.

Dysoxia (as defined above) is oxygen limited cytochrome turn over, which thus comes into play below the second threshold. Therefore to recognize dysoxia, we need to demonstrate changes in intracellular PO_2 accompanied by inverse fluxes in glycolysis. Owing to the difficulties involved in the measurement of these parameters, lactate concentrations have been proposed as a surrogate marker of dysoxia. The reason for this is that under total anaerobic conditions, ATP flux is determined solely by glycolysis and lactate is the end-product of this metabolic pathway. However, glycolytic rate and associated lactate concentrations can alter for reasons other than fluctuations in oxygen supply. Inspection of equation 2 reveals that pyruvate concentrations, NADH/NAD ratio and intracellular pH will influence lactate production independent of tissue PO_2.

Considering each of the above in turn, the amount of pyruvate available to form lactate depends upon the rate of consumption of pyruvate through alternate metabolic pathways – conversion to acetyl CoA, transamination to alanine and conversion to glucose through the Cori cycle. Change in intracellular pH through respiratory alkalosis accelerates glycolysis through activation of phosphofructokinase (PFK). The relative concentrations of ADP and ATP also influence PFK activity and therefore secondarily influence the rate of glycolysis. Increases in intracellular ADP activate glycolysis and vice versa. Alterations in ADP concentrations can result from catecholamine induced stimulation of Na, K-ATPase. The work of Connett et al. [69] and Hotchkiss and Karl [70] examining skeletal muscle lactate production in endotoxic rats also demonstrates that there can be a dissociation between lactate production and tissue PO_2. Similarly, as stated above, lung lactate production was increased in patients with ARDS even in the absence of tissue hypoxia.

Elevations in tissue lactate can thus occur irrespective of the oxygen tension within the cell. However, any elevation in lactate (in the absence of physiological stimulants for lactate production) should be considered abnormal and prompt the search for an underlying pathological process.

∎ Can Tissue Lactate Concentrations be Used to Determine the Mechanism of Elevations in Tissue PCO_2: Flow Stagnation vs Anaerobic Metabolism?

Elevations in tissue PCO_2 during circulatory failure are thought to arise from two processes: an initial rise in tissue PCO_2 due to *flow stagnation*, whereby the PCO_2 is not cleared by the circulation and a delayed rise due to *anaerobic metabolism* if the circulatory failure is severe and persistent [71]. The delayed rise in tissue PCO_2 is due to titration of protons by bicarbonate. The proton release follows anaerobic glycolysis, resulting in generation of lactate. Conventional teaching would suggest that tissue lactate concentrations would be expected to rise only during the phase of anaerobic metabolism. Therefore, measurement of tissue lactate might facilitate the differentiation between the two mechanisms of rise in tissue PCO_2.

However, such an approach may be too simplistic. As discussed before, elevated catecholamine concentrations may lead to lactate generation irrespective of tissue PO_2. Conceptually, catecholamine concentrations could go up during the flow stagnation phase of shock due to a stress response, thus leading to elevated lactate production even in the early stages of circulatory failure. It is likely that tissue lactate might follow a biphasic pattern, an initial small rise followed by a delayed large rise, but this hypothesis has not been tested. It is more likely that trends in tissue lactate concentration rather than absolute values will be more useful in making the distinction between flow stagnation and anaerobic metabolism.

∎ Conclusion

It is now possible to measure lactate concentrations in the tissues either intermittently or continuously. Although clinical outcome studies are lacking, tissue lactate measurements have provided a significant insight into shock physiology, organ function and pathophysiology of critical illness. The notion that lactate is always a marker of tissue hypoxia needs to be dispelled. Elevated tissue lactate is better thought of as a marker of stress, and continued elevation as a persistent stress response. Mizock has put forward the concept of "shock lactate" and "stress lactate", basing his arguments on the lines of evidence spelt out above [72].

Potential applications of tissue lactate measurement (apart from those already mentioned above) include determination of the lactate gap and in the field of transplantation medicine. Persistent ongoing regional ischemia might result in elevated tissue lactate concentration with a relatively normal arterial lactate concentration thus resulting in lactate gap (tissue lactate-arterial lactate). In health, the lactate gap should be negligible, however in organ dysfunction, the lactate gap may be elevated.

The viability of organs pre and post transplant may be determined by their lactate concentrations, thus facilitating precise determination of optimal cold and warm ischemia times.

Nevertheless a number of issues and questions remain. The technique is still in its infancy and our understanding limited. Should we be monitoring one tissue bed or multiple sites in critical illness? No matter which tissues are chosen, the normal values of tissue lactate in humans at these sites are not yet established. The dysoxic threshold in the various tissues is unclear. In those tissues with counter current circulations where there are oxygen gradients, are there lactate gradients as well?

Answers to these questions will improve our understanding and facilitate clinical application of this potential physiological monitor.

References

1. Vincent JL (1990) The relationship between oxygen demand, oxygen uptake, and oxygen supply. Intensive Care Med 16:S145–S148
2. Kellum JA (1998) Lactate and pHi: our continued search for markers of tissue distress. Crit Care Med 26:1783–1784
3. Mizock BA, Falk JL (1992) Lactic acidosis in critical illness. Crit Care Med 20:80–93
4. Bernardin G, Pradier C, Tiger F, Deloffre P, Mattei M (1996) Blood pressure and arterial lactate level are early indicators of short-term survival in human septic shock. Intensive Care Med 22:17–25
5. Friedman G, Berlot G, Kahn RJ, Vincent JL (1995) Combined measurements of blood lactate concentrations and gastric intramucosal pH in patients with severe sepsis. Crit Care Med 23:1184–1193
6. Manikis P, Jankowski S, Zhang H, Kahn RJ, Vincent JL (1995) Correlation of serial blood lactate levels to organ failure and mortality after trauma. Am J Emerg Med 13:619–622
7. Bakker J, Gris P, Coffernils M, Kahn RJ, Vincent JL (1996) Serial blood lactate levels can predict the development of multiple organ failure following septic shock. Am J Surg 171:221–226
8. Marecaux G, Pinsky MR, Dupont E, Kahn RJ, Vincent JL (1996) Blood lactate levels are better prognostic indicators than TNF and IL-6 levels in patients with septic shock. Intensive Care Med 22:404–408
9. Connett RJ, Honig CR, Gayeski TE, Brooks GA (1990) Defining hypoxia: a systems view of VO2, glycolysis, energetics, and intracellular PO2. J Appl Physiol 68:833–842
10. Venkatesh B, Meacher R, Muller M, Morgan T, Fraser J (2001) Monitoring tissue oxygenation during resuscitation of major burns. J Trauma 50:485–494
11. Venkatesh B, Morgan T, Lipman J (2000) Subcutaneous oxygen tensions provide similar information to ileal luminal CO2 tensions in an animal model of hemorrhagic shock. Intensive Care Med 26:592–600
12. Mizock BA (1989) Lactic acidosis. Dis Mon 35:233–300
13. Gutierrez G, Wulf ME (1996) Lactic acidosis in sepsis: a commentary. Intensive Care Med 22:6–16
14. Duke T (1999) Dysoxia and lactate. Arch Dis Child 81:343–350
15. Vincent JL, De Backer D (1995) Oxygen uptake/oxygen supply dependency: fact or fiction? Acta Anaesthesiol Scand Suppl 107:229–237
16. Kreisberg RA (1980) Lactate homeostasis and lactic acidosis. Ann Intern Med 92:227–237
17. Kreisberg RA (1972) Glucose-lactate inter-relations in man. N Engl J Med 287:132–137
18. Rowell LB, Kraning KK 2nd, Evans TO, Kennedy JW, Blackmon JR, Kusumi F (1966) Splanchnic removal of lactate and pyruvate during prolonged exercise in man. J Appl Physiol 21:1773–1783
19. Yudkin J, Cohen RD (1975) The contribution of the kidney to the removal of a lactic acid load under normal and acidotic conditions in the conscious rat. Clin Sci Mol Med 48:121–131
20. Park R, Arieff AI (1980) Lactic acidosis. Adv Intern Med 25:33–68
21. Nordstrom L, Ingemarsson I, Westgren M (1996) Fetal monitoring with lactate. Baillieres Clin Obstet Gynaecol 10:225–242
22. Poole RC, Halestrap AP (1993) Transport of lactate and other monocarboxylates across mammalian plasma membranes. Am J Physiol 264:C761–C782

23. Daniel AM, Shizgal HM, MacLean LD (1978) The anatomic and metabolic source of lactate in shock. Surg Gynecol Obstet 147:697–700
24. Luchette FA, Friend LA, Brown CC, Upputuri RK, James JH (1998) Increased skeletal muscle Na+, K+-ATPase activity as a cause of increased lactate production after hemorrhagic shock. J Trauma 44:796–801
25. James JH, Luchette FA, McCarter FD, Fischer JE (1999) Lactate is an unreliable indicator of tissue hypoxia in injury or sepsis. Lancet 354:505–508
26. Halmagyi DF, Kennedy M, Varga D (1971) Combined adrenergic receptor blockade and circulating catecholamines in hemorrhagic shock. Eur Surg Res 3:378–388
27. Irving MH, Gillett DJ, Varga D, Halmagyi DF (1968) The effect of adrenergic blockade upon shock-induced lactic acidosis in sheep. Br J Surg 55:780–785
28. Halmagyi DF, Irving MH, Gillett DJ, Varga D (1967) Effect of adrenergic blockade on consequences of sustained epinephrine infusion. J Appl Physiol 23:171–177
29. McCarter FD, James JH, Luchette FA, et al (2001) Adrenergic blockade reduces skeletal muscle glycolysis and Na(+), K(+)-ATPase activity during hemorrhage. J Surg Res 99:235–244
30. Luchette FA, Robinson BR, Friend LA, McCarter F, Frame SB, James JH (1999) Adrenergic antagonists reduce lactic acidosis in response to hemorrhagic shock. J Trauma 46:873–880
31. Clutter WE, Bier DM, Shah SD, Cryer PE (1980) Epinephrine plasma metabolic clearance rates and physiologic thresholds for metabolic and hemodynamic actions in man. J Clin Invest 66:94–101
32. Podolin DA, Munger PA, Mazzeo RS (1991) Plasma catecholamine and lactate response during graded exercise with varied glycogen conditions. J Appl Physiol 71:1427–1433
33. Staten MA, Matthews DE, Cryer PE, Bier DM (1987) Physiological increments in epinephrine stimulate metabolic rate in humans. Am J Physiol 253:E322–E330
34. Mazzeo RS, Marshall P (1989) Influence of plasma catecholamines on the lactate threshold during graded exercise. J Appl Physiol 67:1319–1322
35. Levy B, Bollaert PE, Charpentier C, et al (1997) Comparison of norepinephrine and dobutamine to epinephrine for hemodynamics, lactate metabolism, and gastric tonometric variables in septic shock: a prospective, randomized study. Intensive Care Med 23:282–287
36. Meier-Hellmann A, Reinhart K, Bredle DL, Specht M, Spies CD, Hannemann L (1997) Epinephrine impairs splanchnic perfusion in septic shock. Crit Care Med 25:399–404
37. Salak N, Pajk W, Knotzer H, et al (2001) Effects of epinephrine on intestinal oxygen supply and mucosal tissue oxygen tension in pigs. Crit Care Med 29:367–373
38. Shram NF, Netchiporouk LI, Martelet C, Jaffrezic-Renault N, Bonnet C, Cespuglio R (1998) In vivo voltammetric detection of rat brain lactate with carbon fiber microelectrodes coated with lactate oxidase. Anal Chem 70:2618–2622
39. Kenausis G, Chen Q, Heller A (1997) Electrochemical glucose and lactate sensors based on "wired" thermostable soybean peroxidase operating continuously and stably at 37°C. Anal Chem 69:1054–1060
40. Morgan TJ, Clark C, Clagque A (1999) Artifactual elevation of measured plasma L-lactate concentration in the presence of glycolate. Crit Care Med. 27:2177–2179
41. Venkatesh B, Morgan T, Garrett P (2002) The lactate gap: Putting laboratory error to good use. Lancet (in press)
42. Hutchinson PJ, Al-Rawi PG, O'Connell MT, Gupta AK, Pickard JD, Kirkpatrick PJ (2000) Biochemical changes related to hypoxia during cerebral aneurysm surgery: combined microdialysis and tissue oxygen monitoring: case report. Neurosurgery 46:201–205
43. Hutchinson PJ, al-Rawi PG, O'Connell MT, et al (2000) Head injury monitoring using cerebral microdialysis and Paratrend multiparameter sensors. Zentralbl Neurochir 61:88–94
44. Marion DW (1999) Lactate and traumatic brain injury. Crit Care Med 27:2063–2064
45. Ellmerer M, Schaupp L, Trajanoski Z, et al (1998) Continuous measurement of subcutaneous lactate concentration during exercise by combining open-flow microperfusion and thin-film lactate sensors. Biosens Bioelectron 13:1007–1013
46. Marzouk SA, Cosofret VV, Buck RP, Yang H, Cascio WE, Hassen SS (1997) A conducting salt-based amperometric biosensor for measurement of extracellular lactate accumulation in ischemic myocardium. Anal Chem 69:2646–2652

47. Yang Q, Atanasov P, Wilkins E (1999) Needle-type lactate biosensor. Biosens Bioelectron 14:203–210

48. Ignatov SG, Ferguson JA, Walt DR (2001) A fiber-optic lactate sensor based on bacterial cytoplasmic membranes. Biosens Bioelectron 16:109–113

49. Zauner A, Doppenberg EM, Woodward JJ, Choi SC, Young HF, Bullock R (1997) Continuous monitoring of cerebral substrate delivery and clearance: initial experience in 24 patients with severe acute brain injuries. Neurosurgery 41:1082–1091

50. Evans C, Hsu F, Kosaka T (1934) Utilization of blood sugar and formation of lactic acid by the lungs. J Physiol 82:41–60

51. Rochester DF, Wichern WA Jr, Fritts HW Jr, et al (1973) Arteriovenous differences of lactate and pyruvate across healthy and diseased human lung. Am Rev Respir Dis 107:442–448

52. Kellum JA, Kramer DJ, Lee K, Mankad S, Bellomo R, Pinsky MR (1997) Release of lactate by the lung in acute lung injury. Chest 111:1301–1305

53. Roth RA, Reindel JF (1991) Lung vascular injury from monocrotaline pyrrole, a putative hepatic metabolite. Adv Exp Med Biol 283:477–487

54. Walker V, Bennet L, Mills GA, Green LR, Gnanakumaran K, Hanson MA (1996) Effects of hypoxia on urinary organic acid and hypoxanthine excretion in fetal sheep. Pediatr Res 40:309–318

55. Huang CC, Wang ST, Chang YC, Lin KP, Wu PL (1999) Measurement of the urinary lactate:creatinine ratio for the early identification of newborn infants at risk for hypoxic-ischemic encephalopathy. N Engl J Med 341:328–335

56. Naylor JM, Kronfeld DS, Freeman DE, Richardson D (1984) Hepatic and extrahepatic lactate metabolism in sheep: effects of lactate loading and pH. Am J Physiol 247:E747–E55

57. Lautt WW (1985) Mechanism and role of intrinsic regulation of hepatic arterial blood flow: hepatic arterial buffer response. Am J Physiol 249:G549–G56

58. Douzinas EE, Tsidemiadou PD, Pitaridis MT, et al (1997) The regional production of cytokines and lactate in sepsis-related multiple organ failure. Am J Respir Crit Care Med 155:53–59

59. De Backer D, Creteur J, Silva E, Vincent JL (2001) The hepatosplanchnic area is not a common source of lactate in patients with severe sepsis. Crit Care Med 29:256–261

60. Goodman JC, Gopinath SP, Valadka AB, et al (1996) Lactic acid and amino acid fluctuations measured using microdialysis reflect physiological derangements in head injury. Acta Neurochir Suppl (Wien) 67:37–39

61. Goodman JC, Valadka AB, Gopinath SP, Uzura M, Robertson CS (1999) Extracellular lactate and glucose alterations in the brain after head injury measured by microdialysis. Crit Care Med 27:1965–1973

62. Goodman JC, Valadka AB, Gopinath SP, Cormio M, Robertson CS (1996) Lactate and excitatory amino acids measured by microdialysis are decreased by pentobarbital coma in head-injured patients. J Neurotrauma 13:549–556

63. Halestrap AP, Wang X, Poole RC, Jackson VN, Price NT (1997) Lactate transport in heart in relation to myocardial ischemia. Am J Cardiol 80:17A–25A

64. Gorge G, Papageorgiou I, Lerch R (1990) Epinephrine-stimulated contractile and metabolic reserve in postischemic rat myocardium. Basic Res Cardiol 85:595–605

65. Orita H, Fukasawa M, Hirooka S, Minowa T, Uchino H, Washio M (1993) Prevention of postischemic reperfusion injury: the improvement of myocardial tissue blood flow after ischemia by terminal nicorandil-Mg cardioplegia. Surg Today 23:344–349

66. Brooks GA (2001) Lactate doesn't necessarily cause fatigue: why are we surprised? J Physiol 536:1

67. Juel C (1997) Lactate-proton cotransport in skeletal muscle. Physiol Rev 77:321–358

68. O'Keefe GE, Hawkins K, Boynton J, Burns D (2001) Indicators of fatigue and of prolonged weaning from mechanical ventilation in surgical patients. World J Surg 25:98–103

69. Connett RJ, Gayeski TE, Honig CR (1986) Lactate efflux is unrelated to intracellular PO2 in a working red muscle in situ. J Appl Physiol 61:402–408

70. Hotchkiss RS, Karl IE (1992) Reevaluation of the role of cellular hypoxia and bioenergetic failure in sepsis. JAMA 267:1503–1510

71. Schlichtig R, Bowles SA (1994) Distinguishing between aerobic and anaerobic appearance of dissolved CO2 in intestine during low flow. J Appl Physiol 76:2443–2451
72. Mizock BA (2001) The hepatosplanchnic area and hyperlactatemia: A tale of two lactates. Crit Care Med 29:447–449
73. Gaglio G (1886) Die Milchsaure des Blutes und ihre Urssprungsstatten. Arch Anat Physiol Abt 10:400–414
74. Cannon W (1918) Acidosis in shock. Bull Med Paris 1:424–428
75. Clausen S (1922) A method for the determination of small amounts of lactic acid. J Biol Chem 52:262–280
76. Huckabee W (1961) Abnormal resting blood lactate:I. The significance of hyperlactatemia in hospitalised patients. Am J Med 30:833–839
77. Cohen R, Woods H (1976) Clinical and Biochemical Aspects of Lactic Acidosis. Blackwell Scientific Publications, Boston

Oxygen Delivery

Oxygen Delivery and the Critically Ill

M. M. Jonas and C. B. Wolff

"If a treatment cannot ethically be withheld
then clearly no controlled trial can be instituted".
A. B. Hill, 1951 [1]

Introduction

Several well-conducted, randomized clinical trials have unambiguously shown a survival benefit when critically ill patients have early cardiovascular manipulations as a treatment strategy. Increased cardiac output and oxygen delivery (DO_2) in selected patients reduces mortality and morbidity significantly.

The case for optimization of DO_2 in surgical patients has been made sufficiently strongly both by the trials reviewed in this chapter and by the analyses of others, to suggest that optimization of these high risk patients is a treatment known to have a significant positive impact on survival. Further trials involving surgical patients with non-optimized controls may no longer be ethically acceptable or appropriate. Perhaps the focus for research, especially with the new technologies available, needs to be redirected. Future studies need to address which particular parts of the optimization protocols are important, why this is physiologically possible, and whether these goals or alternative strategies are applicable to other, non-surgical, groups of critically ill patients.

Oxygen Delivery

DO_2 represents the total flow of oxygen in the arterial blood. For the whole body this is given as the product of the cardiac output and the arterial oxygen content. The rate of arrival of oxygen has to be greater than the rate of uptake (VO_2). It is less obvious as to what extent the DO_2 must exceed VO_2, except that there must be a gradient of oxygen to permit diffusion from the arterial blood supply into the metabolizing tissue. Tissues differ in the gradient they need. In terms of oxygen extraction (VO_2/DO_2) skeletal muscle and heart manage to extract around 60% of the oxygen delivered, whereas brain only manages around 30%. For the kidney, the extraction is less than 10% unless overall flow is compromised.

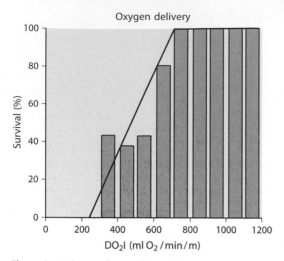

Fig. 1. Survival rates of surgical patients in the first 8 hours post-operatively relating to oxygen delivery index (DO$_2$I). DO$_2$I values above 600 ml/min/m^2 were then used as a therapeutic strategy both during, and subsequently prior to, surgery. The high delivery provided for the increase in oxygen consumption that occurs during surgery (an increase of around 30% in the uncomplicated general surgical postoperative patient) (redrawn after [2])

▌ Clinical Relevance

Shoemaker in a review of his initial studies [2] concluded that, with certain provisos, achieving a targeted DO$_2$ index (DO$_2$I) of 600 ml/min/m^2, reduced mortality and morbidity in high-risk surgical patients. This study retrospectively assessed the relative importance of monitored variables in survivors and non-survivors. The findings were that survival was strongly associated with cardiac output, DO$_2$ and VO$_2$ – i.e., the determinants of oxygen flux. These were patients who had pulmonary artery occlusion pressure (PAOP)-guided volume resuscitation and were mechanically ventilated. In addition hematocrit (Hct) was maintained above 30% and dubutamine was used to increase cardiac output until the target DO$_2$I and other goals were reached.

Figure 1 shows that, for an early series, all patients with a DO$_2$I of 600 ml/min/m^2, or greater, during the 8-hour period following surgery survived. Further series suggested that a predictive index based on DO$_2$I, VO$_2$I and cardiac index (CI) in non-cardiac, high-risk, general surgical patients could predict outcome in 94% of patients [4]. More recent studies have supported this concept, that achieving adequate DO$_2$ as an 'optimizing' procedure preoperatively in high-risk surgical patients, saves lives and reduces morbidity [4–6].

▌ Intravascular Volume and Fluid Transfusion

In Shoemaker's patients, transfusion with colloid for intravascular depletion was accompanied by an increase in CI, mean arterial pressure (MAP), VO$_2$I and DO$_2$I. The observed increase in VO$_2$ implied that there must have been a latent oxygen dept due to an inadequate DO$_2$ to the tissues. Additionally inotrope administration prior to

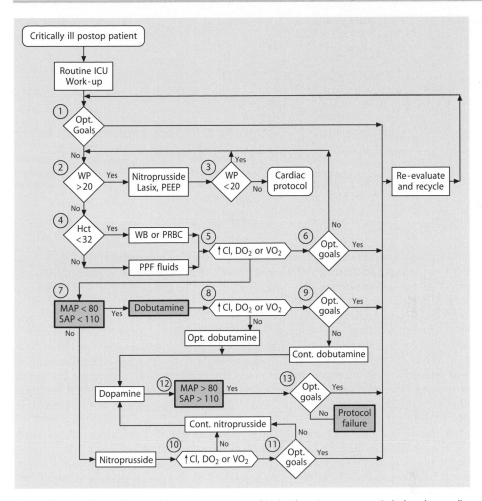

Fig. 2. Shoemaker's overall protocol for the management of high-risk patients postoperatively, based on earlier outcome figures and prior to his pre-operative intervention trial [3]. Optimal goals were CI > 4.5 l/min/m², $DO_2I > 600$ ml O_2/min/m² and $VO_2I > 160$ ml O_2/min/m². PAOP was used as an assessment of intravascular filling. Blood was given to maintain a Hct of 32%, otherwise a volume challenge was used (specifically colloid not crystalloid) and the goals re-assessed. If targeted values were not met, dobutamine was used as the inotrope for low pressure states and nitroprusside when pressures were normal. Dopamine was used for inotrope supplementation (redrawn after [2]). SAP: systolic arterial pressure; WB: whole blood; PRBC: packed red blood cells; WP: wedge pressure

fluid resuscitation lead to marked hemodynamic instability, a situation not found in patients who were adequately filled. These findings emphasize that an adequate blood volume was a prerequisite for other interventions to be effective. But the question of how to assess the adequacy of intravascular expansion is a matter of debate. Shoemaker used PAOP to assess volume adequacy necessitating right heart catheterization. The protocol in Figure 2 outlines the methods used in that trial for optimization.

The use of pulmonary artery catheters for estimation of cardiac output and PAOP for estimation of vascular filling has become increasingly controversial [7].

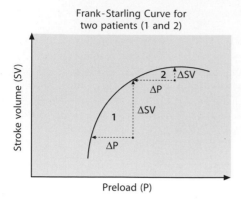

Fig. 3. Two hypothetical patients, 1 and 2 on different portions of their Starling curves. Patient 1 on the steep part of the curve responds with a significant increase in stroke volume as compared with patient 2 on the flat portion for an identical increase in preload

Additionally, several studies have documented the poor correlation of PAOP with left ventricular end-diastolic volume (LVEDV). The implication is that PAOP only provides qualitative assessment of over- or under-filling, i.e., high or low values, intermediate values are difficult to interpret [8, 9]. Increasingly the traditional measures of preload have been considered to be too coarse for an accurate assessment of intravascular filling, especially if used as endpoints for 'titrated' resuscitation – i.e., fluid boluses titrated to a clinical response. This introduces the concept of 'preload responsiveness' where a fluid challenge leads to an increase in cardiac output, and preload unresponsiveness, where a similar challenge gives no change in cardiac output, or even a decrease. The physiological mechanism for the potential hemodynamic response to an increased preload depends on the position of the patient on the Starling curve (Fig. 3).

Dynamic assessment of preload responsiveness requires the ability to estimate cardiac output on a beat by beat basis. Until recently, the majority of cardiac output technologies generated estimates of flow in a time domain too slow to observe dynamic cardiovascular effects in response to fluid challenges. Mythen and Webb [10] used the esophageal Doppler as a semi-continuous guide to plasma volume expansion using colloid boluses. In their study the protocol group received colloid boluses during cardiac surgery to maximize the stroke volume. Outcome was improved in the protocol group, as were indices of splanchnic perfusion. Similar studies are underway using a continuous technology – lithium calibrated, arterial pulse power analysis technology (LiDCO/PulseCO) which has recently become available to calculate continuous DO_2. This system uses an algorithm which calculates cardiac output on a real time basis from the arterial waveform (Jonas et al., unpublished data, [11, 12]). The PulseCO algorithm also measures arterial pressure variations in response to mechanical ventilation. In positive pressure ventilation the increase in intrathoracic pressure transiently decreases preload and therefore cardiac output. These pressure variations have to be measured real time and are represented as stroke volume variation (SVV), systolic pressure variation (SPV), and pulse pressure variation (PPV). Stroke volume variation is the reduction in left ventricular stroke volume (LVSV) associated with reduced venous return during positive pressure ventilation. PPV is defined as the maximum pulse pressure minus the minimum, divided by the average of these two pressures. SPV is the difference between the maximum and minimum systolic pressures following inspiration. These arterial pressure changes give valuable information about preload responsiveness and volemic state [13–15].

Figure 3 can again be used as a physiological explanation, except this time in reverse. The degree to which LVSV decreases during mechanical ventilation is related to the slope of the curve and the inspiratory pressure with its associated reduction in preload. Patient 1 would exhibit far larger arterial pressure variations being on the steeper part of the curve than patient 2 (i.e., patient 1 would be preload responsive and patient 2 being on the flat part of the curve would be unresponsive.) In this mode the ventilator could be used diagnostically as a dynamic test of a patient's cardiovascular performance and Starling relationship by graded alterations in tidal volume and end-expiratory pressure.

Inotropes and Optimization

Subsequent to Shoemaker's studies, Boyd et al. [4] revisited the augmentation of DO_2 in high-risk surgical patients. In this study, both the control and the protocol group blood volume was adjusted with colloid using PAOP as a guide (12–14 mmHg), urine flow (to 100 ml/h), and an assessment of cardiac index was made. Hb was raised to 120 g/l (Hct 32%) and supplementary oxygen given if $SaO_2 < 94\%$. Additionally the protocol group received dopexamine augmentation if DO_2I was less than 600 ml/min/m^2 but stopped if: i) the target was reached; ii) there was chest pain, or ST segment depression; or iii) the heart rate increased by more than 20 beats per min.

Twenty of the 53 patients in the protocol group required dopexamine and, on average, the protocol group patients were close to targeted values. Although there was no significant reduction in length of hospital stay, there were significant reductions in mortality and complications.

The rationale for using dopexamine was its ability to increase cardiac output without increasing cardiac oxygen consumption, coupled with increased renal, hepatic and splanchnic flows. The beneficial effects in the protocol group were attributed to the perioperative increase in DO_2 with dopexamine.

The sparing effect of dopexamine on renal and splanchnic flows may explain the much better effect obtained when improving DO_2I with dopexamine than with epinephrine in a third major study (by Wilson, et al. [5]). Although epinephrine increases cardiac output and therefore DO_2, the question arises as to whether the redistribution of flow is detrimental. It has been shown by an analysis of the study of Koskolou et al. [16] that, in sub-maximal exercise in normal subjects (up to half-maximial exercise), tissues other than muscle suffer no decrement in flow when arterial oxygen content (CaO_2) is normal. However, when CaO_2 is low, blood is diverted away from the non-exercising tissues. This compensation allows the exercising muscle to have the same DO_2 for a given metabolic rate. Epinephrine is known to increase muscle blood flow [17]. The increase in muscle blood flow in patients treated with epinephrine will, however, be surplus to muscle oxygen demand and requirements. It is probable that when DO_2 is increased with epinephrine that mal-distribution of the augmented cardiac output occurs because of muscle vascular bed vasodilatation and splanchnic and renal vasoconstriction. Dopexamine may improve organ function by increasing splanchnic, hepatic and renal flow. It may also improve distribution elsewhere, for example, the immune system.

In the Wilson study [5] the target DO_2 was again 600 ml/min/m^2 and was achieved in a higher proportion of the dopexamine-treated patients (mean DO_2 665 ml/min/m^2) than in the protocol group of Boyd et al. [4], probably because Wilson et al. allowed a heart rate increase of up to 30 beats per min (compared with only 20). Gastro-intestinal complications were virtually absent in the dopexamine group. In contrast, Bennett-Guerrero et al. [18] showed that gastro-intestinal dysfunction was the commonest post-operative problem in patients whose hospital stay was prolonged after having routine moderate-risk elective surgery. It would be tempting to suggest gastro-intestinal dysfunction could result from poor splanchnic oxygen delivery with diversion of blood flow away from the gut. Dopexamine may spare, or enhance, splanchnic blood flow and improve gastro-intestinal function in such patients [19].

▌ Assessment of Results: Empirical and Physiological

Surgical Optimization

Table 1 gives an overview of the mortality and morbidity for the three definitive studies of optimization in high-risk surgical patients discussed in the text. All of the studies show a significant survival benefit with optimization of cardiac preload and DO_2.

A recent UK consensus meeting [6] concluded that "There is a group of surgical patients whose post-operative mortality is 15–30% as compared to the surgical population as a whole whose mortality is 1%. For any given surgical insult, the only factor that can be easily influenced is their cardio-respiratory physiology. If this is optimized, the effects can be dramatic, in terms of improving outcome." Grocott et al. recently completed a meta-analysis of 12 published and peer reviewed papers with an odds ratio which supported the use of goal-directed flow values in the surgical population (unpublished data).

Severe Sepsis and Septic Shock

In the study by Rivers et al. [20], septic patients were given early goal-directed therapy with algorithmic adjustment of central venous pressure (CVP), MAP and central venous oxygen saturation ($ScvO_2$). The target aim was to improve oxygenation and attempt to increase central venous saturation toward normal values.

Table 1. Effects of DO_2 optimization on mortality and morbidity in high-risk surgical patients (see text)

	Mortality		Inotrope	Morbidity
	Control group (%)	Protocol group (%)		
Shoemaker et al. (1988) [3]	35	12.5	Dobutamine	Reduced
Boyd et al. (1993) [4]	22.2	5.7	Dopexamine	Reduced
Wilson et al. (1999) [5]	17	3	Dopexamine/ epinephrine	Least with dopexamine

Severe sepsis is associated with exaggerated oxygen extraction and consumption. A low venous oxygen saturation would reflect an inadequate cardiac output and DO_2 relative to requirements. Normal values for VO_2, CI, DO_2 and venous oxygen saturation were given in an earlier study by the same group in which normal subjects were compared with patients with chronic congestive cardiac failure (CCF) [21]. The chronic CCF patients had adapted to their low cardiac output state and down-regulated their metabolism. These patients increased oxygen extraction to compensate for a low cardiac output. For patients with sepsis the metabolic rate (VO_2) is acutely raised and unlike the CCF group, septic patients are not in a position to down-regulate their metabolism. Rivers et al. [20] used this as a rational and a prompt for early, targeted therapies, to increasing low $ScvO_2$ values.

The relationship between SvO_2 and the provision of an adequate oxygen supply involves some modest calculations and acceptance that there is a relationship between SvO_2 and $ScvO_2$. Oxygen extraction ($E = VO_2/DO_2$) is also equal to (arteriovenous saturation difference)/SaO_2. This is because cardiac output is part of both numerator and denominator. The higher the SvO_2 the less the oxygen extraction. This also means that more oxygen is delivered for a given oxygen consumption. Table 2 gives values for $ScvO_2$ and the arterio-venous oxygen difference (a-v diff.) from [19] for patients in whom early goal-directed therapy aimed to achieve an $ScvO_2$ of 70% or more. Values are also given for control patients not receiving goal-directed therapy and also for the normal subjects studied by the same investigators [21].

The table gives values for E (oxygen extraction) and shows that it is similar for the protocol group and normal subjects. It is possible to calculate also how much DO_2 is required per liter consumption (1/E) and find that the protocol and normal subjects deliver 3.9 and 3.7 liters of oxygen in the arterial blood per liter of oxygen consumed. The control sepsis patients only provided 3.25 liters oxygen per litre consumption. With similar oxygen-carrying capacity this amounts to higher cardiac outputs in normal subjects and protocol patients than in the sepsis control patients. DO_2 and cardiac output are only around 20% greater (3.9/3.25). Despite this apparently marginal difference, Rivers et al. [20] found a highly significant improvement in mortality (30.5% protocol patients; 46.5% controls, $p < 0.01$). Morbidity was also reduced in the protocol patients compared with controls.

Table 2. Mean central venous oxygen saturation ($ScvO_2$) results of Rivers et al. [21] in septic patients, to demonstrate oxygen extraction (E) and the ratio of oxygen delivery (DO_2) to oxygen consumption (1/E) assuming an SaO_2 of 96%. Absolute values of VO_2 and DO_2 depend on absolute value of cardiac output and Hb. Normal values taken from Rady et al. [21] for their control normal subjects (SaO_2 given as 94%)

	$ScvO_2$ (%)	a-v diff. (ml·dl^{-1})	E {=[(a-v) ÷ a]} (%)	$DO_2 ÷ VO_2$ {= 100 ÷ E}
Protocol	70.4	25.6	26.7	3.9
Control	65.3	30.7	32.0	3.25
Normal	67	27	28.9	3.7

a = SaO_2; v = SvO_2; a-v diff. = arterio-venous difference. E = oxygen extraction (%). Similar oxygen extraction values are obtained from textbook values of arterial oxygen content values (arterial 19.1 ml/dl blood and an arterio-venous content difference of 5 ml/dl: namely 26.3%, indicating an oxygen delivery 3.8 times the oxygen consumption

Table 3. Documented values from the studies of Shoemaker et al. [3] and Boyd et al. [4] including calculated values oxygen extraction (E) and 1/E (volume of oxygen delivered per unit volume of oxygen consumption). The hematocrit (Hct) as %, and the mixed venous oxygen saturation (SvO_2) are also given

	Shoemaker et al. 1988 preoptimization – Post-op. values (optimized in protocol group) [3]		Boyd et al. 1993 Pre-op. values (optimized in protocol group) [4]		Boyd et al. 1993 Post-op. values [4]	
	Protocol	Control	Protocol	Control	Protocol	Control
CI (l/min)	4.5	3.95	4.0	2.6	3.5	3.0
DO_2 (ml/min)	598	508	597	399	537	448
VO_2 (ml/min)	148	135	134	126	124	121
Hct (%)	32.6	31.5	36.7	37.3	37.7	36.3
E (%)	24.75	26.59	22.4	31.6	23.1	27
1/E	4	3.8	4.5	3.2	4.3	3.7
SvO_2 (%)	73	71	74	66	74	73

SvO_2, $ScvO_2$, DO_2 and VO_2 in Optimization Studies

Reanalysis of the surgical optimization trials [3–5] and where possible comparisons of DO_2, VO_2 and the DO_2 per unit VO_2 similarly to the above analysis of the Rivers study in sepsis [20] is informative. Representative values are available for Shoemaker et al. [3] and values immediately post-optimization and postoperatively for Boyd et al. [4]. These are given in Table 3. The values for DO_2 given in the Wilson et al. study [5] appeared adequate for both their epinephrine group and their dopexamine group ($DO_2 I > 600$ ml/min/m^2) although VO_2 was not recorded. From Table 3 the protocol groups in both studies [2, 3] achieved a DO_2 close to 600 ml/min/m^2 though this fell in the later stages postoperatively in the patients in the study by Boyd et al. [4].

The DO_2/VO_2 ratio (delivery per unit consumption) was 4 or more in the protocol groups and was lower in the controls. As noted in both studies the protocol groups had much-improved outcomes. The values for SvO_2 do, however, raise a note of caution since they are all above 70%, the target in the Rivers et al. study [20]. This could occur where there was inadequate DO_2, such that the VO_2 is grossly reduced, as was the case in the control groups in both the Shoemaker et al. [3] and the Boyd et al. [4] studies (Table 3).

▌ Conclusion

All of the reviewed studies arrive at the same explicit conclusion, a $DO_2 I > 600$ ml/min/m^2 in surgical patients is associated with a significantly lower mortality. Additionally, augmented DO_2, if achieved early in the course of illness, may influence outcome in refractory situations such as severe sepsis.

New, less invasive, technologies providing the combination of beat by beat measurement of cardiac output, DO_2 and preload responsiveness, offer the opportunity to translate the statistics and findings of these studies into clinical practice.

For the future, further studies are needed to examine the specific roles of types of intravenous fluids, optimum hemoglobin concentration, inotropes and vasodilators in the process of DO_2 optimization. For the present however, in the face of convincing scientific evidence, the question arises, why we are not routinely targeting DO in all critically ill patients?

References

1. Hill AB (1951) The clinical trial. Br Med Bull 7:278–282
2. Shoemaker WC (1990) Monitoring and management of the high risk surgical patient. Care Crit Ill 6:39–47
3. Shoemaker WC, Appel PL, Kram HB, Waxman K, Lee TS (1988) Prospective trial of supranormal values of survivors as therapeutic goals in high risk surgical patients. Chest 94:1176–1186
4. Boyd O, Grounds RM, Bennett D, et al (1993) A randomized clinical trial of the effect of deliberate perioperative increase of oxygen delivery on mortality in high-risk surgical patients. JAMA 270:2699–2707
5. Wilson J, Woods I, Fawcett J, et al (1999) Reducing the risk of major elective surgery: randomised controlled trial of preoperative optimisation of oxygen delivery. Br Med J 318:1099–1103
6. Grocott MPW, Ball JAS (2000) Consensus meeting: management of the high risk surgical patient. Int J Crit Care Med 11 (Special report):1–19
7. Connors AF, Speroff T, Sawson NV, et al (1996) The effectiveness of right heart catheterization in the initial care of critically ill patients. JAMA 276:889–897
8. Godje O, Peyerl M, Seebauer T, et al (1998) Central venous pressure, pulmonary capillary wedge pressure, and intrathoracic blood volumes as preload indicators in cardiac surgical patients. Eur J Cardiothorac Surg 13:533–539
9. Ellis RJ, Mangano DT, Van Dyke DC (1979) Relationship of wedge pressure to end-diastolic volume in patients undergoing myocardial revascularization. J Thorac Cardiovasc Surg 78:605–613
10. Mythen MG, Webb AR (1995) Perioperative plasma volume expansion reduces the incidence of gut mucosal hypoperfusion during cardiac surgery. Arch Surg 130:423–429
11. Band DM, Linton RA, O'Brien TK, Jonas MM, Linton NW (1997) Measurement of cardiac output. J Physiol 498:225–229
12. Linton R, Band DM, Jonas MM, et al (1997) Lithium dilution cardiac output: A comparison with thermodilution. Crit Care Med 25:1796–1800
13. Tavernier B, Makhotine O, Lebuffe G, et al (1998) Systolic pressure variation as a guide to fluid therapy in patients with sepsis-induced hypotension. Anesthesiology 89:1313–1321
13. Michard F, Boussat S, Chemla D, et al (2000) Relation between respiratory changes in arterial pulse pressure and fluid responsiveness in septic patients with acute circulatory failure. Am J Respir Crit Care Med 162:134–138
15. Michard F, Chemla D, Richard C (1999) Clinical use of respiratory changes in arterial pulse pressure to monitor the hemodynamic effects of PEEP. Am J Respir Crit Care Med 159:935–939
16. Koskolou MD, Roach RC, et al (1997) Cardiovascular responses to dynamic exercise with acute anemia in humans. Am J Physiol 273:H1783–H1793
17. Barcroft H, Swan HJC (1953) Sympathetic Control of Human Blood Vessels. Edward Arnold & Co, London
18. Bennett-Guerrero E, Welsby I, Dunn TJ, et al (1999) The use of a postoperative morbidity survey to evaluate patients with prolonged hospitalization after routine, moderate risk, elective surgery. Anesth Analg 89:514–519
19. Smithies M, Yee TH, Jackson L, et al (1994) Protecting the gut and the liver in the critically ill: effects of dopexamine. Crit Care Med 22:789–795
20. Rivers E, Nguyen B, Havstad S, et al (2001) Early goal-directed therapy in the treatment of severe sepsis and septic shock. N Engl J Med 345:1368–1377
21. Rady M, Jafry S, Rivers E, Alexander M (1994) Characterization of systemic oxygen transport in end-stage chronic congestive heart failure. Am Heart J 128:774–781

Monitoring Intensive Care Patients

M. Poeze and G. Ramsay

▋ Introduction

Hemodynamic monitoring is one of the important reasons for patients to be admitted to the intensive care unit (ICU). The first patients were monitored and treated on an ICU during the polio epidemic [1]. Since then major advances have been made in monitoring the critically ill patient, especially after the introduction of intravascular pressure- and flow-recording catheters in the 1970s [1]. Nowadays, intensivists frequently use invasive hemodynamic monitoring, including intra-arterial, pulmonary artery, and central venous catheters to guide therapeutic interventions. Recent studies have directed the intensivist to the use of less-invasive modalities, because of the complications, such as thrombosis and catheter-related sepsis, which are related to the use of invasive techniques [2–5].

Studies aimed at improving the outcome of critically ill and surgical patients have emphasized the importance of better monitoring, better use of monitoring, and early use of monitoring techniques [6]. In patients, who do not yet have complications, but are at an increased risk of developing complications, it seems to be justified to use more invasive hemodynamic monitoring. However, with more widespread use of additional monitoring techniques, a balance should be found between the use of more invasive monitoring techniques with its added information, but also increased complications, and the use of less invasive techniques with fewer complications.

Progress in monitoring technology that has been made in recent decades are related to a change in focus on which parameters should be used. This focus has changed in relation to increasing knowledge concerning the pathophysiology of shock and organ failure. Originally, monitoring was aimed at measuring blood pressure and heart rate. Introduction of invasive monitoring techniques changed this focus to monitoring of cardiac output and pressure-related parameters (wedge pressure) and derived parameters (systemic vascular resistance) – global level of monitoring. Pathophysiological studies, subsequently focused on shock as being an imbalance between oxygen consumption (VO_2) and oxygen delivery (DO_2) in the tissues, instead of a low blood pressure [7]. The use of DO_2 and VO_2 as a goal of hemodynamic optimization instead of pressure-related parameters changed the focus to measuring DO_2 and VO_2 [8]. It appeared that some organ systems are more vulnerable to such an imbalance than other organs. More attention was thus paid to the dysfunction of individual organs during sepsis and shock – organ level of monitoring. The function of the hepatosplanchnic organs was especially used as a monitoring tool. Numerous techniques to assess the function of, and the perfusion through, the hepatosplanchnic organs were developed.

Newer developments focus on the assessment of the microcirculation and mitochondrial function during sepsis and organ failure – cellular level [9]. Techniques for monitoring these systems have been developed, but have, as yet, not been validated for clinical use in septic patients and will not be discussed in this chapter. Several of the monitoring techniques at various levels – from global to regional level – are discussed. The discussion focuses on the use of minimally-invasive and regional monitoring techniques, and addresses technical aspects and the clinical studies published so far.

Global Level of Monitoring: Invasive

Pulmonary Artery Thermodilution Catheter (PAC)

Pulmonary artery, or Swan-Ganz, catheterization was first used in 1970 in patients with acute heart disease. Since that time, this technique has been widely used in cardiac and non-cardiac diseases. The pulmonary artery catheter (PAC) provides global hemodynamic information with accurate assessment of the cardiac output and left ventricular filling pressures. The application of these variables led to new insights into the pathophysiology of shock.

The PAC, which has a balloon at the tip of the catheter, can be advanced through the subclavian, jugular, brachial, or femoral veins. The tip of the PAC lies in the pulmonary artery and closes off one of the branches of this artery when the balloon is inflated (wedge position).

The main variables which can be measured using the PAC are the stroke volume, using a temperature sensor at the tip of the catheter, pulmonary artery pressure (PAP), central venous pressure (CVP), and pulmonary capillary wedge pressure (PCWP) or pulmonary artery occlusion pressure (PAOP), using the balloon at the tip of the catheter. The other variables that can be assessed using the PAC are derived variables and include the cardiac output, systemic and pulmonary vascular resistance (SVR and PVR), left ventricle stroke work index (LVSWI), and right ventricle stroke work index (RVSWI).

In many studies, Swan-Ganz catheter measured parameters are used as 'golden standard', the method to which all other methods are compared. Despite this, the invasive nature of the PAC technique, as well as the validity of the derived parameters, has fostered dissatisfaction with the technique. The complications associated with PAC include thrombosis (0–1.4%), arrhythmia (1.3–1.5%), pneumothorax (1%), and catheter-related sepsis (1%) [2–4]. Moreover, the recent retrospective study by Connors et al. [5] suggested that a significant increase in mortality was associated with the use of the PAC via mechanisms as yet undefined. Subsequently other techniques were developed using less invasive or completely non-invasive methods to determine the cardiovascular status.

Other methods were also deployed to improve the application of the thermodilution method, 'injectionless' cold thermodilution and continuous heat-induced thermodilution [10, 11]. The latter technique uses the traditional thermodilution technique, but uses conduction of warmth instead of cold, and energy conduction instead of fluid. The part of the catheter in the right ventricle is wrapped with warmth filaments. These filaments release warmth into the circulation in a computer-based repetitive on-off sequence. These data are computerized by cross-correlating the input sequence and the measured temperature changes, thereby creating a classical thermodilution curve. The method measures cardiac output continuously, is less influenced by arrhythmia and ventilation, and reduces the volume added during the measurements. 'Injectionless' cold thermodilution also reduces the volume of fluids added [10]. The catheter has an extra balloon proximally on the catheter, into which cold fluid can be injected. After the cold wave has spread from the balloon, the fluid can be withdrawn. This technique significantly reduces the risk of infection.

Double Indicator Dilution Method

Technique. The thermal-dye dilution method (double-dilution method) uses two different injected indicators, i.e., a bolus of ice-cold water and a bolus of indocyanine green (ICG), to create dilution curves. The indicators are injected into a central venous site, similar to the Swan-Ganz thermodilution method and the dilution is measured at one point in the arterial circulation. Usually for this purpose, a specialized fiberoptic-thermistor catheter is inserted through the femoral artery into the descending aorta. The fiberoptic catheter is connected to a fiberoptic densitometer module which measures ICG light absorption at a wave length of 805 NM. Studies have shown that the cardiac output has a good correlation when comparing the thermodilution and dye-dilution method [12].

The principle of the double indicator dilution method is based on the principle that a central venous injected indicator always mixes with the greatest volume available and that after relevant dilution of the indicator it is not possible to re-concentrate. The ice-cold water bolus mingles with the end-diastolic volumes of the right atrium and is then transported further to the right ventricle where it dilutes further into the right-ventricular end-diastolic volume (RVEDV, Fig. 1). The injected indicator then continues through the lungs, the end-diastolic volume of the left atrium and ventricle. The volumes of the vessels between the heart and the lungs play a small role as volume constants in the calculations. Using the cold bolus, the extravascular volumes can be determined. The cold saline bolus can, as a result of heat conduction (convection) also distribute to the extravascular space, depending on the surface and time available for exchange. As the heat exchange area in the lungs

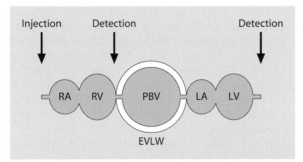

Fig. 1. Schematic depiction of the mixing chambers in the cardiopulmonary system. This schema depicts the flow trajectory of the cold indocyanine green (ICG) bolus through the cardiopulmonary system. The ICG is injection before the right atrium (RA), after which it flows through the right ventricle (RV), pulmonary blood volume (PBV), left atrium (LA), and left ventricle (LV). The ICG remains intravascularly, but the cold bolus extends into the extravascular lung space. When subtracting the volume measured by the ICG from the volume measured, the extravascular lung water volume can be calculated. The measurement sites are the pulmonary artery and the femoral artery. This enables the calculation of the different volumes and cardiac output (see Fig. 2)

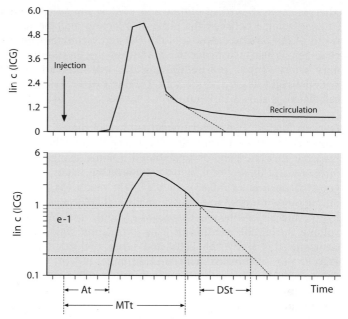

Fig. 2. Schematic depiction of the dilution curves and their analysis for transit times. Specific volumes can be calculated by multiplying the cardiac output by the characteristic transit times: the mean transit times (MTt) and the exponential downslope time (DSt). The result of the CO and the MTt is the volume covered by the relevant indicator, i.e., the volume between the place of injection and the place of measurement. The result of the CO and the DSt is the volume of the largest mixing chamber in the temperature distance covered by the indicator. For example: PBV = DSt dye-dilution arterial times CO thermodilution arterial

is more than 1000 times larger than that of the heart chambers and large vessels, the cold wave also spreads into the extra-vascular volume of the lungs. The ICG dilutes intravascularly only, and, by subtracting the volumes measured by the two different injected indicators, the difference between intra-vascular and extra-vascular volumes can be calculated.

ICG is a non-toxic and well-tolerated dye that binds immediately after injection into the blood stream to plasma proteins, which have a molecular weight of $> 70\,000$ kDa. These plasma proteins remain intravascular for more than 99.9%, even in the presence of severe capillary leakage.

Besides measuring cardiac output, specific volumes can be calculated from each indicators's dilution using the measured mean transit time (MTt) and the exponential downslope time (DSt) (Fig. 2). The MTt is composed of the appearance time, At (time between injection and the time until the first appearance of the indicator), and the mean time difference (dt) between the occurrence of the first indicator and completion of the indicator flow:

$$MTt = At + \frac{\int_0^\infty c \cdot (t - At) \cdot dt}{\int_0^\infty c_i \cdot dt}$$

The resultant of cardiac output and MTt is the volume covered by the indicator, i.e., the volume between the place of injection and the place of measurement. The result of the cardiac output and the DSt represents the volume of the largest mixing chamber. When measuring the MTt from the thermodilution curve in the pulmonary artery (Tdpa) and multiplying this with the cardiac output measured at this site, the right heart end-diastolic volume can be calculated. Other parameters are calculated as shown in Figure 2.

Previous Studies. Two experimental studies in piglets assessed the accuracy and reproducibility of measuring the circulating blood volume [13, 14]. In the first study [13] the measurement of total blood volume using ICG was compared with the measurement of the total blood volume using Evans blue and was found to have a good correlation ($r^2 = 0.83$). In the other study [14] the relation between cardiac output and intrathoracic blood volume (ITBV) was investigated during normo-, hypo-, and hypervolemia. There was a good correlation of the ITBV with the stroke volume during all conditions. This correlation was confirmed in critically ill patients. In this study the ITBV and other preload dependent variables, CVP and PCWP, were compared with preload independent variables, cardiac index (CI), DO_2, and SVR. The authors concluded that ITBV is a suitable indicator of circulating blood volume. In another study in critically ill patients, Haller et al. [15] found an excellent correlation between the cardiac output measured using standard thermodilution and ICG-dilution ($r^2 = 0.91$).

ICG measures plasma volume independently from the disappearance rate from plasma in critically ill patients, unless there is a severe generalized protein capillary leakage [16]. During severe sepsis and inflammation, microvascular damage in the lungs leads to generalized capillary protein leakage. This protein leakage attracts fluid into the interstitium of the lungs, thereby increasing the extravascular lung water (EVLW). Fluid management during critical illness must be aimed at improving perfusion, but may have the disadvantage in severe inflammation that major fluid shifts occur to the extravascular space. To optimize the amount of infusion needed for adequate perfusion and the amount of fluid which can induce failure of the heart, measurement of EVLW can be important. EVLW can be adequately assessed using the double indicator dilution method. Fluid management in critically ill patients using EVLW as a parameter, compared to using CVP, improved outcome (decreased ventilatory days and length of ICU stay). This was associated with a decrease in EVLW in the EVLW-guided treatment group [17]. The predictive value of these double indicator dilution parameters is not known at present.

▌ Global Level of Monitoring: Non-invasive

Doppler Ultrasound

Technique. The Doppler monitor, described in the early 1970s, provides a safe and minimally invasive means of continuously monitoring the global hemodynamic status. The Doppler probe is inserted either into the esophagus (about the size of a nasogastric tube), endotracheal tube, or placed in the suprasternal notch, and measures the blood flow velocity in the descending or ascending aorta, respectively.

Blood flow velocity measurements using ultrasound are based on the Doppler principle: ultrasound is reflected by moving objects (red blood cells) moving towards the transmitted signal causing reflections of a higher frequency. This Doppler shift (ΔF) can be described by:

$$\Delta F = 2 \cdot f_T \cdot v \cdot \frac{\cos \theta}{s}$$

$$v = \frac{2 \cdot \Delta F}{f_T \cdot \cos \theta}$$

The velocity (v) can be calculated using the known ΔF (Hz), the transmitted frequency (f_T), the speed of the ultrasound in the medium (s; 1,540 m/s in body tissue), and the angle between the ultrasound beam and the direction of the object's motion (cos θ). For the measurement of blood flow, transmitted frequencies are usually in the 2 to 16 MHZ range. In using the suprasternal approach, the ultrasound beam is assumed to be in line with the aortic flow, negating any angle effect. Correct placement is judged by achieving a maximum sound pitch and a sharp, well-defined velocity waveform on display. Although this technique has the advantages of being totally non-invasive, significant aortic valve disease will cause turbulence of the blood stream thereby preventing quantification of the flow. Breathing, movement, a short neck, and subcutaneous emphysema, are other problems encountered using this approach.

In the esophageal approach, aortic valve disease has no influence unless severe. The probe can be left *in situ* for up to two weeks. Studies validating Doppler measured cardiac output against simultaneous thermodilution measurements found that it follows changes in cardiac output accurately [18]. The tracheal approach is a relatively new approach and uses endotracheal tubes with the Doppler probe already incorporated, but the number of studies using this technique is limited.

Using the above mentioned approach, the following parameters can be measured using transesophageal Doppler ultrasonography: flow time (FT), peak velocity

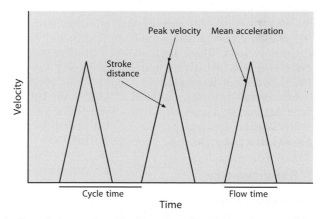

Fig. 3. Schematic depiction of Doppler flow-velocity waveform. The figure shows the schematic depicting of the back-scattered Doppler frequency shifts producing a typical flow-velocity waveform when aiming at the descending aorta. A number of velocity waveform variables can be measured: stroke distance (SD) = area of the waveform, i.e., length of a column of blood traversing the aorta with each ventricular stroke; peak velocity (PV) = velocity at the apex of the waveform; mean accelaration (MA) = value of peak velocity divided by the time to peak velocity

(PV), ventricular ejection time (VET) and heart rate (HR) (Fig. 3). From a normogram using the length, weight, and age of the patient, the cross-sectional area (CSA) of the aorta can be estimated. A newer design combines the Doppler flow velocity measurement with M-mode measurement of the aortic diameter. The parameters, which can be calculated using these parameters are stroke distance (SD = $\int$ VET·v·dt), stroke volume (SD×CSA), cardiac output (SV×HR), and corrected flow time (FTc = FT/$\sqrt{\text{cycle time}}$). The stroke distance is the area of the waveform, which is the length a column of blood travels along the aorta with each ventricular stroke. Assuming that during systole the CSA changes little, the product of SD and the CSA is the volume of blood which is pumped through the vessel with each ventricular stroke. The FTc is a correction of flow time for changes in heart rate and provides an indication of alterations in ventricular filling. The peak velocity is the velocity at the apex of the waveform and is an indicator of left ventricular contractility and function.

Recent developments have made the M-mode and two-dimensional Doppler echocardiography readily available for continuous use in critically ill patients. One of the advantages is that the CSA can be measured during monitoring, which theoretically results in more accurate measurement of the aortic blood flow velocity.

Previous Studies. Most studies concerning the use of Doppler ultrasonography in the ICU compared the measurement of cardiac output with Doppler ultrasonography and the measurement of the cardiac output using thermodilution. Correlation coefficients in these studies varied from 0.58 to 0.98 (mean=0.86) [18–21]. One study showed an increase in the correlation coefficient from 0.53 to 0.89 with increasing experience of the investigator, perhaps explaining some of the lower correlation coefficients [22]. Other studies investigated whether Doppler flowmetry could be used for a non-invasive optimization of left-ventricular filling. One study showed that ventilatory modus could be optimized giving the patients an optimal level of positive end-expiratory pressure (PEEP) without compromising the cardiac performance [23]. In a number of studies the hemodynamic status of surgical patients was optimized during the surgical procedure, attempting to reduce morbidity. Mythen et al. [24] showed that intra-operative optimization of stroke volume was able to reduce post-operative morbidity and length of hospital stay in cardiac surgical patients. These findings were confirmed by Sinclair et al. [25] using the same principle in patients undergoing surgery for a fractured neck of the femur. Thus, reversal of intraoperative hemodynamic abnormalities was associated with a reduced morbidity rate. Poeze et al. [26] showed that unrecognized hemodynamic deterioration in apparently hemodynamically stable patients could be detected using Doppler ultrasonography in post-operative patients with a high predictive power (area under the ROC curve 0.93) [26].

Echocardiography

Echocardiography uses the measurement of stroke volume (difference between end-systolic and end-diastolic ventriclular volume) to measure the cardiac output. Classically two-dimensional models were used, using assumptions of the form of the left ventricle. More recently, 3D models have been used, reconstructing the left ventricle. The use of echocardiography on the ICU is often limited by the availability of the echocardiographic module and the lack of necessary expertise needed to perform this technique frequently.

Bio-impedance

The measurement of stroke volume using the bio-impedance method is based upon the principle that blood is a good conductor of electricity and changes in intrathoracic blood volume during systolic contraction of the left ventricle result in a change in the resistance (impedance) of the chest. However, a considerable variety in the correlation values with thermodilution is found [27]. Moreover, endotracheal tubes, gastric tubes, and intravascular catheters, frequently used in critically ill patients, pose a serious disturbance of a correct signal.

▌ Regional Level of Monitoring

ICG-dilution Measured Splanchnic Blood Flow

Technique. Jorfeldt and Juhlin-Dannefelt originally described the technique for blood flow estimation, but in 1945 Bradley introduced splanchnic blood flow estimation by the Fick principle using a hepatic venous catheter. For this technique, the right jugular vein is used to insert a 7F cournand catheter in a right hepatic vein under portable fluoroscopy. The correct placement of the catheter tip, in a non-wedged position at least 5 cm within the vein, is verified using a small amount of contrast dye. Splanchnic blood flow is measured using a primed-continuous ICG infusion. A bolus of ICG was followed by a continuous infusion for 30 minutes (12 mg followed by 1.1 mg/min). The splanchnic blood flow (Q_{spl}) is calculated with the formula below:

$$Q_{spl} = IR_{ICG} \cdot \frac{C_I}{(C_{art} - C_{hv}) \cdot (1 - Hct)}$$

where IR_{ICG} is the infusion rate of ICG, C_i is the ICG infusate concentration, C_{art} and C_{hv} are the arterial and hepatic venous ICG plasma concentrations, and Hct is the hematocrit.

Blood samples are taken for ICG concentration determination at 20, 25, and 30 minutes of infusion. Triplicate sampling is performed in order to verify that a steady state level of ICG is reached in the blood. Plasma ICG concentrations are measured spectrophotometrically using a wavelength of 805 nm.

Usually this measurement of the splanchnic perfusion is simultaneously performed with measurement of the flow in the leg as a reference point for the splanchnic blood flow. For this purpose, two extra catheters are inserted, one into the femoral artery and one into the femoral vein. Using the same principle the difference between arterial and venous concentration of ICG is used to calculate the leg flow [28].

Previous Studies. A considerable number of studies have been performed regarding total splanchnic blood flow in humans. However, the determinants, clinical course, and impact of splanchnic blood flow abnormalities in patients at risk and patients with multiple organ failure (MOF) have not been well established. Patients with an inflammatory response have an increase in total splanchnic blood flow measured using the Fick principle compared to healthy controls [29]. The oxygen consumption, however, increases to disproportional levels compared to the increase in splanchnic blood flow. Oxygen extraction in the splanchnic area increases as a con-

Table 1. Effects of vasoactive agents on total splanchnic blood flow (TSF) and gastric intramucosal pH (pHi) in septic and non-septic patients

Vasoactive drug	Sepsis	Non-sepsis
Dopamine	↑ TSF = ↓ pHi	↑ TSF
Dobutamine	↑ TSF ↑ pHi	↑ TSF
Dopexamine	↑ TSF = ↓ pHi	↑ TSF = ↓ pHi
Norepinephrine	↑ ↓ TSF	?
Epinephrine	↓ pHi	?

?: unknown; =: unchanged; ↑: increased; ↓: decreased

sequence, but often a oxygen delivery/demand mismatch is present. This mismatch is present during hypotension and normotension and although correction of hypotension increases the blood flow, responses in patients are variable [30]. Surgery is usually accompanied by an increase in splanchnic blood flow due to the stress response, although low flow states in severe hypovolemia may also be present. In low flow states and hypovolemia, splanchnic blood flow decreases while the splanchnic metabolic demand does not change considerably. In these conditions, the above mentioned redistribution to 'less' vital organs in the splanchnic area is induced in order to maintain the perfusion of the heart and the brain. Studies using the ICG-dilution principle have provided extensive information concerning these changes during low and high-flow states. Moreover, numerous recent studies used this technique to evaluate the effects of hemodynamic interventions on splanchnic blood flow. The use of the inotropes and vasopressors, dopamine, dobutamine, dopexamine, norepinephrine and epinephrine has been extensively evaluated in septic and surgical patients [31] (Table 1).

Gastric and Intestinal Tonometry

Technique: The technique of intestinal tonometry was initially described by Fiddian-Green in the mid 1980s in critically ill trauma patients. In tonometry, a balloon-tipped catheter, the tonometer, is placed in the lumen of the stomach, sigmoid colon, or the lumen of the small intestine (usually performed in experimental studies). Using this method the intraluminal PCO_2 ($PiCO_2$ or $PrCO_2$) can be measured, based upon the assumption that ischemia of the splanchnic area is associated with an increased accumulation of PCO_2 in the intraluminal space and that this CO_2 diffuses readily over the gastrointestinal mucosa. Several animal and clinical studies support these assumptions [32]. Intracellular CO_2 will depend on both aerobic metabolism and anaerobic metabolism. When cellular oxygen supply decreases, the production of CO_2 via aerobic metabolism will fall and, below a certain level, anaerobic metabolism will produce lactate and H^+ ions during formation of adenosine triphosphate (ATP). As a result of buffering of the intracellular H^+, CO_2 is produced. This tissue CO_2 is then transported to the lungs by venous blood. During hypoperfusion, this clearance mechanism of CO_2 is hampered and CO_2 will then accumulate in the tissues. The intraluminal PCO_2 is therefore dependent on metabolism, perfusion, and lung physiology [33]. Using the measured intraluminal PCO_2, a pH is calculated using the Henderson-Hasselbalch formula.

Two techniques of measuring intraluminal PCO_2 are available clinically, each with their own advantages and disadvantages: the saline method, and the capnographic method. In the first method, the tonometer balloon is infused with 2.5–4.5 ml of normal saline or phosphate buffered saline. After a calibration period of at least 30 minutes the fluid is withdrawn from the balloon and the intraluminal PCO_2 is measured in this sample with a blood gas analyzer. The advantages of this approach, are the simple applicability, easy availability, and the lower cost compared to the capnographic method. Disadvantages are that in daily care practice errors are observed in 34% of all measurements [34], related to errors in infused volume and inaccurate timing. Moreover, the blood gas analyzer must be calibrated for performance of PCO_2 analyses from variable fluid sources.

Recently the introduction of air tonometry, using a modified capnograph, the Tonocap®, has bypassed some of these practical problems. This method uses air as the equilibrating medium. Air is injected, aspirated, and re-injected on a cycle time of 15 minutes. The PCO_2 of the air from the catheter balloon is measured using the same infra-red technology used in capnographs to measure an expiratory PCO_2. Automated air tonometry has been shown to produce reliable measurements of $PrCO_2$ [35]. In the first study investigating this method, Creteur et al. [36] found a close correlation between saline measured PCO_2 and gas PCO_2. In a study by Graf et al. [37] the gastric air tonometry provided an estimation of the $PrCO_2$ as reliable as the saline tonometry with clinically acceptable precision compared to a predefined $PrCO_2$. In a study by Barry et al. [38], gastric saline and air tonometry were compared *in vivo* in critically ill patients and *in vitro* with variation in temperature and PCO_2, and in both conditions air tonometry (Tonocap®) displayed a lower bias.

Other practical problems are related to the influence of gastric acid secretion on the gastric intramucosal PCO_2. During acid secretion, the CO_2 of the mucosa is 'buffered' by the H^+ of the gastric acid, giving falsely low PCO_2 values. A number of studies have investigated the use of gastric acid secretion inhibition on the tonometric intraluminal PCO_2 giving contradictory results. In a study by Vaisanen et al. the use of ranitidine did not alter the [39] PCO_2 measured in critically ill cardiac surgical patients. However, in a study by Brinkmann et al. [40] injection of pentagastrin and omeprazole significantly changed gastric tonometric intramucosal pH (pHi) in healthy volunteers.

Previous Studies. During recent years, a considerable number of studies have been published using tonometry. A considerable number of these studies have focused on the validity and reproducibility of tonometric derived variables. The validity of gastric pHi was assessed by instilling saline directly into the stomach lumen and by comparing the pHi with directly measured pH by inserting electrodes into the stomach wall. The direct and indirect pHi correlated moderately well.

A number of studies have used tonometry as predictors of morbidity in surgical and medical patient populations. Roumen et al. [41] found that a low pHi after major trauma was an indication of a complicated recovery; in particular, patients who never developed a low pHi had an uncomplicated recovery. Fiddian-Green et al. [42] found that, in high risk patients undergoing abdominal aortic surgery, a colonic pHi < 6.86 was associated with the development of ischemic colitis. In another study [43], this group studied 103 ICU patients and found massive stress ulcer bleeding in patients was associated with a low pHi, whereas patients with pHi >7.24 had no bleeding. Interestingly, gastric juice pH was similar in both groups.

Post-operative surgical patients with a pHi below 7.32 at the end of surgery were found to have a significantly longer length of stay in the ICU and the hospital, and a greater incidence of major complications [44].

Other studies have investigated the relation between pHi or intramucosal PCO_2 and mortality. In a prospective study, Gutierrez et al. [45] were the first to find gastric pHi to differentiate surviving critically ill patients from non-surviving patients. Marik [46] obtained similar results, concluding that indices of oxygenation, including pHi and arterial lactate, are superior to hemodynamic or oxygen-derived variables as predictor of outcome in patients with sepsis. In a study by Bonham et al. [47] patients with severe pancreatitis had a higher risk of death when having a lower pHi. An optimal cut-off point for this increased risk was determined at 7.25. In another study [48], gastric pHi was able to identify the critically ill trauma patient who was at high risk of death and MOF with a cut-off point of 7.10; the patients who did not correct this initial pHi after 24 hours were particularly prone to develop complications. In the study by Poeze et al. [49] in a cohort study of surgical patients, optimal cut-off points for pHi with respect to mortality were calculated using receiver-operator characteristic (ROC) curves. Maximized sensitivity and specificity pre-operatively were at a pHi of 7.35.

Recently, some studies have been published using tonometry as a guide for therapy. The first study to be published using therapy guided by parameters of splanchnic function was by Gutierrez et al. [45]. In their study, the hemodynamic status of critically ill patients was optimized either using pHi guided therapy (aiming at a pHi >7.35) or control therapy after the patients were stratified according to their admission pHi (above or below 7.35). The patients in the pHi-guided therapy group received additional fluids and/or dobutamine until the pHi was over 7.35. For patients admitted with a low pHi, survival was similar in the protocol and control groups, whereas for those admitted with normal pHi, survival was significantly greater in the protocol group than in the control group. Therapy aimed at preventing splanchnic organ hypoxia seemed to improve survival.

Ivatury et al. [50] published a randomized trial comparing pHi guided optimization in critically ill trauma patients with DO_2 guided therapy. The goal of treatment in the pHi guided group was to achieve a pHi of at least 7.30 using fluids and dobutamine. In the other group, the goal of treatment was a DO_2 of at least 600 ml/min/m^2. Survival, as well as the incidence of MOF, were not significantly different between the pHi- and DO_2-guided treatment patients. Although the pHi was significantly higher in the pHi group, the DO_2 was similar among the groups.

The impact of antioxidant, and splanchnic-directed, therapy was investigated by Barquist et al. [51] in critically ill, trauma patients. The patients included had a persistent, uncorrected pHi at 24 hours. Patients were randomized either into a control group, or into a splanchnic therapy group, using xanthine oxidase inhibitor, a hydroxyl radical scavenger, and low-dose isoprotenerol, aiming for a pHi ≥7.25. If this therapy was not sufficient, higher doses of isoprotenerol, dobutamine, nitroglycerine, nitroprusside, and prostaglandin E_1 could be used. There was a 8% mortality rate in the splanchnic therapy group and 29% mortality in the control group (p=0.55). However, a decreased incidence of organ system failure was found in the splanchnic therapy group.

In a randomized, prospective study, patients after elective infrarenal abdominal aortic aneurysm were randomized to receive control treatment or pHi-guided treatment [52]. This pHi-guided therapy used a treatment algorithm including dopamine, norepinephrine, and epinephrine. Mortality was not significantly changed (3% versus 8%), ar morbidity, although more inotropes were used in the treatment group. IIowever, the number of crossovers in the control group was not made clear. In the study group, 45% of patients did not decrease their pHi to a value less than 7.32.

Spies et al. [53] prospectively studied septic shock patients using N-acetylcysteine (NAC) to improve gastric pHi in a double-blind, placebo controlled study. Although the responders (increase in VO_2 >10%) to the NAC had a significantly higher survival ratio than the non-responders, the total treatment group did not have a different mortality ratio from the placebo treated group. However, treatment was only instituted for 90 minutes. In the responder group, the gastric pHi rose significantly, as well the intramucosal PCO_2. Although this study had an excellent set-up and sufficient information is given concerning co-interventions, the number of cross-overs in the total treatment group compared with the control group and *vice versa*, unfortunately, no information is given about the 'spontaneous' responders in the control group.

In the most recent randomized trial specifically aimed at improving a low gastric pHi, Gomersall et al. [54] included critically ill patients. After correcting global hemodynamic and metabolic disturbances, patients were randomized to receive a pHi optimizing therapy or control therapy. The patients receiving pHi-guided therapy received additional fluids and dobutamine infusion when the pHi was below 7.35. No differences in mortality and morbidity were found among the groups. However, no differences were found between the two groups with respect to pHi. Thus, the failure to improve outcome may have been caused by an ability to produce a clinically significant improvement in splanchnic oxygenation.

∎ Organ Specific Tests

Lactulose/rhamnose-intestinal Permeability Test

In clinical studies, intestinal permeability typically is measured by monitoring the urinary excretion of one or more enterally administered agents. These agents should be easily measured, normally not present in the urine, and should not be degradable or metabolized.

Most permeability tests are based upon the conductance of two substances. One agent consists of a relatively small molecule (rhamnose or mannitol), which permeates moderately well through even normal mucosa. The other agent consists of a larger molecule (lactulose) and permeates the normal mucosa only minimally. The measurement of both probes in the urine, and their relationship, gives an indication of the permeability of the mucosa. Originally it was thought that the difference in permeability of the two probes was due to differences in the place of transport, i.e., the paracellular (between adjacent cells) and transcellular (primary permeability of epithelium) routes. However, recent data indicate that such a transcellular 'pore' does not exists. Bjarnason et al. [55] found that the difference in permeability may be explained by the surface available for transport across the mucosa. According to this theory, smaller molecules can be absorbed through paracellular channels along the entire crypt-villus axis, whereas larger molecules can only be absorbed at the bottom of the villus, between cells lining the crypts of the mucosa. During inflammation, an increased absorption of larger molecules can be caused not only by widening of tight-junctions but also by a relative increase in absorptive area for the larger molecules due to villus atrophy. A third mechanism which was recently suggested, is the presence of tissue hyperosmolality at the tip of the villus. This tissue hyperosmolality is caused by the countercurrent mechanism in the villus and is increased during disturbed splanchnic mucosal perfusion.

A large number of studies are now available to support the view that intestinal permeability to lactulose and rhamnose is changed in many forms of critical illness, including high-risk surgery, sepsis, and MOF. After cardiopulmonary surgery, patients with a gastric pHi < 7.32 developed a higher lactulose/rhamnose ratio, while the systemic hemodynamic variables remained stable [56]. In another study, increased levels of endotoxin in the systemic circulation were associated with increased permeability of the gut [56].

Recent studies have focused on the manipulation of intestinal permeability. Sinclair et al. [57] infused dopexamine or dopamine during cardiopulmonary bypass in order to improve intestinal permeability. Compared to dopamine, dopexamine, claimed to induce a selective improvement in splanchnic perfusion, reduced intestinal permeability following surgery. In another study, intestinal permeability was improved in critically ill patients by using enteral nutrition compared to parenteral nutrition [58].

However, a recent study by Hallemeesch and colleaques [59] found that fluid loading during endotoxemia increases the lactulose/rhamnose ratio independent of changes in intestinal permeability. These postmucosal factors make the interpretation of changes in individual patients difficult to predict. Moreover, experimental studies revealed increases in gut permeability without changes in endotoxin/microbial translocation [56].

Lidocaine Metabolism and MEGX Measurements

One approach for measuring liver function as part of the liver-gut axis has been the analysis of lidocaine metabolism. Lidocaine, commonly used as a local anesthetic agent, is metabolized by cytochrome P450 3A to form monoethylglycinexylidide (MEGX) [55]. This de-ethylation of lidocaine is a liver-specific metabolic pathway in the perivenous hepatocytes. Plasma concentrations of MEGX can be measured using fluorescence polarization immunoassay. In clinical practice a dose of 1 mg/kg lidocaine is injected intravenously, and the MEGX concentrations are measured in blood samples drawn immediately before, and 15 minutes after, the lidocaine injection. The amount of lidocaine metabolized is calculated by subtracting the pre-injection MEGX concentration from the post-injection MEGX concentration. Because of the relatively high extraction ratio of lidocaine, this liver function not only depends on hepatic metabolic capacity, but also on hepatic blood flow [60].

In healthy volunteers, the median MEGX concentration is around 75–100 µg/l and values below 25 µg/l are considered to indicate severely disturbed liver function. This test has predominantly been used in selecting liver transplant patients [60, 61], in which lidocaine metabolism seemed to be more useful than ICG metabolism [62]. In critically ill patients, the MEGX test seemed to be useful in predicting mortality [63]. In this study, MEGX concentrations in non-surviving patients dropped from 20 ng/ml on admission to 2.4 ng/mL on day 3, whereas in surviving patients MEGX concentrations remained stable. Igonin et al. [64] showed that low MEGX levels were associated with worsened outcome and increased inflammatory response early in sepsis.

However, other studies have indicated that low MEGX concentrations did not predict reduced splanchnic blood flow in septic patients, due to the high hepatic extraction of lidocaine. Moreover, intrahepatic metabolic compartmentalization may limit the implications of a low lidocaine metabolism.

ICG Clearance Tests

Another specific test of liver function is obtained by measuring the clearance of ICG from the circulation. This test provides information concerning both the function and perfusion of the liver and can be used without the presence of a hepatic vein catheter. It can be measured using an intravascular catheter or by using a non-invasive (transcutaneous sensor) method [65]. The plasma disappearance rate (PDR) indicates how much (%) of the injected ICG disappear from the circulating blood initially per minute due to hepatic elimination and is calculated as follows:

$$PDR = 100 \times \ln 2/t\frac{1}{2}$$

where $t\frac{1}{2}$ is the half life of ICG primary distribution space is the active circulating blood volume (determined by the total blood volume [TBV]). As liver perfusion is also directly dependent on the blood volume, varying blood volumes will result in different value of the PDR even with a constant hepatic ICG elimination. Therefore, ICG clearance is best evaluated using the multiplication of TBV and PDR:

$$CBig = TBV \times PDR$$

$$CPig = TBV \times (1 - Hct) \times PDR$$

where CBig is the ICG blood clearance, and CPig is the ICG plasma clearance

ICG is transported into the gallbladder through a membrane transport mechanism which is energy-dependent. The elimination kinetics are dependent on the liver perfusion, the total circulating blood volume, absorption in the liver cell, intracellular transport, and transport into the gallbladder. Normally, more than 50% of the ICG is extracted by the liver in one passage.

Kholoussy et al. [66] and Pollack et al. [67] found a prognostic correlation between ICG clearance and prognosis for surgical ICU patients. Patients with a PDR below 6% did not survive the post-operative period. In multiple trauma patients, PDR indicated significant liver damage at an early stage [68]. Krenn et al. [69] found that short term PEEP during ventilation in liver transplant patients does not decrease PDR.

Lactate Metabolism and L- and D-lactate Levels

The measurement of lactate in the blood may provide a tool to detect an abnormal circulation. The metabolism of glucose provides a major source of energy. Glucose metabolism can be viewed as a two step process. Glucose is first metabolized to pyruvate through a series of anaerobic reactions that yield two molecules of ATP, i.e., energy. Pyruvate then enters the mitochondria where it is metabolized to CO_2 and H_2O via the Krebs cycle and the electron transport chain (including the cytochrome chain), generating an additional 34 ATP. Under physiological conditions, pyruvate is in equilibrium with lactate and with the oxidized and reduced forms of the cofactor nicotamide adenine dinucleotide (NAD+ and NADH, respectively), facilitated by lactate dehydrogenase (LDH).

During anoxia, the aerobic or mitochondrial metabolism of glucose ceases to function and, as a result, pyruvate accumulates and is converted to lactate [29]. Excess lactate formed during these reactions leaves the cell and accumulates in the extracellular fluid. Increased lactate levels in the blood (hyperlactatemia) can result from increased extracellular lactate concentrations when lactate production exceeds lactate utilization. Some tissues can take up lactate and utilize it; for example, myocardial tissue can take up lactate and convert it into pyruvate. In addition, the liver can take up lactate and convert it into glucose.

The most common cause of hyperlactatemia is global tissue hypoxia. In most cases this is due to systemic perfusion abnormalities. The measurement of blood lactate levels can serve as an indicator of impaired tissue oxygenation, however other possible causes must be ruled out. Numerous experimental and clinical studies have correlated increased lactate levels during circulatory failure with worsened prognosis [33]. Factors which can disturb the interpretation of lactate levels are overproduction or decreased elimination of lactate, the 'washout phenomenon', acute changes in acid-base balance, peripheral and visceral tissue perfusion, and hepatic lactate uptake.

The presence of hyperlactatemia has been suggested to be a marker of disturbed hepatosplanchnic function. The gut is a known producer of lactate during sepsis. Under normal conditions, skeletal muscles release lactate, which is taken up by the liver to a great extent [17]. The liver has a capacity to increase lactate uptake during non-physiological conditions. Lactate production for individual organs is probably a more reliably index of anaerobic metabolism than simple arterial lactate concentration. Lactate production can be calculated from measurements of the organ blood flow and the arterial-venous difference in lactate. However, individual organ production is difficult to measure in the clinical setting. The measurement of hepatic vein lactate concentrations has been used to measure splanchnic lactate metabolism, since the liver has a major impact on blood lactate concentrations. Landow et al. [70] showed that a correlation was present between hepatic vein lactate concentrations and gastric pHi in cardiac surgical patients. A decreased lactate extraction was associated with gastric intramucosal acidosis, increased systemic and hepatic venous lactate concentrations. However, Takala et al. [71] showed that for individual patients this relationship between hepatic venous lactate concentrations and pHi is not so obvious. The increased lactate concentrations in the hepatic vein are not likely correlated to a decreased lactate uptake by the liver but are correlated to an increased splanchnic lactate production. Moreover, the routine insertion of a hepatic vein catheter may impose significant risk to the patient, by increased risk of infection and emboli.

Tenhunen et al. [72] have suggested measuring intestinal intraluminal lactate to have a better idea of the regional lactate metabolism. Others have suggested the measurement of the isomer D-lactate as a marker of splanchnic hypoperfusion. D-lactic acidosis in patients was originally described during short bowel syndrome [73, 74]. Acidosis is caused by the production of D-lactic acid by bacterial fermentation in the gut lumen and its subsequent absorption into the blood. *Klebsiella*, *Escherichia coli*, *Lactobacillus acidophilus* and *Bacteroides* species are known to be capable of synthesizing D-lactate [75]. Although both L-lactate and D-lactate are produced, only the D-isomer accumulates due to the rapid metabolism of L-lactate in the liver. Moreover, although D-lactate dehydrogenase is present in certain lower animal species, in humans only L-lactate dehydrogenase is present. Therefore, D-lactate cannot be metabolized in humans, while D-lactate is excreted in the urine [76]. The site of D-lactic acid production is likely to be the colon, since the colonic bacteria of humans metabolize carbohydrates that have not been metabolized in the small intestine.

During intestinal ischemia, the resident microbial flora of the intestine multiplies rapidly and soon overgrows the ischemic segment [75]. This bacterial proliferation occurs in conjunction with disruption of the mucosal layer of the gut. Both experimental and clinical studies have showed that acute intestinal ischemia causes a rise in D-lactate levels in the systemic circulation [75, 76]. In a study by Murray et al. [75], increased D-lactate levels in the blood were shown to be able to differentiate mesenteric ischemia from other (non-ischemic) abdominal catastrophies with high precision and validity [76]. Poeze et al. [77] showed that in patients undergoing emergency surgery for ruptured abdominal aneurysm, D-lactate levels were highly predictive for the occurrence of intestinal ischemia post-operatively. Recent data show a significant relationship between D-lactate levels and gastric pHi-values [78].

▮ Conclusion

Since the introduction of invasive monitoring technology, numerous new applications have been developed. Both experimental and clinical studies have been performed to test the validity and reproducibility of these techniques. Some, although few, techniques have been tested in randomized clinical trials. A number of studies compare global hemodynamic parameters with regional parameters of perfusion, although no comparison of global volume-related parameters and regional parameters have been performed. More importantly, in this era of evidence based medicine, randomized trials using different techniques need to be performed in order to compare newer techniques to the established means of monitoring critically ill patients.

References

1. Vincent JL, Thijs L, Cerny V (1997) Critical care in Europe. Crit Care Med 13:245–254
2. Rosenwasse RH, Jallo JL, Gretch CC, et al. (1995) Complications of Swan-Ganz catheterization for hemodynamic monitoring in patients with subarachnoid hemorrhage. Neurosurgery 37:872–875
3. Putterman CE (1989) The Swan-Ganz catheter: A decade of hemodynamic monitoring. J Crit Care 4:127
4. Shah KB, Rao TLK, Laughlin S, et al (1984) A review of pulmonary artery catheterisation in 6,245 patients. Anaesthesiology 61:271–275
5. Connors AF, Speroff T, Dawson NV, et al (1996) The effectiveness of right heart catheterization in the initial care of critically ill patients. JAMA 276:889–897
6. Boyd O, Hayes M (1999) The oxygen trail: the goal. Br Med Bull 55:125–139
7. Shoemaker WC, Appel PL, Kram HB (1990) Measurement of tissue perfusion by oxygen transport patterns in experimental shock and in high-risk surgical patients. Intensive Care Med 16:S135–S144
8. Shoemaker WC, Appel PL, Kram HB, Waxman K, Lee TS (1988) Prospective trial of supranormal values of survivors as therapeutic goals in high-risk surgical patients. Chest 94:1176–1186

9. Ince C, van der Sluijs JP, Sinaasappel M, Avontuur JA, Coremans JM, Bruining HA (1994) Intestinal ischemia during hypoxia and experimental sepsis as observed by NADH video-fluorimetry and quenching of Pd-porphine phosphorescence. Adv Exp Med Biol 361:105–110

10. Mihaljevic T, von Segesser LK, Tonz M, Leskosek B, Jenni R, Turina M (1997) Continuous thermodilution measurement of cardiac output: in-vitro and in-vivo evaluation. J Thorac Cardiovasc Surg 42:32–35

11. Greim CA, Roewer N, Thiel H, Laux G, Schulte am Esch J (1997) Continuous cardiac output monitoring during adult liver transplantation: thermal filament technique versus bolus thermodilution. Anesth Analg 85:483–488

12. Schultz RJ, Whitfield GF, LaMura JJ, Raciti A, Krishnamurthy S (1985) The role of physiologic monitoring in patients with fractures of the hip. J Trauma 25:309–316

13. Kisch H, Leucht S, Lichtwarck-Aschoff M, Pfeiffer UJ (1995) Accuracy and reproducibility of the measurement of actively circulating blood volume with an integrated fiberoptic monitoring system. Crit Care Med 23:885–893

14. Lichtwarck-Aschoff M, Beale R, Pfeiffer UJ (1996) Central venous pressure, pulmonary artery occlusion pressure, intrathoracic blood volume, and right ventricular end-diastolic volume as indicators of cardiac preload. J Crit Care 11:180–188

15. Haller M, Zollner C, Briegel J, Forst H (1996) Evaluation of a new continuous thermodilution cardiac output monitor in critically ill patients: a prospective criterion standard study. Crit Care Med 24:716–717

16. Ishihara H, Iakawa T, Hasegawa T, Muraoka M, Tsubo T, Matsuki A (1999) Does indocyanine green accurately measure plasma volume independently of its disappearance rate from plasma in critically ill patients? Intensive Care Med 25:1212–1214

17. Mitchell JP, Schuller D, Calandrino FS, Schuster DP (1992) Improved outcome based on fluid management in critically ill patients requiring pulmonary artery catheterization. Am J Respir Crit Care Med 145:990–998

18. Davies JN, Allen DR, Chant ADB (1991) Non-invasive Doppler-derived cardiac output: a validation study comparing this technique with thermodilution and Fick methods. Eur J Vasc Surg 5:497–500

19. Gardin JM, Dabestani A, Matin K, Allfie A, Russell D, Henry WL (1984) Reproducibility of Doppler aortic blood flow measurments studies on intraobserver, interobserver and day-to-day variability in normal subjects. Am J Cardiol 54:1092–1098

20. Ihlen H, Endresen K, Golf S, Nitter-Hauge S (1987) Cardiac stroke volume during exercise measured by Doppler echocardiography: comparison with the thermodilution technique and evaluation of reproducibility. Br Heart J 58:455–459

21. Krishnamurthy B, McMurray TJ, McClean E (1997) The peri-operative use of the oesophageal Doppler monitor in patients undergoing coronary artery revascularisation. A comparison with the continuous cardiac output monitor. Anaesthesia 52:624–629

22. Lefrant J-Y, Bruelle P, Aya AGM, et al (1998) Training is required to improve the reliability of esophageal Doppler to measure cardiac output in critically ill patients. Intensive Care Med 24:347–352

23. Singer M, Bennett D (1989) Optimisation of positive and expiratory pressure for maximal delivery of oxygen to tissues using oesophageal Doppler ultrasonography. Br Med J 298:1350–1353

24. Mythen MG, Webb AR (1995) Perioperative plasma volume expansion reduces the incidence of gut mucosal hypoperfusion during cardiac surgery. Arch Surg 130:423–429

25. Sinclair S, James S, Singer M (1997) Intraoperative intravascular volume optimisation and length of hospital stay after repair of proximal femoral fracture: randomised controlled trial. Br Med J 315:909–912

26. Poeze M, Ramsay G, Greve JWM, Singer M (1999) Prediction of postoperative cardiac-surgical morbidity and organ failure within 4 hours of ICU admission using esophageal Doppler ultrasonography. Crit Care Med 27:1288–1294

27. Clancy TV, Norman K, Reynolds R, Covington D, Maxwell JG (1991) Cardiac output measurement in critical care patients: Thoracic Electrical Bioimpedance versus thermodilution. J Trauma 31:1116–1120

28. Uusaro A, Ruokonen E, Takala J (1995) Estimation of splanchnic blood flow by the Fick principle in man and problems in the use of indocyanine green. Cardiovasc Res 30:106–112

29. Takala J (1994) Sepsis and human splanchnic metabolism. In: Kinney JM, Tucker HN (eds) Organ Metabolism and Nutrition: Ideas for Future Critical Care. Raven Press Ltd., New York, pp 369–379

30. Takala J (1996) Determinants of splanchnic blood flow. Br J Anaesth 77:50–58

31. Poeze M, Greve JWM, Ramsay G (1999) Is splanchnic perfusion a critical problem in sepsis? In: Baue AE, Berlot G, Gullo A, Vincent JL (eds) Sepsis and Organ Dysfunction. From Basics to Clinical Approach. Springer, Milano, pp 169–181

32. Pastores SM, Katz DP, Kvetan V (1996) Splanchnic ischemia and gut mucosal injury in sepsis and the multiple organ dysfunction syndrome. Am J Gastroenterol 91:1697–1710

33. Anonymous (1996) Third European Consensus Conference in Intensive Care Medicine. Tissue hypoxia. How to detect, how to correct, how to prevent? Am J Respir Crit Care Med 154:1573–1578

34. Brinkert W, Bakker J (1998) Is it time to abandon the pHi concept? Int J Intensive Care 16–21

35. Heinonen PO, Jousela IT, Blomqvist KA, Olkkola KT, Takkunen OS (1997) Validation of air tonometric measurement of gastric regional concentrations of CO_2 in critically ill septic patients. Intensive Care Med 23:524–529

36. Creteur J, De Backer D, Vincent JL (1997) Monitoring gastric mucosal carbon dioxide pressure using gas tonometry: in vitro and in vivo validation studies. Intensive Care Med 87:504–510

37. Graf J, Konigs B, Mottaghy K, Janssens U (2000) In vitro validation of gastric air tonometry using perfluorocarbon FC 43 and 0.9% sodium chloride. Br J Anaesth 84:497–499

38. Barry B, Mallick A, Hartley G, Bodenham A, Vucevic M (1998) Comparison of air tonometry with gastric tonometry using saline and other equilibrating fluids: an in vivo and in vitro study. Intensive Care Med 24:777–784

39. Vaisanen O, Ruokonen E, Parviainen I, Bocek P, Takala J (2000) Ranitidine or dobutamine alone or combined has no effect on gastric intramucosal-arterial PCO_2 difference after cardiac surgery. Intensive Care Med 26:45–51

40. Brinkmann A, Glasbrenner B, Vlatten A, et al (2001) Does gastric juice pH influence tonometric PCO2 measured by automated air tonometry? Am J Respir Crit Care Med 163:1150–1152

41. Roumen RMH, Vreugde JP, Goris RJA (1994) Gastric tonometry in multiple trauma patients. J Trauma 36:313–316

42. Schiedler MG, Cutler NS, Fiddian-Green RG (1987) Sigmoid intramural pH for prediction of ischemic colitis during aortic surgery: a comparison with risk factors and inferior mesenteric artery stumo pressures. Arch Surg 122:881–886

43. Fiddian-Green RG, McGough E, Pittenger G, Rothman E (1983) Predictive value of intramural pH and other risk factors for massive bleeding from stress ulceration. Gastroenterology 85:613–620

44. Mythen M, Webb AR (1994) Intra-operative gut mucosal hypoperfusion is associated with increased post-operative complications and cost. Intensive Care Med 20:99–104

45. Gutierrez G, Palizas F, Doglio G, et al (1992) Gastric intramucosal pH as a therapeutic index of tissue oxygenation in critically ill. Lancet 339:195–199

46. Marik PE (1993) Gastric intamucosal pH. A better predictor of multiorgan dysfunction and death than oxygen-derived variables in patients with sepsis. Chest 104:225–229

47. Bonham MJ, Abu-Zidan FM, Simovic MO, Windsor JA (1997) Gastric intramucosal pH predicts death in severe acute pancreatitis. Br J Surg 84:1670–1674

48. Chang MC, Cheatham ML, Nelson LD, Rutherford EJ, Morris-JAJ (1994) Gastric tonometry supplements information provided by systemic indicators of oxygen transport. J Trauma 37:488–494

49. Poeze M, Takala J, Greve JWM, Ramsay G (2000) Pre-operative tonometry is predictive for mortality and morbidity in high-risk surgical patients. Intensive Care Med 26:1272–1281

50. Ivatury RR, Simon RJ, Islam SI, Fueg A, Rohman M, Stahl WM (1996) A prospective randomized study of end points of resuscitation after major trauma: global oxygen transport indices versus organ-specific gastric mucosal pH. J Am Coll Surg 183:145–154
51. Barquist E, Kirton O, Windsor J, et al (1998) The impact of antioxidant and splanchnic-directed therapy on persistent uncorrected gastric mucosal pH in the critically injured trauma patient. J Trauma 44:355–360
52. Pargger H, Hampl KF, Christen P, Staender S, Scheidegger D (1998) Gastric intramucosal pH-guided therapy in patients after elective repair of infrarenal abdominal aneurysms: is it beneficial? Intensive Care Med 24:769–776
53. Spies CD, Reinhart K, Witt I, et al (1994) Influence of N-acetylcysteine on indirect indicators of tissue oxygenation in septic shock patients: results from a prospective, randomized, double-blind study. Crit Care Med 22:1738–1746
54. Gomersall CD, Joynt GM, Ho KM, Young RJ, Buckley TA, Oh TE (1997) Gastric tonometry and prediction of outcome in the critically ill. Arterial to intramucosal pH gradient and carbon dioxide gradient. Anaesthesia 52:619–623
55. Bjarnason I, MacPherson A, Hollander D (1996) Intestinal permeability: an overview. Gastroenterology 110:967–968
56. Brinkman A, Calzia E, Träger K, Radermacher P (1998) Monitoring the hepato-splanchnic regional in the critically ill patient. Measurement techniques and clinical relevance. Intensive Care Med 24:542–556
57. Sinclair DG, Houldsworth PE, Keogh B, Pepper J, Evans TW (1997) Gastrointestinal permeability following cardiopulmonary bypass: a randomised study comparing the effects of dopamine and dopexamine. Intensive Care Med 23:310–316
58. Hadfield RJ, Sinclair DG, Houldsworth PE, Evans TW (1995) Effects of enteral and parenteral nutrition on gut mucosal permeability in the critically ill. Am J Respir Crit Care Med 152:1545–1548
59. Hallemeesch MM, Lamers WH, Soeters PB, Deutz NEP (2000) Increased lactulose/rhamnose ratio during fluid load is caused by increased urinary lactulose excretion. Am J Physiol 278:G83–G88
60. Oellerich M, Ringe B, Gubernatis G, et al (1989) Lignocaine metabolite formation as a measure of pre-transplant liver function. Lancet 25:640–642
61. Schinella M, Guglielmi A, Veraldi GF, Boni M, Frameglia M, Caputo M (1994) Evaluation of the liver function of cirrhotic patients based on the formation of monoethylglycine xylidide (MEGX) from lidocaine. Eur J Clin Chem Clin Biochem 31:553–557
62. Oda Y, Kariya N, Nakamoto T, Nishi S, Asada A, Fujimori M (1995) The monoethylglycinexylidide test is more useful for evaluating liver function than indocyanine green test: case of a patient with remarkably decreased indocyanine green half-life. Ther Drug Monit 17:207–210
63. Maynard ND, Bihari DJ, Dalton RN, Beale R, Smithies MN, Mason RC (1997) Liver function and splanchnic ischemia in critically ill patients. Chest 111:180–187
64. Igonin AA, Armstrong VW, Shipkova M, Kukes VG, Oellerich M (2000) The monoethylglycinexylidide (MEGX) test as a marker of hepatic dysfunction in septic patients with pneumonia. Clin Chem Lab Med 38:1125–1128
65. Sakka SG, Reinhart K, Meier-Hellmann A (2000) Comparison of invasive and noninvasive measurements of indocyanine green plasma disappearance rate in critically ill patients with mechanical ventilation and stable hemodynamics. Intensive Care Med 26:1553–1556
66. Kholoussy AM, Pollack D, Matsumoto T (1984) Prognostic significance of indocyanine green clearance in critically ill surgical patients. Crit Care Med 12:115–116
67. Pollack DS, Sufian S, Matsumoto T (1979) Indocyanine green clearance in critically ill patients. Surg Gynecol Obstet 149:853–854
68. Gottlieb ME, Stratton HH, Newell JC, Shah DM (1984) Indocyanine green. Its use as an early indicator of hepatic dysfunction following injury in man. Arch Surg 119:264–268
69. Krenn CG, Krafft P, Schaefer B, et al (2000) Effects of positive end-expiratory pressure on hemodynamics and indocyanine green kinetics in patients after orthotopic liver transplantation. Crit Care Med 28:1760–1765
70. Landow L (1993) Splanchnic lactate production in cardiac surgery patients. Crit Care Med 21:S84–S91

71. Takala J, Uusaro A, Parviainen I, Ruokonen E (1996) Lactate metabolism and regional lactate exchange after cardiac surgery. New Horiz 4:483–491
72. Tenhunen JJ, Kosunen H, Alhava E, Tuomisto L, Takala J (1999) Intestinal luminal microdialysis: a new approach to assess gut mucosal ischemia. Anesthesiology 91:1807–1815
73. Oh MS, Phelps KR, Traube M, Barbosa-Saldivar JL, Boxhill C, Carroll HJ (1979) D-lactic acidosis in a man with the short-bowel syndrome. N Engl J Med 301:249–252
74. Hove H, Mortensen PB (1995) Colonic lactate metabolism and D-lactic acidosis. Dig Dis Sci 40:320–330
75. Murray MJ, Barbose JJ, Cobb CF (1993) Serum D(-)-lactate levels as a predictor of acute intestinal ischemia in a rat model. J Surg Res 54:507–509
76. Murray MJ, Gonze MD, Nowak LR, Cobb CF (1994) Serum D(-)-lactate levels as an aid to diagnosing acute intestinal ischemia. Am J Surg 167:575–578
77. Poeze M, Froon AHM, Greve JWM, Ramsay G (1998) D-lactate as an early marker of intestinal ischaemia after ruptured abdominal aneurysm repair. Br J Surg 85:1221–1224
78. Poeze M, Solberg B, Greve JWM, Ramsay G (2000) Gastric pHi and PrCO2 are related to D-lactate and not to L-lactate levels. Intensive Care Med 26:S343 (Abst)

Gastric Mucosal Tonometry in Daily ICU Practice

T. Uhlig, G. Pestel, and K. Reinhart

▌ Introduction

As a guide to therapy for critically ill patients, reliable monitoring parameters are indispensable to maintain homeostasis. Invasive techniques like direct hemodynamometry or pulmonary catheterization, laboratory parameters like blood lactate or results from blood gas analysis, mixed venous saturation (SvO_2) or base excess, provide important information, facilitating adequate fluid therapy, or therapy with inotropes if necessary. All methods mentioned have to be interpreted cautiously in light of their quality as global parameters. Conclusive data about regional oxygen debt is not possible. The regional blood flow of the splanchnic region has gained special interest in recent years; it has even been called the "canary of the body" [1]. The need to monitor this eminently sensitive area is therefore undisputed.

▌ Tonometry in Clinical Practice

Apart from experimental methods, tonometry is the method of choice for the intensive care clinician. Tonometry is a voltage measurement, a method which reflects a partial pressure equilibration of a gas, e.g., CO_2, between two compartments after a defined equilibration period. Boda and Muranyi suggested 'gastrotonometry' for the monitoring of artificial respiration in 1959. This method did not receive wide acceptance, because "gastric PCO_2 may be misleadingly high ... in severe shock accompanied by an excessive slowing of the circulation" [2]. Measurement of intramucosal CO_2 as a monitoring parameter, by means of a nasogastric tube, was reintroduced twenty years later in clinical trials [3–5] using gastric intramucosal pH (pHi) as the tonometric variable of choice. pHi, derived from measured gastric intramucosal CO_2 and hypothesized equivalence of gastric mucosal and arterial bicarbonate, has been established as an outcome variable in several studies [6–9]. The normal value of pHi has been defined inconsistently in literature; 'normal' values of 7.32 [5] or 7.35 [6], or even 7.39 [10] have been documented. All these results were determined by means of cumbersome liquid tonometry. The use of saline as a carrier has been criticized [11, 12], because of variation in the results with different blood gas analyzers [13] and because of non-agreement of regional bicarbonate and systemic bicarbonate [14]. In clinical practice, the long equilibration time was regarded as a problem in monitoring intensive care patients. A relevant monitoring device has to mirror quickly the changing clinical conditions in intensive care unit (ICU) patients.

Gas Tonometry

Some essential methodical obstacles of tonometry seem to have been resolved [15, 16] with the introduction of recirculating gas tonometry. The catheter balloon is filled with air, instead of liquid. A sample of the gas in the balloon is drawn at regular intervals; CO_2 partial pressure (PCO_2) is measured by infrared sensor, tested, and displayed. The values obtained by recirculating gas tonometry and liquid tonometry are comparable [17, 18], and the superiority in precision of recirculating gas tonometry over liquid tonometry is undoubted. The fast and reproducible measurement of values with moderate invasiveness is acceptable. For methodical reasons the difference between gastric intramucosal and arterial PCO_2, the PCO_2-gap, is considered as the parameter of choice instead of pHi. However, the superiority of the PCO_2-gap does not remain unchallenged [19, 20]. As for pHi, there is no accepted opinion about normal values of PCO_2-gap; in the literature, values ranging from 2–4 [2], 6 [17], 7 [21], 8 [22] up to 10 mmHg [23] have been documented. Experimental results yielded the anaerobic threshold in metabolism at a PCO_2-gap of 25–35 mmHg [24]. Recently it was stated that even PCO_2-gaps up to 40 mmHg may not be predictive of compromised splanchnic perfusion [19]. Interestingly, in an older experimental study [25], laboratory animals survived a PCO_2-gap up to 118 mmHg provided that a period of four hours was not exceeded.

Empirical Results

In an observational study, 42 patients were enrolled (unpublished data). They were divided into three groups:
1. Patients undergoing elective surgery with an estimated high volume input and output (n = 15).
2. Patients undergoing neurosurgical procedures (n = 11).
3. Multiple trauma cases from the emergency room (n = 16).

The patients were allocated into two groups for the evaluation of intramucosal PCO_2 ($PiCO_2$) (Fig. 1). Thirt-five patients without complications were compared with seven patients with complications. A complication was defined as death, unplanned reoperation, and reintubation. Systemic inflammatory response syndrome (SIRS) and allied disorders were not judged to be a complication due to their high incidence in surgical ICUs [29]. All raw $PiCO_2$ values were recorded, regardless of the state of ventilation, sedation, or nutrition. To compare different $PiCO_2$-levels in stable ICU patients, the PCO_2-gap was chosen as the tonometric parameter. The PCO_2-gap was computed by subtracting the arterial PCO_2 value from the documented $PiCO_2$ value. We further studied the group of 35 patients without complications, to elucidate the course of tonometric parameters in these surgical ICU patients, by dividing the PCO_2-gaps of these 35 patients into 24-hour-segments.

Clinical Recommendations

Clinical impressions suggest that there might be a tolerable corridor above the experimentally found normal value of 10 mmHg for PCO_2-gap, i.e., a $PiCO_2$ of 50 mmHg, in normoventilated patients. We compared the segments of PCO_2-gap

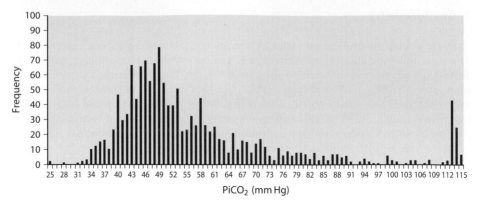

Fig. 1. Intramucosal carbon dioxide tensions (PiCO$_2$) in critically ill patients: Distribution of frequencies

below 10 mmHg with those segments with a PCO$_2$-gap above 10 mmHg. For the comparison with the segments of PCO$_2$-gap below 10 mmHg we chose only segments with a PCO$_2$-gap between 10 and 20 mmHg, because we wanted to compare segments with PCO$_2$-gap-fluctuations of 10 mmHg only. Comparisons were made concerning volume therapy (crystalloids, colloids) given, need for inotropes (dopamine, dobutamine, norepinephrine, epinephrine), and need for transfusions of packed red cells and fresh frozen plasma. In patients without complications, documented PiCO$_2$ values had a lower mean and a lower standard deviation (49.7±11.4; median 49) compared to patients with complications (57.5±19.3; median 51). A histogram of PiCO$_2$ values of patients with complications shows a marked asymmetric shift to the right compared to patients without complications. In the seven patients with complications, 29.9% (n=428) of 1429 measured values where above 60 mmHg, whereas in 35 patients without complications only 11.9% (n=578) of 4869 measured values exceeded the value of 60 mmHg. In patients without complications, PiCO$_2$ values above 80 mmHg were quite rare, whereas in patients with complications, PiCO$_2$ values between 81 and 100 mmHg appeared in 5.7% of all measured values, and values between 101 and 120 mmHg appeared in 6.7%. As the frequency distribution of PiCO$_2$ implies a large variability in PiCO$_2$ values measured, we wondered what the 24-hour-segments of PCO$_2$-gap would look like in individual patients. In our 35 patients without complications, we found 156 segments of 24-hour-measurements of PCO$_2$-gap. Only 21 segments of these 156 (13.5%) always had PCO$_2$-gap values between 0 and 10 mmHg, which had been detected experimentally as a normal value for PCO$_2$-gap. Eighteen segments out of the 156 (11.5%) had PCO$_2$-gap values between 10 and 20 mmHg. One hundred seventeen segments out of the 156 (75%) had PCO$_2$-gap values in a wide range of more than 10 mmHg, and were therefore not used for comparison. We compared the 21 segments of PCO$_2$-gap below 10 mmHg with 18 segments of PCO$_2$-gap between 10 and 20 mmHg, to check whether different therapeutic strategies might explain different PCO$_2$-gap values in patients, in whom no difference in outcome was seen. Interestingly, no difference between a PCO$_2$-gap course below 10 mmHg and PCO$_2$-gap between 10 and 20 mmHg could be found irrespective of fluid therapy, inotropic support, and transfusion therapy.

■ Some Critical Recommendations

Despite the obvious advantages of monitoring the splanchnic region, gastric mucosal tonometry is not widely established as yet. Still unsolved is the question as to whether arterial bicarbonate can be equated with gastric mucosal bicarbonate. If arterial and gastric mucosal bicarbonate are identical, then pHi would indeed be intramucosal pH and could be accepted as a monitoring parameter of the splanchnic region. This precautionary thought applies as well to the analysis of the so called pH-gap – the difference between gastric mucosal and arterial pH. This pH-gap has been postulated to be superior to pHi [30]; however this postulate was criticized for mathematical and methodical reasons [31]. To clarify these questions, a study checked the hypothesis that calculated pHi and arterial acid-base-status were independent of each other [5]. The results of the study showed that pHi is influenced by changes in the acid-base-status in arterial blood, which is not a regional but a systemic variable. Another hypothesis was checked – whether pH-gap and PCO_2-gap, would provide the same information [5]. This could not be confirmed, as at increasing pH differences the deviation of the PCO_2-gap rises depending on the arterial PCO_2. This inaccuracy can be avoided simply, by using the gastric mucosal–arterial PCO_2 difference, which has been considered as a parameter of choice [5, 32]. We used 'raw' $PiCO_2$ for trend monitoring because values are easy to obtain, are expressed rapidly, and displayed immediately. To determine PCO_2-gap non-invasively, end tidal CO_2 determination has been proposed recently [33] for brief monitoring procedures. However, this method proved to be difficult in the intensive care context for clinical and technical reasons. Various states of ventilation may have a different impact on PCO_2-gap as a monitoring variable for splanchnic perfusion [20]. To rule out the possibility that alteration in $PiCO_2$ are due to altered ventilation patterns, arterial blood gas analysis still remains indispensable. But, as arterial blood gas analysis should be mandatory when ventilation parameters are changed, the PCO_2-gap can be assessed reliably in addition to 'raw' $PiCO_2$ values. With the Tonocap® device, semi-continuous monitoring of gastric mucosal PCO_2 has been made possible. Repeated measurements and registration of 'raw' $PiCO_2$ within a short time permit trend monitoring. We computed a mean of 49.7 with a standard deviation of 11.4 in the frequency distribution of 'raw' $PiCO_2$ in 35 intensive care patients without complications, and a mean of 57.5 with a standard deviation of 19.3 in patients with complications. In these seven patients with complications, the curve of the $PiCO_2$ frequency distribution obviously shifts to the right with 29.9% of measured values above 60 mmHg. Whether shifting of the $PiCO_2$ curve is the CO_2 counterpart of documented shifting of spectrophotometrically assessed gastric mucosal microvascular hemoglobin oxygen saturation in septic patients [34], is only a hypothesis at present.

Whether a PCO_2-gap of 10 mmHg should be the parameter of choice has been questioned; in a study of 114 injured patients [35] a threshold value of PCO_2-gap of 18 mmHg was found to predict multiorgan dysfunction syndrome and death. So the question is, whether in a clinical setting besides a physiological normal value, perhaps a higher tolerable value exists which makes attention mandatory, but has no impact on therapy. In our study, we found that patients with a PCO_2-gap between 10 and 20 mmHg were no worse off, needed no more therapy, and could be transferred to the ward without complications. This 'tolerable corridor' corresponds to a $PiCO_2$ value of 50 to 60 mmHg in normoventilated patients. Such a 'tolerable corridor' would agree with recent experimental findings, where the anaerobic threshold was proposed for a PCO_2-gap of 25–35 mmHg [24] and a PCO_2-gap up to 50 mmHg was proposed as the level where one could be sure of critical flow reduction in the splanchnic circulation [19]. Clinically a PCO_2-gap below 25 mmHg was considered as the target to avoid hypoxia [36].

▌ Conclusion

In summary, ICU patients with complications have both a higher $PiCO_2$ and a wider standard deviation as compared to patients without complications. The time profile of the aberration from normal $PiCO_2$ normal values is at least as meaningful as a single elevation in $PiCO_2$ values in judging the clinical situation. Above physiological values of $PiCO_2$ or PCO_2-gap there seems to be a 'tolerable corridor'. Clinical course may be assessed by $PiCO_2$ profiles. Further studies need to clarify this, and define $PiCO_2$ profiles in various patient groups to elucidate the clinical impact of $PiCO_2$ guided therapy.

References

1. Dantzker DR (1993) The gastrointestinal tract. The canary of the body? JAMA 270:1247–1248
2. Boda D, Muranyi L (1959) Gastrotonometry: An aid to the control of ventilation during artificial ventilation. Lancet 273:181–182
3. Fiddian-Green RG, McGough E, Pittenger G, Rothman E (1983) Predictive value of intramural pH and other risk factors for massive bleeding from stress ulceration. Gastroenterology 85:613-620
4. Grum CM, Fiddian-Green RG, Pittenger GL, Grant BJB, Rothman ED, Dantzker DR (1984) Adequacy of tissue oxygenation in intact dog intestine. J Appl Physiol 56:1065–1069
5. Fiddian Green RG, Baker S (1987) Predictive value of stomach wall pH for complications after cardiac operations: Comparison with other monitoring. Crit Care Med 15:153–156
6. Doglio GR, Pusajo JF, Egurrola MA, et al (1991) Gastric mucosal pH as a prognostic index of mortality in critically ill patients. Crit Care Med 19:1037–1040
7. Gutierrez G, Palizas F, Doglio G, et al (1992) Gastric intramucosal pH as a therapeutic index of tissue oxygenation in critically ill patients. Lancet 339:195–199
8. Marik PE (1993) Gastric mucosal pH. A better predictor of multiorgan dysfunction syndrome and death than oxygen-derived variables in patients with sepsis. Chest 104:225–229
9. Mythen MG, Webb AR (1994) Intraoperative gut mucosal hypoperfusion is associated with increased post-operative complications and costs. Intensive Care Med 20:99–104
10. Parviainen I, Vaisanen O, Ruokonen E, Takala J (1996) Effect of nasogastric suction and ranitidine on the calculated gastric mucosal pH. Intensive Care Med 22:319-323
11. Riddington D, Venkatesh B, Clutton-Brock T, Bion J, Venkatesh KB (1994) Measuring carbon dioxide tension in saline and alternative solutions: quantification of bias and precision in two blood gas analysers. Crit Care Med 22:96–100
12. Takala J, Parviainen I, Siloaho M, Ruokonen E, Hämäläinen E (1995) Measuring carbon dioxide tension in saline. Crit Care Med 23:1609–1610
13. Takala J, Parviainen I, Siloaho M, Ruokonen E, Hämäläinen E (1994) Saline PCO2 is an important source of error in the assessment of gastric mucosal pH. Crit Care Med 22:1877–1879
14. Schlichtig R, Mehta N, Gayowski TJP (1996) Tissue arterial pCO2 difference is a better marker of ischemia than intramural pH (pHi) or arterial pH-pHi difference. J Crit Care 11:51–56
15. Guzman JA, Kruse JA (1996) Development and validation of a technique for continuous monitoring of gastric mucosal pH. Am J Respir Crit Care Med 153:694–700
16. Temmesfeld-Wollbrück B, Szalay A, Olschewski H, Grimminger F, Seeger W (1997) Advantage of buffered solutions or automated capnometry in air-filled balloons for use in gastric tonometry. Intensive Care Med 23:423–427

17. Creteur J, DeBacker D, Vincent JL (1997) Monitoring gastric mucosal carbon dioxide pressure using gas tonometry. Anesthesiology 87:504–510
18. Janssens U, Graf J, Koch KC, Hanrath P (1998) Gastric tonometry: In vivo comparison of saline and air tonometry in patients with cardiogenic shock. Br J Anaesth 81:676–680
19. Kellum JA, Rico P, Garuba AK, Pinsky MR (2000) Accuracy of mucosal pH and mucosal-arterial carbon dioxide tension for detecting mesenteric hypoperfusion in acute canine endotoxemia. Crit Care 28:462–466
20. Guzman JA, Kruse JA (1999) Gut mucosal-arterial PCO2 gradient as an indicator of splanchnic perfusion during systemic hypo- and hypercapnia. Crit Care Med 27:2760–2765
21. Schaffartzik W (1995) Die intramukosale CO2-Messung. Anästhesiol Intensivmed Notfallmed Schmerztherap 30 (Suppl):14–17
22. Bennet-Guerrero E, Panah MH, Bodian CA, et al (2000) Automated detection of gastric luminal partial pressure of carbon dioxide during cardiovascular surgery using the Tonocap. Anesthesiology 92:38–45
23. Nöldge-Schomburg G, Armburster K, Geiger K, Zander R (1995) Der Normalwert des intramukosalen CO2-Partialdrucks. Anästhesiol Intensivmed Notfallmed Schmerztherap 30 (Suppl):18–19
24. Schlichtig RA, Bowles SA (1994) Distinguishing between aerobic and anaerobic appearance of dissolved CO2 in intestine during low flow. J Appl Physiol 76:2443–2451
25. Myers MB, Cherry G, Gesser J (1972) Relationship between surface pH and PCO2 and the vascularity and viability of intestine. Surg Gyn Obstet 134:787–789
26. Marik PE, Varon J (1998) The hemodynamic derangements in sepsis. Implication for treatment strategies. Chest 114:854–860
27. Russel JA (1999) Catecholamines and the splanchnic circulation. Crit Care Med 27:242–243
28. Kettler D (1994) Permissive anaemia compared with blood transfusion in patients with cardiac disease: another point of view. Current Opin Anaesthesiol 7:1–4
29. Muckart DJ, Bhagwanjee S (1997) American College of Chest Physicians/Society of Critical Care Medicine Consensus Conference definitions of the systemic inflammatory response syndrome and allied disorders in relation to critically injured patients. Crit Care Med 25:1787–1795
30. Fiddian-Green RG (1995) Gastric intrmucosal pH, tissue oxygenation and acid-base balance. Br J Anaesth 74:591–606
31. Gomersall CD, Joynt GM, Ho KM, Young RJ, Buckley TA, Oh TE (1997) Gastric tonometry and prediction of outcome in the critically ill. Anaesthesia 52:619–623
32. Russell JA (1997) Gastric tonometry: does it work? Intensive Care Med 23:3–6
33. Lebuffe G, Decoene C, Pol A, Prat A, Vallet B (1999) Regional capnometry with air automated tonometry detects circulatory failure earlier than conventional hemodynamics after cardiac surgery. Anesth Analg 89:1084–1090
34. Temmesfeld-Wollbrück B, Szalay A, Mayer K, Olschowski H, Seeger W, Grimminger F (1998) Abnormalities of gastric mucosal oxygenation in septic shock. Am J Respir Crit Care Med 157:1586–1592
35. Miller PR, Kincaid EH, Meredith JW, Chang MC (1998) Threshold values of intramucosal pH and mucosal-arterial CO2 gap during shock resuscitation. J Trauma 45:868–872
36. Vallet P, Tavernier B, Lund N (2000) Assessment of tissue oxygenation in the critically ill. Eur J Anaesth 17:221–229

Coagulopathies

Thrombotic Microangiopathies

C. Adrie and E. Azoulay

▌ Introduction

Since the first description in 1925, thrombotic microangiopathies (TMA) have led to one of the most exciting fields of ongoing research to elucidate the pathophysiologic mechanisms responsible for this disorder. We shall review some of the classic clinical knowledge and more recent breakthroughs in the understanding of the mechanisms involved and the controversial treatments.

▌ Thrombotic Thrombocytopenic Purpura (TTP) and Hemolytic Uremic Syndrome (HUS): a Single Entity?

The term TMA encompasses the spectrum of classical thrombotic thrombocytopenic purpura (TTP) described first by Moschowitz [1] and hemolytic uremic syndrome (HUS) described three decades later by Gasser et al. [2]. Both share the same histologic lesion, widening of the subendothelial space and microvascular thrombosis, and a similar pathophysiologic process, leading to thrombocytopenia and hemolytic anemia through platelet consumption and erythrocyte disruption in the injured microvasculature [3, 4]. The diagnosis classically relies on the pentad of symptoms: hemolytic anemia with presence of schistocytes and negative Coombs test, thrombocytopenia, fever, central nervous systems (CNS) abnormalities, and renal dysfunction.

Because they share the same histologic lesion, HUS and TTP are now believed to be a variable expression of the same disease called TMA [3]. The different clinical manifestations of HUS and TTP are essentially related to the different distribution of the vascular process. Therefore, in children with glomerular and pre-glomerular vascular involvement, the dominant clinical manifestations are the consequence of renal dysfunction. In adults, the microangiopathic process electively affects the brain with neurological symptoms dominating the clinical picture. However, wide differences still remain between the two classic different clinical expressions with numerous overlaps (Table 1).

Several classifications have been proposed to identify subsets of patients with TMA with similar clinical characteristics. For instance, Drummond [5] and then Remuzzi [3] tried to propose a more complete classification as follows:
▌ infantile and childhood TMA,
▌ hereditary and recurrent TMA,
▌ postinfectious TMA,

Table 1. Classic clinical aspects differentiating HUS and TTP. Table represents the main differences between the two usual expressions of thrombotic microangiopathies. Because of the similarities, HUS and TTP have been recognized as a single entity. This explains the often overlapping and indistinguishable clinical presentation

	Hemolytic-uremic syndrome (HUS)	Thrombotic thrombocytopenic purpura (TTP)
▌ Main organ dysfunction	Renal dysfunction	CNS abnormalities
▌ Spontaneous Outcome	Favorable	Mortality rate > 90%
▌ Plasmapheresis	?	+ + + +
▌ Causes	Mainly enteropathogenic *Escherichia coli* (serotype O157/H7 + +)	Idiopathic related to HIV, connective diseases, cancer, etc.
▌ Age	Children	Adults
▌ Antibiotic	–	+ + +
▌ Von Willebrand factor-cleaving protease activity	Normal	Decreased
▌ Factor H	Decreased in some patients	Normal?

CNS: central nervous system; HIV: human immunodeficiency virus

▌ TMA accompanying systemic diseases and, finally,
▌ those associated with pregnancy, or with the use of drugs such as oral contraceptives, cyclosporine A, or antineoplastic drugs etc.

▌ TMA: Recent Advances in Pathophysiology

Different triggering factors may be involved such as bacterial viral infection, pregnancy, drug therapy, chemotherapy and bone marrow transplantation. Triggering probably induces endothelial damage which is thought to be the initial step. Unusual, large molecular weight von Willebrand factor (vWf) multimers are normally found in the Weibel-Palade bodies of endothelial cells and in platelet alpha granules. These multimer, but not the normal, plasma vWf forms, can induce aggregation of platelets under high shear stress. Systemic endothelial cell injury may lead to excessive release of these unusual, large polymers of vWf that cannot be processed to smaller forms by a specific enzyme [6, 7] (Fig. 1). As a result, they can be measured in plasma of patients during the remission phase and are absent during acute or relapse probably because of their 'consumption' by the shear stress-induced platelet aggregation [8]. Recently, Furlan et al. [9] showed that non-familial TTP is due to the presence of an inhibitor of vWf-cleaving factor, whereas the familial form seems to be caused by a constitutional deficiency of the protease. This appeared to be related to the presence of inhibitory IgG antibodies [10]. Interestingly, the vWf-cleaving factor activity was found to be normal in non familial HUS [9].

Other autoantibodies have already been associated with TTP such as antiplatelet antibodies, anti-CD16 which is a membrane polypeptide and is expressed in platelets as well as many other cells [11], and anti-endothelial cell antibodies [12]. Immune injury to vascular endothelial cells could expose thrombogenic subendothelial surfaces, induce apoptosis [13], and finally release vWf from intracellular stores, which could potentiate platelet agglutination through some secondary interaction,

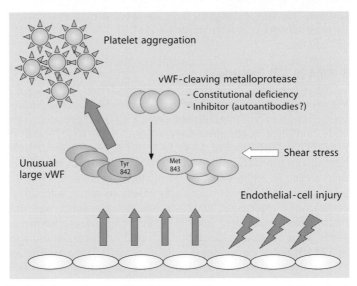

Platelet aggregation

vWF-cleaving metalloprotease
- Constitutional deficiency
- Inhibitor (autoantibodies?)

Shear stress

Unusual
large vWF

Tyr
842

Met
843

Endothelial-cell injury

Fig. 1. Pathophysiology of thrombotic microangiopathy (TMA). Deficit in metalloprotease. Endothelial injury leads to the release of unusually large molecular weight von Willebrand factor (vWf) multimers, which, jointly with high shear stress, induces a massive platelet aggregation. These large vWf multimers are normally released by the endothelium and proteolyzed by the vWf-cleaving protease. This enzyme has been shown to be constitutionally deficient in the familial form of TTP patients and inhibited by IgG autoantibodies in non-familial forms [9, 10]

such as high shear rate or platelet antibodies. Together, these autoantibodies suggest a dysregulation of the immune system and represent the substratum for the use of immune modulatory approaches of this disease.

Two distinct verotoxins, verotoxin-1 and -2, also known as shiga-like toxins because of their close homology with the toxin produced by *Shigella dysenteriae* (serotype 1), cause the human disease. These toxins are closely related exotoxins encoded in the DNA of bacteriophages and incorporated into the genome of a restricted number of *Escherichia coli* serotypes. Verotoxin is formed by a biologically active subunit A, and a number of B subunits by which the toxin binds to specific glycolipid receptors. The distribution of verotoxin receptors may determine the localization of microvascular lesions [14].

Transient hypocomplementemia with evidence of alternative pathway activation has been reported in typical, diarrhea-associated cases of HUS where the etiology is likely to have been verocytotoxin-producing *Escherichia coli* [15]. Usually the reduction in plasma concentrations is mild and reversible. By contrast, a few cases demonstrate persistently low complement C3 and in some of these, there are low plasma concentrations of the complement regulator, factor H. Investigation of these patients, linkage analysis in familial HUS, and more recently reports of mutations in the factor H gene in sporadic cases, together indicate an important association between factor H and a clinically recognizable subgroup of HUS [16]. This factor represents the most abundant complement regulator in plasma. It also operates attached to host surfaces, including endothelium. It accelerates the decay of C3bBb, the C3 convertase of the alternative pathway, and, with factor I as a cofactor, it cleaves and inactivates C3b. Thus, factor H with other complement regulators located on host cells or in the soluble phase prevents indiscriminate complement activation. Certain pathogens have evolved with the ability to bind factor H and thereby subvert complement attack [16].

TMA in ICU Patients

We recently studied a series of 30 patients requiring admission to the intensive care unit (Coppo et al., unpublished data) (ICU). There were 19 males and 11 females with simplified acute physiology score (SAPS) II [17] and logistic organ dysfunction (LOD) [18] score of 37.3±18.7 and 6.8±0.7, respectively. TMA was related to human immunodeficiency virus (HIV) infection in nine cases, systemic lupus erythematosus in eight, two were idiopathic, seven were related to drug intake, transplantation, or pregnancy. In eight cases, an acute infectious disease was the only cause found. Moreover, an acute infectious episode was diagnosed in twelve patients who already had another underlying disease known to be related to TMA. Thus, acute infectious diseases, suspected or documented, appear to act as a trigger of TMA whether or not there is another underlying association.

The description of the organ failure according to the LOD definition is represented in Table 2. Twenty seven patients (90%) presented with CNS involvement, ranging from headache to seizure or focal deficits through confusion. Seven patients required hemodialysis and 17 mechanical ventilation mostly because of CNS manifestations. Of note, two septic patients required inotropic support despite adequate fluid administration and thus met the definition criteria for septic shock as already described in another case report [19]. The latter may be difficult to distinguish from TMA since severe sepsis may share some identical non-specific signs and clinical symptoms.

Plasma Administration: Infusion or Exchange?

Plasma infusion has been described as a very efficient way to treat TTP since 1977 [20]. Concomitantly, Bukowsky et al. [21] showed that plasmapheresis was also an efficient means of plasma administration. Up to 1987, both routes of plasma administration were considered to be equivalent allowing complete remission in 60 to

Table 2. Organ failure at admission as described in the logistic organ dysfunction (LOD) score [18]. We defined four groups depending on the associated condition: HIV (human immunodeficiency virus) disease, SLE (systemic lupus erythematosus), infection (when only an acute infection was diagnosed), and others (miscellaneous such as drugs, malignant diseases, post-partum or idiopathic)

Organ failure	Infection (n=7)	HIV disease (n=9)	SLE (n=6)	Others (n=8)	Total (n=30)
Cardiovascular	0	1	0	1	2
Renal	4	5	0	2	11
Neurologic	5	6	2	2	15
Hepatic	1	3	0	0	4
Hematological	5	6	4	6	21
Pulmonary	1	0	0	2	3

80% of the cases [22]. Subsequently, Rock et al. [23], in a randomized study, showed that patients given plasma infusion alone had a lower response at nine days and a higher mortality at six months as compared to the patients with plasma exchange therapy (37 vs. 21%, respectively). However, there was a marked disparity in the volume of plasma delivered, being three times higher in the plasma exchange group (with particularly low volume administered in the plasma infusion group: 30 ml/kg for the first day and then 20 ml/kg/d). In contrast, retrospective studies showed that when matching volumes were delivered, the outcome was similar [24]. Indeed, several other groups also believe that high doses of plasma infusion are a safe, readily available, and reasonable alternative to expensive and time-consuming plasma exchange, particularly in TMA induced by *Escherichia coli* O157:H7 [4, 25, 26]. The fact that benefit is seen with plasma infusion only argues for a missing or altered factor in the circulation [7].

There are no scientific studies that have precisely determined the optimal plasma exchange schedule and duration of plasma administration, which remain empirical. Plasma administration, either by infusion or exchange, represents the cornerstone of therapy in the adult with HUS and in patients with all ages with TTP [27, 28] but its usefulness remains controversial in children with HUS [3].

▍ TMA and Anti-infectious Therapy

Since the first reports of HUS associated with bacteria of the family Enterobacteriaceae such as *Escherichia coli* (Serotype O157:H7) and *Shigella dysenteriae* (Serotype 1) [29–31], a large number of other infectious agents have been recognized to induce TMA (Coppo et al., unpublished data). Furthermore, non-bacterial agents such as herpes virus [32, 33], HIV [34] or other viruses [35], and fungal agents [36] have also been associated with TMA. Clearly, a large variety of non specific infectious agents, besides verotoxin-secreting Enterobacteriaceae, may play a key role in triggering TMA and inducing relapse or refractoriness (Coppo et al., unpublished data, [37]). This supports active antiinfectious treatment against the responsible infection.

However, this may not always be the case. Recently, Wong et al. [38] showed that antibiotic treatment of children with *Escherichia coli* O157:H7 increases the risk of the HUS probably by causing Shiga-toxin release from the injured bacteria in the intestine, making the toxin more available for absorption. Therefore, the use of antibiotic should be strongly discouraged in children with gastrointestinal infections until the results of stool culture are available. Similarly, despite the absence of an association between treatment and antimotility drugs or opioid narcotics and the risk of HUS in this study [38], these drugs should be avoided in children with diarrhea, because of their reported association with complications of *Escherichia coli* O157:H7 infection and with the prolongation of symptoms [39–41].

▍ Corticosteroids?

Although Bell et al. [27], in a retrospective study, found that steroids alone may be beneficial in TTP patients, it must be emphasized that only non-severe patients were managed with steroids alone (i. e., patients who did not show evidence of neurological involvement). Whether they may be of some benefit in addition to plasma therapy remains hypothetical [7]. An appropriate randomized study to assess the role of steroids has not been carried out (especially in association with plasma administration). However, as evidence supporting an immune-mediated basis for the disorder continues to accumulate, steroid therapy increases in acceptance, at least in non-septic patients.

▊ Platelet Transfusions?

Platelet transfusions may be dangerous in patients with TMA. Patients have been observed to have abrupt, striking deterioration after platelet transfusion, consistent with the exacerbation of thromboses [42, 43]. However, the severity of the disease at presentation has not been compared among patients who do or do not receive platelet transfusion and it is likely that platelet transfusions were administered to the more severely ill patients. Thus it was not clear whether the platelet transfusion was directly responsible for the unfavorable outcome. Moreover, the doses of plasma administered during plasma exchange were not specified. Other teams have reported no observed adverse effect following platelet transfusions when they are required for an invasive procedure [44, 45]. However, until such a procedure is validated on a larger series of patients, the use of platelets should be avoided and be restricted to patients presenting a refractory life threatening thrombocytopenia and/or requiring surgery or any kind of invasive procedure [44].

▊ Antiplatelet Agents?

These drugs have been extensively used in the treatment of TMA. The rationale for this is based on the formation of platelet aggregates and the consideration that inhibition and down-regulation of platelet responses would be of benefit, although the literature is variable with regard to demonstrating platelet activation in TMA [7]. There is no clear evidence for recommending their use in TMA [45].

▊ Conclusion

In this mini review, we intended to give a little glimpse of the recent advances in these fields and to apprehend some controversies of this rare but interesting disease that may require ICU admission. Plasma administration either by infusion or exchange remains the cornerstone of treatment for this disease. However, much progress remains to be made to better understand the pathophysiology of this disease process.

References

1. Moschowitz E (1924) Hyaline thrombosis of the terminal arterioles and capillaries: a hitherto undescribed disease. Proc N Y Pathol Soc 24:21–24
2. Gasser C, Gautier E, Steck A, Siebenmann RE, Oechslin R (1955) Hämolytisch-urämische Syndrome: Bilaterale Nierenrindennekrosen bei akuten erworbenen hämolytischen Anämien. Schweiz Med Wochenschr 85:905–909

3. Remuzzi G (1987) HUS and TTP: variable expression of a single entity. Kidney Int 32:292–308
4. Ruggenenti P, Lutz J, Remuzzi G (1997) Pathogenesis and treatment of thrombotic microangiopathy. Kidney Int Suppl 58:S97–101
5. Drummond KN (1985) Hemolytic uremic syndrome – then and now. N Engl J Med 312:116–118
6. Moake JL (1998) von Willebrand factor in the pathophysiology of thrombotic thrombocytopenic purpura. Clin Lab Sci 11:362–364
7. Rock GA (2000) Management of thrombotic thrombocytopenic purpura. Br J Haematol 109:496–507
8. Moake JL (1997) Studies on the pathophysiology of thrombotic thrombocytopenic purpura. Semin Hematol 34:83–89
9. Furlan M, Robles R, Galbusera M, et al (1998) von Willebrand factor-cleaving protease in thrombotic thrombocytopenic purpura and the hemolytic-uremic syndrome. N Engl J Med 339:1578–1584
10. Tsai HM, Lian EC (1998) Antibodies to von Willebrand factor-cleaving protease in acute thrombotic thrombocytopenic purpura. N Engl J Med 339:1585–1594
11. Tandon NN, Rock G, Jamieson GA (1994) Anti-CD36 antibodies in thrombotic thrombocytopenic purpura. Br J Haematol 88:816–825
12. Leung DY, Moake JL, Havens PL, Kim M, Pober JS (1988) Lytic anti-endothelial cell antibodies in haemolytic-uraemic syndrome. Lancet 2:183–186
13. Dang CT, Magid MS, Weksler B, Chadburn A, Laurence J (1999) Enhanced endothelial cell apoptosis in splenic tissues of patients with thrombotic thrombocytopenic purpura. Blood 93:1264–170
14. Remuzzi G, Ruggenenti P (1995) The hemolytic uremic syndrome. Kidney Int 48:2–19
15. Monnens L, Molenaar J, Lambert PH, Proesmans W, van Munster P (1980) The complement system in hemolytic-uremic syndrome in childhood. Clin Nephrol 13:168–171
16. Taylor CMT (2001) Hemolytic-uremic syndrome and complement factor H deficiency: clinical aspects. Semin Thromb Hemost 27:185–190
17. Le Gall JR, Lemeshow S, Saulnier F (1993) A new Simplified Acute Physiology Score (SAPS II) based on a European/North American multicenter study. JAMA 270:2957–2963
18. Le Gall JR, Klar J, Lemeshow S, et al (1996) The Logistic Organ Dysfunction system. A new way to assess organ dysfunction in the intensive care unit. ICU Scoring Group. JAMA 276:802–810
19. Pene F, Papo T, Brudy-Gulphe L, et al (2001) Septic shock and thrombotic microangiopathy due to Mycobacterium tuberculosis in a nonimmunocompromised patient. Arch Intern Med 161:1347–1348
20. Byrnes JJ, Khurana M (1977) Treatment of thrombotic thrombocytopenic purpura with plasma. N Engl J Med 297:1386–1389
21. Bukowski RM, Hewlett JS, Harris JW, et al (1976) Exchange transfusions in the treatment of thrombotic thrombocytopenic purpura. Semin Hematol 13:219–232
22. Shepard KV, Bukowski RM (1987) The treatment of thrombotic thrombocytopenic purpura with exchange transfusions, plasma infusions, and plasma exchange. Semin Hematol 24:178–193
23. Rock GA, Shumak KH, Buskard NA, et al (1991) Comparison of plasma exchange with plasma infusion in the treatment of thrombotic thrombocytopenic purpura. Canadian Apheresis Study Group. N Engl J Med 325:393–397
24. Novitzky N, Jacobs P, Rosenstrauch W (1994) The treatment of thrombotic thrombocytopenic purpura: plasma infusion or exchange? Br J Haematol 87:317–320
25. Fakhouri F, Vincent F, Legendre C (2000) Pathological and therapeutic distinctions in HUS/TTP. Lancet 355:497
26. Ruggenenti P, Galbusera M, Cornejo RP, Bellavita P, Remuzzi G (1993) Thrombotic thrombocytopenic purpura: evidence that infusion rather than removal of plasma induces remission of the disease. Am J Kidney Dis 21:314–318
27. Bell WR, Braine HG, Ness PM, Kickler TS (1991) Improved survival in thrombotic thrombocytopenic purpura-hemolytic uremic syndrome. Clinical experience in 108 patients. N Engl J Med 325:398–403

28. Dundas S, Murphy J, Soutar RL, et al (1999) Effectiveness of therapeutic plasma exchange in the 1996 Lanarkshire Escherichia coli O157:H7 outbreak. Lancet 354:1327–1330
29. Remuzzi G, Ruggenenti P (1998) The hemolytic uremic syndrome. Kidney Int Suppl 66:S54–S57
30. Moake JL (1994) Haemolytic-uraemic syndrome: basic science. Lancet 343:393–397
31. Boyce TG, Swerdlow DL, Griffin PM (1995) Escherichia coli O157:H7 and the hemolytic-uremic syndrome. N Engl J Med 333:364–368
32. Jeejeebhoy FM, Zaltzman JS (1998) Thrombotic microangiopathy in association with cytomegalovirus infection in a renal transplant patient: a new treatment strategy. Transplantation 65:1645–1648
33. Satoh K, Takahashi H, Nagai K, Shibata A (1988) Thrombotic thrombocytopenic purpura and herpes zoster infection. Ann Intern Med 108:154–155
34. Hymes KB, Karpatkin S (1997) Human immunodeficiency virus infection and thrombotic microangiopathy. Semin Hematol 34:117–125
35. Wasserstein A, Hill G, Goldfarb S, Goldberg M (1981) Recurrent thrombotic thrombocytopenic purpura after viral infection. Clinical and histologic simulation of chronic glomerulonephritis. Arch Intern Med 141:685–687
36. Miniero R, Nesi F, Vai S, et al (1997) Cryptococcal meningitis following a thrombotic microangiopathy in an unrelated donor bone marrow transplant recipient. Pediatr Hematol Oncol 14:469–474
37. Creager AJ, Brecher ME, Bandarenko N (1998) Thrombotic thrombocytopenic purpura that is refractory to therapeutic plasma exchange in two patients with occult infection. Transfusion 38:419–423
38. Wong CS, Jelacic S, Habeeb RL, Watkins SL, Tarr PI (2000) The risk of the hemolytic-uremic syndrome after antibiotic treatment of Escherichia coli O157:H7 infections. N Engl J Med 342:1930–1936
39. Cimolai N, Carter JE, Morrison BJ, Anderson JD (1990) Risk factors for the progression of Escherichia coli O157:H7 enteritis to hemolytic-uremic syndrome. J Pediatr 1990:589–592
40. Cimolai N, Morrison S, Carter JE (1992) Risk factors for the central nervous system manifestations of gastroenteritis-associated hemolytic-uremic syndrome. Pediatrics 90:616–621
41. Cimolai N, Basalyga S, Mah DG, Morrison BJ, Carter JE (1994) A continuing assessment of risk factors for the development of Escherichia coli O157:H7-associated hemolytic uremic syndrome. Clin Nephrol 42:85–89
42. Harkness DR, Byrnes JJ, Lian EC, Williams WD, Hensley GT (1981) Hazard of platelet transfusion in thrombotic thrombocytopenic purpura. JAMA 246:1931–1933
43. Gordon LI, Kwann HC, Rossi EC (1987) Deleterious effects of platelet transfusion and recovery in patients with thrombotic microangiopathy. Semin Hematol 24:194–201
44. Coppo P, Lassoued K, Mariette X, et al. (2001) Effectiveness of platelet transfusions after plasma exchange in adult thrombotic thrombocytopenic purpura: a report of two cases. Am J Hematol 68:198–201
45. Georges JN (2000) How I treat patients with thrombotic thrombocytopenic purpura-hemolytic uremic syndrome. Blood 96:1223–1229

Pro-hemostatic Therapy for Prevention and Treatment of Bleeding

M. Levi, R. Vink, and E. de Jonge

▌ Introduction

The hemostatic system is able to swiftly convert fluid blood to a solid clot when there is a disruption of vascular integrity and bleeding occurs. Simultaneously, another important feature of hemostasis is to maintain blood fluidity within the blood vessel to guarantee adequate circulation throughout the body. These two paradoxical functions of the coagulation system can only be executed when, under physiological circumstances, there is a balance between low-level ongoing basal coagulation activation and permanent anticoagulation by both physiological anticoagulant mechanisms and fibrin removal as a function of the fibrinolytic system. Pharmacological agents may interfere in this balance, for example by inhibiting coagulant activity or promoting anticoagulant mechanisms, and indeed this type of treatment has proven to be effective in the prevention and treatment of thrombotic disease. Similarly, other agents are capable of promoting hemostasis or fibrin formation, or can block fibrinolytic activity. These so-called 'pro-hemostatic agents' may be useful in the prevention and treatment of bleeding in patients with coagulation defects, but also in patients with an *a priori* normal coagulation system, who experience severe (post-operative) bleeding or are to undergo procedures known to be associated with major blood loss [1]. In this chapter, we will discuss the aims and potential risks of pro-hemostatic therapy, the various agents with a pro-hemostatic potential and the efficacy of pro-hemostatic drugs to reduce perioperative blood loss or treat excessive (postoperative) bleeding.

▌ Aims and Potential Risks of Pro-hemostatic Therapy

Most experience with pro-hemostatic therapy has been accumulated in the prevention and treatment of bleeding in patients with congenital and acquired coagulation defects. Indeed, specific correction of a hemostatic defect is highly effective in this situation, as, for example, has been shown in the management of hemophilia with coagulation factor concentrates. There is, however, increasing evidence that promoting hemostatic function may be of benefit also in patients with less specific abnormalities or even a normal coagulation status and who encounter severe bleeding or are at high risk for bleeding [2, 3]. Interestingly, there seems not to be a strong need in general to specifically target a factor or pathway in the coagulation or fibrinolytic system that is causally related to the hemostatic defect, since interference in one part of the system may be able to compensate for a defect in another part. A good illustration is the proven efficacy of antifibrinolytic agents in the prevention and treatment of bleeding in patients with mild hemophilia or von Willebrand's disease [4].

It is important to focus on the general aim of pro-hemostatic interventions. In patients with severe bleeding the arrest of blood loss, and stabilizing the patient's hemodynamics, is obviously more important than normalizing laboratory tests. In case of prevention of expected (peri-operative) bleeding, the main focus should not be on the reduction of blood loss per se, but rather on the prevention of transfusion requirements. Allogeneic transfusion is associated with undesirable immunologic and (at least theoretical) blood-borne infectious complications and is related to increased post-operative morbidity and even mortality. Hence, when assessing efficacy of pro-hemostatic interventions, these clinically more relevant outcomes, rather than the amount of blood loss, should be taken into account.

The safety of pro-hemostatic therapy also deserves some consideration. Interfering in the balance between coagulant and anticoagulant mechanisms can indeed result in undesirable adverse effects. The best illustration may be the higher risk of bleeding in patients receiving anticoagulant therapy. Conversely, pro-hemostatic agents may, at least theoretically, predispose for thrombotic complications. The occurrence of such complications, which are fortunately relatively rare, seems to be very much dependent on considerate clinical use of this therapy. In fact, the expected benefit of the application of pro-hemostatic agents in distinct clinical situations should be balanced with the risk of thrombosis in that particular patient population. Ideally, the benefit/risk ratio should be evaluated in properly controlled clinical trials.

▌ Pro-hemostatic Agents

Platelets, Plasma, and Coagulation Factor Concentrates

Platelet transfusion may be considered in patients with severe thrombocytopenia and bleeding or at risk for bleeding [5]. Platelet concentrates usually contain a mixture of the platelet preparation of a blood donation from 5–6 donors (equals 5–6 units). After platelet transfusion, the platelet count should rise with at least 5×10^9/l per unit of platelets transfused. A lesser response may be present in patients with fever, a consumptive coagulopathy, or splenomegaly, or may indicate alloimmunization of the patient after repeated transfusion. Platelet transfusion is particularly effective in patients with a thrombocytopenia due to impaired platelet production or increased consumption, whereas in disorders of enhanced platelet destruction (for example immune thrombocytopenia) alternative therapies, such as steroids or human immunoglobin, may provide better results. Basic guidelines for platelet transfusion are given in Table 1.

Fresh or frozen plasma contains all coagulation factors and may be used to replenish congenital or acquired deficiencies in these factors. For more specific therapy or if the transfusion of large volumes of plasma is not desirable, fractionated plasma of purified coagulation factor concentrate is available [2, 5]. Suggested guidelines for the use of fresh frozen plasma are given in Table 2.

Prothrombin complex concentrates (PCCs) contain the vitamin K-dependent coagulation factors II, VII, IX and X. Hence, these concentrates may be used if immediate reversal of coumarin therapy is required. Also, PCCs may be used if a global replenishment of coagulation factors is necessary and large volumes of plasma

Table 1. Suggested transfusion guidelines for platelet concentrates

▌ Platelet count $< 10 \times 10^9$/l
▌ Platelet count $< 50 \times 10^9$/l with demonstrated bleeding or a planned surgical/invasive procedure
▌ Documented platelet dysfunction (e.g. prolonged bleeding time) with (microvascular) bleeding or undergoing a surgical/invasive procedure and (assumed) insufficient efficacy of other interventions (e.g. desmopressin)
▌ Bleeding patients or patients undergoing a surgical procedure who require more than 10 U of packed red cells

Table 2. Suggested transfusion guidelines for fresh frozen plasma

▌ Correction of multiple or specific coagulation factor deficiencies in bleeding patients or if a surgical/invasive procedure is planned
  – congenital deficiencies of a specific factor (provided specific factor concentrates are not available, e.g. factor XI)
  – acquired deficiencies, e.g. related to liver disease, massive transfusion or disseminated intravascular coagulation

▌ Volume replacement in case of severe bleeding to avoid massive transfusion of gelatin or crystalloid solutions
▌ Thrombocytopenic thrombotic purpura

are not tolerated. One should realize, however, that in such cases only a selected number of coagulation factors is administered and important deficiencies of, for example factor V, or fibrinogen are not treated.

Cryoprecipitate is fractionated plasma, which mainly contains von Willebrand factor, factor VIII, and fibrinogen. However, due to the problems in the production of cryoprecipitate, particularly with regard to the standards to prevent the transmission of infectious agents, in most parts of the Western world cryoprecipitate is not available anymore.

For a selected number of clotting factors, purified concentrates, containing only that specific factor, are available. These concentrates are particularly useful in case of an isolated (usually congenital) deficiency of a single clotting factor, such as factor VIII concentrate for the treatment of hemophilia A. These concentrates may consist of clotting factors that are purified by affinity chromatography of plasma, however, recombinant coagulation factors are increasingly used [6].

One should realize that plasma and clotting factor concentrates derived from plasma are obtained from human donors. Potentially, this carries the risk of transmission of blood borne diseases, and despite all kind of measures to prevent this complication, at present these risks are not annihilated. Hence, the use of these products should be limited as much as possible, especially if no strict indication is present and alternative treatment is available.

Desmopressin

De-amino D-arginine vasopressin (DDAVP, desmopressin) is a vasopressin analog that, despite minor molecular differences (Fig. 1), has retained its antidiuretic properties but has fewer vaso-active effects [7]. DDAVP induces release of the contents

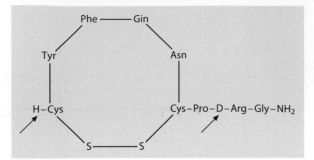

Fig. 1. Structure of DDAVP (desmopressin). The arrows indicate the modification of the original vasopressin molecule, i.e., replacement of the amino-group from the cysteine by hydrogen and substitution of L-arginine by R-arginin. These minimal molecular changes have major functional consequences, rendering the molecule much less vaso-active while retaining antidiuretic and pro-hemostatic properties

of the endothelial cell associated Weibel Palade bodies, including von Willebrand factor [8]. Hence, the administration of DDAVP results in a marked increase in the plasma concentration of von Willebrand factor (and associated coagulation factor VIII) and, by yet unexplained additional mechanisms, a remarkable potentiation of primary hemostasis as a consequence. DDAVP can be administered parenterally by different routes (intravenously [IV], subcutaneously, and intranasally) but is mostly administered by IV administration, which results in an immediate pro-hemostatic effect. DDAVP is used for the prevention and treatment of bleeding in patients with von Willebrand disease or mild hemophilia A, and further in patients with an impaired function of primary hemostasis, such as in patients with uremia, liver cirrhosis or in patients with aspirin-associated bleeding [1, 9, 10].

A rare but important adverse effect of DDAVP is the occurrence of acute myocardial infarction, particularly in patients with unstable coronary artery disease, probably due to the remaining vaso-active effect of the drug. Hence, in these patients the use of DDAVP is contraindicated. The antidiuretic effect of DDAVP is clinically not very significant and may be dealt with by fluid restriction for some time. An exception to this rule is children, who may experience severe dilution hyponatremia after the administration of DDAVP, and should be monitored clinically for 24 hours after its administration.

Recombinant Factor VIIa

Based on the current insight that activation of coagulation *in vivo* predominantly proceeds by the tissue factor/factor VII(a) pathway (Fig. 2), recombinant factor VIIa (NovoSeven®) has been developed as a pro-hemostatic agent and is now available for clinical use [11]. Indeed, recombinant factor VIIa appears to exert potent pro-hemostatic effects. Most experience with recombinant factor VIIa has been accumulated in patients with severe coagulation defects that are difficult to treat, such as patients with antibodies to coagulation factors and excessive bleeding [12, 13]. In addition, in patients with severe thrombocytopenia or disorders of primary hemostasis that fail to respond to conventional treatment, recombinant factor VIIa has been applied. In most of these situations administration of recombinant factor VIIa was shown to be effective in controlling bleeding, although most of the reports are uncontrolled series. Recombinant factor VIIa acts primarily by a tissue factor-dependent mechanism, which

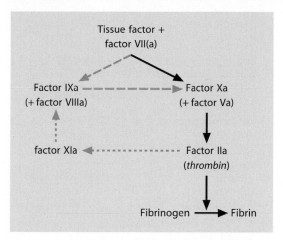

Fig. 2. Schematic representation of the *in vivo* function of coagulation. The initiation of coagulation is mediated by the tissue factor/factor VIIa complex. The principal route of thrombin generation proceeds by the direct activation of factor X and subsequent prothrombin to thrombin conversion (black arrows). Additional factor Xa is formed by an alternative pathway, due to tissue factor/factor VIIa-mediated activation of factor IX and the activation of factor X by this activated factor IX (and co-factor VIII) (gray arrows). A third amplifying pathway consist of the thrombin-mediated activation of factor XI, which can subsequently activate factors IX and X (dotted arrows). From this scheme the pro-hemostatic action of recombinant factor VIIa can be understood

limits its action to the site of bleeding, although some tissue factor-independent effects (potentially on the platelet surface) may play a role as well [14–16]. At present, a more general use of this agent for bleeding patients without an apparent coagulation defect is the subject of a number of ongoing clinical trials. One of these trials, in patients who underwent abdominal prostatectomy, demonstrated that the administration of recombinant factor VIIa was associated with a 50% reduction in perioperative blood loss, thereby completely eliminating the need for blood transfusion [17]. Preliminary results of other trials in liver surgery and trauma patients show promising results as well. Although so far only a very limited number of thrombotic complications of recombinant factor VIIa treatment have been reported in these trials, the safety of this strategy in a general, elderly population with potential co-morbidity remains to be established. Lastly, but importantly, the very high costs of recombinant factor VIIa, might limit its widespread use in clinical practice.

Anti-fibrinolytic Agents

Agents that exert anti-fibrinolytic activity are aprotinin and the group of lysine analogs [4]. The pro-hemostatic effect of these agents proceeds not only by the inhibition of fibrinolysis (thereby shifting the procoagulant/anticoagulant balance towards a more procoagulant state), but also due to a protective effect on platelets, as has been demonstrated at least for aprotinin x. The mechanism of this platelet-protective effect has, besides a potential prevention of plasmin-mediated loss of platelet receptors, not been elucidated. Whether the pro-hemostatic effect of the anti-fibrinolytic agents will eventually result in a higher incidence of thromboembolic complications is still a matter of debate (see further), however, this has so far not been shown in straightforward clinical trials.

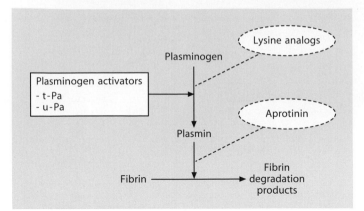

Fig. 3. Schematic representation of the fibrinolytic system and point of impact of antifibrinolytic agents. Lysine analogs bind to lysine binding sites on fibrin, thereby competing with plasminogen binding to fibrin. The conversion of plasminogen to plasmin by plasminogen activators is several-fold less efficient if plasminogen cannot bind to fibrin. Aprotinin directly binds to plasmin and blocks the proteolytic site of this protease. t-PA: tissue plasminogen activator; u-PA: urokinase plasminogen activator

Aprotinin is a 58 amino acid polypeptide, mainly derived from bovine lung, parotid gland or pancreas [4]. Aprotinin directly inhibits the activity of various serine proteases, including plasmin, coagulation factors or inhibitors, and constituents of the kallikrein-kinin and angiotensin system. This rather non-specific mode of action of aprotinin is frequently considered as a disadvantage for its use, however, the interactions of aprotinin with proteases other than plasmin have never been demonstrated to cause clinically important adverse effects. The clinically most important side effect of aprotinin is a rarely occurring, but sometimes serious, allergic or anaphylactic reaction. The use of aprotinin is contra-indicated in ongoing systemic intravascular activation of coagulation, as in disseminated intravascular coagulation (DIC), and in patients with renal failure.

Lysine analogs, i.e., ε-aminocaproic acid and tranexamic acid are potent inhibitors of fibrinolysis [1]. The antifibrinolytic action of lysine analogs is based on the competitive binding of these agents to the lysine-binding sites of a fibrin clot, thereby competing with the binding of plasminogen (Fig. 3). Impaired plasminogen binding to fibrin delays the conversion of plasminogen to plasmin and subsequent plasmin-mediated fibrinolysis, which then proceeds at an inefficient and slow rate. Subtle molecular variations between different lysine analogs may have important consequences for their fibrinolysis-inhibiting capacity. Indeed, tranexamic acid (Cyklokapron®) is at least ten times more potent than ε-aminocaproic acid (Amicar®). The use of lysine analogs is contra-indicated in situations with ongoing systemic activation of coagulation (such as in DIC) and furthermore in macroscopic hematuria, since the inhibition of urinary fibrinolysis due to the high concentrations of the antifibrinolytic agent in the urine may result in deposition of urinary tract-obstructing clots.

Other Pro-hemostatic Agents

Conjugated estrogen preparations may cause an improvement in primary hemostasis. However, except for a limited number of mostly uncontrolled studies in patients with uremic thrombocytopathy, and preliminary observations in patients who undergo liver transplantation, there is no sound evidence for the use of these agents to prevent or treat peri-operative bleeding.

Fibrin sealant, usually consisting of a combination of human fibrinogen and bovine thrombin may be used as a topical hemostatic agent. Although a number of controlled studies have shown the efficacy of this treatment in various surgical situations, there is no evidence that application of fibrin sealant results in a reduction in intraoperative or postoperative blood loss or other clinically significant outcome measures. Besides, fibrinogen is usually derived from human donor plasma, which may carry the risk of transmission of blood borne diseases. Moreover, the bovine origin of the thrombin may result in the formation of anti-coagulation factor antibodies that may cross-react with human coagulation factors, resulting in a potentially severe bleeding tendency.

▌ Reduction of Peri-operative Blood Loss by Interventions in the Coagulation System

Peri-operative blood loss may be due to surgical causes or to a defective hemostasis, and in some complicated situations a combination of these causes may be present [2, 3]. This may lead to excessive bleeding, resulting in enhanced transfusion requirements, a longer duration of operation, or even the need for re-exploration and a prolongation of the intensive care or hospital stay. Even if it is not certain that a coagulation disorder is the most important factor in the enhanced blood loss, interventions in the hemostatic system may be beneficial to prevent excessive bleeding and associated complications. This has been extensively investigated in particular in cardiac surgery and liver transplantation. In fact, the efficacy and safety of pro-hemostatic interventions in other types of surgery has not convincingly been shown in clinical trials with appropriate methodology.

Cardiac surgery, in particular coronary artery bypass surgery and heart valve replacement, is frequently associated with major blood loss. Besides the involvement of large vessels in the surgical area, other mechanisms may contribute to enhanced bleeding. These mechanisms include: 1) the loss of platelets and impairment of platelet function, due to cardiopulmonary by-pass, 2) hemodilution with associated decreased plasma concentrations of coagulation factors, 3) incomplete neutralization of heparin given during cardiopulmonary by-pass; and 4) an inadequate function of the fibrinolytic system, for which besides the observed enhanced release of plasminogen activators from the vessel wall, no clear explanation is presently available. A number of pharmacological agents have been used in an effort to diminish bleeding associated with cardiopulmonary by-pass [18].

A large number of studies have focused on the potential beneficial effect of aprotinin on the prevention of (excessive) bleeding in patients undergoing cardiac surgery. Randomized, controlled trials invariably showed that administration of aprotinin resulted in a reduction of perioperative blood loss, postoperative chest tube drainage, the number of transfused units and the number of patients receiving any transfusion. Most studies showed at least a 40% reduction in perioperative blood loss in patient with various *a priori* risks for the development of excessive peri-operative bleeding (low risk patients, re-operations, patients undergoing prosthetic valve implantation in combination with coronary artery by-pass grafting, etc.), and a 50% reduction in transfusion requirements. However, these figures need to be interpreted with caution because of the substantial inter-center variations in blood-saving techniques and transfusion practice, for example due to different 'transfusion triggers'. Furthermore, a number of clinical studies revealed that aprotinin reduced the incidence of re-thoracotomy due to excessive bleeding, however, the number of patients in the trials was not sufficiently high to reach statistical significance. Recently, several meta-analyses have been performed summarizing the placebo-controlled clinical trials with aprotinin [19–22]. These meta-analyses show a mean reduction in blood loss of 400 ml and a three-fold lower need to give any transfusion in cardiac surgery patients that had received aprotinin. Moreover, the two most recent meta-analyses show that the use of aprotinin results in a three-fold reduction in the incidence of re-exploration and the results of one of these studies indicate a two-fold reduction in mortality as compared with placebo. The dose of aprotinin used in most studies was relatively high, i. e., 280 mg (2×10^6 IU) loading dose over 30 minutes after the induction of anesthesia, followed by a 70 mg/hr (0.5×10^6 IU) continuous infusion for the duration of the operation and occasionally a dose of 280 mg (2×10^6 IU) added to the priming fluid of the cardiopulmonary by-pass circuit. Lower doses of aprotinin have been used as well in a variety of studies. A meta-analysis of studies comparing the higher and the lower dose of aprotinin shows that the higher dose is more effective in reducing blood loss and transfusion requirements, but that there is no statistically significant difference in the incidence of re-thoracotomy and mortality [19].

The potential blood loss-reducing effect of another anti-fibrinolytic therapy, i. e., with lysine-analogs, has also been investigated in a number of clinical trials. Generally, ε-aminocaproic acid showed insufficient efficacy as compared to tranexamic acid and most studies have focused on the latter agent. Tranexamic acid reduced bleeding after cardiac surgery, resulting in reduced transfusion requirements and a smaller number of patients that needed any transfusion. The effects of high dose tranexamic acid (up to 10 gram peri-operatively) resulted in a 40% reduction in blood loss and a 50% reduction in the number of transfused units in most controlled clinical trials. The above mentioned meta-analyses of all studies with lysine-analogs showed a 40% reduction in the number of patients that received any blood product and an about 2.5-fold reduction in the incidence of re-exploration [19, 20].

A number of recent studies have been initiated directly comparing aprotinin and tranexamic acid. A meta-analysis of these trials appears to indicate a higher efficacy of aprotinin as compared with lysine analogs, although the differences in the most important clinical endpoints, i. e., mortality and re-thoracotomy, did not reach statistical significance. Also, it should be noted that the use of aprotinin may result in a severe anaphylactic reaction, whereas lysine analogs are devoid of such serious adverse events. Lastly, aprotinin is much more expensive as compared with lysine analogs.

Placebo-controlled trials have provided evidence that the administration of desmopressin reduces peri-operative blood loss (15–40%) and decreases transfusion requirements (30%) in patients undergoing coronary artery by-pass surgery [8]. However, these favorable findings were not confirmed in other trials that showed no beneficial effect of desmopressin in the prevention of (excessive) peri-operative blood loss. The differential effects of desmopressin treatment may have been caused by varying patient selection criteria in the different clinical trials. A number of meta-analyses of all controlled clinical trials with desmopressin in cardiac surgery show a beneficial effect on blood loss and transfusion requirements, whereas the percentage of patients that need any transfusion, the incidence of re-exploration, and mortality are not statistically affected by desmopressin [19]. Subgroup analysis of the various clinical trials show that desmopressin might be particularly effective in case of the preoperative use of aspirin, which is not uncommon in patients undergoing cardiac surgery. The effect of desmopressin, however, appears to be relatively small as compared with aprotinin and tranexamic acid, although direct comparisons are scarce.

A lot of discussion based on surprisingly few solid scientific data is currently ongoing on the issue whether the beneficial effect of therapy for the prevention of (excessive) peri-operative blood loss might be offset by a potentially harmful net procoagulant effect, associated with graft occlusion and thrombotic complications. In one study, patients treated with aprotinin during their coronary artery by-pass surgery appeared to have more vein graft occlusions at coronary angiography one year post-operatively (20.5 versus 12.7% in patients that had not received aprotinin). Also, clinical end-points such as perioperative myocardial infarction were not in favor of aprotinin treatment [23]. However, all these data came from a retrospective analysis of a multicenter trial, in which in only one center all patients had received aprotinin and the result may thus have been caused by other, center-dependent factors. Other, though mostly uncontrolled, studies had not shown an increase in clinically important thrombotic events upon the use of aprotinin, however, these studies were small and did not systematically study these adverse effects, e.g., by means of coronary angiography. The earlier mentioned meta-analyses did not indicate a statistically significant increase in the incidence of peri-operative myocardial infarction in patients receiving aprotinin or lysine analogs. Hence, at this time a potential prothrombotic and graft-occluding effect of these interventions has not been firmly established.

Major liver surgery and in particular orthotopic liver transplantation may be associated with excessive blood loss. Factors which, in addition to surgical causes, contribute to this complication are impaired synthesis of coagulation proteins by the diseased liver, a pre-existing thrombocytopenia and thrombocytopathy, and impaired clearance of activated coagulation and fibrinolytic factors during the brief anhepatic phase. A small number of relatively small randomized controlled trials show that the administration of either aprotinin or tranexamic acid results in the reduction of blood loss and transfusion requirements [24, 25]. However, studies on the appropriate dose of these agents have yielded conflicting results and the definitive place of these pro-hemostatic agents in extensive liver surgery needs to be established. Initial experience with recombinant factor VIIa (see before) seems to show a beneficial effect of this agent in patients undergoing liver transplantation.

▌ Management of Excessive (Postoperative) Bleeding

Severe bleeding is a frequently occurring clinical condition. Bleeding may happen spontaneously but may also occur in the course of an operative treatment or in the postoperative phase and may become the predominant feature of the patient's illness. A central issue in a patient who has excessive bleeding during or after surgery is the decision whether the bleeding is a result of a systemic hemostatic defect or a local problem in surgical hemostasis. This distinction may sometimes be difficult, unless there are clear signs of a generalized bleeding tendency, such as simultaneous bleeding from various locations and sites of intravenous cannulation. Even in that case, however, the primary cause might be a local surgical problem, with secondary coagulation defects for example as a result of massive transfusion therapy (see further). In all cases of severe bleeding a global coagulation screening (i.e., platelet count, activated partial thromboplastin time (aPTT), prothrombin time (PT) should be carried out as soon as possible. If these tests show abnormal results, a brief trial of therapy with replacement of deficient hemostatic factors should be provided. However, unless there is prompt cessation of bleeding, this should not delay the decision to apply local interventions or (re-)operate if even the smallest suspicion of a local problem exists.

Systemic coagulation defects in severely bleeding patients with a previously normal coagulation system may in general be caused by two different mechanisms: 1) loss of platelets and coagulation factors due to bleeding and dilution of these elements upon massive transfusion of red cells and plasma substitutes; and 2) consumption of platelets and coagulation factors in the framework of DIC [5, 26].

Patients with severe blood loss may require massive fluid replacement therapy with blood substitutes such as crystalloid, colloid, dextran and starch solutions. The use of these synthetic plasma volume expanders in excess of 1 liter/hour is, however, in some cases associated with an impairment of primary hemostasis (most probably due to interference with von Willebrand factor function) and the plasma coagulation system (due to dilution). This has in particular been established for dextrans and gelatin-based plasma volume expanders [27]. Hence, the disproportionate use of these products may result in a deterioration of the hemostatic capability of a patient and potentially aggravate the bleeding. Therefore, if there is need for massive expansion of circulating volume in bleeding patients or patients at risk for bleeding, these preparations should be used in combination with fresh frozen plasma.

Transfusion with large amounts of packed red cells without concomitant replacement of platelets and coagulation factors may cause a generalized dilution coagulopathy [28]. This might be easily monitored by a decrease in platelet count to usually $50–100\times10^9$/l and a prolongation of global clotting times (aPTT and PT). Although there is no evidence from clinical studies to support this practice, it is generally recommended that in bleeding patients who need massive transfusion of red cells, for every 2–3 units of red cells, 1 unit of plasma is administered. In the absence of other factors that may cause a coagulation defect, this will result in a (near) normalization of coagulation times. Regarding the low platelet count, a more conservative strategy appears to be justified. A prospective trial showed no benefit of prophylactic transfusion of platelets in patients that received more than 12 units of red cells in a short period of time. However, retrospective analyses show that in bleeding patients with a platelet count lower than 50×10^9/l, transfusion of platelets is effective. Hence, the threshold for platelet transfusion in patients with bleeding can be held at 50×10^9/l, unless a defective platelet function is suspected. In that case a platelet transfusion at higher platelet counts could be considered [5].

Pharmacotherapeutic interventions to improve hemostasis may in some exceptional cases be contemplated, although there is not a lot of evidence from clinical trials to support this strategy. These interventions may consist of antifibrinolytic treatment, such as the administration of aminocaproic acid, tranexamic acid, or aprotinin. From a theoretical viewpoint it is not useful to combine these antifibrinolytic therapies. Lysine analogs have been shown to be helpful in the management of patients with upper gastro-intestinal bleeding, although this may be less relevant with the current possibilities of local hemostatic therapy in these patients. The administration of recombinant factor VIIa has shown impressive effects in patients with excessive bleeding in a small series of case-reports, but the safety and efficacy of this approach will definitively need further study.

▌ Conclusion

Pro-hemostatic therapy aims at an improvement of hemostasis, which may be achieved by amelioration of primary hemostasis, stimulation of fibrin formation, or inhibition of fibrinolysis. These treatment strategies may be applied to specifically correct a defect in one of the pathways of coagulation, but have in some situations also been shown to be effective in reducing bleeding in patients without a primary defect in coagulation. Pro-hemostatic interventions appear to be effective in reducing peri-operative blood loss and reducing transfusion requirements in specific situations and may be helpful adjuncts in the management of severe spontaneous and post-operative bleeding. The theoretical risk of a higher incidence of thrombotic complications associated with the use of pro-hemostatic therapy seems to be low in clinical practice, although there is a need for more systematic and adequately controlled clinical observations to better establish the efficacy and safety of pro-hemostatic interventions.

References

1. Mannucci PM (1998) Hemostatic drugs. N Engl J Med 339:245–253
2. Levi M, van der Poll T (2000) Hemostasis and coagulation. In: Norton JA, Bollinger RA, Chang AE, Lowry SF (eds) Surgery: Scientific Basis and Current Practice. Springer, New York, pp 161–176
3. Francis JL (1992) The use of drugs to reduce blood loss during surgery. Hematol Rev 7:85–99.
4. Marder VJ, Butler FO, Barlow GH (1994) Antifibrinolytic therapy. In: Colman RW, Hirsh J, Marder VJ, Salzman EW (eds) Hemostasis and Thrombosis: Basic Principles and Clinical Practice. J.W. Lippincott, Philadelphia, pp 795–814
5. Edmunds LH, Salzman EW (1994) Hemostatic problems, transfusion therapy, and cardio-pulmonary bypass in surgical patients. In: Colman RW, Hirsh J, Marder VJ, Salzman EW (eds) Hemostasis and Thrombosis: Basic Principles and Clinical Practice. J.W. Lippincott, Philadelphia, pp 1031–1045
6. Limentani SA, Roth DA, Furie BC, Furie B (1993) Recombinant blood clotting proteins for hemophilia therapy. Semin Thromb Hemost 19:62–72
7. Richardson DW, Robinson AG (1985) Desmopressin. Ann Intern Med 103:228–239
8. Mannucci PM (1997) Desmopressin (DDAVP) in the treatment of bleeding disorders: the first 20 years. Blood 90:2515–2521
9. Mannucci PM, Remuzzi G, Pusinri F, et al (1983) De-amino-8-D-arginine vasopressin shortens the bleeding time in uremia. N Engl J Med 308:8–12
10. Agnelli G, Parise P, Levi M, Cosmi B, Nenci GG (1995) Effects of desmopressin on hemostasis in patients with liver cirrhosis. Haemostasis 25:241–247
11. Hedner U (1998) Recombinant activated factor VII as a universal haemostatic agent. Blood Coagul Fibrinolysis 9 (suppl 1):S147–S152
12. Roberts HR (1998) Clinical experience with activated factor VII: focus on safety aspects. Blood Coagul Fibrinolysis 9 (suppl 1):S115–S118
13. Friederich PW, Wever PC, Briet E, Doorenbos CJ, Levi M (2001) Succesful treatment with recombinant factor VIIa of therapy-resistant severe bleeding in a patient with acquired von Willebrand disease. Am J Hematol 66:292–294

14. ten Cate H, Bauer KA, Levi M, et al (1993) The activation of factor X and prothrombin by recombinant factor VIIa in vivo is mediated by tissue factor. J Clin Invest 92:1207–1212
15. Friederich PW, Levi M, Bauer KA, et al (2001) Ability of recombinant factor VIIa to generate thrombin during inhibition of tissue factor in human subjects. Circulation 103:2555–2559
16. Hoffman M, Monroe DM, Roberts HR (1998) Activated factor VII activates factors IX and X on the surface of activated platelets: thoughts on the mechanism of action of high-dose activated factor VII. Blood Coagul Fibrinolysis 9 (suppl 1):S61–S65
17. Friederich PW, Geerdink MG, Spataro M, et al (2000) The effect of the administration of recombinant activated factor VII (NovoSeven) on perioperative blood loss in patients undergoing transabdominal retropubic prostatectomy: the PROSE study. Blood Coagul Fibrinolysis 11 (suppl 1):S129–132
18. Harker LA (1986) Bleeding after cardiopulmonary surgery. N Engl J Med 314:1446–1448.
19. Levi M, Cromheecke ME, de Jonge E, et al (1999) Pharmacological strategies to decrease excessive blood loss in cardiac surgery: a meta-analysis of clinically relevant endpoints. Lancet 354:1940–1947
20. Munoz JJ, Birkmeyer NJ, Birkmeyer JD, O'Connor GT, Dacey LJ (1999) Is epsilon-aminocaproic acid as effective as aprotinin in reducing bleeding with cardiac surgery?: a meta-analysis. Circulation 99:81–89
21. Fremes SE, Wong BI, Lee E, et al (1994) Metaanalysis of prophylactic drug treatment in the prevention of postoperative bleeding. Ann Thorac Surg 58:1580–1588
22. Laupacis A, Fergusson D (1997) Drugs to minimize perioperative blood loss in cardiac surgery: meta-analyses using perioperative blood transfusion as the outcome. The International Study of Peri-operative Transfusion (ISPOT) Investigators. Anesth Analg 85:1258–1267
23. van der Meer J, Hillege HL, Kootstra GJ, et al (1993) Prevention of one-year vein-graft occlusion after aortocoronary-bypass surgery: a comparison of low-dose aspirin, low-dose aspirin plus dipyridamole, and oral anticoagulants. The CABADAS Research Group of the Interuniversity Cardiology Institute of The Netherlands. Lancet 342:257–264
24. Lentschener C, Benhamou D, Mercier FJ (1997) Aprotinin reduces blood loss in patients undergoing elective liver resection. Anest Analg 84:875–881
25. Porte RJ, Molenaar IQ, Begliomini B, et al (2000) Aprotinin and transfusion requirements in orthotopic liver transplantation: a multicentre randomised double-blind study. EMSALT Study Group. Lancet 355:1303–1309
26. Levi M, ten Cate H (1999) Disseminated intravascular coagulation. N Engl J Med 341:586–592
27. de Jonge E, Levi M, Berends F, et al (1998) Impaired haemostasis by intravenous administration of a gelatin-based plasma expander in human subjects. Thromb Haemost 79:286–290
28. Lim RC, Olcott C, Robinson AJ (1973) Platelet response and coagulation changes following massive blood replacement. J Trauma 18:577–581

Coagulopathy in Trauma Patients

M. Lynn, I. Jeroukhimov, and Y. Klein

▌ Introduction

Massive hemorrhage is a major cause of trauma-related mortality. It has been shown that uncontrolled bleeding is the second most common cause of death after central nervous system (CNS) injuries in the pre-hospital setting [1], and the first responsible for early in-hospital mortality (first 48 hours) from major trauma [2].

Coagulopathy, when presenting with hypothermia and metabolic acidosis is associated with high mortality and was shown to be the most common cause of bleeding-related mortality early in the postoperative period [3]. Severe injury by itself, as well as multiple subsequent pathophysiologic events, is the cause of hemostatic failure in these patients. The pathogenesis of severe posttraumatic coagulopathy is complex. Virtually every aspect of the normal coagulation cascade is affected in the cold and acidotic trauma patient [4]. In the past decades, many surgeons emphasized the role of prevention or early treatment of this deadly triad. Damage control surgery with planned re-operations was advocated. Immediate control of surgical bleeding as well as vigorous early correction of hypothermia and aggressive resuscitation improved survival of these patients [5]. Nevertheless, ongoing diffuse bleeding in this environment continuous to be an ominous sign and predictor of early trauma-related mortality [3, 6, 7].

▌ Physiology of Hemostasis

Under normal conditions, hemostasis is achieved by an interaction of blood vessels, formed elements of the blood, and a number of enzymatic cascade reactions. When a vessel is injured, subendothelial tissues and collagen are exposed. This provides sites to which platelets can adhere and aggregate, with the release of granules (platelet factor 4, thromboglobulin, thrombospondin, platelet-derived growth factor [PDGF], fibrinogen, von Willebrand factor) and dense granules (ADP, serotonin) [8]. With the release of platelet granule contents, particularly ADP, further platelet aggregation occurs at the site of injury. The endothelial cells at the site of injury also produce thromboxane A_2, which stimulates platelet aggregation, locally; this very potent constrictor of smooth muscle leads to vasoconstriction. Platelet activation also leads to platelet procoagulant activity through surface coagulation factors (factor Va). These events result in the formation of a platelet plug within minutes of vessel injury. Ultimately, however, the production of a stable fibrin clot, through a series of enzymatic reactions, is necessary for adequate hemostasis.

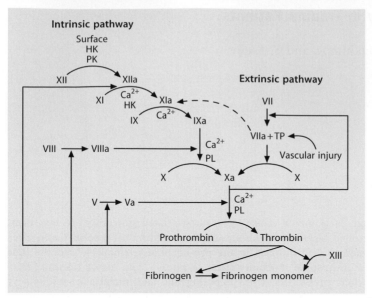

Fig. 1. Coagulation cascade. HK: high molecular weight kininogen; PK: prekalliklein; Ca^{2+}: calcium, PL: platelet factor 3

The process leading to clot formation involves interactions among the phospholipid surfaces, enzymes, and substrates. There are two pathways by which coagulation occurs: intrinsic and extrinsic (Fig. 1). The intrinsic pathway begins with the interaction of factor XII with prekallikrein and high-molecular-weight kininogen. Factor XII becomes factor XIIa, which in turn converts factor XI to factor XIa. Activated factor XI then activates factor IX to factor IXa in the presence of calcium. Activated factor IXa forms a complex with activated factor VIIIa, calcium ion, and phospholipids to activate factor X. Activated factor Xa is able to convert prothrombin to thrombin, which changes fibrinogen into fibrin. Factor XIII converts fibrin monomers into a cross-linked fibrin clot in the presence of calcium. In the extrinsic pathway, the initial step involves the interaction of subendothelial tissue factor and collagen with factor VII. In the presence of calcium, the factor VII-subendothelial complex is formed and activates factor X. Activated factor Xa then converts prothrombin to thrombin, and the reaction proceeds to the formation of fibrin.

To oppose the tendency toward blood coagulation, and to maintain the fluid characteristics of blood in the intravascular space, the fibrinolytic system must function properly [9]. The main reaction of the fibrinolytic pathway is the activation of plasminogen to plasmin by plasminogen activators, which include tissue plasminogen activator (tPA) and urokinase. Plasmin is a powerful proteolytic enzyme that breaks down fibrin into soluble fragments. Like many other enzymatic reactions, the fibrinolytic system is closely regulated. A major inhibitor of plasminogen activation is plasminogen activator inhibitor (PAI)-1, which is found in low concentration in plasma, but increases after trauma or operation. The major inhibitor of plasmin is α_2-antiplasmin, which circulates at relatively high concentrations and can neutralize large amounts of plasmin. The plasminogen activators, mainly tPA, and their predominant inhibitor, PAI-1, circulate at low concentrations and are readily cleared from the circulation. Small changes in their production or elimination significantly change the balance of their activities in the plasma.

▌ Pathogenesis of Coagulopathy in Trauma Patients

Coagulopathy occurring in severely injured patients is multifactorial. Four major events have been recognized as contributing to post-traumatic coagulopathy: Hemodilution, consumption of clotting factors, hypothermia, and metabolic derangements [10]. Dilutional thrombocytopenia is the most common coagulation abnormality in trauma patients, and is particularly common in patients receiving more than 1.5 times their blood volume in transfusions. Only about 35 to 40% of platelets remain in circulation after replacement of one blood volume. Dilution of procoagulant factors occurs as a decrease in the concentration of clotting factors owing to the transfusion of packed red blood cells (RBCs) or crystalloid solutions. Dilution of procoagulant factors has not been defined on a numerical basis *per se*, although it is an acknowledged feature of fluid resuscitation. Hiippala et al. [11] studied the dilution of platelets and factors in patients who received packed RBCs and noted that fibrinogen was the most vulnerable of the factors measured. The fibrinogen concentration decreased to 1.0 g/l (normal being 1.5 to 3.5 g/l) after the replacement of 142% of the calculated blood volume with packed RBCs. Other factors are also subject to dilution, the ultimate result of which is a significant coagulopathy. The principal anticoagulant factors antithrombin III, protein C, and protein S are also diluted as a result of massive transfusion [12]. During the massive transfusion of factor-depleted red cell concentrates, the levels of anticoagulant factors probably decrease in a manner similar to the dilution of procoagulant factors, as described by Hiippala et al. [11]. The consequence of a decrease in antithrombin III in this setting is not directly known.

The severely bleeding patient is at high risk of hypothermia, which has a tremendous adverse effect on the normal coagulation mechanism. Hypothermia affects hemostasis at various levels. Platelet function is diminished as a result of both quantitative and qualitative changes. Hypothermia alters the enzymatic kinetics in the coagulation cascade and prolongs coagulation. Hypothermia also influences the dynamic equilibrium of the fibrinolytic system. Historically, thrombocytopenia was initially observed to occur during hypothermia and was implicated as an important disturbance in hypothermia bleeding. Early studies performed by Villalobos and associates [13], found that platelet sequestration contributed to hypothermia-induced bleeding. Labeled canine platelets were sequestered in the liver and spleen during hypothermia, an effect that was quickly reversed by rewarming. Hessel and coworkers [14] also demonstrated that platelet sequestration contributed to hypothermic bleeding. Although canine models demonstrated thrombocytopenia as an important cause of bleeding, studies in other species found that other effects on platelets were important as well [15, 16].

Morphologically, human platelets exposed to cold exhibit increased adhesiveness and aggregation. These changes include the loss of normal discoid morphology, platelet swelling, and development of pseudopods. Valeri and coworkers [16] demonstrated that during hypothermia in baboons, the production of thromboxane B_2 by platelets was decreased, which correlated with increased bleeding time. Michelson and associates [15] demonstrated that the expression of platelet surface molecules was affected by hypothermia in normal human volunteers. The time-dependent upregulation of platelet surface GMP-140 expression (reflecting-a-granule secretion) was abolished by hypothermia at 22 °C. Similarly, the von Willebrand factor receptor, GPIb-IX complex, was nearly abolished by hypothermia at the same temperature. There was also a marked reduction in the number of platelet aggregates emerging from a standardized wound in volunteers. Upon rewarming to 37 °C, however, the decreases in thromboxane B_2, surface receptor expression, and platelet aggregation were all reversible.

Although earlier studies have attributed the bleeding abnormality to causes such as thrombocytopenia, platelet dysfunction, or a dilutional effect, recent research has focused on the coagulation cascade. When clotting tests were performed at temperatures below 37 °C, it was observed that temperature was an important factor determining the clotting-study results. Reed and colleagues [17] showed that as the assaying temperature was decreased from 37 to 25 °C, clotting times were prolonged significantly. Prothrombin time was significantly increased at all temperatures below 35 °C. Similarly, the activated partial thromboplastin time (aPTT) was significantly prolonged at temperatures below 33 °C. Similar results have been demonstrated by other researchers [18–20]. Such disparity between hypothermic coagulopathy and clotting studies was further illustrated by Reed and colleagues [20] in an animal study. By performing clotting studies at incrementally lower temperatures (from 37 to 25 °C) in blood obtained from normothermic rats, they found that the prothrombin time, aPTT, and thrombin time were all significantly prolonged. In contrast, in the same study when clotting tests were performed at 37 °C in blood obtained from hypothermic rats, no significant abnormalities were demonstrated. Their studies suggested that altered enzyme kinetics in the coagulation cascade is a major effect of hypothermia. Functionally, these altered enzymatic activities are important, and the coagulopathic changes have been compared with specific clotting-factor deficiencies. *In vitro* studies by Johnston and associates [21] at temperatures less than 33 °C showed that hypothermia is equivalent to factor-deficiency states under normothermic conditions, despite the presence of normal clotting-factor levels. At 33 °C with normal clotting-factor levels, the clotting process is functionally equivalent to a factor-IX deficiency of 33% of its normal level.

Just as hypothermia has an impact on platelet function and the coagulation cascade, it also exerts an effect on the fibrinolytic system. Fibrinolysis is increased in hypothermic dogs [22]. Yenari and coworkers [23] showed more clot lysis at lower temperatures. This was attributed to the impairment of intrinsic inhibitors of fibrinolysis such as PAI or a_2-antiplasmin.

Patients with massive injuries may also develop systemic clotting factor depletion and diffuse coagulopathy due to the body's continuous attempts to form clots at multiple injury sites. Fibrinolysis is activated by clotting, and teleologically serves to clear thrombi from the microvasculature and to limit the formation of thrombus. Massive clotting factor activation due to multiple injuries may result in uncontrolled fibrinolysis, and a cycle of clotting factor activation with further production of antithrombins [24].

Shock eventually results in intracellular metabolic derangements in oxygen and substrate utilization that lead to metabolic acidosis. Studies demonstrate a strong correlation between the development of coagulation abnormalities and the duration of hypotension. There are also studies demonstrating that hypoperfusion is associated with consumptive coagulopathy and microvascular bleeding independent of the amount of blood loss [25]. In one study, shock-induced acidosis lasting greater than 150 min independently resulted in significant prolongation of the aPTT and decreases in factor V activity [26].

A number of specific injuries may lead to rapid development of a coagulopathic state. Brain injury, and subsequent breakdown of the blood-brain barrier, may result in release of tissue thromboplastin from the damaged tissue into systemic circulation [27]. Severe pulmonary contusion also may produce similar phenomena with release of tissue thromboplastin into systemic circulation. Regardless of the source, the release of thromboplastin causes an intravascular activation of the extrinsic cascade, activation of thrombin, and formation of fibrin clots. Vigorous fibrinolysis resolubilizes the clots, manifested as an elevation in D-dimer levels. As a result, coagulation factors and fibrinogen are depleted and a disseminated intravascular coagulation (DIC) picture develops. Severe liver injury may result in coagulopathy by several different mechanisms. Sometimes this injury may be severe enough to cause inability to produce sufficient amount of coagulation factors [28]. Resuscitation of patient with severe liver injury may require large amount of crystalloids, which leads to hemodilution and, as a consequence, dilutational coagulopathy.

▌ Diagnosis

Coagulopathy in a trauma patient can usually be easily recognized. The mainstay of diagnosis is the clinical assessment of ongoing bleeding. Physical examination is an important diagnostic modality, and oozing from cut surfaces, intravascular catheter sites, or mucous membranes should be sought. Laboratory studies are drawn in abundance on these patients, most commonly platelet count, prothrombin time, aPTT, and fibrinogen level.

Hypothermia is a significant independent contributor to coagulopathy. Care should be taken when interpreting laboratory studies of coagulation function in the hypothermic patient. The standard assays used to assess clotting function, such as the aPTT, prothrombin time, and bleeding time, are all performed at a standardized temperature of 37 °C. Although this provides useful quantitative information regarding clotting factors, it does not take into account the qualitative dysfunction due to hypothermia. This fact was demonstrated in a recent study by Rohrer and Natale [29], which showed a dramatic increase in mean prothrombin time and aPTT with a decreasing assay temperature in pooled plasma from normal volunteers. Rohrer and Natale concluded that the contribution of hypothermia to a bleeding diathesis might potentially be overlooked on the basis of testing at standardized temperatures. An additional weak point of the main coagulation tests is the significant time interval required for their completion. Indeed, in most centers the usual period to obtain standard prothrombin time and aPTT may be as long as one hour [24].

Thromboelastography (TEG) is a promising new technology in predicting hemorrhage that can be performed at bedside. TEG measures the viscoelastic properties of blood [30]. Clot forming consists of the interaction of platelets with fibrin; thus, platelet and clotting factor interactions are not independent. TEG uses a warm cup containing a fixed piston that does not touch the sidewalls. Approximately 0.4 ml of blood is placed in the cup, which rotates around the piston until a bridging clot has formed. A paper tracing provides the amount of power required to maintain the rotational movement of the cup. TEG examines whole blood coagulation, and provides information on how fast the clot forms, the speed of clot growth, clot strength, and whether clot strength is maintained or breaks down early. These are the key elements in determining the likelihood of platelet and clotting factor deficiencies, as well as increased fibrinolysis [31]. This device has influenced both blood utilization and reoperation rates in cardiac surgery, and its successful use is being increasingly reported in the trauma literature [32].

▌ Treatment

Therapy of patients with coagulopathy after major trauma should be rapidly initiated and aggressively pursued throughout all the steps of resuscitation and treatment. The management begins with ensuring adequate help and equipment (e.g., blood warmers, blood filters, pressure gauges) are available for rapid administration of fluid, blood, and blood products. The patient needs dependable, large-bore venous access. The blood bank should be informed as early as possible that large amounts of blood and blood products are needed.

When exsanguinating trauma patients undergo surgery, all attempts should be directed to rapid cessation of surgical bleeding and control of contamination. Any attempts to repair all the injuries and restore continuation of the gastrointestinal tract in a hypothermic, profoundly coagulopathic and acidotic patient should be avoided. Packing of diffusely bleeding surfaces with multiple laparotomy pads and temporary abdominal closure followed by rapid transfer of the patient to an intensive care unit (ICU) is no longer controversial, but standard of care. Priorities in ICU focus on restoring the global physiologic function of the patient.

The major goal is to arrest the vicious circle of hypothermia, coagulopathy, and acidosis. Hypothermia is ideally treated by prevention. All measures must be initiated to prevent additional heat loss. Routine use of environment and fluid warmers will help to decrease further decline of body temperature. Despite attempts to minimize ongoing heat loss and passively rewarm the patient, hypothermia may develop and in some instances require invasive procedures (body-cavity lavage or extracorporeal circulatory rewarming) to increase body temperature [33].

Recognition and prompt treatment of hypoperfusion is also vital. Aggressive fluid and blood replacement therapy is necessary to minimize and reverse cellular shock and correct metabolic acidosis. Blood and blood product therapy is essential to these patients. The administration of whole blood does not result in dilution of procoagulant factors, as whole blood contains stable concentrations of all factors but V and VIII, which though decreased, are still present in sufficient concentrations to support normal clotting. Prophylactic administration of blood components does not decrease transfusion requirements [25]. Optimally, therapy should be directed by abnormalities in coagulation laboratory tests. However, when massive exsanguination is seen and large volumes of packed RBCs required, both clinical and laboratory coagulopathy is usually noted. In this situation, delay in initiation of blood component therapy for conformation of coagulopathy by laboratory studies is detrimental. Transfusing of clotting factors and platelets until the consumptive process resolves is an essential first step in treatment. Clinically, treatment of coagulopathic bleeding is critically compromised by current coagulation monitoring technologies. These tests are time consuming; 40 to 60 minutes elapses before results are obtained. If clotting factors are needed, an additional 30 to 40 minutes is required for thawing and transport. The entire blood volume of the bleeding trauma patient may have been exchanged during that time interval, making the results of the laboratory tests obsolete. More than that, one should keep in mind that the significance of coagulopathy in hypothermic patients is mainly underestimated by standard coagulation tests. In different studies it has been shown that as assaying temperature was decreased from 37 °C to below 35 °C, the prothrombin time was significantly increased as well as the aPTT and the thrombin time [17–19]. Therefore, when standard coagulation tests are performed at a temperature of 37 °C they may not reveal the real state of abnormality.

It has been recommended that rules dictating the empiric transfusion of a certain number of platelet units or units of plasma after a specific level of red cell transfusion should be abandoned. Although we would agree with this recommendation in principle, the practice of damage control surgery requires recognition and treatment of coagulopathy even faster than stat laboratory turnaround time permits [10]. For this reason, practice should base the diagnosis of coagulopathy on clinical grounds if laboratory studies are not available. Specifically, if patients show oozing from cut surfaces, intravenous lines, or other visible signs of overt coagulopathy, platelets and fresh frozen plasma are transfused at that time while awaiting results of laboratory studies.

Recently, a new adjunct to the treatment of coagulopathy in trauma patients has been reported [38] and is undergoing controlled animal trials. Recombinant activated factor VIIa (rFVIIa) was developed as a potential pro-hemostatic agent for the treatment of bleeding episodes in patients with hemophilia A and B with inhibitors to factors VIII and IX respectively). RFVIIa is identical in structure and activity to human Factor VII [34].

The mechanism of action of rFVIIa is activation of factors XI and X, inducing thrombin burst and faster formation of the fibrin clots at the site of vascular injury (Fig. 2). rFVIIa basically bypasses all the intrinsic pathway of the coagulation cascade and shortens time required for completion of secondary clot formation.

Martinowitz et al. reported the use of rFVIIa in moribund trauma patients [38]. In their experience, the drug has been administered to cold and coagulopathic patients, where standard medical and surgical technique has failed to control diffuse bleeding. Hemorrhage ceased in almost all patients. No thromboembolic events

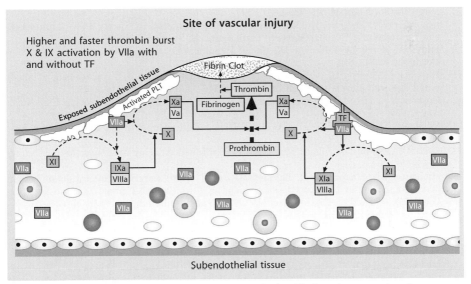

Fig. 2. Mechanism of action of recombinant factor VIIa. PLT: platelets; TF: tissue factor; a: activated

were observed. Preliminary animal studies have been reported recently with promising results [39, 40].

Conclusion

Refractory coagulopathy in trauma patients is a common event and associated with high mortality when combined with hypothermia and acidosis. The diagnosis of coagulopathy is made on a clinical basis. TEG may be a new aid for fast diagnosis of coagulation abnormalities. The mainstay of treatment is immediate bleeding control, rapid termination of surgery, and early and aggressive correction of hypothermia and metabolic derangements. A new adjunct (rFVIIa) is being studied in controlled animal models with promising results.

References

1. MacKenzie EJ, Fowler CJ (2000) Epidemiology. In: Mattox KL, Feliciano DV, Moore EE (eds) Trauma. Fourth Edition, MacGraw-Hill, New York, pp 21–39
2. Sauaia A, Moore FA, Moore EE, et al (1995) Epidemiology of trauma death: a reassessment. J Trauma 38:185–193
3. Hoyt DB, Bulger EM, Knudson MM, et al (1994) Death in the operating room: An analysis of multicenter experience. J Trauma 37:426–432
4. Rotondo MF, Zonies DH (1997) The damage control sequence and underlying logic. Surg Clin N Am 77:761–777
5. Johnson JW, Gracias VH, Schwab CW, et al (2000) Evolution in damage control for exanguinating penetrating abdominal injury. J Trauma 51:261–269
6. Moore EE (1996) Staged laparotomy for hypothermia, acidosis, and coagulopathy syndrome. Am J Surg 172:405
7. Rotondo MF, Schwab CW, McGonigal MD, et al (1993) Damage control: an approach to improve survival in exanguinated penetrating abdominal injury. J Trauma 35:375–382
8. Patt A, McCroscey BL, Moore EE (1988) Hypothermia-induced coagulopathies in trauma. Surg Clin North Am 68:775–785
9. Bell WE (1979) Physiology of the fibrinolytic enzyme system. In: Sherry S (ed) Thrombosis and Thrombolysis. Hoechst-Roussel Pharmaceuticals, Somerville, p 192
10. Eddy VA, Morris JA, Cullinane DC (2000) Hypothermia, coagulopathy, acidosis. Surg Clin North Am 80:845–854
11. Hiippala ST, Myllyla GJ, Vahtera EM (1995) Hemostatic factors and replacement of major blood loss with plasma-poor red cell concentrates. Anesth Analg 81:360–365
12. Goskowicz R (1999) The complication of massive blood transfusion. Anesth Clin North Am 17:959–975
13. Villalobos TJ, Adelson E, Borila TG (1955) Hematologic changes in hypothermic dogs. Proc Soc Exp Biol Med 89:192–196
14. Hessell FA, Schmer G, Dillard DH (1980) Platelet kinetics during deep hypothermia. J Surg Res 28:23–34
15. Michelson AD, MacGregor H, Barnard MR, et al (1994) Reversible inhibition of human platelet activation by hypothermia in vivo and in vitro. Thromb Hemost 71:633–640
16. Valeri CR, Feingold H, Cassidy G, et al (1987) Hypothermia-induced reversible platelet dysfunction. Ann Surg 205:175–181
17. Reed RL, Bracey AWJ, Hudson JD, et al (1990) Hypothermia and blood coagulation: dissociation between enzyme activity and clotting factor levels. Circ Shock 32:141–152
18. Rohrer MJ, Natale AM (1992) Effect of hypothermia on the coagulation cascade. Crit Care Med 20:1402–1405
19. Gubler KD, Gentillello LM, Hassantash SA, Maier RV (1994) The impact of hypothermia on dilutional coagulopathy. J Trauma 36:847–851

20. Reed RL, Johnson TD, Hudson JD, Fischer RP (1992) The disparity between hypothermic coagulopathy and clotting studies. J Trauma 33:465–470
21. Johnston TD, Chen Y, Reed RL (1994) Functional equivalence of hypothermia to specific clotting factor deficiencies. J Trauma 37:413–417
22. Yoshihara H, Yamamoto T, Mihara H (1985) Changes in coagulation and fibrinolysis occurring in dogs during hypothermia. Thromb Res 37:503–512
23. Yenari MA, Palmer JT, Bracci PM, Steinberg GK (1995) Thrombolysis with tissue plasminogen activator (tPA) is temperature dependent. Thromb Res 77:475–481
24. Gentilello LM, Pierson DJ (2001) Trauma critical care. Am J Respir Crit Care Med 163:604–607
25. Reed RL II, Ciavarella D, Heimbach DM, et al (1986) Prophylactic platelet administration during massive transfusion: a prospective, randomized, double-blind clinical study. Ann Surg 203:40–48
26. Harke H, Rahman S (1980) Haemostatic disorders in massive transfusion. Bibl Haematol 46:179–188
27. Goodnight SH, Kenoyer G, Rapoport ST, et al (1974) Defibrination after brain tissue destruction. N Engl J Med 290:1043–1047
28. Rotondo MF, Reilly PM (2000) Bleeding and coagulation complications. In: Mattox KL, Feliciano DV, Moore EE (eds) Trauma. Fourth Edition. McGraw-Hill, New York, pp 1274–1275
29. Rohrer M, Natala A (1992) Effect of hypothermia on the coagulation cascade. Crit Care Med 20:1402–1405
30. Chandler W (1995) The thromboelastograph and the thromboelastograph technique. Semin Thromb Hemost 21(suppl 4):1–6
31. Spiess BD (1995) Perioperative coagulation monitoring. In: Spiess BD, Counts RB, Gould SA (eds) Perioperative Transfusion Medicine, 1st ed. Williams & Wilkins, Baltimore, pp 250–254
32. Kaufmann CR, Dwyer KM, Crews JD, et al (1997) Usefulness of thromboelastography in assessment of trauma patient coagulation. J Trauma 42:716–720
33. Peng RY, Bongard FS (1999) Hypothermia in trauma patients. J Am Coll Surg 188:685–696
34. Bernstein DE, Jeffers L, Erhardtsen E, et al (1997) Recombinant factor VIIa corrects prothrombin time in cirrhotic patients: a preliminary study. Gastroenterology 113:1930–1937
35. Hender U, Ignerslev J (1998) Clinical use of recombinant FVIIa. Trans Sci 19:163–176
36. Arkin S, Cooper HA, Hutter JJ, et al (1998) Activaited recombinant human coagulation factor VII therapy for intracranial hemorrhage in patients with hemophylia A and B with inhibitors: results of Novoseven emergency use program. Hemostasis 28:93–98
37. Poon MC, Demers C, Jobin F, et al (1999) Recombinant factor VIIa is effective for bleeding and surgery in patients with Glanzmann thrombastenia. Blood 94:3951–3953
38. Martinowitz U, Kenet G, Segal E, et al (2001) Recombinant activated factor VII for adjunctive hemorrhage control in trauma. J Trauma 51:431–439
39. Lynn M, Jeroukhimov I, Jewelewicz D, et al (2002) Early use of recombinant factor VIIa improves mean arterial pressure and may potentially decrease mortality in experimental hemorrhagic shock – a pilot study. J Trauma (in press)
40. Martinowitz U, Holcomb JB, Pusateri AE (2001) Intravenous rFVII administered for hemorrhage control in hypothermic coagulopathic swine with grade V liver injury. J Trauma 50:721–729

Head Trauma

Traumatic Brain Injury: Severity and Outcome

B. van Baalen, E. Odding, and A. I. R. Maas

▎ Introduction

Traumatic brain injury (TBI) has been termed a silent epidemic [1]. In the USA, approximately 95 per 100 000 inhabitants sustain a fatal, or severe enough injury to require hospital admission, each year [2]. In the Federal Republic of Germany, the annual incidence of severe TBI is estimated at 10 000 [3]. In the Netherlands, the incidence is 79 per 100 000 inhabitants [4]. Whilst this incidence is lower, compared to other causes of brain injury, such as stroke, the long-term effects and socio-economic costs are equal or even higher, as TBI primarily affects younger age groups.

Classification at the two ends of the spectrum of TBI, i.e., at the beginning (initial severity) and at the end (final outcome), may be considered important for a variety of reasons. Classification of initial severity and estimation of risk of complications is important when determining what level of care, and which facilities individual patients require. In studies where treatment effect is investigated, or results of treatment presented, the initial severity is a major prognostic factor that has to be considered. Classifying patients in the initial period is essential when specific therapies require targeting to a subset of the population. Likewise, the results of therapy in the acute or subacute (rehabilitation) phase, or accuracy of prognostic studies can only be evaluated if the final outcome is measured accurately.

In rehabilitation medicine, the main goal is to prognosticate for future outcome in order to develop treatment strategies. Functional outcome expressed as the extent of disability and handicap after sustaining a TBI covers a wide range from very minor to very severe. Spontaneous recovery to pre-traumatic level of functioning may occur but, especially in the more severe cases, a complex array of long-term sequelae may persist. All areas of life may be affected by TBI, resulting in various cognitive, social, behavioral, emotional, and/or physical problems. The set of relevant domains is large and there is no direct relation between neurological impairments and long-term disabilities. Most studies focus on functional outcome at six to twelve months post injury (using the Glasgow Outcome Scale [GOS] and the Disability Rating Scale [DRS]), and much less is known about the lifelong consequences of TBI.

Whatever the focus of interest, outcome in TBI is usually assessed by healthcare professionals, and seldom includes self-assessment. Yet, self-assessment is an essential part in determining quality of life in patients surviving TBI. Quality of life assessment has proven particularly useful in the fields of oncology and cardiovascular disease, but its usefulness and applicability in TBI is still under investigation. Outcome assessment should not so much reflect the interest of health care professionals, but rather integrate the various components of the outcome spectrum, including aspects of physical well-being, activities of daily life, neuropsychological impairment, and social reintegration as perceived by health care professionals, as well as by patients themselves and their caregivers. Nevertheless, the focus of outcome will vary according to the time after injury and the specific focus of interest.

The aim of the present chapter is to review currently employed methods for classifying initial severity and final outcome in TBI. This review was carried out to answer our question about the optimal set of measurement tools needed for a prospective study on the determinants of (future) disability and handicap. We therefore focus on the most used and/or best-documented scales.

▌ Classification of Initial Severity

TBI is a heterogeneous disease, encompassing a wide range of pathologies, including diffuse axonal injury, focal contusions, and space occupying intra- and extradural hematomas. Following the primary damage due to the initial impact, secondary brain damage ensues due to intrinsic pathophysiologic mechanisms and development of mass lesions, and is frequently exacerbated by systemic insults. Patients with TBI may be classified according to clinical severity, mechanism of injury, or morphologic changes. Presence of TBI and clinical severity, thereof, is evidenced by the presence and duration of post-traumatic amnesia, and in more severe cases by the degree and duration of a depressed level of consciousness. Post-traumatic amnesia can be measured reliably with the Galveston Orientation and Amnesia Test (GOAT), and the level of consciousness by the Glasgow Coma Scale (GCS).

Galveston Orientation and Amnesia Test

The presence of post-traumatic amnesia is a prerequisite for the diagnosis of TBI. The duration of post-traumatic amnesia is related to the severity of injury and has shown a robust correlation with treatment costs and general outcome [5]. The duration of post-traumatic amnesia can be measured accurately with the GOAT. The GOAT is a short mental status exam devised to evaluate the extent and duration of confusion and amnesia following TBI. Standardized questions are asked relating to orientation to person, to time, to place, and to the ability to recall events, just prior to and after injury. In administering GOAT, each patient starts with 100 points and points are deducted for errors made in answering the questions. A score of 76 to 100 on the GOAT may be considered as normal, a score of 66 to 75 as borderline, patients with a score below 75 may be considered to still be in a state of post-traumatic amnesia. A graph of serial scores obtained over time depicts the recovery of the TBI patient from the phase of post-traumatic amnesia [6]. Inter-rater reliability has been demonstrated. Post-traumatic amnesia, as measured by the GOAT, appears to be able to predict specific functional capacity in the population of TBI-patients. This predictive value can be enhanced by taking age into account [7].

Glasgow Coma Scale

The GCS is widely accepted as a standardized method for evaluating level of consciousness in patients with acute neurological disorders [8]. The GCS is comprised of three response scores (eye opening [E], motor score [M], verbal score [V]), which for purposes of research and classification may be summated to a total EMV score (3–15). Coma is commonly defined as GCS score ≤8 [9] and inability to open the eyes. TBI patients with a GCS ≤8 on admission are classified as severe TBI, patients with an admission GCS of 9 to 13 as moderate. Formerly, moderate TBI was defined as a GCS of 9–12, but recently it has been suggested that patients with a GCS of 13 should be included in the moderate TBI group, as the risk of complications is equal to patients with a GCS score of 9 to 12 [13]. Within the mild traumatic brain injury (i.e., GCS 14 or 15) patients may be recognized to be at high, moderate, or low risk of developing intra-cranial mass lesions.

Inter and intra-rater reliability in the use of GCS is high. The GCS score has been shown to be highly associated with acute morbidity and mortality, but less strongly with long-term functional outcome [10].

Mechanism of Injury

According to the mechanism of injury, patients may be differentiated as closed versus penetrating head injury. This makes sense, since outcome differs significantly with the lesions sustained. In closed head injury, acceleration/deceleration forces, such as frequently occur in road traffic accidents (RTA) cause diffuse injuries, and more local impact causes contusions. In penetrating head injury, the penetrating object primarily causes local destruction and, depending on the kinetic energy transmitted to the tissue, more widespread devastating injuries. In civilian situations penetrating head injury is predominantly caused by gunshot wounds, often self-inflicted. The risk of infection and epilepsy are more prominent features in penetrating head injury. Outcome in penetrating head injury is much poorer than in closed head injury. Within the Traumatic Coma Data Bank study including patients with only severe injuries, overall mortality in the closed head injury group was 32.5% [11] and in patients with penetrating head injury 88% [12]. Poorer outcome in penetrating head injury is primarily determined by mortality. In penetrating head injury, sequelae are primarily caused by physical disabilities versus more severe cognitive impairment in patients with closed head injury.

Morphology

Assessment of clinical severity of injury according to the GCS is impaired by the fact that many patients today already arrive in the hospital sedated, paralyzed, and ventilated. In a survey performed by the European Brain Injury Consortium on severe and moderate TBI, the full GCS was testable in only 77% of patients on admission to hospital [13]. For these reasons interest has focused on more technical examinations, such as computerized tomography (CT) or magnetic resonance imaging (MRI), for classifying TBI. In the acute phase, MRI, though more sensitive, is impractical. CT examinations permit evaluation of structural damage, detection of mass lesions, traumatic subarachnoid hemorrhage, and may show evidence of raised intra-cranial pressure (ICP). In 1991 Marshall et al. [12], analyzing the US Traumatic Coma Data Bank, proposed a scale for classifying TBI according to CT findings. This scale differentiates patients into six categories, according to the presence or absence of abnormalities, obliteration of basal cisterns, presence of midline shift, and mass lesions. A clear correlation between CT classification and outcome has been shown. Although the composition of the scale has not been scientifically validated, in practice it has proven validity and demonstrated prognostic significance. Whether a different classification system for penetrating head injury is required remains to be investigated.

▮ Determination of Outcome

The focus of interest on outcome varies according to the fields of interest of the health care professional. Acute care physicians, focusing primarily on treatment results, desire a simple general outcome scale. In this field the GOS and DRS are commonly used. In rehabilitation medicine, it has become common practice to classify the consequences of disease according to the International Classification of Disabilities and Handicaps (ICIDH) [14, 15]. The first version, developed in 1980, classified impairments, disabilities, and handicaps. In December 1999, the 'Beta-2 draft' of the second version was published. The ICIDH-2 provides a description of situations with regard to human functioning and disability. It is organized in three dimensions:
1) body level, named body functions and structure;
2) individual level, named activities; and
3) society level, named participation.

The body functions are the physiological or psychological functions of body systems, and the body structures are anatomical parts of the body. Impairments are problems in body functions or structure as a significant deviation or loss. An activity is the performance of a task or action. Activity limitations are difficulties an individual may have in the performance of activities. Participation is an individual's involvement in the life situations in relation to health conditions, body functions and structures, activities, and contextual factors (contextual factors represent the background of an individual's life and living). Participation restrictions are problems an individual may have in the manner or extent of involvement in life situations. What is often called 'functional outcome' should encompass at least the relevant domains of the dimensions activity and participation.

The question in TBI rehabilitation is what these relevant domains are. One study classified 55% of patients, 3 to 7 years post-traumatic, as having a cognitive disability, while 45% had emotional and behavioral disabilities [4]. There were fewer problems with locomotor, and personal care functions. It is not difficult to imagine that these cognitive, behavioral and emotional problems may have a major impact on family and social relations, and the ability to lead a gainful life. And, not only does the injury affect the patient himself but it can also have large effects on the lives of the people in the immediate environment of the patient like partner, children, or parents. In our opinion, future scientific research should focus on these aspects.

Having defined the area of functional outcome, one must establish the manner in which to measure its aspects. The complexity of relevant outcomes, combined with the limited resources for research, has led to the use of assessment tools not specifically developed and validated for the TBI population. The current state of the art leads both researchers and clinical managers to question how function and progress of patients with TBI should be assessed.

▌ General Outcome Scales

Glasgow Outcome Scale

The GOS is widely accepted as a measure of general outcome after TBI; prognostic studies have focused on GOS at discharge or six months after injury, and the GOS dichotomized into unfavorable/favorable outcome has been uniformly utilized as a primary outcome measure in clinical trials. The full GOS encompasses five outcome categories: death, vegetative state, severe disability, moderate disability, and good recovery [16]. Overall recovery is categorized on the basis of the following determinants: consciousness, independence in the home, independence outside the home, work, social & leisure activities, and family & friendships. The GOS has been criticized because there are no guidelines for dealing with commonly encountered problems, such as the effects of extra-cranial injury, epilepsy, and pre-injury unemployment [17, 18] and because of relative insensitivity in patients with more favorable outcomes. GOS-ratings tend to plateau at 6 months, and therefore the instrument will be insensitive to the gains shown by patients after this period [7]. Several schemes for extending the GOS, allowing for further differentiation in the upper categories have been suggested [19–22]. Detailed criteria for assessing the extended GOS (GOSE) have been proposed by Wilson et al [23]. The GOSE subdivides the upper three categories of the scale (severe disability, moderate disability and good recovery) into an upper level and a lower level [24]. Traditionally, outcome assessed by the GOS, has been assigned after a short interview, usually unstructured and not involving a written protocol. This open-ended format encourages impressionistic use of the scale, sometimes causing variable results between individual assessors [20] and there is evidence of systematic bias between different professional groups [17]. Assessment of the GOS and GOSE using a standard format with a written protocol is practical and reliable [24]. A disadvantage in using the structured interview, however, is the inability to correct for pre-injury deficits. In the original assessment of the GOS, a patient was assigned to the category good recovery if he attained the same level of functioning as pre-trauma. The structured interview format does not allow for taking such aspects into consideration and is limited to a description of the present situation. Consequently, although permitting more standardized assessment, the use of the proposed structured interviews may carry some risk of underestimating the actual degree of recovery in comparison to the pre-trauma level.

Disability Rating Scale

Although termed a disability rating scale, the DRS includes determination of the level of consciousness and degree of social adaptability, and hence is better classified as a general outcome measure. The DRS was developed as an instrument to provide quantitative information to chart the progress of severe head injury patients from coma to community, particularly through the mid-zone of the recovery spectrum, between early arousal from coma and early sentient functioning [25]. It measures changes in the following categories:
▌ level of arousal and awareness – identical to the GCS
▌ cognitive ability to deal with problems of feeding, toileting, and grooming
▌ degree of physical dependence on others
▌ psychosocial adaptability as reflected primarily by the ability to do useful work as independently as possible in a socially relevant context.

For each category, points are given for the disability present, and summation of these permits defining 10 outcome categories: no disability (0), mild disability (1), partial disability (2–3), moderate disability (4–6), moderately severe disability (7–11), severe disability (12–6), extremely severe disability (17–21), vegetative state (22–24), extremely vegetative state (25–29), death (30). The DRS is a reliable and valid measure, which has been shown to be associated with long-term disability after moderate and severe TBI [18, 26, 27, 28]. In addition, it proved to be significantly associated with neurophysiologic measures of brain dysfunction as reflected in brain evoked potential abnormality scores [29, 30]. It has, however, not been shown to be superior to the GOS; in fact, results of a recent study evaluating the relative value of GOS and DRS showed the GOS to provide a more complete assessment of disability than the DRS [31].

Measures of Disabilities

A disability refers to any restriction or lack of ability to perform an activity within the manner or the range that is considered normal for a human being. Disability represents a disturbance at the level of the acting person and may arise as a direct consequence of impairment. Disability may result from (psychological) response of the individual to a physical, sensory or other impairment [14, 15]. Various assessment scales for disabilities have been utilized in TBI, primarily in rehabilitation medicine. These scales include the Barthel Index, the Rancho Los Amigos Levels of Cognitive Functioning Scale (LCFS), the Functional Independence Measure (FIM) and Functional Assessment Measure (FAM), as well as the Neurobehavioral Rating Scale (NRS).

Barthel Index

The Barthel Index was initially developed to follow progress in self-care and mobility skills during in-patient rehabilitation of stroke patients, and to indicate the amount of care required. It has evolved into one of the commonly employed measures for physical disabilities in rehabilitation in general [32]. It is an index of daily living [33], registering the actual performance of a patient. The five outcome categories are: extremely severely disabled (0–4), severely disabled (5–9), disabled (10–14), mildly disabled (15–19), and not disabled (20). The index is, however, limited in scope; it does not take psychological status, social functioning, or household activities, into account. Consequently, a ceiling effect prevents the detection of further relevant improvements in TBI-patients [34]. The reliability and validity of the Barthel Index in neurological disease has been primarily established in stroke research but not in TBI research.

Rancho Los Amigos Levels of Cognitive Functioning Scale

The LCFS was originally designed as a description of the eight stages of cognitive functioning through which brain injured patients typically progress in hospital and acute rehabilitative care [35]. The eight levels of functioning cover much of the observable range of psychosocially relevant behaviors [36]. The scale ranges from no response, in which the patient is in deep coma and completely unresponsive, to purposeful and appropriate functioning, where the patient is alert and oriented, able to recall and integrate past and recent events, and is aware of, and responsive to, their environment). Although this scale reflects common trends in recovery, it does not clarify the status of the individual patient's cognitive processes at a particular time [37]. There is some debate about the usefulness of the LCFS in TBI-research. Some state that, because the reliability and validity of the LCFS is less than of the DRS, it should not be used [26]. Others argue that because of the simplicity and clinical utility of the LCFS, and its widespread use in the United States, it is an asset to any data set [9].

Functional Independence Measure and Functional Assessment Measure

The FIM was developed to resolve the longstanding problem of lack of uniform measurement and data on disability and rehabilitation outcomes. The FIM is an 18-item ordinal scale, measuring changes in functional status within an individual over the course of a comprehensive medical rehabilitation program [38]. The areas examined include: self-care, sphincter control, mobility, locomotion, communication, and social cognition. The FIM item-scores range from 1 (needs total assistance, performing less than 25% of the task) to 7 (completely independent). Good reliability across a wide variety of settings, raters, and patients has been reported [38–45]. Because of the complex functional sequelae of TBI, ceiling effects of the FIM have been reported. The psychosocial and cognitive disabilities, common in TBI, have therefore led to an extension of the FIM, the FAM [46]. The twelve FAM-items are swallowing, car transfer, community access, reading, writing, speech in-

Table 1. Reliability coefficients for measures of disability and handicap found in the literature. X: no data available

	Inter-rater	Intra-rater	Other
Disability measures			
Glasgow Outcome Score (GOS)	K=0.89	X	Sensitivity to change 33%
Extended Glasgow Outcome Score (GOSE)	K=0.85	X	X
Barthel Index	0.95	0.89	X
Barthel Index (Dutch)	K=0.88	X	X
Disability Rating Scale (DRS)	0.89	X	Sensitivity to change 71%
Functional Independence Measure (FIM)	0.95	0.95	X
FIM+Functional Assessment Measure (FAM)	ICC>0.60	X	X
Level of Cognitive Functioning Scale (LCFS)	0.89	0.82	X
Neurobehavioral Rating Scale (NRS)	0.89	X	X
Frenchay Activities Index (FAI)	0.8	0.83	Internal consistency α=0,78–0,87
Handicap measures			
Wimbledon Self Report Scale (WSRS)	X	0.94	X
Supervision Rating Scale (SRS)	K=0.64 ICC=0.86	X	X
Sickness Impact Profile (SIP)	0.92	0.75–0.92	Internal consistency α=0.91–0.95
SIP68	X	ICC=0.97	Internal consistency α=0,90–0,92
Rand-36	X	0.60–0.81	Internal consistency α=0,62–0,96
Coop/Wonca	X	0.67–0.82	Sensitivity to change
Community Integration Questionnaire (CIQ)	X	X	X

telligibility, emotional status, adjustment to limitations, employability, orientation, attention, and safety judgment. The scores, like the FIM-items, range from 1 to 7.

Neurobehavioural Rating Scale

The NRS is a modification of the Brief Psychiatric Rating Scale [47]. This 27-item scale has been developed for head trauma patients, and measures common behavioral and psychiatric symptoms after TBI [48, 49]. Examples of these symptoms are inattention/reduced alertness, somatic concern, disorientation, anxiety, conceptual disorganization, agitation, and motor retardation. Ratings are made on a 7-point scale from non-present to extremely severe. Satisfactory inter-rater reliability has been reported, and both severity and chronicity of closed head injury was reflected in the NRS. Brief structured interviews or observations in a naturalistic setting can be used to administer the NRS.

▎ Measures of Handicap

Handicap is defined by the disadvantages experienced by the individual at the level of the interaction with the social environment. The WHO-model emphasizes that for the same type of impairment and degree of disability, the level of handicap can vary considerably from individual to individual depending on personal background, pre-morbid lifestyle, and circumstances after the illness. It is therefore clear that derivation of a standard against which to measure handicap is not easy [50]. Measures of handicap are strongly related to health-related quality of life assessment. Berger et al. [51] have discussed the literature on quality of life after TBI. In terms of quality of life domains, they identified the physical, psychological, social, and especially cognitive aspects of quality of life. This review highlighted the lack of standardized definitions and multidimensional assessment of quality of life in TBI.

In measuring handicaps and quality of life, disease specific instruments may be identified in contrast to more generic measures. Generic measures include the Sickness Impact Profile (SIP), the SF-36, the Wimbledon Self Report Scale (WSRS), and the Coop/Wonca charts. More disease specific scales include the Supervision Rating Scale (SRS), Community Integration Questionnaire (CIQ) and the Aachener Life Quality Inventory.

Sickness Impact Profile

The SIP is a multidimensional general health status instrument, which measures perceived changes in behaviour judged by the patient as the consequence of being sick. The test-retest reliability of the SIP in terms of various reliability measures was investigated using different interviewers, forms, administration procedures, and a variety of subjects who differed in terms of type and severity of dysfunction. The results provided evidence of feasibility of collecting reliable data using the SIP under these various conditions. The SIP is comprised of 136 items which are all statements regarding behavior. Respondents are asked to check those items that apply to their situation on the day they fill out the list and that are related to their health status [52]. The 136 items are divided over 12 categories and result in three scores: the physical SIP-score, the psychosocial SIP-score and the total SIP-score. The SIP has been used in many studies addressing a wide variety of objectives and involving many study populations from various countries [53–56]. The SIP has been used in several studies of TBI [57–61]. Modifications to make the SIP more sensitive for TBI-patients were shown to be inferior to the original SIP [62]. The time needed to assess the SIP has been regarded as an obstacle to routine use [63, 64]. In order to make the SIP less time-consuming, but maintaining its widely accepted internal properties, a short generic version was developed. This so-called SIP-68 was developed in the Netherlands and contains 68 items, which are divided over six sub-scales: somatic autonomy, mobility control, psychic autonomy and communication, social behavior, emotional stability, and mobility range. These six sub-scales together were able to predict total SIP136-scores almost perfectly. Pearson's correlation coefficient for the total-scores SIP136–SIP68 is 0.97 in the TBI population [65]. No studies on TBI patients using this short form have been published so far.

Rand-36-item Health Survey 1.0/MOS SF-36

The Rand-36 is a multidimensional questionnaire measuring health-related quality of life. It is suitable for use in the general population in patients with various conditions [66]. The Rand-36 comprises eight sub-scales: physical functioning, role limitations as a result of physical problems, bodily pain, general health perception, social functioning, role limitations as a result of emotional problems, mental health, and health change. It has been tested extensively and has shown good psychometric properties [67–69]. Floor and ceiling effects have been reported. Although some health concepts, like sleep, cognitive functioning, health distress, self-esteem, eating, and communication are not measured specifically, the scales of the Rand-36 have been shown to be associated with these concepts [70].

Wimbledon Self Report Scale

The WSRS provides a measure of emotional state and detects mood disorders. It was standardized on a hospitalized population in which the majority of patients had neurological disorders, and it provides a general appraisal of mood state rather than being limited to specific symptoms of anxiety and/or depression. Intra-rater reliability is high (Table 1). The WSRS consists of 30 adjectives and phrases describing feelings (e.g., nervous, rejected, happy, desperate) in which the participant rates the frequency of occurrence in the previous week on a 4-point scale, ranging from 'never' to 'almost always' [71].

The Coop/Wonca Charts

The Dartmouth Coop Functional Health Assessment Charts/Wonca (Coop/Wonca) is a short, self-completed questionnaire and was developed for patients in primary care, specifically for use in office practices [72–74]. Additionally, it has been used in other settings, including hospital in-patients, patients in day-care and in nursing homes, and in the general population. The Coop/Wonca is intended to measure the patient's functional status by assessing the actual performance (or capacity to perform) of a wide range of physical, social, and work activities that are normal for people in good health [75]. The following dimensions are assessed: physical function, emotional status, role function, social function, health change, overall health, and pain. In the Netherlands the Coop/Wonca Charts have proved valid and reliable and their sensitivity to change has been demonstrated [76].

Supervision Rating Scale

The Supervision Rating Scale (SRS) measures the level of supervision that a patient receives from caregivers. The SRS rates levels of supervision on a 13-point ordinal scale that can optionally be grouped into five ranked categories (independent, overnight supervision, part-time supervision, full-time supervision, and full-time direct supervision). SRS ratings are strongly associated with ratings on the DRS and GOS [25]. No report of its use or specific validity in TBI has been found since its original publication.

Community Integration Questionnaire

The assessment of community integration, i.e., the degree to which TBI victims return to life in their families, neighborhoods, and communities, in spite of impairments and disabilities, is essential to any TBI-outcome study. The CIQ is a 15-item scale with three sub-scales assessing home integration, social integration, and productive activity in persons with TBI. Home integration includes five items associated with domestic activities, housework, caring for children, shopping, etc. Social integration includes six items related to visiting friends and engaging in leisure activities among others. Higher scores indicate greater integration [77]. The productive activity domain contains four items involved with work, school, volunteer activities and the use of transportation, which is found to be the most reliable and sensitive sub-scale. In its current format, the CIQ is a measure of the community integration of persons with TBI that appears useful for research and rehabilitation program evaluation. However, the establishment of pre-injury community integration status, and the association of CIQ-scores with impairment and disability have not been investigated. No validity studies have been reported [78].

The Aachener Life Quality Inventory

The Aachener Life Quality Inventory was developed for evaluative and predictive purposes from the SIP, more specifically focusing on patients with brain damage. It concerns a patient self-report and relative rated form, also available as an interview. It has been tested for psychometric criteria in neurological patients including those with TBI. This inventory, containing 117 items and measuring eight dimensions, has primarily been used in Germany, and to our knowledge an English version is not yet available [79].

▌ Discussion and Recommendations for Future Research

Classifying TBI, in terms of initial severity as well as long-term outcome, can be considered important. When attempting to classify TBI, the ultimate goal of the assessment should be kept in mind. In the early assessment of initial severity, clinical assessment and CT-classification are used for allocation of resources, for reasons of prognosis, and for inclusion/exclusion criterion for clinical studies. In this regard it has been stated that patients with a GCS < 9, classified as severe, should receive ICP monitoring and be admitted to a specialized center. But, does this mean that other patients with moderate injury require a different approach? Results of recent studies have shown that moderate TBI is not such a benign disease as previously thought; mortality rates of 11 to 15% are reported [13]. The coexistence of moderate TBI with extra-cranial injury is associated with a doubling of predicted mortality throughout the injury severity ranges studied [80]. Relevant questions when considering allocation of resources, necessity for referral, and admission to an intensive care unit (ICU) are: what are the risks of developing problems, such as mass lesion, raised ICP, secondary insults, or compromised cerebral perfusion pressure; and is it possible that such complications can be detected earlier, prevented, and treated in the appropriate situation? Such an approach would favor calculation of an individualized risk assessment, rather than an overall classification. In TBI trials, the treatment under investigation should be targeted not only at patients with the pathophysiologic mechanism against which a new therapy is active, but equally importantly, at a population where the chance of demonstrating improvement is possible and realistic. From a point of view of clinical trial design and from a prognostic perspective, it should be realized that the TBI-population includes patients with an *a priori* poor chance of survival, as well as patients with an *a priori* high chance of favorable outcome. Although classifying patients with TBI according to clinical condition or according to CT parameters is valid, a different approach, and one which in our opinion deserves more attention, is attempting to classify patients according to prognostic estimates; identifying patients with a certain risk profile. These risk profiles may relate to different endpoints, such as risk of secondary insult, risk of intra-cranial mass lesion, and hence for an evidence based allocation of intensive care facilities to appropriately targeted patients, or to overall outcome measures, permitting better comparisons between series concerning treatment results and affording opportunities for quality assurance.

Further studies on prognostic modeling in TBI, cross validating prognostic equations over various databases are necessary to permit classification of patients according to prognostic profiles. Such an approach would further be of value in analysis of future clinical trials on neuroprotective agents and provide possibilities of targeting such therapies to a population in whom effect might be demonstrated. Furthermore, such an approach could be utilized in targeting and evaluating the effect of specific rehabilitation programs in TBI. Whatever the endpoint chosen, a prerequisite is that such an endpoint is appropriate and clearly defined with evaluation performed at a specific time. Physical and neurological recovery is greatest in the first six months post-injury. Overall outcome measures, such as the GOS, the GOSE or the DRS, are appropriate when evaluating results of early management, and based on results obtained it would seem valid to perform such estimation at six months post injury, as indeed is generally accepted. However, following the first six-month period other problems become more apparent, both in the patient and their relatives, particularly concerning aspects of social reintegration and perceived quality of life. Even in mildly injured TBI patients, major problems may occur even years after injury. Assessment of long-term functional outcome would ideally require a lifelong follow-up, but this is not a realistic goal for scientific research. Given the available data showing that most problems are revealed during the first three years post-injury, a follow-up of three years would appear appropriate for determining long-term functional outcome.

▌ Conclusion

Future research on outcome in TBI should focus on determinants of outcome:
1) In intensive care medicine to identify patients with a certain risk profile. Dependent on which endpoint is chosen (risk of complications, allocation of intensive care facilities, outcome), various databases in TBI research are necessary.
2) In rehabilitation medicine to identify those patients who will have greatest chance of benefiting from intensive rehabilitation programs; more research is needed to determine the long-term functional outcome in TBI, the socio-economic costs involved in the long term, and the influence of behavioral problems on family cohesion.

Validation of generic outcome measures is required in the TBI-population; the relative value of various outcome measures needs to be determined, and furthermore the usefulness and applicability of measures for health related quality of life in TBI is required. Such measures should permit differentiation in patient perceived, caregiver perceived and significant other perceived quality of life. To this end more disease specific scales are required.

References

1. Goldstein M (1990) Traumatic brain injury: A silent epidemic. Ann Neurol 27:327
2. National Center for Injury Prevention and Control (1999) Epidemiology of traumatic brain injury in the United States. At: http//www.cdc.gov/ncipc/dacrrdp/tbi.htm
3. Lehr D, Baethmann A, Reulen HJ, et al (1997) Management of patients with severe head injury in the preclinical phase: A prospective analysis. J Trauma 42 (suppl 5):S71–S75
4. Van Balen HGG, Mulder Th, Keyser A (1996) Towards a disability-oriented epidmiology of traumatic brain injury. Disabil Rehabil 18:181–190
5. Hall KM, Johnston MV (1994) Outcomes evaluation in TBI rehabilitation. Part 2: measurement tools for a nationwide data system. Arch Phys Med Rehabil 75 (suppl):SC10–SC18
6. Levin HS, O'Donnell VM, Grossman RG (1979) The Galveston Orientation and Amnesia Test. A practical scale to assess cognition after head injury. J Nerv Ment Dis 167:675–684
7. Zafonte RD, Mann NR, Millis SR, Black KL, Wood DL, Hammond F (1997) Posttraumatic amnesia: Its relation to functional outcome. Arch Phys Med Rehabil 78:1101–1106
8. Teasdale G, Jennet B (1974) Assessment of coma and impaired consciousness: a practical scale. The Lancet 2:81–84
9. Hall KM (1997) Establishing a national traumatic brain injury information system based upon a unified data set. Arch Phys Med Rehabil 78:S5–S11
10. Zasler ND (1997) Prognostic indicators in medical rehabilitation of traumatic brain injury: a commentary and review. Arch Phys Med Rehabil 78:S12–S16
11. Marshall LF, Marshall SB, Klauber MR, et al (1991) The diagnosis of head injury requires a classification based on computed axial tomography. J Neurotrauma 9 (suppl 1):S287–S292
12. Aldrich EF, Eisenberg HM, Saydjari C, et al (1992) Predictors of mortality in severely head-injured patients civilian gunshot wounds: A report from the NIH Traumatic Coma Data Bank. Surg Neurol 38:418–423
13. Murray GD, Teasdale GM, Braakman R, et al (1999) The European Brain Injury Consortium survey of head injuries across Europe. Acta Neurochir (Wien) 141:223–236
14. World Health Organization (1980) International Classification of Impairments, Disabilities, and Handicaps. World Health Organization, Geneva
15. World Health Organization (1997) ICIDH-2: International Classification of Impairments, Activities and Participation. A manual of Dimensions of Disablement and Functioning. Beta-1 draft for field trials. World Health Organization, Geneva
16. Jennett B, Bond M (1975) Assessment of outcome after severe brain damage. A practical scale. The Lancet 1:480–485

17. Anderson SI, Housley AM, Jones PA, Slattery J, Miller JD (1993) Glasgow Outcome Scale: an interrater reliability study. Brain Injury 7:309–317
18. Boake C (1996) Supervision Rating Scale: a measure of functional outcome from brain injury. Arch Phys Med Rehabil 77:765–772
19. Smith RM, Fields FRJ, Lenox JL, Morris HO, Nolan JJ (1979) A functional scale of recovery from severe head trauma. Clin Neuropsychol 1:48–50
20. Maas AIR, Braakman R, Schouten HJA, Minderhoud JM, Van Zomeren AH (1983) Agreement between physicians on assessment of outcome following severe head injury. J Neurosurg 58:321–325
21. Livingston MG, Livingston HG (1985) The Glasgow Assessment Schedule: clinical and research assessment of head injury outcome. Int Rehabil Med 7:145–149
22. Horne G, Schremitsch E (1989) Assessment of the survivors of major trauma accidents. Aust N Z J Surg 59:465–470
23. Wilson JTL, Pettigrew LEL, Teasdale GM (1998) Structured interviews for the Glasgow Outcome Scale and the Extended Glasgow Outcome Scale. J Neurotrauma 15:587–597
24. Jennett B, Snoek J, Bond MR, Brooks N (1981) Disability after severe head injury: Observations on the use of the Glasgow Outcome Scale. J Neurol Neurosurg Psych 44:285–293
25. Rappaport M, Hall KM, Hopkins K, Belleza T, Cope DN (1982) Disability Rating Scale for severe head trauma: coma to community. Arch Phys Med Rehabil 63:118–123
26. Gouvier WD, Blanton PD, LaPorte KK, Nepomuceno C (1987) Reliability and validity of the Disability Rating Scale and the Levels of Cognitive Functioning Scale in monitoring recovery from severe head injury. Arch Phys Med Rehabil 68:94–97
27. Heinemann, AW, Linacre JM, Wright BD, Hamilton BB, Granger C (1994) Prediction of rehabilitation outcomes with disability measures. Arch Phys Med Rehabil 75:133–143
28. Fleming JM, Maas F (1994) Prognosis of rehabilitation outcome in head injury using the disability rating scale. Arch Phys Med Rehabil 75:156–163
29. Rappaport M, Hall K, Hopkins K, Belleza T, Berrol S, Reynolds G (1977) Evoked brain potentials and disability in brain-damaged patients. Arch Phys Med Rehabil 58:333–338
30. Rappaport M, Hall K, Hopkins K, Belleza T (1981) Evoked potentials and head injury: 1. Rating of evoked potential abnormality. Clin Electroencephalogr 12:154–166
31. Pettigrew LEL, Wilson JTL, Teasdale GM (1998) Assessing disability after head injury: improved use of the Glasgow Outcome Scale. J Neurosurg 89:939–943
32. Wade DT (1996) Measurement in Neurological Rehabilitation. Oxford University Press, Oxford
33. Collin C, Wade DT, Davis S, et al (1988) The Barthel ADL Index: a reliability study. Int Disabil Stud 10:61–63
34. Heyink J (1997) The Barthel Index. In: Hutchinson A, Bentzen N, König-Zahn C (eds) Cross Cultural Health Outcome Assessment: a User's Guide. European Research Group on Health Outcomes, pp 99–103
35. Hagen C (1982) Language cognitive disorganization following closed head injury: a conceptualization. In: Trexler LE (ed) Cognitive Rehabilitation: Conceptualization and Intervention. Plenum Press, New York, pp 131–151
36. Lezak MD (1995) Neuropsychological Assessment (3rd edn). Oxford University Press, New York
37. Sohlberg MM, Mateer CA (1989) Introduction to Cognitive Rehabilitation. Guilford Press, New York
38. Granger CV, Hamilton BB, Keith RA, Zielezny M, Sherwin FS (1986) Advances in functional assessment for medical rehabilitation. Top Geriatr Rehabil 1:59–74
39. Hamilton BB, Granger CV, Sherwin FS, et al (1987) A uniform national data system for medical rehabilitation. In: Fuhrer MJ (ed) Rehabilitation Outcomes: Analysis and Measurement. Brookes, Baltimore, pp 137–147
40. Hamilton BB, Laughlin JA, Granger CV, et al (1991) Interrater agreement of the seven level functional independence measure. Arch Phys Med Rehabil 72:790 (Abst)
41. Ottenbacher KJ, Hsu Y, Granger CV, Fiedler RC (1996) The reliability of the functional independence measure: a quantitative review. Arch Phys Med Rehabil 77:1226–1232
42. Smith-Knapp K, Corrigan JD, Arnett JA (1996) Predicting functional independence from neuropsychological tests following traumatic brain injury. Brain Injury 10:651–661

43. Granger CV, Cotter AC, Hamilton BB, et al (1990) Functional assessment scales: study of persons with multiple sclerosis. Arch Phys Med Rehabil 71:870–875
44. Granger CV, Cotter AC, Hamilton BB, et al (1993) Functional assessment scales: a study of persons after stroke. Arch Phys Med Rehabil 74:133–138
45. Granger CV, Divan N, Roger BS, et al (1995) Functional assessment scales: a study of persons after traumatic brain injury. Am J Phys Med Rehabil 74:107–113
46. Willer B, Rosenthal M, Kreutzer JS, Gordon WA, Rempel R (1993) Assessment of community integration following rehabilitation for traumatic brain injury. J Head Trauma Rehabil 8:75–87
47. Overall JE, Gorham DR (1962) The brief psychiatric rating scale. Psychol Rep 10:799–812
48. Levin HS, High WM, Goethe KE, et al (1987) The neurobehavioral rating scale: assessment of the behavioural sequelae of head injury by the clinician. J Neurol Neurosurg Psychiatry 50:183–193
49. Corrigan JD, Dickerson J, Fisher E, Meyer P (1990) The Neurobehavioural Rating Scale: replication in an acute, inpatient rehabilitation setting. Brain Injury 4:215–222
50. Powell JH, Beckers K, Greenwood RJ (1998) Measuring progress and outcome in community rehabilitation after brain injury with a new assessment instrument- the BICRO-39 scales. Arch Phys Med Rehabil 79:1213–1225
51. Berger E, Leven F, Pirente N, Boullon B, Neugebauer E (1999) Quality of life after traumatic brain injury: A systematic review of the literature. Restor Neurol Neurosci 14:93–102
52. Pollard WE, Bobbit RA, Bergner M, Martin DP, Gilson BS (1976) The sickness impact profile: reliability of a health status measure. Med Care 14:146–155
53. Bergner M, Bobbitt RA, Kressel S, et al (1976) The Sickness Impact Profile: conceptual formulation and methodology for the development of a health status measure. Int J Health Serv 6:393–415
54. Krenz C, Larson EB, Buchner DM, Canfield CG (1988) Characterizing patient dysfunction in Alzheimer's-Type dementia. Med Care 26:453–461
55. Hart CG, Evans RW (1987) The functional status of ESRD patients as measured by the Sickness Impact Profile. J Chron Dis 40:1175–1305
56. Dego R (1984) Pitfalls in measuring the health status of Mexican Americans: comparative validity of the English and Spanish Sickness Impact Profile. Am J Pub Health 74:569–573
57. Corrigan JD, Smith-Knapp K, Granger CV (1998) Outcomes in the first 5 years after traumatic brain injury. Arch Phys Med Rehabil 79:298–230
58. Smith JL, Magill-Evans J, Brintnell S (1998) Life satisfaction following traumatic brain injury. Can J Rehabil 11:131–140
59. Van Balen HGG, Mulder Th (1996) Beyond the stereotype: an epidemiological study on the long-term sequelae of traumatic brain injury. Clin Rehabil 10:259–266
60. Moore AD, Stambrook M, Gill DD, Lubusko AA (1992) Differences in long-term quality of life in married and single TBI patients. Can J Rehabil 6:89–98
61. Fleming JH, Strong J, Ashton R (1998) Cluster analysis of self-awareness levels in adults with traumatic brain injury and relationship to outcome. J Head Trauma Rehabil 13:39–51
62. Temkin N, McLean A, Dikmen S, Gale J, Bergner M, Almes MJ (1988) Development and evaluation of modifications to the Sickness Impact Profile for head injury. J Clin Epidemiol 41:47–57
63. Wilkin D, Hallam L, Doggett MA (1992) Measures of Need and Outcome for Primary Health Care. Oxford University Press, Oxford
64. Keith RA (1994) Functional status and health status. Arch Phys Med Rehabil 75:478–483
65. De Bruin AF, Diederiks JPM, Witte de LP, Stevens FCJ, Philipsen H (1994) The development of a short generic version of the Sickness Impact Profile. J Clin Epidemiol 47:407–418
66. Ware JE, Sherbourne CD (1992) The MOS 36-Item Short-Form Health Survey (SF-36). I: Conceptual framework and item selection. Med Care 30:473–483
67. Brazier JE, Harper R, Jones NMB, et al (1992) Validating the SF-36 health survey questionnaire: a new outcome measure for primary care. Br Med J 305:160–164
68. Ware J, Snow KK, Kosinski M, et al (1993) SF-36 Health Survey: Manual and Interpretation Guide. The Health Institute, New England Medical Center Hospitals, Boston

69. McHorney CA, Ware JE, Raczek AE (1993) The MOS-36-Item Short-Form Health Survey (SF-36). II: Psychometric and clinical tests of validity in measuring physical and mental health constructs. Med Care 31:247–263

70. Hanestad BR (1997) The MOS SF-36/RAND 36-Item Health Survey 1.0/HSQ. In: Hutchinson A, Bentzen N, König-Zahn C (eds) Cross Cultural Health Outcome Assessment: a User's guide. European Research Group on Health Outcomes, pp 60–67

71. Coughlan AK, Storey P (1988) The Wimbledon Self-Report Scale: emotional and mood appraisal. Clin Rehabil 2:207–213

72. Nelson E, Wasson J, Kirk J, et al (1987) Assessment of function in routine clinical practice: description of the COOP Chart method and preliminary findings. J Chronic Dis 40 (suppl 1):55S–63S

73. Scholten JHG, Van Weel C (1992) Functional Status Assessment in Family Practice: the Dartmouth COOP Functional Health Assessment Charts/WONCA. Meditekst, Lelystad

74. Weel C van, König-Zahn C, Touw-Otten FWMM, et al (1995) Measuring Functional Health Status with the COOP/WONCA Charts. A Manual. NCH series 7 Northern Centre of Health Care Research, Groningen

75. Nelson EC, Landgraf JM, Hayes RD, et al (1990) The functional status of patients: how can it be measured in physician's offices? Med Care 28:1111–1126

76. König-Zahn C (1997) The COOP/WONCA Charts. In: Hutchinson A, Bentzen N and König-Zahn C (eds) Cross Cultural Health Outcome Assessment: a User's Guide. European Research Group on Health Outcomes, pp 48–53

77. Willer B, Ottenbacher KJ, Coad ML (1994) The community integration questionnaire. A comparitive examination. Am J Phys Med Rehabil 73:103–11

78. Dijkers M (1997) Measuring the long-term outcomes of traumatic brain injury: A review of the community integration questionnaire. J Head Trauma Rehabil 12:74–91

79. Hütter BO, Glisbach JM (1999) Das Aachener Lebensqualitätsinventar (ALQI) für Patienten mit Hirnschädigung: Erste Ergebnisse zu methodischen Gütekriterien. Zeitschrift für Neuropsychologie 10:38

80. McMahon CG, Yates DW, Campbell FM, Hollis S, Woodford M (1999) Unexpected contribution of moderate traumatic brain injury to death after major trauma. J Trauma 47:891–895

Biochemical and Molecular Mechanisms after Severe Traumatic Brain Injury in Children

P. M. Kochanek, R. P. Berger, and L. W. Jenkins

▌ Introduction

Secondary damage after severe traumatic brain injury (TBI) in infants and children represents the key target for the development and application of novel therapies. Our group at the Safar Center for Resuscitation Research and the Children's Hospital of Pittsburgh has put considerable effort into defining the mechanisms involved in the evolution of damage after severe TBI in pediatric patients and has also worked to develop and use experimental models of TBI to evaluate both novel diagnostic tools and putative therapies. In this chapter, we outline some of our most recent findings on a number of exciting fronts. First, we will update our work at the bedside that takes advantage of the cerebrospinal fluid (CSF) bank that we have accumulated from infants and children with severe TBI. The CSF bank, funded by the Centers for Disease Control and Prevention in the USA, is a unique resource that includes over 1000 CSF samples from nearly 100 pediatric victims of severe TBI. The CSF bank has become instrumental in studying biochemical and molecular mechanisms in our critically ill patients. For a review of the initial investigations of secondary injury mechanisms in pediatric TBI by our group, we suggest two recent reviews [1, 2]. The investigations by our group discussed in this chapter represent the more recent studies (Fig. 1).

These clinical studies include a series of recent reports describing:
▌ the time course of neuronal and astrocytic cell death in infants and children after severe TBI and
▌ the roles of oxidative stress, the endogenous neuroprotectants and mediators of regeneration, in secondary brain injury.

After this update, we will return to the bench to describe a step beyond gene chip technology, and discuss the novel work by Jenkins et al. [3] demonstrating the first application of proteomics to an experimental model of TBI in immature 17-day-old rat pups.

▌ Neuron Specific Enolase (NSE) and S100B in Clinical TBI

In prior studies by our group, we characterized a number of biochemical and molecular markers that had considerable potential to mediate detrimental affects in the secondary injury cascade after severe TBI in infants and children [1]. These studies shed light on the secondary injury cascade and uncovered important differ-

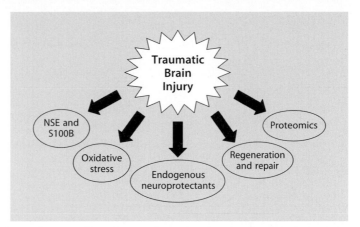

Fig. 1. Cartoon depicting the specific areas addressed in this chapter including clinical studies of recently reported work using cerebrospinal fluid (CSF) to describe: 1) the time course of astrocytic and neuronal (or astrocyte and neuron) death in infants and children after severe traumatic brain injury (TBI) assessed by the astrocyte marker S-100B and neuron specific enolase (NSE); 2) recent investigation of the role of oxidative stress; 3) the participation of the endogenous neuroprotectants, adenosine, procalcitonin and adrenomedullin; 4) identification of increases in several known mediators of regeneration; 5) the novel work in our center demonstrating the first application of proteomics to an experimental model of TBI

ences in the biochemical and molecular events in infant and children who are victims of non-inflicted versus inflicted head trauma. In each of these studies, the inflicted head trauma patients – victims of child abuse including the shaken baby syndrome – demonstrated a unique pattern of often remarkably high levels of mediators of secondary damage [1], such as glutamate and quinolinic acid, and low levels of endogenous neuroprotectants such as bcl-2 [9].

However, one important, more basic study remained to be carried out, namely using our bank of serially collected CSF samples to try to identify the time course of both neuronal and astrocyte death after injury. To achieve this goal, two biochemical markers were selected: neuron-specific enolase (NSE) and S100B [4–8]. NSE is a glycolytic enzyme localized primarily to the neuronal cytoplasm, while S100B is a calcium-binding protein localized to astroglial cells. The physiologic function of S100B is not entirely understood, but its levels are increased in the presence of central nervous system (CNS) lesions [8]. Both of these markers have been extensively studied in adults.

In recent work, we [10] studied CSF samples (n=35) from ten infants and children, five with severe non-inflicted TBI and five with severe inflicted TBI. Lumbar CSF samples from five children evaluated for meningitis were used as a comparison group. NSE was increased in both non-inflicted and inflicted TBI versus the comparison group in 34 of 35 samples. NSE was increased over 30-fold (117.1 ng/ml vs. 3.5 ng/ml). After non-inflicted TBI, a transient peak in NSE was seen at ~11 hours after injury. In contrast, after inflicted head trauma, an early increase in NSE was followed by a sustained and delayed peak ~63 hours after injury (Fig. 2). A single, early peak in S100B was observed in patients with non-inflicted and those with inflicted TBI.

Thus, markers of both neuronal and astroglial death are markedly increased in CSF after severe non-inflicted and inflicted TBI. Inflicted TBI produced a unique

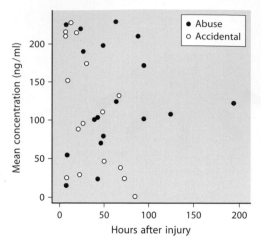

Fig. 2. Graph of mean cerebrospinal fluid (CSF) concentration of neuron specific enolase (NSE), a marker of neuronal death, versus hours after injury in infants and children who were victims of severe traumatic brain injury (TBI) from either child abuse (closed circles) or accidents (open circles). After non-inflicted TBI, a transient peak in NSE was seen at ∼11 hours after injury. In contrast, after inflicted head trauma (child abuse), the early increase in NSE was followed by a sustained and delayed peak at a ∼63 hours. This delayed peak in NSE may reflect delayed neuronal death, which may represent an important therapeutic target in either child abuse victims or infants (see text for details). (From [10] with permission)

time course of NSE, presumably representing two waves of neuronal death, the second of which may represent apoptosis. It is also possible that young age, rather than the mechanism of injury, is responsible for the delayed neuronal death. Recent studies in experimental TBI have suggested important age-related differences in the contribution of apoptosis to neuronal death [11]. Since most of the infants with severe TBI represented in our CSF bank are victims of abuse, we cannot currently address the question as to whether this finding is a result of difference in age or injury mechanism. In either case, the second wave of cell death is an important finding since delayed neuronal death may represent an important therapeutic target in certain infants with severe TBI and may help further our understanding of the biochemical differences between inflicted and non-inflicted TBI.

▌ Markers of Oxidative Stress in Clinical TBI

Studies at the bench, spanning from neuronal culture to experimental models of TBI strongly suggest that oxidative damage is one of the key final common pathways of neuronal death [12–14]. Oxidative damage to membrane lipid, proteins, and nucleic acids all may play important roles in neuronal dysfunction and death. Recently, Baylr et al. [15, 16], used our established CSF bank to perform a comprehensive study identifying markers of oxidative damage, assessing the status of both total oxidative reserve and specific antioxidants, including both ascorbate and glutathione. F_2-isoprostane, a stable and reliable marker of lipid peroxidation of arachidonate, in CSF from infants and children, was markedly increased early after TBI, suggesting rapid lipid peroxidation. Levels were significantly increased versus control and peaked on the first day after injury [15]. However, evidence for ongoing oxidative stress after severe TBI in infants and children was suggested by the fact that progressive depletion in total antioxidant reserve, and both ascorbate and glutathione concentrations, was seen over the initial week after injury. Finally, increases in ascorbate radical in CSF were demonstrated using electron paramagnetic resonance spectroscopy after clinical TBI.

These findings raise several important points. First, although cause and effect was not addressed, they suggest a possible role for oxidative stress in the evolution of secondary damage after clinical pediatric TBI. Second, they suggest that markers of lipid peroxidation such as F2-iosprostane and/or oxidative stress, such as total antioxidant reserve, could serve as surrogate markers of the ability of therapies to attenuate posttraumatic oxidative stress. The potential value of this should not be dismissed. Two large clinical trials of therapies targeting oxidative damage after severe TBI in adults, the tirilizad and polyethylene glycol-conjugated superoxide dismutase (PEG-SOD) trials, both failed to reveal a benefit; however, no demonstration of efficacy of either agent against oxidative damage *in vivo* was shown [17, 18]. This may be particularly important since limitations in the ability of both agents to penetrate the brain have recently been suggested [19]. Third, the marked depletion of CSF ascorbate is particularly concerning, since this is being observed in the face of standard of care, which includes administration of vitamins in conventional hyperalimentation. It is very possible that standard approaches to care are inadequate in this regard. Further study is needed. The potential utility of these assays at the bedside could be valuable for a wide variety of therapies such as hypothermia, anti-excitotoxic agents, or other treatments, since oxidative damage has been suggested to be a final common pathway for a large number of cascades. Finally, current studies by our group to determine the time course and magnitude of oxidative damage in non-inflicted versus inflicted TBI are underway.

Endogenous Neuroprotectants in Clinical TBI

In prior reports and reviews by our group, increases in CSF levels were seen for a number of biochemical and molecular markers of putative endogenous neuroprotectants. For example, Clark et al. [9] reported increased CSF concentrations of the anti-apoptotic mitochondrial protein bcl-2 after severe TBI in infants and children. Surprisingly, the increase in bcl-2 was not observed in victims of inflicted TBI. We suggested that unique aspects of child abuse could account for this finding. First, it was possible that massive injuries to the brain in many of these victims might overwhelm the ability to allow for the gene induction and synthesis of this protein after injury. Alternatively, chronic brain injury, seen in many victims of child abuse, might alter the sequence of molecular events after the severe insult that resulted in presentation.

One other putative endogenous neuroprotectant that we previously identified was adenosine [1, 20, 21]. Adenosine, formed from the breakdown of adenosine triphosphate (ATP), is both a powerful anti-excitotoxic agent and a potent vasodilator. Sharples et al. [22] and more recently Adelson et al. [23] reported early hypoperfusion after severe TBI in infants and children. A variety of etiologies has been suggested for the early reduction in posttraumatic cerebral blood flow (CBF) including spreading depression, local compression, endothelial swelling, vasospasm from mediators such as endothelin, among other mechanisms (reviewed in [1]). We speculated that adenosine might be one of several putative endogenous agents pro-

duced in response to early hypoperfusion. Recent work in our laboratory has identified two additional endogenous vasodilators that may represent retaliatory agents
elaborated in response to the early posttraumatic hypoperfusion, namely, procalcitonin and adrenomedullin.

Procalcitonin is a 116 amino acid pro-peptide of the hormone calcitonin, produced from alternative processing of the calcitonin/calcitonin-gene-related-peptide
(CGRP) gene [24]. Procalcitonin and CGRP are potent vasodilating neuropeptides.
They may be produced as a compensatory, endogenous neuroprotective response to
ischemic stress. Procalcitonin and CGRP both belong to the insulin gene superfamily and demonstrate homologous relationships to adrenomedullin [25]. Adrenomedullin also possesses vasodilatory properties [26]. The molecular similarities between procalcitonin, CGRP, and adrenomedullin suggest the possibility of overlapping functional properties between these molecules.

Han et al. [27] recently quantified procalcitonin concentrations in CSF samples
from 28 infants and children with severe TBI and 22 controls. Initial CSF procalcitonin concentration in patients with severe TBI was increased over three-fold versus
controls (0.41 ng/ml versus 0.12 ng/ml). Univariate analysis revealed significant *inverse* associations between CSF procalcitonin concentration and both time after injury and child abuse as a mechanism of injury, while multivariate analysis showed
an independent, inverse association between CSF procalcitonin and only child
abuse (p = 0.05). Figure 3 graphically depicts these inverse associations, and shows
that the marked increase in CSF procalcitonin peaks early after TBI and that this
robust post-injury increase in CSF procalcitonin is remarkably attenuated in victims of child abuse. The failure to produce similar increases in CSF procalcitonin
after inflicted, versus non-inflicted, TBI mirrors our previously discussed observation that the endogenous neuroprotectant bcl-2 is not induced in the setting of in-

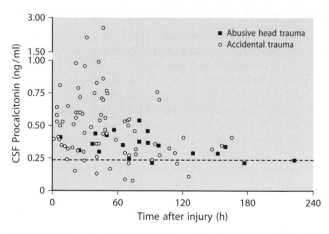

Fig. 3. Plot of cerebrospinal fluid (CSF) procalcitonin concentration (ng/ml) from children with severe traumatic
brain injury (TBI), versus time. Each point (n = 99) represents a single measurement of CSF procalcitonin in victims of child abuse (closed squares) or non-inflicted trauma (open circles). CSF procalcitonin was inversely associated with both time after injury and child abuse using univariate regression analysis. An independent, inverse
association between CSF procalcitonin concentration and child abuse (p = 0.05) was demonstrated by multivariate analysis. The dotted line represents the highest CSF procalcitonin concentration (0.24 ng/ml) observed from
the control population. (From [27] with permission)

flicted TBI. Procalcitonin is thus the second mediator that we have studied in CSF to have an inverse association with child abuse. The significance of this observation remains to be determined though one may infer that procalcitonin also possesses neuroprotective properties. The lower CSF procalcitonin concentration among victims of child abuse could, as previously discussed, result from the possibility that child abuse victims sustain such overwhelming brain injury that endogenous compensatory neuroprotectants are not synthesized. Alternatively, since many victims of child abuse are not brought to medical attention for hours or even days after injury, the peak CSF levels may have been missed. Finally, once again, we cannot rule out age-related differences in the CSF procalcitonin response, since most of the infants sustaining TBI in our series were victims of child abuse.

In collaboration with Dr. Naoto Minamino and his group at the National Cardiovascular Center Research Institute in Osaka, Japan, we also recently measured CSF levels of adrenomedullin after severe TBI in infants and children [28]. Adrenomedullin is a recently discovered 52-amino-acid peptide that is a potent vasodilator produced in brain in experimental models of cerebral ischemia [29]. Infusion of adrenomedullin increases regional CBF and reduces infarct volume after vascular occlusion in rats [30] and thus, like bcl 2 and procalcitonin, may represent an endogenous neuroprotectant. Total adrenomedullin concentration was measured using a radioimmunometric assay in 66 CSF samples from 21 pediatric patients during the initial 10 days after severe TBI. Adrenomedullin concentration was markedly increased in CSF of infants and children after severe TBI vs control. Overall, a 4.5-fold increase was observed vs control; however, as much as a 800-fold increase was seen in some patients. Unlike procalcitonin, we did not demonstrate a significant inverse association between adrenomedullin concentration and inflicted head trauma.

A variety of studies in experimental and clinical TBI have revealed marked blood flow reductions after severe injury. Our recent clinical data discussed above strongly support the existence of mediators that could mount an endogenous retaliatory vasodilatory response. Whether these mediators are successful in producing the recovery in blood flow that so often accompanies favorable recovery, or possibly mediate delayed hyperemia that may contribute to brain swelling, remains to be determined. In addition, we and other groups are using experimental models of TBI to determine the effect of augmenting early posttraumatic cerebral blood flow [31–33].

▌ Markers of Regeneration in Clinical TBI

Little is known about the composition, timing, and magnitude of the regenerative response after severe TBI in either adults or children. Knowledge of this response could be of particular value in the setting of TBI in infants and children, since focal insults are amenable to rehabilitation and brain plasticity may represent a considerable opportunity for repair during development.

Recently, investigators in our group have detected increases in a number of putative molecules involved in the regenerative response to TBI, including nerve growth factor [34], vascular endothelial growth factor (VEGF) [35], and hepatocyte growth factor [36]. In light of the overlap with the prior discussion of putative mediators involved in the recovery of posttraumatic cerebral blood flow, we will limit or discussion to our investigation of VEGF.

VEGF is a key regulator of angiogenesis in the tissue response to injury [37]. VEGF is induced by hypoxemia and has been shown to be increased in brain in a variety of experimental injury paradigms, including TBI [38]. In neuronal culture, VEGF has been shown to exhibit a direct neuroprotective effect [39], and it is strongly associated with angiogenesis in many models of CNS injury [38]. VEGF production has been linked to stimulation of adenosine A2b receptors. This suggests the possibility of a linkage between posttraumatic hypoxia/ischemia, ATP breakdown, adenosine formation and subsequent retaliatory vasodilation and stimulation of angiogenesis.

Shore et al. [35] recently reported increases in VEGF in CSF after severe TBI in infants and children. VEGF levels peaked at 91.6 ng/dl, about six times control. The peak in VEGF levels occurred at 22.5 hr after TBI. Also consistent with our theory, a multivariate regression model, revealed that the increases in VEGF were significantly associated with increases in adenosine. Temporally, it appeared overall that peak CSF VEGF followed peak adenosine concentration. The increase in VEGF in CSF after clinical TBI may represent evidence that the biochemical signals for regeneration, particularly angiogenesis, are set into motion as early as one day after injury. Recent studies outside of the central nervous system describe remarkably rapid vascular regeneration and remodeling. This suggests that such events may be important even in the intensive care unit (ICU). Similarly, the coupled increases in VEGF and adenosine suggest a remarkable, albeit logical, linkage between the mechanisms of vasodilatation and angiogenesis in the injured brain. These findings may begin to open up new therapeutic opportunities. As stem cell biology and other tools develop to facilitate the reconstitution of damaged brain regions, restoration of the cerebral circulation will need to be considered and knowledge of the endogenous angiogenic factors involved is likely to be essential.

▌ Proteomics Application to Experimental TBI in the Developing Rat Brain

Recently, a flurry of excitement and new investigation has rightfully emerged as a result of the development of genomics and gene chip technology. Characterization of the time course and patterns of gene expression in a disease such as severe TBI could be of great relevance. For example, the sequence of molecular participants in executing delayed neuronal death could be unraveled as could the specific interactions between this cascade and other mechanisms. Similarly, one could envisage defining, in both experimental models, and ultimately in patients, the time course for the initiation of repair, regeneration, and plasticity, which could help direct the optimal initiation of therapies and interventions targeting these mechanisms. One major limitation of genomic strategies is that they quantify messenger ribonucleic acid (mRNA). Recently, Fey and Larsen [40] reported that the correlation between mRNA and protein expression is frequently less than 50%, even when protein synthesis is not pathologically altered. This is likely to be an even greater problem in the setting of tissue injury. Obviously, knowledge of the consequences of injury on cellular proteins would provide insight into the successful induction of new genes and information on the structural integrity of the cellular architecture.

In an attempt to circumvent this problem, tools have been developed to facilitate global cellular protein analyses (proteomics). Over twenty years ago, two dimensional (2D) gel electrophoresis was developed [41]. This method separates proteins based on both charge and molecular weight. We recently reported the first application of this proteomics method to a model of experimental TBI [3]. Protein changes were assessed in the hippocampus, a key site of secondary damage, of immature (post-natal day 17) rats at 24 hours after TBI. Six injured rats were compared to an equal number of shams. Injury was produced using the controlled cortical impact model modified for use in immature rats [42]. Using 2D gel electrophoresis and classical silver staining methods, approximately 1500 high copy protein spots were identified. From these 1500 protein spots roughly 600 proteins matched across gel pairs with the remaining proteins representing unmatched proteins. These may represent proteolytic degradation fragments or posttranslationally modified proteins. Remarkably, a 10-fold decrease or increase was noted for about 10% of the total proteins resolved. Changes in important cytoskeletal and cell signaling proteins were identified from a subset of 50 proteins identified by gel matching with existing data bases. For example, significant reductions in the important cytoskeletal proteins actin and both alpha- and beta-tubulin were detected. Similarly, significant reductions in the phosphatidylinoitol transfer protein alpha were also observed, suggesting the possibility of important alterations in cell signaling via the protein kinase C pathway. Finally, a 60% increase in Cu-Zn SOD was observed, which may represent part of the attempted endogenous induction of antioxidant defenses. Based on the clinical studies discussed earlier in this report, it appears that the induction of protein antioxidant defenses, such as SOD, is frequently inadequate after severe TBI.

Finally, the 2D gel format provided an additional opportunity to begin to unravel the complex signaling cascades of secondary changes in cellular proteins. In addition to the study of protein degradation and induction with conventional silver stain methodology, immunoblot analysis of the proteins separated on these 2D gels, using new commercial antibodies that recognize specific phosphorylatation sequences, facilitated the unique assessment of protein modification of substrate protein function. The term 'function proteomics' has been applied to this approach. This approach allows the investigation of many 'low copy' proteins that may not be identified by silver stains but have important roles in the evolution of secondary damage and repair. For example, protein kinase B is an important enzyme that phosphorylates and inactivates a number of molecular participants in the cell-death cascade, such as Bad, caspase-9, and forkhead transcription factors (reviewed in [43]). Using an antibody in our TBI model that specifically identifies the protein kinase B phosphorylation sequence revealed reduced PKB phosphorylation of some of these proteins. This is consistent with reduced survival signaling after TBI [3]. Clearly, further application of this powerful functional proteomics approach could provide unprecedented insight into the mechanism of cell injury, survival, and repair after TBI.

▌ Conclusion

In these studies bridging the ICU and the bench, we have first demonstrated that the serial collection and subsequent biochemical and molecular analysis of CSF samples can serve as an important tool to help define the time course of cell death and identify key participants in secondary brain damage. We also described some of our work beginning to characterize both the endogenous neuroprotectants and markers of regeneration. It is clear that infants who are victims of inflicted head trauma exhibit a unique pathobiology, with enhanced and sustained biochemical evidence of secondary damage and concomitantly deficient endogenous defenses. Finally, we have taken the first step to attempt to simultaneously define the global spectrum in changes in structural and effector proteins after TBI by applying conventional and functional proteomics methodology to an experimental model of TBI in the developing rat brain. Successful translation of this method to the bedside represents the next logical step to unravel the complex events in clinical TBI. We hope that a greatly improved understanding of this complex disease will lead to the targeted application of novel therapies.

Acknowledgement. We thank Drs. Hülya Baylr, Valerian Kagan, Yong Han, Courtney Robertson, Paul Shore, Robert Clark, P. David Adelson, Naoto Minamino, and Edwin Jackson for important contributions to the individual studies reviewed in this manuscript. We also thank Keri Janesko and Grant Peters for technical support of the CSF bank and the proteomics studies, respectively. We also wish to thank the Centers for Disease Control and Prevention (University of Pittsburgh Center for Injury Research and Control CIRCL/CDC), the National Institutes of Health (NS 30318, NS 40049, NS 01809), and the General Clinical Research Center of Children's Hospital of Pittsburgh (M01 RR00084) for support. We thank Christopher Edwards for preparation of figures and Janice Hasch and Marci Provins-Chonko for assistance with manuscript preparation.

References

1. Kochanek PM, Clark RSB, Ruppel RA, et al (2000) Biochemical, cellular and molecular mechanisms in the evolution of secondary damage after severe traumatic brain injury in infants and children: Lessons learned from the bedside. Pediatr Crit Care Med 1:4–19
2. Kochanek PM, Clark RSB, Ruppel RA, Adelson PD, Dixon CE, Jenkins L (2001) Pediatric traumatic brain injury: From bench to bedside and back In: Marwah J, Dixon E, Banik N (eds) Traumatic CNS Injury. Prominent Press, Scottsdale, pp 251–272
3. Jenkins LW, Peters GW, Dixon CE, et al (2001) Proteomic changes using large format 2D gel electrophoresis and pH 3–10 IPG strips 24 hours after CCI in 17 postnatal day (PND) rats. J Neurotrauma 18:1151 (Abst)
4. Karkela J, Bock E, Kaukinen S (1993) CSF and serum brain-specific creatine kinase isoenzyme (CK-BB), neuron specific enolase (NSE) and neural cell adhesion molecule (NCAM) as prognostic markers for hypoxic brain injury after cardiac arrest in man. J Neur Sci 116:100–109
5. Skogseid I, Nordby H, Urdal P, Paus E, Lilleaas F (1992) Increased serum creatine kinase BB and neuron specific enolase following head injury indicated brain damage. Acta Neurochir 115:106–111
6. Vazquez M, Rodriguez-Sanchez F, Osuna E, et al (1995) Creatine kinase BB and neuron specific enolase in cerebrospinal fluid in the diagnosis of brain insult. Am J Forensic Med Pathol 16:210–214
7. Yamazaki Y, Yada K, Morii S, Kitahara T, Ohwada T (1995) Diagnostic significance of serum neuron-specific enolase and myelin basic protein assay in patients with acute head trauma. Surg Neurol 43:267–271
8. Hardemark H, Ericsson N, Kotwica Z, et al (1989) S-100 protein and neuron specific enolase in CSF after experimental traumatic or focal ischemic brain damage. J Neurosurg 71:727–731
9. Clark RSB, Kochanek PM, Adelson PD, et al (2000) Increases in Bcl-2 protein in cerebrospinal fluid and evidence for programmed-cell death in infants and children following severe traumatic brain injury. J Pediatrics 137:197–204

10. Berger RP, Janesko KL, Wisniewski SR, et al (2002) Neuron-specific enolase and S100B in cerebrospinal fluid after severe traumatic brain injury in infants and children. Pediatrics (in press)

11. Bittigau P, Sifringer M, Pohl D, et al (1999) Apoptotic neurodegeneration following trauma is markedly enhanced in the immature brain. Ann Neurol 45:724–735

12. Kontos HA, Wei EP (1986) Superoxide production in experimental brain injury. J Neurosurg 64:803–807

13. Shohami E, Beit-Yannai E, Horowitz M, Kohen R (1997) Oxidative stress in closed head injury: Brain antioxidant capacity as an indicator of functional outcome. J Cereb Blood Flow Metab 17:1007–1019

14. Tyurin VA, Tyurina YY, Borisenko GG, et al (2000) Oxidative stress following traumatic brain injury in rats: Quantitation of biomarkers and detection of free radical intermediates. J Neurochem 75:2178–2189

15. Baylr H, Kagan VE, Tyrina YY, et al (2001) Assessment of antioxidant reserve and oxidative stress in cerebrospinal fluid after severe traumatic brain injury in infants and children. Pediatr Res Suppl 49:43A (Abst)

16. Baylr H, Marion DW, Kagan VE, et al (2002) Marked gender effect of lipid peroxidation after traumatic brain injury in adult patients. Crit Care Med (Abst, in press)

17. Muizelaar JP, Marmarou A, Young HF, et al (1993) Improving the outcome of severe head injury with oxygen radical scavenger polyethylene glycol-conjugated superoxide dismutase: A phase II trial. J Neurosurg 78:375–382

18. Marshall LF, Maas AIR, Marshall SB, et al (1998) A multicenter trial on the efficacy of using tirilizad mesylate in cases of head injury. J Neurosurg 89:519–525

19. Hall ED, Andrus PK, Smith SL, et al (1997) Pyrrolopyrimidines: novel brain-penetrating antioxidants with neuroprotective activity in brain injury and ischemia models. J Pharmacol Exp Ther 281:895–904

20. Robertson CL, Bell MJ, Kochanek PM, et al (2002) Increased adenosine in cerebrospinal fluid after severe traumatic brain injury in infants and children: Association with severity of injury and excitotoxicity. Crit Care Med (in press)

21. Clark RSB, Carcillo JA, Kochanek PM, et al (1997) Cerebrospinal fluid adenosine concentration and uncoupling of cerebral blood flow and oxidative metabolism after severe head injury in humans. Neurosurgery 41:1284–1293

22. Sharples PM, Stuart AG, Matthews DS, Aynsley-Green A, Eyre JA (1995) Cerebral blood flow and metabolism in children with severe head injury. Part 1: Relation to age, Glasgow coma score, outcome, intracranial pressure, and time after injury. J Neurol Neurosurg Psychiatry 58:145–152

23. Adelson PD, Clyde B, Kochanek PM, Wisniewski SR, Marion DW, Yonas H (1997) Cerebrovascular response in infants and young children following severe traumatic brain injury: A preliminary report. Pediatr Neurosurg 26:200–207

24. Dragunow M, Sirimanne E, Lawlor PA, Williams C, Gluckman P (1992) Accumulation of calcitonin-gene related peptide-like immunoreactivity after hypoxic-ischaemic brain injury in the infant rat. Mol Brain Res 14:267–272

25. Wimalawansa SJ (1997) Amylin, calcitonin gene-related peptide, calcitonin, and adrenomedullin: A peptide superfamily. Crit Rev Neurobiol 11:167–239

26. Kitamura K, Kangawa K, Kawamoto M, et al (1993) Adrenomedullin: a novel hypotensive peptide isolated from human pheochromocytoma. Biochem Biophys Res Commun 192:553–560

27. Han YH, Carcillo JA, Ruppel RA, et al (2002) Cerebrospinal fluid procalcitonin is increased after traumatic brain injury in children. Pediatr Crit Care Med (in press)

28. Robertson CL, Minamino N, Ruppel R, et al (2001) Increased adrenomedullin in cerebrospinal fluid after traumatic brain injury in infants and children. J Neurotrauma 18:861–868

29. Wang X, Yue T, Barone FC, et al (1995) Discovery of adrenomedullin in rat ischemic cortex and evidence for its role in exacerbating focal brain ischemic damage. Proc Natl Acad Sci USA 92:11480–11484

30. Dogan A, Suzuki Y, Koketsu N, et al (1997) Intravenous infusion of adrenomedullin and increase in regional cerebral blood flow and prevention of ischemic brain injury after middle cerebral artery occlusion in rats. J Cereb Blood Flow Metab 17:19–25

31. Kochanek PM, Hendrich KS, Melick JA, et al (2001) Adenosine-receptor agonists attenuate posttraumatic cerebral Hypoperfusion in rats: Perfusion MRI assessment. J Neurotrauma 18:1184 (Abst)
32. Armstead WM (1999) Role of endothelin-1 in age-dependent cerebrovascular hypotensive responses after brain injury. Am J Physiol 277:H1884–H1894
33. Kelly DF, Kozlowski DA, Haddad E, Echiverri A, Hovda DA, Lee SM (2000) Ethanol reduces metabolic uncoupling following experimental head injury. J Neurotrauma 17:261–272
34. DeKosky ST, Ikonomovic MD, Wisniewski SR, et al (1999) Post-trauma levels of cytokines and growth factors in adult and pediatric CSF. J Neurotrauma 16:994 (Abst)
35. Shore PM, Jackson EK, Janesko KL, et al (2001) Vascular endothelial growth factor is increased in CSF after traumatic brain injury in children. J Neurotrauma 18:1186 (Abst)
36. Fink EL, Satchell MA, Kochanek PM, et al (2002) Cerebrospinal fluid analysis of hepatocyte growth factor concentration in infants and children after traumatic brain injury. Crit Care Med (Abst, in press)
37. Ferrara N (1999) Molecular and biological properties of vascular endothelial growth factor. J Mol Med 77:527–543
38. Nag S, Takahashi JL, Kilty DW (1997) Role of vascular endothelial growth factor in blood-brain barrier breakdown and angiogenesis in brain trauma. J Neuropathol Exp Neurol 56:912–921
39. Jin KL, Mao XO, Greenberg DA (2000) Vascular endothelial growth factor: Direct neuroprotective effect in in vitro ischemia. Proc Natl Acad Sci USA 97:10242–10247
40. Fey SJ, Larsen PM (2001) 2D or not 2D. Curr Opin Chem Biol 5:26–33
41. O'Farrell PH (1975) High resolution two-dimensional electrophoresis of proteins. J Biol Chem 250:4007–4021
42. Adelson PD, Skinner JC, Davis DS, et al (2000) A model of focal TBI in the neonatal rat. J Neurotrauma 17:969 (Abst)
43. Jenkins L, Dixon CE, Peters G, Gao W, Zhang X, Kochanek PM (2001) Cell signaling: serine/threonine protein kinases and traumatic brain injury. In: Clark RSB, Kochanek PM (eds) Brain Injury. Kluwer Academic Publishers, Boston

Monitoring of Intracranial Pressure and Cerebral Compliance

G. Citerio and I. Piper

▌ Introduction

Traumatic brain injury (TBI) is a common form of trauma. For example, in the UK, head injury occurs in more than 500,000 persons per annum of which about 10% are diagnosed as severe, 15% moderate, and the remainder as minor, head injury [1, 2]. Head trauma is a significant cause of death and disability, especially in young males (median age <30) and is associated with raised intracranial pressure (ICP). Raised ICP is defined as pressure greater than 20 mmHg and appears most commonly in the more than 50% of patients with severe head injury who remain comatose after resuscitation. These features have been confirmed in a recent Italian prospective data collection on patients with severe head injury admitted to intensive care [3]. In this study, the most frequent intracranial complications were raised ICP (defined as ICP>20 mmHg for at least 15 minutes, 69%), and intractable ICP (defined as ICP>30 mmHg for more than 30 minutes despite maximal therapy, 33%).

Over the past 50 years there has been active and wide ranging research into the causes and consequences of raised ICP. In particular, the introduction during the 1970s of continuous ICP monitoring led to renewed activity in both clinical and experimental research into the physiology and pathophysiology of maintaining craniospinal volume and pressure. This interest has not been just in monitoring pressure but also in using information derived from pressure monitoring to help both predict raised ICP and to determine the underlying cause.

ICP is a reflection of the relationship between alterations in craniospinal volume and the ability of the craniospinal axis to accommodate added volume. The craniospinal axis is essentially a partially closed box with container properties including both viscous and elastic elements. The elastic or, its inverse, the compliant, properties of the container will determine what added volume can be absorbed before intracranial pressure begins to rise. So an understanding of raised ICP encompasses an analysis of both intracranial volume and craniospinal compliance.

This chapter reviews the relationship of raised ICP to outcome and its significance as part of the development of the primary injury. This section is followed by a review of both the historical and current concepts underlying our present understanding of the physiology and pathophysiology of maintaining intracranial pressure and volume.

▮ Raised Intracranial Pressure in TBI: Relationship to Outcome

Raised ICP has been found to be associated with a poorer outcome from injury, with the higher the level of ICP, particularly the peak ICP level, correlating with the expected prognosis for mortality and morbidity [4–7]. An extensive body of clinical data now indicates that lowering elevated ICP reduces the risk of herniation and ensures adequate cerebral perfusion, thus maximizing the likelihood of recovery [8–10].

Variations in the type of ICP monitor, site of placement, treatment thresholds, patient referral characteristics, and outcome measures, can all combine to produce a large variability both in measured ICP and outcome, irrespective of whether ICP is monitored or how it is treated. Another source of variation in terms of raised ICP is the inherent variability of the head injured population, with outcome being dependent on a number of other factors. For example, mass lesions are generally accompanied by elevations in ICP and are associated with a poorer outcome, while diffuse injuries tend to have lower ICP levels yet are associated with a similar poor outcome [9].

Data from large prospective trials carried out from single centers and from well controlled multi-center studies have provided the most convincing evidence for a direct relationship between ICP and outcome [10, 11–13]. Narayan et al. [10], in a prospective study in 133 severely head injured patients, demonstrated that the outcome prediction rate was increased when the standard clinical data such as age, Glasgow Coma Score (GCS) on admission, and pupillary response with extraocular and motor activity, were combined with ICP monitoring data. Marmarou et al. [12], reporting on data of 428 patients from the National Institute of Health's Traumatic Coma Data Bank, showed that following the usual clinical signs of age, admission motor score, and abnormal pupils, the proportion of hourly ICP recordings greater than 20 mmHg was the next most significant predictor of outcome. Outcome was classified by the Glasgow Outcome Score (GOS) at six month follow up. These authors also found, using step-wise logistic regression, that following ICP, an arterial pressure below 80 mmHg was a significant predictor of outcome. Jones et al. [13] prospectively studied 124 adult head injured patients during intensive care using a computerized data collection system capable of minute by minute monitoring of up to 14 clinically indicated physiological variables. These authors found that ICP above 30 mmHg, arterial pressure below 90 mmHg, and cerebral perfusion pressure (CPP) below 50 mmHg, significantly affected patient morbidity. Recently, Stocchetti et al. [14] selected a cohort of 138 severe TBI patients, in which there was digitally recorded intracranial and arterial pressures. The severity of intracranial hypertension was related to poorer results at 6 months.

Although in the past there have been differing opinions about the contribution of continuous ICP monitoring to reduction in mortality and morbidity following head injury, there is now sufficient evidence to dispel any doubt about the value of ICP monitoring towards improving outcome and allowing more informed decisions to be made about patient management.

Over the past decade, guidelines for head injury treatment have been developed in the USA by the Brain Trauma Foundation (BTF), a non-profit organization, in collaboration with the Joint Section on Neurotrauma and Critical Care of The American Association of Neurological Surgeons (AANS) and the Congress of Neurological Surgeons [15]. For ICP monitoring, technological recommendations state: "the ventricular catheter connected to an external strain gauge is the most accurate, low cost, and reliable method of monitoring intracranial pressure (ICP). It also allows therapeutic cerebrospinal fluid (CSF) drainage. ICP transduction via fiberoptic or strain gauge devices placed in ventricular catheters provide similar benefits, but at a higher cost. Parenchymal ICP monitoring with fiberoptic or strain gauge catheter tip transduction is similar to ventricular ICP monitoring, but has the potential for measurement drift. Subarachnoid, subdural, and epidural monitors (fluid coupled or pneumatic) are currently less accurate" [15].

▌ Control of Intracranial Volume and Pressure: Historical Concepts

The history of ICP issues has been well reviewed [16–18] and starts from the doctrine named after Monro [19] and Kellie [20], which proposed that the brain and its contained blood were incompressible, enclosed in a rigid and inextensible skull, of which the total volume remained constant. In its original form, the Monro-Kellie doctrine did not take into account the CSF as a component of the cranial compartment. The concept of reciprocal volume changes between blood and CSF was introduced in 1846 by Burrows [21] and later extended in the early twentieth century by Weed and McKibben [22, 23] to allow for reciprocal changes in all the craniospinal constituents. Cushing [24–26], then a research worker for Kocher, described in both experimental and clinical studies the close relationship between increases in ICP and blood pressure and proposed that the blood pressure rose in order to maintain adequate blood supply to the hind brain, the stimulus to this vasopressor response believed to be medullary ischemia [27, 28].

At about this time, a false confidence developed in the lumbar CSF pressure technique (lumbar puncture) which caused Cushing's findings to be challenged. Reports emerged [29–31] that some patients showing clinical signs of brain compression had normal lumbar CSF pressures and that in other patients, elevations in blood pressure were found at times when ICP was well below the level of the blood pressure. Partly because of this apparent dissociation between ICP and clinical symptoms, emphasis switched away from ICP measurement towards the relationship between craniospinal volume and pressure, particularly the importance of the elastic properties of the craniospinal system. Ryder et al. [32] were the first to characterize the craniospinal volume-pressure relationship as a non-linear quantity describing it as a hyperbolic function, which implies an increase in elastance as pressure increases. Furthermore, it was partly the work of Ryder et al. [33] that restored confidence in ICP measurement, by demonstrating a differential pressure between intraventricular and lumbar CSF pressure recording. This phenomenon was reported as early as 1895 by Bayliss and colleagues [34] who noted that it was impossible to obtain valid ICP measurements below the tentorium during later stages of progressive supratentorial brain compression.

It was not until the 1960s when Lundberg [35] published his now classic monograph, that interest in clinical ICP measurement was rekindled. Using ventricular fluid pressure recording in patients with brain tumors, Lundberg was the first to delineate the frequency with which raised ICP occurs clinically, at times reaching pressures as high as 100 mmHg. Lundberg also described three types of spontaneous pressure wave fluctuation: "A" waves or plateau waves of large amplitude (50–100 mm Hg) with a variable duration (5–20 min); "B" waves which are smaller (up to 50 mm Hg), sharper waves with a dominant frequency of 0.5–2 per minute;

and finally "C" waves which are small (up to 20 mmHg) rhythmic oscillations with a frequency of 4–8 per minute. This work was then extended to include head injuries [36, 37], intracranial hemorrhage [38], post-hypoxic brain damage [39] and benign intracranial hypertension [40]. ICP can, therefore, increase under an assortment of experimental and clinical circumstances, the frequency often being underestimated by the lumbar pressure recording technique. For this reason, lumbar pressure recordings have been completely abandoned.

∎ Control of Intracranial Volume and Pressure: Current Concepts

Following on from this earlier work, the research carried out in the 1970s and early 80s provides much of the basis for our current concepts of ICP and craniospinal compliance. The ICP rise is, unfortunately, a delayed phenomenon and describes the exhaustion of intracranial compensatory mechanisms. Therefore, earlier indicators of an impending imbalance of the system could help the clinician in the untimely detection of a potentially dangerous situation.

Marmarou [41], interested in CSF dynamics, was the first to provide a full mathematical description of the craniospinal volume-pressure relationship, developing a mathematical model of the CSF system which produced a general solution for the CSF pressure. The model parameters were subsequently verified experimentally in an animal model of hydrocephalus. As a corollary from this study, Marmarou demonstrated that the non-linear craniospinal volume-pressure relationship could be described as a straight line segment relating the logarithm of pressure to volume, which implies a monoexponential relationship between volume and pressure. Marmarou termed the slope of this relationship the pressure-volume index (PVI), which is the notional volume requored to raise ICP tenfold. PVI is expressed by the formula:

$$PVI = \Delta V / (\log_{10} Po/Pm) \qquad \text{(Eqn 1)}$$

where ΔV expresses the volume, in ml, added or withdrawn from the ventricular system, Po is the initial pressure and Pm the final pressure.

Unlike elastance (change in pressure per unit change in volume, dP/dV), or its inverse, compliance (change in volume per unit change in pressure, dV/dP), the PVI characterizes the craniospinal volume-pressure relationship over the whole physiological range of ICP.

The PVI is calculated from the pressure change resulting from a rapid injection or withdrawal of fluid from the CSF space, and has found widespread use both clinically and experimentally as a measure of lumped craniospinal compliance [42–45]. In the clinical setting, PVI measures are obtained by first removing 2 ml of CSF and recording the reduction in pressure. By this technique, the PVI can be estimated, and after deciding upon a peak pressure that should not be exceeded, a maximum volume injection can be calculated. Ordinarily, the PVI measures are obtained by repeated withdrawal and injection of 2 ml and the average PVI is calculated from multiple injections (Fig. 1). Injection of fluid into the CSF space is not performed when ICP is high; in these cases, PVI is obtained only from withdrawal of known quantities of fluid.

Any factor increasing in volume within the craniospinal axis will deplete available compensatory exchange space (decompensation), reduce compliance, and even-

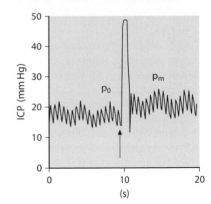

Fig. 1. Example of a computer recorded pressure-volume index (PVI) test. PVI measures are obtained by repeated withdrawal and injection of 2 ml and the average PVI is calculated from multiple injections. p_o: initial pressure; p_m: final pressure

tually lead to increased ICP. Shapiro and Marmarou [44] found that a PVI reduced by 80% of control values, was predictive of raised ICP in pediatric head injury. Tans and Poortvliet [46], also using the PVI in patients, state that the values of 10 and 13 ml are key values, with lower values indicating that active ICP reduction and improvement in compliance are required.

Marmarou's mathematical model developed an improved understanding not only of lumped intracranial compliance but also of the inter-relationships of the static and dynamic processes of formation, storage and absorption of CSF. Clearly, the balance between formation and storage is critical, and if the absorption of CSF is hindered, perhaps as a result of increased CSF outflow resistance, this will result, once the storage capacity of CSF becomes exhausted, in raised ICP. There is a clear relationship between CSF pressure and cerebral venous pressure (CVP) and Davson [47] showed that by withdrawing CSF at the estimated rate of CSF production (approx 0.3 ml/min), it is possible to determine the baseline CVP. This value can then be substituted into the steady-state ICP equation:

$$ICP = \text{formation rate} \times \text{outflow resistance} + \text{venous pressure} \qquad \text{(Eqn 2)}$$

Marmarou has extended Davson's work and his general solution for ICP allowed the derivation of an equation for CSF outflow resistance based on a bolus injection technique [41, 42]. Through a single volume injection (Vo) and noting the starting pressure (Po), peak pressure resulting from the volume injection (Pp) and the pressure (P2) on the return trajectory at a time (t2, usually 2 minutes), the outflow resistance (Ro) can be calculated.

In head injury management, the usefulness of knowing CSF outflow resistance stems from the premise that increased CSF outflow resistance is one possible 'non-vascular' cause of raised ICP. In general terms, causes of raised ICP can be categorized into 'vascular' and 'non-vascular' mechanisms. Vascular mechanisms would include active cerebral vasodilatation due to stimuli such as increased CO_2 levels or decreased arterial inflow pressure (assuming intact pressure autoregulation) or passive distension of cerebral vessels in the absence of autoregulation, or by venous outflow obstruction. Non-vascular mechanisms would include increases in brain bulk due to increased brain water content (edema) or to an increasing intracerebral, extradural or subdural mass. A further non-vascular mechanism would be an increase in CSF outflow resistance possibly due to obstruction in the normal CSF

pathway which results in dilation of the channels proximal to the site of the obstruction.

CSF outflow resistance measurement is used less often in head injury research
but is generally accepted as valuable in the diagnosis of diseases associated with
disturbances in CSF-dynamics, such as hydrocephalus. Using these bolus techniques, Marmarou and colleagues have extended their utility in head injury by demonstrating that through measurement of the PVI and CSF outflow resistance, it is
possible to calculate the percentage contribution of CSF and vascular factors to the
elevation of ICP [48]. This important study has shown that the CSF contribution to
ICP in severely head injured patients accounts for only about 30% of the ICP rise
while the majority of ICP is attributable to vascular mechanisms.

However, the use of the PVI method is not without disadvantages:

▌ With this technique there is an increased, but not quantified, risk of infection.
Causes include: manipulation of the route of access to the CSF system to test the
PVI, obtain CSF samples or to recalibrate the pressure transducer that poten-
tially may expose the patient to a higher risk of infection.

▌ Variability exists between measurements due to the difficulty of manually injecting consistent volumes of fluid at a constant rate of injection. As a result an
average of repeated measures is usually required.

▌ The procedure is time consuming and requires highly trained personnel.

As a consequence of these limitations, PVI tests are not routinely used in the clinical setup.

▌ Continuous Cerebral Compliance Monitoring: Novel Technology

To resolve these methodological disadvantages, a new form of ICP monitoring has
recently been developed (Spiegelberg Brain Compliance Monitor, Spiegelberg, Ham-
burg). This system, in theory, may improve the prediction of raised ICP. The new
technology uses a double lumen ICP catheter with a small microballoon at its tip
(Fig. 2) to add, and cyclically remove, small volumes (0.2 ml) into the ventricular
system. Measuring the ICP response to this added volume allows the minute-by-
minute calculation of 'compliance', a measure of brain stiffness, which may help
predict ICP before it rises to levels damaging to brain function.

Piper et al. [49, 50] evaluated this new device in the clinical setting and reported
on the results of testing the method against a manual volume pressure response
method in 10 patients with hydrocephalus. In this comparison study, 19 pairs of
compliance measurements were obtained from 10 patients. The compliance values
obtained ranged from 0.141 to 1.407 ml/mmHg. There was a good correlation between the two methods ($r^2 = 0.85$). The average bias in compliance between the two
methods was 0.11 ml/mmHg (95% CI for the bias = 0.0438, 0.1788) with the new
method reading higher compliance than the manual method. The published results
indicate that the new automatic method of compliance measurement correlates well
with an independent and classical measurement of compliance.

Assessment of a new form of health care technology to be used in the neuro-intensive care of patients must also be made against existing forms of monitoring.
However, no single center has sufficient expertise for all the available forms of
monitoring. Although frameworks exist for collaboration across multiple centers

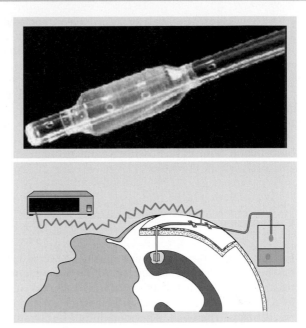

Fig. 2. Details of the double lumen ICP catheter for continuous compliance determination. In the upper part, the photograph shows a ventricular catheter with a small microballoon at its tip. This allows small volumes (0.2 ml) to be added to, and cyclically removed from, the ventricular system. The system is controlled by an external unit connected to the ventricular catheter, as presented in the lower part of the figure

for investigating new drug therapies, these studies are limited only to infrequent collection of basic physiological and demographic data. For this reason, Ian Piper has set up the "Brain-IT" (Brain Monitoring with Information Technology) network, a collaborative framework of basic scientists, clinicians and small enterprises working within the field of brain injury with a specific interest in developing and assessing standardized methods for collection and analysis of neuro-intensive care monitoring data (http://www.brainit.gla.ac.uk) [51].

Preliminary results of this multicenter experience with the Spiegelberg Brain Compliance Monitor are now available [52]. Continuous intraventricular ICP and compliance were monitored in 71 patients and archived to computer. Data from 8 European centers have been recruited to date, and include a total of 70 days of ICP and compliance monitoring data collected from 16 head injured patients, 34 patients with hydrocephalus, 13 following debulking of a tumor, and 8 patients post-subarachnoid haemorrhage (SAH).

ICP was analyzed when compliance was divided into bands from 0 to 1 ml/mmHg in increments of 0.2. Receiver-operator characteristic (ROC) analysis was used to identify compliance thresholds associated with raised ICP. Head injury and SAH patients spent the greatest time (33 and 22%, respectively) with compliance between 0.4 to 0.6 ml/mmHg (median ICPs were 17 ± 4 and 15 ± 5 mmHg, respectively). A power analysis of the database showed sufficient numbers of patients have been recruited in the hydrocephalus group and a ROC analysis determined that a mean compliance value of 0.809 (lower and upper 95% CI = 0.725 and 0.894) was a critical threshold for raised ICP greater than 10 mmHg.

A compliance threshold for raised ICP associated with hydrocephalus has thus been defined. This study, when complete, will identify compliance thresholds for raised ICP in the other patient groups as a pre-requisite to the design and implementation of a controlled trial testing whether treating these thresholds improves patient management and outcome.

However, in the management of brain-injured patients within neuro-intensive care, a single physiological parameter such as ICP is rarely measured in isolation. Minute by minute multi-parameter monitoring is now commonly employed with the use of a number of invasive and non-invasive technologies used to measure brain blood flow, oxygen delivery, and pathophysiological levels of certain neuro-chemicals within the brain.

▌ Conclusion

ICP is a cornerstone of the monitoring of severe head injured patients. Raised ICP has been found to be associated with a poorer outcome from injury and, for this reason, control of ICP maximizes the likelihood of recovery. Unfortunately the rise in ICP is a phenomenon that describes the exhaustion of intracranial compensatory mechanisms. Therefore, determination of intracranial compliance could provide the clinician with an earlier indicator of an impending imbalance of the system and could help detect potentially dangerous situations. The classical method for determining the intracranial compliance at the bedside, as described by Marmarou, is not routinely used due to its disadvantages: it is a time consuming procedure that requires highly trained personnel and manipulation of the ventricular system. Continuous monitoring of compliance measurement was not possible previously. Recently, a double lumen ICP catheter with a small microballoon at its tip has been developed for continuous, automated monitoring of the intracranial compliance. A multicenter study, part of the Brain-IT collaboration, is ongoing to define the inherent variability of compliance, using this method, in different populations of patients, including TBI. Using this information, critical compliance thresholds for raised ICP can be defined. These thresholds can then be tested in a subsequent prospective clinical trial. Updates on the Compliance Study Protocol can be obtained from the Brain-IT web site: http://www.brainit.gla.ac.uk/brainit/.

References

1. Miller JD, Jones PA, Dearden NM, Tocher JL (1992) Progress in the management of head injury. Br J Surg 79:60–64
2. Pickard JD, Czosnyka M (1993) Management of raised intracranial pressure. J Neurol Neurosurg Psychiatry 56:845–858
3. Citerio G, Stocchetti N, Cormio M, Beretta L (2000) Neuro-Link, a computer-assisted database for head injury in intensive care. Acta Neurochir (Wien) 142:769–776
4. Becker DP, Miller JD, Ward JD, et al (1977) The outcome from severe head injury with early diagnosis and intensive management. J Neurosurg 47:491–502
5. Marshall LF, Smith RW, Shapiro HM (1979) The outcome with aggressive treatment in severe head inuries. Part 1: The significance of intracranial pressure monitoring. J Neurosurg 50:20–25
6. Miller JD, Becker DP, Ward JD, et al (1977) Significance of intracranial hypertension in severe head injury. J Neurosurg 47:503–516

7. Pitts LH, Kaktis JV, Juster R, Heilbrun D (1980) ICP and outcome in patients with severe head injury. In: Shulman K, Marmarou A, Miller JD, Becker DP, Hochwald GM, Brock M (eds) Intracranial Pressure IV. Springer, Heidelberg, pp 5–9

8. Eisenberg HM, Gary HE Jr, Aldrich EF, et al (1990) Initial CT findings in 753 patients with severe head injury. A report from the NIH Traumatic Coma Data Bank. J Neurosurg 73:688–698

9. Miller JD, Butterworth JE, Gudeman SK, et al (1981) Further experience in the management of severe head injury. J Neurosurg 54:289–299

10. Narayan RK, Kishore PRS, Becker DP, et al (1982) Intracranial pressure: to monitor or not to monitor: a review of our experience with severe head injury. J Neurosurg 56:650–659

11. Saul TG, Ducker TB (1982) Effect of intracranial pressure monitoring and aggressive treatment on mortality in severe head injury. J Neurosurg 56:498–503

12. Marmarou A, Anderson RL, Ward JD, et al (1991) Impact of ICP instability on outcome in patients with severe head trauma. J Neurosurg 75 (suppl 5):s59–s66

13. Jones PA, Andrews PJD, Midgley S, et al (1994) Measuring the burden of secondary insults in head-injured patients during intensive care. J Neurosurg Anaesth 6:4–14

14. Stocchetti N, Rossi S, Buzzi F, et al (1999) Intracranial hypertension in head injury: management and results. Intensive Care Med 25:371–376

15. Bullock R, Chesnut RM, Clifton G, et al (1996) Guidelines for the management of severe head injury. Brain Trauma Foundation, American Association of Neurological Surgeons, Joint Section on Neurotrauma and Critical Care. J Neurotrauma 1996 13:641–734

16. Masserman JH (1935) Intracranial hydrodynamics: Central nervous system shock and edema following rapid fluid decompression of ventriculo-subarachnoid spaces. J Nerv Ment Dis 80:138–158

17. Stern WE (1963) Intracranial fluid dynamics. The relationship of intracranial pressure to the Monro-Kellie doctrine and the reliability of pressure assessment. J R Coll Surg Edinb 9:18–36

18. Langfitt TW, Weinstein JD, Kassell NF, Simeone FA (1964) Transmission of increased intracranial pressure I: within the craniospinal axis. J Neurosurg 21:989–997

19. Monro A (1783) Observations on the Structure and Function of the Nervous System. Creech and Johnston, Edinburgh

20. Kellie G (1824) An account of the appearances observed in the dissection of two of three individuals presumed to have perished in the storm of the third and whose bodies were discovered in the vicinity of Leith on the morning of the 4th, November 1821, with some reflections on the pathology of the brain. Trans Med Chir Soc Edinb 1:84–169

21. Burrows G (1846) On Disorders of the Cerebral Circulation and on the Connection between Affections of the Brain and Diseases of the Heart. Longmans, London

22. Weed LH, McKibben PS (1919) Pressure changes in cerebrospinal fluid following intravenous injection of solutions of various concentrations. Am J Physiol 48:512–530

23. Weed LH (1929) Some limitations of the Monro-Kellie hypothesis. Arch Surg 18:1049–1068

24. Cushing H (1901) Concerning a definite regulatory mechanism of the vasomotor centre which controls blood pressure during cerebral compression. Johns Hopkins Hospital Bulletin 12:290–292

25. Cushing H (1902) Some experimental and clinical observations concerning states of increased intracranial tension. Am J Med Sci 124:375–400

26. Cushing H (1903) The blood pressure reaction of acute cerebral compression, illustrated by cases of intracranial haemorrhage. Am J Med Sci 125:1017–1044

27. Jennet WB (1961) Experimental brain compression. Arch Neurol 4:599–607

28. Johnston IH, Rowan JO (1974) Raised intracranial pressure and cerebral blood flow: 3. Venous outflow tract pressures and vascular resistances in experimental intracranial hypertension. J Neurol Neurosurg Psychiatry 37:392–402

29. Browder J, Meyers R (1936) Observations on behavior of the systemic blood pressure, pulse and spinal fluid pressure following craniocerebral injury. Am J Surg 31:403–427

30. Smyth CE, Henderson WR (1938) Observations on the cerebrospinal fluid pressure on simultaneous ventricular and lumbar punctures. J Neurol Psychiatry 1:226–237

31. Evans JP, Espey FF, Kristoff FV, Kimball FD, Ryder HW (1951) Experimental and clinical observations on rising intracranial pressure. Arch Surg 63:107–114

32. Ryder HW, Espey FF, Kristoff FV, Evans PP (1951) Observations on the interrelationships of intracranial pressure and cerebral blood flow. J Neurosurg 8:46–58
33. Ryder HW, Espey FF, Kimbell FD, et al (1953) The elasticity of the craniospinal venous bed. J Lab Clin Med 42:944
34. Bayliss WM, Hill L, Gulland GL (1895) On intracranial pressure and the cerebral circulation. J Physiol 18:334–362
35. Lundberg N (1960) Continuous recording and control of ventricular fluid pressure in neurosurgical practice. Acta Psychiatr Neurol Scand 36 (suppl):149
36. Lundberg N, Troupp H, Lorin H (1965) Continuous recording of the ventricular fluid pressure in patients with severe acute traumatic brain injury. J Neurosurg 22:581–590
37. Johnston IH, Johnston JJ, Jennett WB (1970) Intracranial pressures following head injury. Lancet 2:433–436
38. Richardson A, Hide TAH, Eversden ID (1970) Long-term continuous intracranial pressure monitoring by means of a modified subdural pressure transducer. Lancet 2:687–689
39. Langfitt TW, Kumar VS, James HE, Miller JD (1974) Continuous recording of intracranial pressure in patients with hypoxic brain damage. In: Brierley JS, Meldrum BS (eds) Brain Hypoxia. Heinemann, London, pp 118–135
40. Johnston IH, Paterson A (1972) Benign intracranial hypertension: aspects of diagnosis and treatment. In: Cant J S (ed) Optic Nerve. Himpton, London, pp 155–165
41. Marmarou A (1973) A theoretical and experimental evaluation of the cerebrospinal fluid system. PhD Thesis, Drexel University
42. Marmarou A, Shulman K, LaMorgese J (1975) Compartmental analysis of compliance and outflow resistance of the cerebrospinal fluid system. J Neurosurg 43:523–534
43. Shapiro K, Fried A, Takai F, Kohn I (1985) Effect of the skull and dura on neural axis pressure-volume relationships and CSF hydrodynamics. J Neurosurg 63:75–81
44. Shapiro K, Marmarou A (1982) Clinical applications of the pressure-volume index in treatment of pediatric head injuries. J Neurosurg 56:819–825
45. Maset AL, Marmarou A, Ward JD, et al (1987) Pressure-volume index in head injury. J Neurosurg 67:832–840
46. Tans JT, Poortvliet DC (1983) Intracranial volume-pressure relationship in man. Part 2: Clinical significance of the pressure-volume index. J Neurosurg 59:810–816
47. Davson H (1967) Physiology of the Cerebrospinal Fluid. Churchill, London
48. Marmarou A, Maset AL, Ward JD, et al (1987) Contribution of CSF and vascular factors to elevation of ICP in severely head-injured patients. J Neurosurg 66:883–890
49. Piper IR, Spiegelberg A, Bernardo A, et al (1997): A comparative study of the Spiegelberg Compliance Device with a manual volume injection method: A Clinical Evaluation. In: Proceedings of the 10th International Symposium on Intracranial pressure and Neuromonitoring, Williamsburg, USA (Abst)
50. Piper I, Spiegelberg A, Whittle I, Signorini D, Mascia L (1999) A comparative study of the Spiegelberg compliance device with a manual volume-injection method: a clinical evaluation in patients with hydrocephalus. Br J Neurosurg 13:581–586
51. Piper I, Contant C, Citerio G (2000) Brain Monitoring With Information Technology. The BRAIN IT group experience. Minerva Anestesiol 66 (suppl 1/5):17–21
52. Piper IR, Yau Y, Contant C, et al (2000) Multi-centre assessment of the Spiegelberg compliance monitor: Preliminary results. Acta Neurochir Suppl 76:491–494

The MRC CRASH Trial

I. Roberts

Introduction

Worldwide, many millions of people are treated each year for severe head injury. A substantial proportion die, and many more are permanently disabled [1]. Road traffic crashes alone account for an estimated five million head injuries each year [2]. Reliable assessment of the net benefits and hazards of various interventions for the treatment and rehabilitation of head injuries could be of considerable public health importance.

For such a common problem, if a widely practicable treatment could be shown to reduce the absolute risk of death and disability by 'just' a few percent, then this might affect the treatment of hundreds of thousands of patients each year, protecting thousands from death or long term disability. But in order to detect reductions of this magnitude, both moderate random errors and moderate biases must be avoided [3]. This means that randomized controlled trials of treatments for head injury should be large enough to avoid moderate random errors and designed in such a way that moderate biases are also avoided [3]. However, most head injury trials are small. A year 2000 survey of the size and quality of randomized trials in head injury found that the average number of randomized participants was 82, and the largest trial included only 1,156 participants (Fig. 1) [4]. None of the trials would have been large enough to detect reliably the difference between a 20% and a 15% risk of death or disability. The paucity of head injury trials is underscored by the fact that the total number of randomized participants in all of the available trials in head injury combined (16,613) is less than that in some individual trials in heart disease and stroke.

Corticosteroids in Head Injury

Corticosteroids have been used in the treatment of severe head injury for over thirty years, although recently their value has been questioned because of the failure to reliably demonstrate effectiveness in randomized trials [5]. Nevertheless, throughout the world, corticosteroids continue to be used widely, albeit inconsistently. Two 1996 British surveys, of nursing staff at 39 neurosurgical intensive care units (ICUs), and of medical directors at 44 neurosurgical ICUs, found that corticosteroids were used in the treatment of head injury in 49% and 14% of units respectively [6, 7].

If a treatment as simple and widely practicable as corticosteroids produced just a moderate benefit, this could be worthwhile. For example, if corticosteroids re-

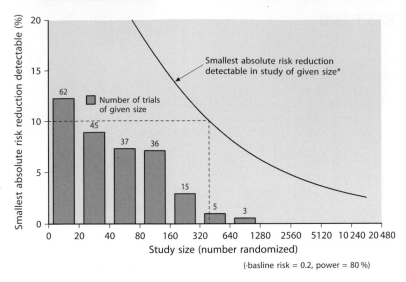

Fig. 1. Histogram of trial size and smallest absolute risk reduction detectable of existing randomized-controlled trials in head injury

duced the absolute risk of death by 2% (e.g., from 15% to 13% dead), and reduced the risk of permanent disability by a similar amount, then treatment of 500,000 patients would avoid 10,000 deaths and prevent 10,000 permanent disabilities. Such a benefit would be impossible to demonstrate reliably without evidence from large randomized trials. If 10,000 patients were randomly allocated to receive a corticosteroid infusion and 10,000 to placebo infusion, then a 2% absolute reduction in the risk of death or disability should be detectable, and a 3% reduction would certainly be detectable. By contrast, a trial involving only 2,000 patients would probably miss such differences. Reliable refutation of benefit is of equal importance, as it would protect those currently treated with corticosteroids from any adverse effects. So far, all of the randomized trials of corticosteroids in head injury have been small: the largest included only a few hundred patients, and even in aggregate they have involved only about 2,000 patients [8]. Existing trials are too small to demonstrate or refute the possibility of moderate but clinically important benefits or harm from corticosteroids. As a result, the use of corticosteroids in head injury has waxed and waned over time with extensive practice variations.

Evidence of benefit from corticosteroids in acute spinal cord injury has renewed interest in their role in brain injury. The Second US National Acute Spinal Cord Injury Study (NASCIS 2) compared 24 hours of corticosteroid (methylprednisolone) with placebo in 333 patients with acute spinal cord injury [9]. At six months, patients receiving corticosteroids rather than placebo within eight hours of injury had greater improvement in motor function, and in sensation to pinprick and touch. Similar results were reported in a Japanese trial of the same regimen involving 151 patients [9]. More recent trials of methylprednisolone in acute spinal cord injury have indicated slightly more neurological recovery with 48 than with 24 hours of treatment [7]. On the basis of these results, high dose methylprednisolone is now widely used in the management of acute spinal cord injury.

The dose of corticosteroid used in randomized trials in acute spinal cord injury was based on results from animal studies showing that methylprednisolone can reduce post-traumatic neuronal degeneration following spinal cord injury with 30 mg per kilogram of body weight being required for maximal effect. High dose methylprednisolone has also been shown to reduce post-traumatic neuronal degeneration and improve outcome in animal head injury models. Hall found that 30 mg/kg methylprednisolone enhanced recovery in mice that were subjected to moderately severe brain injury when given five minutes post injury [10]. To date, there have been only two small randomized trials of high dose (30 mg/kg) methylprednisolone in head injury [11, 12]. In both there was a non-significant reduction in the risk of death in the methylprednisolone treated group, but because the trials were small, the effectiveness of high dose methylprednisolone in the treatment of head injury remains uncertain (pooled risk difference 3% lower mortality, 95% confidence interval 14% lower to 9% higher).

Results from animal studies also suggest that early administration of corticosteroid is important for maximal effect. Because axonal disruption after acute central nervous system (CNS) trauma does not occur for several hours, there may be an early phase when neurological deficit is reversible [13]. Timing of corticosteroid administration has also been shown to be important in acute spinal cord injury [9]. However, the administration of corticosteroids in many of the existing trials in head injury may have been outside this window of opportunity.

∎ The CRASH Trial: The First Large, Simple Trial in Head Injury

The CRASH trial (corticosteroid randomization after significant head injury) is a large, simple, randomized, placebo controlled trial of the early administration of a 48-hour infusion of corticosteroid (methylprednisolone) on the risk of death and disability following head injury [14]. The results of the trial will inform clinical decision making in an area of increasing public health importance. Reliable demonstration of a benefit from corticosteroids has the potential to avoid thousands of deaths and disabilities. Similarly, because corticosteroids are currently given to patients with head injury throughout the world, the reliable refutation of any benefit would protect thousands of patients from possible side effects. However, to detect or refute improvements of only a few percent in outcome, many thousands of acute head injury patients must be randomized between corticosteroid and placebo infusions. Such large numbers will be possible only if hundreds of doctors and nurses collaborate in the participating emergency departments. Management of the increasing global burden of head injury must be addressed in a similar way to that adopted so successfully in ischemic heart disease. Prevention and the understanding of basic pathophysiology must be complemented by well-conducted large, simple trials.

∎ Conclusion

The global epidemic of head injuries is only just beginning. At present, over a million people die each year, and a similar number are disabled from brain injuries, often with profound effects on the quality of life of the affected individuals and their carers. Road traffic crashes account for most of the deaths and car use is rapidly increasing in many countries. It is estimated that by 2020, road traffic crashes will have moved from ninth to third in the world disease burden ranking, as measured in disability adjusted life years, and second in the developing countries. The identification of effective treatments for head injury is of global health importance. With over 2000 patients recruited, the CRASH trial is already the largest randomized controlled trial in head injury conducted to date and recruitment is set to continue for another four years. However, the trial will only reach the recruitment target of 20,000 patients if hundreds of doctors and nurses worldwide join the trial and help to make it a success). Trial recruitment is ongoing and new collaborators are welcome.

References

1. Murray CJL, Lopez AD (1996) Global health statistics: a compendium of incidence, prevalence and mortality estimates for over 200 conditions. Harvard University Press, Boston
2. Murray CJL, Lopez AD (1997) Alternative projections of mortality and disability by cause 1990–2020: Global Burden of Disease Study. Lancet 349:1498–1504
3. Peto R, Collins R, Gray R (1995) Large-scale randomised evidence: large simple trials and overviews of trials. J Clin Epidemiol 48:23–40
4. Dickinson K, Bunn F, Wentz R, Edwards P, Roberts I (2000) Size and quality of randomised controlled trials in head injury: review of published studies. Br Med J 320:1308–1311
5. Task Force of the American Association of Neurological Surgeons and Joint Section in Neurotrauma and Critical Care (1995) Guidelines for the management of severe head injury. Brain Trauma Foundation, New York
6. Jeevaratnum DR, Menon DK (1996) Survey of intensive care of severely head injured patients in the United Kingdom. Br Med J 312:944–947
7. Matta B, Menon D (1996) Severe head injury in the United Kingdom and Ireland: A survey of practice and implications for management. Crit Care Med 24:1743–1748
8. Alderson P, Roberts I (1997) Corticosteroids in acute traumatic brain injury: a systematic review of randomised trials. Br Med J 314:1855–1859
9. Bracken MB (2001) Pharmacological interventions for acute spinal cord injury. Cochrane Database Syst Rev: CD001046
10. Hall ED (1985) High dose glucocorticoid treatment improves neurological recovery in head-injured mice. J Neurosurg 62:882–887
11. Giannotta SL, Weiss MH, Apuzzo MLJ, Martin E (1984) High dose glucocorticoids in the management of severe head injury. Neurosurgery 15:497–501
12. Stubbs DF, Stiger TR, Harris WR (1989) Multinational controlled trial of high-dose methylprednisolone in moderately severe head injury. In: Capildeo R (ed) Steroids in Diseases of the Central Nervous System. John Wiley & Sons, Chichester, pp 163–168
13. Teasdale G (1991) The treatment of head trauma: implications for the future. J Neurotrauma 8 (suppl 1):53–60
14. CRASH: Corticosteroid randomization after significant head injury. At: *http://www.crash.lshtm.ac.uk*

Neurological Challenges

Assessing Consciousness in Critically Ill Patients

S. Laureys, S. Majerus, and G. Moonen

Introduction

An accurate and reliable evaluation of the state of consciousness in intensive care unit (ICU) patients is of primordial importance for their appropriate management. Altered states of consciousness are commonly encountered in ICUs. Even excluding neurological and neurosurgical ICUs, altered states of consciousness are the primary reason for adult ICU admission in 3 to 7% of cases [1]. Additionally, secondary alterations of consciousness due to encephalopathy, seizures, and cerebrovascular accidents are known to occur in one-eighth of unselected patients admitted to a medical ICU, and even more frequently in those with sepsis [2, 3]. Up to one-fifth of patients develop an acute confusional state in the ICU [4].

Consciousness is a multifaceted concept that can be divided into two major components: the *level* of consciousness (i.e., arousal, wakefulness, or vigilance) and the *content* of consciousness (i.e., awareness of the environment and of the self) [5] (Fig. 1). Arousal is maintained by a diffuse system of upper brainstem and thalamic neurons (called the reticular activating system) and its connections to the cerebral hemispheres. Therefore, depression of either brainstem or global hemispherical function may cause reduced wakefulness. Brainstem reflexes are a key to the assessment of the functional integrity of the brainstem's reticular activating system. Awareness is thought to be dependent upon the functional integrity of the cerebral cortex and its reciprocal subcortical connections; each of its many aspects resides to some extent in anatomically defined regions of the brain [6].

Unfortunately, at present, consciousness cannot be measured objectively by any machine; its estimation requires the interpretation of several clinical signs. Many scoring systems have been developed for the quantification and standardization of the assessment of consciousness. The present chapter will discuss the possibilities and pitfalls of a behavioral assessment of consciousness in patients and review the most frequently used 'consciousness scales' in the ICU.

Clinical Evaluation of Consciousness

Both arousal and awareness are not on-off phenomena but are part of a large continuum. At the patient's bedside, arousal is assessed by the presence of spontaneous or stimulation-induced eye opening. It ranges from alert *waking* (spontaneous eye opening), *sleep* (eye opening following moderate external stimuli), through *stupor* (eye opening following vigorous external stimuli) and *coma* (no eye opening). Awareness refers to the collective thoughts and feelings of an individual. Clinically,

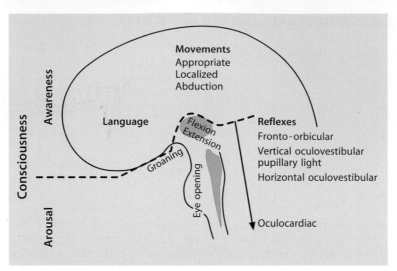

Fig. 1. A simplified scheme of consciousness and of its two major components: arousal and awareness. Note: the gray area represents the reticular activating system encompassing the brainstem and thalamus; the arrow near the brainstem denotes the progressive disappearance of brainstem reflexes during rostral-caudal deterioration

we are limited to the appraisal of the patient's potential to perceive the external world and to voluntary interact with it (i.e., perceptual awareness). In practice, this is evaluated by careful and repeated examination of the capacity to formulate reproducible, voluntary, purposeful and sustained behavioral responses to auditory, tactile, visual or noxious stimuli. By asking the patient to say or write their name we can assess awareness of self (self-consciousness); another – much more difficult – possibility is to evaluate patient self recognition in a mirror [7]. The patient needs to be aroused in order to perform the cognitive processes required for awareness. Hence, patients in a coma are unaware because they cannot be aroused. However, as illustrated by patients in a vegetative state, arousal is only a necessary, and not a sufficient, condition for awareness. Indeed, patients in a vegetative state are aroused (as shown by preserved spontaneous eye opening and sleep-wake cycles) but show no sign of awareness.

Consciousness is intimately related to higher functions such as perception, attention, working memory, declarative memory, cognition, mental imagery, motivation, emotion, and language. Visual, auditory or somatosensory deficits in our patients may seriously reduce their perceptual awareness. Attention forms a component of perception in that it accounts for the selection and directed concentration on processing certain information with the exclusion of other competing stimuli or data. Sensory signals reach the level of consciousness only if they become the target of selective attention, and only these find their way to declarative memory [8]. Lesions of the parietal lobe, either of the cortex or of subjacent white matter, may result in hemi-neglect, hemi-inattention and a tendency not to use the contralateral hand and arm. Consciousness is bound to the information-containing elements of the explicit memory trace and is recovered along with the memory. Working memory is the short-term retention of a limited number of items held in consciousness for immediate use. Conscious recollection is constantly occurring and provides us with a sense of familiarity and continuity. In contrast, patients without current explicit memory are "isolated in a single moment of being ... without a past or future, stuck in a constantly changing, meaningless moment" [9]. Motivational and emotional drives help to determine behavior, once the stimulus has been received, and to assess its significance relevant to competing internal and external factors. Language is a highly developed cognitive activity allowing for internal conversation and conceptual formulation. Thinking, like consciousness, is difficult to define satisfactorily. The act of thinking depends on all the components of consciousness previously mentioned and also includes an awareness of one's own cognitive activity. Confusion is a disorder of the content of consciousness. Any impairment of cognitive function may cause confusion, i.e., impaired perception, attention, understanding, action, or coherence of thought. It may also be the presenting sign in isolated focal dysfunction such as aphasia or visuospatial agnosia. Delirium is synonymous with an acute confusional state accompanied by fluctuating agitation and increased arousal [10].

Consciousness Scales

Glasgow Coma Scale

Teasdale and Jennett published the Glasgow Coma Scale (GCS) in the *Lancet* in 1974 as an aid in the clinical assessment of post-traumatic unconsciousness [11]. It was devised as a formal scheme to overcome the ambiguities that arose when information about comatose patients was presented and groups of patients compared. The GCS has three components: the eye (E), verbal (V), and motor (M) response to external stimuli. The best or highest responses are recorded. The scale consisted of 14 points, but was later adapted to 15, with the division of the motor category 'flexion to pain' into two further categories (Fig. 2). So far, more than 1500 publications have appeared to its use (MEDLINE search performed in December 2001, limited to title and abstract word). It is a component of the Acute Physiology and Chronic Health Evaluation (APACHE) II score, the (Revised) Trauma Score, the Trauma and Injury Severity Score (TRISS) and the Circulation, Respiration, Abdomen, Motor, Speech (CRAMS) Scale, demonstrating the widespread adoption of the scale.

The presence of spontaneous eye opening "indicates that the arousal mechanisms of the brainstem are active" [11]. As stated above, preserved arousal does not imply the presence of awareness. Patients in a vegetative state have awakened from their coma but remain completely unaware of their environment and self. Most comatose patients who survive will eventually open their eyes, regardless of the severity of their cerebral injuries [12]. Indeed, less than 4% of head-injured patients never open their eyes before they die [13]. The eye opening in response to speech tests the reaction "to any verbal approach, whether spoken or shouted, not necessarily the command to open the eyes" [11]. Again, this response is observed in vegetative patients who can be awakened by non-specific auditory stimulation. In these patients, it is recommended to differentiate between a reproducible response to command and to non-sense speech. Eye opening in response to pain should be tested by a stimulus in the limbs, because the grimacing associated with supraorbital or jaw-angle pressure may cause eye closure.

After arousing the patient, the presence of verbal responses indicates the restoration of a high degree of interaction with the environment (i.e., awareness). An ori-

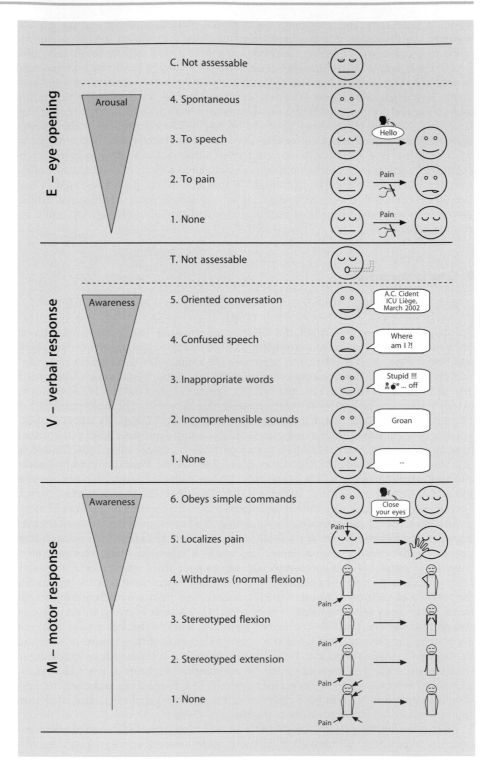

ented conversation implies awareness of the self (e.g., the patient can answer the question: "What is your name?") and environment (e.g., the patient correctly answers the questions: "Where are we?" and "What year/month is it?"). Confused speech is recorded when the patient is capable of producing language, for instance phrases and sentences, but is unable to answer the questions about orientation. When the patient presents intelligible articulation but exclaims only isolated words in a random way (often swear words, obtained by physical stimulation rather than by a verbal approach) this is scored as 'inappropriate speech'. Incomprehensible sounds refer to moaning and groaning without any recognizable words. This rudimentary vocalization does not necessitate awareness and is thought to depend on subcortical functioning as it can be observed in anencephalic children and vegetative patients.

The motor response first assesses whether the patient obeys simple commands, given in verbal, gestural, or written form. A non-specific sound stimulus may induce a reflex contraction of the patient's fingers or alternatively such a reflex response can result from the physical presence of the examiner's fingers against the palm of the patient (i.e., grasping reflex). Before accepting that the patient is truly obeying commands, it is advised to test that the patient will also release and squeeze again to repeated commands. If there is no response a painful stimulus is applied. First, pressure is applied to the fingernail bed with a pencil. If flexion is observed stimulation is then applied to other sites (applying pressure to the supraorbital ridge, pinching the trapezium or rubbing the sternum) to differentiate between localization (i.e., a stimulus at more than one site causes a limb to move so as to attempt to remove it by crossing the midline), withdrawal flexion (i.e., a rapid flexion of the elbow associated with abduction of the shoulder) or 'abnormal' flexion (i.e., a slower stereotyped flexion of the elbow with adduction of the shoulder that can be achieved when stimulated at other sites). Stereotyped flexion responses are the most common of the motor reactions observed in severely brain-injured patients; they are also the most enduring [14]. Extensor posturing is more easily distinguished and is usually associated with adduction, internal rotation of the shoulder, and pronation of the forearm. The term 'decerebrate rigidity' should be avoided because it implies a specific physioanatomical correlation. Abnormal flexion and extension motor responses often co-exist [15]. It is important to appreciate that it is the best response that should be scored and that abduction movements reflect some residual awareness while stereotyped postures do not. The presence of asymmetrical responses are significant in indicating that there is a focal as well as a diffuse disturbance of brain function, and this should be noted separately. The side showing the impaired response locates the site of the focal brain damage and the level of the best response of the better side reflects the extent of general depression in brain function. The scale of responses to pain is applicable to the movements of the arms. The movements of the legs are not only more limited in range, but may take place on the basis of a spinal withdrawal reflex (e.g., in brain death, a spinal reflex may still cause the legs to flex briskly in response to pain applied locally [16]).

It is very tempting to sum the three components of the GCS (E-V-M) into a total score, ranging from 3 to 15. However, given the increased use of intubation, ventilation, and sedation of patients with impaired consciousness before arrival at special-

---

Fig. 2. Glasgow Coma Scale (GCS). (Adapted from [11] with permission)

ists units, and even before arrival at hospital [17], patients might wrongly be scored as GCS 3/15 rather than being more appropriately reported as impossible to assess or score. In a recent study of 1005 patients with head injuries in European centers, assessment of each of the three components of the GCS was possible only in 61% of patients before hospital, in 77% on arrival at the first hospital, in 56% on arrival in the neurosurgical unit, and in 49% 'post-resuscitation' [18]. The inappropriate scoring of absent responsiveness as 3, has led to some data indicating that the mortality of patients with a score of 3 is apparently lower than that of those with a score of 4. Summing GCS components has also been criticized on a purely mathematical basis. Because there are only four units assigned to the eye responses, versus five to the verbal and six to the motor responses, the scale incorporates a numerical skew toward motor response. This problem can be tackled by weighting individual scores for eye, verbal and motor responses in such a way that each has a minimum contribution of one and a maximum of five [19]. This approach, however, is too complicated for practical use. Moreover, this effort to provide mathematical parity for the three components has abutted against studies that have stressed the particular importance of the motor portion of the GCS. Indeed, the motor score is more important than either of the other two components in predicting the magnitude of neurological injury for patients with severe head injury [20], while verbal and eye scores are more pertinent in patients who are not, in fact, comatose. It is a widespread but erroneous usage to define mild brain injury as a summed score ranging from 13–15, moderate injury, 9–12, and severe injury, 3–8. Indeed, in the persistent vegetative state, patients open their eyes spontaneously (E4) and may make moaning sounds (V2) or flex abnormally to pain (M3), while their condition hardly reflects 'moderate' brain injury. For clinical purposes, summation of the GCS is too imprecise [21]. To achieve a total score of 6 to 12 there are more than 10 simple combinations of variables, each with very different clinical profiles. In Glasgow, patients are always described by the three separate responses and never by the total [22]. It is, therefore, good practice to communicate the GCS in terms such as 'patient scored E2, VT, M4' and only sum its three components for research applications.

Glasgow Liège Scale

One of the most frequently expressed reservations regarding the GCS has been its failure to incorporate brainstem reflexes. A number of investigators have disagreed with Teasdale and Jennett that spontaneous eye opening is sufficiently indicative of brainstem arousal systems activity and have proposed coma scales that include brainstem responses [23]. Many coma scales that include brainstem indicators have been proposed (e.g., the Comprehensive Level of Consciousness Scale [24], the Clinical Neurologic Assessment Tool [25], the Bouzarth Coma Scale [26], the Maryland Coma Scale [27]) but none have known a widespread use. These scales generally have been more complex than the GCS.

A simpler system is the Glasgow Liège Scale (Fig. 3). It was developed in 1982 in Liège and combines the Glasgow Scale with a quantified analysis of five brain stem reflexes: fronto-orbicular, vertical oculocephalic, pupillary, horizontal oculocephalic, and oculocardiac [28]. The fronto-orbicular reflex is considered present when percussion of the glabella produces contraction of the orbicularis oculi muscle. The oculocephalic reflexes (doll's head) are scored as present when deviation of at least one eye can be induced by repeated flexion and extension (vertical) or horizontal

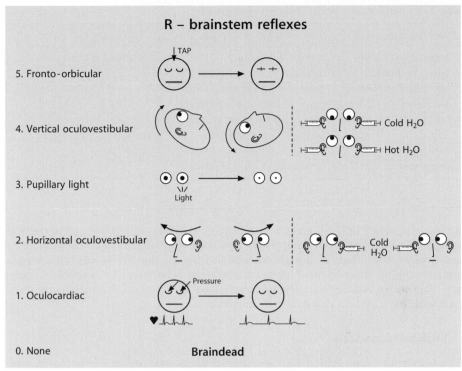

Fig. 3. Glasgow-Liège Scale (GLS). Note: when oculocephalic reflexes (doll's eyes) cannot be tested or are absent, the (vertical and horizontal) oculovestibular reflexes (ice water testing) should be evaluated. (Adapted from [28] with permission)

neck movement (horizontal). If the reflexes are absent or cannot be tested (e.g., immobilized cervical spine), an attempt is made to elicit ocular motion by external auditory canal irrigation using iced water (i.e., oculovestibular reflex testing). With cold-water irrigation of the head at $30°$ elevation from the horizontal, the eyes deviate tonically toward the ear irrigated (horizontal). When cold water is injected simultaneously into both ears canals, the eyes deviate tonically downwards; the reverse occurs with bilateral irrigation of warm water (vertical). The oculocardiac reflex is scored as present when pressure on the eyeball causes the heart rate to slow down. As for the GCS, the best response determines the brainstem reflex score (R). The selected reflexes disappear in descending order during rostral-caudal deterioration. The disappearance of the last reflex, the occulo-cardiac, coincides with brain death.

Reaction Level Scale

The Reaction Level Scale (RLS85) was developed in Sweden in 1985 as an eight-grade scale for the assessment of patients in the ICU [29]. Its numeric values are not necessarily separated by steps of equal value. The information content of the GCS and the RLS85 is similar, though their construction differs (Table 1). By combining eye, verbal, and motor responses into a single-line ordinal scale it has a bet-

Table 1. Reaction Level Scale (RLS85). (From [29] with permission)

Clinical descriptor	Responsiveness	Score
▌Alert	No delay in response	1
▌Drowsy or confused	Responsive to light stimulation	2
▌Very drowsy or confused	Responsive to strong stimulation	3
▌Unconscious	Localizes but does not ward off pain	4
▌Unconscious	Withdrawing movements on pain stimulation	5
▌Unconscious	Stereotype flexion movements on pain stimulation	6
▌Unconscious	Stereotype extension movements on pain stimulation	7
▌Unconscious	No response on pain stimulation	8

ter discriminatory ability, greater accuracy, and higher inter-observer agreement than the GCS [23] and can be applied to patients who are intubated or whose eyes are swollen shut. There is a high correlation between the two scales, indicating a similar ranking order of neurologic defect severity. The Swedish Societies of Intensive Care, Anesthesiology and Neurosurgery have recommended replacement of the GCS with the RLS85 in that country's hospitals.

Innsbruck Coma Scale

The Innsbruck Coma Scale (ICS), also developed for assessment of victims of trauma, was published in 1991 [30]. The total score is analogous to that of the GCS in having a number of separate assessments that are scored separately but can be added for an aggregate score (Table 2). Its eight items allow for a maximal score of 23. It is similar to the GCS, but excludes verbal response and contains pupillary size and reaction, movement and position of the eyes, and oral automatisms. An anomaly is that the score rates dilated fixed pupils of greater severity (lower score) than midposition nonreactive pupils [31]. Thus, a patient with brain death (where midposition pupils are generally the rule) would achieve a better score than one who is not brain dead.

Edinburgh-2 Coma Scale

The Edinburgh-2 Coma Scale (E2CS) is a single-line scoring system [32]. The best response is the one that is used in tabulating the score which is inversely related to consciousness (Table 3). The disadvantage of this score is that it cannot be applied to patients who are unable to give an oral response.

▌Pitfalls Encountered in ICU Patients

Untrained or inexperienced observers produce unreliable scoring of consciousness [33]. In one study, one in five ICU workers was mistaken when asked to make judgments as to whether patients were 'conscious' or 'unconscious', [34]. Consciousness needs considerable skill to evaluate and the observer should be aware of the pitfalls encountered in ICU settings. It is also well known that the preceding score of the

Table 2. Innsbruck Coma Scale (ICS). (From [30] with permission)

Item	Factor	Score
Eye opening	Spontaneous	3
	To acoustic stimuli	2
	To painful stimuli	1
	None	0
Reaction to acoustic stimuli	Turning towards stimuli	3
	Better-than-extension movements	2
	Extension movements	1
	None	0
Reaction to pain	Defensive movements	3
	Better-than-extension movements	2
	Extension movements	1
	None	0
Body posture	Normal	3
	Better-than-extension movements	2
	Extension movements	1
	None	0
Pupil size	Normal	3
	Narrow	2
	Dilated	1
	Completely dilated	0
Pupil response to light	Sufficient	3
	Reduced	2
	Minimum	1
	None	0
Position and movements of the eyeballs	Fixing of the eyes	3
	Sway of eyeballs	2
	Divergent	1
	Divergent fixed	0
Oral automatisms	Spontaneous	2
	To external stimuli	1
	None	0

Note: Maximum total score is 23.

Table 3. Edinburgh-2 Coma Scale (E2CS). (From [32] with permission)

Stimulation (maximal)	Response (best)	Score
Two sets of questions:	Answers correctly to both	0
1. Month?	Answers correctly to either	1
2. Age?	Incorrect for both	2
Two sets of commands:	Obeys correctly to both	3
1. Close and open hands	Obeys correctly to either	4
2. Close and open eyes	Neither correct	5
Strong pain	Localizing	6
	Flexion	7
	Extension	8
	None	9

patient frequently influences the examiner when rating the patient's present state of consciousness. Therefore, scoring should be done in a 'blinded' manner.

Obviously, problems arise when the eyes are swollen shut, either following peri-orbital edema, direct ocular trauma, facial injury, craniotomy, cranial nerve VII injury, or neuromuscular blockade. In these circumstances, enforced closure of the patient's eyes should be recorded on his chart by marking 'C' (=eyes closed) [35]. In deep coma, flaccid eye muscles will show no response to stimulation yet the eyes remain open if the lids are drawn back. Such opening should be recorded as unresponsive. It is important to stress that although opening of the eyes implies arousal, it does not necessarily mean that the patient is aware.

Continued speechlessness may be due to causes other than unawareness (e.g., neuromuscular blockade, intubation via the oropharynx or through a tracheostomy, fractured mandible or maxillae, edematous tongue, deafness, foreign language, dysphasia, confusion or delirium). The evaluation of verbal responses is also biased when patients are sedated, alcohol or drug intoxicated, or too young to speak. As discussed above, the use of early intubation and administration of neuromuscular paralyzing agents in the pre-hospital phase of care has rendered verbal and motor responses unmeasurable in these cases. Early treatment was uncommon when the GCS was first described, but has since gained greater acceptance. The RLS85, which does not include a verbal response criterion, is the most notable alternative for scoring intubated patients. Several other techniques have been proposed to designate the verbal score in intubated patients. Some have proposed to assign an arbitrary score of one point to all intubated patients [36]. Others have created a pseudo-score by averaging the testable scores and adding this calculated score to the sum in lieu of the verbal score [37]. Linear regression predication of the verbal scores based on the other two scores has also been utilized [38].

The best alternative is to report separate responses, using a non-numerical designation of 'T' (=intubated) when the verbal score cannot be assessed and not to sum the responses [17]. The patient's verbal response may also be impaired as a result of a single focal lesion of the speech areas in the dominant hemisphere, that is, aphasia. The assessment of such a patient's language ability requires a specialized evaluation (i.e., written instructions and written replies in the case of motor dysphasia). The level of verbal response should still be indicated but an appropriate note may be made that the impairment is considered to be due to dysphasia ('D'=dysphasia) [35]. Motor responses cannot be reliably monitored in cases of spinal cord, plexus or peripheral nerve injury or in the presence of splint or immobilization devices. As previously stated, one must take care not to interpret a grasp reflex or postural adjustment as a response to command.

In most scoring systems, awareness is assessed as the level of obedience to commands. This approach cannot be applied to cases where the patient is clinically or pharmacologically paralyzed yet alert (e.g., locked-in syndrome, severe polyneuropathy, or use of neuromuscular blocking agents) or those with psychogenic unresponsiveness. It is important to stress that special effort should be made to identify and exclude these rare causes of pseudo-coma. The GCS has also been critiqued for lacking reliability in monitoring levels of consciousness in patients with moderate brain injury [23]. More detailed scales are recommended for the assessment of awareness in these patients [39, 40]. Finally, we remain with a theoretical limitation to the certainty of our clinical assessment of consciousness, since we can only infer the presence or absence of conscious experience in another person [41]. Finally, as consciousness is a subjective first person experience, we remain with a theoretical limitation as to the certainty of our clinical assessment of consciousness (since the clinician can only infer the presence or absence of conscious experience in another person) [41].

▌ Conclusion

Despite its drawbacks, the GCS remains the most universally utilized consciousness scale worldwide. The eye opening score (E) directly relates to the level of consciousness (i.e., arousal) but does not test the content of consciousness (i.e., awareness). In minor and moderate brain-injured patients, the verbal (V) and motor (M) score covaries with the level of awareness of self and environment. The observation of a verbal response (except for groaning and moaning) or of a localizing or abduction movement witnesses the presence of awareness. Stereotyped flexion or worse denotes severe brain dysfunction. Appending the brainstem reflexes (R), such as in the GLS, permits a better evaluation of the brainstem arousal systems. Finally, even if the GCS is the most widely used and validated tool to evaluate the state of consciousness, it also is the most frequently misused. One recent study showed that 51% of patients were incorrectly assessed [42]. It is also important to stress that for clinical use, patients should be characterized by the three separate scores (E, V, M and R) and never by the total sum. If eye or verbal responses cannot be evaluated, this should be indicated by marking a 'C' (eyes closed) or 'T' (intubated), respectively. By virtue of its simplicity the GCS seems destined to be used in intensive care and emergency medicine for some time.

Acknowledgements. This work was supported by grants from the Fonds National de la Recherche Scientifique de Belgique (FNRS), the Special Funds for Scientific Research of the University of Liège and by the Queen Elisabeth Medical Foundation. SL and SM are respectively Postdoctoral Researcher and Research Fellow at the FNRS.

References

1. Groeger JS, Strosberg MA, Halpern NA, et al (1992) Descriptive analysis of critical care units in the United States. Crit Care Med 20:846–863
2. Bleck TP, Smith MC, Pierre-Louis SJ, et al (1993) Neurologic complications of critical medical illnesses. Crit Care Med 21:98–103
3. Papadopoulos MC, Davies DC, Moss RF, Tighe D, Bennett ED (2000) Pathophysiology of septic encephalopathy: a review. Crit Care Med 28:3019–3024
4. Dubois MJ, Bergeron N, Dumont M, Dial S, Skrobik Y (2001) Delirium in an intensive care unit: a study of risk factors. Intensive Care Med 27:1297–1304
5. Plum F, Posner JB (1983) The Diagnosis of Stupor and Coma. FA Davis, Philadelphia
6. Llinas R, Ribary U, Contreras D, Pedroarena C (1998) The neuronal basis for consciousness. Philos Trans R Soc Lond B Biol Sci 353:1841–1849
7. Gallup GG Jr (1997) On the rise and fall of self-conception in primates. Ann N Y Acad Sci 818:72–82
8. Moscovitch M (1995) Models of consciousness and memory. In: Gazzaniga MS (ed) The Cognitive Neurosciences. Bradford Book MIT Press, Cambridge, pp:1341–1356
9. Sacks O (1985) The Man who Mistook his Wife for a Hat. Summit Books, New York
10. American Psychiatric Association. Task Force on DSM-IV (2000) Diagnostic and statistical manual of mental disorders: DSM-IV-TR. American Psychiatric Association, Washington, DC

11. Teasdale G, Jennett B (1974) Assessment of coma and impaired consciousness. A practical scale. Lancet 2:81–84
12. Jennett B (1972) Prognosis after severe head injury. Clin Neurosurg 19:200–207
13. Bricolo A, Turazzi S, Feriotti G (1980) Prolonged posttraumatic unconsciousness: therapeutic assets and liabilities. J Neurosurg 52:625–634
14. Born JD (1988) The Glasgow-Liège Scale. Prognostic value and evaluation of motor response and brain stem reflexes after severe head injury. Acta Neurochir 95:49–52
15. Bricolo A, Turazzi S, Alexandre A, Rizzuto N (1977) Decerebrate rigidity in acute head injury. J Neurosurg 47:680–689
16. Ivan LP (1973) Spinal reflexes in cerebral death. Neurology 23:650–652
17. Marion DW, Carlier PM (1994) Problems with initial Glasgow Coma Scale assessment caused by prehospital treatment of patients with head injuries: results of a national survey. J Trauma 36:89–95
18. Murray LS, Teasdale GM, Murray GD, et al (1993) Does prediction of outcome alter patient management? Lancet 341:1487–1491
19. Bhatty GB, Kapoor N (1993) The Glasgow Coma Scale: a mathematical critique. Acta Neurochir 120:132–135
20. Jagger J, Jane JA, Rimel R (1983) The Glasgow coma scale: to sum or not to sum? Lancet 2:97
21. Bozza Marrubini M (1984) Classifications of coma. Intensive Care Med 10:217–226
22. Teasdale G, Jennett B, Murray L, Murray G (1983) Glasgow coma scale: to sum or not to sum. Lancet 2:678
23. Segatore M, Way C (1992) The Glasgow Coma Scale: time for change. Heart Lung 21:548–557
24. Stanczak DE, White JG 3rd, Gouview WD, et al (1984) Assessment of level of consciousness following severe neurological insult. A comparison of the psychometric qualities of the Glasgow Coma Scale and the Comprehensive Level of Consciousness Scale. J Neurosurg 60:955–960
25. Crosby L, Parsons LC (1989) Clinical neurologic assessment tool: development and testing of an instrument to index neurologic status. Heart Lung 18:121–129
26. Bouzarth WF (1968) Neurosurgical watch sheet for craniocerebral trauma. J Trauma 8:29–31.
27. Salcman M, Schepp RS, Ducker TB (1981) Calculated recovery rates in severe head trauma. Neurosurgery 8:301–308
28. Born JD (1988) The Glasgow-Liège Scale (GLS). Act Neurochir (Wien) 91:1–11
29. Starmark JE, Stalhammar D, Holmgren E, Rosander B (1988) The Reaction Level Scale (RLS85). Manual and guidelines. Acta Neurochir (Wien) 91:12–20
30. Benzer A, Mitterschiffthaler G, Marosi M, et al. (1991) Prediction of non-survival after trauma: Innsbruck Coma Scale. Lancet 338:977–978
31. De'Clari F (1991) Innsbruck coma scale. Lancet 338:1537
32. Sugiura K, Muraoka K, Chishiki T, Baba M (1983) The Edinburgh–2 coma scale: a new scale for assessing impaired consciousness. Neurosurgery 12:411–415
33. Rowley G, Fielding K (1991) Reliability and accuracy of the Glasgow Coma Scale with experienced and inexperienced users. Lancet 337:535–538
34. Teasdale G, Jennett B (1976) Assessment and prognosis of coma after head injury. Acta Neurochir (Wien) 34:45–55
35. Teasdale G (1975) Acute impairment of brain function–1. Assessing 'conscious level'. Nurs Times 71:914–917
36. Marshall LF, Becker DP, Bowers SA, et al. (1983) The National Traumatic Coma Data Bank. Part 1: Design, purpose, goals, and results. J Neurosurg 59:276–284
37. Grahm TW, Williams FC Jr, Harrington T, Spetzler RF (1990) Civilian gunshot wounds to the head: a prospective study. Neurosurgery 27:696–700
38. Meredith W, Rutledge R, Fakhry SM, Emery S, Kromhout-Schiro S (1998) The conundrum of the Glasgow Coma Scale in intubated patients: a linear regression prediction of the Glasgow verbal score from the Glasgow eye and motor scores. J Trauma 44:839–844
39. Majerus S, Van der Linden M, Shiel A (2000) Wessex Head Injury Matrix and Glasgow/Glasgow-Liège Coma Scale: A validation and comparison study. Neuropsych Rehab 10:167–184

40. Ansell BJ, Keenan JE (1989) The Western Neuro Sensory Stimulation Profile: A tool for assessing slow to recover head injured patients. Arch Phys Med Rehabil 70:104–108
41. Bernat JL (1992) The boundaries of the persistent vegetative state. J Clin Ethics 3:176–180
42. Crossman J, Bankes M, Bhan A, Crockard HA (1998) The Glasgow Coma Score: reliable evidence? Injury 29:435–437.

The Brain in Post-anoxic Coma: Predicting Outcome

G. B. Young

Introduction

About 40% of patients with cardiac arrest can be resuscitated with restoration of spontaneous circulation and respiration. The overall 1 year survival rate of initially unconscious survivors resuscitated from cardiac arrest has been variably quoted to be between 10 and 25% [1, 2]. Anoxic-ischemic encephalopathy is the principal cause of mortality in at least 30–40% of those who die; only 3–10% return to their previous lifestyle, including employment [3]. Under 1% survive in a persistent vegetative state (PVS) [4]. Since primary cardiac arrest is so common, the problems of assessment and management of anoxic-ischemic encephalopathy are of great importance to the intensivist and emergency physician.

Pathology and Pathogenesis

From experimental studies, it is clear that ischemia is the essential component in producing neuronal death in cardiac arrest. Hypoxia alone, even with arterial oxygen concentrations of <25 mmHg, does not produce neuronal death [5]. Thus, the term 'generalized ischemic encephalopathy' is more accurate pathophysiologically. The mechanisms for neuronal death include: release of excitotoxic neurotransmitters, activation of N-methyl-D-aspartate receptors with calcium influx into neurons, peroxynitrite production, failure of clearance of hydrogen ions, and lactate and free radical production on reperfusion [6].

Certain neurons show a 'selective vulnerability' to ischemic insults. The large cell layers (3, 5 and 6) of the neocortex, the CA1 and end folium (CA4–6) of the hippocampus are especially vulnerable. Other relatively vulnerable regions include the Purkinje cells of the cerebellum, the putamen, caudate and thalamus. If the patient survives for a sufficient time, the neurons are replaced by a gliotic reaction. Transsynaptic degeneration may affect thalamic nuclei and brainstem nuclei such as the inferior olivary complex. If the insult is sufficiently severe, all neurons may die, producing brain death [7].

It is, thus, not surprising that patients who are comatose after cardiac arrest often show intact central respiratory drive and brainstem functions (some of the latter may be enhanced as 'release phenomena'), even though the vulnerable regions (frequently all cell layers of the neocortex) may have no viable neurons. Such patients would be doomed to survive in a state no better than a PVS.

Assessment of Prognosis

Clinical Predictors

Several clinical studies have shown that it is possible to predict a poor outcome in a subset of patients. 'Poor outcome' includes PVS, but also conditions with various degrees of awareness and disability, including dementia and motor deficits. This is less definitive than a prediction of an outcome no better than PVS, a condition from which withdrawal of care would not be so controversial. Coma lasting more than 3 days carries a greater than 90% risk of poor outcome [8]. Levy and colleagues [9], in their series of 210 patients with anoxic-ischemic encephalopathy, found that independent existence did not occur with absence of pupillary light reflexes at the time of initial evaluation. Most patients, however, recover all of their testable brainstem reflexes within a few hours. The motor response is fairly highly predictive; in the study of Levy et al. only one of 93 patients with no response or decorticate or decerebrate posturing to stimulation at 24 hours recovered awareness. The use of paralyzing and sedative drugs can preclude accurate assessment, however. A number of algorithms have been constructed for prediction at postarrest days 3, 7 and 14. Longstreth's group [2] found the following four variables on admission gave a positive predictive value for awakening of 0.84: motor response, pupillary light response, spontaneous eye movements, and serum glucose. False prediction of not wakening occurred in 16 (10%) patients, but 12 of these could not live independently. Edgren and colleagues [3] found predictive accuracy at resuscitation for poor outcome ranged from 52–84%. At 3 days, clinical predictors for poor outcome using the Glasgow and Glasgow-Pittsburgh Coma Scales were reliable for poor outcome (severe cerebral disability, PVS or death) with absence of motor response being the best predictor. Myoclonic status epilepticus in coma has a 96% (CI 80–100%) association with a bad outcome [10]. Unless there is considerable compromise of brainstem function, one cannot make a certain, early prediction of an outcome of PVS or death in coma using clinical predictors alone. Severe cerebral disability may not be definitive enough; prediction of PVS, persistent coma or death would be more useful. An editorial comment recommended a further prospective study, and that 4–6 weeks should elapse before a decision is made to withdraw care [11]. This seems excessively long, when there are better predictors of an outcome no better than PVS.

It is also difficult to reliably predict a favorable outcome in initially comatose survivors of cardiac arrest; 29% (CI 13–49%) with intact brainstem reflexes and 78% of those with a Glasgow Coma Scale (GCS) score of >8 had a good outcome [10].

Electrophysiological Predictors

Electrophysiological tests allow a 'real-time' assessment of cerebral cortical function in patients who cannot respond clinically. The tests are portable, safe and inexpensive and directly examine cortical-thalamic neuronal function. They have advantages over blood-flow and most metabolic studies in these regards.

Event-Related Potentials. The cortical N20 response to median nerve stimulation (Fig. 1) approaches the ideal prognostic test [12]. The absence of the N20 response from median nerve stimulation is specific but is not especially sensitive for a hopeless prognosis. The lack of this response shows nearly 100% specificity for an outcome no better than a PVS, but 50% of patients with a preserved N20 response die

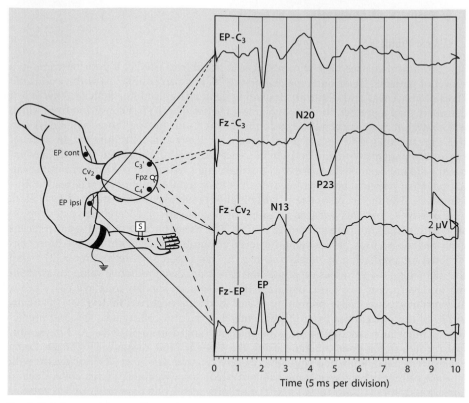

Fig. 1. Technique used in recording median nerve somatosensory-evoked potential (SSEP) which defines Erb's point (EP) over the brachial plexus, the N13 peak (generated in the medulla), the N20 and P23 cortical evoked potentials from the primary somatosensory cortex. (From [30] with permission)

without recovery of awareness. Connolly et al.'s [13] application of 'cognitive event-related potentials' seems promising for selecting those patients who show processing and discrimination of cognitively meaningful signals. The population of ischemic encephalopathy patients needs to be examined with these techniques.

Electroencephalogram (EEG). EEGs performed after the first day of arrest may show deteriorating patterns associated with a fatal outcome. This is supported by experimental models, in which it has been shown that the phenomenon of 'delayed neuronal death' may take more than 24 hours to develop [14]. The following EEG patterns found after cardiac arrest are usually associated with a poor neurological outcome: generalized suppression; generalized burst-suppression; generalized periodic patterns, especially with epileptiform activity; and alpha or alpha-theta pattern coma [15]. These are illustrated in Figures 2–5.

We have had at least one patient with incomplete suppression, >10 but <20 µV, but none with <10 µV amplitudes, who recovered conscious awareness. There are no reports of recovery of conscious awareness in a child or adult with an isoelectric EEG that was recorded more than 24 hours after restoration of circulation. Autopsy reports show severe cortical damage [16]. Thus an isoelectric EEG, recorded more

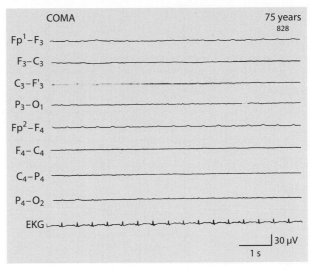

Fig. 2. Generalized suppression followed cardiac arrest and severe ischemic encephalopathy. The patient died without recovering consciousness. (From [21] with permission)

than 24 hours from cardiac resuscitation and normal blood pressure, is a reliable indication of an outcome no better than PVS.

Burst-suppression again has not been well defined in published studies, and, in many cases, burst-suppression is lumped with other patterns. A fatal outcome occurred in all 14 patients with various generalized burst-suppression patterns in the series of Brenner et al. [17], and in all 27 children with unspecified burst-suppression in the series of Pampligioni and Harden [18]. However, occasional survivors are found, especially in those without epileptiform discharges in the bursts [19]. The presence or absence of simple or even fairly complex movements (e.g., tongue thrusting, grimacing) does not alter the usually unfavorable outcome. When generalized epileptiform activity occurs within the bursts, patients rarely recover consciousness [20, 21]. Similarly, generalized epileptiform discharges, either as periodic, stereotyped phenomena or as burst of discharges, as the only EEG activity on an otherwise totally suppressed background, are almost always associated with lack of recovery of awareness. The electroencephalographer should be aware that drugs, especially midazolam and propofol, commonly used in intensive care units (ICUs), may produce a burst-suppression pattern.

After cardiac arrest, the occurrence of generalized epileptiform activity, either as sequential spikes or spike and wave, single or generalized epileptiform discharges as part of a burst-suppression pattern, or generalized periodic or pseudoperiodic complexes has been associated with a fatal outcome without recovery of consciousness. This is often associated with myoclonus or eye opening accompanying the bursts of epileptiform activity [22]. However, Mori and Tsuruta [23] reported such a case with a favorable recovery. There is a striking similarity of these patterns to the stages 3, 4, or 5 of the sequential changes of status epilepticus of other causes, as described by Treiman et al. [24] (Treiman's five stages include: 1. Discrete seizures: epileptiform activity occurs in discrete epochs separated by post-ictal slow frequency waves; 2. Merging seizures: epileptiform activity persists throughout, but

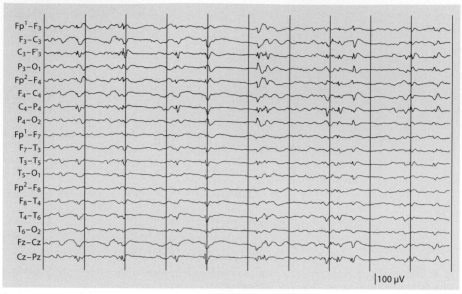

A

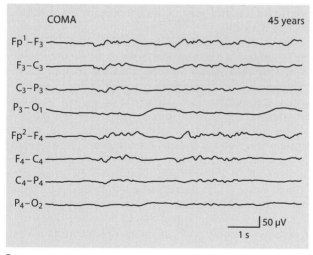

B

Fig. 3. A shows a generalized burst-suppression pattern with sharply contoured epileptiform potentials within the bursts. **B** shows a burst-suppression pattern with slow frequency waves but without epileptiform activity. (From [21] with permission)

the discharges wax and wane in frequency and amplitude; 3. Continuous seizures: spikes and spike-waves are rhythmic and relatively constant throughout the seizures; 4. Continuous with flat periods: ongoing epileptiform activity is interrupted by generalized attenuation of voltage from 0.5–8 seconds; 5. Periodic epileptiform discharges on a flat background: high voltage, repetitive epileptiform discharges occur regularly against a flat or suppressed background). The mortality rate of pa-

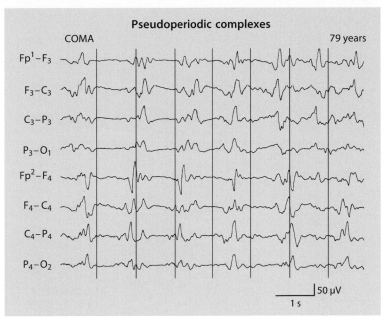

Fig. 4. Generalized pseudoperiodic epileptiform complexes appear against a suppressed background in a comatose patient following cardiac arrest. No myoclonus was noted. (From [15] with permission)

tients with such seizures without cardiac arrest ranges from 6–35% [25]. Thus, it is important to differentiate the (usually) fatal status epilepticus following cardiac arrest from the status epilepticus of seizure disorders. If this cannot be done clinically, or with EEG, other tests to confirm the non-viability of the cortex, such as somatosensory testing, sequential EEGs, or evolutionary changes from continuous EEG monitoring may be valuable.

Following cardiac arrest, alpha pattern coma consists of diffuse or frontally predominant, continuous rhythms in the alpha (8–13 Hz) frequency band. Unlike normal alpha pattern, it is not responsive to eye opening or stimulation. There is no fundamental difference in the etiologies, clinical picture and prognostic significance among alpha, theta, and a mixture of alpha and theta patterns, and they can be combined for practical purposes [26]. Patients usually remain vegetative or die without recovering conscious awareness. However, again, some patients may make a satisfactory recovery. Thus, finding an alpha pattern coma following cardiac arrest is not, in itself, prognostically definitive, but should be regarded as a 'transitional pattern'. By six days post-arrest, the pattern usually evolves into a prognostically definitive pattern in over 90% of cases [27]. Those who die without recovering consciousness develop a burst-suppression pattern without reactivity and those who survive have more continuous rhythms and develop electrographic reactivity to stimulation. Alternatively, somatosensory-evoked potential testing may establish the prognosis sooner.

Apart from complete EEG suppression after 24 hours from cardiac arrest, no other single EEG pattern has a 100% association with an outcome no better than PVS. The value of single recordings, taken in isolation, is limited to various probabilities, but never to certainty of poor outcome. The predictive value of the EEG is greatly en-

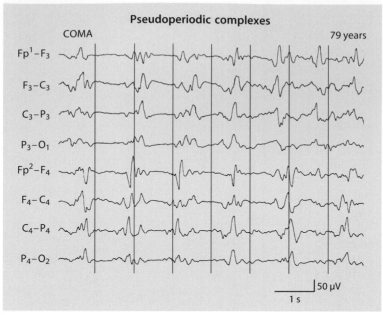

Fig. 5. The top EEG shows a diffuse alpha-theta pattern coma, 1 day after cardiac arrest. The bottom EEG, recorded 5 days later, shows a burst-suppression pattern. The patient remained in coma until death. (From [27] with permission)

hanced, however, if serial or continuous EEGs are done over several days to note trending or evolution, reactivity and variability [28]. Further, if other factors, including even partial absence of cranial nerve reflexes, absence of EEG reactivity and variability are included, the odds ratios for mortality without recovery of consciousness are markedly increased [21]. More research into the prognostic value of continuous and serial EEG studies and the use of combined variables will be valuable. A carefully performed, prospective, multi-centered study with sufficient numbers should provide information that will better define the optimal prognostic role of EEG, evoked potentials and various clinical factors individually and in combination.

Biochemical/Metabolic/Blood Flow Prognostic Tests

Nuclear magnetic resonance (NMR) spectroscopy allows a non-invasive, *in vivo* examination of high energy phosphate in both neurons and glia. Following severe anoxic insult, there is a decrease of 40–60%. It is difficult-to-impossible in an individual case to know the proportion of loss due to neuronal death. N-acetyl aspartate (NAA) and N-acetylaspartylglutamate are compounds found only in neurons [29]. These can be detected by NMR spectroscopy. Although absence of these N-acetylaspartyl compounds is conceivably reversible, preliminary evidence indicates that NAA reduction by 7 days shows a strong correlation with neuronal loss (Nakano et al., unpublished data). This technology holds considerable promise for prognosis following cardiac arrest, but conclusive studies are needed.

Measurement of brain-derived creatine kinase (CK), neuronal specific enolase, lactate and other chemicals in the cerebrospinal fluid has been incompletely assessed. There appears to be considerable overlap between values in survivors and non-survivors. There is also some concern in performing lumbar punctures in patients who may develop raised intracranial pressure (ICP). In severe hypoxic-ischemic encephalopathy, ATP stores are reduced, as revealed by *in vivo* NMR spectroscopy [29]. After the condition stabilizes, cerebral blood flow (CBF) is consistently reduced; cerebral oxygen and glucose metabolism are also diminished to about 40–60% of normal. The measured metabolic activity reflects both neuronal and glial function and for this reason seems less specific than electrophysiological evaluation. Also, the technology is not commonly available.

Management

Patients resuscitated from cardiac arrest require immediate, high quality intensive care. Along with optimal general care, it is important to minimize ongoing or subsequent brain damage by:

- preventing hyperglycemia and hyperthermia;
- maintaining adequate blood pressure: because of loss of autoregulation, adequate systemic blood pressure is essential; on the other hand, hypertension may lead to cerebral edema;
- achieving normal arterial concentrations of oxygen and carbon dioxide: excessive oxygen may contribute to increased free radical damage; hypocapnia reduces cerebral perfusion and hypercapnia raises ICP.

Myoclonic seizures often respond to intravenous valproate which can be given as a loading dose of 30 mg/kg. These steps protect the brain and allow for later application of prognostic tests.

Conclusion

Patients with anoxic-ischemic encephalopathy after cardiac arrest should be vigorously supported in an ICU while prognostic determination is implemented. Clinical guidelines are of limited value. In those patients who remain comatose (providing there are no confounders such as sedating or paralyzing drugs) with absent pupillary light reflexes and either no response or decerebrate or decorticate responses, the neurological prognosis is poor. In others, those with intact brainstem function, ancillary tests are needed for prognosis.

The most specific test thus far is the short latency somatosensory-evoked potential (N20 response with median nerve stimulation). This test is sensitive to a poor outcome only 50% of the time. It is suggested that EEG trending is of help in those patients who remain comatose with intact brainstem function and preserved N20 responses. Those who progress to suppression or a burst-suppression pattern from previous patterns after 5 days are unlikely to recover awareness. This requires the proviso that there are no confounders such as sepsis or sedative drugs. Further work needs to be done on developing prognostic guidelines.

References

1. Thomassen A, Wernberg M (1979) Prevalence and prognostic significance of coma after cardiac arrest outside intensive care and coronary care units. Acta Anesth Scand 23:143–148
2. Longstreth W, Diehr P, Inui TS (1983) Prediction of awakening after out-of-hospital cardiac arrest. N Engl J Med 308:1378–1382
3. Edgren E, Hedstand U, Kelsey S, Sutton-Tyrell K, Safar P (1994) Assessment of neurological prognosis in comatose survivors of cardiac arrest. Lancet 343:1052–1053
4. Stephenson HE, Reid CL, Hinton W (1952) Some common denominators in 1200 cases of cardiac arrest. Ann Surg 137:731–740
5. Pearigen P, Gwinn R, Simon RP (1996) The effects of in vivo hypoxia on brain injury. Brain Res 725:184–191
6. Dawson VL, Dawson TM, Bartley DA, Uhl GR, Snyder SH (1993) Mechanisms of nitric oxide-mediated neurotoxicity in primary brain cultures. J Neurosci 13:2651–2661
7. Korein J, Maccario M (1969) On the diagnosis of cerebral death: a prospective study. Electroenceph Clin Neurophysiol 27:700
8. Bell JA, Hodgson HJF (1974) Coma after cardiac arrest. Brain 97:361–372
9. Levy DE, Caronna JJ, Singer BH, et al (1985) Predicting outcome from hypoxic-ischemic coma. JAMA 253:1420–1426
10. Bassetti C, Bomio F, Mathis J, Hess CW (1996) Early prognosis in coma after cardiac arrest: a prospective clinical electrophysiological, and biochemical study of 60 patients. J Neurol Neurosurg Psychiatry 61:610–615
11. Saltman L, Marori M (1994) Coma after cardiac arrest: will he recover all right? Lancet 343:1052–1053
12. Zandbergen ED, de Haan RJ, Stoutenbeek CP, et al (1998) Systematic review of early prediction of poor outcome in anoxic-ischaemic coma. Lancet 352:1808–1812
13. Connolly JF, Phillips NA, Stewart SH, Blake WG (1992) Event-related potential sensitivity to acoustic and semantic properties of terminal words in sentences. Brain Lang 43:1–18
14. Kirino T (1982) Delayed neuronal death in the gerbil hippocampus following ischemia. Brain Res 239:57–69
15. Young GB (2000) The EEG in coma. J Clin Neurophysiol 17:473–485
16. Brierley JB, Adams JH, Graham DI, Simpson JA (1971) Neocortical death after cardiac arrest. Lancet ii:560–565
17. Brenner RP, Schwartzman RJ, Richey ET (1975) Prognostic significance of episodic low amplitude or relatively isoelectric EEG patterns. Dis Nerv Syst 36:582–589
18. Pampiglioni G, Harden A (1968) Resuscitation after cardiopulmonary arrest. Lancet 1:1261–1264
19. Chen R, Bolton CF, Young GB (1996) Prediction of outcome in patients with anoxic coma: A clinical and electrophysiological study. Crit Care Med 24:672–678
20. Synek VM (1988) Prognostically important coma patterns in diffuse anoxic and traumatic encephalopathies in adults. J Clin Neurophysiol 5:161–174
21. Young GB, Kreeft JH, McLachlan RS, Demelo J (1999) EEG and clinical associations with mortality in comatose patients in a general intensive care unit. J Clin Neurophysiol 16:354–360
22. Simon RP, Aminoff MJ (1986) Electrographic status epilepticus in fatal anoxic coma. Ann Neurol 20:351–355
23. Mori E, Tsuruta H (1983) Transient eye opening with EEG burst-suppression pattern in postanoxic encephalopathy. Arch Neurol 40:189–190
24. Treiman DM, Walton NY, Kendrick C (1990) A prospective sequence of electroencephalographic changes during generalized convulsive status epilepticus. Epilepsy Res 5:49–60
25. Hauser WA (1983) Status epilepticus: Frequency, etiology and neurological sequelae. In: Delgado-Escueta AV, Wasterlain CG, Treiman DM, Porter RJ (eds) Advances in Neurology Vol 34: Status Epilepticus: Mechanisms of Brain Damage and Treatment. Raven Press, New York, pp 3–14
26. Synek VM, Synek BJL (1984) "Theta pattern coma" a variant on alpha pattern coma. Clin EEG 15:116–121

27. Young GB, Blume WT, Campbell VC, et al. (1994) Alpha, alpha-theta and theta coma: a clinical outcome study utilizing serial recordings. Electroenceph Clin Neurophysiol 91:93–99
28. Holmes GL, Lombroso CT (1993) Prognostic value of background patterns in neonatal EEG. J Clin Neurophysiol 10:323–352
29. Younkin DP (1993) Magnetic resonance spectroscopy in hypoxic-ischemic encephalopathy. Clin Invest Med 16:116–121
30. Rothstein TL (2000) The role of evoked potentials in anoxic-ischemic coma and severe brain trauma. J Clin Neurophysiol 17:486–497

The Rationale for Human Selective Brain Cooling

B. A. Harris and P. J. D. Andrews

▌ Introduction

Human selective brain cooling seems to have received relatively little attention from clinicians although it is pertinent to a number of specialities. This is possibly because much of the research has been undertaken in the field of thermal physiology in animals and volunteers, and the relevance of this to clinical practice has not been perceived.

▌ Brain Cooling Mechanisms

The human brain is purported to have three cooling mechanisms: cooling of venous blood by the skin which in turn cools the arterial (carotid) blood supply to the brain; cooling by heat loss through the skull; and cooling by heat loss from the upper airways (which is abolished by endotracheal intubation) [1–3]. The last two mechanisms can produce selective brain cooling, i.e., a reduction in brain temperature below that of arterial blood from the trunk. These mechanisms work by cooling cerebral venous blood, which in itself achieves brain cooling but also may lead to cooling of cerebral arterial blood. Even if arterial blood temperature remains the major determinant of brain temperature these two mechanisms are potentially clinically important, because factors which enhance or inhibit them will have an effect on brain temperature.

Zenker and Kubik [3] showed it is anatomically possible for the skull and upper airways to cause selective brain cooling in humans. Evaporation of sweat from the scalp and face and secretions from the nose cools blood in, for example, emissary, diploic, ophthalmic, and facial veins. This cooled venous blood is transferred via the dural venous sinuses to the dura mater. The dura mater may transmit the cooling to the cerebrospinal fluid (CSF), which in turn influences parenchymal temperature by direct contact and via arteries extending over long distances within the subarachnoid space, pial vascular network and parenchyma. In addition, some authors believe that the cavernous sinus, which is cooled by veins from the face and by heat loss from the upper airways, is involved in brain cooling by countercurrent heat exchange with the internal carotid, which changes direction in the sinus thus augmenting the surface available for heat exchange [4–8]. Some animals have a more developed version of this countercurrent heat exchanger, the carotid rete, which plays a major part in selective brain cooling [9].

▌ The Complementary Nature of Selective Brain Cooling Mechanisms

Brain cooling by heat loss through the skull and through the upper airways appear to be anatomically complementary since between them they almost completely encircle the brain with cool venous blood and cool air (Fig. 1). The anatomy which makes heat loss through the skull possible, e.g., the dural venous sinuses, surrounds the brain under the skull from the front round to, and into, the back of the brain. Under the base of the brain lies the anatomy for cooling via the upper airways, i.e., the nose, paranasal sinuses, and cavernous sinus. Around the brainstem lies the vertebral venous plexus which may be cooled via the vertebral artery as a result of nose breathing [7].

These selective brain cooling mechanisms may also be physiologically complementary. Niinimaa et al. [10] investigated the switching point from nasal to oronasal breathing during submaximal exercise in 30 men and women. Nasal resistance and the perception of effort in breathing "predicted the switching point with only 68.9% accuracy, suggesting that there may be determinants other than those investigated in the present study." We suggest that during exercise the balance alters between heat loss through the skull and heat loss through the upper airways. As head sweating increases with increasing exercise so it becomes possible to switch to oronasal breathing, thus reducing the work of the increased breathing which exercise requires, but without compromising brain temperature.

▌ Brain Cooling and Evolution

Falk [11] showed that as the brains of early humans grew in size, their emissary veins developed in tandem, which supports the radiator theory that as humans evolved and developed bigger brains they must have developed an increased venous cooling capacity. Climate has also played a part in the development of brain cooling

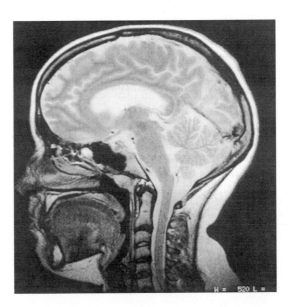

Fig. 1. Dural venous sinuses, paranasal sinuses, nose and turbinates

mechanisms, such that nose size and shape [12–14] and paranasal sinus size [15, 16] seem to be logically related, in terms of brain cooling, to the climates that populations came from (Harris, unpublished).

▌ Selective Brain Cooling by Heat Loss through the Skull: Mechanisms and Human Evidence

For temperature transfer from the inner brain, convection is more important than conduction [3, 17, 18]. Cooling by convection is achieved by changes in the direction and rate of venous bloodflow. Cabanac and Brinnel [5] demonstrated that blood in the mainly valveless emissary veins flowed rapidly away from the scalp in moderately hyperthermic humans, delivering blood cooled by evaporation from the sweating face and scalp to the brain. In normothermia, the flow was either undetectable, or reversed (i.e., from brain to scalp) and much slower. Caputa et al. [19] and Hirashita et al. [20] have shown similar flow patterns in the angularis oculi and ophthalmic veins. Caputa and Cabanac's finding that "dehydration results in active inhibition of sweating on the body but not on the forehead, where evaporation is needed for selective cooling of the brain" [21] suggests that this brain cooling mechanism is important by comparison with body cooling. Cabanac and Brinnel speculate "that the reversal of blood flow in the emissary veins depends upon pressure gradient reversal between internal and external jugular venous systems due to skin vasodilatation during hyperthermia." [5]. Head up positions increase the venous pressure gradient across the skull by gravity and also therefore increase emissary flow and enhance selective brain cooling [22]. In addition, low intrathoracic pressure on inspiration causes blood to drain freely from the jugular veins and the vertebral venous plexus [23]. This facilitates the flow of venous blood from the brain and it is unlikely to be coincidental that the flow to the jugular veins is greatest on inspiration when the cooling effect of heat loss from the upper airways is also greatest. Yawning may potentiate the effect [24].

▌ Selective Brain Cooling by Heat Loss from the Upper Airways: Mechanisms and Human Evidence

Mechanisms

The superior sagittal and cavernous sinuses receive venous drainage from the nose [25] and it is through these that brain cooling via the upper airways may be achieved. du Boulay et al. [7] believe that the proximity of the carotid artery to the trachea, larynx, and pharynx is also a factor and that "vertebral artery blood to the brainstem might ... be cooled by proximity to the vertebral venous plexus conducting cooled blood from around the pharynx." It has been suggested that the nose may be more important for temperature regulation than respiration, because of its heat transfer ability and because turbinate complexity in different mammals is related to body insulation [26]. This view gains support from the fact that the nose has thermoregulatory responses and controls. Nasal mucosal blood flow decreases in response to skin cooling and increases in response to skin warming and to rises in core temperature [26, 27]. Nervous control of heat and moisture exchange is regulated by the hypothalamus [28].

Heat loss by evaporation and convection from the upper airways takes place mainly in the nose [29] and can account for over 10% of body heat loss in humans [30] due to the net heat loss with each breath. Evaporative heat loss occurs because forming water vapor from nasal secretions uses thermal energy [31]. Convective heat loss results from air turbulence and flow resistance caused by the shape of the nose, changes in nasal mucosal blood flow, and the rhythmic action of the nasal valve with respiration [32].

The increased work that nose breathing requires by comparison with oral breathing, particularly in babies who are obligatory nose breathers, and the fact that 85% of adults preferentially nose breathe [33], with sole oral breathing being very rare [34], suggests that nose breathing is important physiologically. Brain cooling would be a physiological justification for the extra work since conditioning of inspired air is achievable by mouth breathing. However, the importance of the other functions of the nose cannot be discounted, for example immune protection to the lower airways [30] and the effect of nasally produced nitric oxide (NO) no on lung function [32].

Human Evidence

Mariak et al. [35] demonstrated selective brain cooling by heat loss from the upper airways in humans using intracranial temperature measured, "on the midline between the cribriform plate and the frontal lobes", in four conscious, intubated patients under conditions of mild hyperthermia (esophageal temperatures variously 36.9–37.5 °C). When airflow through the upper respiratory tract was reinstated by extubation, brain temperature above the cribriform plate fell by 0.4–0.85 °C and in three patients dropped below esophageal temperature. Once the temperatures had stabilized, the patients were asked to breathe intensively for three minutes, in through their noses and out through their mouths. This caused a decrease of 0.20–0.30 °C in the temperature above the cribriform plate.

Prior to extubation, subdural and tympanic temperatures were similar to the temperature above the cribriform plate; after extubation they paralleled esophageal temperature, not demonstrating a particular drop, but having their upward courses deflected despite maintenance of external warming. Mariak et al. [35] comment that because cooling did not affect tympanic temperature it was likely to be limited to the frontal and basal regions of the brain. The lack of subdural temperature drop could also indicate that the effect of cooling diminishes with distance from the nasopharynx. Nevertheless, the deflection in rise of all these temperatures on extubation suggests that heat loss from the upper airways does have more global effects.

▌ Selective Brain Cooling in Hyperthermia, Normothermia, and Fever

Some authors propose that selective brain cooling only occurs during hyperthermia and not during normothermia or fever [2, 36]. In normothermia, it is supposed that selective brain cooling is not necessary because the brain can be cooled sufficiently by arterial blood from the trunk [2]. However, although they do not point this out, Mariak et al. [35] demonstrate selective brain cooling in normothermia in humans. Towards the end of their study, esophageal temperature in one patient was 36.8 °C and in another 37 °C, in both cases brain temperature was about 0.2 °C lower. Therefore, selective brain cooling can occur in normothermia in humans but the differential appears to be smaller than in hyperthermia.

A raised temperature can be due to hyperthermia or fever. Hyperthermia exists when the thermoregulatory set point is normal but temperature regulation has malfunctioned or is overcome by circumstances and unable to keep body temperature at the set point, for example in exercise and heatstroke [37]. Selective brain cooling in exercise hyperthermia permits a higher core body temperature which increases muscle efficiency [24, 38]. In fever, it is commonly believed that the thermoregulatory set point has been reset at a higher than normal level and consequently heat conserving mechanisms have been activated [37, 39]. This is a defense mechanism which it is argued would be illogical for selective brain cooling to overcome. Nevertheless, selective brain cooling with reversal of blood flow in the ophthalmic and angularis oculi veins has been shown in two feverish humans [20, 38]. Mariak et al. [36] did not demonstrate selective brain cooling in a retrospective study of feverish neurosurgical patients. However, they give no information on intubation and the only data showing both parenchymal brain temperature and esophageal temperature are in a patient with severe cerebral trauma, Glasgow Coma Scale (GCS) 6, who it is reasonable to assume was intubated. (Rectal temperature is not an appropriate measure for demonstrating selective brain cooling [40]). In feverish animals (with a rete) selective brain cooling by heat loss from the upper airways was reduced when temperature was rising to give protection and increased when the protective effect of temperature rise had occurred and temperature was on the way down again [41]. This is a beautifully logical thermoregulatory response and there seems to be no reason why it should not also occur in humans.

▌ Effect of Nasal Airflow on Mood – the Vascular Theory of Emotional Efference

"The vascular theory of emotional efference [VTEE] states that facial action can alter the volume of air inhaled through the nose, which in turn influences brain temperature and affective states. Cooling enhances positive affect, whereas warming depresses it" [8]. The logic is that because brain cooling is important, processes that facilitate it, such as heat loss from the upper airways, have evolved to be pleasant, and impeding factors unpleasant. These subjectively felt effects are "mediated by temperature-dependent changes in the release and synthesis of emotion-related neurochemicals" [8].

There is support for this theory from experimental studies in animals and humans. In rats, Berridge and Zajonc [42] found that hypothalamic cooling caused the same behavior as pleasurable electrical stimulation. In humans it has been shown that facial actions influence frontopolar artery temperature and affect. Smiling, for example, reduced temperature, put subjects in a good mood and increased the volume of air inhaled through the nose compared with facial actions associated with negative emotions [8, 43]. Prevention of nasal breathing generated negative affect and increased temperature [8]. The effects of facial action and prevention of nasal breathing appear to be localized to the head [8].

Despite the caveats attached to this research, the basic relationships that the VTEE predicts do appear to exist, which has implications for all those whose upper respiratory tract is bypassed.

▌ Clinical Relevance of Selective Brain Cooling

Some examples of the clinical relevance of selective brain cooling are given here but it is likely to be important in other fields also, ear, nose and throat (ENT), and psychology for example.

In Infants

Nose breathing is more work for infants than adults and yet they exhibit "reluctance to use a less resistive oral airway for breathing until the facility is acquired at about 5–6 months" [33]. We believe that selective brain cooling explains why nose breathing is so important to infants despite the work it requires. du Boulay et al. [6] suggest that selective brain cooling might be the explanatory link between pyrexia, prone position, and heavy wrapping as risk factors for sudden infant death syndrome (SIDS) [6, 7]. We believe that selective brain cooling also explains why mouth breathing increases the risk of SIDS and dummy use reduces it [44] by about 1.5–4 times [45–47]. We would suggest too that the increase in nasal congestion in a lying position [48] and the enhanced efficiency of selective brain cooling in a head up position [22] are of significance in the context of SIDS.

In Upper Airway Bypass

Nasal airflow may have significant effects on the brain and affect, which are as yet not fully understood but may be important and subtle, particularly in the severely ill in whom even small improvements in physiology can make an additive difference. Therefore, there may be an argument for restoring nasal airflow in anyone who has an endotracheal tube or tracheostomy.

After Brain Injury

In the search for ways to improve outcome after brain injury, temperature, and methods of manipulating it for therapeutic purposes, has been the subject of considerable research effort. Systemic and head selective hypothermia have both been shown to convey neuroprotection after brain injury in animals [49, 50]. However, a sufficiently powered randomized controlled trial of systemic hypothermia in humans showed no evidence of differences in outcome between hypothermic and normothermic groups measured at six months [51]. Patients in the hypothermic group had lower white blood cell counts and it appears that this group experienced an increase in morbidity from infection which may have negated any benefits of hypothermia (personal communication). Suppression of immune response and increases in infection are recognized side-effects of systemic hypothermia [52, 53]. Selective head cooling has had little effect on brain temperature in adults [54, 55].

On the other hand, pyrexia is common in humans after a severe neurological insult [56] and even mild pyrexia has a detrimental effect on the compromised brain [5–59]. Given this, and the risks and difficulties associated with hypothermia, it would be worth paying more attention to reducing pyrexia after brain injury and selective brain cooling could provide brain specific ways of doing this.

Heat Loss through the Skull after Brain Injury

The cooling caps used for selective head cooling work largely by conduction and cause scalp skin vasoconstriction. Capitalizing on the normal physiological mechanisms for selective brain cooling by heat loss through the skull, i.e., convective cooling without vasoconstriction, might have more success. For example, keeping the head wet and blowing dry, tepid air over it. A 30 °C head up position enhances the efficiency of selective brain cooling through emissary vein blood flow from scalp to brain [22]; fortunately this is the position in which brain injured patients are commonly nursed.

Heat Loss from the Upper Airways after Brain Injury

We are beginning a randomized, controlled, crossover trial of airflow through the upper respiratory tract of brain-injured, intubated patients with frontal lobe brain temperature monitoring. We wish to find out if it is possible to lower brain temperature and/or produce selective brain cooling in patients for whom this heat loss mechanism is not otherwise available.

A Cautionary Note on the Manipulation of Selective Brain Cooling

If immune response to body temperature is modulated by the brain [60, 61], then even making the brain alone hypothermic may cause immune depression and increased infection. In addition, if immune defense is accelerated and more efficient at raised temperatures [62], reducing brain temperature to normal in fever may increase morbidity and mortality from infection.

▌ Conclusion

There is evidence that selective brain cooling in humans exists, that it is a rational thermoregulatory mechanism, and that it has clinical significance which needs further exploration. There is much more to discover, for example about its action in fever, its influence on affect and psychological well-being, and its interactions with the immune system and with neurotransmitter function.

Acknowledgement. We wish to express particular thanks to the staff of the ICU at the Western General Hospital, Edinburgh for their support of our research.

References

1. Brengelmann GL (1993) Specialized brain cooling in humans? FASEB J 7:1148–1153
2. Cabanac M (1993) Selective brain cooling in humans: "fancy" or fact? FASEB J 7:1143–1146
3. Zenker W, Kubik S (1996) Brain cooling in humans – anatomical considerations. Anat Embryol (Berl) 193:1–13
4. Cabanac M, Caputa M (1979) Natural selective cooling of the human brain: evidence of its occurrence and magnitude. J Physiol 286:255–264
5. Cabanac M, Brinnel H (1985) Blood flow in the emissary veins of the human head during hyperthermia. Eur J Appl Physiol Occup Physiol 54:172–176
6. du Boulay GH, Lawton M, Wallis A (1998) The story of the internal carotid artery of mammals: from Galen to sudden infant death syndrome. Neuroradiology 40:697–703

7. du Boulay G, Lawton M, Wallis A (2000) Selective brain cooling in animals: internal carotid's significance for sudden infant death syndrome. Ambulatory Child Health 6 (suppl 1):36–38

8. McIntosh DN, Zajonc RB, Vig PS, Emerick SW (1997) Facial movement, breathing, temperature, and affect: implications of the vascular theory of emotional efference. Cognition and Emotion 11:171–195

9. Baker MA (1982) Brain cooling in endotherms in heat and exercise. Annu Rev Physio 44:85–96

10. Niinimaa V, Cole P, Mintz S, Shepard RJ (1980) The switching point from oral to oronasal breathing. Respir Physiol 42:61–71

11. Falk D (1992) Braindance. Henry Holt and Co, New York

12. Hall RL, Hall DA (1995) Geographic variation of native people along the Pacific Coast. Hum Biol 67:407–426

13. Carey JW, Steegmann AT (1981) Human nasal protrusion, latitude, and climate. Am J Phys Anthropol 56:313–319

14. Wolpoff MH (1969) Climatic influence on the skeletal nasal aperture. Am J Phys Anthropol 29:405–424

15. Koertvelyessy T (1972) Relationships between the frontal sinus and climatic conditions: a skeletal approach to cold adaptation. Am J Phys Anthropol 37:161–172

16. Shea BT (1977) Eskimo craniofacial morphology, cold stress and the maxillary sinus. Am J Phys Anthropol 47:289–300

17. Hayward JN, Baker MA (1969) A comparative study of the role of the cerebral arterial blood in the regulation of brain temperature in five mammals. Brain Res 16:417–440

18. Cabanac M, Germain M, Brinnel H (1987) Tympanic temperatures during hemiface cooling. Eur J Appl Physiol Occup Physiol 56:534–539

19. Caputa M, Perrin G, Cabanac M (1978) Ecoulement sanguin réversible dans la veine ophtalmique: mécanisme de refroidissement sélectif du cerveau humain. C R Acad Sci 287:D1011–D1014

20. Hirashita M, Shido O, Tanabe M (1992) Blood flow through the ophthalmic veins during exercise in humans. Eur J Appl Physiol 64:92–97

21. Caputa M, Cabanac M (1988) Precedence of head homoeothermia over trunk homoeothermia in dehydrated men. Eur J Appl Physiol 57:611–615

22. Nagasaka T, Brinnel H, Hales JR, Ogawa T (1998) Selective brain cooling in hyperthermia: the mechanisms and medical implications. Med Hypotheses 50:203–211

23. Eckenhoff JE (1970) The physiologic significance of the vertebral venous plexus. Surg Gynecol Obstet 131:72–78

24. Dean MC (1988) Another look at the nose and the functional significance of the face and nasal mucous membrane for cooling the brain in fossil hominids. J Human Evolution 17:715–718

25. Gray RF, Hawthorne M (1992) Synopsis of Otolaryngology, 5th ed. Butterworth–Heinemann Ltd, Oxford

26. Cole P (1982) Modification of inspired air. In: Proctor DF, Andersen IB (eds) The Nose: Upper Airway Physiology and the Atmospheric Environment. Elsevier Biomedical Press, Oxford, pp 351–370

27. White MD, Cabanac M (1995) Nasal mucosal vasodilatation in response to passive hyperthermia in humans. Eur J Appl Physiol Occup Physiol 70:207–212

28. Eccles R (1982) Neurological and pharmacological considerations. In: Proctor DF, Andersen IB (eds) The Nose: Upper Airway Physiology and the Atmospheric Environment. Elsevier Biomedical Press, Oxford, pp 191–214

29. Irlbeck D (1998) Normal mechanisms of heat and moisture exchange in the respiratory tract. Respir Care Clin North Am 4:189–98

30. Drake-Lee A (1997) The physiology of the nose and paranasal sinuses. In: Gleeson M (ed) Scott-Brown's Otolaryngology: Vol 1 Basic Sciences (6th ed). Butterworth-Heinemann Ltd, Oxford, pp 1/6/1–1/6/21

31. Houdas Y, Ring E (1982) Human Body Temperature: Its Measurement and Regulation. Plenum Press, New York

32. Djupesland MD, Chatkin JM, Qian W, Haight JS (2001) Nitric oxide in the nasal airway: a new dimension in otorhinolaryngology. Am J Otolaryngol 22:19–32
33. Cole P (1982) Upper respiratory airflow. In: Proctor DF, Andersen IB (eds) The Nose: Upper Airway Physiology and the Atmospheric Environment. Elsevier Biomedical, Oxford, pp 163–182
34. Proctor D (1982) The upper airway. In: Proctor DF, Andersen IB (eds) The Nose: Upper Airway Physiology and the Atmospheric Environment. Elsevier Biomedical Press, Oxford, pp 23–44
35. Mariak Z, White MD, Lewko J, Lyson T, Piekarski P (1999) Direct cooling of the human brain by heat loss from the upper respiratory tract. J Appl Physiol 87:1609–1613
36. Mariak Z, Jadeszko M, Lewko J, Lebkowski W, Lyson T (1998) No specific brain protection against thermal stress in fever. Acta Neurochir (Wien) 140:585–590
37. Webb AR, Shapiro MJ, Singer M, Suter PM (1999) Hyperthermia and pyrexia. In: Oxford Textbook of Critical Care. Oxford University Press, New York, pp 796–811
38. Cabanac M (1998) Selective brain cooling and thermoregulatory set point. J Basic Clin Physiol Pharmacol 9:3–13
39. Kluger MJ (1994) Fever and antipyresis. In: Zeisberger E, Schönbaum E, Lomax P (eds) Thermal Balance in Health and Disease: Recent Basic Research and Clinical Progress. Advances in Pharmacological Sciences Series. Birkhäuser Verlag, Basel, pp 342–52
40. Maloney SK, Fuller A, Mitchell G, Mitchell D (2001) Rectal temperature measurement results in artefactual evidence of selective brain cooling. Am J Physiol 281:R108–114
41. Kuhnen G (1994) Selective brain cooling during fever? In: Zeisberger E, Schönbaum E, Lomax P (eds) Thermal Balance in Health and Disease: Recent Basic Research and Clinical Progress. Advances in Pharmacological Sciences Series. Birkhäuser Verlag, Basel, pp 353–358
42. Berridge KC, Zajonc RB (1991) Hypothalamic cooling elicits eating: differential effects on motivation and pleasure. Psycholog Sci 2:184–189
43. Zajonc RB, Murphy ST, Inglehart M (1989) Feeling and facial efference: implications of the vascular theory of emotions. Psychol Rev 96:395–416
44. L'Hoir MP, Engelberts AC, van Well GTJ, et al (1999) Dummy use, thumb sucking, mouth breathing and cot death. Eur J Pediatr 158:896–901
45. Mitchell EA, Taylor BJ, Ford RP, et al (1993) Dummies and the sudden infant death syndrome. Arch Dis Child 68:501–504
46. Fleming PJ, Blair PS, Bacon C, et al (1996) Environment of infants during sleep and risk of the sudden infant death syndrome; results of 1993–5 case-control study for confidential inquiry into stillbirths and deaths in infancy. Br Med J 313:191–195
47. Arnestad M, Anderson M, Rognum TO (1997) Is the use of dummy or carry-cot of importance for sudden infant death? Eur J Paediatr 156:968–970
48. Stradling JR (1996) The upper respiratory tract. In: Weatherall DJ, Ledingham JGG, Warrell DA (eds) The Oxford Textbook of Medicine. Vol. 2. (3rd ed) Oxford University Press, Oxford, pp 2609–2612
49. Dietrich WD (1992) The importance of brain temperature in cerebral injury. J Neurotrauma 9:S475–S485
50. Barone FC, Feuerstein GZ, White RF (1996) Brain cooling during transient focal ischemia provides complete neuroprotection. Neurosci Biobehav Rev 21:31–44
51. Clifton GL, Miller ER, Choi SC, et al (2001) Lack of effect of induction of hypothermia after acute brain injury. N Engl J Med 344:556–563
52. Clardy CW, Edwards KM, Gay JC (1985) Increased susceptibility to infection in hypothermic children: possible role of acquired neutrophil dysfunction. Pediatr Infect Dis 4:379–382
53. Schubert A (1995) Side effects of mild hypothermia. J Neurosurg Anesthesiol 7:139–147
54. Mellergård P (1992) Changes in human intracerebral temperature in response to different methods of brain cooling. Neurosurgery 31:671–677
55. Corbett RJT, Laptook AR (1998) Failure of localized head cooling to reduce brain temperature in adult humans. NeuroReport 9:2721–2725
56. Kilpatrick MM, Lowry DW, Firlik AD, Yonas H, Marion DW (2000) Hyperthermia in the neurosurgical intensive care unit. Neurosurgery 47:850–856

57. Ginsberg MD, Busto R (1998) Combating hyperthermia in acute stroke: a significant clinical concern. Stroke 29:529–534
58. Jones PA, Andrews PJ, Midgley S, et al (1994) Measuring the burden of secondary insults in head-injured patients during intensive care. J Neurosurg Anesthesiol 6:4–14
59. Reith J, Jorgensen HS, Pedersen PM, et al (1996) Body temperature in acute stoke: relation to stroke severity, infarct size, mortality, and outcome. Lancet 347:422–425
60. Mariak Z (1999) How does the immune system communicate with the brain? Neurologica I Neurochirurgia Polska 33:665–674
61. Zeisberger E, Roth J (1993) Neurobiological concepts of fever generation and suppression. Neuropsychobiology 28:106–109
62. Kluger MJ (1991) Fever: role of pyrogens and cryogens. Physiol Rev 71:93–127

Septic Encephalopathy

G. B. Young

▌ Introduction

Of in-patients with positive blood cultures, we found that over 70% had some evidence of brain dysfunction [1]. Forty-six percent of these were in the intensive care unit (ICU), with the rest on the wards. The encephalopathy associated with systemic infections is a diffuse disturbance in cerebral function. Septic encephalopathy is a diagnosis of exclusion: there should be no clinical or laboratory evidence of direct central nervous system (CNS) infection (e.g., meningitis, macroscopic intracranial abscess or empyema), head trauma, fat embolism, adverse reactions to medications, sedative or paralyzing drug effects.

▌ Pathology and Pathophysiology

In fatal cases, watershed brain infarctions from sustained hypotension are rarely encountered, however, the brain may show microscopic abnormalities [2]. Eight of 12 of our patients with post-mortem examinations had disseminated microabscesses. The cerebral cortex is the most commonly involved site, but deep structures and even the spinal cord may be affected. Other less common lesions include multiple microscopic infarctions, brain purpura, and central pontine myelinolysis [2]. Some cases may show no abnormality on gross or light microscopic examination.

The mechanism of sepsis-associated encephalopathy is uncertain. In advanced cases it is likely multifactorial, given the variety of pathological findings. The early, fully reversible cases are not likely associated with structural change and are probably 'metabolic' in nature. Other mechanisms, in addition to the metabolic disturbances, operate in more advanced cases. The following mechanisms have been proposed:

Microvascular Disorder. The blood-brain barrier, which normally rigidly maintains a homeostatic environment for brain cells, becomes leaky in a dynamic, patchy manner within the first few hours of endotoxemia in experimental animals [3]. In addition the differential flux of chemicals across the blood-brain barrier is altered, e.g., in sepsis aromatic amino acids are more readily transported than branched chain amino acids from blood to brain. Reduced cerebral blood flow (CBF) and increased cerebrovascular resistance are found in human cases of septic encephalopathy; microthromboses may also occur. Most, if not all of these phenomena likely relate to the production of cytokines (tumor necrosis factor [TNF] and interleukins [IL]-1 and -2) and their effects on endothelial nitric oxide (NO) synthase (eNOS) production. Inhibition of eNOS leads to impairment of the microcirculation of the brain and other organs by causing vasoconstriction [4]. Free radical production may also alter capillary permeability.

Free Radical-excitotoxic Injury. Endotoxin lipopolysaccharides (LPS) trigger increases in interferon (IFN)-γ, inducible/inflammatory nitric oxide synthase (iNOS) in non-neuronal (glial and microglial) cells and reactive oxygen and nitrogen species [5]. In the face of depleted antioxidants (glutathione and ascorbate), augmented extra-cellular glutamate in the brain's extracellular fluid (increased release and reduced reuptake), there is a setting for neuronal and glial cell loss [6]. This results from reactive oxygen species (ROS), intra-neuronal peroxynitrite production, and covalent modification of lipids and proteins in neurons and glia. Thus neuronal and glial death may occur in advanced sepsis.

Amino Acids and Neurotransmitter Imbalance. Humans with sepsis, and animal models of sepsis, both show an increased ratio of aromatic to branched-chain amino acids [7]. This correlates with a reduction in the concentrations of norepinephrine, dopamine, and serotonin in the brains of septic rats.

Brain Micro-abscesses. These (mentioned above) are of uncertain significance with respect to the pathogenesis of encephalopathy [2]. They are not detected in life unless one finds retinal microabscesses (a rarity in our experience). There is no good way of knowing when they occur in the course of sepsis, but, based on the surrounding reaction in the brain, they are probably not all agonal. If they do occur, they could contribute, directly or indirectly, in causing further neuronal damage because of the release of the above-mentioned cytokines and other inflammatory mediators.

Failure of Other Organs. Hepatic or renal failure may, in themselves, cause an encephalopathy. Since septic encephalopathy often precedes multi-organ failure (MOF), this secondary mechanism would not explain the early encephalopathy of sepsis. MOF likely plays a contributory role in producing brain dysfunction in advanced sepsis, however.

Other. There are a number of factors that are yet to be explored, such as the production of gamma-amino butyric acid (GABA), GABA receptors in the brain, benzodiazepine-like substances (with inhibitory or sedating properties) and quinolinic acid, which are elevated in hepatic dysfunction [8–10]. We should not forget iatrogenically-induced encephalopathy, as drugs often show delayed clearance in sepsis, and variations in osmolality and reduced serum phosphate concentration may be produced by feeds.

Clinical Features

The principal neurological findings of septic encephalopathy relate to altered mental status [11]. Mildly encephalopathic patients demonstrate a fluctuating confusional state and inappropriate behavior. Inattention and writing errors (including spelling, writing full sentences, orientation of writing on the page) are common. More severely affected patients show delirium, an agitated confusional state, or coma.

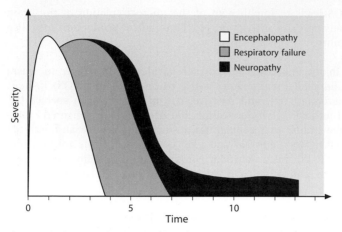

Fig. 1. Typical course of nervous system complications in sepsis: encephalopathy, difficulty weaning from the ventilator, and then polyneuropathy. In the severe form this may take months, but could be weeks in milder forms. (From [11] with permission)

The most common motor sign is paratonic rigidity or *gegenhalten*, a resistance to passive movement of limbs that is velocity-dependent: the resistance that is felt with movements at normal rate disappears when the limb is moved slowly [11]. Asterixis, multifocal myoclonus, seizures and tremor are relatively infrequent. Cranial nerve functions are (almost) invariably spared.

Clinical or laboratory evidence of peripheral nerve dysfunction, critical illness polyneuropathy, is found in 70% of our encephalopathic patients [11]. The neuropathy is axonal in type and takes many months to resolve. It is later in onset than the encephalopathy and is much slower to recover than the brain dysfunction [11]. Clinically one finds decreased movement and the loss of deep tendon reflexes. Motor function is usually more affected than sensation, so that the patient may grimace without other movement when a nail bed is squeezed. In severe cases, the polyneuropathy may affect the phrenic nerves, creating problems in weaning the patient from the ventilator [12].

The relative time course of the encephalopathy, the failure to wean from the ventilator (often due to critical illness polyneuropathy or myopathy) and the resolution of critical illness polyneuropathy is illustrated in Figure 1.

▌ Laboratory Investigations

The electroencephalogram (EEG) serves as the most sensitive test for sepsis-associated encephalopathy [13]. It may show mild, diffuse, reversible slowing in bacteremia, even if the neurological examination is normal. The severity of the EEG abnormality is parallel to the impairment in mental status. As the encephalopathy worsens, mild slowing in the theta (>4 to <8 Hz) range is followed by diffuse delta (≤4 Hz) waves, then generalized triphasic waves, and finally by suppression or a generalized burst-suppression (alternating diffuse reductions in voltage with burst of higher voltage waves) pattern. The relationships of EEG classifications to severity of encephalopathy and mortality are illustrated in Figures 2 and 3.

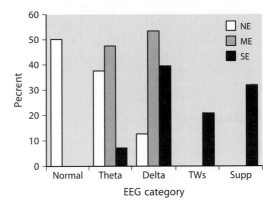

Fig. 2. Histogram showing the percentages of patients with no clinical encephalopathy with bacteremia (NE), mild septic encephalopathy (ME), and severe septic encephalopathy (SE) with electroencephalographic (EEG) classifications: normal, theta (mild generalized slowing), delta (severe slowing), triphasic waves (TWs) and generalized suppression or burst-suppression (Supp). (From [13] with permission)

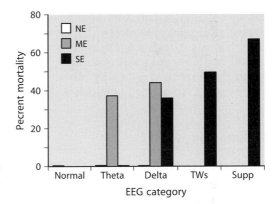

Fig. 3. Histogram of mortality for the various EEG and encephalopathic states described in Figure 2. (From [13] with permission)

In our experience with bacteremia, the mortality is directly related to the severity of the EEG abnormality: 0% with normal, 19% with theta, 36% with delta, 50% with triphasic waves, and 67% with suppression or burst-suppression.

Computed tomographic (CT) brain scans are normal [2]. Cerebrospinal fluid (CSF) analysis shows only a mild elevation of protein concentration in some, not all, of the patients and normal cell counts and glucose concentrations, even in patients with brain microabscesses at autopsy [1].

We find no significant correlation of severity of encephalopathy with any specific bacteria, but there is a trend for patients with multiple bacteria on blood culture and with *Candida albicans* to have more severe brain dysfunction and a higher mortality rate [1].

The following biochemical tests show a direct proportional change with the severity of the encephalopathy: serum urea, creatinine, bilirubin, and alkaline phosphatase. The degree of renal impairment is rarely sufficient to account for the brain dysfunction [1]. Hepatic failure is, however, usually difficult to assess clinically or to quantify biochemically. Encephalopathic septic patients have greater elevation of aromatic amino acids and lower concentrations of branched chain amino acids in plasma than do non-encephalopathic patients [14]. This is similar to the unbalanced ratio found in hepatic failure. In sepsis, however, it may relate mainly to altered metabolism of amino acids in muscle and liver.

Management

First one must establish the diagnosis. It is especially important to perform a lumbar puncture on obtunded patients with systemic inflammatory response syndrome (SIRS), to rule out meningitis. Seizures (uncommon) should be treated with standard anti-epileptic medications such as phenytoin.

Patients usually die of the severity of the systemic illness or of failure of organs other than the brain [1]. Clinicians and nurses should be watchful for early encephalopathy, as it can be a presenting feature of sepsis. Prompt, specific treatment of the septic illness (appropriate anti-microbial therapy, drainage of abscesses, etc.) with prevention of MOF will save lives, as mortality is directly related to the severity of sepsis and the number of failed organs [15]. With the administration of a mixture of amino acids with high concentrations of branched-chain amino acids, Freund and colleagues successfully reversed septic encephalopathy in five patients [16]. This short-term improvement is gratifying, but this treatment may not be helpful for advanced cases with MOF. Potential future therapies may prevent or lessen the severity of sepsis by affecting cytokine or free radical production, the expression of cell adhesion molecules, or NO generation.

Conclusion

Septic encephalopathy is a diffuse disturbance in cerebral function that occurs in the context of systemic inflammatory response. It is usually a reversible encephalopathy, but some advanced cases may have structural damage to the brain. In severe cases, septic encephalopathy is associated with difficulty weaning from the ventilator (due to neuropathy or myopathy) and a protracted axonal polyneuropathy (critical illness polyneuropathy). The EEG is helpful in grading the severity of the encephalopathy. Thus far, there is no specific treatment for the encephalopathy itself. The brain will usually recover if the other organs of the body regain their function.

References

1. Young GB, Bolton CF, Austin TW (1990) The encephalopathy associated with septic illness. Clin Invest Med 13:297–304
2. Jackson AC, Gilbert JJ, Young GB, Bolton CF (1985) The encephalopathy of sepsis. Can J Neurol Sci 12:303–307
3. du Moulin GC, Paterson D, Hedley-White J, Broitman SA (1985) *E. coli* peritonitis and bacteremia cause increased blood-brain barrier permeability. Brain Res 340:261–268
4. Spain DA, Wilson MA, Bar-Natan MF, Garrison RN (1994) Nitric oxide synthetase inhibition aggravates intestinal microvascular vasoconstriction and hypoperfusion of bacteremia. J Trauma 36:720–725

5. Papadopoulos MC, Davies DC, Moss RF, et al (2000) Pathophysiology of septic encephalopathy: a review. Crit Care Med 28:3019–3024
6. Zhao ML, Liu JS, He D, et al (1998) Inducible nitric oxide synthase expression is selectively induced in astrocytes isolated from the adult human brain. Brain Res 813:402–405
7. Freund HR, Muggia-Sullam M, Peiser J, Melamed E (1985) Brain neurotransmitter profile is deranged during sepsis and septic encephalopathy in the rat. J Surg Res 38:267–271
8. Schafer DF, Jones EA (1982) Hepatic encephalopathy and the gamma-aminobutyric-acid neurotransmitter system. Lancet I:18–20
9. Millen KD, Szauter KM, Kaminsky-Russ (1990) "Endogenous" benzodiazepine activity in body fluids of patients with hepatic encephalopathy. Lancet 336:81–83
10. Moroni F, Lombardi G, Carlà V, et al (1986) Increase in the content of quinolinic acid in cerebrospinal fluid and frontal cortex of patients with hepatic failure. J Neurochem 47:1667–1671
11. Bolton CF, Young GB, Zochodne DW (1993) The neurological complications of sepsis. Ann Neurol 33:94–100
12. Zochodne DW, Bolton CF, Wells GA, et al (1987) Critical illness polyneuropathy: a complication of sepsis and multiple organ failure. Brain 110:819–842
13. Young GB, Bolton CF, Archibald YM, Austin TW, Wells GA (1992) The electroencephalogram in sepsis-associated encephalopathy. J Clin Neurophysiol 9:145–152
14. Sprung CL, Cerra FB, Freund HR (1991) Amino acid alterations and encephalopathy in the sepsis syndrome. Crit Care Med 19:753–757
15. Pine RW, Wertz MJ, Lennard ES (1983) Determinants of organ malfunction or death in patients with intra-abdominal sepsis. Arch Surg 118:242–249
16. Freund HR, Ryan JA, Fischer JE (1978) Amino acid derangements in patients with sepsis: treatment with branched chain amino acid rich infusions. Ann Surg 188:423–430

Critical Care Management of Refractory Status Epilepticus

J. Claassen, L.J. Hirsch, and S.A. Mayer

▌ Introduction

Status epilepticus is defined as continuous or repetitive seizure activity persisting for at least 30 minutes without recovery of consciousness between attacks. Though differing to some degree, most authors define refractory status epilepticus as generalized status epilepticus that continues clinically or electrographically despite first and second line therapy. Definitions differ primarily regarding the required number of failed anticonvulsant drugs (two [1–5] or three [6–9]), and whether a minimum duration of persistent seizure activity is required (ranging from none [1, 5, 7–9] to one [3] or two [2, 4] hours). Status epilepticus can be classified according to clinical and electroencephalogram (EEG) findings (Fig. 1).

▌ Pathophysiology

Generalized Convulsive Status Epilepticus (GCSE).
Episodes of GCSE often start with discrete tonic-clonic seizures, evolving to more continuous motor activity, finally leading to the disappearance of all motor activity despite ongoing seizure activity, also known as 'subtle status epilepticus', 'non-convulsive status epilepticus (NCSE)', or 'electromechanical dissociation' [10, 11]. During the initial phase ('phase of compensation'), cerebral metabolism and blood flow are increased, but physiological mechanisms are sufficient to prevent cerebral tissue damage. Therapeutic interventions are most promising when initiated during this period [12]. With ongoing seizure activity, physiological demands surpass the capabilities of cerebral compensatory mechanisms resulting in hypoxia, metabolic cellular failure, and neuronal injury, worsened by loss of cerebral autoregulation [10, 11]. Increased autonomic stimulation persists and cardiorespiratory functions may progressively fail. Uncontrolled status epilepticus can lead to the development of additional seizure foci in the brain.

Non-convulsive Status Epilepticus.
NCSE is defined as continuous or repetitive electrographic seizure activity for at least 30 minutes associated with alteration in mental status or behavior [13]. NCSE has only recently been recognized as a neurological emergency, and to some degree the discussion of this phenomenon is complicated by differences in terminology [14–16]. The above definition combines 'the wandering confused' NCSE patient, who has a good prognosis, with the comatose intensive care unit (ICU) patient with an acute brain insult, who has a poor prog-

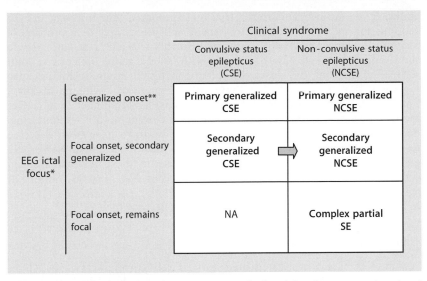

Fig. 1. Proposed classification scheme of status epilepticus in severely obtunded and comatose patients based on the clinical syndrome and electroencephalograph (EEG) findings. Convulsive status epilepticus (CSE) implies bilateral rhythmic tonic-clonic activity; non-convulsive (NCSE) involves altered mental status, with or without subtle motor manifestations (facial twitching, nystagmus). Determination of the EEG ictal focus is based on current EEG observations, recent history and imaging, and prior history of epilepsy. Primary generalized onset convulsive and non-convulsive status epilepticus (i.e., absence or petit mal SE, or 'spike wave stupor') are very amenable to treatment and are rarely life threatening. Arrow indicates that when untreated, secondary generalized convulsive status epilepticus (GCSE) often evolves into NCSE (i.e., 'subtle' generalized convulsive SE). Complex partial status epilepticus can be clinically indistinguishable from secondary generalized NCSE. Note that simple partial status epilepticus (i.e., epilepsia partialis continua) does not apply (NA) to this classification scheme of ICU patients

nosis (Fig. 1). For all practical purposes, these two patient groups should be considered separately, since the former category responds well to therapy and usually returns to baseline. This chapter focuses only on the latter group, encountered primarily in the ICU. In addition to impaired consciousness or mentation, these patients may have minimal facial twitching or nystagmoid eye movement. The sequence of pathophysiological events in NCSE is not well understood, but morbidity and mortality are high [5, 14, 16].

Complex Partial Status Epilepticus (CPSE). CPSE closely resembles 'subtle' generalized status epilepticus, and in patients who present delayed with incomplete documentation of neurological findings at first presentation, the two conditions can be difficult to differentiate even with EEG monitoring.

∎ Epidemiology

Status epilepticus is a life-threatening condition which affects 120,000 to 200,000 people annually in the United States [17], and 9 to 31% of these patients will be refractory to first and second line therapy [6, 18, 19]. NCSE occurs in about 14% of patients after control of GCSE [14]. The results of the Veterans Affairs (VA) Cooperative Study [18], a randomized trial that compared four different first-line interventions for, indicate that refractory status epilepticus may be a problem of greater magnitude than is generally appreciated. In this trial, 38% of patients with 'overt' status epilepticus and 82% of patients with 'subtle' status epilepticus continued to seize after receiving full doses of two anticonvulsant drugs. In the unexplained comatose ICU patient, excluding those with seizures or twitching at any point in time, the exact frequency of NCSE may be considerably higher than conventionally thought (8% on routine EEG [20]), and only continuous EEG monitoring reliably documents this phenomenon. Non-convulsive seizures have been described in up to 34% of patients in neurological ICUs, and 76% of these had NCSE [21]. Etiologies of refractory status epilepticus are similar to those for status epilepticus in general, frequently being stroke or central nervous system (CNS) tumor (20%), epilepsy (20%), toxic-metabolic encephalopathy (19%), CNS infection (19%), hypoxia-ischemia (12%), and traumatic brain injury (TBI, 5%) [22].

Predictors of Refractoriness

Few studies have investigated predictors of refractoriness [19, 22–24]. Failure of first- and second-line therapy has been associated with delayed treatment and prolonged seizure duration. Non-structural causes for status epilepticus such as hypoxia-ischemia, metabolic encephalopathy, and CNS infection [23, 24], are more refractory to therapy. NCSE and focal motor seizures at onset have also been identified as independent risk factors for refractoriness in status epilepticus [19]; secondary-generalized seizures tend to be particularly resistant to treatment [8].

Outcome

Outcome in refractory status epilepticus is extremely poor; mortality is almost 50% [2, 5, 22, 25, 26] and only a third of patients return to their pre morbid functional baseline [5, 19]. There are conflicting data on the morbidity and mortality associated with NCSE [5, 14–16], but poor prognosis is associated with NCSE in the setting of acute brain disease [5, 14]. In one small preliminary study, de novo epilepsy developed in 45% of NCSE survivors [27]. Similar to status epilepticus in general, mortality in refractory status epilepticus is associated with older age [22, 28, 29], etiology (e.g., hypoxia, stroke, subarachnoid hemorrhage) [10, 22, 23, 28–32], long seizure duration [22, 23, 29, 30], and high Acute Physiology and Chronic Health Evaluation-II (APACHE-II) scale [5, 22]. EEG documentation of NCSE [14], ictal discharges [33], and periodic lateralized epileptiform discharges [33], have been associated with poor outcome and mortality after GCSE.

▌ Complications of Refractory Status Epilepticus

Morbidity after status epilepticus may result from neurological deficits caused by the seizures themselves (e.g., resulting in cerebral hypoxia), acute brain disease (e.g., the stroke or tumor causing status epilepticus), or secondary medical complications and prolonged hospitalization. Acute systemic effects of GCSE include hyperglycemia, lactic acidosis, massive catecholamine release, cardiac arrhythmia, hyperpyrexia, increased central venous pressure (CVP), and increased cardiac output [11, 34]. Later consequences of prolonged status may include cardiorespiratory failure, hypoglycemia, hyponatremia, pulmonary edema, aspiration, cardiac arrhythmia, tachycardia, hypotension, hyperpyrexia, lactic and respiratory acidosis, rhabdomyolysis, shoulder dislocation, and rib fractures [11, 34]. Refractory status epilepticus is associated with a number of serious medical complications, even after controlling for hospital length of stay, including fever, pneumonia, hypotension, bacteremia, and anemia treated with blood transfusions [19, 35].

Management

Anticonvulsive Therapy

Standard Treatment for Status Epilepticus. In accordance with evidence from prospective, double-blind, multicenter studies [12, 18, 36], lorazepam is the first-line treatment of choice for status epilepticus, with a success rate of 65% [18]. Though second-line therapy has not been prospectively evaluated, phenytoin or fosphenytoin are the most frequently recommended (Table 1) [9]. Once patients fail to respond to two anticonvulsant drugs, seizure activity is extremely difficult to control. In the VA Cooperative Study [18], 38% of patients with 'overt' status epilepticus and 82% of patients with 'subtle' status epilepticus continued to seize after receiving two anticonvulsant drugs, and only 2% and 5%, respectively, stopped seizing after receiving a third agent [37]. The earlier anticonvulsants are started, the easier status epilepticus is controlled [12]. If therapy is begun within 30 minutes of onset, 80% will respond to the first line anticonvulsant drug, whereas if therapy is not begun within two hours only 40% will respond [23].

Traditional Treatment Approach for Refractory Status Epilepticus. Treatment of refractory status epilepticus has not been studied in a prospective trial, and guidelines give a spectrum of options. Intravenous (IV) therapy is the preferred mode of administra-

Table 1. Treatment dosages in management of status epilepticus

	Loading dose (mg/kg)	Maximum bolus rate (mg/min)	Continuous IV start dose (mg/kg/h)	Continuous IV dose range (mg/kg/h)	Enzyme inducer*
IV anticonvulsant drugs					
Lorazepam	0.1	2 mg	NA	NA	–
Phenytoin	18–20	<50	NA	NA	+
Fosphenytoin	18–20	150	NA	NA	+
Phenobarbital	10–20	75–100	NA	NA	+
Valproic Acid	15–60**	20	NA	NA	–
Continuous IV anticonvulsant drugs					
Midazolam	0.2–0.5[†]	4	0.1	0.1–2.0	–
Propofol	1–2[†]	?	2	2–15	–
Pentobarbital	5–20[†]	25	1	1–5	–

* Other important enzyme inducers include primidone and carbamazepine; ** in the presence of enzyme-inducing drugs, larger doses (40–60 mg/kg) are needed to establish and maintain therapeutic levels; [†] repeat bolus if seizures do not stop; NA, not applicable

tion, due to more controlled, and generally more rapid, achievement of therapeutic serum levels; oral medications should be avoided whenever possible. After failure of benzodiazepines and phenytoin/fosphenytoin, the traditional treatment algorithm prescribes loading with phenobarbital at this point, followed by continuous IV pentobarbital if that fails [7]. Response rates to third-line agents range between 2 [18] and 58% [19], depending on first- and second-line doses, length of status epilepticus duration prior to third-line agents, and the etiology of the status epilepticus. However, almost every patient will stop seizing with pentobarbital infusion [38, 39]. One advantage of barbiturates is the extensive experience with these drugs. Pentobarbital infusion lowers cerebral oxygen demand, intracranial pressure (ICP), and lipid peroxidation. However, barbiturates are heavily sedating and have a long half life, which may prolong the duration of mechanical ventilation and recovery to an alert state after the seizures have stopped. Furthermore, they may cause considerable hypotension [22], myocardial depression, infections, and ileus [25].

Newer Treatment Options for Refractory Status Epilepticus. Recently, a large number of new anticonvulsant medications have emerged, and some of these may be promising for therapy of refractory status epilepticus (Fig. 2). So far, most experience exists with continuous infusions of midazolam [3–6, 22] and propofol [4, 22, 40, 41]. In a systematic review, no difference in mortality (48%) could be found comparing 193 patients with refractory status epilepticus treated with continuous IV propofol, continuous IV midazolam or continuous IV pentobarbital [22]. This study also did not demonstrate any differences between propofol and midazolam for clinical endpoints such as acute treatment failure, breakthrough seizures, or post-treatment seizures when compared to continuous IV pentobarbital. By contrast, pentobarbital had a lower frequency of acute treatment failure and breakthrough seizures, but this was confounded by the fact that pentobarbital was more often infused with a titration goal of EEG background suppression and the lack of continuous EEG monitoring in most pentobarbital treated patients [22]. Hypotension also occurred more often with pentobarbital (titrated to EEG background suppression) than with propofol or midazolam (usually

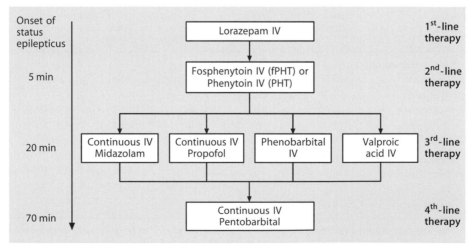

Fig. 2. Treatment algorithm for refractory status epilepticus

not titrated to EEG background suppression) [6, 22, 25, 40]. There is some preliminary evidence in a small retrospective series that propofol is associated with a higher mortality than midazolam [4]. In all patients treated with continuous infusions of an anticonvulsant drug, these drips should be continued for at least 24 hours after seizures are stopped [9], before a gradual taper is started (midazolam or propofol should be tapered over 6–24 hours). Possibly, higher doses and a longer period of continuous infusion anticonvulsant drugs may improve seizure control. However, published experience with these medications is limited, and no evidence-based treatment recommendations can be given at this point.

Valproic acid is an alternative non-continuous IV medication for the patient with refractory status epilepticus [42]. Major advantages include less sedation (intubation may be avoided), minimal hypotension and respiratory depression [42], and established therapeutic levels. Due to the interaction between phenytoin and valproic acid, both heavily protein bound anticonvulsant drugs, it is important to follow unbound (free) levels, especially of phenytoin, to avoid toxicity.

Occasionally in highly refractory patients with refractory status epilepticus, oral medications are added (via the nasogastric tube or percutaneous endoscopic gastrostomy [PEG]), including levetiracetame, topiramate, gabapentin, and carbamazepine. Particularly during tapering of continuous IV anticonvulsant drugs, these medications may be helpful to prevent breakthrough and withdrawal seizures. A number of other medications have been used successfully (continuous IV thiopental, continuous IV lorazepam, lidocaine, inhalational agents [e.g., isoflurane], ketamine, paraldehyde, electroconvulsive therapy), but have not proven to be effective or safe, or data are insufficient to evaluate efficacy and safety. Patients should not be paralyzed so that possible convulsive movements are not missed.

Serum levels of the following anticonvulsants should be obtained daily; therapeutic ranges for ICU patients are in parenthesis: phenytoin (10 to 25 µg/ml), free phenytoin, of particular importance in long term ICU patients and patients with a low albumin (1.0 to 2.5 µg/ml), valproic acid (60 to 140 µg/ml), phenobarbital (20 to 40 µg/ml), and carbamazepine (6 to 12 µg/ml). Serum levels in the ICU do not reflect steady state pharmacokinetics, but rather the blood concentration at a single time point.

Diagnostic Procedures

Electroencephalography. EEG is the diagnostic cornerstone in the management of refractory status epilepticus (Fig. 3). Recent advances in computer technology have made continuous digital EEG monitoring possible for the routine management of ICU patients and have largely replaced intermittent paper recordings. Advantages of digital EEG include post hoc remontaging, post hoc filter adjustments, quantitative analysis, data management and storage, seizure and spike detection, and off site EEG reading (e.g, via an intra- or internet connection). Without continuous EEG monitoring, the response of anticonvulsant drug treatment can be difficult to interpret, since subclinical electrographic seizure activity can be detected in up to 48% of patients after control of convulsive status epilepticus [14]. Using continuous EEG monitoring, frequent breakthrough seizures (56%) and withdrawal seizures (68%) have been reported in refractory NCSE patients treated with continuous IV midazolam [5], which were usually electrographic only. During the taper of continuous IV anticonvulsant drugs, EEG monitoring is crucial to detect recrudescence of subclinical seizure activity.

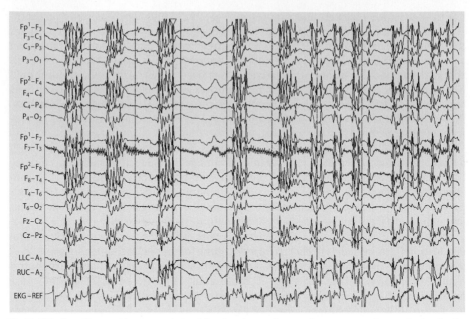

Fig. 3. EEG of an 87 year old women admitted for altered mental status. Frequent runs of generalized polyspike wave discharges are evident, consistent with an electrographic seizure in progress

EEG findings in the aftermath of status epilepticus include a range of periodic epileptiform discharges (PED) that do not meet formal seizure criteria [43, 44]. These PEDs are characterized by a spike or sharp wave followed by a slow wave that occur every 1 to 2 seconds, and may be lateralized (PLEDs), generalized (GPEDs), or bilateral but independent (BIPLEDs). They may occur in patients with acute focal brain injury in the absence of seizures, but also appear frequently in the aftermath of prolonged, untreated seizures [43, 44], and have been associated with poor outcome in status epilepticus [33, 45]. There is controversy regarding the interpretation and therapeutic implications of these EEG findings. Recently authors have used serial EEG data [44, 46], single-photon-emission computed tomography (SPECT) [47], and (18)F-fluorodeoxy-glucose (FDG)-positron emission computed tomography (PET) findings [48] to argue that PEDs following status epilepticus may be ictal. Others classify PEDs as part of an ictal-interictal continuum [45, 49]. In a retrospective study of status epilepticus, PLEDS on the initial EEG were associated with refractory status epilepticus [19], most likely reflecting the longer duration of status epilepticus in these patients.

In a prospective randomized trial for refractory status epilepticus, titration of continuous IV anticonvulsant drugs will possibly use EEG endpoints (e.g., no seizures, burst suppression, or complete suppression). In a systematic review comparing continuous IV propofol, continuous IV midazolam, and continuous IV pentobarbital, no effect on mortality could be identified for different titration goals [22].

Neuroimaging. Computed tomography (CT) and magnetic resonance imaging (MRI) are mandatory to identify underlying structural pathology in the workup of patients with refractory status epilepticus. CT or MRI findings may be seen as a consequence of status epilepticus and should not automatically be classified as the underlying cause of status epilepticus. These findings include small amounts of subarachnoid blood, small hemorrhagic 'contusions', small T2-hyperintensities in the gray and white matter, particularly after prolonged partial status epilepticus, and some degree of cerebral edema [50]. Secondary deterioration may be difficult to detect particularly in the sedated patient, however, any clinical deterioration (e.g., new neurological findings) warrants re-imaging.

Modern neuroimaging tools have furthered the understanding of status epilepticus but their role for the management of patients with refractory status epilepticus is limited. Imaging abnormalities in prolonged seizures include focal signal hyperintensities on fluid attenuated inversion recovery (FLAIR) MRI sequences [51]. Diffusion weighted imaging (DWI) using apparent diffusion coefficient (ADC) maps, demonstrated abnormalities in the affected cortex possibly related to associated cytotoxic edema [52]. The radiologic characteristics of status epilepticus may resemble those of ischemic stroke (on MRI, cortical enhancement on DWI and T2; on CT, decreased attenuation, effacement of sulci, and loss of gray-white differentiation), but can be differentiated based on the non-vascular distribution, increased flow on magnetic resonance angiography, leptomeningeal enhancement on post contrast MRI findings [53]. Proton magnetic resonance spectroscopy reveals elevated lactate, decreased N-acetylaspartate, and elevated choline [51, 54]. EEG triggered functional MRI may reveal focal signal increase [51]. Ictal SPECT may show focal hyperperfusion [55].

Conclusion

Status epilepticus is commonly refractory to at least two anticonvulsant medications. Refractory status epilepticus is often caused by acute brain disease (stroke, tumor, infection, trauma), less often epilepsy related, and carries a high morbidity

Table 2. General ICU management of the patient with refractory status epilepticus

Access
- Intubation for airway protection
- Intravenous access (central venous line desirable)
- Arterial catheter

Diagnostic tests
- Arterial blood gasses obtained frequently (or at least pulse oximetry)
- Routine blood tests (including: calcium, magnesium, lactate, glucose)
- EKG
- Lumbar puncture if patient is febrile or cause of status epilepticus is not clear (including: HSV-PCR, cryptococcus antigen, cultures)
- Pregnancy test in women
- CT and MRI

Basic interventions
- Fever: cooling blanket and antipyretics
- Hyperglycemia: insulin drip
- Deep venous thrombosis: prophylaxis

HSV, herpes simplex virus; CT, computerized tomography; MRI, magnetic resonance imaging; EKG, electrocardiogram

and mortality. Continuous EEG monitoring is mandatory for the management of this disease. The traditional treatment of choice for refractory status epilepticus is phenobarbital followed by continuous infusions of pentobarbital if that fails. Newer medications available for the treatment of refractory status epilepticus include IV valproic acid, and continuous midazolam and propofol infusions. Because pentobarbital always seems to be effective and phenobarbital fails to control status epilepticus in a substantial number of patients, continuous IV propofol, continuous IV midazolam, and valproic acid can be considered as alternative third-line anticonvulsants (Fig. 2). If seizures are refractory to the third-line agent, pentobarbital can be considered as the 'ultimate step'. The most frequent management error for refractory status epilepticus is delayed diagnosis, undertreatment allowing prolonged status epilepticus, and not adding a third or fourth agent soon enough. So far treatment preferences are based on retrospective series. Treatment of choice will have to be determined in a randomized controlled trial.

References

1. Jagoda A, Riggio S (1993) Refractory status epilepticus in adults. Ann Emerg Med 22:1337–1348
2. Stecker MM, Kramer TH, Raps EC, O'Meeghan R, Dulaney E, Skaar DJ (1998) Treatment of refractory status epilepticus with propofol: clinical and pharmacokinetic findings. Epilepsia 39:18–26
3. Hanley DF, Kross JF (1998) Use of midazolam in the treatment of refractory status epilepticus. Clin Ther 20:1093–1105
4. Prasad A, Worrall BB, Bertram EH, Bleck TP (2001) Propofol and midazolam in the treatment of refractory status epilepticus. Epilepsia 42:380–386
5. Claassen J, Hirsch LJ, Emerson RG, Bates JE, Thompson TB, Mayer SA (2001) Continuous EEG monitoring and midazolam infusion for nonconvulsive refractory status epilepticus. Neurology 57:1036–1042
6. Bleck TP (1993) Advances in the management of refractory status epilepticus. Crit Care Med 21:955–957
7. Working Group on Status Epilepticus (1993) Treatment of convulsive status epilepticus: recommendations of the Epilepsy Foundation of America's Working Group on Status Epilepticus. JAMA 270:854–859
8. Cascino GD (1996) Generalized convulsive status epilepticus. Mayo Clin Proc 71:787–792
9. Lowenstein DH, Alldredge BK (1998) Status epilepticus. N Engl J Med 338:970–976
10. Shorvon S (1999) Status epilepticus: Its Clinical Features and Treatment in Children and Adults. Cambridge University Press, Cambridge
11. Shorvon S (2000) Emergency treatment of epilepsy: acute seizures, serial seizure clusters and status epilepticus. In: Shorvon S (ed) Handbook of Epilepsy Treatment. Blackwell Science Ltd, Oxford, pp 173–194
12. Alldredge BK, Gelb AM, Isaacs SM, et al (2001) A comparison of lorazepam, diazepam, and placebo for the treatment of out-of-hospital status epilepticus. N Engl J Med 345:631–637
13. Kaplan PW (1999) Assessing the outcomes in patients with nonconvulsive status epilepticus: nonconvulsive status epilepticus is underdiagnosed, potentially overtreated, and confounded by comorbidity. J Clin Neurophysiol 16:341–352
14. DeLorenzo RJ, Waterhouse EJ, Towne AR, et al (1998) Persistent nonconvulsive status epilepticus after the control of convulsive status epilepticus. Epilepsia 39:833–840
15. Kaplan PW (1996) Nonconvulsive status epilepticus in the emergency room. Epilepsia 37:643–650
16. Krumholz A, Sung GY, Fisher RS, Barry E, Bergey GK, Grattan LM (1995) Complex partial status epilepticus accompanied by serious morbidity and mortality. Neurology 45:1499–1504

17. DeLorenzo RJ, Hauser WA, Towne AR, et al (1996) A prospective, population-based epidemiologic study of status epilepticus in Richmond, Virginia. Neurology 46:1029–1035
18. Treiman DM, Meyers PD, Walton NY, et al (1998) A comparison of four treatments for generalized convulsive status epilepticus. Veterans Affairs Status Epilepticus Cooperative Study Group. N Engl J Med 339:792–798
19. Mayer SA, Claassen J, Lokin J, Fitzsimmons BF, Mendehlson F (2002) Predictors of refractory status epilepticus. Arch Neurol (in press)
20. Towne AR, Waterhouse EJ, Boggs JG, et al (2000) Prevalence of nonconvulsive status epilepticus in comatose patients. Neurology 54:340–345
21. Jordan KG (1992) Nonconvulsive seizures (NCS) and nonconvulsive status epilepticus (NCSE) detected by continuous monitoring in the Neuro ICU (NICU-CEEG). Neurology 42:194 (Abst)
22. Claassen J, Hirsch LJ, Emerson RG, Mayer SA (2002) Treatment of refractory status epilepticus with pentobarbital, propofol, or midazolam: A systematic review. Epilepsia (in press)
23. Lowenstein DH, Alldredge BK (1993) Status epilepticus at an urban public hospital in the 1980s. Neurology 43:483–488
24. De Lorenzo RJ, Towne AR, Waterhouse EJ, Morton LD, Garnett LK, Ko D (2001) Refractory status epilepticus: clinical presentations, mortality, and risk factors. Epilepsia 42:144 (Abst)
25. Yaffe K, Lowenstein DH (1993) Prognostic factors of pentobarbital therapy for refractory generalized status epilepticus. Neurology 43:895–900
26. Krishnamurthy KB, Drislane FW (1996) Relapse and survival after barbiturate anesthetic treatment of refractory status epilepticus. Epilepsia 37:863–867
27. Shneker BF, Fountain NB (2001) Epilepsy as chronic sequel of nonconvulsive status epilepticus. Epilepsia 42:147 (Abst)
28. Logroscino G, Hesdorffer DC, Cascino G, Annegers JF, Hauser WA (1997) Short-term mortality after a first episode of status epilepticus. Epilepsia 38:1344–1349
29. Waterhouse EJ, Garnett LK, Towne AR, et al (1999) Prospective population-based study of intermittent and continuous convulsive status epilepticus in Richmond, Virginia. Epilepsia 40:752–758
30. Aminoff MJ, Simon RP (1980) Status epilepticus. Causes, clinical features and consequences in 98 patients. Am J Med 69:657–666
31. Towne AR, Pellock JM, Ko D, DeLorenzo RJ (1994) Determinants of mortality in status epilepticus. Epilepsia 35:27–34
32. Dennis LJ, Claassen J, Connolly ES, et al (2002) Nonconvulsive status epilepticus after subarachnoid hemorrhage. Neurosurgery (in press)
33. Jaitly R, Sgro JA, Towne AR, Ko D, De Lorenzo RJ (1997) Prognostic value of EEG monitoring after status epilepticus: a prospective adult study. J Clin Neurophys 14:326–334
34. Wijdicks EFM (1997) Status epilepticus. In: Wijdicks EFM (ed) The Clinical Practice of Critical Care Neurology. Lippincott-Raven, Philadelphia, pp 279–289
35. Claassen J, Lokin JK, Fitzsimmons BFM, Mendelsohn FA, Mayer SA (2002) Predictors of functional disability and mortality after status epilepticus. Neurology 58:139–142
36. Leppik IE, Derivan AT, Homan RW, Walker J, Ramsay RE, Patrick B (1983) Double-blind study of lorazepam and diazepam in status epilepticus. JAMA 249:1452–1454
37. Treiman DM, Walton NY, Collins JF, Point P (1999) Treatment of status epilepticus if first drug fails. Epilepsia 40:243 (Abst)
38. Rashkin MC, Youngs C, Penovich P (1987) Pentobarbital treatment of refractory status epilepticus. Neurology 37:500–503
39. Lowenstein DH, Aminoff MJ, Simon RP (1988) Barbiturate anesthesia in the treatment of status epilepticus: clinical experience with 14 patients. Neurology 38:395–400
40. Brown LA, Levin GM (1998) Role of propofol in refractory status epilepticus. Ann Pharmacotherapy 32:1053–1059
41. Walker MC, Smith SJM, Shorvon SD (1995) The intensive care treatment of convulsive status epilepticus in the UK. Anaesthesia 50:130–135
42. Sinha S, Naritoku DK (2000) Intravenous valproate is well tolerated in unstable patients with status epilepticus. Neurology 55:722–724
43. Treiman DM. Electroclinical features of status epilepticus (1995) J Clin Neurophys 12:343–362

44. Garzon E, Fernandes RM, Sakamoto AC (2001) Serial EEG during human status epilepticus: evidence for PLED as an ictal pattern. Neurology 57:1175–1183
45. Nei M, Lee J-M, Shanker VL, Sperling MR (1999) The EEG and prognosis in status epilepticus. Epilepsia 40:157–163
46. Treiman DM, Walton NY, Kendrick C (1990) A progressive sequence of electroencephalographic changes during generalized convulsive status epilepticus. Epilepsy Res 5:49–60
47. Assal F, Papazyan JP, Slosman DO, Jallon P, Goerres GW (2001) SPECT in periodic lateralized epileptiform discharges (PLEDs): a form of partial status epilepticus? Seizure 10:260–265
48. Handforth A, Cheng JT, Mandelkern MA, Treiman DM (1994) Markedly increased mesiotemporal lobe metabolism in a case with PLEDs: further evidence that PLEDs are a manifestation of partial status epilepticus. Epilepsia 35:876–81
49. Pohlmann-Eden B, Hoch DB, Cochius JI, Chiappa KH (1996) Periodic lateralized epileptiform discharges – a critical review. J Clin Neurophysiol 13:519–530
50. Yaffe K, Ferriero D, Barkovich AJ, Rowley H (1995) Reversible MRI abnormalities following seizures. Neurology 45:104–108
51. Lazeyras F, Blanke O, Zimine I, Delavelle J, Perrig SH, Seeck M (2000) MRI, (1)H-MRS, and functional MRI during and after prolonged nonconvulsive seizure activity. Neurology 55:1677–1682
52. Chu K, Kang DW, Kim JY, Chang KH, Lee SK (2001) Diffusion-weighted magnetic resonance imaging in nonconvulsive status epilepticus. Arch Neurol 58:993–998
53. Lansberg MG, O'Brien MW, Norbash AM, Moseley ME, Morrell M, Albers GW (1999) MRI abnormalities associated with partial status epilepticus. Neurology 52:1021–1027
54. Petroff OA, Prichard JW, Behar KL, Alger JR, Shulman RG (1984) In vivo phosphorus nuclear magnetic resonance spectroscopy in status epilepticus. Ann Neurol 16:169–177
55. Beattie JL, Passaro EA, Kutluay E (2001) Ictal SPECT in nonconvulsive status epilepticus. Epilepsia 42:70 (Abst)

Neurocognitive Impairment in Survivors of ARDS

R. O. Hopkins

Introduction

Critically ill, mechanically ventilated patients in the intensive care unit (ICU) consume a considerable proportion of medical resources [1]. As intensive care treatment has improved due to advances in medical technology and knowledge, more critically ill patients are surviving. Most outcome studies following intensive care treatment have focused on survival as the major ICU outcome variable. During the past two decades, other outcome variables have emerged as important measures of recovery including physical recovery, respiratory symptoms, pulmonary function, health-related quality of life (HRQL), neurocognitive function, and affect. Recent studies indicate that critically ill patients experience impaired HRQL and psychosocial impairments following treatment in the ICU [1–3]. Reports also indicate that mechanically ventilated patients reported anxiety [4] and painful or unpleasant experiences due to respiratory treatment [5]. Forty percent of ICU survivors were unable to return to work due to physical and/or psychosocial problems [6]. One limitation of most outcome research on ICU survivors is the heterogeneity of the patient groups, so outcome data for specific ICU patient populations, such as survivors of acute respiratory distress syndrome (ARDS), is limited.

Acute Respiratory Distress Syndrome

Severe acute lung injury (ALI) and profound arterial hypoxemia characterize ARDS, which is often refractory to supplemental oxygen. The American-European Consensus Conference on ARDS [7] defined criteria for ARDS. ARDS was defined as acute onset of an illness accompanied by an ARDS risk factor, PaO_2/FiO_2 ratio <200 mmHg, bilateral infiltrates on chest radiographs, and no evidence of left atrial hypertension. Chest radiographs show widespread alveolar infiltrates and physiologic abnormalities, including severe hypoxemia, right-to-left blood shunting, and decreased pulmonary compliance [8]. ARDS is often accompanied by multiple organ dysfunction including central nervous system (CNS) dysfunction. ARDS may occur in response to various direct or indirect insults to the lung, including sepsis, trauma, massive transfusions, aspiration, pneumonia, and other medical or surgical conditions [9]. Hudson and colleagues compared risk factors to the incidence of ARDS, and found that patients with sepsis syndrome and multiple transfusions had the highest incidence of ARDS [10].

The incidence of ARDS in the United States is approximately 5 per 100,000 cases per year [11]. Despite progress in supportive care, ARDS mortality rates vary between 40% and 90%, [8, 12, 13] and have been reported to be as high as 90% in patients with both ARDS and sepsis [14]. However, recent studies have suggested that mortality associated with ARDS is declining. A retrospective review of all ARDS cases found that ARDS mortality rates declined between 1983 and 1993 from 68 to 36% [15].

A number of studies have looked at a variety of factors that may predict mortality following ARDS. Montgomery and colleagues found that sepsis syndrome was the leading cause of mortality in ARDS patients [12]. Lee et al. [16] used APACHE II scores, lung injury scores (LIS), and sepsis to predict mortality following ARDS and found that sepsis was the only predictor of mortality. Similarly, the mortality rate for patients with risk factors and ARDS was 69% compared to 19% for patients with risk factors alone [10]. One report found that the patients' response to treatment of hypoxemia on the first day determined mortality in 68–75% of ARDS cases [17]. Finally, a study of ARDS patients found a 65% mortality in patients with a history of alcohol abuse compared to 36% for non-alcoholics [18].

▌ Pulmonary Function

Initial outcome studies of ARDS used survival as the major outcome variable (see above). Only limited information exists concerning intermediate outcomes, including pulmonary function. An early report in a small group of ARDS survivors noted that those patients who reported dyspnea, either at rest or on exertion, were either unable to return to work or had to change occupation as a result of their pulmonary insult [19]. Elliot et al. [20] reported impaired pulmonary function, including impaired lung diffusion capacity for carbon monoxide (D_{LCO}). Prior studies have reported impaired pulmonary function [9], and severe restrictive impairments and abnormalities in D_{LCO} following ARDS [21]. Alternatively, pulmonary function was impaired initially, progressively improved to 6 months, with no further improvement after 6 months [22]. Current research indicates that a large percentage of ARDS survivors experience persistent reductions in D_{LCO} and restrictive lung deficits that range in severity from mild to severe. Alternatively some ARDS patients' lung volumes and flow appear to return to normal limits. However, these studies suggest that many ARDS survivors have persistent pulmonary function test abnormalities that persist over time.

▌ Health Related Quality of Life (HRQL)

During the past two decades, quality of life has emerged as an important measure of recovery from a variety of disease states, and to evaluate patient outcomes. For example, activities of daily living were severely impaired at the time of hospital discharge but ARDS patients had no limitations in activities of daily living at one year [23]. Physical recovery following ARDS appears to be complete 6 to 12 months post discharge, however, impairments in HRQL persist. McHugh et al. [24] assessed HRQL in ARDS survivors, and found that pulmonary function and total health improved dramatically at three months, stabilized at six months, with mild but continued improvement at 1 year. Age was related to improved HRQL, with patients less than 40 years old reporting improvement in HRQL while those over 40 years old did not show improvements [24]. A prospective study of ARDS survivors reported decreased HRQL, including impairments in physical health, social role, pain and physical role, but not in emotional or mental health, bodily pain and general health [23]. Other investigators following ARDS [25] and ALI [26] have reported similar findings. Davidson and colleagues compared ARDS patients to trauma patients matched for injury severity and found that the ARDS patient had significantly worse HRQL and reported more respiratory symptoms than controls [27].

▌ Neuropsychological Outcome

Neurocognitive and psychological outcome have only recently been assessed in survivors of ARDS. However, qualitative data from previous ARDS studies indicate that the patients were reporting neurocognitive complaints including impaired memory, nightmares, anxiety, and sleep disruption [26]. The first report of neurocognitive outcome was a study of two patients with Hantavirus pulmonary syndrome (HPS) who met the American Thoracic Society (ATS) criteria for ARDS [28]. The HPS patients experienced severe hypoxemia and concomitant neurocognitive impairments at hospital discharge and one year post-hospital discharge. Both patients demonstrated cognitive impairments, including verbal and non-verbal memory impairments, with some cognitive deficits that improved at 1-year follow-up, whereas other deficits persisted. One patient had impaired abstract reasoning, decreased mental processing speed and severe verbal and visual memory deficits. At one year, her speed of processing and abstract reasoning skills improved, but she still exhibited significant memory impairments. Blood gas data showed that her mean PaO_2 was 60.9±13.9 mmHg. The second patient had impairments in memory, math, visual-spatial skills, and slow mental processing speed. Blood gas data showed that his mean PaO_2 was 55.9±11.1 mmHg. At one year he exhibited little change [28]. This study indicated that hantavirus syndrome with severe HPS and hypoxemia can result in persistent impairments in neurocognitive function.

Hopkins et al. [23] assessed neurocognitive outcome in 55 ARDS survivors using a prospective within subjects design. The risk factors for the ARDS survivors included sepsis, pneumonia, trauma, aspiration, pancreatitis, and near drowning. There were 25 males and 30 females in the group, with a mean age of 45.5±16.0 years (range = 16 to 78 years) and mean education level of 12.8±2.0 years (range = 8 to 18 years). The mean APACHE II score was 18 ± 6.5 and a mean length of stay in the respiratory ICU of 27.7 days. None of the ARDS survivors had traumatic brain injuries, demyelinating diseases, encephalitis, strokes, or previous episodes of anoxia.

Excluding those patients who died during the first year, the follow-up rate at one year was 94%. A battery of neuropsychological tests was administered that assessed intelligence, memory, attention, executive function, mental processing speed, and visual-spatial abilities. At the time of hospital discharge, 100% of the patients experienced cognitive impairments, including problems with memory, attention, concentration, and global loss of cognitive function. At one-year follow-up, 30% of the patients experienced impaired general intelligence and 78% at least one of the following; impaired memory, attention, concentration and/or mental processing speed (48%) [23]. At one year, only 19% had impaired intellectual function. Forty percent of the ARDS patients had impaired executive function and 42% of patients experienced decreased speed of mental processing. ARDS patients reported that they had problems remembering appointments, what to buy at the grocery store, and what they read. ARDS survivors reported difficulty remembering and following directions, that they forget they are cooking until they smell food burning, and forget their destination when driving [23].

Continuous oxygen saturation data were automatically collected through the connection of bedside pulse oximetry to a clinical data management computer. The oxygen saturations were sampled every 2 min and a 15 min floating median was recorded. In the ARDS patients, pulse oximetry was measured for a total of 31,665 h, with a mean of 609±423 h. The patients' mean saturation's (<90% = 122±144 h, <85% = 13±18 h, and <80% = 1±3 h) showed that the patients were hypoxemic for a significant amount of time. Hypoxemia was significantly correlated with neurocognitive outcome including attention, memory, intelligence, speed of processing, visual-spatial skills (block design), and executive function at one year. No correlations were found between neurocognitive outcome and markers of illness severity such as APACHE II, mean PaO_2, mean inspired fraciton of oxygen (FiO_2), length of mechanical ventilation, ICU length of stay, or hospital length of stay [23].

A study that retrospectively assessed neuropsychological performance in 33 ARDS survivors compared them with a cohort of 24 critically ill control patients matched for risk factors of sepsis and trauma [29]. The subjects were administered a battery of neurocognitive tests and the results indicated cognitive impairments similar to those reported by Hopkins and colleagues [23]. The ARDS survivors had significantly greater impairments in attention, visual processing, psychomotor speed, and cognitive flexibility compared to the critically ill control patients. The authors conclude: "Factors specific to the disease process or complications of ARDS may be responsible for some neuropsychiatric sequelae observed in these patients." [29].

A recent study by Rothenhausler and colleagues [30] retrospectively assessed 46 ICU survivors who met the ARDS criteria of the American-European Consensus Conference [7] for cognitive performance, and employment status, as well as HRQL. The patients were assessed an average of 6.4±3.2 years post ICU discharge (median = 6.0 years). The patients' mean age was 41.5±14.7 years, with a mean LIS of 3.2±0.3, mean APACHE II score of 22.8±5.9, and were in the ICU for an average of 32.3±21.1 days. The patients were assessed by the SKT (Syndrom Kurztest) test, a brief measure of attention and memory and psychosocial interview. Twenty-four percent of the patients had cognitive impairments most prominently on measures of attention, however 41% of the patients were disabled from work. Given that the patients' mean age was 41 years and assuming a normal life expectancy, the loss of income to these patients and their families, not to mention the financial impact to society, is high. All of the patients with cognitive impairments were disabled, indicating that the cognitive impairments contribute significantly to the inability to work. All of the patients were impaired for HRQL when compared to normative population data. The patients with cognitive deficits reported the lowest HRQL. Of interest is the fact that disability was found in 41% of the patients whereas cognitive impairments were only reported in 24% of the patients. The SKT assesses attention and memory but not other cognitive functions such as mental processing speed, mental flexibility, executive function, psychomotor speed, or visual-spatial abilities, to name a few. Thus, the 17% of patients with disability may have had other cognitive impairments that were not assessed in this study [30]. The cognitive impairments were not related to markers of illness severity such as APACHE II scores, use of extracorporeal membrane oxygenation (ECMO), day intubated, or risk factors, which is similar to the findings of a previous study [23]. Long-term survivors of ARDS continue to report decreased HRQL, cognitive impairments and inability to return to work.

Psychological Outcome

The interplay between systemic medical illness and mood disorders has been reported in the literature for years. Evidence that mood disorders are associated with medical illness is accumulating and the data suggest that there is a wide variability in the prevalence rates [31]. One study found that illness severity and degree of functional disability were associated with the development of depressive illness [32]. It is estimated that depression affects 12.6% of patients seen in a general medical practice, however, affective changes appear to be more common in patients with pulmonary disorders. Depression occurs at rates as high as 43% in patients with chronic obstructive pulmonary disease (COPD) and 40% in patients with obstructive sleep apnea syndrome [33]. Patients with COPD frequently report depression [34, 35] and anxiety [36, 37]. Similar findings have been found in patients with obstructive sleep apnea syndrome [38, 39]. Several studies have assessed psychological outcome in ARDS survivors. For example, Wienert and colleagues [26] found that 15 months after the diagnosis of ALI, 75% of the patients reported symptoms of depression and 15 months later 2.25% of the ARDS patients still had scores indicating depression [26]. Hopkins et al. [23] assessed affect using the Beck Depression Inventory (BDI) and Beck Anxiety Inventory (BAI). The ARDS patients BDI and BAI at one year were within normal limits, indicating that overall the ARDS patients do not report clinical levels of depression or anxiety. Although the total ARDS group had normal BDI and BAI scores, 48% of the patients reported elevated symptoms of anxiety and depression (BDI and BAI scores greater than 10) [23].

Treatment in the ICU can be extremely stressful and ICU survivors have reported distressing memories of the ICU [26]. In a retrospective study, Schelling and colleagues [25] assessed 80 ARDS patients for adverse ICU experiences and their effect on the development of posttraumatic stress disorder [25]. The ARDS patients were administered questionnaires to assess posttraumatic stress disorder and the number of adverse ICU experiences they remembered. The ARDS patients reported traumatic experiences during ICU therapy including nightmares, anxiety and pain, which were associated with posttraumatic stress disorder and impaired HRQL. Those patients that reported two or more adverse experiences developed significant posttraumatic stress disorder and reported worse general health compared to the patients who reported no or one adverse experience. Like previous studies, this study found decreased HRQL, and the development of posttraumatic stress disorder in a substantial number of the ARDS patients who reported adverse ICU experiences [25].

A second study by the German group was carried out to validate the use of a measure of posttraumatic stress disorder using a structured psychiatric interview in ARDS patients using a retrospective cohort design [40]. The Post-Traumatic Stress Syndrome 10-Question Inventory proved to be a reliable and valid instrument for use in assessing the development of posttraumatic stress disorder in ARDS survivors. They found that 23% of ALI survivors developed posttraumatic stress disorder 2 years after ICU discharge, and there was a significant relationship between traumatic memories and the development of posttraumatic stress disorder [40]. These results indicate that a subset of ARDS patients may experience depression, anxiety, and posttraumatic stress disorder that may impact on cognitive function and employment.

▌ Etiology of Neurocognitive Impairment

We do not fully understand the etiology(s) of ARDS-induced brain injury, but hypoxemic episodes and/or reduced cerebral perfusion are undoubtedly implicated. One possible cause of the cognitive impairments is hypoxia or hypoxemia. Our previous study has shown that cognitive sequelae were associated with hypoxia due to ARDS as measured by continuous pulse oximetry [23]. Other pulmonary disorders characterized by hypoxia result in cognitive impairments including COPD [34–36, 41], following cardiac and/or respiratory arrest [42–44] and obstructive sleep apnea syndrome [45, 46]. Hypoxia has been shown to cause impaired attention and concentration, memory, and visual-spatial deficits similar to what we observed in the ARDS survivors. Hypoxia may also result in neuropathological changes like hippocampal atrophy [42–44, 47]. The degree of cognitive impairment appears to parallel the degree of morphologic abnormality as demonstrated by quantitative magnetic resonance image (MRI) analysis [47]. Given that ARDS patients often experience prolonged periods of hypoxia along with the known sensitivity of the temporal lobe limbic structures to hypoxia, it is possible that ARDS survivors may develop cognitive impairments similar to those observed in other patients who have experienced hypoxia.

An alternative explanation for the cognitive impairments following ARDS are toxic or metabolic effects, such as cytokines and inflammation, and associated disorders (e.g., sepsis) that may result in brain injury. Severe sepsis is associated with acute organ dysfunction due to generalized inflammatory and procoagulant response to infection [48]. For example Capuron and associates [49] found that memory impairments were commonly associated with infectious diseases [49]. Patients with sepsis in a randomized, double-blind, placebo-controlled clinical trial [50] were given activated protein C (APC, drotrecogin alfa activated) for 96 hours. APC inhibits thrombosis and inflammation and is an important modulator of coagulation and inflammation associated with severe sepsis [51]. Bernard and colleagues [50] found that APC significantly reduced mortality in patients with severe sepsis. It is unknown if treatment with APC may also reduce cognitive dysfunction. Interestingly, a study that induced cytokine activation in healthy male volunteers using intravenous injection of *Salmonella abortus equi* endotoxin, found increased levels of anxiety, depressed mood, and decreased verbal and non-verbal memory [52]. The cognitive and psychological changes were positively correlated with endotoxin-induced cytokine secretion. A study of patients with chronic fatigue syndrome with elevated cytokine levels found that the cytokine levels were related to self-reported cognitive difficulties (e.g. attention, concentration, and memory), and to anxiety and depression [53].

A study that assessed long-term outcome following sepsis and multiple organ failure (MOF) found that three out of five patients experienced cognitive impairment [54]. In addition, inflammatory processes have be implicated in the pathogenesis of degenerative changes and cognitive impairments associated with Alzheimer's Disease [55]. A study that assessed the effects of chronic inflammation in rats resulted in damage to the basal forebrain, temporal lobe and hippocampus, as well as a significant impairment in spatial memory [56]. The toxic or metabolic effects on brain function following ARDS are largely unknown. It is also possible that the combination of hypoxemia and sepsis in ARDS survivors results in more severe impairments than either hypoxemia or sepsis alone.

■ Conclusion

ARDS is a life-threatening illness with a high mortality rate. ARDS survivors exhibit impaired HRQL, cognitive impairments due to brain injury, and some ARDS survivors report increased depression, anxiety, and posttraumatic stress disorder. Impaired HRQL appears to be related to the severity of the ARDS, underlying disease, and impairments in pulmonary function. Symptoms of posttraumatic stress disorder and depression are related to ICU treatment, administration of sedative and neuromuscular agents, and adverse memories of the ICU. Cognitive impairment, including memory, executive function and mental processing speed due to disease processes are also related to decreased HRQL and work disability. The cognitive impairments experienced by our ARDS survivors make it difficult to return to work in jobs that require processing of complex cognitive information, rapid response times, and make large demands on the memory system. The cognitive impairments appear to persist for years following ARDS, indicating that they may be permanent. Further research is warranted to establish the etiology(s) of the brain injury observed in ARDS survivors. Research should be designed to determine whether treatments that decrease illness severity (i.e., treatment of hypoxia, inflammation, cytokines, ischemia, emboli, etc.), new sedative drugs that increase calm alertness (i.e., zyprexa) that may decrease ICU stress, and treatment with antidepressants or interventions to help patients cope with ICU stress, may improve cognitive function, HRQL, depression, and decrease the incidence of posttraumatic stress disorder in ARDS survivors.

References

1. Spicher E, White DP (1987) Outcome and function following prolonged mechanical ventilation. Arch Intern Med 147:421–425
2. Konopad E, Noseworth TW, Johnston R, Shustack A, Grace M (1995) Quality of life measures before and one year after admission to an intensive care unit. Crit Care Med 23:1653–1659
3. Tian ZM, Miranda DR (1995) Quality of life after intensive care with the sickness impact profile. Intensive Care Med 21:422–428
4. McCartney JR, Boland RJ (1994) Anxiety and delirium in the intensive care unit. Crit Care Clin 19:673–680
5. Bergbom-Engberg I, Haljamae H (1989) Assessment of patients' experience of discomforts during respirator therapy. Crit Care Med 17:1068–1072
6. Goldstein RL, Campion EW, Thibault GE, Mulley AG, Skinner E (1989) Functional outcomes following medical intensive care. Crit Care Med 14:783–788
7. Bernard GR, Artigas A, Brigham KL, et al (1994) The American-European consensus conference on ARDS: Definitions, mechanisms, relevant outcomes, and clinical trial coordination. Am J Respir Crit Care Med 149:818–824
8. Murray JF, Matthay MA, Luce JM, Flick MR (1988) An expanded definition of the adult respiratory distress syndrome. Am Rev Respir Dis 138:720–723
9. Suchyta M, Clemmer T, Elliott CG, Orme JJ, Weaver L (1993) The adult respiratory distress syndrome. A report of survival and modifying factors. Chest 104:647–648
10. Hudson LD, Milberg JA, Anardi D, Maunder RJ (1995) Clinical risks for development of acute respiratory distress syndrome. Am J Respir Crit Care Med 151:293–301
11. Thomsen GE, Morris AH (1995) Incidence of the adult respiratory distress syndrome in the state of Utah. Am J Respir Crit Care Med 152:965–971
12. Montgomery AB, Stager MA, Carrico CJ, Hudson LD (1985) Causes of mortality in patients with the adult respiratory distress syndrome. Am Rev Respir Dis 132:485–489
13. Petty TL, Ashbaugh DG (1971) The adult respiratory distress syndrome: Clinical features factors influencing prognosis, and principles of management. Chest 60:233–239

14. Fein AM, Lippman M, Holzman H, Eliraz A, Goldberg SK (1983) The risk factors, incidence, and prognosis of the adult respiratory distress syndrome following septicemia. Chest 83:40–42
15. Milberg JA, Davis DR, Steinberg KP, Hudson LD (1995) Improved survival of patients with acute respiratory distress syndrome (ARDS): 1983–1993. JAMA 273:306–309
16. Lee J, Turner S, Morgan CJ, Keogh BF, Evans TW (1994) Adult respiratory distress syndrome: has there been a change in outcome predictive measures? Thorax 49:596–597
17. Gondos T, Szabo K, Jokkel G, Penzes I (1991) Outcome prediction in adult respiratory distress syndrome using discriminant analysis of cardiorespiratory data. Acta Med Hug 48:51–60
18. Moss M, Bucher B, Moore FA, Moore EE, Parsons PE (1996) The role of chronic alcohol abuse in the development of acute respiratory distress syndrome in adults. JAMA 275:50–54
19. Halvey A, Sirik Z, Adam YG, Leewinsohn G (1984) Long-term evaluation of patients following the Adult Respiratory Distress Syndrome. Respir Care 29:132–137
20. Elliott CG, Rassmusson BY, Crapo RO, Morris AH, Jensen RL (1987) Prediction of pulmonary function abnormalities after adult respiratory distress syndrome (ARDS). Am Rev Respir Dis 135:634–638
21. Peters JI, Bell RC, Prihoda TJ, Harris G, Andrews C, Johansen WG (1989) Clinical determinants of abnormalities in pulmonary function in survivors of the adult respiratory distress syndrome. Am Rev Respir Dis 139:1163–1168
22. Hudson LD (1994) What happens to survivors of the adult respiratory distress syndrome? Chest 105:26S (Abst)
23. Hopkins RO, Weaver LK, Pope D, Orme JF Jr, Bigler ED, Larson-Lohr V (1999) Neuropsychological sequelae and impaired health status in survivors of severe acute respiratory distress syndrome. Am J Respir Crit Care Med 160:50–56
24. McHugh LG, Milberg JA, Whitcomb ME, Schoene RB, Maunder RJ, Hudson LD (1994) Recovery of function in survivors of the acute respiratory distress syndrome. Am J Respir Crit Care Med 150:90–4
25. Schelling G, Stoll C, Haller M, et al (1998) Health-related quality of life and post-traumatic stress disorder in survivors of the acute respiratory distress syndrome (ARDS). Crit Care Med 25:651–659
26. Wienert CR, Gross C, Kangas JR, Bury CR, Marinelli WA (1997) Health-related quality of life after acute lung injury. Am J Respir Crit Care Med 156:1120–1128
27. Davidson TA, Caldwell ES, Curtis JR, Hudson LD, Steinberg KP (1999) Reduced quality of life in survivors of acute respiratory distress syndrome compared with critically ill control patients. JAMA 281:354–360
28. Hopkins RO, Larson-Lohr V, Weaver LK, Bigler ED (1998) Neuropsychological impairments following hantavirus pulmonary syndrome. J Int Neuropsychological Soc 4:190–196
29. Marquis KA, Curtis JR, Caldwell ES, et al (2000) Neuropsychologic sequelae in survivors of ARDS compared with critically ill control patients. Am J Respir Crit Care Med 16:A383 (Abst)
30. Rothenhausler HB, Ehrentraut S, Stoll C, Schelling G, Kapfhammer HP (2001) The relationship between cognitive performance and employment and health status in long-term survivors of the acute respiratory distress syndrome: results of an exploratory study. Gen Hosp Psychiatry 23:90–96
31. Popkin MK, Andrews JE (1997) Mood disorders secondary to systemic medical conditions. Semin Clin Neuropsychiatry 2:296–306
32. Jackson R, Baldwin B (1993) Detecting depression in elderly medically ill patients: the use of the Geriatric Depression Scale compared with medical and nursing observations. Age Ageing 22:349–353
33. Reynolds CF, Kupfer DJ, McEachran AB, Taska LS, Sewitch DE, Coble PA (1984) Depressive psychopathology in male sleep apneics. J Clin Psychiatry 45:287–290
34. Krass I, Dyksterhuis JE, Rubin H, Patel K (1975) Correlation of psycholophysiologic variables with vocational rehabilitation outcome in patients with chronic obstructive pulmonary disease. Chest 67:433–440
35. Prigatano GP, Parsons O, Levin DC, Wright E, Hawryluk G (1983) Neuropsychological test performance in mildly hypoxemic patients with chronic obstructive pulmonary disease. J Consult Clin Psychology 51:108–116

36. Heaton RK, Grant I, McSweeny AJ, Adams KM, Petty TL (1983) Psychologic effects of continuous and nocturnal oxygen therapy in hypoxemic chronic obstructive pulmonary disease. Arch Intern Med 143:1941–1947

37. Prigatano G, Wright D, Levin D (1984) Quality of life and its predictors in patients with mild hypoxemia and chronic obstructive pulmonary disease. Arch Intern Med 144:1613–1619

38. Beutler LE, Ware JC, Karacan I, Thornby JI (1981) Differentiating psychological characteristics of patients with sleep apnea and narcolepsy. Sleep 4:39–47

39. Klonoff H, Fleetham J, Raylor R, Clark C (1987) Treatment outcome of obstructive sleep apnea. J Nervous Mental Dis 175:208–212

40. Stoll C, Kapfhammer HP, Rothenhausler HB, et al (1999) Sensitivity and specificity of a screening test to document traumatic experiences and to diagnose post-traumatic stress disorder in ARDS patients after intensive care treatment. Intensive Care Med 25:697–704

41. Grant I, Heaton R, McSweeny A, Adams K, Timms R (1982) Neuropsychological findings in hypoxemic chronic obstructive pulmonary disease. Arch Intern Med 142:1470–1476

42. Hopkins RO, Kesner RP, Goldstein M (1995) Memory for novel and familiar spatial and linguistic temporal distance information in hypoxic subjects. J Int Neuropsychological Soc 1:454–468

43. Kesner RP, Hopkins RO (2001) Short-term memory for duration and distance in humans: Role of the hippocampus. Neuropsychology 15:58–68

44. Press GA, Amaral DG, Squire LR (1986) Hippocampal abnormalities in amnesic patients revealed by high-resolution magnetic resonance imaging. Nature 341:54–57

45. Findley LJ, Barth JT, Powers DC, Wilhor SC, Boyd DG, Suratt PS (1986) Cognitive impairments in patients with obstructive sleep apnea and associated hypoxemia. Chest 90:686–690

46. Bedard M, Montplaisir J, Richer F, Roulea I, Malo J (1991) Obstructive sleep apnea syndrome: Pathogenesis of neuropsychological deficits. J Clin Exp Neuropsychiatry 13:950–964

47. Hopkins RO, Gale SD, Johnson SC, Anderson CV, Bigler ED, Blatter DD (1995) Severe anoxia with and without concomitant brain atrophy and neuropsychological impairments. J Int Neuropsychology Soc 1:501–509

48. Bone RC, Grodzin CJ, Balk RA (1997) Sepsis: a new hypothesis for pathogenesis of the disease process. Chest 112:235–243

49. Capuron L, Lamarque D, Dantzer R, Goodall G (1999) Attentional and mnemonic deficit associated with infectious disease in humans. Psychol Med 29:291–297

50. Bernard GR, Vincent JL, Laterre PF, et al (2001) Efficacy and safety of recombinant human activated protein C for severe sepsis. N Engl J Med 344:699–709

51. Esmon CT (1992) The protein C anticoagulant pathway. Arterioscler Thromb 12:135–145

52. Reichenberg A, Yirmiya R, Schuld A, et al (2001) Cytokine-associated emotional and cognitive disturbances in humans. Arch Gen Psychiatry 58:445–452

53. Patarca-Montero R, Antoni M, Fletcher MA, Klimas NG (2001) Cytokine and other immunologic markers in chronic fatigue syndrome and their relation to neuropsychological factors. Appl Neuropsychol 8:51–64

54. Sieser A, Schwarx S, Brainin M (1992) Critical illness polyneuropathy: clinical aspects and long-term outcome. Wien Klin Wochenschr 104:294–300

55. McGeer PL, Akiyama H, Itagaki S, McGeer EG (1989) Immune system response in Alzheimer's disease. Can J Neurol Sci 16:516–527

56. Hauss-Wegrzyniak B, Dobrzanski P, Stoehr JD, Wenk GL (1998) Chronic neuroinflammation in rats reproduces components of the neurobiology of Alzheimer's disease. Brain Res 780:294–303

Abdominal Crises

Immunomodulatory Treatment of Severe Acute Pancreatitis

T. Dugernier, M. S. Reynaert, and P. F. Laterre

▌ Introduction

Severe acute pancreatitis is characterized by multiple-system organ failure (MOF) that emerges early after onset of disease, and local complications, in particular pancreatic infection, that usually supervene later in the course of the attack.

Despite advances in intensive care therapy, better delineation of surgical indications, and refinements in percutaneous, endoscopic, and operative procedures for drainage of infected necrotic areas, the course of severe acute pancreatitis remains taxed with a prohibitive morbidity and mortality. Organ dysfunction occurs in one in four patients with acute pancreatitis and the mortality associated with severe acute pancreatitis still ranges between 10 to 60% depending primarily upon the presence of sterile or infected pancreatic necrosis [1]. The two major determinants of outcome are the intensity of early MOF and the extent of (peri)pancreatic necrosis, as a third of the mortality can be ascribed to the former, while infected pancreatic necrosis, whose incidence is closely related to the volume of necrotic areas, accounts for the bulk of deaths [1].

Besides the premature intra-acinar activation of pancreatic proenzymes and a local microcirculatory impairment, the excessive stimulation of immune effector cells has been increasingly postulated as a critical pathophysiological mechanism creating an intense local inflammatory response and secondary retroperitoneal tissue injury [2]. In addition, the amplification of the local inflammatory necrotizing process through the activation of a complex network of proinflammatory pathways and mediators acting in concert and the secondary induction of exaggerated systemic inflammatory response have emerged as the central mechanism of early distant organ damage in recent years (Fig. 1). In the past decade, an improved knowledge of the pathophysiological mechanisms underlying local and remote tissue injury have oriented, at last, care that was exclusively supportive and empirical to a more directed therapeutic approach to severe acute pancreatitis. Early endoscopic sphincterotomy to dislodge impacted stones in severe acute biliary pancreatitis, antibioprophylaxis or/and selective digestive decontamination (SDD) to reduce the incidence of pancreatic infection, and early nutritional support by the jejunal route to promote gut barrier function and to lessen potential bacterial translocation, are all components of this new therapeutic strategy. However, in part because patients seek medical attention long after initiating events have occurred, reduction of pancreatic exocrine secretion and antiprotease therapy has failed to convey any benefit in clinical studies despite encouraging results in experimental pancreatitis, and direct manipulation of the glandular microcirculation has never been attempted in humans [3]. Thus, a specific treatment able to interfere early with the major determinants of outcome of these patients is still eagerly awaited.

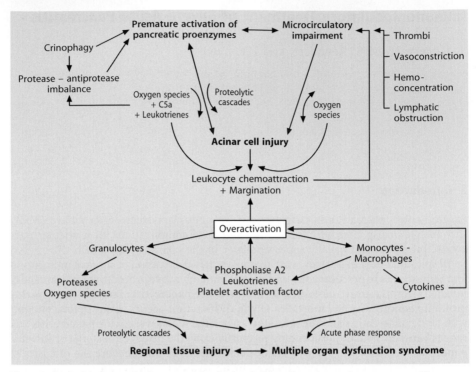

Fig. 1. Pathophysiological mechanisms underlying local and distant tissue damage in acute pancreatitis

In this context modulation of the inflammatory response to initial acinar cell injury is expected theoretically to prevent distant organ damage, to limit the extent of the local necrotizing process that creates the culture medium for bacterial proliferation, and ultimately to improve survival.

This chapter will focus on the experimental and clinical evidence of the role of excessive stimulation of immune effector cells in mediating local and remote tissue injury in severe acute pancreatitis and also will address the results of immunomodulating therapy in both experimental pancreatitis and the clinical setting.

▎ Role of Overactivation of Leukocytes in Experimental Acute Pancreatitis

Despite considerable progress in understanding the pathophysiology of acute pancreatitis, the mechanisms of development of this disease remain obscure, in particular those leading from a localized pancreatic necrosis and inflammation into a systemic response and MOF. Historically the progression of pancreatitis has been attributed to premature activation of digestive enzymes in acinar cells, resulting in glandular autodigestion and subsequent spillage into the circulation. The key role has been devoted to trypsin which, if uninhibited, is able to activate both pancreatic proenzymes and the inflammatory cascade systems leading to the release of large amounts of vasoactive substances thought to be responsible for remote organ dysfunction.

However, acute pancreatitis involves a complex cascade of events and there are likely numerous local and systemic mediators of tissue damage (Fig. 1).

Interleukin (IL)-1 and tumor necrosis factor (TNF) are the 'first-order' mediators in the host response to acute cell injury. Although essential for normal defense against noxious stimuli and control of both cellular function and interactions in an autocrine or paracrine fashion, tissue overproduction and secondary systemic spill-over of these cytokines may result in local and widespread deleterious effects. Rinderknecht first hypothesized that cytokines may play a fundamental role in the pathophysiology of acute pancreatitis and that the complicated course and fatal outcome of some of these patients was not primarily due to autodigestion of the pancreas by prematurely activated enzymes, but to excessive leukocyte stimulation following the initial acinar cell injury [2].

Only a few immune effector cells are present in the interstitium of the normal pancreas and TNF mRNA and its protein product are normally not detectable in the gland [4]. In a number of different experimental models, gene induction of IL-1 and TNF and protein production occurred prior to significant changes in pancreatic histology as early as 30 minutes after initiation of pancreatitis and peaked hours after onset of the attack [4, 5]. Actually, production of both cytokines started first in the pancreatic parenchyma and then was observed after a significant delay within the systemic circulation and in specific distant organs including the lungs, liver, and spleen [4]. These data suggest that tissue resident and infiltrating activated inflammatory cells, rather than circulating leukocytes, play the major role in organ-specific cytokine production [4]. The rise and fall of these cytokines mimicked the development and resolution of the disease. Cytokine concentrations were several orders of magnitude higher in the pancreatic tissue than in the serum, indicating a site of production located in the gland [4]. These findings were corroborated by Grewal et al. [6] who showed higher levels of TNF in the portal vein of animals than time-matched concentrations obtained from the hepatic vein or peripheral blood. In a pancreatitis model of graded severity that was induced with a combination of caerulein and controlled intraductal infusion of glycodeoxycholic acid, the time course of leukocyte accumulation in the pancreas and distant organs was determined by technetium-99m-labeled white blood cells (WBC) and tissue myeloperoxidase activity [7]. In severe grades of pancreatitis, marked leukocyte accumulation and myeloperoxidase activity were found in the pancreas and in the lung as early as 3 hours after induction of the attack. Microscopic studies substantiated these findings and demonstrated an early glandular invasion by monocytes and polymorphonuclear (PMN) cells in necrotizing pancreatitis [5]. Using immunohistochemistry and depletion of specific leukocyte populations, most IL-1 and TNF seemed to be produced by macrophages, infiltrating monocytes and PMNs even if pancreatic acinar cells were shown also to synthesize and release TNF, platelet activating factor (PAF) and chemokines such as monocyte chemoattractant protein (MCP)-1 and RANTES [8–10].

Levels of the proximal cytokines correlated with the severity of pancreatitis and outcome as well as with the development of remote organ dysfunction [4]. The production of IL-1 and TNF triggers several proinflammatory cascades locally and at distant sites, upgrades the expression of adhesion molecules on vascular endothelium in the gland and remote organs, and finally recruits and activates inflammatory cells, in particular neutrophils, that first invade the pancreas within 2–3 h after induction of the attack and subsequently infiltrate distant organs. This excessive stimulation of immune effector cells results in the release of a variety of potentially damaging inflammatory mediators including other cytokines, chemokines, activated oxygen species, proteases, phospholipase A2, PAF, leukotrienes, nitric oxide (NO), and adhesion molecules whose serum, pancreatic, and distant tissue levels or activities were closely associated with the severity of pancreatic, and remote, damage [8, 10–12].

Together with this proinflammatory axis the body mounts anti-inflammatory mechanisms through the release of cytokines with downregulating features (e.g., IL-4, IL-10, transforming growth factor [TGF]-β, IL-1 receptor antagonist [IL-1ra], soluble TNF receptors) in an attempt to restore a delicate balance between pro- and anti-inflammatory mediators. In severe cases it can be envisaged that depending upon this balance, the array of mediators contributes to a spiral of events which aggravate local and remote tissue damage and perpetuate cellular activation through complex signaling and numerous positive feedback circuits that involve several types of cells to sustain and amplify the activity of the inflammatory response. In particular, decreased pancreatic and generalized microcirculatory perfusion and secondary ischemia may be attributed in part to excessive leukocyte-endothelium interaction in postcapillary venules.

The pivotal and deleterious role of these proximal proinflammatory cytokines is further compounded with the mode of cell death they mediate, as the latter may impact significantly on the severity of the attack. Using a perfused human pancreas, although neither IL-1 nor TNF was able to induce biochemical or histological evidence of acute pancreatitis, acinar cells when they were exposed to concentrations that are typically found in the gland during pancreatitis, became apoptotic instead of undergoing necrosis [8, 13]. Actually TNF concurrently induces pro- and anti-apoptotic mechanisms in acinar cells. Anti-apoptotic mechanisms are mediated by activation of the transcription factor nuclear factor-κB (NF-κB) and several mitogen-activated protein kinases (MAPK) [14]. Whereas complete TNF neutralization inhibited apoptosis, the administration of pro-apoptotic substances has been shown to decrease the severity of experimental pancreatitis [8, 15]. So, although not involved in the early stage of acinar cell injury, these proximal proinflammatory cytokines released by both pancreatic acinar cells and resident/infiltrating macrophages, recruit and activate inflammatory cells in the area and induce both apoptotic and necrotic cell death in a variable proportion. Although the role of apoptosis during this disease remains unclear, several lines of evidence indicate that the severity of acute pancreatitis is closely related to the degree of necrosis in the pancreas whereas an inverse relationship can be found with apoptosis [15]. The latter may thus be protective as, contrary to necrosis, it does not trigger the inflammatory response.

As none of the 'first-line' proinflammatory cytokines are able *per se* to induce acute pancreatitis what remains unclear are the links between the etiological factor, the initial acinar cell injury due to the combined effects of the oxidative stress, the premature activation of pancreatic zymogens, and the microcirculatory impairment and the secondary local excessive stimulation of leukocytes as well as the signaling mechanism responsible for the delayed and specific manner in which the remote organs become involved through activation of mononuclear cells throughout the body. Inasmuch as the systemic manifestations of severe acute pancreatitis closely resemble, clinically and histologically, those associated with Gram-negative sepsis the pattern of TNF and IL-1 elevation was unchanged in pancreatitis induced in germ-free rats as well as in endotoxin-resistant CD14-knockout mice [16]. These observations ruled out endotoxin as the sole inducer of the early cytokine surge in acute pancreatitis. Rather, both activated oxygen species and inappropriately-activated pancreatic enzymes may trigger the inflammatory response through either unrelated or dependent NF-κB mechanisms (Fig. 2).

The transcription factor NF-κB, upon its nuclear translocation from the cytoplasm, is involved in the transcription of a variety of genes including most of the aforementioned proinflammatory substances. Within minutes of initiation of hormone-induced pancreatitis, NF-κB activation and degradation of its inhibitory protein IκB have been demonstrated first in acinar cells and then in infiltrating pancreatic inflammatory cells as well as in peritoneal and alveolar macrophages [17]. A

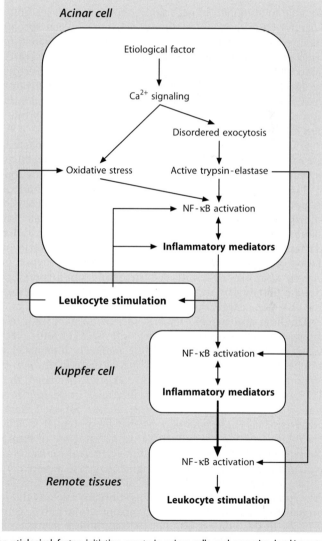

Fig. 2. Possible links between the etiological factor, initiating events in acinar cells and excessive local/remote leukocyte stimulation

biphasic nuclear translocation of the transcription factor was observed: the transient and early phase of NF-κB activation implicated acinar cells and the second wave involved inflammatory cell infiltration into the pancreas which produce cytokines such as TNF-α and IL-1β known to activate NF-κB. Activation of NF-κB in acinar cells resulted in upregulation of certain cytokines which mediate both acinar cell death and inflammation. Thus, NF-κB activation could be the link between the initial acinar cell injury and the inflammatory and cell death responses, the hallmarks of severe acute pancreatitis (Fig. 2) [17].

Oxidative stress appears early in the course of acute pancreatitis and parallels the severity of the attack [18]. Activated oxygen species generated either by damaged mitochondria or trypsin-mediated xanthine oxidase (XO) activation, then by the microcirculatory disturbances, and later by leukocytes at sites of inflammation, are able to stimulate signal transduction pathways leading to NF-κB activation [11]. Therefore, the early production of activated oxygen species in acinar cells may play an important role in the induction of the inflammatory reaction by mobilizing P-selectin and, in parallel, by activating the genes of several cytokines and adhesion molecules through NF-κB (Fig. 2) [11]. In addition, besides their direct cytotoxicity by attacking biological membranes, the release of activated oxygen species causes a dramatic increase in the level of intracellular free calcium with subsequent activation of phospholipase A2 and secondary increased production of chemotactic factors such as leukotrienes and PAF.

Finally, activated oxygen species have been demonstrated to inactivate antiproteases, in particular α1-antitrypsin, and thus, may facilitate the deleterious effect of activated pancreatic proteases in the cellular micro environment.

Pancreatic proteases, including trypsin, elastase, and carboxypeptidase A, when inappropriately activated have been shown to stimulate directly, albeit by an unknown molecular mechanism, tissue macrophages and monocytes to produce inflammatory cytokines [19, 20]. This process was dependent, at least for pancreatic elastase and to a lesser extent carboxypeptidase A, on NF-κB activation and degradation of its inhibitory protein IκB-β [20]. In vivo experiments extended these findings by showing the ability of systemically administered pancreatic elastase to precipitate pulmonary and hepatic dysfunction along with up-regulation of TNF, IL-1 and IL-6 gene expression in these target organs [21, 22].

The lung and hepatic injuries incited by pancreatic elastase were histologically indistinguishable from acute lung injury (ALI) and liver damage associated with sepsis or pancreatitis and could be markedly attenuated in animals devoid of the p55 TNF receptor or through p38 MAP kinase inhibition, thereby excluding a direct noxious effect of the protease [21, 22]. Furthermore, the pulmonary and hepatic TNF and IL-1 mRNA production increased in healthy rats after systemic administration of sterile and cytokine-free ascites obtained from rats with bile salt pancreatitis [23]. These data suggest that the potential inciting event that initiates the proinflammatory cascade may lie in the presence of free activated proteases in the interstitium of the pancreas and the peritoneal cavity. Thus, the systemic release of pancreatic elastase may be the signal from the pancreas that triggers systemic and tissue resident mononuclear cells to produce inflammatory mediators through nuclear translocation of NF-κB in target organs such as the lungs, spleen and liver, so propagating the local pancreatic inflammation into a generalized systemic disease (Fig. 2). In this context, Kupffer cells are both a major target for activation by cytokines or proteases reaching the liver from the pancreas through the portal vein or lymphatics and a major secondary source of inflammatory mediators and noxious substances, thereby amplifying the systemic inflammatory response (Fig. 2). Kupffer cell blockade, or bypassing this organ with a portocaval shunt during experimental pancreatitis, protected the lungs from alveolar macrophage activation, secondary neutrophil recruitement, and subsequent lung damage but did not modify the severity of local pancreatic injury [24]. The pathway of transfer of this activating enzymatic signal, i.e., the portal vein, the lymphatic system or direct absorption from the peritoneal circulation, remains obscure.

Other relevant, but NF-κB independent, potential mechanisms for leukocyte attraction, migration, and activation both locally and at distant sites include trypsin-generated C5a and leukotrienes as well as activated type I phospholipase A2 released by acinar cells and type II of neutrophil origin that catalyze the release of PAF from membrane phospholipids.

▍ Immunomodulation in Acute Pancreatitis: Experimental Studies

Further evidence of the prominent and detrimental role of excessive leukocyte stimulation in mediating local and remote tissue damage has been provided by multiple studies examining the blockade of proinflammatory mediators. Studies using prophylactic or delayed antagonism of TNF-α, with either anti-TNF polyclonal antibody or recombinant TNF receptor, demonstrated an attenuation in severity of pancreatitis biochemically and histologically, lowered serum IL-1 and IL-6, decreased acute lung and liver injury, and improved survival [25].

Interestingly, two studies tempered these findings: blockade of TNF using goat anti-TNF antiserum in a murine model of pancreatitis increased pancreatic and pulmonary edema, and delaying antagonism of TNF until circulating cytokines were elevated but not yet maximal, was more effective than prophylactic blockade [25, 26]. These results point to a potential regulatory effect of TNF either on the local immune system or on the mode of acinar cell death. Thus, mediators that can have harmful effects if produced in excessive quantities may nevertheless have beneficial immunomodulatory effects so that neutralizing their activity at the wrong moment may be deleterious.

Studies that examined inhibition of IL-1β used a recombinant form of the natural receptor antagonist to IL-1 (IL-1ra) and showed similar results as with the blockade of TNF with regards to attenuation of local/remote tissue damage and survival. The use of knock-out mice devoid of active receptors for IL-1 or TNF further confirmed that inhibition of either cytokine was nearly equivalent in terms of decreased severity and improved outcome [27]. Preventing the activity of both cytokines concurrently had no additional effect on the degree of pancreatitis but did attenuate the systemic inflammatory response and was associated with an additional but modest decrease in mortality [27]. Intracellular influx of calcium ion is known to act as a signal for TNF release and its subsequent action at distant sites. Treatment of rats with a calcium channel blocker prior to the induction of pancreatitis inhibited serum TNF-α expression, reduced the severity of acute pancreatitis both locally and distantly, and improved survival [28]. Preventing the production of IL-1 and TNF by using an anti-inflammatory cytokine such as IL-10, or by strategies that interfere with cytokine transcription, translation, intracellular processing, and cytokine release, was equally successful as blocking their action [29].

Intervening in the events upstream to cytokine production or downstream to the proinflammatory cascade yielded similar results. Blockade of NF-κB activation with the antioxidant N-acetylcysteine (NAC) or macrophage pacification through inhibition of p38 MAPK phosphorylation attenuated local and remote tissue injury and improved survival [29, 30]. Compounds with PAF antagonistic properties have been showed to improve pancreatic histology and to attenuate leukocyte infiltration and the increased pulmonary capillary permeability [31]. One of the major effects by which cytokine upregulation mediates distant injury is by adhesion molecule overexpression on endothelial cells. Strategies that interfere with neutrophil migration such as depletion of circulating neutrophils, the use of antineutrophil antibody that prevent their adhesion to endothelium, and antichemokine therapy based on monoclonal antibody against IL-8 or knock-out animals with deletion of the MIP-1a/ RANTES receptor CCR1 were demonstrated to decrease the severity of ALI [12, 32]. Similarly, intercellular adhesion molecule (ICAM)-1 knock-out mice or animals treated with monoclonal antibody specific to the ICAM-1 receptor were protected against acute pancreatitis and subsequent lung injury, pointing to the importance of neutrophil recruitment in the pathogenesis of pancreatitis and distant tissue damage [33].

Finally therapeutic modalities designed to boost antioxidant defenses such as NAC or transgenic copper/zinc superoxide dismutase (SOD) yielded beneficial results in caerulein-induced pancreatitis, which put emphasis on the deleterious role of the oxidative stress [11, 30].

So, ample experimental evidence has accumulated that, regardless of the initiating factor or etiology, excessive production of macrophage- and neutrophil-derived pro-inflammatory substances such as TNF, IL-1, and PAF play a key role in pancreatic damage and in the end-organ dysfunction accompanying severe acute pancreatitis. Combined, these studies have shown how these mediators are intimately related in their production and activity. To date, the antagonism of none of these individual mediators has been shown to be superior to others in animal studies. It should be emphasized that regardless of the model of acute pancreatitis, anti-mediator therapy was administered in all these experiments either prophylactically or within a short time period after induction of the attack. Although these studies suggest that downmodulation of the inflammatory response is beneficial in experimental pancreatitis, only a blockade prior to distant organ dysfunction associated with the peak of cytokine is protective, suggesting only a narrow therapeutic window.

❚ Role of Overactivation of Leukocytes during Clinical Acute Pancreatitis

Because of the rapid onset of the attack, the inevitable delay of a patient's presentation at the hospital, and the inaccessibility of human pancreatic tissue, the pathogenetic mechanisms involved in the initiation of acinar cell and remote tissue injury have been studied in several animal models of experimental pancreatitis with biochemical, morphological, and pathophysiological similarities to various aspects of human disease. Although the induction of pancreatitis in laboratory animals has been invaluable to elucidate the pathophysiology/cellular biology of this disease and to test novel treatment modalities, caution should be exercised in translating experimental results into humans. The clinical and pathogenetic relevance of these models to clinical pancreatitis should be questioned as none recreates the human situation: 1) agents commonly employed to induce experimental pancreatitis are not known to cause human disease; 2) the time-course of the illness is different from the human counterpart as necrotizing acute pancreatitis in animals has a very high early mortality; 3) there is a striking difference in the timing of initiation of treatment. Therapy in humans for this disease is usually not started within the first 24 h while even experimental studies that delayed treatment after induction of the attack assumed a parallel time-course of the disease process with regards to dynamics of trypsinogen activation, elevation of proinflammatory cytokines and development of pancreatic necrosis or organ dysfunction, and very few included animals with manifest pancreatic necrosis and remote organ dysfunction before therapy was started.

The majority of the clinical work on the overactivation of leukocytes during clinical acute pancreatitis has focused on two primary objectives: to establish the role of inflammatory mediators in producing the remote organ dysfunction associated with the disease and to find early markers of severity. Most investigators observed the appearance of cytokines or other mediators in patients hospitalized with acute pancreatitis of variable severity and correlated their levels with end-organ failure, overall mortality, and local severity as defined by the presence of necrosis or the emergence of regional complications. Although tissue levels, and not serum concentrations, are responsible for most of the biologic effects of these inflammatory mediators, in particular cytokines, all but two clinical studies, unlike animal experiments, either assessed mediator levels exclusively in serum usually with commercially prepared ELISA kits or studied their *in vitro* production by leukocytes isolated from the systemic circulation of patients with the disease.

The degree and duration of both IL-6 and IL-8 elevation in the systemic compartment paralleled closely and were shown to bear strong relationship with local and remote injury and outcome [34, 35]. IL-8 is known as a proinflammatory chemokine whose primary target cell is the neutrophil where it causes degranulation and the release of activated oxygen species and potentially damaging enzymes, notably elastase and group II phospholipase A2. It is not surprising, therefore, that a positive correlation was found between IL-8 and neutrophil elastase and that increased plasma concentrations of the latter, a marker of the intensity of neutrophil activation, could be detected in patients with a severe attack as early as at the time of admission [35]. Similarly, although the serum concentration of group II phospholipase A2 did not differ significantly with respect to systemic complications in patients with severe pancreatitis, increasing serum levels of this enzyme were found to reflect the ongoing systemic inflammatory response syndrome (SIRS) and lend support to the pathophysiological role of activated PMNs [36]. Scintigraphy with leukocytes tagged with technetium-99 m-HM-PAO demonstrated an early leukocyte infiltration into the pancreas that was correlated with the severity of the attack [37]. Cell adhesion proteins play a pivotal role in leukocyte adhesion to postcapillary venular endothelium and subsequent transendothelial migration. Proinflammatory cytokines enhance the expression of these molecules on the cell surface of leukocytes and endothelial cells with consecutive shedding of truncated forms into the circulation. Elevated plasma levels of soluble isoforms of E-selectin and ICAM-1 were found in patients with severe acute pancreatitis and were comparable to those in patients with sepsis [38, 39]. The highest concentrations were associated with the development of pancreatic necrosis and MOF, further indicating that interactions between activated leukocytes and endothelium may play a significant role in local and distant tissue damage during this disease.

Contrary to the animal, and in contrast with IL-6 and IL-8 whose production is primarily induced in various cells by the 'first-order' proinflammatory cytokines, only a minority of patients will demonstrate IL-1 or TNF in their serum at any time during hospitalization [34, 40, 41]. However these studies were potentially flawed by the inevitable delay between onset of symptoms and admission to hospital which might have precluded the detection of an early but transient systemic rise of these proximal proinflammatory cytokines. To circumvent this problem post-endoscopic retrograde pancreatography (ERP) pancreatitis was used as a human model to describe the time course of the release of cytokines and their antagonists from the very outset of the attack [42]. Nine out of 70 patients (13%) developed acute pancreatitis and in only one of them was the attack classified as severe. IL-8 and IL-1ra were the earliest detectable cytokines and their serum concentrations peaked 12 h after the insult whereas IL-6 levels peaked at 24 h. In contrast IL-1β was not found in the systemic circulation and the TNF system did not seem involved as indicated by the lack of detectable changes in TNF even when samples were taken as early as 1 h after ERP.

In vitro studies based on serial cultured leukocytes that were isolated from the peripheral circulation of patients with acute pancreatitis and from normal volunteers, showed that IL-6 and IL-8 production was higher in patients with pancreatitis and, among the latter, those with a complicated local course or organ failure possessed circulating leukocytes which were comparatively hyperstimulated as assessed by the release of TNF, IL-6, and IL-8 [40, 43].

These findings suggested a possible role for cytokines in the mediation of local and systemic injury in acute pancreatitis as these studies avoided the pitfalls of circulating cytokine determination by immunoassays including interference with cytokine inhibitors, breakdown by proteolytic enzymes released from the inflamed pancreas, the short half-life of these mediators in the circulation, and the preponderant action at the autocrine and paracrine level.

Furthermore, the absence of detectable cytokines in peripheral blood does not exclude local production in the inflamed organ with occasional spilling into the circulation. Only two studies conducted in human acute pancreatitis addressed cytokine levels in other compartments than the systemic circulation. Montravers and co-workers, albeit in a limited number of patients with ALI complicating severe acute pancreatitis, observed high TNF and IL-6 levels both in plasma and the thoracic lymph whereas levels of IL-1 remained within the normal range in both compartments. A significant lymph to plasma gradient was consistently recorded for IL-6 during the period of the study and lymph IL-6 levels were correlated with the lung injury score (LIS) [44]. Mayer and co-workers measured cytokine levels once in 24 ascites samples and nine lesser sac aspirates obtained from 20 patients with severe acute pancreatitis by fine needle aspiration or at surgery [45]. Local concentrations of IL-1, IL-6, and IL-10 were significantly higher than corresponding peak serum values while no significant difference could be demonstrated for IL-1ra. Peak serum levels of all mediators were significantly higher in severe, compared with mild, attacks and in non-survivors compared with survivors. Taken together, these results suggest, if not a pancreatic, at least a splanchnic production of these inflammatory mediators including the proximal proinflammatory cytokines.

After exposure to these 'first-order' proinflammatory mediators, target cells downregulate rapidly their responsiveness either by shedding the receptors into the circulation (IL-1ra, soluble TNF receptor) or by synthesizing and releasing anti-inflammatory cytokines (IL-4, IL-10). The blood levels of these mediators which have a longer half-life than TNF and IL-1 reflect the degree of inflammation and may be considered as an index of TNF/IL-1 activity. So, elevated concentrations of soluble TNF receptors in plasma were found in the early stage of acute pancreatitis and were associated with the severity of the attack, the development of pancreatic necrosis, MOF, and death [34, 46]. Increased serum IL-1ra, comparable to levels found in sepsis, was demonstrated in clinical acute pancreatitis and was associated with severity and MOF [38]. As IL-1ra was the single cytokine whose pancreatic concentration did not exceed peak serum value, a local imbalance in IL-1β/IL-1ra was inferred to be involved in the pathogenesis of severe local damage [45]. To date the most comprehensive study of both components of the cytokine cascade during clinical severe acute pancreatitis has been reported by a French group of investigators [41]. They profiled serial serum pro- and anti-inflammatory cytokines at inclusion and during the ICU stay in 50 patients with severe acute pancreatitis. They demonstrated that besides an early surge of proinflammatory cytokines, notably IL-6, a striking rapid and sustained release of anti-inflammatory mediators as assessed by plasma IL-10 and IL-1ra occurred in all patients. Thus, local and remote tissue damage which are assumed to be mediated by proinflammatory cytokines was documented despite the early release of anti-inflammatory mediators. This finding raises the unsolved question of the balance between the two components of the cytokine cascade that should still be addressed locally and at distant sites during clinical acute pancreatitis.

Of note, although IL-10 and IL-6 plasma concentrations were associated with outcome by univariate analysis, the cytokine levels offered no additional prognostic information compared with physiologic scores and were unable to predict death accurately in individual patients.

▌ Relevance of Immunomodulation to Clinical Acute Pancreatitis

The dominant roles excessive leukocyte stimulation and inflammatory mediators play in the pathogenesis of pancreatic necrosis and systemic damage during acute pancreatitis is now becoming much better understood. There is little doubt that preventing the release or the effects of IL-1, TNF, or PAF dramatically alters the expected course of experimental pancreatitis. The question remaining is whether similar antagonism of the cytokine network during clinical acute pancreatitis would benefit patients with this disease. In the absence of a deep understanding of the intra-acinar cell initiating events that trigger the damage and, as many (if not all) patients arrive in hospital long after these events, it seems obvious that a strategy of damage prevention is impractical. Rather a logical strategy of damage control is to downregulate the inflammatory response by blocking the production or the effects of the inflammatory mediators which are believed to be responsible for most of the local and distant injury in this disease.

Although these therapeutic options provide exciting areas of investigation, to date the clinical evidence in support of their benefits remains limited and controversial. So far only two immunomodulating trials have been conducted in human acute pancreatitis. The first randomized, placebo-controlled study tested in 144 patients the prophylactic administration of IL-10, given as a single bolus injection, for the prevention of post-endoscopic retrograde cholangio-pancreatography (ERCP) pancreatitis [47]. IL-10 was injected 30 minutes before the start of the procedure. Although no difference was observed in plasma cytokines (IL-6, IL-8 and TNF) IL-10 reduced significantly the incidence of post-ERCP pancreatitis. In the group of patients with hyperamylasemia IL-10 pre-treatment was able to limit the increase in TNF plasma levels, which suggested that this immunomodulatory cytokine might limit local tissue damage by downregulating the production of proinflammatory mediators. In the second randomized controlled trial, 290 patients with predicted severe acute pancreatitis received placebo or lexipafant, an imidazolyl derivative that has an affinity for the PAF receptor seven times more avid than PAF itself, by continuous infusion for up to 7 days [48]. Although patients were included within 72 h of the onset of symptoms, 44% already had organ failure on entry into the study. As the majority of organ failures had occurred before initiation of treatment, a putative beneficial effect of PAF antagonist could not be demonstrated on the small numbers of new organ failures. In addition, at the end of the treatment period there was no difference in organ failure score between the two groups and neither the incidence of local complications nor the mortality rate were influenced by the therapy.

One lesson that has been learned from the experimental studies and this limited clinical experience is the importance of the timing of immunomodulating treatment. Sepsis and acute pancreatitis share in common inflammatory mediators and clinical manifestations of MOF. As sepsis is often heralded by the emergence of organ failure(s) and acute pancreatitis by onset of pain, the latter has been considered at first glance as an ideal candidate for immunomodulation. Nevertheless, a therapeutic window allowing for the antagonism of cytokines or mediators downstream in the inflammatory cascade remains to be demonstrated in clinical acute pancreatitis. What remains unclear is why a minority of patients progresses from a limited local inflammation to extensive pancreatic necrosis, MOF and death, although presumably it is patients in whom the inflammatory cascade spirals out of control who may benefit from mediator blockade and it is this subset that should be identified rapidly as early therapy is mandatory to be effective. Even if, unlike sepsis, few patients who present shortly after the onset of pain exhibit organ dysfunction at that time, the cytokine surge has already started and the incidence of local/remote tissue damage rises rapidly in the next 48–72 h. Unfortunately an early and accurate selection on an individual basis of those who will develop MOF is impossible in the clinical setting so that a timely initiation of immunotherapy before the emergence of extensive tissue damage remains questionable.

Other questions require careful consideration before acceptance of this therapeutic approach: What are the kinetics of cytokine tissue levels, in particular the balance and the interrelation between pro- and anti-inflammatory mediators and between the latter and activated pancreatic enzymes?; Will mediator blockade and its timing affect the risk of infection, particularly infected pancreatic necrosis, in this high risk population?; and unlike animals will it influence the mode of acinar cell death?; Owing to the narrow therapeutic window should therapy be targeted to a further step in the inflammatory cascade induced by the 'first-line' cytokines?

▌ Conclusion

Whatever the etiological factors, the clinical course of acute pancreatitis follows a similar pattern once the process has been initiated, which indicates common pathophysiological mechanisms. Although the initiating events at the cellular and molecular levels are still poorly understood, the earliest lesions occur within the acinar cells and include alteration in calcium signaling, disordered luminal exocytosis, and oxidative stress. At the time the patients seek medical attention, it is the interplay between aberrant activation of digestive enzymes within the acinar cells, microcirculatory disturbances, and secondary excessive leukocyte stimulation that accounts for the local inflammatory necrotizing process and subsequent remote organ injury. Although the relative contibution of these three pathophysiological mechanisms remains unknown there is a growing experimental and clinical evidence that inflammatory mediators play a pivotal role, if not in pancreatic necrosis, at least in the propagation of a local disease process into MOF. Logically, these findings may boost immunomodulating therapy in the clinical management of patients with acute pancreatitis. However, given the multiplicity, inherent redundancy, and pleiotropy of mediators/mechanisms involved in the attack, precise targets for specific interventions are difficult to ascertain. Indiscriminate use or overreliance on the simplistic approach of proximal cytokine blockade may rather yield disappointing results or even harmful effects, just as protease inhibitors did in the past.

References

1. Beger HG, Bittner R, Block S, Büchler M (1986) Bacterial contamination of pancreatic necrosis. A prospective clinical study. Gastroenterology 91:433–438
2. Rinderknecht H (1988) Fatal pancreatitis, a consequence of excessive leukocyte stimulation? Int J Pancreatol 3:105–112
3. Büchler M, Malfertheiner P, Uhl W, et al (1993) Gabexate mesilate in human acute pancreatitis. Gastroenterology 104:1165–1170
4. Norman J, Fink G, Denham W, et al (1997) Tissue specific cytokine production during experimental acute pancreatitis: a probable mechanism for distant organ dysfunction. Dig Dis Sci 42:1783–1788
5. Fink GW, Norman J (1996) Intrapancreatic interleukin 1 gene expression by specific leukocyte populations during acute pancreatitis. J Surg Res 63:369–373
6. Grewal HP, Kotb M, Mohey El din A, et al (1994) Induction of tumor necrosis factor in severe acute pancreatitis and its subsequent reduction after hepatic passage. Surgery 115:213–221
7. Werner J, Dragotakes S, Fernandez-del Castillo C, et al (1998) Technetium-99m-labeled white blood cells: a new method to define the local and systemic role of leukocytes in acute experimental pancreatitis. Ann Surg 227:86–94
8. Gukovskaya AS, Gukovsky I, Zaninovic V, Song M, Sandoval D, Gukovsky S (1997) Pancreatic acinar cells produce, release and respond to tumor necrosis factor-alpha. Role in regulating cell death and pancreatitis. J Clin Invest 100:1853–1862
9. Yang B, Demaine A, Kingsnorth A (2000) Chemokines MCP-1 and RANTES in isolated rat pancreatic acinar cells treated with CCK and ethanol in vitro. Pancreas 21:22–31
10. Sandoval D, Gukovskaya A, Reavey P, et al (1996) The role of neutrophils and platelet-activating factor in mediating experimental pancreatitis. Gastroenterology 111:1081–1091
11. Telek G, Ducroc R, Scoazec J-Y, Pasquier C, Feldmann G, Rozé C (2001) Differential upregulation of cellular adhesion molecules at the sites of oxidative stress in experimental acute pancreatitis. J Surg Res 96:56–67
12. Osman MO, Kristensen JU, Jacobsen N, et al (1998) A monoclonal anti-interleukin 8 antibody (WS-4) inhibits cytokine response and acute lung injury in experimental severe acute necrotising pancreatitis in rabbits. Gut 43:232–239
13. Denham W, Yang J, Fink G, et al (1998) TNF but not IL-I decreases pancreatic acinar cell survival without affecting exocrine function; a study in the perfused human pancreas. J Surg Res 74:3–7
14. Malaka D, Vasseur S, Bödeker H, et al (2000) Tumor necrosis factor alpha triggers antiapoptotic mechanisms in rat pancreatic cells trough pancreatitis-associated protein I activation. Gastroenterology 119:816–828
15. Bathia M, Wallig MA, Hofbauer B, et al (1998) Induction of apoptosis in pancreatic acinar cells reduces the severity of acute pancreatitis. Biochem Biophys Res Com 19:476–483

16. Eubanks JW, Sabek O, Kotb M, et al (1998) Acute pancreatitis induces cytokine production in endotoxin-resistant mice. Ann Surg 227:904–911

17. Gukovsky I, Gukovskaya A, Blinman T, Zaninovic V, Pandol S (1998) Early NF-κB activation is associated with hormone-induced pancreatitis. Am J Physiol 275:G1402–G1414

18. Tsai K, Wang SS, Chen TS, et al (1998) Oxidative stress: an important phenomenon with pathogenetic significance in the progression of acute pancreatitis. Gut 42:850–855

19. Lundberg A, Eubanks J, Henry J, et al (2000) Trypsin stimulates production of cytokines from peritoneal macrophages in vitro and in vivo. Pancreas 21:41–51

20. Jaffray C, Mendez C, Denham W, Carter G, Norman J (2000) Specific pancreatic enzymes activate macrophages to produce tumor necrosis factor-alpha: role of nuclear factor Kappa B and inhibitory Kappa B proteins. J Gastrointest Surg 4:370–378

21. Jaffray C, Yang J, Norman J (2000) Elastase mimics pancreatitis-induced hepatic injury via inflammatory mediators. J Surg Res 90:95–101

22. Jaffray C, Yang J, Carter G, Mendez C, Norman J (2000) Pancreatic elastase activates pulmonary nuclear factor kappa B and inhibitory kappa B, mimicking pancreatitis-associated adult respiratory distress syndrome. Surgery 128:225–231

23. Denham W, Yang J, Norman J (1997) Evidence for an unknown component of pancreatic ascites that induces adult respiratory distress syndrome through an interleukin-1 and tumor necrosis factor-dependent mechanism. Surgery 122:295–302

24. Gloor B, Blinman T, Rigberg D, et al (2000) Kupffer cell blockade reduces hepatic and systemic cytokine levels and lung injury in hemorrhagic pancreatitis in rats. Pancreas 21:414–420

25. Norman J, Fink G, Messina J, Carter G, Franz M (1996) Timing of tumor necrosis factor antagonism is critical in determining outcome in murine lethal acute pancreatitis. Surgery 120:515–521

26. Guice KS, Oldham KT, Rezmick DG, Kunkel SL, Ward PA (1991) Anti-tumor necrosis factor antibody augments edema formation in caerulein-induced acute pancreatitis. J Surg Res 51:495–499

27. Denham W, Yang J, Fink G, et al (1997) Gene targeting demonstrates additive detrimental effects of interleukin I and tumor necrosis factor during pancreatitis. Gastroenterology 113:1741–1746

28. Hughes CB, El-Din A, Kotb M, Gaber L, Gaber A (1996) Calcium channel blockade inhibits release of TNF alpha and improves survival in a rat model of acute pancreatitis. Pancreas 13:22–28

29. Yang J, Denham W, Tracey K, et al (1998) The physiologic consequences of macrophage pacification during severe acute pancreatitis. Shock 10:169–175

30. Demols A, Van Laethem J-L, Quertinmont E, et al (1998) N-Acetylcysteine decreases severity of acute pancreatitis in mice. Pancreas 20:161–169

31. Imrie CW (1999) The possible role of platelet-activating factor antagonist therapy in the management of severe acute pancreatitis. Bailliere's Clin Gastroenterol 13:357–364

32. Gerard C, Frossard J-L, Bhatia M, et al (1997) Targeted disruption of the B-chemokine receptor CCRI protects against pancreatitis-associated lung injury. J Clin Invest 100:2022–2027

33. Frossard JL, Saluja A, Bhagat L, et al (1999) The role of intercellular adhesion molecule 1 and neutrophils in acute pancreatitis and pancreatitis-associated lung injury. Gastroenterology 116:694–701

34. de Beaux AC, Goldie AS, Ross JA, Carter DC, Fearon KC (1996) Serum concentrations of inflammatory mediators related to organ failure in patients with acute pancreatitis. Br J Surg 83:349–353

35. Gross V, Andreesen R, Leser HG, et al (1992) Interleukin-8 and neutrophil activation in acute pancreatitis. Eur J Clin Invest 22:200–203

36. Hietaranta A, Kemppainen E, Puolakkainen P, et al (1999) Extracellular phospholipases A2 in relation to systemic inflammatory response syndrome (SIRS) and systemic complications in severe acute pancreatitis. Pancreas 18:385–391

37. Schölmerich J, Schümichen C, Lausen M, et al (1991) Scintigraphic assessment of leukocyte infiltration in acute pancreatitis using technetium-99m-hexamethyl propylene amine oxine as leukocyte label. Dig Dis Sci 36:65–71

38. Hynninen M, Valtonen M, Markkanen H, et al (1999) Interleukin 1 receptor antagonist and E-selectin concentrations: a comparison in patients with severe acute pancreatitis and severe sepsis. J Crit Care 14:63–68

39. Kaufmann P, Smolle K, Brunner G, Demel U, Tilz G, Krejs G (1999) Relation of serial measurements of plasma-soluble intercellular adhesion molecule-1 to severity of acute pancreatitis. Am J Gastroenterol 94:2412–2416

40. de Beaux AC, Ross JA, Maingay JP, Fearon KC, Carter DC (1996) Proinflammatory cytokine release by peripheral blood mononuclear cells from patients with acute pancreatitis. Br J Surg 83:1071–1075

41. Brivet F, Emilie D, Galanaud P, et al (1999). Pro- and anti-inflammatory cytokines during acute severe pancreatitis: an early and sustained response, although unpredictable of death. Crit Care Med 27:749–755

42. Messmann H, Vogt W, Falk W, et al (1998) Interleukins and their antagonists but not TNF and its receptors are released in post-ERP pancreatitis. Europ J Gastroent Hepatol 10:611–617

43. McKay CJ, Gallagher G, Brooks B, Imrie CW, Baxter JN (1996) Increased monocyte cytokine production in association with systemic complications in acute pancreatitis. Br J Surg 83:919–923

44. Montravers P, Chollet-Martin S, Marmuse JP, Gougerot-Picidalo MA, Desmonts JM (1995) Lymphatic release of cytokines during acute lung injury complicating severe pancreatitis. Am J Respir Crit Care Med 152:1527–1533

45. Mayer J, Rau B, Gansauger F, Beger H (2000) Inflammatory mediators in human acute pancreatitis; clinical and pathophysiological implications. Gut 47:546–552

46. Kaufmann P, Tilz G, Lueger A, Demel U (1997) Elevated plasma levels of soluble tumor necrosis factor receptor (sTNFRp60) reflect severity of acute pancreatitis. Intensive Care Med 23:841–848

47. Devière J, Le Moine O, Van Laethem J-L, et al (2001) Interleukin 10 reduces the incidence of pancreatitis after therapeutic endoscopic retrograde cholangiopancreatography. Gastroenterology 120:498–505

48. Johnson C, Kingsnorth A, Imrie C, et al (2001) Double blind, randomised, placebo controlled study of a platelet activating factor antagonist, lexipafant, in the treatment and prevention of organ failure in predicted severe acute pancreatitis. Gut 48:62–69

Abdominal Perfusion Pressure as a Prognostic Marker in Intra-abdominal Hypertension

M. Malbrain

▌ Introduction

Elevated intra-abdominal pressure (IAP) is a continuum from intra-abdominal hypertension (IAH) to abdominal compartment syndrome (ACS) and has considerable impact on end-organ function [1]. However, no data are available on IAP from large prospective clinical trials. Many thresholds have been proposed as the critical value for IAP in guiding decompression. Recent publications have improved our understanding of the pathophysiological mechanisms. We are now aware that even slight elevations in IAP of 10 mmHg may have a tremendous impact on end-organ function [1]. However, it is probably not the absolute value of IAP but the acuity of increase in IAP or the trend over time that is predictive for outcome. Most of the published studies relate to the hemodynamically stable patient or laboratory animal without prior insult. Extrapolation of these results to a critically ill patient or to a trauma patient who may have experienced episodes of shock and resuscitation and hence of ischemia-reperfusion (I/R) injury, may be incorrect. Co-morbidities play an important role in aggravating the effects of raised IAP such as pre-existing chronic renal failure, massive hemorrhage, hypovolemia, positive end-expiratory pressure (PEEP), or pre-existing cardiomyopathy, and these may reduce the threshold of IAH that causes clinical manifestations of ACS. Indeed, the critical IAP value differs from patient to patient and from time to time. A prognostic parameter that could help us in following these patients and guiding therapy would be very helpful. This chapter will focus on abdominal perfusion pressure (APP), defined as mean arterial pressure (MAP) minus IAP, as such a possible parameter.

▌ Rationale

Many organs are capable of maintaining blood flow relatively constant over a wide range of perfusion pressures. The efficiency of this process differs from organ to organ and is greatest in the brain and kidneys. However, virtually all organs exhibit this sort of autoregulation. In most cases, blood flow is preserved within the mean pressure range of 60 to 160 mmHg. For the kidney, autoregulation has also been described in relation to the constant glomerular filtration rate (GFR) in response to variations in perfusion pressure. Adapting the renal vascular resistance of the preglomerular vasculature is the key-factor for autoregulation mediated by mechanisms intrinsic to the kidneys, which may reside in the vascular wall [2].

The etiology of renal impairment in IAH with decreases in renal blood flow, GFR, urine output, and tubular dysfunction is probably multifactorial and due to endocrine, hemodynamic, and direct effects [1]. Figure 1 shows the different cardiovascular pathophysiologic mechanisms of IAH. An increase in antidiuretic hormone (ADH) production, and changes in the renin-angiotensin-aldosterone pathways with a rise in renin and aldosterone levels, atrial natriuretic peptide and circulating catecholamines has been noted [3]. In some studies, endothelin came forward as a possible auto./paracrine mechanism that decreases renal blood flow and GFR by constricting preglomerular vessels [4]. A direct hydrostatic effect by mechanical compression of both pre- and postglomerular vasculature resulting in increased renal vascular resistance together with a drop in cardiac output are probably the most likely causes, although persistence of renal impairment has been described when cardiac output is kept normal by dobutamine and fluids [1]. Other factors that may contribute include compression of the renal vein causing outflow obstruction which may rise intra-parenchymal pressures, resulting in the shunting of blood away from the renal cortex [1, 5–8]. Within this concept, renal decapsulation was popular some decades ago in selective renal compartment syndrome, but has been abandoned since [9]. Compression of the ureters has been ruled out since the placement of ureteral stents did not resolve renal impairment (Sugrue, unpublished data). The changes in renal function and diuresis usually resolve with early

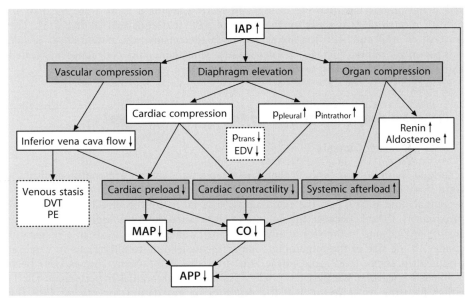

Fig. 1. Cardiovascular implications of intra-abdominal hypertension (IAH). Cardiac preload is diminished due to a direct compressive effect on the vessels and the heart. Cardiac contractility is diminished due to cardiac compression and raised intrathoracic pressures mediated by diaphragm elevation which erroneously increases central venous pressure (CVP) and pulmonary capillary wedge pressure (PCWP). Organ compression and compression of the venous capacitance vessels in the abdomen result in elevated afterload either by a direct effect or by the mediation of renin-angiotensin aldosteron and endothelin. Finally, cardiac output (CO) and mean arterial pressure (MAP) drop resulting in a low abdominal perfusion pressure (APP), which then may lead to splanchnic hypoperfusion. DVT: deep venous thrombosis; PE: pulmonary embolism; EDV: end-diastolic volume; Ptrans: transmural pressure

decompression [1, 6, 7], although some reports did not show improvement in renal function after decompression [10]. In an interesting, and one of the few, prospective studies, Sugrue et al. [10] analyzed outcomes in 49 consecutive patients with IAH who underwent temporary abdominal closure (TAC). The study showed, a bit surprisingly, no improvement in renal function after decompression, although 10 patients experienced brisk diuresis. A possible mechanism may be the development of a renal compartment syndrome with ongoing IAH causing acute tubular necrosis, which needs more time to recuperate. Recently, the same group was the first to prospectively show in a logistic regression model that IAP, together with age, hypotension, and sepsis, were independent risk factors for renal impairment in a sample of 263 patients after abdominal surgery [11]. Ulyatt [12] proposed renal perfusion pressure (RPP) together with the filtration gradient (FG) as key-factors in the development of renal failure. The FG is the mechanical force across the glomerulus and equals the difference between the glomerular filtration pressure (GFP) and the proximal tubular pressure (PTP), hence:

$$FG = GFP - PTP \qquad \text{(Eqn 1)}$$

In IAH, PTP equals IAP and GFP can be estimated by MAP–IAP. The FG can then be calculated by the formula:

$$FG = MAP - 2(IAP) \qquad \text{(Eqn 2)}$$

Therefore, changes in absolute IAP value will have a greater effect on renal function and urine production than the changes in MAP. Cheatham et al. were the first to publish a retrospective study on the value of APP that equals MAP–IAP [13]. The concept of APP and RPP highlights the need to consider the abdomen as a sole compartment rather than an isolated cavity. Cheatham and colleagues suggested using an APP of 50 mmHg or more as a resuscitation endpoint [13].

■ Pathophysiology: Analogy with Cerebral Perfusion Pressure?

Intra-abdominal Contents

A unique feature of the brain is that the intracranial contents are confined within a rigid bony cage (the skull). The intracranial contents are 85% brain cells, 10% cerebrospinal fluid (CSF), and the remaining 5% is taken by the blood volume of approximately 150 ml. Because the volume of the cranial cavity is limited by its bony casing, any change in the size of any intracranial compartment leads to a reciprocal change in the size of the remaining compartments leading to alterations in cerebral perfusion pressure (CPP) and intracranial pressure (ICP). Many studies have been published regarding the best treatment options for intracranial hypertension (ICH) either focusing on lowering ICP (by diuretics or evacuation) or raising CPP (by maintaining correct MAP with fluids or vasopressors). In analogy with the head, the abdomen can be considered as a closed box (like the skull) with partially rigid sides (spine and pelvis) with an anchorage above (costal arch) and partially flexible sides (abdominal wall and diaphragm), filled with organs (equivalent to the brain in the skull) including the small and large intestine, liver, kidneys, spleen, and perfused by the mesenteric arteries with a mesenteric and venous capacitance blood volume. These abdominal organs are surrounded by a third space filled with peritoneal fluid (equivalent to the CSF in our analogy) [1]. In real life, things are complicated by the moveable diaphragm, the shifting costal arch, the contractions of the abdominal wall, and the intestines that may be empty or filled with air, liquid, or fecal mass.

IAP Measurement

Since the abdomen and its contents can be considered as relatively non-compressive and primarily fluid in character, the pressure values follow the hydrostatic laws of Pascal, and the IAP can be measured in nearly every part of the abdomen [1]. The degree of flexibility of the walls and the specific gravity of its contents determine pressure at a given point at a given position (prone, supine, etc.). The IAP is the steady state pressure concealed within the abdominal cavity. The IAP shifts with respiration as evidenced by an inspiratory increase (diaphragmatic contraction) and an expiratory decrease (relaxation) [14]. Different direct and indirect measurement methods have been suggested. Measurement of IAP by an indwelling catheter in the urinary bladder has been promoted as the gold standard [1, 15–17]. The highly compliant wall of the bladder acts as a passive diaphragm and intrinsic bladder pressure does not rise when its volume is between 50 and 100 ml. Since most patients in the ICU have a central venous or arterial line connected to a pressure transducer and a Foley bladder catheter in place, it takes less than 5 min to calculate the IAP [1]. A major problem with this technique is that it is intermittent, that it poses a risk for needle stick injury, and that it interferes with urinary output estimation [1]. Recent data show that IAP is a physiologic parameter that fluctuates over time, so ideally continuous measurement together with APP, in analogy with ICP and CPP, would be the best way to monitor IAP. Unfortunately, due to a lack of clinical awareness such a device has not yet been developed.

Finally, a quick idea of the IAP can be obtained in a patient without a pressure transducer, by using his own urine as transducing medium [1]. The Foley catheter is clamped just above the urine collection bag (as distal as possible), so that the transparent tubing fills with urine (this may be a total of 20 to 30 ml according to the length), if insufficient urine is available 50 ml of saline can be injected through the culture aspiration port. After declamping, the tubing of the Foley catheter is then held at a 90° angle to the pelvis to a position of 30 to 40 cm above the symphysis pubis (used as zero reference). The meniscus of urine (or saline in an anuric patient) should show respiratory variation. The IAP is indicated by the level of urine or saline in the tube and is equivalent to the height in cm from the pubic bone of this urine or saline column. Confirmation of correct measurement can be made by inspecting the respiratory variations and by applying pressure on the abdomen that should increase the meniscus as IAP increases. The conversion ratio from cm of urine or saline to cm of H_2O is close to $1:1$; from cmH_2O to mmHg is $1:1.36$. This easy and rapid estimation of IAP can only be done in a patient with a compliant bladder without spasm and a sufficient urine output so that the bladder is not fully emptied, in the latter case saline could be injected instead.

We recently tested two prototypes (Holtech Medical, Copenhagen, Denmark) for IAP measurement using the patients' own urine as pressure transmitting medium (data on file). A 50 ml container fitted with a bio-filter for venting is inserted between the Foley catheter and the drainage bag. The container fills with urine during drainage; when the container is elevated, the 50 ml urine flows back into the patient's bladder, and IAP can be read from the position of the meniscus in the clear manometer tube between the container and the Foley catheter. The first prototype consisted of a 50 ml plastic bag with a bio-filter, inserted between the Foley catheter and the urine collection bag; a major drawback was occasional blocking of the bio-filter, leading to overestimation of IAP in some cases. Another drawback was the occasional presence of air-bubbles in the manometer tube, producing multiple menisci leading to misinterpretation of IAP. In addition, the volume of urine flowing back into the bladder was not well defined. Prototype 2 was adapted to correct for the drawbacks of prototype 1, using a rigid 50 ml reservoir with a large bio-filter surface. In total 60 paired measurements were performed in five patients with prototype 1 (IAPproto1) and 119 paired measurements were performed in seven patients with prototype 2 (IAPproto2) and these measurements were compared with the gold standard via an indwelling bladder catheter using a pressure transducer (IAPves). There was a good correlation between IAPves and IAPproto1: IAPves = $0.592 \times$ IAPproto1 + 3.666 mmHg ($r^2 = 0.71$, p < 0.0001), but the bias was considerable. The analysis according to Bland and Altman showed that IAPproto1 consistently underestimated IAPves with a mean difference or bias of -1.5 ± 2.9 (SD) mmHg (95% confidence interval (CI) -2.2 to -0.7); the limits of agreement (LA) were -7.3 to 4.4 mmHg (95% CI -8.6 to -6 for the lower LA (LLA) and 3.1 to 5.7 mmHg for the upper LA (ULA)); these intervals are large and thus reflect poor agreement. Modification of prototype 1 led to a major improvement in the quality and reproducibility of the IAP measurement: IAPves = $0.9 \times$ IAPproto2 + 1.17 mmHg ($r^2 = 0.96$, p < 0.0001). The analysis according to Bland and Altman showed that IAPproto2 was almost identical to IAPves with a mean difference or bias of 0.17 ± 0.8 (SD) mmHg (95% CI 0.03 to 0.3); with small limits of agreement -1.4 to 1.7 mmHg (95% CI -1.6 to -1.1 for the LLA and 1.5 to 2 mmHg for the ULA); these intervals are small and thus reflect good agreement. This non-invasive technique, using the patients' own urine as transducing medium, can reduce nursing time and costs to a minimum. IAP measurement can easily be done 2-hourly together, and without interfering, with urine output measurements. The risk of infection and needle stick injury is also reduced.

IAP

As the intra-abdominal volume increases, initially compensation takes place and the IAP will remain non-pathologically stable up to a given point at which decompensation begins with a dramatic rise in IAP from that point (Fig. 2) [19]. From a theoretical viewpoint, the abdominal compliance curve would therefore look like the intracranial compliance curve. Abdominal pressure-volume curves have been studied extensively in animals and in post-mortem studies, and these may not reflect real-life compliance in humans (Sugrue, unpublished data). The abdomen exhibits a great tolerance to increasing volume with little initial rise as seen during laparoscopy where up to 5 liters of air are insufflated without a significant impact on IAP (limited to 12–15 mmHg). The critical point being somewhere around 7 to 8 liters as demonstrated by Sugrue et al. [18] who found that the mean volume of gas required to generate an IAP of 20 mmHg was 8.8 ± 4.3 l. Over time, adaptation can occur and this critical point will be different from patient to patient and depends upon underlying etiologies and predisposing conditions. Co-morbidities, such as pre-existing chronic renal failure, massive hemorrhage, hypovolemia, PEEP or pre-existing cardiomyopathy, play an important role in aggravating the effects of raised IAP and may reduce the threshold of IAH that causes clinical manifestations of ACS [1]. In most cases, it is the acuity of increase in IAP that is important and

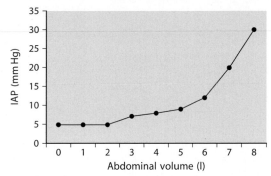

Fig. 2. Theoretical abdominal pressure-volume curve. As the abdominal volume increases in the first part of the curve, compensation occurs and intra-abdominal pressure (IAP) rises little. In the second part of the abdominal pressure-volume curve, compensation is increasingly ineffective up to a critical point (IAPcrit). Beyond this point of the curve, a small increase in intra-abdominal volume will cause a great rise in IAP. For a patient on this point of the curve meticulous care is mandatory with monitoring of IAP and abdominal perfusion pressure (APP) to avoid abdominal hypoperfusion with catastrophic bowel ischemia, bacterial translocation, multiple organ failure, and death. Similarly small decreases in volume will result in large decreases in IAP

not necessarily the absolute increase [1, 7, 19, 20]. Chronic ACS has been described in morbidly obese patients, in patients with cirrhosis and chronic ascites (where up to 20 l of ascites only account for IAP's of 15 mmHg), and in pregnancy. Hence we can classify IAH into 4 groups:

- hyperacute IAH that lasts only *seconds or minutes* as with laughing, straining, coughing, sneezing, during defecation, or physical activity;
- acute IAH that is mainly due to trauma or intra-abdominal hemorrhage of any cause and leads to ACS within a couple of *hours*;
- subacute IAH such as occurs with most medical causes in the ICU that lead to IAH within a couple of *days* and results from a combination of etiologic factors and predisposing conditions;
- chronic IAH such as with morbid obesity, intra-abdominal tumor (large ovarian cyst, fibroma, etc.), chronic ascites (liver cirrhosis or chronic ambulatory peritoneal dialysis (CAPD)), or pregnancy. In such cases, the abdominal wall adapts progressively over *months or years* to the increase in IAP and allows time for the body to adapt, so that IAH-complications do not occur [1].

Getting back to our abdominal compliance curve we can identify three parts (Fig. 2). In the first part, compensation takes place and IAP will remain stable, at a critical volume level with corresponding critical IAP (IAPcrit). IAP will further rise exponentially, a small increase in abdominal volume even caused by an initially harmless insult (ileus, colonic dilatation, ascites, small hemorrhage) may be sufficient to cause a dramatic increase in IAP and subsequent decrease in APP. Similarly, any small decrease in abdominal volume achieved by simple methods (gastric suctioning, rectal enema, ascites evacuation, furosemide, sitting the patient up by shifting the bed to a 30° position), may result in a substantial decrease in IAP. As stated earlier, the APP equals MAP minus IAP. The aim of treatment should therefore be to maintain APP above 60 or at least 50 mmHg; this should be achieved with an adequate MAP and the lowest IAP possible.

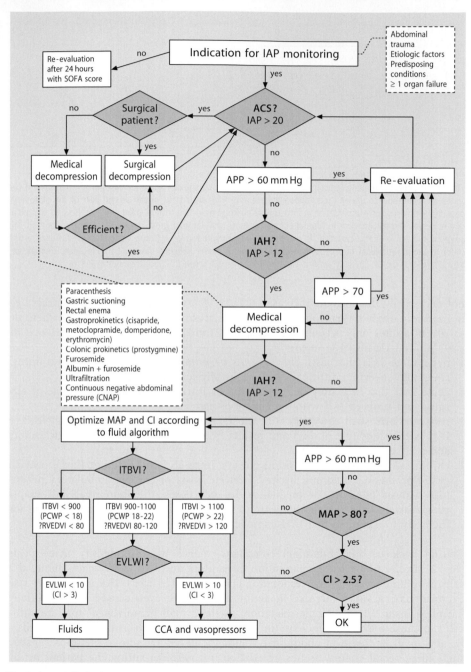

Fig. 3. Intra-abdominal pressure (IAP) monitoring and intra-abdominal hypertension (IAH) treatment algorithm. In the absence of correct blood volume measurements, traditional filling pressures can be used adapting the thresholds according to the degree of IAH, values are given between brackets as a directive. Since no clear-cut thresholds cut be obtained from the literature, values for right ventricular end-diastolic volume index (RVEDVI) are preceded by a question-mark. APP: abdominal perfusion pressure; MAP: mean arterial pressure; CI: cardiac index; ITBVI: intrathoracic blood volume index; EVLWI: extravascular lung water index

If measures aimed at reducing IAP fail to maintain adequate APP, then the MAP should be increased in analogy with CPP. To achieve this, careful volume loading and vasopressors can be given. Figure 3 shows an algorithm that will be discussed further in detail under the caption therapeutic implications. Burch and co-authors [21] defined a grading system of IAH/ACS to guide therapy: Grade I (7 to 11 mmHg), grade II (11 to 18 mmHg), grade III (18 to 25 mmHg) and grade IV (> 25 mmHg). It was suggested that most of the patients with grade III and all of the patients with grade IV should undergo surgical abdominal decompression [21]. In all grades adequate intravascular volume should be maintained whilst avoiding overfilling. Since increased IAP is a continuum ranging from moderate IAH to severe ACS we propose the following grading system: grade 0 (IAP 0–7 mmHg: normal condition); grade I (IAP 8–11 mmHg: equivocal, at risk for IAH); grade II (IAP 12–15 mmHg: moderately increased IAP or moderate IAH); grade III (IAP 16–20 mmHg: severely increased IAP or severe IAH); grade IV (IAP 21–25 mmHg: very severely increased IAP or moderate ACS); grade V (IAP > 25 mmHg: dangerously increased IAP or severe ACS). The cut-offs are based on our evolving understanding of the pathophysiological implications of raised IAP and the repeated revision of critical IAP. While we would have waited for pressures above 30 or 35 mmHg a few years ago, more and more surgeons are now convinced that the abdomen should be opened at much lower IAPs [13].

Indications for IAP Monitoring in the ICU

Obviously any patient who is at risk of developing IAH should be monitored. But there is the problem, who is at risk? Reading the literature there seems to be consensus that any patient who stays in the intensive care unit (ICU) after abdominal surgery should be monitored, especially if they are mechanically ventilated. It also became clear that any patient with acute renal failure is a good candidate for IAP monitoring [1, 13]. So, briefly, since IAH has an impact on every organ within and outside the abdomen any patient that develops one or more organ failures should be monitored. A practical way to do this would be to monitor organ function daily by means of a scoring system like the multiple organ dysfunction (MOD) score or the sequential organ failure assessment (SOFA) and to initiate IAP monitoring once organ failure starts. Definite evidence for this approach has been lacking until now. As Sugrue recently stated in his MD thesis (submitted to University of New South Wales, Liverpool, Australia): the lack of clinical awareness of the value of IAP is a major clinical challenge. A recent article published on behalf of the SOFA group of the European Society of Intensive Care [22], on acute renal failure in ICU makes no mention of IAP as predictor or cause of renal impairment in ICU patients. In a way this apathy to IAP is not totally unexpected. In the advent of the results of forthcoming large multicenter trials we need to be very cautious and stay alert. Therefore, every ICU patient merits our careful attention especially if predisposing conditions like sepsis or septic shock with capillary leakage, acidosis, coagulopathy, multiple transfusions, liver dysfunction with ascites or hypothermia and etiologic factors like massive fluid resuscitation, ileus, abdominal infection, hemoperitoneum, abdominal surgery or pneumoperitoneum are present [1].

■ Literature Data

Retrospective Studies

Performing a Medline search using 'abdominal perfusion pressure' as the search item, only one study could be identified dealing with the effects of APP [13]. In this 25 month retrospective study, all patients admitted to the surgical and trauma ICU were screened for IAH, defined as IAP above 15 mmHg, on admission and then twice daily. Once IAH was diagnosed, IAP measurements were obtained every 4 hours together with MAP, with APP calculated as MAP minus IAP. ACS was defined as an IAP above 25 mmHg together with signs and symptoms of end-organ failure. During their stay the lowest values for APP, MAP, pH and urinary output were noted together with the highest value for IAP, base deficit or excess (BE) and arterial lactate. A total of 149 consecutive patients were screened and data analysis was limited to 144 mainly trauma patients (68%; 30% were surgical patients, and 2% obstetrical). A total of 2298 IAP measurements were performed. Mean IAP was quite high, 22 ± 8 mmHg, and on average IAP was monitored for 3 ± 2 days during which 16 ± 4 measurements were performed. Mortality was high since only 47% survived the development of IAH and only 27% the subsequent progression to ACS. The mean values for the above stated resuscitation endpoints differed significantly between survivors and non-survivors ($p < 0.0001$). However, when the worst values were entered in a multiple regression logistic model it was found that APP was superior to any other resuscitation endpoint in its ability to predict the patient survival from IAH. These values were typically encountered at the time of abdominal decompression or shortly before the patient's death. Figure 4 plots the top three endpoints in a relative operating characteristic (ROC) curve. The area under the ROC curve (AUROC) was 0.73 for APP, 0.62 for MAP and 0.29 for IAP. Analysis of different thresholds for APP showed that maintenance of an APP of at least

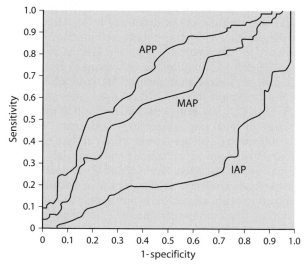

Fig. 4. ROC curve analysis of predictors of survival from intra-abdominal hypertension. APP: abdominal perfusion pressure; MAP: mean arterial pressure; IAP: intra-abdominal pressure. (From [13] with permission)

50 mmHg had the best sensitivity (76%) and specificity (57%) as a predictor for patient survival.

This study [13] also compared the impact of the evolution of treatment options during the two halves of the study period. In the second half, mean IAP values were lower confirming the development of an intolerance for high IAP values. With lower IAP and earlier decompression, fewer patients developed ACS (43 versus 64%) and mortality was decreased (28 versus 44%). This study puts some interesting light on the management of IAH and prevention of ACS. The IAP value lacks sensitivity and specificity to be used as a good endpoint and APP seems a better predictor since it not only addresses the severity of IAH but also the adequacy of tissue perfusion. However, this study is limited by its retrospective nature, the authors could have applied this concept during the second half of the study period after publication of the first abstract. The authors also report their results of resuscitation endpoint variables either as mean or as worst value; however, they do not provide data on a time scale. In other words, if the worst value occurs just before death it is of no use in predicting outcome. An ideal prognostic parameter should be routinely and reproducibly measurable, and rapidly and universally available. Furthermore, it should be obtained on admission or at least within the first 24 to 72 hours. It would be interesting to see a separation in the plots of daily mean APP values between survivors and non-survivors over time. Patients were not treated following a strict protocol and indication for decompression was left to each surgeon's individual decision and it is not stated in the article whether it was either based on high IAP or low APP. If APP is considered as a resuscitation endpoint then patients with normal or high APP (as is in hypertensive patients), but high IAP, would not undergo decompression? In a comment, the authors [13] state that the first goal must be to decompress in the presence of elevated IAP, the second goal would then be to maintain normal APP. In the ROC curve analysis shown in Figure 4 there is also the problem of mathematical coupling of APP, MAP and IAP; the curves thus compare the same parameters and, furthermore, the resuscitation endpoints predict different things since APP predicts survival and IAP mortality, so they should be analyzed in separate ROC curves, one for survival and another for mortality. This will be explained in the following paragraphs.

▋ Prospective Studies

Abdominal Banding

Even today, surgeons continue to try to pack intestinal loops into a cavity which is too small to receive them. They sometimes even close the abdomen by means of plastic plates and metal wires, the so-called 'ventre au fils' even if this happens at the expense of a tense abdomen and increased IAP. And, once the swollen intestines are finally back in place, some surgeons even apply an abdominal velcro belt in order to prevent incisional hernia. This practice should be discouraged, and surgeons urged to open the abdomen simply on the basis of an IAP-value without obvious clinical signs of ACS and to leave it open. Recent data are indeed in favor of a moratorium to be placed on the postoperative use of these velcro belts in mechanically ventilated, hemodynamically unstable ICU patients. We studied the effects of abdominal banding on the resuscitation endpoints suggested by Cheatham (data on file published in part) [23, 24]. We performed 19 measurements in eight patients at baseline and during the four stages of the study, after stabilization for 30 min at each stage. Baseline: normal IAP (10.8±3.3 mmHg) and zero PEEP (ZEEP);

▌ stage 1: increased IAP (17.3±3 mmHg, abdominal compression by banding) and ZEEP;
▌ stage 2: increased IAP (18.3±3 mmHg) and PEEP (15±2.5 cmH$_2$O) set at IAP-level from stage 1;
▌ stage 3: normal IAP (11.6±3.1 mmHg, abdominal decompression by removing belt) and same PEEP-level as stage 2;
▌ stage 4: normal IAP (10±3 mmHg) and ZEEP (return to baseline).

The evolution of the variables during the different study stages is plotted in Figure 5. Analysis of these data first shows that APP, FG, IAP, intramucosal pH (pHi), and CO$_2$-gap change more rapidly than global indices of perfusion such as MAP, arterial pH, BE and HCO$_3$-values that basically remain stable; the former may thus be better resuscitation endpoints. Second, the combination of IAH with PEEP (stage 2) had the most deleterious effects, abdominal decompression on the other hand quickly normalized the study variables. Third, it has to be noted that in stage 3 (decompression with PEEP) MAP tended to deteriorate further, probably because of a drop in systemic vascular resistance (SVR) due to re-opening of the venous capacitance vessels in the abdomen; despite this APP and FG return to normal levels. These results are in accordance with the findings of Cheatham et al.; the effects are reversible but are most likely to pose a risk in patients with underlying disease, insufficient filling status, and limited myocardial reserve [1, 6, 7, 25–31].

Single Center Pilot Study

Over a 12 month period 405 patients, hospitalized in a 7-bed mixed ICU, were screened for increased IAP >12 mmHg with the standardized intravesical pressure recording method [1, 7, 32]. Data for computation of severity scores were collected within the first 24 hours of ICU admission, and maximal IAP and lowest APP values were recorded within the first 72 hours. The SAPS-II was 35.1±17.4, APACHE-II 16.4±9.2, MOD score 3.4±3.3 and SOFA 3.9±3, IAP 8.1±4.6 mmHg, MAP 79.7±22.5 mmHg and APP 71.6±23.7 mmHg. Figure 6 shows the difference in two resuscitation endpoints with regard to hospital outcome. In patients who died in the hospital, the APP was significantly lower (60.8±23.1 mmHg) than in patients who survived (75.7±22.6 mmHg), p<0.0001); as was MAP (72.2±21.5 versus 82.5±22.2 mmHg, p<0.0001). The IAP was significantly higher in patients who died (11.4±5.3 versus 6.9±3.6 mmHg; p<0.0001). The incidence of IAH was 17.5% (cut-off 12 mmHg), 8.9% (cut-off 15 mmHg) and the incidence of ACS (cut-off 20 mmHg) was 2%. Within the group of patients with IAH (IAP>12 mmHg), however, there was no significant difference between survivors and non-survivors in MAP (72.4±29.6 versus 68.8±18.9 mmHg) and APP (57.7±30.1 versus 52.6±19.7 mmHg); although there was a trend towards lower values in non-survivors. Within this group of IAH patients IAP tended to be higher in non-survivors (16.2±3.9 versus 14.7±2.6 mmHg) although this also did not reach statistical significance. Figure 7 plots the Kaplan-Meier survival curves according to IAP and APP quartiles. The higher the IAP, the higher the hospital mortality (panel A): 11.5% in the first IAP quartile (IAP±5 mmHg, mean IAP 3.2±1.4 mmHg); 18.8% in the second IAP quartile (IAP >5 and ≤7.8 mmHg, mean IAP 7.2±0.7 mmHg);

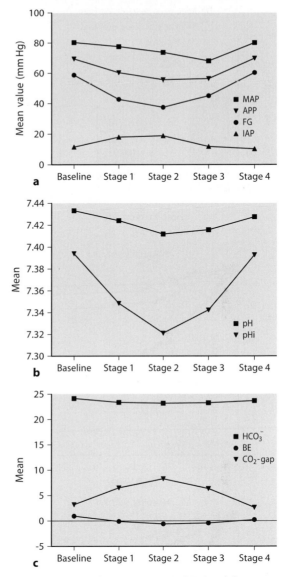

Fig. 5. Effects of abdominal compression, application of positive end-expiratory pressure (PEEP) and decompression on cardiovascular function and blood gas-derived variables at baseline and during different study stages after stabilization for 30 min in each stage. Baseline: normal intra-abdominal pressure (IAP) and zero PEEP (ZEEP); stage 1: increased IAP (abdominal banding) and ZEEP (=abdominal compression); stage 2: increased IAP and PEEP (cm H_2O) set at IAP (mmHg) (=synergy between IAH and PEEP); stage 3: normal IAP (= abdominal decompression) and same PEEP level as stage 2; stage 4: normal IAP and ZEEP (=return to baseline). In total 19 measurements were done at each stage in 8 patients. Panel **a:** Evolution of IAP, mean arterial pressure (MAP), abdominal perfusion pressure (APP) and filtration gradient (FG) ($p < 0.0001$ for all comparisons between different stages by one-way ANOVA). Panel **b:** Effects on arterial pH (pH) and intramucosal pH (pHi) ($p < 0.009$ for pHi for all comparisons between different stages by one-way ANOVA, $p = NS$ for pH). Panel **c:** Effects on arterial bicarbonate (HCO_3^-), base excess (BE) and CO_2^- gap (regional CO_2 minus arterial CO_2) ($p < 0.0001$ for CO_2^- gap for all comparisons between different stages by one-way ANOVA, $p = NS$ for HCO_3^- and BE)

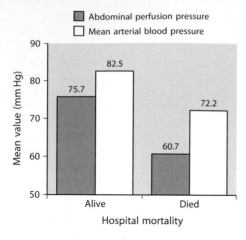

Fig 6. Clustered bar plot with mean values for abdominal perfusion pressure (APP) and mean arterial pressure (MAP) in survivors and non-survivors from a prospective single center sample of 405 mixed ICU patients (p < 0.0001 for all comparisons by independent samples student's *t* test)

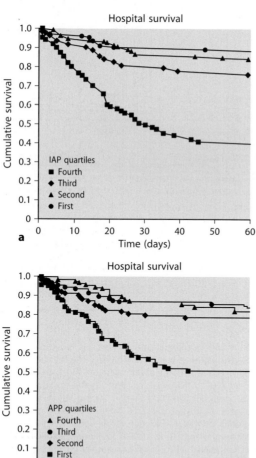

Fig. 7. Kaplan-Meier curves from a prospective single center sample of 405 mixed ICU patients. Panel **a:** Cumulative hospital survival curves for intra-abdominal pressure (IAP) quartiles. Panel **b:** Cumulative hospital survival curves for abdominal perfusion pressure (APP) quartiles

27% in the third IAP quartile (IAP >7.8 and ≤10 mmHg, mean IAP 9.5±0.5 mmHg) and 60.4% in the fourth IAP quartile (IAP >10 mmHg, mean IAP 14.7±3.7 mmHg). The lower the APP, the higher hospital mortality (panel B): 17.5% in the fourth (APP>86 mmHg, mean APP 104.3±16 mmHg), 17% in the third (APP > 68 and ≤86 mmHg, mean APP 76.6±4.9 mmHg), 22.9% in the second (APP >56 and ≤68 mmHg, mean APP 62.8±3.4 mmHg) and 51.5% in the first APP quartile (APP ≤56 mmHg, mean APP 44.8±10.2 mmHg).

Figure 8 plots the ROC curve examining the three endpoints with SAPS-II as predictors for hospital mortality (panel A). The AUROC is 0.883 for SAPS-II (95% CI=0.847–0.918), 0.758 for IAP (95% CI=0.705–0.812), 0.31 for APP (95% CI=0.249–0.371), and 0.358 for MAP (95% CI=0.296–0.421) (panel A). This seems to be quite opposite to the results found by Cheatham et al. [13] (Fig. 4). However, when we examine the same endpoints for hospital survival (panel B) we find comparable results, the AUROC is then 0.69 for APP (95% CI=0.629–0.751), 0.642 for MAP (95% CI=0.579–0.704) and 0.242 for IAP (95% CI=0.188–0.295). This means

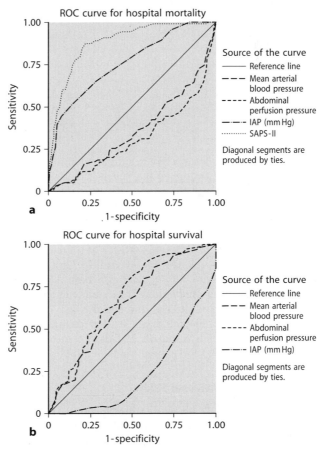

Fig. 8. ROC curves. The sample was a prospective population of 405 mixed ICU patients. Panel **a:** analysis of predictors of mortality from intra-abdominal hypertension (IAH). Panel **b:** analysis of predictors of survival from IAH

Table 1. Sensitivity and specificity for predicting patient survival (Cheatham study [13]) and mortality from intra-abdominal hypertension (single center pilot study [32] and the multicenter Critically Ill and Abdominal Hypertension (CIAH) study [33])

	Sensitivity			Specificity		
	Cheatham	Pilot	CIAH	Cheatham	Pilot	CIAH
APP						
40 mmHg	0.53	0.14	0.14	0.78	0.98	0.95
50 mmHg	0.76	0.39	0.53	0.55	0.91	0.85
60 mmHg	0.92	0.55	0.79	0.25	0.76	0.62
MAP						
60 mmHg	0.23	0.34	0.4	0.87	0.87	0.87
70 mmHg	0.57	0.58	0.69	0.6	0.64	0.61
80 mmHg	0.83	0.74	0.85	0.21	0.42	0.41
IAP						
9 mmHg		0.65	0.91		0.72	0.26
12 mmHg		0.44	0.75		0.93	0.59
15 mmHg	0	0.23	0.47	0.96	0.97	0.75
20 mmHg	0.08	0.06	0.17	0.84	0.99	0.92
25 mmHg	0.19			0.66		
30 mmHg	0.27			0.28		
35 mmHg	0.48			0.21		
40 mmHg	0.6			0.12		

that the studied endpoints predict different things. It seems logical that the higher the APP or MAP the higher the survival, and the higher the SAPS-II or IAP the lower the survival and the higher the mortality. Therefore, the AUROC should be examined for hospital mortality for SAPS-II and IAP and for survival for MAP and APP. The conclusions of Cheatham stating that APP and MAP are superior in predicting survival than IAP should be revised. The correct interpretation of the data by Cheatham show that the AUROC for IAP for hospital mortality is 0.709 which is quite similar to that for APP for survival (0.726). Stated otherwise: a low IAP would be as good a predictor for survival as a high APP. Analysis of different thresholds for APP in the pilot study show that maintenance of an APP of at least 60 mmHg had the best sensitivity (55%) and specificity (76%) as a predictor for patient survival, whereas maintenance of an MAP at 70 mmHg had the best sensitivity (58%) and specificity (64%). A cut-off of IAP at 9 mmHg had the best sensitivity (65%) and specificity (72%) for patient outcome (Table 1).

Multicenter International Study

In January 2001, 257 newly admitted patients, hospitalized in different ICUs were included prospectively in the Critically Ill and Abdominal Hypertension (CIAH) international multicenter study [33]. Patients were screened for IAH (defined as IAP ≥ 12 mmHg, normal being 0–5 mmHg) with a standardized intravesical pressure recording method. The IAP was recorded twice daily together with fluid balance, and SOFA score. There were 46.7% medical, 28% elective surgery, 16.7% emergency surgery, and 8.6% trauma patients. The major study endpoint was hospital mortality. Data have been collected from 13 centers: Belgium (90 patients from 5 centres), Italy (82 patients from 4), Australia (33 patients from 1), Israel (20 patients from 1), Brazil (20 patients from 1) and Austria (12 patients from 1). The body mass index (BMI) was 25.7±5.2, M/F ratio 2/1, age 61.7±11.4, APACHE-II score 17.4±8.4, SAPS-II score 39.8±17. SOFA score on day 1 was 6.3±3.8 with 1.1±1 organ failures. The IAP (on day 1) was 9.9±4.9 mmHg, the maximal IAP by day 3 (IAPmax) was 12.9±5.4 mmHg, and mean IAP during the first 3 days was 9.9±4.4 mmHg. The ICU stay was 9.9±11.4 days, and hospital (HOS) stay was 27.9±23.6 days. An IAPmax above 12 mmHg was present in 136 patients (52.9%), above 15 mmHg in 84 (32.7%) and above 20 mmHg in 29 (11.3%). The incidence of IAH (and mean IAPmax) in medical patients was 49.2% (12.8±5.6) versus 50% (12.7±4.9) in elective, 74.4% (14.7±5.5) in emergency surgery, and 40.9% (10.8±4.8) in trauma patients. Mean IAPmax was not different among countries. IAPmax correlated well with (cumulative) fluid balance and SOFA score, and all three parameters were significantly higher from day 1 to 7 in patients who died. Hospital mortality was 34.6%; 58 medical patients died (48.3%), 8 elective surgery (11.1%), 19 emergency surgery (44.2%), and 4 trauma patients (18.2%). Figure 9 shows the difference in two resuscitation endpoints with regard to hospital outcome. In patients who died in the hospital the APP was significantly lower (54.2±15.5 mmHg) than in patients who survived (69±23 mmHg, p<0.0001); as was MAP (68.3±14.9 versus 81.3±22.5 mmHg, p<0.0001). The IAP was significantly higher in patients who died (15.1±5.6 versus 11.8±5 mmHg, p<0.0001). Within the group of patients with IAH (IAP >12 mmHg) there was also a significant (p<0.001) difference between survivors and non-survivors in MAP (80.8±22.4 versus 67.9±13.5 mmHg) and APP (64.9±22.6 versus 51.8±13.5 mmHg). Within this group of IAH patients, IAP was not significantly different in non-survivors (17.1±4.9 versus 16.6±3.7 mmHg) confirming the superiority of APP as an outcome predictor.

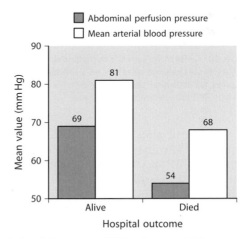

Fig. 9. Clustered bar plot with mean values for abdominal perfusion pressure (APP) and mean arterial pressure (MAP) in survivors and non-survivors from a prospective multicenter sample of 257 mixed ICU patients. Preliminary data analysis was limited to 145 cases where paired measurements were available (p<0.0001 for all comparisons by independent samples student's *t* test)

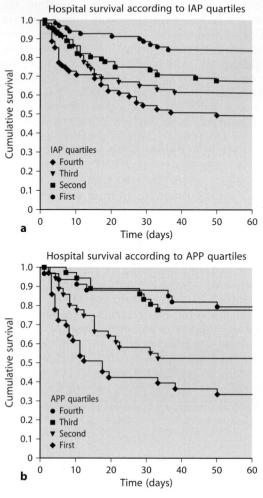

Fig. 10. Kaplan-Meier curves from a prospective multicenter sample of 257 mixed ICU patients. Panel **a:** cumulative hospital survival curves for intra-abdominal pressure (IAP) quartiles. Panel **b:** cumulative hospital survival curves for abdominal perfusion pressure (APP) quartiles (preliminary data analysis was limited to 145 cases where APP measurements were available)

Figure 10 plots the Kaplan-Meier survival curves according to IAP and APP quartiles. The higher the IAP the higher the hospital mortality (panel A): 16.2% in the first IAP quartile (IAP ≤ 9 mmHg, mean IAP$= 6.9 \pm 1.7$ mmHg); 33.8% in the second IAP quartile (IAP >9 and ≤ 12 mmHg, mean IAP$=11 \pm 0.7$ mmHg); 38.6% in the third IAP quartile (IAP >12 and IAP ≤ 16 mmHg, mean IAP$= 14.4 \pm 1.2$ mmHg) and 52.5% in the fourth IAP quartile (IAP >16 mmHg, mean IAP$= 20.5 \pm 3.7$ mmHg). The lower the APP, the higher the hospital mortality (panel B): 20% in the fourth (APP >74 mmHg, mean APP$= 92.8 \pm 19.2$ mmHg), 24.3% in the third (APP >58.2 and ≤ 74 mmHg, mean APP$= 66 \pm 5$ mmHg), 47.2% in the second (APP >49 and ≤ 58.2 mmHg, mean APP$= 53.3 \pm 2.9$ mmHg) and 67.6% in the first APP quartile (APP ≤ 49 mmHg, mean APP 41.7 ± 6.2 mmHg). Figure 11 plots

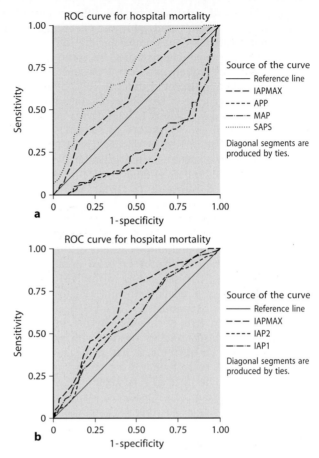

Fig. 11. ROC curves. The sample was a prospective population of 257 mixed ICU patients. Panel **a:** Analysis predictors of mortality from intra-abdominal hypertension (IAH) (preliminary data analysis was limited to 144 cases where all 4 variables were available). SAPS: simplified acute physiology score; IAPmax: maximal IAP value by day 3; APP: abdominal perfusion pressure; MAP: mean arterial pressure. Panel **b:** Analysis of predictors of mortality from intra-abdominal hypertension (data analysis included all 257 cases). IAP1: mean IAP value on day 1; IAP2: mean IAP value on day 3

the ROC curve for hospital mortality for the three endpoints and SAPS-II. The AUROC is 0.718 for SAPS-II (95% CI=0.635–0.801), 0.678 for IAP (95% CI=0.611–0.745) (panel A). Converting to the AUROC for survival this gives 0.731 for APP (95% CI=0.646–0.815), and 0.708 for MAP (95% CI=0.622–0.795). The maximal IAP value by day 3 has the best prediction for outcome with an AUROC 0.678 (95% CI=0.611–0.745) compared to 0.611 for IAP on day 2 (95% CI=0.540–0.683) and 0.598 for IAP on day 1 (95% CI=0.526–0.670) (panel b). Analysis of the different thresholds shown in Table 1 shows that maintenance of an APP of at least 60 mmHg has the best sensitivity (79%) and specificity (62%) as a predictor for patient survival, whereas maintenance of a MAP of 70 mmHg has the best sensitivity (69%) and specificity (61%). A cut-off of IAP at 12 mmHg has the best sensitivity (75%) and specificity (59%) for patient outcome. Table 1 also compares the results for specificity and sensitivity for the different cut-offs for IAP, APP and MAP obtained from Cheatham's study [14], the pilot single center study and the multicenter international CIAH study. Comparing the different AUROC for APP and IAP obtained from the above cited studies, we come to the same conclusion, namely that IAP and APP are equally important parameters (APP being slightly superior) in predicting patient outcome with an AUROC of around 0.7.

The trend over time of IAP showed a lowering of IAP by day 3 in survivors with a ΔIAP (IAP on day 3 minus IAP on day 1) of -0.6 ± 3.4 mmHg in survivors versus 0.7 ± 4.9 mmHg in non-survivors (p<0.0001); this was also the case for ΔSOFA (SOFA on day 3 minus SOFA on day 1): -1.1 ± 2.2 in survivors versus 0.2 ± 2.9 in non-survivors (p<0.0001). In univariate analysis, admission scoring systems, IAP-max, IAPmean, (cumulative) fluid balance on days 2, 3 and 4, ΔIAP, ΔSOFA and organ failure were significantly (p<0.001) related to hospital mortality. Multivariate regression analysis showed that ΔIAP (p=0.034), ΔSOFA (p<0.0001), IAPmax (p=0.048) were the only independent predictors for hospital mortality while severity scores and mean IAP value were not.

In conclusion, the preliminary results of this recent prospective multicenter clinical trial show that IAH can be expected in about 50% of cases. The incidence differs from 40.9 to 74.4% according to the ICU population studied, being highest in emergency surgery patients; and from 11.3 to 52.9% according to the cut-off used. IAH, together with (cumulative) fluid balance and organ failure, are predictors for hospital mortality. It is not necessarily the absolute value of IAP but the trend of IAP over time (ΔIAP) and its relation with positive fluid balance and ΔSOFA that seems predictive for outcome. A zero or negative fluid balance together with a drop in IAP and SOFA score by day 3 are strong predictors for good outcome. Analysis of ROC curves show that APP is slightly superior to IAP however these data were limited to a subgroup of 145 patients. Maintaining an APP above 60 mmHg and an IAP below 12 mmHg seems the best way to obtain a good outcome.

Discussion

As Cheatham and colleagues [13] noted, ROC curves help us to evaluate a test for its overall discriminatory power to predict survival from non-survival. ROC curves graph the sensitivity of a diagnostic test (true positive portion) versus 1 minus the specificity (false positive portion). A test with absolute discriminatory power, i.e., that always predicts survival or non-survival has an area under the ROC curve of 1, and a test that predicts survival no more often than by chance has an area under the ROC curve of 0.5. However, by interpreting these curves one has to be careful in what one wants to compare. For instance, since Cheatham looked at hospital survival, it is clear that we expect survival to be better in patients with higher APPs and higher MAPs, however we suspect lower survivals with higher IAPs [13]. In order to be consistent, we should look at the ROC curve for hospital mortality instead of survival if we are dealing with a continuous variable that affects outcome adversely the higher the variable value, as is the case with regard to IAP and also, for instance, for SAPS-II. In fact what we really want to learn from the ROC curves is an answer to the question "Is my study parameter any better than chance in predicting outcome?". If we interpret the results correctly we learn from Cheatham's study that IAP is as good at predicting mortality (with AUROC of 0.709 instead of the suggested 0.291) than APP in predicting survival (with AUROC of 0.726).

■ Therapeutic Implications

As stated in Cheatham's study [13] we no longer have to wait for high IAP levels above 25–30 mmHg at which the classic clinical manifestations of ACS become evident as we used to 10 years ago. We should intervene already at the relatively low level of 10 mmHg at which subtle changes take place, that remain undetectable by global indices of perfusion but yet compromise splanchnic perfusion [23, 24]. Based on the above mentioned results with regard to sensitivity and specificity the cut-offs of 12 mmHg in medical and 15 mmHg in surgical patients seem reasonable in defining IAH, and, in these patients, medical decompression should be encouraged before attempting surgical decompression. Whether this critical level remains the same in all patients or whether it depends upon the grading of the response (chronic versus acute versus subacute versus hyperacute), underlying and predisposing conditions, filling status, etiologic factors, or co-morbidities remains a subject for further study.

Merging the results of the above-mentioned retro- and prospective studies with the available literature data on the pathophysiologic implications of IAH (Fig. 1) we propose an algorithm for dealing with patients with IAH (Fig. 3). During the patients' ICU stay the indication for IAP monitoring has to be assessed daily. Once the indication has been posed, the primary goal should be to decompress whenever ACS is present. In a postoperative patient, the easiest way is to go back to the operating room and to perform surgical decompression with temporary abdominal closure. If the primary reason for admission is medical (for instance a ventilated decompensated chronic obstructive pulmonary disease (COPD) patient with secondary sepsis) it will be much harder to convince the surgeon to decompress, moreover no literature data are available with regard to the benefits of this procedure. If medical decompression is ineffective, one can always opt for a surgical approach. If decompression is successful the secondary goal then becomes to maintain APP within normal levels (>60 mmHg). The patient should then be screened for IAH (>12 mmHg). If IAH is not present the patient can be re-evaluated on a regular basis (e.g., IAP monitoring every 6 hours); if IAH is present with low APP further medical decompression should be attempted and the disappearance of IAH should be checked afterwards. If medical decompression fails and APP drops below 60 mmHg, abdominal perfusion should be optimized by guiding MAP >80 mmHg and cardiac index (CI) >2.5 l/min/m^2. Figure 3 also shows the algorithm for guiding fluid therapy in IAH. Since our traditional filling pressures such as central venous pressure (CVP) and pulmonary capillary wedge pressure (PCWP) are of no use in IAH due to their mathematical coupling to intrathoracic pressure, other preload markers should be used [1, 24, 30]. The right ventricular end-diastolic volume index (RVEDVI) obtained by volumetric thermodilution and the intra-thoracic blood volume index (ITBVI) and extra-vascular lung water index (EVLWI) obtained by dye indicator dilution have all been proved to be better markers of preload in IAH [1, 24, 30]. If MAP or CI are insufficient in the presence of low APP, fluids should be administrated if ITBVI is low (<1100 ml/m^2) and if there is no risk of pulmonary capillary leakage (EVLWI <10 ml/kg); in other cases catecholamines and vasopressors should be administered. In the absence of correct blood volume values the thresholds should be revised for PCWP, with 18 mmHg being the absolute minimum (the higher the IAP the higher the PCWP threshold). A simple rule is that any IAP value above 10 mmHg rises PCWP with IAP minus 10 mmHg. So if the PCWP is 23 and IAP is 17 mmHg then the real transmural PCWP would be somewhere around 23 minus 7 or 16 mmHg, and fluids should be administered. Ideally pleural pressures should be monitored by means of an esophageal balloon in order to obtain correct transmural pressures but previous work has shown that there seems to be a linear relation between IAP and pleural pressure. The effect of PEEP on PCWP can be calculated as the PEEP above 10 divided by 2; the effects of PEEP under 15 cmH$_2$O on IAP are negligible [1, 7]. In the acute phase of shock in a patient with IAH, liberal administration of fluids is non-debatable; however, in view of the results of the CIAH study fluids should be administered cautiously after initial stabilization and the administration of vasopressors (in order to limit on-going fluid resuscitation) should not be delayed. This is in accordance with other studies indicating that achieving at least one day of zero or negative fluid balance by day 3 is a good independent predictor of survival in patients with septic shock [33, 34].

▊ Conclusion

A few years ago, most of the data related to IAP was from anecdotal reports, animal studies, and small retrospective or prospective human studies mainly from the surgical literature. The recent results from a large retrospective trial and the preliminary results from the single center pilot studies in Belgium and Italy [35] and the large international multicenter trial in mixed ICUs indicate the strong clinical relevance of IAP in the general ICU population. The concept of IAP is not new in medicine, its effects were known two centuries ago! The idea of focussing on APP instead of IAP alone, in analogy with CPP, is tempting but still in its infant stage and further prospective validation needs to be done [13]. Little by little, the mystery of IAH is unraveled and transgresses the boundaries of acute and chronic illness, and of medical and surgical specialties [36]. More and more data are being gathered proving the superiority of APP as a resuscitation endpoint and outcome predictor; however, as always in science, further studies need to be done to confirm these preliminary results.

Acknowledgements. The writer wishes to thank all the ICU nurses of the Ste-Elisabeth Hospital in Brussels for their time and patience in the routine measurement of IAP and their positive feedback, especially from Koen and Olivier in the refinement of the measurement method. The writer is also indebted to his wife Ms Bieke Depré for her patience, advice and technical assistance with the preparation of this manuscript.

References

1. Malbrain MLNG (2001) Intra-abdominal pressure in the intensive care unit: Clinical tool or toy? In: Vincent JL (ed) Yearbook of Intensive Care and Emergency Medicine. Springer, Berlin, pp 547–585
2. Dworkin LD, Brenner BM (1996) The renal circulations. In: Brenner BM (ed) The Kidney, 5th edn. WB Saunders, Philadelphia, pp 247–285
3. Le Roith D, Bark H, Nyska M, Glick SM (1982) The effect of abdominal pressure on plasma antidiuretic hormone levels in the dog. J Surg Res 32:65–69
4. Hamilton BD, Chow GK, Inman SR, Stowe NT, Winfield HN (1998) Increased intra-abdominal pressure during pneumoperitoneum stimulates endothelin release in a canine model. J Endourol 12:193–197

5. Bradley SE, Bradley GP (1947) The effect of increased intra-abdominal pressure on renal function in man. J Clin Invest 26:1010–1022
6. Cheatham ML (1999) Intra-abdominal hypertension and abdominal compartment syndrome. New Horiz 7: 96–115
7. Malbrain MLNG (2000) Abdominal pressure in the critically ill. Curr Opin Crit Care 6:17–29
8. Shenasky JH, Gillenwater JY (1972) The renal hemodynamic and functional effects of external counterpressure. Surg Gynecol Obstet 134:253–258
9. Stone HH, Fulenwider JT (1977) Renal decapsulation in the prevention of post-ischemic oliguria. Ann Surg 186:333–355
10. Sugrue M, Jones F, Janjua KJ, Deane SA, Bristow P, Hillman K (1998) Temporary abdominal closure: a prospective evaluation of its effects on renal and respiratory function. J Trauma 45:914–921
11. Sugrue M, Jones F, Deane SA, Bishop G, Bauman A, Hillman K (1999) Intra-abdominal hypertension is an independent cause of postoperative renal impairment. Arch Surg 134:1082–1085
12. Ulyatt DB (1992) Elevated intra-abdominal pressure. Australian Anaesth: 108–114
13. Cheatham ML, White MW, Sagraves SG, Johnson JL, Block EFJ (2000) Abdominal perfusion pressure: a superior parameter in the assessment of intra-abdominal hypertension. J Trauma 49:621–627
14. Overholt RH (1931) Intraperitoneal pressure. Arch Surg 22:691–703
15. Kron JL, Harman PK, Nolan SP (1984) The measurement of intra-abdominal pressure as a criterion for abdominal re-exploration. Ann Surg 199:28–30
16. Iberti TJ, Lieber CE, Benjamin E (1989) Determination of intra-abdominal pressure using a transurethral bladder catheter: clinical validation of the technique. Anesthesiology 70: 47–50
17. Cheatham ML, Safcsak K (1998) Intraabdominal pressure: a revised method for measurement. J Am Coll Surg 186:594–595
18. Sugrue M, Buist MD, Lee A, Sanchez DJ, Hillman KM (1994) Intra-abdominal pressure measurement using a modified nasogastric tube: description and validation of a new technique. Intensive Care Med 20:588–590
19. Schein M, Wittmann DH, Aprahamian CC, Condon RE (1995) The abdominal compartment syndrome: the physiological and clinical consequences of elevated intra-abdominal pressure. J Am Coll Surg 180:745–753
20. Bloomfield J-GL, Ridings PC, Blocher CR, Marmarou A, Sugerman HJ (1997) A proposed relationship between increased intra-abdominal pressure, intrathoracic, and intracranial pressure. Crit Care Med 25:496–503
21. Burch JM, Moore EE, Moore FA, Franciose R (1996) The abdominal compartment syndrome. Surg Clin North Am 76:833–842
22. De Mendonca A, Vincent JL, Suter PM, et al (2000) Acute renal failure in the ICU: risk factors and outcome evaluated by the SOFA score. Intensive Care Med 26:915–921
23. Malbrain MLNG, Debaveye Y, Bertieaux S (2000) Effects of abdominal compression and decompression on cardiorespiratory function and regional perfusion. Intensive Care Med 26 (suppl 3):S264 (Abst)
24. Malbrain MLNG, De Coninck J, Debaveye Y, Delmarcelle D (2001) Optimal preload markers in intra-abdominal hypertension. Intensive Care Med 27 (suppl 2):S202 (Abst)
25. Richardson JD, Trinkle JK (1976) Hemodynamic and respiratory alterations with increased intra-abdominal pressure. J Surg Res 20:401–404
26. Luca A, Cicera I, Barcia-Pagan JC, et al (1993) Hemodynamic effects of acute changes in intra-abdominal pressure in patients with cirrhosis. Gastroenterology 104:222–227
27. Steinman M, da Silva LE, Coelho IJ, et al (1998) Hemodynamic and metabolic effects of CO_2 pneumoperitoneum in an experimental model of hemorrhagic shock due to retroperitoneal hematoma. Surg Endosc 12:416–420
28. Kitano Y, Takata M, Sasaki N, Zhang Q, Yamamoto S, Miyasaka K (1999) Influence of increased abdominal pressure on steady-state cardiac performance. J Appl Physiol 86:1651–1656

29. Chang MC, Miller PR, D'Agostino R, Meredith JW (1998) Effects of abdominal decompression on cardiopulmonary function and visceral perfusion in patients with intra-abdominal hypertension. J Trauma 44: 440–445

30. Cheatham ML, Safcsak K, Block EF, Nelson LD (1999) Preload assessment in patients with an open abdomen. J Trauma 46:16–22

31. Ridings PC, Bloomfield GL, Blocher CR, Sugerman HJ (1995) Cardiopulmonary effects of raised intra-abdominal pressure before and after intravascular volume expansion. J Trauma 39: 1071-1075

32. Malbrain MLNG (1999) Abdominal pressure in the critically ill: measurement and clinical relevance. Intensive Care Med 25:1453-1458

33. Malbrain MLNG, for the CIAH study group (2001) Incidence of intra-abdominal hypertension in the ICU and its relation with fluid balance, organ failure and 28 day mortality. Intensive Care Med 27 (suppl 2):S176 (Abst)

34. Alsous F, Khamiees M, DeGirolamo A, Amoateng-Adjepong Y, Monthous CA (2000) Negative fluid balance predicts survival in patients with septic shock. Chest 117:1749–1754

35. Pelosi P, Brazzi L, Gattinoni L (2001) Measuring intra-abdominal pressure in the intensive care setting. In: Vincent JL (ed) Yearbook of Intensive Care and Emergency Medicine. Springer, Berlin, pp 586–595

36. Ivatury RR, Sugerman HJ (2000) Abdominal compartment syndrome: A century later, isn't it time to pay attention? Crit Care Med 28:2137–2138

Intra-abdominal Pressure and Chest Wall Interaction

M. Del Turco, F. Giunta, and V. M. Ranieri

▌ Introduction

Acute lung injury (ALI) is characterized by of a reduction in functional residual capacity (FRC) and an increase in static elastance of the respiratory system [1]. Such increase in static elastance of the respiratory system is mostly due to alterations in the mechanical properties of the lung because of the leading role of the underlying pulmonary injury. However, recent studies [2, 3] have reported that chest wall elastance may also be increased in patients with ALI probably through the increase in abdominal pressure. This chapter will

- ▌ discuss the physiology of the abdomen-chest wall interaction,
- ▌ describe the gold standard technique to measure intra-thoracic and abdominal pressures, and
- ▌ discuss the mechanisms and potential clinical implications of increased intra-abdominal pressure (IAP).

▌ Physiology of Abdomen-chest Wall Interaction

The chest wall operates in series with the lung being divided into two parallel pathways, the rib cage and the diaphragm-abdomen. The diaphragm forms the caudal distensible boundary of the chest cavity and is mechanically coupled to the abdominal wall and contents. The abdomen mechanically behaves like a closed fluid system and transmission of abdominal pressure is nearly homogeneous. The average density of abdominal contents is similar to that of water, and, therefore, under static conditions the walls are subjected to a surface pressure gradient that approximates a hydrostatic gradient. The change in pressure across the chest wall, when the muscle are relaxed (static condition), with the airway closed, is considered the change in pleural pressure, which is the surface pressure between the opposite surface of the thorax separated by the visceral and parietal pleural.

Pleural pressure exhibits a hydrostatic pressure gradient along the height of the lungs and it is higher in gravity-dependent portions of the pleural space, being similar to the alveolar pressure at end expiration. The degree of lung distension is greater in the non-dependent than in the dependent portion of the chest wall. In the upright posture, at the end of a normal expiration, the pressure beneath the dome of the diaphragm and at the surface of the lungs above the diaphragm is approximately -3 or -4 cmH$_2$O. In the upright posture, gravity acts in the inspiratory direction on the abdomen-diaphragm and in the expiratory direction on the rib cage, and the hydrostatic effect of the abdomen is greater at small than at large vol-

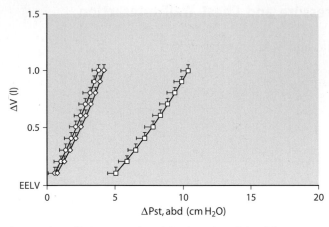

Fig. 1. Volume (ΔV)-pressure ($\Delta Pst,abd$) relationship of the abdomen in patients undergoing cardiac surgery (*open circle*), and patients with medical (*open diamond*) and surgical (*open square*) acute respiratory distress syndrome (ARDS). From [4] with permission. EELV: end-expiratory lung volume

umes [4, 5]. In the supine position gravity has a marked expiratory action on the abdomen-diaphragm, and the abdominal container exerts a pressure of approximately 10 cmH$_2$O displacing the diaphragm upward with a consequent decrease in FRC and stiffness of the chest wall [4, 5]. In both supine and upright postures, rib cage compliance decreases as volume is reduced below FRC [4, 5].

Mutoh et al. [6], studied the effect of abdominal distension on lung and chest wall mechanics in anesthetized and paralyzed mechanically ventilated pigs, demonstrated that abdominal distension, by changing pleural pressure, may alter the part of the chest wall near the diaphragm-abdomen reducing FRC and impairing the alveolar-arterial O$_2$ difference. The same authors studied the respiratory effects of large volume infusion in pigs and found that fluid overload, by causing abdominal distension and increasing the pleural pressure in dependent lung, may alter chest wall mechanics [7].

▍ Measurements of Intra-thoracic and Abdominal Pressure

Bladder Pressure to Measure Abdominal Pressure

Although IAP can be measured by direct (intra-peritoneal pressure) [8] or indirect (caval pressure [9], gastric pressure [10] and bladder pressure [11]) methods, measurement of IAP by an indwelling catheter in the urinary bladder is considered the method of choice since an animal study showed that direct (via a peritoneal catheter) and indirect (via a urinary bladder catheter) were equal for pressure ranging from 5 to 70 mmHg [11].

The use of bladder pressure as an estimate of abdominal pressure was originally described by Kron et al. [12] and Iberti et al. [13]. This method may put the patient at increased risk of urinary tract infection, and healthcare providers at risk of needle stick injuries, while the revision of Kron's original technique, reported by Cheatham and Safcsak [11], is considered simple, minimally invasive, and can be easily performed at the bedside.

A standard intravenous infusion set is connected to 1000 ml of normal saline, two stop-cocks, a 60 ml Luer lock syringe and a disposable pressure transducer. An 18′ guage is inserted into the culture aspiration port of the Foley catheter and the needle is removed. The infusion catheter is attached to the first stop-cock via arterial pressure tubing. The zero reference point is the symphysis pubis and the mid-axillary line when the patient is completely supine. The Foley catheter is clamped distal to the culture aspiration port and 50 ml of saline is instilled into the bladder. After equilibration the patient's IAP is measured [11]. Intra-bladder pressure cannot be measured in cases of bladder trauma or when the bladder is compressed.

Esophageal Pressure to Measure Intra-thoracic Pressure

Pleural pressure may be estimated by the measurement of intra-esophageal pressure (Pes) since the esophagus is a compliant and easily accessible intra-thoracic structure surrounded by two pleural layers and changes in pleural pressure are directly transmitted to the hollow viscus. Measurement of Pes is usually obtained by a validated technique [14], inserting trans-nasally a thin-walled balloon catheter into the esophagus from the nose. An occlusion test is performed, occluding the airway opening at end-expiration and allowing the subject to perform a series of 3 to 5 spontaneous occluded inspiratory efforts. This maneuver is important to confirm the proper intra-esophageal positioning of the balloon. This conventional balloon technique appears not to be valid in the supine position, probably because in the supine position there is a horizontal gradient in changes of pleural surface with the greater values towards the lung base.

▍ Abdominal Distension and Clinical Implication

Elevated IAP has been shown to produce multiple adverse effects, involving both intra-abdominal and extra-abdominal organ systems, a syndrome often referred to as intra-abdominal hypertension (IAH). Bradley and coworkers [15] demonstrated that increasing IAP to 20 mmHg in human volunteers reduced renal blood flow and glomerular filtration rate (GFR). The consequences of IAH include cardiovascular, renal, abdominal visceral (gut dysfunction and bacterial translocation), neurological, and respiratory abnormalities with the development of an abdominal compartment syndrome (ACS) [16, 17]. ACS is defined as the pathologic state caused by an acute increase in IAP above 20–25 mmHg that adversely affects end-organ function or that can cause serious wound complications in which abdominal decompression has beneficial effects [18]. The ACS occurs when the pressure within the abdomen increases to the point that vascular inflow is compromised and the function and viability of the tissue within the compartment are threatened. The ACS develops with acute and rapid (60 minutes) elevations in IAP [19]; frequently IAH and ACS cannot be separated from the underlying disease.

The exact IAP value that defines IAH and ACS still remains subject to debate, but levels of IAP as low as 10 mmHg can cause organ dysfunction [20] and decompression should be performed at levels of IAP above 20–25 mmHg [21]. Burch et al. [22] defined a grading system of IAH-ACS to guide therapy: Grade I 10–15 cmH$_2$O, Grade II 15–25 cmH$_2$O, Grade III 25–35 cmH$_2$O, Grade IV >35 cmH$_2$O. Patients with grade III and IV IAH should undergo abdominal decompression.

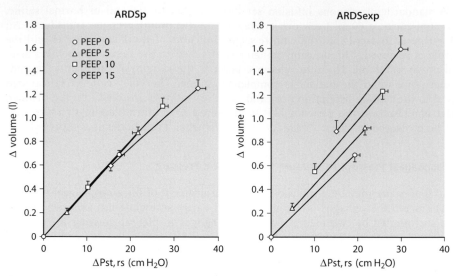

Fig. 2. Volume (ΔV)-pressure (ΔPst,rs) relationship in patients with pulmonary (ARDSp) and extra-pulmonary (ARDSexp) acute respiratory distress syndrome (ARDS). From [5] with permission. PEEP: positive end-expiratory pressure

IAH can develop in both medical and surgical patients [23] and it is frequent after major abdominal trauma [21]. Conditions associated with elevation of IAP are abdominal infection, such as necrotizing pancreatitis, intra-peritoneal or retro-peritoneal hemorrhage, grossly edematous bowel secondary to massive fluid resuscitation, ileus and intra-abdominal sepsis; abdominal surgery for these diseases, in which there is abdominal closure under excessive tension; laparoscopy with CO_2 pneumo-perito-neum, and extrinsic compression of the abdomen (pneumatic anti-shock garment). Massive fluid resuscitation can also lead to increased IAH by increasing interstitial fluid volume (capillary leak), particularly in patients with sepsis [7]. Ischemia-reperfu-sion, release of vasoactive substances and oxygen-derived free radicals, and temporary mesenteric venous obstruction may also ensuing visceral and retroperitoneal edema.

Recent data seem to suggest the clinical utility of abdominal perfusion pressure (APP, MAP-IAP) as a clinical resuscitation endpoint and predictor of survival during treatment for IAH and ACS. Cheatham and coworkers [24] studied 144 surgical patients treated for IAH in a retrospective study and found that the abdominal perfusion gradient seemed to be the best predictor of patient outcome when compared with IAP or other traditional resuscitation endpoints (MAP, arterial pH, base deficit, arterial lactate, and hourly urinary output). The value of abdominal perfusion shows not only the severity of IAH, but also the adequacy of tissue perfusion, indicating the need for compressive laparotomy. A target APP of 50 mmHg is identified as the resuscitation endpoint in predicting outcome from IAH.

Abdominal Distension and the Respiratory System

Any increase in abdominal pressure may directly and indirectly affect the respiratory system, lung, and chest wall. Diaphragmatic elevation leads to direct pulmonary compression [6] thus explaining the reduction in FRC observed in obese patients

[25] or during anesthesia [26]. Abdominal distension may affect chest wall mechanics indirectly by the downward displacement of the static pressure-volume relationship of the chest wall at lower lung volume and directly by changes in chest wall configuration [27].

Recently the role of the abdomen has been shown to influence lung and chest wall mechanics in patients with ALI [2, 3]. Ranieri and coworkers [2] showed that patients with ALI following major abdominal surgery have a stiffer chest wall than patients with 'medical' ALI due to abdominal distension. Gattinoni and coworkers [3] found that in 'primary' ALI (ALI associated with predominant consolidation), there is a decreased lung compliance with normal chest wall and the application of PEEP caused minimal alveolar recruitment. On the other hand, when ALI is characterized by interstitial edema and alveolar collapse ('secondary' ALI), lung is preserved and chest wall compliance is decreased because abdominal distension and PEEP recruits previously collapsed alveoli.

Abdominal Distension and the Cardiovascular System

Elevation in IAP leads to a reduction in cardiac output [28, 29], even at IAP values of 10 to 15 mmHg. The diminished cardiac output results from decreased preload and increased after-load and reduced cardiac contractility at IAP greater than 30 mmHg [30]. The reduction in preload is due to a reduction in venous return, which results in reduced stroke volume and compensatory increase in heart rate. This results from increased venous resistance within the abdomen and thorax, leading to reduced caval and retroperitoneal venous flow (lower-extremity venous outflow). At an IAP of 10 mmHg, venous return may be enhanced by the mobilization of blood from the capacitance vessels within the abdomen. This can explain the slight increase in cardiac output with small increases in IAP (autotransfusion obtained by military antishock trouser [MAST]) [31]. Systemic vascular resistance (SVR) also rises (increased afterload), secondary to the reduction in cardiac output and direct arteriolar compression within the abdomen. Increased thoracic pressure and diaphragmatic elevation are responsible for reduction in ventricular compliance which, combined with the increased systemic afterload, reduces cardiac contractility. Paradoxically, the decreased preload is accompanied by higher central venous pressure (CVP) and pulmonary capillary wedge pressure (PCWP), caused by greater intra-thoracic pressure (pleural pressure) due to diaphragmatic elevation. These variables (CVP and PCWP), commonly used as indicators of preload, in this condition are not correlated significantly with CI and a better predictor of preload than CVP and PCWP is right ventricular end diastolic volume index (RVEDVI), a volumetric estimate of preload independent of zero-pressure references [32].

Abdominal Distension and Renal Function

Oliguria can be seen at an IAP of 15–20 mmHg, whereas increases to 30 mmHg lead to anuria [15, 18]. The etiology of renal dysfunction is multi-factorial and may due to a decrease in cardiac output by the mechanisms described above and/or by mechanical compression of parenchymal and renal veins, causing an increase in renal vascular resistance and outflow obstruction, reducing effective renal plasma flow. The changes in renal and systemic hemodynamics lead to increased circulating levels of anti-diuretic hormone (ADH) with further increases in renal vascular resistances and sodium and water retention [33]. Although urine flow rate is subject to several factors that may alter its value, decompression, with a subsequent increase in urine output, has been described by several authors [34]. As a result, oliguria, associated with increased IAP, was the first criteria to be described as an indication for surgical abdominal decompression.

Abdominal Distension and Central Nervous System

The acutely increased IAP produces a significant increase in intra-cranial pressure (ICP) and decrease in cerebral perfusion by augmenting pleural pressure, causing a functional obstruction to cerebral venous outflow via the jugular venous system [35, 36]. The same phenomenon may be involved in patients with severe obesity, suffering from idiopathic intracranial hypertension (pseudotumor cerebri) due to chronically increased IAP [37]. However, the association between acutely elevated IAP and ICP has been shown to influence neurological morbidity only in patients with head injuries [35, 36].

Abdominal Distension and Abdominal Viscera

Under normal conditions, the intestinal epithelial barrier acts as a selective route of entry, allowing movement of necessary molecules through the epithelium and preventing the entry of potentially pathogenic organism or their products. Several factors may contribute to the decrease in splanchnic blood flow from increased IAP as a direct mechanical compression of the splanchnic veins (increased splanchnic vascular resistance), myogenic reflexes within the splanchnic vasculature and mesenteric vasoconstriction induced by vasoactive hormones released with increased IAP [38]. The gut is extremely sensitive to increases in IAP: mesenteric blood flow may be reduced with IAPs as low as 10 mmHg [20], and during IAH, intestinal perfusion decreases, leading to a reduction in tissue oxygen tension at the mucosa, anaerobic metabolism and acidosis [39]. As previously noted, the increased visceral edema, secondary to resuscitation (fluid overload), may lead to a vicious circle of worsening perfusion and bowel ischemia [7]. The gut hypoperfusion resulting from increased IAP, has been proposed as a possible mechanism for the loss of the mucosal barrier and the subsequent development of bacterial translocation, sepsis and multiple organ failure (MOF) [19, 38]. These phenomena may occur at much lower abdominal pressures than those at which the classical manifestations of ACS become evident [19]. Global indices of tissue perfusion (blood pressure, pulse rate, arterial pH, and lactate) have not been demonstrated to be useful to reflect alterations in regional perfusion, whereas IAP and gastric tonometry are considered early signs of tissue hypoperfusion [39].

References

1. Marini JJ (1990) Lung mechanics in the adult respiratory distress syndrome. Clin Chest Med 11:673–690
2. Ranieri VM, Brienza M, Santostasi S, et al (1997) Impairment of lung and chest wall mechanics in patients with acute respiratory distress syndrome. Role of abdominal distension. Am J Respir Crit Care Med 156:1082–1091
3. Gattinoni L, Pelosi P, Suter PM, Pedoto A, Vercesi P, Lissoni A (1998) Acute respiratory distress syndrome caused by pulmonary and extrapulmonary disease. Different syndromes? Am J Respir Crit Care Med 158:3–11

4. Agostoni E (1986) Static behavior of the respiratory system. In: Macklem PT, Mead J (eds) Handbook of Physiology. Sect. 3: The Respiratory System. Vol 3: Mechanics of Breathing. Part 1. American Physiology Society, Bethesda, pp 113–130

5. Agostoni E (1986) Passive Mechanical properties of the chest wall. In: Macklem PT, Mead J (eds) Handbook of Physiology. Sect. 3: The Respiratory System. Vol 3: Mechanics of brething. Part 2. American Physiology Society, Bethesda, pp 429–442

6. Mutoh T, Lamm WJ, Embree LJ, Hildebrandt J, Albert PK (1991) Abdominal distension alters regional pleural pressures and chest wall mechanics in pigs in vivo. J Appl Physiol 70(6):2611–2618

7. Mutoh T, Lmm WJ, Embree LJ, Hildebrandt J, Albert PK (1992) Volume infusion produces abdominal distension, lung compression, and chest wall stiffening in pigs. J Appl Physiol 72(2):575–582

8. Iberti TJ, Kelly KM, Gentili DR, Hirsch S, Benjamin E (1987) A simple technique to accurately determine intra-abdominal pressure. Crit Care Med 15:1140–1142

9. Lacey SR, Bruce J, Brooks SP, et al (1987) The different merits of various method of indirect measurement of intaabdominal pressure as a guide to closure of abdominal wall defect. J Pediatr Surg 22:1207–1211

10. Sugrue M, Buist MD, Lee A, Sanchez DJ, Hillman KM (1994) Intra-abdominal pressure measurement using a modified nasogastric tube: description and validation of a new technique. Intensive Care Med 20:588–590

11. Cheathman ML, Safcsak K (1998) Intraabdominal pressure: a revised method for measurement. J Am Coll Surg 186:594–595

12. Kron JL, Harman PK, Nolan SP (1984) The measurement of intra-abdominal pressure as a criteriion for abdominal re-exploration. Ann Surg 199:28–30

13. Iberti TJ, Liber CE, Benjamin E (1989) Determination of intra-abdominal pressure using a transurethral bladder catheter: clinical validation of the technique. Anesthesiology 70:47–50

14. Baydur A, Behrakis PK, Zin WA, Jaeger M, Milic-Emili J (1982) A simple method for assessing the validity of the esophageal balloon technique. Am J Respir Crit Care 126:788–791

15. Bradley SE (1947) The effect of increased intra-abdominal pressure on renal function in man. J Clin Invest 26:1010

16. Ivatury RR (1996) Intra-abdominal hypertension: the abdominal compartment syndrome. In: Ivatury RR, Cayten CG (eds) The Textbook of Penetrating Tauma. Williams and Wilkins, Baltimore, pp 939–951

17. Simon RJ (1994) Intra-abdominal hypertension in patients with catastrophic abdominal trauma: the benefit of prophylaxis and aggressive control. Crit Care Med 22:A72 (Abst)

18. Morris JA, Eddy VA, Blinman TA, Rutherford EJ, Sharp KW (1993) The staged laparotomy for trauma: issues in unpacking and reconstruction. Ann Surg 217:576–586

19. Diebel NL, Dulchavsky SA, Brown WJ (1997) Splanchnic ischemia and bacterial translocation in the abdominal compartment syndrome. J Trauma 43:852–855

20. Diebel LN, Wilson RF, Dulchavsky SA, Saxe J (1992) Effect of increased intra-abdominal pressure on hepatic arterial, portal venous, and hepatic microcirculatory blood flow. J Trauma 33:279–283

21. Ivatury RR, Porter JM, Simon RJ, et al (1998) Intra-abdominal hypertensiion after life-threatening penetrating abdominal trauma: prophylaxis, incidence, and clinical relevance to gastric mucosal PH and abdominal compartment syndrome. J Trauma 44:1016–1023

22. Burch JM, Moore EE, Moore FA, Franciose R (1996) The abdominal compartment syndrome. Surg Clin North Am 76:833–842

23. Saggi BH, Sugarman HJ, Ivatury RR, Bloomfield GL (1998) Abdominal compartment syndrome. J Trauma 45:597–609

24. Cheatham ML, White MW, Sagraves SG, Johnson JL, Block EF (2000) Abdominal perfusion pressure: a superior parameter in the assessment of intra-abdominal hypertension. J Trauma 49:621–627

25. Pelosi P, Croci M, Ravagnan I, et al (1997) Respiratory system mechanics in sedated, paralyzed, morbidly obese patients. J Appl Physiol 82(3):811–818

26. Froese AB, Bryan AC (1974) Effects of anesthesia and paralysis on diaphragmatic mechanics in man. Anesthesiology 41:242–255

27. Fahy BG, Barnas GM, Flowers JL, Nagle SE, Njoku MJ (1995) The effects of increased abdominal pressure on lung and chest wall mechanics during laparoscopic surgery. Anesth Analg 81:744–750

28. Cullen DJ, Coyle JP, Teplick R, Long MC (1989) Cardiovascular, pulmonary, and renal effects of massively increased intra-abdominal pressure in critically ill patients. Crit Care Med 17:118–121

29. Ridings PC, Bloomfield GL, Blocher GR, Sugerman HJ (1995) Cardiopulmonary effects of raised intra-abdominal pressure before and after intravascular volume expansion. J Trauma 39:1071–1075

30. Robotham JL, Wise RA, Bromberger-Barnea B (1985) Effects of changes in abdominal pressure on left ventricular performance and regional blood flow. Crit Care Med 13:803–808

31. Kelman GR (1972) Cardiac output and arterial blood-gas tension during laparoscopy. Br J Anaesth 44:1155–1161

32. Cheatham ML, Safcsak K, Block EF, Nelson LD (1999) Preload assessment in patients with an open abdomen. J Trauma 46:16–22

33. Bloomfield GL, Blocher GR, Falchry IF, Sica DA, Surgerman HJ (1997) Elevated intra-abdominal pressure increases plasma renin activity and aldosterone levels. J Trauma 42:997–1003

34. Cheatham ML (1999) Intra-abdominal hypertension and compartment syndrome. New Horiz 2:96–115

35. Bloomfield GL, Ridings PC, Blocher GR, Marmarou A, Sugerman JH (1997) A proposed relationship between increased intraabdominal, intrathoracic, and intracranial pressure. Crit Care Med 25:496–503

36. Saggi BH, Bloomfield Gl, Sugarman JH, et al (1999) Treatment of intracranial hypertension using nonsurgical abdominal decompression. J Trauma 46:646–651

37. Sugerman HJ, DeMaia EJ, Felton WL 3rd, Nakatsuka M, Sismarnis A (1997) Increased intra-abdominal pressure and cardiac filling pressure in obesity associated pseudotumor cerebri. Neurology 49:507–511

38. Sugerman HJ, Bloomfield GL, Saagi BW (1999) Multisystem organ failure secondary to increased intraabdominal pressure. Infection 27:61–66

39. Sugrue M, Jones F, Lee A, et al (1996) Intraabdominal pressure and gastric intramucosal pH: is there an association? World J Surg 20:988–991

Renal Failure

The Kidney in Sepsis

T. Whitehouse and M. Singer

▌ Introduction

The kidney is, if not the forgotten organ, then perhaps the least investigated in the critically ill patient. However, other than offering the patient the best intensive care management possible, with appropriate maintenance of pressure and flow through judicious use of fluids and vasoactive drug support, there is no specific treatment available to reverse kidney dysfunction [1]. The introduction of biocompatible membranes has made renal replacement therapy (RRT) an easy, safe and routine procedure on most ICUs. Except in cases of deliberate treatment withdrawal, death from acute renal failure is now very rare. Acute renal failure is thus often regarded as a relatively minor, easily supported distraction, compared with the weightier cardiorespiratory problems that preoccupy the intensivist.

Acute renal failure induced by sepsis remains an enigma. Unexplained features include the absence of significant histological change, despite anuria and biochemical derangement, and the lag-time for recovery of renal function which may take up to several months despite early resolution of systemic inflammation and restoration of a normal circulatory profile. Impressively, severe renal failure is usually reversible to such a degree that most patients become independent of RRT. This is fortunate as, depending on patient mix and acute renal failure definition, the rate of acute renal failure associated with sepsis varies between 9–40% of ICU admissions [2, 3], a workload that would overwhelm chronic dialysis units if life-long RRT were required. A recent audit of Scottish ICUs showed the percentage of patients requiring long-term RRT was just 1.6% in the absence of pre-morbid renal impairment [4].

Renal failure developing in the ICU carries a poor prognosis [5] while combined renal and respiratory failure carries a considerably worse prognosis than respiratory failure alone [6]. In the absence of disease-modifying therapies, it is impossible to measure the impact on mortality for preventing acute renal failure. 'Renal salvage' with furosemide, while having some theoretical benefits on reducing tubular cell energy consumption [7], and flushing of debris out of tubules and ducts, has never been shown convincingly to improve either renal function or survival. Similarly, the use of dopamine to increase renal flow is probably not advantageous [8, 9], and may be detrimental.

Understanding of the pathophysiology underlying sepsis-induced acute renal failure remains scanty. In this chapter, we shall cover what little is known about mechanisms underlying sepsis-induced renal failure and discuss the likely involvement of nitric oxide (NO). We postulate the final common pathway may lie within the mitochondrion whose role is to supply high-energy phosphate bonds in the form of ATP. Control of mitochondrial respiration is a physiological function of NO. In sepsis, NO is over-produced in quantities that may significantly inhibit oxidative phosphorylation. Lack of available energy stores to drive the kidney's excretory, secretory and absorptive functions may prompt cellular shutdown – a state of 'hibernation' from which the kidney awakens upon patient recovery. Through this mechanism it may avoid cell death (necrotic and/or apoptotic) from occurring to an extent sufficient to compromise eventual recovery. The term "acute renal success" was first coined by Thurau and Boylan in 1976 [10] with respect to the role of the juxtaglomerular apparatus and the macula densa in urinary concentration ability. It may also be appropriate to use this phrase when referring to sepsis-induced acute renal failure.

▌ Anatomy and Physiology

Although comprising only 0.5% of total body weight, the kidneys in health receive 25% of total cardiac output. This is the greatest blood flow per unit weight of tissue found in the body and ensures adequate clearance. In this process, the entire circulating volume is filtered and reabsorbed twice an hour. Daily urinary production is the overspill of the excess between filtration and subsequent reabsorption of approximately 180 litres of plasma per day.

The building blocks of the kidney are the nephrons, the constituent parts being glomerulus, proximal tubule, loop of Henlé, distal tubule and collecting ducts. Glomerular filtration depends upon renal plasma flow, the balance of hydrostatic and oncotic pressures across the capillary, and the permeability of the Bowman's capsule. To maintain filtration pressure, a complex interplay of mediators appears to balance afferent and efferent arteriolar tone. The renin-angiotensin system, the sympathetic system, prostaglandins, and NO have all been implicated [11].

Human kidneys have two populations of nephrons, superficial and juxtamedullary. Delivery of sodium chloride (NaCl) to the thick ascending limb of the loop of Henlé and the distal convoluted tubule of the nephron is determined by glomerular filtration rate (GFR) and proximal tubular function. Although most sodium (85%) is reabsorbed in the proximal tubule, absorption of sodium in the thick ascending limb of the loop of Henlé and urea delivery from the medullary collecting duct ensures the generation of a graduated medullary interstitial hypertonicity. The formation of this gradient allows fine-tuning of blood osmolarity by the absorption of water in the collecting ducts under the control of vasopressin (anti-diuretic hormone, ADH). At the same time, the complex arrangement of blood vessels ensures a high flow to the glomeruli (predominantly in the cortex) to ensure clearance, and a much lower flow to the medulla to favour reabsorption. The arrangement of nephrons and capillaries that gives the kidney its ability to concentrate urine also makes it vulnerable to hypoxia at times of stress. At its weakest point – the corticomedullary junction – lie the Na/K-ATP pumps responsible for sodium reabsorption and maintenance of the osmotic gradient.

Histological Changes Seen in Sepsis

Although the term 'acute tubular necrosis' (ATN) is colloquially applied to the renal dysfunction of sepsis, histology fails to reveal either necrosis or signs of tubular damage [12]. In one paper [13], rhesus monkeys were given endotoxin, either as a 10 mg/kg bolus or by prolonged infusion at a rate of 10 mg/kg/hr. Only minor morphological changes were seen in those animals receiving the endotoxin bolus, while those receiving endotoxin infusion showed sequestration of neutrophils and monocytes in the peritubular capillaries and, to a lesser extent, in the glomeruli; however, no sequestration was seen in the tubules. These changes were associated with occasional fibrin deposits and extensive endothelial cell damage with focal capillary disruption. Only in the advanced stages, when the endotoxin infusion had been running for 22 hours in animals not resuscitated with fluid, were changes seen that included prominent interstitial edema and focal necrosis of tubular epithelium. Endothelial cell changes seen in the glomeruli were far less severe than those observed in the peritubular capillaries.

Histological data from septic patients are even less common. In an important post-mortem study of patients dying of multiple organ failure (MOF), Hotchkiss et al. [12] observed;

> "histologic findings in kidneys from control patients revealed no acute changes. Surprisingly, despite the high prevalence of clinical renal dysfunction (65%) ... only one septic patient had evidence of kidney necrosis. No renal tubular nor glomerular cell apoptosis was seen in any septic patient. Hence, in patients without pre-existing renal disease, renal histology did not reflect the severity of renal injury indicated by the decrease in kidney function." Also noteworthy was the lack of comment on the presence of microvascular thrombosis.

The presence of normal-looking kidneys under light microscopy points towards a lack of overt inflammatory activity that could be responsible for renal dysfunction. However, this feature is not simply isolated to sepsis. Early studies of biopsies taken at post mortem and from patients with 'ATN' failed to find overt tubular necrosis [14, 15], though subsequent studies using electron microscopy did reveal some ultrastructural changes [16]. This latter study examined biopsies taken from 24 patients diagnosed with ATN following sepsis, post-partum hemorrhage, surgery, or trauma. Despite the wide range of underlying causes, cellular disintegration was very rare in both recovering and active ATN. They further noted that apoptosis was not present in the proximal tubules of the controls and was rare in acute renal failure (1.6–2.1% of cells studied).

Regional Differences in Renal Perfusion and Oxygenation

In health, the renal cortex has a much higher blood flow than the medulla [17]. This is partly to ensure adequate plasma clearance by the glomeruli. Furthermore, to maintain an osmotic gradient within the medulla, a lower flow must exist here so that the solutes that constitute the gradient are not washed out. In an organ as sensitive to relative hypovolemia, it would be logical to assume a vascular component would contribute to sepsis-induced acute renal failure. However, one recent study [18] failed to ameliorate organ failure in an animal model by aggressive resuscitation with albumin.

Characterization of intra-renal hemodynamics is hampered by current technology. Laser-Doppler studies exist [19, 20], but are only able to express changes in regional flow (or, more precisely, flux) rather than absolute values. Second, the laser-

Doppler probes only measure over a minute surface area and are affected by proximity or otherwise to blood vessels. Linking absolute flow to tissue PO_2 may allow estimation of regional oxygen delivery (DO_2). However, all that can be noted at present is that tissue PO_2 differences between cortex and medulla tends to converge under septic conditions. Assuming passive diffusion of oxygen between vessels and tissue, the rise in medullary tissue PO_2 in sepsis noted by several authors [20, 21] may be due to changes in flow and/or cellular dysoxia.

Hypotension is a common accompaniment of sepsis due to a combination of hypovolemia, vasodilatation, a variable degree of myocardial depression, and vascular hyporeactivity. At the very least, hypotension will decrease the pressure gradient across the glomerulus and hence the filtration pressure within the capsule. However, this cannot be the sole cause of acute renal failure, as it may develop in the absence of any obvious hemodynamic perturbation. The septic insult also leads to production of a range of cytokines and vasoactive mediators that produce regional microcirculatory pockets of vasodilatation and vasoconstriction. The acute stress response initiated by shock results in activation, among others, of the sympathetico-adrenal system (with increased levels of catecholamines), the renin-angiotensin system, and a rise in vasopressin. The multi-modal effects of vasopressin could have advantageous, deleterious and, ultimately, unpredictable effects on renal function. A review by Holmes et al. [22] summarized that plasma vasopressin levels at 10–20 pg/ml could cause antidiuresis through V2 receptors (V2R) receptors. However, by acting through V1 receptors (V1R), a diuresis could be achieved at any level (between 1 and 1000 pg/ml). These receptors were also responsible for decreasing renal blood flow. Similarly, stimulation of the sympathetic system leads not only to an outpouring of epinephrine that may enhance renal flow, but also norepinephrine that causes vasoconstriction.

In sepsis, changes thus occur at both macrocirculatory and microcirculatory levels. Intra-renal hemodynamics have not been characterized in man while a confounding feature in many animal models is the co-existence of hypovolemia due to inadequate resuscitation. This may account in part for the wide variation in reported results [23], not to mention differences in the type of model chosen, animal species, choice and degree of insult and number/severity of surgical procedures. Even in hyperdynamic models, variable renal blood flow responses have been seen [24, 25], suggesting that selective renal vasoconstriction maintains a normal renal blood flow in the face of an increasing cardiac output [24].

Several studies have characterized the oxygen gradient that exists within the kidney [19, 26–28]. Absolute values of cortical and medullary PO_2 vary between groups; as with intra-renal hemodynamics, this may also be contingent upon variations within the model and measuring technique (Table 1). There is, however, general agreement that the corticomedullary region has the lowest tissue PO_2 value. The juxtamedullary and outer medullary areas contains a high density of energy dependent Na^+/K^+ATPase pumps that require high oxygen extraction. The PO_2 at any point is the balance between local DO_2 and oxygen consumption (VO_2). Regions of low tissue PO_2 may then be assumed to have low DO_2 and/or high oxygen extraction. Inhibition of Na^+/K^+ATPase pumps by a loop diuretic (furosemide) caused a rise in medullary PO_2; this may also contribute to a reduction in tubular damage [29]. This was tested in human volunteers using blood oxygenation level-dependent magnetic resonance imaging (BOLD MRI) [30]. Unstimulated medullary kidney cells have a lower VO_2 compared with cortical cells but are able to raise their VO_2 to comparable levels when stimulated by endotoxin [31].

Table 1. Regional renal tissue oxygen values for various models. (1 kPa = 7.5 mmHg)

Cortex	Medulla	Reference
5.60 ± 0.53 kPa	4.53 ± 0.80 kPa	[26]
8.13 ± 0.93 kPa	2.13 ± 0.53 kPa	[19]
5.1 kPa	1.27 kPa	[45]
3.0 ± 0.17 kPa	2.02 ± 0.17 kPa	[21]

▍ Nitric Oxide and the Kidney

NO may be an important regulator of renal VO_2. The value for half-maximal NO-mediated inhibition of respiration was virtually identical to that found in isolated mitochondria [32]. A direct correlation has long been recognized between sodium excretion and VO_2. This is probably a reflection of the large proportion of VO_2 expended on sodium excretion compared with other renal cellular functions. Blocking NO production with the NO synthase (NOS) inhibitor L-NMMA increased sodium excretion in dogs [33]. In theory, changes in sodium excretion may be closely linked to the rate of mitochondrial respiration.

Over-production of NO has been implicated in the organ dysfunction developing in septic animal models although human data remain scanty. All three isoforms of NOS are produced in the kidney: neuronal (nNOS), inducible (iNOS) and endothelial (eNOS) [34]. Endotoxemia causes expression of iNOS and increases the activity of eNOS but does not affect nNOS [35]. The excessive vasodilatation and hypotension associated with circulatory shock are reversed by inhibitors of the iNOS, though without necessarily improving the accompanying organ dysfunction [36, 37]. NO is involved in all areas implicated in the development of acute renal failure, namely intra-renal flow distribution, control of cellular respiration and VO_2, and apoptosis and cell death.

Distribution of Blood Flow

Brezis et al. [19] showed how the NO donor sodium nitroprusside increased flow to the renal medulla and elevated medullary tissue PO_2. Administration of a loop diuretic under these conditions did not cause a further rise in medullary PO_2 as opposed to untreated kidneys. The same group found that an endotoxin infusion resulted in maintained total renal flow, an increase in cortical flow, but no change in outer medullary flow [20]. These changes were blocked by the relatively non-specific NOS inhibitor, N^G-nitro-L-arginine methyl ester (L-NAME). Furthermore, pre-treatment 24 hours prior with a single dose of endotoxin globally reduced systemic and renal flows although, again, the effect was attenuated by L-NAME. In addition, other vasoactive mediators may act on renal blood flow via NO production; for example, vasopressin administration appeared to increase renal blood flow, an effect blocked by L-NAME [22].

Control of Cellular Respiration

At low concentrations for short periods, NO reversibly inhibits mitochondrial complex IV (cytochrome c oxidase) by competing with oxygen [38]. Complex IV is a key enzyme involved in generation of ATP and the only step in the whole oxidative phosphorylation pathway at which oxygen is consumed. Indeed, this one enzyme accounts for approximately 90% of total body VO_2. NO is thus considered to be an important physiological regulator of VO_2 in health. In pathological states such as sepsis, the larger amounts of NO produced over long durations may produce a longer-acting, if not irreversible, inhibition of the electron transport chain. This may be related to production of peroxynitrite ($ONOO\bullet^-$) formed through reaction of NO with superoxide generated in excess by mitochondria at the level of complex III as a consequence of downstream inhibition by NO.

Apoptosis

NO is an important mediator for inducing apoptosis [39]. Although apoptosis has not been shown to be a histological feature of acute renal failure in sepsis, it should be borne in mind that apoptotic cells are rapidly cleared; further studies may be needed before excluding loss of cells as a contributory factor to acute renal failure.

Renal Mitochondrial Dysfunction in Sepsis

A number of animal models have been used to investigate mitochondrial function in sepsis [40]. Little consistency is seen in short-term models though studies lasting in excess of 12 hours usually show decreased mitochondrial activity. Few studies have been performed on renal tissue or cells. Fry's group found no uncoupling of mitochondrial respiration [41] nor significant alterations in State 3 and State 4 respiratory rates [42] in liver and kidney mitochondria isolated from endotoxic rats five hours after injection. However, Mela performed a series of investigations on mitochondrial function and ultrastructural change in rat and guinea pig models. Kidney and brain mitochondrial oxygen utilization and ATP synthesis were significantly depressed 24 hrs after induction of sepsis [43]. High-dose steroids prevented this deterioration in mitochondrial function and completely abolished the 60% mortality seen in untreated animals [44]. Preliminary data from our long-term fecal peritonitis rat model confirm a decrease in renal cellular respiration.

Conclusion

The pathophysiology underlying acute renal failure remains a conundrum. Treatment directed at correcting hypovolemia and improving systemic blood flow may still not avert renal dysfunction. The acute renal failure seen in sepsis and other shock conditions may be a deliberate attempt by the organ to preserve its long-term integrity in the face of a short-term insult. Teleologically, this makes sense. The ability of an organism to survive the initial acute insult, only to be killed in the medium term by irrecoverable renal failure runs counter to evolutionary theory. It may be that, by reducing the amount of intracellular work, the kidney could reduce its ATP utilization, thereby maintaining ATP levels above the trigger for cell death (apoptosis or necrosis). Once the organism recovers, then the 'milieu interieur' would be suitable for renal function to resume. The mitochondria may be an important target in sepsis, and may underlie the dysfunction noted in both biochemistry and urine output.

References

1. O'Leary MJ, Bihari DJ (2001) Preventing renal failure in the critically ill. There are no magic bullets-just high quality intensive care. Br Med J 322:1437–1439
2. Rangel-Frausto MS, Pittet D, Costigan M, et al (1995) The natural history of the systemic inflammatory response syndrome (SIRS). A prospective study. JAMA 273:117–123
3. Levy EM, Viscoli CM, Horwitz RI (1996) The effect of acute renal failure on mortality. A cohort analysis. JAMA 275:1489–1494
4. Noble JS, MacKirdy FN, Donaldson SI, Howie JC (2001) Renal and respiratory failure in Scottish ICUs. Anaesthesia 56:124–129
5. de Mendonca A,Vincent JL, Suter PM, et al (2000) Acute renal failure in the ICU: risk factors and outcome evaluated by the SOFA score. Intensive Care Med 26:915–921
6. Sweet SJ, Glenney CU, Fitzgibbons JP, Friedmann P, Teres D (1981) Synergistic effect of acute renal failure and respiratory failure in the surgical intensive care unit. Am J Surg 141:492–496
7. Brezis M, Agmon Y, Epstein FH (1994) Determinants of intrarenal oxygenation. I. Effects of diuretics. Am J Physiol 267:F1059–F1062
8. Bellomo R, Chapman M, Finfer S, Hickling K, Myburgh J (2000) Low-dose dopamine in patients with early renal dysfunction: a placebo-controlled randomised trial. Australian and New Zealand Intensive Care Society (ANZICS) Clinical Trials Group. Lancet 356:2139–2143
9. Galley HF (2000) Renal-dose dopamine: will the message now get through? Lancet 356:2112–2113
10. Thurau K, Boylan JW (1976) Acute renal success. The unexpected logic of oliguria in acute renal failure. Am J Med 61:308–315
11. Thijs A, Thijs LG (1998) Pathogenesis of renal failure in sepsis. Kidney Int Suppl 66:S34–S37
12. Hotchkiss RS, Swanson PE, Freeman BD, et al (1999) Apoptotic cell death in patients with sepsis shock and multiple organ dysfunction. Crit Care Med 27:1230–1251
13. Richman AV, Okulski EG, Balis JU (1981) New Concepts in the pathogenesis of acute tubular necrosis associated with sepsis. Ann Clin Lab Sci 11:211–219
14. Finckh ES, Jeremy D, Whyte HM (1962) Structural renal damage and its relation to clinical features in oliguric renal failure. Q J Med 31:429–446
15. Brun C, Munk O (1957) Lesions of the kidney in acute renal failure following shock. Lancet 1:603–609
16. Olsen TS, Olsen HS, Hansen HE (1985) Tubular ultrastructure in acute renal failure in man: epithelial necrosis and regeneration Virchows. Arch A Pathol Anat Histopathol 406:75–89
17. Brezis M, Rosen S (1995) Hypoxia of the renal medulla – its implications for disease. N Engl J Med 332:647–655
18. Camacho MT, Totapally BR, Torbati D, Wolfsdorf J (2001) Pulmonary and extrapulmonary effects of increased colloid osmotic pressure during endotoxemia in rats. Chest 120:1655–1662
19. Brezis M, Heyman SN, Epstein FH (1994) Determinants of intrarenal oxygenation. II. Hemodynamic effects. Am J Physiol 267:F1063–F1068
20. Heyman SN, Darmon D, Goldfarb M, et al (2000) Endotoxin-induced renal failure. i. A role for altered renal microcirculation. Exp Nephrol 8:266–274
21. James PE, Bacic G, Grinberg OY, et al (1996) Endotoxin-induced changes in intrarenal PO_2 measured by in vivo electron paramagnetic resonance oximetry and magnetic resonance imaging. Free Radic Biol Med 21:25–34
22. Holmes CL, Patel BM, Russell JA, Walley KR (2001) Physiology of vasopressin relevant to management of septic shock. Chest 120:989–1002
23. Khan RZ, Badr KF (1999) Endotoxin and renal function: perspectives to the understanding of septic acute renal failure and toxic shock. Nephrol Dial Transplant 14:814–818
24. Ravikant T, Lucas CE (1977) Renal blood flow distribution in septic hyperdynamic pigs. J Surg Res 22:294–298
25. Cronenwett JL, Lindenauer SM (1978) Distribution of intrarenal blood flow during bacterial sepsis. J Surg Res 24:132–141

26. Liss P, Nygren A, Revsbech NP, Ulfendahl HR (1997) Intrarenal oxygen tension measured by a modified clark electrode at normal and low blood pressure and after injection of x-ray contrast media. Pflugers Arch 434:705–711

27. Leichtweiss HP, Lubbers DW, Weiss C, Baumgartl H, Reschke W (1969) The oxygen supply of the rat kidney: measurements of intrarenal PO_2. Pflugers Arch 309:328–349

28. Lubbers DW, Baumgartl H (1997) Heterogeneities and profiles of oxygen pressure in brain and kidney as examples of the PO_2 distribution in the living tissue. Kidney Int 51:372–380

29. Heyman SN, Rosen S, Epstein FH, Spokes K, Brezis ML (1994) Loop diuretics reduce hypoxic damage to proximal tubules of the isolated perfused rat kidney. Kidney Int 45: 981–985

30. Epstein FH, Prasad P (2000) Effects of furosemide on medullary oxygenation in younger and older subjects. Kidney Int 57:2080–2083

31. James PE, Jackson SK, Grinberg OY, Swartz HM (1995) The effects of endotoxin on oxygen consumption of various cell types in vitro: an EPR oximetry study. Free Radic Biol Med 18:641–647

32. Koivisto A, Pittner J, Froelich M, Persson AE (1999) Oxygen-dependent inhibition of respiration in isolated renal tubules by nitric oxide. Kidney Int 55:2368–2375

33. Seeliger E, Persson PB, Boemke W, et al (2001) Low-dose nitric oxide inhibition produces a negative sodium balance in conscious dogs. J Am Soc Nephrol 12:1128–1136

34. Millar CG, Thiemermann C (1997) Intrarenal haemodynamics and renal dysfunction in endotoxaemia: effects of nitric oxide synthase inhibition. Br J Pharmacol 121:1824–1830

35. Bachmann S, Bosse HM, Mundel P (1995) Topography of nitric oxide synthesis by localizing constitutive NO synthases in mammalian kidney. Am J Physiol 268:F885–F898

36. Schwartz D, Brasowski E, Raskin Y, et al (2001) The outcome of non-selective vs selective nitric oxide synthase inhibition in lipopolysaccharide treated rats. J Nephrol 14:110–114

37. Wray GM, Millar CG, Hinds CJ, Thiemermann C (1998) Selective inhibition of the activity of inducible nitric oxide synthase prevents the circulatory failure but not the organ injury/ dysfunction caused by endotoxin. Shock 9:329–335

38. Brown GC (2000) Nitric oxide as a competitive inhibitor of oxygen consumption in the mitochondrial respiratory chain. Acta Physiol Scand 168:667–674

39. Beltran B, Mathur A, Duchen MR, Erusalimsky JD, Moncada S (2000) The effect of nitric oxide on cell respiration: A key to understanding its role in cell survival or death. Proc Natl Acad Sci USA 97:14602–14607

40. Singer M, Brealey D (1999) Mitochondrial dysfunction in sepsis. In: Brown GC, Nicholls DG, Cooper CE (eds) Mitochondria and Cell Death-Biochemical Society Symposium. Portland Press, London, pp 149–166

41. Asher EF, Garrison RN, Ratcliffe DJ, Fry DE (1983) Endotoxin cellular function and nutrient blood flow. Arch Surg 118:441–445

42. Garrison RN, Ratcliffe DJ, Fry DE (1982) The effects of peritonitis on murine renal mitochondria. Adv Shock Res 7:71–76

43. Mela L (1981) Direct and indirect effects of endotoxin on mitochondrial function. Prog Clin Biol Res 62:15–21

44. Mela L, Miller LD (1983) Efficacy of glucocorticoids in preventing mitochondrial metabolic failure in endotoxemia. Circ Shock 10:371–381

Hepatorenal Failure

K. Lenz, C. Kapral, and N. P. Linz

▌ Introduction

The hepatorenal syndrome is a fully reversible impairment of renal function in patients with severe hepatic failure (Table 1). Before hepatorenal syndrome can be diagnosed, primary causes such as hypovolemia, infection, nephrotoxins and other renal diseases must be excluded [1]. Hepatorenal syndrome causes no morphological changes in the kidney, although morphological alterations in the course of oligoanuria may reveal a transition from intermediary to irreversible kidney damage with necrosis of the tubule. In patients with hepatorenal syndrome who are scheduled for liver transplantation, this may raise the relevant issue of simultaneous kidney transplantation.

The prognosis of hepatorenal syndrome depends on the restoration of liver function and intrahepatic pressures. Therefore, as a rule the prognosis is poor. It also depends on how rapidly hepatorenal syndrome develops (Table 2). The prognosis is especially poor in patients who develop hepatorenal syndrome within two days (hepatorenal syndrome type I).

Table 1. Diagnostic criteria for hepatorenal syndrome

Major criteria
- ▌ Low glomerular filtration rate, as indicated by serum creatinine ≥1.5 mg/dl or 24-h creatinine clearance < 40 ml/min
- ▌ Absence of shock, severe infection, fluid losses and treatment with nephrotoxic drugs
- ▌ Proteinuria lower than 500 mg/day
- ▌ No sustained improvement in renal function (decrease in serum creatinine to 1.5 mg/dl or less or increase in creatinine clearance to 40 ml/min or more) following the expansion of volume with 1.5 l of a saline based plasma expander

Additional criteria
- ▌ Urine volume less than 1000 ml/day
- ▌ Urine sodium less than 10 mval/l
- ▌ Urine osmolality greater than plasma osmolality
- ▌ Serum sodium concentration lower than 130 mval/l

All major criteria must be present for the diagnosis of hepatorenal syndrome. Minor criteria are not necessary but may provide useful supportive evidence

Table 2. Types of hepatorenal syndrome

▌ Type I hepatorenal syndrome: Patients with a rapidly progressive reduction of renal function as defined by a doubling of the initial serum creatinine to a level greater than 2.5 mg/dl or 50% reduction of the initial 24 h creatinine clearance to a level of less than 20 ml/min in less than two weeks
▌ Type II hepatorenal syndrome. Patients in whom renal failure does not progress, according to the previously mentioned criteria

▌ Pathophysiology and Diagnosis

Hepatorenal syndrome is diagnosed after other causes of renal failure secondary to impairment of renal function (serum creatinine >2.5 mg/dl) have been excluded in patients with simultaneous liver damage, poor elimination of sodium (fractional excretion <1%) and a normal urine report [2]. A prerenal component is excluded by infusion of a crystalloid solution (e.g., 500 ml of 0.9% NaCl). The reduced glomerular filtration rate is due to poor renal circulation on the one hand, and reduced filtration fraction on the other.

Several factors are considered to induce the impairment in renal function. Enhanced portal blood flow with vasodilatation in the splanchnic region may be a useful mechanism of maintaining normal liver function. Thus, the liver function of patients who were transplanted because of liver failure was found to be dependent on *in vitro* liver circulation [3]. The enhanced blood flow further increases pressure in the liver. Elevated pressure in the liver, secondary to swelling during the course of glutamine infusion via the superior mesenteric artery, led to a reduction in renal circulation and the glomerular filtration rate (GFR). This is due to direct hepatorenal interactions [4]. The intrahepatic increase in pressure leads to enhanced activity of sympathetic efferences from the liver, which, transposed in the lumbar spinal marrow, cause enhanced renal sympathetic activity (hepatorenal reflex) [5]. This usually leads to renal vasoconstriction. Denervation of the kidney eliminates this activation of renal sympathetic activity and thereby reduces the impairment of renal function. This may also be caused by hepatic vagal denervation [6]. In a clinical study, Solus Herruzo et al. [7] were able to interrupt this hepatorenal reflex in patients with portal hypertension and thereby improve renal function.

Vasodilation in the splanchnic region causes a redistribution of blood and activation of baroreceptors in the aortic arch. Such activation is reinforced by compliance disorders in the venous system, and the efficacy of volume therapy is reduced [8]. The activation of baroreceptors also leads to stimulation of the sympathetic system and the renin-angiotensin-aldosterone system (RAAS), as well as to the non-osmotic release of anti-diuretic hormone (ADH). This results in further renal vasoconstriction, further re-absorption of sodium in the proximal tubule, and increased re-absorption of water in the collecting tubules. The increased sympathetic activity abolishes autoregulation of the kidney, because of which renal circulation becomes pressure dependent even in the presence of physiological blood pressure. The reason is that the level at which renin starts to be released is shifted to below a mean arterial blood pressure of 110 mmHg [9, 10].

Even in the dormant phase of alcoholic liver disease, vasoactive substances in the liver are known to be produced in large quantities when the production of cytokines is increased. In the presence of endotoxin stimulation, such activation is disproportionately increased. Even in cases of non-alcoholic liver disease, the strong infiltration of endotoxins might play a role. Thus, patients who had hepatorenal syndrome prior to liver transplantation revealed significantly higher concentrations of interleukin (IL)-2 and IL-6 as well as tumor necrosis factor (TNF) in comparison with patients who had no hepatorenal syndrome before liver transplantation [11]. Furthermore, increased endothelin concentrations have been observed, and regulatory disorders of the adenosine system have also been discussed [12].

In animal experiments, bile acids lead to changes in circulation. In humans, however, this appears to be of significance only in the presence of extreme bilirubin levels. Very high concentrations may additionally lead to reversible damage of the tubule. Increased intraabdominal pressure secondary to ascites also activates the renal sympathetic system and thus worsens renal circulation.

▌ Therapeutic Approach

These pathophysiological features have led to a variety of therapeutic approaches in patients with hepatorenal syndrome. It would be reasonable to assume that renal function is improved by substances that abolish renal vasoconstriction. However, the experiments with prostaglandin performed thus far have produced very diverse results [13]. Likewise, dopamine was observed to induce improvements in cirrhotic patients with relatively good renal function, but not in patients with massively impaired renal function [14, 15].

A lumbar sympathetic blockade was shown to improve renal function in patients with hepatorenal syndrome [7]. The use of substances that reduce portal vein pressure, e.g., ornipressin and terlipressin, resulted in improved renal function in several clinical studies [16, 17]. Likewise, the placement of a portosystemic shunt may alleviate hepatorenal syndrome [18, 19]. It is not certain whether acetylcysteine also improves renal function by this mechanism [20].

The activation of baroreceptors is reduced by normalizing the redistribution of blood with the use of substances that mainly induce vasoconstriction in the splanchnic region. The splanchnic region of flow has a very high density of V1 receptors, so that vasopressin derivatives, such as ornipressin and vasopressin, cause redistribution from the splanchnic region and thereby improve renal circulation [21, 22]. Whether these substances also normalize venous compliance is not known. The substances are especially effective when used in combination with a volume exchange agent [17]; this is strongly indicative of the fact that there is no effect on venous compliance. Human albumin has been the almost exclusive agent for volume exchange, and has been administered in combination with vasopressin derivatives to improve renal function. The extent to which other phenomena (e.g., nitric oxide [NO] binding, antioxidative effects), apart from the volume effect, play a role is not known at the present time.

In animal experiments, the abolition of autoregulation was normalized by the administration of vasopressin. This might also be important with regard to the clinical effects of terlipressin and ornipressin. In experimental studies, in the presence of a high sympathetic tonus, renal function and the elimination of sodium were further improved by a combination of vasopressin and atrial natriuretic peptide (ANF). In experimental portal hypertension, a combination of ANF and vasopressin derivatives was found to have an additive effect on renal function [23]. Clinical studies on this issue are confirming the results [24].

In tense ascites, puncture of the ascites improves renal function. However, care should be taken to ensure that the paracentesis does not induce hypovolemia, which in turn, would worsen renal function. Therefore, a large-volume puncture of ascites should always be coupled with sufficient volume substitution.

The release of cytokines, such as TNF, can be reduced with pentoxifylline [25]. The administration of pentoxifylline was shown to prevent renal failure in patients with alcoholic fatty liver hepatitis. In addition, terlipressin administration decreased iNOS expression and improved circulatory and liver dysfunction in endotoxin challenged rats with cirrhosis [26] Acetylcysteine also had a beneficial effect on renal function by reducing the activation of vasoactive substances [27]. Antibiotics were found to reduce NO-induced vasodilatation in patients with cirrhosis [28]; the phenomenon is attributed to decreased endotoxemia. The use of the liver support system, MARS (molecular adsorbent recirculating system), was observed to improve renal function in patients with hepatorenal syndrome [29, 30]. One cause might be the stabilization of circulation that goes along with this treatment. The reasons for this effect are not known. One hypothesis is based on albumin dialysis and its consequent elimination of substances that act on the circulation, as well as the improved albumin binding capacity, which causes substances that act on the circulation to be bound to albumin. MARS results in the removal of bile acids, which might also develop circulatory activity in the presence of extreme hyperbilirubinemia.

▌ Conclusion

All these therapies have been shown to improve, but not normalize, renal function in patients with hepatorenal syndrome. Some patients, whose renal function is not improved in spite of these measures, need extracorporeal measures to bridge the time until liver transplantation. Successful liver transplantation is currently the only effective long-term treatment for the hepatorenal syndrome.

References

1. Arroyo V, Gines P, Gerbes AL, et al (1996) Definition and diagnostic criteria of refractory ascites and hepatorenal syndrome in cirrhosis. Hepatology 23:164–173
2. Moore K (1997) The hepatorenal syndrome Clin Sci 92:433–443
3. Cardoso JE, Gautreau C, Jeyaraj PR, et al (1994) Augmenation of portal blood flow improves function of human cirrhotic liver. Hepatology 19:375–380
4. Lang F, Tschernko E, Schulze E, et al (1991) Hepatorenal reflex regulationg kidney function. Hepatology 14:590–594
5. Kostreva DR, Castaner A, Kampine JP (1980) Reflex effects of hepatic baroreceptors on renal and cardiac sympathetic nerve activity. Am J Physiol 238:R390–R394
6. Levy M, Wexler MJ (1987) Hepatic denervation alters first phase urinary sodium excretion in dogs with cirrhosis. Am J Physiol 253:F664–F671
7. Solis-Herruzo JA, Duran A, Favela V, et al (1987) Effects of lumbar sympathetic block on kidney function in cirrhotic patients with hepatorenal syndrome. J Hepatol 5:167–173
8. Hadengue A, Moreau R, Gaudin C, Bacq Y, Chamigneulle B, Lebrec D (1992) Total effective compliance in patients with cirrhosis: A study to the response to acute blood volume expansion. Hepatology 15:809–815
9. Kirchheim HR, Ehmke H (1994) Vasoactive hormones: modulators of renal function. Clin Invest 72:685–687
10. Persson PB, Ehmke H, Nafz B, Kirchheim RH (1990) Sympathetic modulation of renal autoregulation by carotid occlusion in conscious dog. Am J Physiol 258:F364–F370

11. Burke GW, Cirocco R, Roth D, et al (1993) Activated cytokine pattern in hepatorenal syndrome: Fall in levels after successful orthotopic liver transplantation. Transplant Proc 25:1876–1877

12. Gerbes AL, Gülber V, Bilzer M (1998) Endothelin and other mediators in the pathophysiology of portal hypertension. Digestion 59 (suppl 2):8–10

13. Wong F, Massie D, Hsu P, Dudley F (1994) Dose dependent effects of oral misoprostol on renal function in alcoholic cirrhosis. Gastroenterology 106:658–663

14. Peschl L (1978) Klinische und experimentelle Untersuchungen über die Wirkung von Dopamin auf die Hämodynamik und Funktion von Niere und Leber. Wien Klein Wochenschr 86:1–33

15. Bennet WM, Keeffe E, Melnyk C, et al (1975) Response to dopamine hydrochloride in the hepatorenal syndrome. Arch Intern Med 135:964–970

16. Lenz K, Hörtnagl H, Druml W, et al (1991) Ornipressin in the treatment of functional renal failure in decompensated liver cirrhosis. Gastroenterology 101:1060–1067

17. Guevara M, Gines P, Fernandez-Esparach G, et al (1998) Reversibility of hepatorenal syndrome by prolonged administration of ornipressin and volume expansion. Hepatology 27:35–41

18. Guevara M, Gines P, Bnadi JC, et al (1998) Transjugular intrahepatic portosystemic shunt in hepatorenal syndrome: effects on renal function and vasoactive systems. Hepatology 28:590–592

19. Brensing KA, Textor J, Perz J, et al (2000) Long term outcome after transjugular intrahepatic portosystemic stent-shunt in non transplant cirrhotics with hepatorenal syndrome: A phase II study. Gut 47:288–295

20. Holt S, Goodier D, Marley R (1999) Improvement in renal function in hepatorenal syndrome with N-acetylcysteine. Lancet 353:294–295

21. Heinemann A, Wachter CH, Fickert P, Trauner M, Stauber RE (1998) Vasopressin reverses mesenteric hyperemia and vasoconstrictor hyperresponsivness in anesthetized portal hypertensive rats. Hepatology 27:646–654

22. Schmid GP, Abbound FM, Wendling MG, et al (1994) Regional vascular effects of vasopressin: plasma levels and circulatory responses. Am J Physiol 227:998–1004

23. Ganger DR, Gottstein J, Blei AT (1988) Hemodynamic and renal effects of atrial natriuretic factor in portal hypertensive rats. Potentiation by Phe-Ile-Orn-vasopressin. J Pharmacol Exp Ther 246:941–945

24. Gadano A, Moreau R, Vachiery F, et al (1997) Natriuretic response to the combination of atrial natriuretic peptide and terlipressin in patients with cirrhosis and refractory ascites. J Hepatol 26:1229–1234

25. Akriviadis E, Botla R, Briggs W, Han S, Reynolds T, Shakil O (2000) Pentoxifyllin improves short term survival in severe acute alcoholic hepatitis: A double blind, placebo controlled trial. Gastroenterology 119:1637–1648

26. Barriere E, Tazi KA, Poirel O, Lebrec D, Moreau R (2001) Terlipressin administration decreases iNOS expression and improves circulatory and liver dysfunction in endotoxin-challenged rats with cirrhosis. J Hepatol 34 (Suppl 1):61 (Abst)

27. Fernando B, Marley R, Holt S, et al (1998) N-acetylcysteine prevents development of the hyperdynamic circulation in the portal hypertensive rat. Hepatology 28:689–694

28. Chin-Dusting JPF, Rasaratnam B, Jennings GLR, Dudley FJ (1997) Effect of fluoroquinolone on the enhanced nitric oxide induced peripheral vasodilation seen in cirrhosis. Ann Intern Med 127:985–988

29. Sorkine S, Abraham RB, Szold O, et al (2001) Role of molecular adsorbent recycling system (MARS) in the treatment of patients with acute exacerbation of chronic liver failure. Crit Care Med 29:1332–1336

30. Mitzner S, Stange J, Klammt S, et al (2000) Improvement of hepatorenal syndrome with extracorporeal albumin dialysis MARS: Results of a prospective, randomized, controlled trial. Liver Transplant 6:277–286

Acute Renal Failure in the Critically Ill Patient: Is there a Magic Bullet?

H. L. Corwin

Introduction

Acute renal failure has been a clinical challenge over the last five decades. In 1972, Stott and colleagues [1] reflecting on the high mortality from acute renal failure over the preceding two decades, posed the question "Why the persistently high mortality in acute renal failure?". Over the subsequent 30 years, the same question has been repeatedly asked; in 1983, "Persistent high mortality in acute renal failure: Are we asking the right questions?" [2]; in 1986, "Acute renal failure – The continuing challenge" [3]; and in 1996, "Still lethal after all these years" [4]. Although there have been more optimistic reports recently [5–7], the fact remains that, in spite of the advances in all aspects of medical care over the last 50 years, acute renal failure in 2002 still carries a mortality of 50 to 60%, little changed from the 1950s [5, 8, 9]. This chapter will focus on the current state of therapy for acute renal failure.

Incidence

Acute renal failure, acute tubular necrosis (ATN) in particular, is a hospital phenomenon. Community acquired acute renal failure is uncommon, with an incidence of 1% of hospital admissions [10]. In a general hospital population, the incidence of hospital acquired acute renal failure is between 2 and 5% [11, 12]. In the intensive care unit (ICU), the incidence of acute renal failure ranges from 7 to 23% [13–16]. In contrast to other clinical settings, the predominant etiology of acute renal failure seen in the ICU is ischemic ATN or nephrotoxic injury [17, 18]. As many as 60% of acute renal failure patients in the ICU require dialysis, reflecting the severity of injury in this setting [13, 14].

Outcome

The presence of acute renal failure is associated with an increase in mortality. For example, the relative risk of death increases to 6.2 if acute renal failure develops during hospitalization [11]. The mortality rate of critically ill patients in the ICU with acute renal failure approaches 80% [17]. Those patients requiring dialysis have a particularly poor prognosis, with a mortality of close to 90%. While it is apparent that a high mortality is associated with severe forms of acute renal failure such as ATN, it is important to appreciate that pre-renal failure is also associated with an increase in the risk of dying [10–12]. Mortality is related to the level of serum creatinine, which in turn directly reflects the severity of the acute renal failure [12].

It is rare in the 1990s for patients to die 'of' acute renal failure, rather they die 'with' acute renal failure. This has led to the suggestion that acute renal failure is an 'epiphenomenon' in the critically ill patient unlikely to recover [4]. While this extreme view is open to question, it is clear that acute renal failure in the ICU is inseparable from multiple organ failure (MOF).

Mortality in acute renal failure is influenced by the failure of other organ systems [19, 20]. In the ICU patient, the kidney is the third most common organ to fail, following cardiac and respiratory failure [19]. Acute renal failure with no other organ damage is rare in the ICU patient [12, 19, 20]. Failure of one or more additional organs is seen in over 90% of acute renal failure patients with most episodes of acute renal failure occurring following other organ failure. The kidney is the first organ to fail in only 22% of acute renal failure patients [19]. The incidence of acute renal failure in cardiac failure is 44% and following respiratory failure is 27%. Seventy four percent of acute renal failure patients have cardiac failure, respiratory failure, or both. While there is some debate as to which other organ system failures are most important (cardiac and respiratory failure in particular), the onset of any organ system failure adversely affects prognosis. Isolated acute renal failure carries a mortality of less than 10%, however mortality very quickly rises to greater than 70% with three additional failed organs [10, 20]. The presence of respiratory failure and acute renal failure is a particularly lethal combination [19, 21]. Although the relative contribution of individual factors to mortality is debatable, it is clear that mortality in acute renal failure is directly related to the number of other organ systems which are dysfunctional. However, the most important factor responsible for death in patients with acute renal failure remains the underlying cause of the acute renal failure [22, 23]. As many as 70% of deaths, at least in part, may be attributable to the underlying disease [22].

The relationship between organ failure and mortality depends not only on the number of failed organs but also on the temporal relationship of the organ failure to the onset of acute renal failure [14]. The presence of organ failure prior to the onset of acute renal failure carries a higher mortality than organ failure which develops after the onset of acute renal failure (70 vs 55%). This is consistent with the observation that the underlying cause of the acute renal failure is most often responsible for death [22, 23] and that delayed acute renal failure (developing during the ICU course) has a worse prognosis than initial acute renal failure [13].

▌ Therapy

The therapeutic approach to the patient with acute renal failure can be separated into those measures directed towards preventing acute renal failure or modifying the clinical course of established acute renal failure and those directed towards the treatment of the consequences of established acute renal failure, i.e., dialysis therapy.

Prevention of Acute Renal Failure

A number of studies have attempted to identify risk factors for developing acute renal failure in the hospital [11, 24] and in the ICU [14–16, 25]. Pre-renal factors are particularly important. The importance of pre-renal factors is not surprising since pre-renal failure represents a shift from renal compensation to hemodynamic stress to a de-compensated state where the kidney is at risk for more severe renal injury [26]. The degree of acute renal failure is related to the number and severity of acute insults sustained, all of which are additive [24]. The predominance of pre-renal physiology among the risk factors for acute renal failure, highlights the importance of maintaining adequate renal perfusion to protect the kidney against injury. Maintaining adequate intra-vascular volume and avoiding renal insults as much as possible remain the mainstay of prevention of renal injury.

Mannitol treatment prior to ischemic injury has been found to afford some degree of renal protection in a variety of experimental models of acute renal failure [27–29]. Mannitol is thought to protect against injury by reducing tubular obstruction, increasing renal blood flow (via increased prostaglandin production), and acting as a free radical scavenger. On the other hand, the clinical efficacy of mannitol has been less convincing. Most of the studies evaluating the effect of mannitol on acute renal failure have been uncontrolled. Mannitol has been shown to reverse oliguria in some patients if given early enough in the course of acute renal failure, although renal function may not improve [30, 31].

Mannitol is widely used in patients with hemoglobinuria and myoglobinuria due to crush injuries or other pigment injury. In these situations, mannitol is usually combined with fluid resuscitation and alkalinization of urine appears to be effective in preventing acute renal failure [32]. The relative importance of mannitol in this treatment regimen is not clear. Similarly, pretreatment with mannitol has been widely used as a mean to protect against contrast-induced acute renal failure [33]. However, more recent data suggest that mannitol does not protect the kidney against contrast-induced acute renal failure and may aggravate the damaging effect of contrast on renal function in patients with diabetes-induced renal insufficiency [34]. There are limited controlled data supporting the efficacy of prophylactic mannitol in preventing acute renal failure in patients undergoing general or vascular surgery [35, 36].

The evidence for a protective effect of 'loop' (of Henle) diuretics in experimental acute renal failure is less consistent than with mannitol [27–29]. The clinical use of loop diuretics in acute renal failure has been extensively studied. Most of the studies have been in patients with established acute renal failure (as opposed to prophylactic or early acute renal failure). High dose furosemide has been reported to decrease both the length of oliguria and the need for dialysis, but no effect on mortality has been demonstrated [37, 38]. Other studies, while showing increased urine flow, demonstrated no improvement in oliguria, dialysis or mortality [39, 40]. Only one of fifteen studies, using survival as an end point, has demonstrated an improvement in mortality with the use of diuretics in acute renal failure [28, 29]. On the other hand, patients with 'early' acute renal failure may be more likely to survive if they respond to diuretics by increasing their urine output [28]. This most likely reflects the selection of patients with less severe acute renal failure, rather than any effect of the diuretic *per se*.

There has been growing interest in the use of continuous infusions of loop diuretics in critically ill patients, including those with acute renal failure [41, 42].

There are data to suggest that this method of diuretic delivery may overcome diuretic 'tolerance' or 'resistance' in selected patients. Continuous infusion of loop diuretics is possibly a safer and more effective alternative to bolus injection of these drugs in refractory patients particularly those in the ICU.

In the 35 years since the renal effects of low dose dopamine were first demonstrated, it has become one of the most widely used therapies in ICUs around the world [43]. Although there is abundant evidence that low dose dopamine will result in a significant increase in urine output, there are few data to suggest that there is any renal protective effect. This lack of data on the efficacy of renal dose dopamine on outcome, however, has done little to dim the enthusiasm for its use.

Dopamine, a natriuretic hormone, increases sodium excretion by diminishing reabsorption, primarily in the proximal tubules [44, 45]. Dopamine acting via generation of cyclic AMP, decreases the activity of the Na^+/H^+ exchanger in the luminal membrane, a transporter that plays an important role in the entry of filtered sodium into the cell [46]. Low dose dopamine (0.5–3 µg/kg/min), dilates the interlobular arteries and both the afferent and efferent arterioles [47, 48]. These vascular effects result in a relatively large increase in renal blood flow with a lesser or no elevation in glomerular filtration rate (GFR) [49]; the relative lack of increase in GFR is due to the dilatation of efferent arterioles, which minimizes the rise in intraglomerular pressure.

Much of the clinical interest in low dose dopamine was stimulated by several uncontrolled studies in the early 1980s suggesting that dopamine alone, or in combination with furosemide, was effective in inducing a diuresis [50–53]. The effect of low dose dopamine on renal function and outcome are less clear. In a study of patients with acute renal failure due to malaria, the combination of dopamine and furosemide was more effective than dopamine alone in improving acute renal failure in patients with moderate renal insufficiency (serum creatinine 2 to 4 mg/dl). However, this combination had no effect once the serum creatinine reached 6 mg/dl [54]. On the other hand, dopamine is no more effective than saline in preventing contrast-induced acute renal failure in patients with chronic renal failure [55]. More recent studies confirm the ability of low dose dopamine to induce a diuresis but offer little support to the belief that low dose dopamine is effective in preventing acute renal failure in most clinical circumstances [56–58]. As is seen with diuretics, the increase in urine output seen with low dose dopamine may not always translate into improved survival. Recently, in a study of nearly 400 patients with oliguria and septic shock, 147 patients non-randomly received either low dose dopamine (44%), high dose dopamine (32%), or no dopamine (24%) [59]. The incidence of acute renal failure and the subsequent need for dialysis was similar among the three patient groups. Similarly, in a study of 256 patients (from the placebo arm of a multicenter intervention trial), 91 treated with low dose dopamine, there was no significant reduction in the relative risk of either death or dialysis associated with low dose dopamine [60].

It is important to recognize that the use of low dose dopamine is not 'risk free'. In addition to its cardiac effects, low dose dopamine has been associated with hastening the onset of gut ischemia [61]. Dopamine may also have effects on hormones and immune function, although the significance of these are unclear [62].

Over the last decade, editorials have discouraged the routine use of low dose dopamine and stressed the need for controlled clinical trials [63, 64]. Recently a randomized trial of over 300 patients conducted by the ANZICS Clinical Trials Group demonstrated that low dose dopamine did not confer any renal protection [65].

This result is supported by a recent meta-analysis of dopamine in acute renal failure which evaluated 24 studies with over a total of 1000 patients [66]. No clinical benefit was associated with the use of low dose dopamine. At this point we may need to face the fact that it may not be lack of data but rather lack of effect that is the difficulty. As has been pointed out, the dream of preventing renal failure with dopamine may not ever come true [64].

The above are the therapies which have been clinically studied most extensively. However, a number of other agents have been studied in experimental models and in some clinical settings. These include: calcium channel blockers, endothelin antagonists, atrial natriuretic peptide, urodilantin, anti-intercellular adhesion molecule-1 (ICAM-1) antibodies, as well as others (see [67] for review). These agents work on different points in the pathophysiology of acute renal failure. Although some of these agents have shown benefit in experimental models none have demonstrated broad clinical utility at this point and are still under investigation.

Treatment of Acute Renal Failure

As many as two thirds of patients who develop acute renal failure, particularly ATN, will require dialysis [14]. Through the mid to late 1980s over 90% of dialysis for acute renal failure was hemodialysis [68]. Over the last 5 years, however, the use of continuous dialysis techniques in critically ill patients (both acute and chronic) has increased. Patients with acute renal failure who undergo dialysis have a high mortality. Mortality approaches 90% in critically ill patients who require dialysis [69, 70]. Several studies have examined the factors that influence (or are associated with) survival in patients with acute renal failure who require dialysis [71, 72]. The failure of other organs is closely linked with poor outcome.

The question – whether early, more intensive dialysis results in improved survival in acute renal failure – has been debated for over 35 years. Early studies have supported this hypothesis [73, 74]. However, these studies relied on historical control populations. For example, in a study of 500 acute renal failure patients those who received 'prophylactic' dialysis to keep their blood urea nitrogen (BUN) less than approximately 100 mg/dl had a reduction in mortality (42 to 29%) compared to an earlier time period during which dialysis was not initiated until the BUN rose above approximately 175 mg/dl [74].

Only two prospective controlled trials have addressed the value of intensive dialysis for acute renal failure. In a study of war casualties [75], intensive dialysis to maintain a pre dialysis creatinine of 5 mg/dl, as compared to 10 mg/dl, resulted in improved patient survival and fewer complications. The small number of patients in this study and its restricted scope limit its applicability to the general acute renal failure population. More recently, the results of a controlled trial of intensive dialysis of acute renal failure patients in a general hospital setting was reported [76]. Intensive dialysis was defined as dialysis sufficient to maintain the BUN below 60 mg/dl and serum creatinine below 5 mg/dl (versus 100 mg/dl and 9 mg/dl respectively). This usually required daily hemodialysis. There was no improvement in either survival or complication rate with the more intensive dialysis regimen. However, this study also had a small number of patients. More recent data suggests that it is the delivered dialysis (Kt/V) that is the important variable in influencing acute renal failure outcome [77].

Hemodialysis may have other effects in the patient with acute renal failure that impact on outcome. The interaction of blood with the hemodialysis membrane is a complex process which can result in the activation of a variety of systems in the body including complement, coagulation, and white blood cells (see [78] for review). This interaction of blood and artificial membrane is referred to as biocompatibility (or incompatibility). Derivatives of cellulose are the most commonly used dialysis membranes. These cellulose membranes, cuprophane in particular, have been implicated in blood-membrane interactions. There are now synthetic polymer membranes available which are more biocompatible than the cellulose membranes. The activation of the 'inflammatory' cascades and the resultant production of mediators, e.g., cytokines, are in turn responsible for a number of both acute and chronic clinical sequelae. There is clinical and experimental evidence, for example, to suggest that dialysis itself may impact on the rate of recovery from acute renal failure. Other sequelae of membranes which are not biocompatible include: fever, hypotension, immune dysfunction and susceptibility to infection, pulmonary dysfunction, malnutrition. Two prospective, controlled trials have examined the effects of membrane biocompatibility on the clinical course of acute renal failure [79, 80]. Both studies demonstrated a trend (albeit not statistically significant) towards improved survival in the acute renal failure patients dialyzed with biocompatible membranes.

Continuous renal replacement therapy (CRRT) encompasses a wide variety of techniques used to support the patient with acute renal failure (although has been used in other settings), which are applied over a 24 hour period. As initially proposed by Kramer et al. [81] in the late 1970s, continuous arterio-venous hemofiltration (CAVH) was a simple technique driven by a patient's own blood pressure; however, over the years this has been replaced by a variety of more complicated pump-driven systems.

Until recently, hemodialysis was the mainstay of renal replacement therapy in patients with acute renal failure. Up through the mid 1980s well over 90% of acute renal failure related dialysis was hemodialysis, the remainder being either intermittent hemofiltration or peritoneal dialysis. In the mid 1970s the use of CRRT for acute renal failure (other than peritoneal dialysis) was first reported. Initially, CAVH or continuous arterio-venous hemodiafiltration (CAVHD) was used; however, this has now been supplanted in many institutions by pump-driven continuous venovenous hemofiltration (CVVH) and hemodiafiltration (CVVHD). By the end of the 1980s continuous hemofiltration accounted for at least 20% of acute renal failure dialysis [68].

In contrast to hemodialysis, which is excellent at removing low molecular weight compounds (less than 500 daltons), CAVH/CVVH is effective at removing larger molecular weight compounds (up to 20000 to 30000 daltons). This latter property may offer advantages for treating patients with sepsis and/or MOF.

As the experience with CRRT has grown, it has been clearly demonstrated that CRRT achieves metabolic control as good or better than conventional dialysis [82–85]. Clearances with continuous therapy approach 25 l/day with CVVH to 40 l/day with CVVHD. On the other hand, hemodialysis has an approximate clearance of 20 l/day and peritoneal dialysis has a clearance of 5 to 10 l/day. Only with intense hemodialysis is control of azotemia comparable to CVVH achieved [86]. The removal of excess volume is particularly facilitated by CRRT. It also offers advantages for the patient who is hemodynamically unstable and would, therefore, not be able to tolerate conventional dialysis therapy.

The ability of CRRT to clear 'middle molecules' (up to 30000 daltons) has raised the possibility that this form of renal replacement therapy may be uniquely suited for the patient with sepsis or MOF. Many mediators potentially involved in the inflammatory response associated with sepsis and MOF are of a molecular size which would make them susceptible to removal by CRRT. There are experimental and clinical data suggesting that these mediators are removed by CRRT [87]. However, the significance of this mediator removal is not clear since serum levels do not fall in spite of the clearances observed [87–89].

There have been several studies evaluating the effect of continuous hemofiltration in experimental septic shock [90–93]. In a variety of animal models, significant improvement in hemodynamic and pulmonary parameters are associated with this therapy that are independent of changes in volume ('0' balance hemofiltration). Overall, the experimental data are consistent with a beneficial effect associated with the removal of circulating factors by continuous hemofiltration in septic animals. However, the impact of continuous renal replacement therapy on the outcome of sepsis in the ICU has still not been demonstrated [94].

As yet, there are no controlled clinical data on continuous hemofiltration in sepsis/septic shock or MOF. Continuous hemofiltration has been used in these clinical settings for patients with and without acute renal failure [87]. The available data are uncontrolled and often retrospective. However, improvements in both cardiovascular and respiratory parameters have been demonstrated to follow initiation of continuous hemofiltration. In some studies this improvement has been associated with the removal of circulating factors, e.g., myocardial depressant factor, in the ultra filtrate, although in other studies it is difficult to rule out an effect related to volume removal. An impact on survival remains to be demonstrated. Recently, encouraging results were reported in a small study employing high volume hemofiltration in the treatment of patients with sepsis [95]. Important features of the technique used by these investigators include early hemofiltration initiation after ICU admission, as well as use of high blood flows (450 ml/min) for a 4 hour period followed by conventional continuous hemofiltration.

Given the complexity of sepsis and the immune cascade, it is probably a naive hope that the non-specific removal of mediators will be the answer. Further data are clearly still necessary before the precise role of hemofiltration in the therapy of sepsis is established.

Whether or not the advantages of CRRT translate into better outcomes is still unclear. Over the last 5 years, in 19 clinical series the mortality in 1131 critically ill patients treated with CRRT was 60% [96]. During the same time period, in eight clinical series, a total of 482 patients treated with hemodialysis had a mortality of 65% [96]. Direct comparisons of hemodialysis and CRRT are few and in general involve historical controls, making it difficult to draw meaningful comparisons. Overall there is a trend, albeit not statistically significant, towards improved survival with CRRT [82]. Survival rates with CRRT comparable to rates seen with conventional dialysis are noted often, despite higher severity of illness. Patients with intermediate severity of illness (APACHE 19 to 29) were more likely to survive if treated with CRRT, however there was no effect at the extremes of severity of illness [85]. The patients receiving CRRT who survived, had shorter ICU and hospital stays than survivors treated with hemodialysis. There do not appear to be differences in survival rates observed among the different forms of CRRT (CAVH, CVVH, CAVHD, CVVHD) [85]. However, survival may be improved by higher ultrafiltration rates [97]. There has been a recent randomized trial comparing intermittent and continuous dialysis in 166 patients with acute renal failure [98]. In this study, intermittent dialysis was in fact associated with better outcomes, however the groups were not balanced and when this was corrected for no significant differences in outcomes between the two therapies were noted.

The answer to the question whether to choose CRRT or intermittent hemodialysis for the critically ill patient with acute renal failure is still unclear. The data available suggest that continuous therapy is at least comparable with hemodialysis. The amount of dialysis delivered rather than simply modality of dialysis may be the important variable impacting outcome of patients with acute renal failure. To the extent that control of volume is important for a particular patient, CRRT is the therapy of choice in the ICU.

A clear consensus on the optimal time to initiate dialysis is still lacking. However, the data available certainly support an aggressive strategy for the initiation of dialysis. To the extent possible, dialysis therapy should anticipate the complications of acute renal failure as they develop, rather than be driven by the necessity for emergency treatment of these complications, e.g., hyperkalemia, severe acidosis, volume overload.

∎ Conclusion

It is clear that there is still no 'magic bullet' for acute renal failure. Diuretics are effective in converting patients to non-oliguric acute renal failure, however there are few clinical data supporting the contention that they protect the kidney or alter the course of established acute renal failure. If diuretics are used to increase urine output in acute renal failure, continuous infusion may be a good alternative to bolus therapy. Similarly, the use of low dose dopamine is well out of proportion to the data supporting the effectiveness of the therapy. Renal dose dopamine (usually in combination with a loop diuretic) will induce a diuresis in many patients with acute renal failure, but does not protect the kidney. As with diuretics, the increase in urine output does not necessarily translate into improved outcome. The use of low dose dopamine should be discouraged. In spite of the disappointment with pharmacologic therapy for acute renal failure, thus far, there is reason for optimism. There has been, and continues to be, an explosion in our understanding of the pathogenesis of acute renal failure as well as the factors leading to renal recovery. This is now leading to the development of novel therapies specifically directed at those factors involved in the pathogenesis of acute renal failure [67]. As these therapies move from the laboratory to the bedside, the ability to prevent acute renal failure and/or alter the course of established acute renal failure will hopefully finally improve.

References

1. Stott RB, Cameron JS, Ogg CS, Bewick M (1972) Why the persistently high mortality in acute renal failure? Lancet 2:75–79
2. Butkus DE (1983) Persistent high mortality in acute renal failure: Are we asking the right questions? Arch Intern Med 143:209–212
3. Cameron JS (1986) Acute renal failure – the continuing challenge. Q J Med 59:337–343
4. Prough DS (1996) Still lethal after all these years. Crit Care Med 24:189–190
5. McCarthy JT (1996) Prognosis of patients with acute renal failure in the intensive-care unit: A tale of two eras. Mayo Clin Proc 71:117–126
6. Conlon PJ, Schwab SJ (1996) Renal failure in the intensive care unit: An old tale gets better. Mayo Clin Proc 71:205–207

7. Biesenbach G, Zazgornik J, Kaiser W, Grafinger P, Stuby U, Necek S (1992) Improvement in prognosis of patients with acute renal failure over a period of 15 years: An analysis of 710 cases in a dialysis center. Am J Nephrol 12:319–325

8. Brivet FG, Kleinknecht DJ, Loirat P, Landais PJM (1996) Acute renal failure in intensive care units – causes, outcome, and prognostic factors of hospital mortality: a prospective multicenter study. Crit Care Med 24:192–198

9. Swann RC, Merrill JP (1953) The clinical course of acute renal failure. Medicine 32:215–283

10. Kaufman J, Dhakal M, Patel B, Hamburger R (1991) Community acquired acute renal failure. Am J Kidney Dis 17:191–198

11. Shusterman N, Strom BL, Murray TG, et al (1987) Risk factors and outcome of hospital acquired acute renal failure. Am J Med 83:65–71

12. Hou SH, Bushinsky DA, Wish JB, et al (1983) Hospital acquired renal insufficiency: a prospective study. Am J Med 72:243–248

13. Brivet FG, Kleinknecht DJ, Loirat P, Landais PJM (1996) Acute renal failure in intensive care units – causes, outcome, and prognostic factors of hospital mortality: a prospective multicenter study. Crit Care Med 24:192–198

14. Groeneveld ABJ, Tran JJ, Van der Meulen J, et al (1991) Acute renal failure in the medical intensive care unit:predisposing, complicating factors and outcome. Nephron 59:602–610

15. Menashe PI, Ross SA Gottieb JE (1988) Acquired renal insufficiency in critically ill patients. Crit Care Med 16:1106–1109

16. Wilkins RG, Faragher EB (1983) Acute renal failure in an intensive care unit: incidence, prediction and outcome. Anaesthesia 38:628–634

17. Chertow GM, Christiansen CL, Cleary PD, et al (1995) Prognostic stratification in critically ill patients with acute renal failure requiring dialysis. Arch Intern Med 155:1505–1511

18. Cosentino F, Chaff C, Piedmonte M. Risk factors influencing survival in ICU acute renal failure. Nephrol Dial Transplant 9 (suppl 4):179–182

19. Gillespie DJ, Marsh HMM, Divertie MB, Meadows JA (1986) Clinical outcome of respiratory failure in patients requiring prolonged (>24 hours) mechanical ventilation. Chest 90:364–369

20. Chertow GM, Lazarus JM, Paganini EP, et al (1998) Predictors of mortality and the provision of dialysis in patients with acute tubular necrosis. J Am Soc Nephrol 9:692–698

21. Corwin HL, Bonventre JV (1989) Factors influencing survival in acute renal failure. Semin Dial 2:220–225

22. Woodrow G, Turney JH (1992) Cause of death in acute renal failure. Nephrol Dial Transplant 7:230–234

23. Liano F (1994) Severity of acute renal failure: The need of measurement. Nephrol Dial Transplant 9 (suppl 4):229–238

24. Rasmussen HH, Ibels LS (1982) Acute renal failure: Multivariate analysis of causes and risk factors. Am J Med 73:211–218

25. Jochimsen F, Schafer JH, Maurer A, Distler A (1990) Impairment of renal function in medical intensive care: Predictability of acute renal failure. Crit Care Med 18:480–485

26. Badr KF, Ichikawa I (1988) Prerenal failure: A deleterious shift from renal compensation to decompensation. N Engl J Med 319:623–629

27. Luke RG, Briggs JD, Allison ME, Kennedy AC (1970) Factors determining response to mannitol in acute renal failure. Am J Med Sci 259:168–174

28. Conger JD (1993) Drug therapy in acute renal failure. In: Lazarus JM, Brenner BM (eds) Acute renal failure. Churchill Livingston, New York, pp 527–552

29. Levinsky NG, Bernard DB (1988) Mannitol and loop diuretics in acute renal failure. In: Brenner BM, Lazarus JM (eds) Acute Renal Failure. Churchill Livingston, New York, pp 841–856

30. Barry KG, Malloy JP (1962) Oliguric renal failure: Evaluation and therapy by the intravenous infusion of mannitol. JAMA 179:510–515

31. Eliahou HE (1964) Mannitol therapy in oliguria of acute onset. Br Med J 1:807–811

32. Better OS, Stein JH (1990) Early management of shock and prophylaxis of acute renal failure in traumatic rhabdomyolysis. N Engl J Med 322:825–829

33. Anto HR, Chou SY, Porush JG, Shapiro WB (1981) Infusion intravenous pyelography and renal function: Effects of hypertonic mannitol in patients with chronic renal insufficiency. Arch Intern Med 141:1652–1656

34. Weisberg LS, Kurnik PB, Kurnick BRC (1994) Risk of radiocontrast nephropathy in patients with and without diabetes mellitus. Kidney Int 45:259–265

35. Gubern JM, Sancho JJ, Simo J, Sitges-Serra A (1988) A randomised trial on the effect of mannitol on post-operative renal function in patients with obstructive jaundice. Surg 103:39–44

36. Paul MD, Mazer D, Byrick RJ, Rose DK, Goldstein MB (1986) Influence of mannitol and dopamine on renal function during elective infrarenal aortic clamping in man. Am J Nephrol 6:427–434

37. Cantarovich F, Locatelli A, Fernandez JC (1971) Frusemide in high doses in the treatment of acute renal failure. Post Grad Med J 47:13–19

38. Cantarovich F, Galli C, Benedetti L (1973) High dose frusemide in established acute renal failure. Br Med J 4:449–455

39. Kleinknecht D, Ganeval D, Gonzalez-Duque LA, Fermanian J (1976) Furosemide in acute oliguric renal failure. A controlled trial. Nephron 17:51–58

40. Brown CB, Ogg CS, Cameron JC (1981) High dose frusemide in acute renal failure: A controlled trial. Clin Nephrol 15:90–96

41. Martin SJ, Danziger LH (1994) Continuous infusion of loop diuretics in the critically ill: A review of the literature. Crit Care Med 22:1323–1329

42. Barter DC (1998) Diuretic therapy. N Engl J Med 339:387–395

43. Goldberg LI, McDonald RH, Zimmerman AM (1963) Sodium diuresis produced by dopamine in patients with congestive heart failure. N Engl J Med 269:1060–1064

44. Denton MD, Chertow GM, Brady HR (1996) Renal-dose dopamine for the treatment of acute renal failure: scientific rationale, experimental studies and clinical trials. Kidney Int 50:4–14

45. Seri I, Cone BC, Gullans SR, et al (1990) Influence of Na$^+$ intake on dopamine-induced inhibition of renal cortical Na$^+$-K$^+$-ATPase. Am J Physiol 258:F52–F60

46. Felder CC, Campbell T, Albrecht F, Jose PA (1990) Dopamine inhibits Na$^+$-H$^+$ exchanger activity in renal BBMV by stimulation of adenylate cyclase. Am J Physiol 259:F297–F303

47. Steinhausen M, Weis S, Fleming J, et al (1986) Response of in vivo renal microvessels to dopamine. Kidney Int 30:361–370

48. Szelip HM (1991) Renal dose dopamine: Fact or fiction. Ann Intern Med 115:153–154

49. Olsen NV, Hansen JM, Ladefoged SD, et al (1990) Renal tubular reabsorption of sodium and water during infusion of low-dose dopamine in normal man. Clin Sci 78:503–507

50. Henderson IS, Beattie TJ, Kennedy AC (1980) Dopamine hydrochlorine in oliguric states. Lancet 2:827–829

51. Parker S, Carlon GC, Isaacs M, Howland WS, Kahn RC (1981) Dopamine administration in oliguria and oliguric renal failure. Crit Care Med 9:630–632

52. Lindner A (1983) Synergism of dopamine and furosemide in diuretic resistant oliguric acute renal failure. Nephron 33:121–126

53. Graziani G, Cantaluppi A, Casati S, et al (1984) Dopamine and frusemide in oliguric acute renal failure. Nephron 37:39–42

54. Lumlertgul D, Keopling M, Sitprija V (1989) Furosemide and dopamine in malaria acute renal failure. Nephron 52:40–46

55. Weisberg LS, Kurnik PS, Kurnik BR (1993) Dopamine and renal blood flow in radiocontrast induced nephropathy in humans. Ren Fail 15:61–67

56. Baldwin L, Henderson A, Hickman P (1994) Effect of postoperative low dose dopamine on renal function after elective major vascular surgery. Ann Intern Med 120:744–747

57. Flancbaum L, Choban PS, Dasta JF (1994) Quantitative effects of low dose dopamine on urine output in oliguric surgical intensive care unit patients. Crit Care Med 22:61–66

58. Duke GJ, Breidis JH, Weaver RA (1994) Renal support in critically ill patients: Low dose dopamine or low dose dobutamine. Crit Care Med 22:1919–1925

59. Marik PE, Iglesias J, and the NORASEPT II study investigators (1999) Low dose dopamine does not prevent acute renal failure in patients with septic shock and oliguria. Am J Med 107:387–390

60. Chertow GM, Sayegh MH, Allegren RL, Lazarus JM (1996) Is the administration of dopamine associated with adverse or favorable outcomes in acute renal failure? Am J Med 101:49–53

61. Segal JM, Phang T, Walley KR (1992) Low dose dopamine hastens onset of gut ischemia in a porcine model of hemorrhagic shock. J Appl Physiol 73:1159–1164

62. Devins SS, Miller A, Herndon BL (1992) Effects of dopamine on T-lymphocyte proliferative responses and serum prolactin concentrations in critically ill patients. Crit Care Med 20:1644–1649

63. Szerlip HM (1991) Renal-dose dopamine: Fact and fiction. Ann Intern Med 115:153–154

64. Vincent JL (1994) Renal effects of dopamine: Can our dream ever come true? Crit Care Med 22:5–6

65. ANZICS Clinical Trials Group (2000) Low-dose dopamine in patients with early renal dysfunction: A placebo controlled randomised trial. Lancet 356:2139–2143

66. Kellum JA, Decker JM (2001) Use of dopamine in acute renal failure: A meta-analysis. Crit Care Med 29:1526–1531

67. Lameire N, Vanholder R (2001) Pathophysiologic features and prevention of human and experimental acute tubular necrosis. J Am Soc Nephrol 12:S20–S32

68. Biesenbach G, Zazgornik J, Kaiser W, Grafinger P, Stuby U, Necek S (1992) Improvement in prognosis of patients with acute renal failure over a period of 15 years: An analysis of 710 cases in a dialysis center. Am J Nephrol 12:319–325

69. Speigel DM, Ullian ME, Zerbe GO, Berl T (1991) Determinants of survival and recovery in acute renal failure patients dialysed in intensive care units. Am J Nephrol 11:44–47

70. Muku L, Latimer RG (1988) Acute hemodialysis in the surgical intensive care unit. Am Surgeon 54:548–552

71. Lohr JW, McFarlane MJ, Grantham JJ (1988) A clinical index to predict survival in acute renal failure requiring dialysis. Am J Kidney Dis 11:254–259

72. Lein J, Chan V (1985) Risk factors influencing survival in acute renal failure treated by hemodialysis. Arch Intern Med 145:2067–2069

73. Fischer RP, Griffen WO, Reiser M, Clark DS (1966) Early dialysis in the treatment of acute renal failure. Surg Gynecol Obstet 123:1019–1023

74. Kleinknecht D, Jungers P, Chanard J, Barbanel, Ganeval D (1972) Uremic and non-uremic complications in acute renal failure: Evaluation of early and frequent dialysis on prognosis. Kidney Int 1:190–196

75. Conger JD (1975) A controlled evaluation of prophylactic dialysis in post-traumatic acute renal failure. J Trauma 15:1056–1063

76. Gillum DM, Dixon BS, Yanover MJ, et al (1986) The role of intensive dialysis in acute renal failure. Clin Nephrol 25:249–255

77. Schiffl H, Lang SM, König, Held E (1997) Dose of intermittent hemodialysis and outcome of acute renal failure: A prospective randomized study. J Am Soc Nephrol 8:209A (Abst)

78. Hakim RM (1993) Clinical implications of hemodialysis membrane biocompatibility. Kidney Int 44:484–494

79. Schiffl H, Lang SM, König A, Strasser T, Haider MC, Held E (1994) Biocompatible membranes in acute renal failure: Prospective case-controlled study. Lancet 344:570–572

80. Hakim RM, Wingard RL, Parker RA (1994) Effect of the dialysis membrane in the treatment of patients with acute renal failure. N Engl J Med 331:1338–1342

81. Kramer P, Kaufhold G, Grone HJ, et al (1980) Management of anuric intensive care patients with arteriovenous hemofiltration. Int J Artif Organs 3:225

82. Van Bommel EFH, Leunissen KML, Weimer W (1994) Continuous renal replacement therapy for critically ill patients: An update. Intensive Care Med 9:265–280

83. Bellomo R, Parkin G, Love J, Boyce N (1992) Use of continuous haemodiafiltration: An approach to the management of acute renal failure in the critically ill. Am J Nephrol 12: 240–245

84. Bellomo R, Boyce N (1993) Acute continuous hemodiafiltration: A prospective study of 110 patients and a review of the literature. Am J Kidney Dis 21:508–518

85. Bellomo R, Farmer M, Parkin G, Wright C, Boyce N (1995) Severe acute renal failure: A comparison of acute hemodiafiltration and conventional dialytic therapy. Nephron 71:59–64

86. Clark WR, Mueller BA, Alaka KJ, Macias WL (1994) A comparison of metabolic control by continuous and intermittent therapies in acute renal failure. J Am Soc Nephrol 4:1413–1420
87. Schetz M, Ferdinande P, Van den Berghe G, Verwaest C, Lauwers P (1995) Removal of pro-inflammatory cytokines with renal replacement therapy: Sense or nonsense? Intensive Care Med 21:169–176
88. Bellomo R (1995) Continuous hemofiltration as blood purification in sepsis. New Horiz 3:732–737
89. Bellomo R, Tipping P, Boyce N (1993) Continuous veno-venous hemofiltration with dialysis removes cytokines from the circulation of septic patients. Crit Care Med 21:522–526
90. Grootendorst AF, van Bommel EFH, van der Hoven B, van Leengoed LAMG, van Osta ALM (1992) High volume hemofiltration improves right ventricular function in endotoxin-induced shock in the pig. Intensive Care Med 18:235–240
91. Gomez A, Wang R, Unruh H, et al (1990) Hemofiltration reverses left ventricular dysfunction during sepsis in dogs. Anesthesiology 73:671–685
92. Stein B, Pfenninger E, Grunert A, Schmitz JE, Deller A, Kocher F (1991) The consequences of continuous haemofiltration on lung mechanics and extravascular lung water in a porcine endotoxic shock model. Intensive Care Med 17:293–298
93. Stein B, Pfenninger E, Grunert A, Schmitz JE, Hudde M (1990) Influence of continuous haemofiltration on haemodynamics and central blood volume in experimental endotoxic shock. Intensive Care Med 16:494–499
94. De Vaiese AS, Vanholder RC, De Sutter JH, et al (1998) Continuous renal replacement therapies in sepsis: Where are the data? Nephrol Dial Transplant 13:1362–1364
95. Honore PM, Jamez J, Wauthier M, et al (2000) Prospective evaluation of short term, high volume, isovolemic hemofiltration on the hemodynamic course and outcome of patients with intractable circulatory failure resulting from septic shock. Crit Care Med 28:3581–3587
96. Bellomo R, Ronco C (1995) Acute renal failure in the intensive care unit: Which treatment is best? In: Bellomo R, Ronco R (eds) Acute Renal Failure in the Critically Ill. Springer, Berlin, pp 385–406
97. Ronco C, Bellomo R, Homel P, et al (2000) Effects of different doses in continuous veno-venous haemofiltration on outcomes of acute renal failure: A prospective randomised trial. Lancet 355:26–30
98. Mehta RL, McDonald B, Gabbai FB, et al (2001) A randomized clinical trial of continuous versus intermittent dialysis for acute renal failure. Kidney Int 60:1154–1163

Particular Aspects

Perioperative Management of the Severely Burned Patient

E.R. Sherwood and L.C. Woodson

▌ Introduction

Burn care has improved markedly since the end of World War II. Important innovations include aggressive fluid resuscitation, early excision and grafting of burn wounds, more effective antibiotics, advances in enteral nutritional support and the development of multidisciplinary burn centers. Most patients with burns involving 80% or more of the total body surface area will survive if promptly treated. A recent study identified three risk factors that are predictive of increased mortality following thermal injury: age greater than 60 years, burns over more than 40% of the total body surface area, and the presence of inhalation injury [1]. Mortality increased in proportion to the number of risk factors present. Significant coexisting disease or delays in resuscitation also increased the mortality rate.

Modern burn care depends on coordination of a multidisciplinary team. The current standard of surgical treatment calls for early excision and grafting of nonviable burn wounds. This approach decreases the incidence of serious infection and reduces the systemic inflammatory response by removing necrotic tissue. The effects of inflammatory mediators on metabolism and cardiopulmonary function reduce physiologic reserve and the patient's tolerance to the stress of surgery deteriorates with time. Assuming adequate resuscitation, extensive surgery is best tolerated soon after injury when the patient is most fit. However, it must be recognized that the initial resuscitation of patients with large burns results in large fluid shifts and may result in hemodynamic instability, electrolyte abnormalities, and respiratory insufficiency. Reynolds and colleagues reported that more than half of the deaths resulting from burn injuries occurred due to failed resuscitation [2]. Effective management of patients with extensive burn injuries requires an understanding of the pathophysiologic changes associated with large burns and careful evaluation to assure that resuscitation has been optimized.

Major burn injury results in pathophysiological changes in virtually all organ systems (Table 1). Assessment of acute burn patients requires special attention to airway management and pulmonary support, vascular access, adequacy of resuscitation, and associated injuries. Much of the morbidity and mortality associated with burn injuries are related to the size of the injury. The extent of the burn injury is expressed as the total body surface area (TBSA) burned.

Knowledge of the burn depth is also critical to anticipating physiological insult as well as planned surgical treatment. First degree or superficial second-degree burns may heal without scarring or deformity and do not require surgical excision. Deeper second degree and third degree burns require surgical debridement and grafting with associated surgical blood loss. Accurate estimates of blood loss are

Table 1. Perioperative challenges in the acute burn patient

▌ Compromised airway	▌ Decreased colloid osmotic pressure
▌ Pulmonary insufficiency	▌ Edema
▌ Altered mental status	▌ Dysrhythmia
▌ Associated injuries	▌ Impaired temperature regulation
▌ Limited vascular access	▌ Altered drug response
▌ Rapid blood loss	▌ Renal insufficiency
▌ Impaired tissue perfusion due to:	▌ Immunosuppression
– Hypovolemia	▌ Infection/sepsis
– Decreased myocardial contractility	
– Anemia	

Table 2. Calculation of expected blood loss during excision and grafting of burn wounds

Surgical procedure	Predicted blood loss
<24 h since burn injury	0.45 ml/cm^2 burn area
1–3 days since burn injury	0.65 ml/cm^2 burn area
2–16 days since burn injury	0.75 ml/cm^2 burn area
>16 days since burn injury	0.5 ml/cm^2 burn area
presence of infected wounds	>1 ml/cm^2 burn area

crucial in planning preoperative management of burn patients. With extensive wound excision or debridement, large amounts of blood can be lost rapidly. Adequate preparation in terms of monitors, vascular access and availability of blood products is essential. Surgical blood loss depends on area to be excised (cm^2), the time elapsed since injury and the presence of infection [3] (Table 2). Blood loss from skin graft donor sites will also vary depending on whether it is an initial or repeat harvest. Skin grafts obtained from previously harvested sites bleed more vigorously than fresh sites due to hyperemia and neovascularization of the previously harvested areas.

▌ Effect of Burn Injury on the Airway and Pulmonary Function

Burn injuries to the face and neck can distort anatomy and reduce the range of mobility in ways that make direct laryngoscopy difficult or impossible. Specific alterations include impaired mouth opening and decreased range of motion of the neck. Edema of the tongue, oropharynx, and larynx may be severe. Facial swelling due to direct burn injury and the interstitial accumulation of resuscitation fluids in the immediate postburn period can make airway manipulation difficult. The tissue injury and sloughing present after severe facial burns may impair the ability to mask ventilate the patient. All of these factors can make airway management in the burn patient challenging.

The level of respiratory support required by burned patients must also be assessed. Support may range from supplemental blow-by or mask oxygen to tracheal intubation and mechanical ventilation with high positive end-expiratory pressure

(PEEP) and increased inspired oxygen fraction (FiO$_2$) requirements. Lung injury can occur from smoke inhalation, systemic inflammation, or aggressive fluid resuscitation. Common sequelae include upper airway injury with stridor and bronchospasm, and lower airway obstruction from mucus plugs and epithelial casts. Pulmonary edema due to acute lung injury (ALI) or volume overload may necessitate the need for high PEEP and FiO$_2$ requirements. For patients with very high PEEP requirements or markedly elevated peak inspiratory pressures, it must be determined whether a standard anesthesia machine ventilator is adequate to support the patient. The use of an intensive care unit (ICU) ventilator may be necessary in some cases. If the patient is intubated at the time of the preoperative evaluation it is essential to know what the indications for intubation were so that an appropriate plan for postoperative support can be made.

There is general recognition that smoke inhalation injury increases morbidity and mortality for burn patients [4]. Several factors are predictive of inhalation injury. These include exposure to a closed space fire, a period of unconsciousness at the accident scene, burns including the face and neck, singed facial or nasal hair, hoarseness, dysphagia, oral and/or nasal soot deposits, and carbonaceous sputum. The presence of an inhalation injury in combination with a cutaneous burn increases the volume of fluid required for resuscitation by as much as 44% [5]. Numerous studies have also shown an increased incidence of pulmonary complications such as pneumonia, respiratory failure, or acute respiratory distress syndrome (ARDS) in patients with burns and inhalation injury when compared to those with burns alone [6]. Sequelae of inhalation injury include upper airway distortion and obstruction from direct thermal injury as well as impaired pulmonary gas exchange due to effects of toxic gases on lower airways and pulmonary parenchyma. These two components of the inhalation injury have separate time courses and pathophysiological consequences. Foley described findings of 335 autopsies performed on patients who died from extensive burns [7]. Intra-oral, palatal, and laryngeal burns were not uncommon among patients with inhalation injuries. The most common sites of laryngeal injury were the epiglottis and vocal folds where their edges were exposed. In contrast, thermal necrosis below the glottis and upper trachea was not observed in any of these patients. The lower airways are nearly always protected from direct thermal injury by the efficiency of heat-exchange in the oro- and nasopharynx unless the injury involves steam or an explosive blast.

Carbon monoxide and cyanide are two major toxic components of smoke. The burn patient with evidence of inhalation injury should be evaluated for the presence of toxicity resulting from these compounds. Carbon monoxide binds hemoglobin 200 times more avidly than oxygen [8]. Therefore, carbon monoxide markedly impairs the association of oxygen with hemoglobin and decreases oxygen carrying capacity. Carbon monoxide also shifts the oxyhemoglobin dissociation curve to the left thus decreasing the release of oxygen into tissues. These factors result in decreased oxygen delivery (DO$_2$) to tissues and, at critical levels, lead to anaerobic metabolism and metabolic acidosis. Signs and symptoms of carbon monoxide poisoning include headache, mental status changes, dyspnea, nausea, weakness, and tachycardia. Patients suffering carbon monoxide poisoning have a normal PaO$_2$ and oxygen saturation by routine pulse oximetry. They are not cyanotic. Carboxyhemoglobin must be detected by co-oximetry. Carboxyhemoglobin levels above 15% are toxic and those above 50% are often lethal. The major treatment approach is administration of 100% oxygen and, in severe cases, hyperbaric treatment to increase the partial pressure of oxygen in blood [9].

Cyanide is also a component of smoke resulting from the burning of some plastic products [10]. Cyanide directly impairs the oxidative apparatus in mitochondria and decreases the ability of cells to utilize oxygen in metabolism. These alterations result in conversion to anaerobic metabolism and the development of metabolic acidosis. Signs and symptoms are non-specific and include headache, mental status changes, nausea, lethargy, and weakness. Hydrogen cyanide levels above 100 ppm are generally fatal. Treatment includes nitrates to increase methemoglobin levels. Methemoglobin competes with cytochrome oxidase for cyanide. However, excessive levels of methemoglobin lead to decreased oxygen carrying capacity and may be toxic. Administration of sodium thiosulfate will cause production of thiocyanate, which decreases the toxicity of cyanide and increases its elimination.

▌ Airway Management

If injuries do not preclude conventional airway management, standard induction and intubation procedures are appropriate. Hu and colleagues reported that gastric emptying was not delayed in patients with severe burns so that a rapid sequence induction is not necessary [11]. However, attention should be given to gastric residuals during enteral feeding. Development of sepsis can slow gastric emptying which can result in retained fluids in the stomach and risk of aspiration.

When burns include the face and neck, swelling and distortion may make direct laryngoscopy difficult or impossible. In addition, loss of mandibular mobility may impair airway manipulation and make mask ventilation difficult. Fiberoptic intubation while maintaining spontaneous ventilation is a safe and reliable technique under these conditions.

Since most anesthetics cause collapse of pharyngeal tissues and airway obstruction, they are unsuitable for fiberoptic intubation in patients whose airway would be difficult to manage with a mask [12]. Ketamine, however, is unique among anesthetic drugs because it maintains spontaneous ventilation and airway patency [13].

Airway management using a laryngeal mask airway (LMA) has also been used successfully during burn surgery for children. McCall and coworkers [14] reported their experience with 141 general anesthetics administered to 88 pediatric burn patients. Nineteen (13.5%) of the procedures were complicated by respiratory events such as unseating, desaturation, and partial laryngospasm that required intervention. Two of these events required intraoperative intubation without sequelae.

▌ Effect of Burn Injury on the Circulation

Thermal injury has profound effects on the systemic circulation and hemodynamic management is a major component of perioperative care. It is critical to assess the adequacy of post-burn fluid resuscitation and the hemodynamic status of the patient. Important variables include blood pressure, heart rate, urine output, central venous pressure, base deficit, and blood lactate levels. In patients with pulmonary artery catheters, cardiac output, mixed venous oxygen saturation (SvO_2), cardiac and pulmonary filling pressures and DO_2 parameters provide important information regarding the hemodynamic status of the burn patient. In addition, determination of blood hemoglobin level, fluid requirements, and the need for vasopressors or inotropes are important for developing an effective anesthetic plan. Patients suffering burn injury exhibit two distinct phases of cardiovascular response. Initially, a state of burn shock develops in response to the massive tissue injury. If resuscitation is adequate, this phase is followed by a hyperdynamic state characterized by tachycardia and increased cardiac output. The latter stage is primarily a response to systemic inflammation and the hypermetabolic state that ensues.

After massive thermal injury, a state of burn shock develops due to intravascular hypovolemia and, in most cases, myocardial depression. Decreased cardiac output, increased systemic vascular resistance (SVR) and tissue hypoperfusion characterize burn shock [15–16]. Intravascular hypovolemia results from alterations in microvascular permeability in both burned and unburned tissues leading to the development of interstitial fluid accumulation. The net effect of these changes is the development of massive edema during the first 24 to 48 hours after thermal injury with a concomitant loss of intravascular volume. The hypotension associated with burn injury is also due, in part, to myocardial depression. The inflammatory response to thermal injury results in the release of inflammatory mediators such as tumor necrosis factor (TNF)-α and interleukin-1 (IL-1). TNF-α and IL-1 are known to have myocardial suppressant effects [17]. These factors, and other possibly unrecognized factors, are responsible for the depression in myocardial function that often results from burn injury.

Several fluid resuscitation protocols that utilize various combinations of crystalloids, colloids, and hypertonic fluids have been developed. Isotonic crystalloid resuscitation is employed in most burn centers and generally provides adequate volume resuscitation. However, compared to colloids and hypertonic solutions, crystalloid resuscitation may require larger volumes and cause more tissue edema and hypoproteinemia. Therefore, interest has developed in analyzing colloid and hypertonic resuscitation regimens. Overall, colloid resuscitation within the first 24 hours of burn injury has not improved outcome compared to crystalloid resuscitation [18]. Furthermore, a recent meta-analysis indicated that mortality is higher in burned patients receiving albumin as part of the initial resuscitation protocol [19]. Because of the added cost with little benefit, colloid solutions have not been used routinely in the United States for initial volume resuscitation in burned patients. The use of hypertonic saline, either alone or in conjunction with colloids, has been advocated also in the initial resuscitation of burned patients. Among the potential benefits are reduced volume requirements to attain similar levels of intravascular resuscitation and tissue perfusion compared to isotonic fluids [20]. Theoretically, the reduced volume requirements would decrease the incidence of pulmonary and tissue edema thus reducing the incidence of pulmonary complications and the need for escharotomy. Hypertonic saline dextran solutions have been shown to expand intravascular volume by mobilizing fluids from intracellular and interstitial fluid compartments. Although hypertonic saline dextran solutions will transiently de-

Table 3. Criteria for adequate fluid resuscitation

▌ Normalization of blood pressure	▌ Gastric intramucosal pH (>7.32)
▌ Urine output (1–2 ml/kg/hr)	▌ Central venous pressure
▌ Blood lactate (<2 mM/l)	▌ Cardiac index (CI) (4.5 l/min/m^2)
▌ Base deficit (<-5)	▌ Oxygen delivery index (DO$_2$I) (600 ml/min/m^2)

crease fluid requirements, both clinical and experimental studies have not shown an overall decrease in total resuscitation fluid needs [21–22].

Several parameters have been used to assess the adequacy of volume resuscitation in burned patients (Table 3). Regardless of the parameter used, a critical factor is early volume resuscitation and establishment of tissue perfusion. Traditionally, urine output (0.5–1 ml/kg/hr) and normalization of blood pressure (mean arterial blood pressure of greater than 70 mmHg) have been used as endpoints to indicate adequate volume replacement. However, recent studies indicate that these parameters may be poor predictors of adequate tissue perfusion. Jeng and colleagues showed that attaining urine outputs of greater than 30 ml/hr and mean blood pressures of greater than 70 mmHg correlated poorly with other global indicators of tissue perfusion [23]. Other recent studies have shown that normalization of blood pressure, heart rate and urine output do not correlate with improved outcome [24]. Therefore, in the pre-operative assessment of the burn patient, the anesthesiologist should not base the cardiovascular assessment strictly on these parameters.

Blood lactate and base deficit provide indirect indices of global tissue perfusion. Lactic acid is a byproduct of anaerobic metabolism and is an indicator of either inadequate DO_2 or impaired oxygen utilization. In the absence of conditions such as cyanide poisoning or sepsis that alter oxygen utilization at the cellular level, lactate production serves as a marker of oxygen balance. Serum lactate levels have also served as a useful marker of fluid resuscitation and tissue perfusion in burn patients [25]. A recent study showed serum lactate to be the most predictive index of adequate tissue perfusion. Lactate levels of less than 2 mM/l in the first 24–72 hours after burn injury correlated with increased survival [26]. Base deficit is another indirect indicator of global tissue perfusion. Base deficit provides a readily obtained and widely available indicator of tissue acidosis and shock. Base deficit has been shown to correlate closely with blood lactate and provide a useful indicator of inadequate DO_2. A retrospective study by Kaups and colleagues showed that base deficit was an accurate predictor of fluid requirements, burn size, and mortality rate [27].

Invasive cardiovascular monitors are not used routinely in burned patients to guide volume resuscitation. Most patients can be adequately resuscitated without their use. However, a small subset of patients such as those with underlying cardiovascular disease or those that do not respond normally to volume resuscitation may benefit from invasive monitoring. Some recent investigations have focused on the use of cardiac index and DO_2 as useful endpoints to guide volume resuscitation [28–29]. Bernard and colleagues have shown that patients surviving large burn injuries had higher cardiac indices and more effective DO_2 than non-survivors [30]. Some investigators have proposed the use of supranormal DO_2 as a means of assuring adequate tissue perfusion [31–32]. The preselected goals were a cardiac index of 4.5 l/m^2 and DO_2 index of 600 $ml/min/m^2$. These values represent approximately 150% of normal cardiac index and DO_2 values. Attaining supraphysiologic cardiac output and DO_2 has been shown to improve outcome in some studies. Schiller and colleagues [33] demonstrated that maintaining hyperdynamic hemodynamics using fluids and inotropes improved survival in burn patients. However, other investigations, including a meta-analysis, have shown that achieving supraphysiological levels of cardiac output and DO_2 did not improve mortality or decrease the incidence of organ failure in trauma and burn patients [34–36]. The use of inotropes to attain supraphysiological oxygen transport could be detrimental in some cases. One study that employed dobutamine to drive cardiac output and elevate DO_2 in trauma patients demonstrated increased mortality [37].

▌ Blood Transfusion

Unless significant co-existing injuries exist, blood loss is usually not a major factor in the immediate management of burn patients. However, significant blood loss is common during excision and grafting of burn wounds. The amount of blood loss is determined by the age of the burn, the body surface area involved and whether infection is present (Table 2). In general, more blood loss will result as the time from initial injury increases and if wounds are infected. Controversy exists regarding transfusion triggers and targets. Some authors advocate allowing hematocrits to drop to 15–20% prior to transfusion in otherwise healthy patients undergoing limited excision, and transfusing at a hematocrit of 25% in patients with pre-existing cardiovascular disease [38]. The same group proposed maintaining hematocrits near 25% in patients with more extensive burns and near 30% if the patients have pre-existing cardiovascular disease. A small study by Sittig and Deitch showed fewer transfused units and no increase in adverse hemodynamic or metabolic effects in patients transfused at a hemoglobin of 6–6.5 g/dl compared to patients maintained at a hemoglobin near 10 g/dl [39]. However, in general, few data exist regarding the optimum management strategy for blood transfusion during burn wound excision. Assessment of blood transfusion needs is best determined by evaluating the clinical status of the patient.

▌ Effect of Burn Injury on Renal Function

Acute renal failure is a relatively common complication following thermal injury. The incidence of acute renal failure following burn injury has been reported to range from 0.5–30% and is most dependent on the severity of the burn and the presence of inhalation injury [40]. The development of acute renal failure is an indicator of poor prognosis with mortality rates as high as 85% reported by some investigators [41]. Jeschke and colleagues [42] have reported a mortality rate of 56% in pediatric burn patients suffering acute renal failure. Holm and colleagues [41] observed that acute renal failure could be divided into early and late categories. Early acute renal failure was defined as occurring within five days of burn injury. The most common apparent causes were hypotension and myoglobinuria. Acute renal failure occurring five days after injury was defined as late. Sepsis was the most common cause with a small number of cases resulting from the administration of nephrotoxic drugs. Factors that decrease the incidence of acute renal failure and associated mortality include adequate fluid resuscitation, early wound excision, and prevention of infection. Regardless of the cause, it is critical to assess renal function in burn patients in order to develop a comprehensive anesthetic plan. Important areas of analysis include urine output, dialysis dependence, volume status, and electrolytes. Also, diuretic therapy should be noted. Scheduled doses of diuretics may need to be continued during the perioperative period to maintain urine output.

Thermoregulation in Burn Patients

Maintenance of proper body temperature is critical for optimizing wound healing and recovery in severely burned patients. Because the skin is in direct contact with the environment, it plays an important role in thermal regulation. Of course, patients with large body surface area burns have had much of their skin removed. This ablates some or all of the insulating properties of skin. However, Wallace and colleagues have shown that burn patients perceive changes in ambient temperature as effectively as normal controls [43]. An increase in the gradient of ambient temperature to skin temperature results in heat loss that ultimately results in a sensation of cold. Changes in metabolic rate correlate most with the patient's sensation of cold discomfort rather than ambient temperature. Burn patients respond with a brisk increase in heat generation and metabolic rate during periods of perceived cold discomfort [43]. In burn patients, the central threshold for sensing and responding to cold stimuli is higher and the increase is proportional to the size of the burn. The work of Caldwell and colleagues predicts that the temperature set point will increase by 0.03 °C per % total body surface area burned [44]. This increase in temperature threshold appears to be due to the hypermetabolic state and the presence of pyrogenic inflammatory mediators such as TNF-α, IL-1 and IL-6 that are present after thermal injury.

Conclusion

Patients that have suffered severe thermal injury present a significant challenge. These patients exhibit alterations in cardiovascular, pulmonary, and thermoregulatory function. The primary challenges include maintenance of adequate perfusion and hemodynamic stability. In most cases, hemodynamic management requires invasive monitoring and aggressive volume management. Airway management requires thorough examination and planning. Burn patients commonly require special approaches such as awake fiberoptic intubation in order to safely secure the airway. A variety of anesthetic techniques can be safely and effectively employed in severely burned patients. The specific technique employed is dependent on the type and severity of injury, the physiological status of the patient and the experience of the practitioner. Keys to the effective management of these critically injured patients are constant monitoring, diligence, and effective cooperation among the operating room and ICU staff.

References

1. Ryan CM, Schoenfeld DA, Thorpe WP, Sheridan RL, Cassem EH, Tompkins RG (1998) Objective estimates of the probability of death from burn injuries. N Engl J Med 338:362–366
2. Reynolds EM, Ryan DP, Sheridan RL, Doody DP (1995) Left ventricular failure complicating severe pediatric burn injuries. J Pediatr Surg 30:264–269
3. Desai MH, Herndon DN, Broemeling L, Barrow RE, Nichols RJ, Rutan RL (1990) Early burn wound excision significantly reduces blood loss. Ann Surg 211:753–759
4. Thompson PB, Herndon DN, Traber DL, Abston S (1986) Effect on mortality of inhalation injury. J Trauma 26:163–165
5. Navar PD, Saffle JR, Warden GD (1985) Effect of inhalation injury on fluid resuscitation requirements after thermal injury. Am J Surg 150:716–720

6. Hollingsed TC, Saffle JR, Barton RG, Craft WB, Morris SE (1993) Etiology and consequences of respiratory failure in thermally injured patients. Am J Surg 166:592–597
7. Foley FD (1969) The burn autopsy. Am J Clin Path 52:1–13
8. Ernst A, Zibrak JD (1998) Carbon monoxide poisoning. N Engl J Med 339:1603–1608
9. Tibbles P, Perrotta P (1994) Treatment of carbon monoxide poisoning: A critical review of human outcome studies comparing normobaric oxygen with hyperbaric oxygen. Ann Emerg Med 24:269–276
10. Clark CJ (1982) Measurement of toxic combustion products in fire survivors. J Royal Soc Med 153:41–44
11. Hu OY, Ho ST, Wang JJ, Lin CY (1993) Evaluation of gastric emptying in severe, burn-injured patients. Crit Care Med 21:527–531
12. Mathru M, Esch O, Lang J, et al (1996) Magnetic resonance imaging of the upper airway: Effects of propofol anesthesia and nasal continuous positive airway pressure in humans. Anesthesiology 84:275–278
13. Lang J, Herbert M, Esch, Chaljuh G, Mathru M (1997) Magnetic resonance of the upper airway: Ketamine preserves airway potency compared to propofol anesthesia in human volunteers. Anesth Analg 84:542 (Abst)
14. McCall VE, Fischer CG, Schomaker E, Young VM (1999) Laryngeal mask airway use in children with acute burns: intraoperative airway management. Paediatr Anaesth 9:515–520
15. Deitch EA (1990) The management of burns. N Engl J Med 323:1249–1253
16. Horton JW, Baxter CR, White DJ (1989) Differences in cardiac responses to resuscitation from burn shock. Surg Gynecol Obstet 168:201–213
17. Muller-Werdan U, Engelmann H, Werdan K (1998) Cardiodepression by tumor necrosis factor-alpha. Eur Cytokine Netw 9:689–691
18. Alderson P, Schierhout G, Roberts I, Bunn F (2000) Colloids versus crystalloids for fluid resuscitation in critically ill patients. Cochrane Database Syst Rev 2:CD000567
19. The Albumin Reviewers (2000) In: Alderson P, Bunn F, Lefebvre C, Li Wan Po A, Li L, Roberts I, Schierhout G (ed) Human albumin solution for resuscitation and volume expansion in critically ill patients. Cochrane Database Syst Rev 2:CD001208
20. Guha SC, Kinsky MP, Button B, et al (1996) Burn resuscitation: crystalloid versus colloid versus hypertonic saline hyperoncotic colloid in sheep. Crit Care Med 24:1849–1857
21. Elgjo GI, Poli de Figueiredo LF, Schenarts PJ, Traber DL, Traber LD, Kramer GC (2000) Hypertonic saline dextran produces early (8–12 hrs) fluid sparing in burn resuscitation: a 24-hr prospective, double-blind study in sheep. Crit Care Med 28:163–171
22. Suzuki K, Ogino R, Nishina M, Kohama A (1995) Effects of hypertonic saline and dextran cardiac functions after burns. Am J Physiol 268:H856–H864
23. Jeng JC, Lee K, Jablonski K, Jordan MH (1997) Serum lactate and base deficit suggest inadequate resuscitation of patients with burn injuries: application of a point-of-care laboratory instrument. J Burn Care Rehabil 18:402–405
24. Dries DJ, Waxman K (1991) Adequate resuscitation of burn patients may not be measured by urine output and vital signs. Crit Care Med 19:327–329
25. Porter JM, Ivatury RR (1998) In search of the optimal end points of resuscitation in trauma patients: a review. J Trauma 44:908–914
26. Holm C, Melcer B, Horbrand F, Worl HH, von Donnersmarck GH, Muhlbauer W (2000) Haemodynamic and oxygen transport responses in survivors and non-survivors following thermal injury. Burns 26:25–33
27. Kaups KL, Davis JW, Dominic WJ (1998) Base deficit as an indicator or resuscitation needs in patients with burn injuries. J Burn Care Rehabil 19:346–348
28. Schiller WR, Bay RC, Garren RL, Parker I, Sagraves SG (1997) Hyperdynamic resuscitation improves survival in patients with life-threatening burns. J Burn Care Rehabil 18:10–16
29. Holm C, Melcer B, Horbrand F, von Donnersmarck GH, Muhlbauer W (2000) The relationship between oxygen delivery and oxygen consumption during fluid resuscitation of burn-related shock. J Burn Care Rehabil 21:147–154
30. Bernard F, Gueugniaud PY, Bertin-Maghit M, Bouchard C, Vilasco B, Petit P (1994) Prognostic significance of early cardiac index measurements in severely burned patients. Burns 20:529–531

31. Bishop MH, Shoemaker WC, Appel PL, et al (1995) Prospective, randomized trial of survivor values of cardiac index, oxygen delivery, and oxygen consumption as resuscitation endpoints in severe trauma. J Trauma 38:780–787

32. Fleming A, Bishop M, Shoemaker W, et al (1992) Prospective trial of supranormal values as goals of resuscitation in severe trauma. Arch Surg 127:1175–1179

33. Schiller WR, Bay RC, Garren RL, Parker I, Sagraves SG (1997) Hyperdynamic resuscitation improves survival in patients with life-threatening burns. J Burn Care Rehabil 18:10–16

34. Heyland DK, Cook DJ, King D, Kernerman P, Brun-Buisson C (1996) Maximizing oxygen delivery in critically ill patients: a methodologic appraisal of the evidence. Crit Care Med 24:517–524

35. Gattinoni L, Brazzi L, Pelosi P, et al (1995) A trial of goal-oriented hemodynamic therapy in critically ill patients. SvO2 Collaborative Group. N Engl J Med 333:1025–1032

36. Durham RM, Neunaber K, Mazuski JE, Shapiro MJ, Baue AE (1996) The use of oxygen consumption and delivery as endpoints for resuscitation in critically ill patients. J Trauma 41:32–39

37. Hayes MA, Timmins AC, Yau EH, Palazzo M, Hinds CJ, Watson D (1994) Elevation of systemic oxygen delivery in the treatment of critically ill patients. N Engl J Med. 330:1717–1722

38. Mann R, Heimbach DM, Engrav LH, Foy H (1994) Changes in transfusion practices in burn patients. J Trauma 37:220–222

39. Sittig KM, Deitch EA (1994) Blood transfusions: for the thermally injured or for the doctor? J Trauma 36:369–372

40. Davies DM, Pusey CD, Rainford DJ, Brown JM, Bennett JP (1979) Acute renal failure in burns. Scand J Plast Reconstr Surg 13:189–192

41. Holm C, Horbrand F, von Donnersmarck GH, Muhlbauer W (1999) Acute renal failure in severely burned patients. Burns 25:171–178

42. Jeschke MG, Barrow RE, Wolf SE, Herndon DN (1998) Mortality in burned children with acute renal failure. Arch Surg 133:752–756

43. Wallace BH, Caldwell FT Jr, Cone JB (1994) The interrelationships between wound management, thermal stress, energy metabolism, and temperature profiles of patients with burns. J Burn Care Rehabil 15:499–508

44. Caldwell FT Jr, Wallace BH, Cone JB (1994) The effect of wound management on the interaction of burn size, heat production, and rectal temperature. J Burn Care Rehabil 15:121–129

Hypertensive Crises

J. Varon, P. E. Marik, and R. E. Fromm Jr.

▌ Introduction

Hypertension is a common clinical problem. Physicians across the world of multiple specialties are likely to encounter patients with hypertensive urgencies and emergencies. Various terms have been applied to these conditions; all characterized by acute elevations in blood pressure [1]. Prompt, but careful consideration of therapy is necessary to limit morbidity and mortality. Unfortunately, accelerated hypertension is amongst the most misunderstood and mismanaged of 'acute' medical problems seen in critical care medicine. Many healthcare providers concentrate on rapidly reducing an elevated blood pressure without understanding the pathophysiological principles involved and potential consequences.

▌ Terminology and Definitions

The Joint National Committee on Prevention, Detection, Evaluation, and Treatment of High Blood Pressure has classified hypertension in stages according to the degree of elevation of blood pressure [2].

- ▌ Stage 1: patients have a systolic BP of 140–159 mmHg or a diastolic BP of 90–99 mmHg.
- ▌ Stage 2: individuals have a systolic BP of 160–179 mmHg or a diastolic BP of 100–109 mmHg.
- ▌ Stage 3: includes a systolic BP pressure equal or greater than 180 mmHg or a diastolic BP equal or greater to 110 mmHg. This stage is also termed severe or accelerated hypertension.

A number of different terms have been applied to severe acute elevations of blood pressure [1]. However, most authors have defined hypertensive crises or emergencies as a sudden increase in systolic and diastolic blood pressure associated with end-organ damage. The end-organs considered include: the central nervous system (CNS), the heart, and/or the kidneys. The term, hypertensive urgencies, has been applied to patients with severely elevated blood pressures without current acute end-organ damage, but for whom the potential for injury exists. Table 1 lists those clinical conditions which meet the diagnostic criteria of hypertensive crises. It is important to note that the clinical differentiation between hypertensive emergencies and hypertensive urgencies depends on the presence of target organ damage, rather than the absolute level of blood pressure.

Table 1. Hypertensive emergencies

▌Hypertensive encephalopathy
▌Dissecting aortic aneurysm
▌Acute pulmonary edema with respiratory failure
▌Acute myocardial infarction/unstable angina
▌Eclampsia
▌Acute renal failure
▌Microangiopathic hemolytic anemia

Another frequently encountered term, 'malignant hypertension', has been defined as a syndrome characterized by elevated blood pressure accompanied by encephalopathy, retinopathy or nephropathy [2]. However, the authors consider this term to be misleading and prefer to avoid its use. Postoperative hypertension has arbitrarily been defined as systolic blood pressure greater than 190 mmHg and/or diastolic blood pressure 100 mmHg on two consecutive readings following surgery.

A systolic pressure greater than 169 mmHg, or a diastolic greater than 109 mmHg, in a pregnant woman is considered a hypertensive emergency requiring immediate pharmacological management [3]. The special situations of pregnancy-induced hypertension (PIH) are sufficiently complex to require a detailed discussion in their own right and, thus, will not be reviewed in this chapter.

▌ Epidemiology, Etiology, Pathogenesis

Hypertension is extremely common in the modern world. Sixty million United States inhabitants suffer from this disorder [2]. More than 90% of these patients have essential hypertension; three quarters of those affected do not have their blood pressure well controlled.

The incidence of hypertensive crises is higher among African-Americans and the elderly. The majority of patients presenting with hypertensive crises will have been previously diagnosed as hypertensive, and will have had inadequate blood pressure control. The incidence of postoperative hypertensive crises varies depending on the population examined, being reported in 4–35% of patients shortly after the surgical procedure [4]. Like other forms of accelerated hypertension, a prior history of hypertension is common.

The pathophysiology of hypertensive crises is thought to be due to an abrupt increase in systemic vascular resistance (SVR) likely related to humoral vasoconstrictors. With severe elevations of blood pressure, endothelial injury occurs and fibrinoid necrosis of the arterioles may ensue. This vascular injury leads to deposition of platelets and fibrin, and a breakdown of the normal autoregulatory function. The resulting ischemia prompts further release of vasoactive substances completing a vicious cycle.

It should be appreciated that most patients who present to hospital with an elevated blood pressure are 'chronically hypertensive' with a rightward shift of the pressure/flow (cerebral and renal) autoregulation curve [5]. Furthermore, most patients with severe hypertension (diastolic pressure ≥120 mmHg) have no acute end-organ damage. Rapid antihypertensive therapy in this setting may be associated with significant morbidity.

▌ Clinical Manifestations

The manifestations of hypertensive crises are those of end-organ dysfunction. It is important to recognize that the absolute level of blood pressure may not be as important as the rate of increase. For example, patients with long-standing hypertension may tolerate systolic blood pressures of 200 mmHg or diastolic increases up to 150 mmHg without developing hypertensive encephalopathy, while children or pregnant women may develop encephalopathy with diastolic blood pressures greater than 100 mmHg.

Headache, altered level of consciousness and less severe degrees of CNS dysfunction are the classic manifestations of hypertensive encephalopathy. Advanced retinopathy with arteriolar changes, hemorrhages and exudates, as well as papilledema, are commonly seen on examination of fundi in patients with hypertensive encephalopathy. Cardiovascular manifestations of hypertensive crises may include angina or acute myocardial infarction. Cardiac decompensation may lead to symptoms of dyspnea, orthopnea, cough, fatigue, or frank pulmonary edema. Severe injury to the kidney may lead to renal failure with oliguria and or hematuria.

One syndrome warranting special consideration is aortic dissection. Propagation of the dissection is dependent not only on the elevation of the blood pressure itself, but also on the rate of rise of the pressure waveform of left ventricular ejection. For this reason, specific therapy aimed at both targets (blood pressure and rate of pressure rise) is utilized for these cases (see below).

▌ Initial Evaluation of the Patient with Hypertensive Crises

The key to successful management of patients with severely elevated blood pressure is to differentiate hypertensive crises from hypertensive urgencies. This is accomplished by a targeted medical history and physical examination supported by appropriate laboratory evaluations. Prior hypertensive crises, anti-hypertensive medications prescribed, and blood pressure control should be ascertained. Particular enquiry should include the use of monoamine oxidase inhibitors and recreational drugs (i.e., cocaine, amphetamines, phencyclidine). The blood pressure in all limbs should be measured. In obese patients appropriately sized cuffs should be used. Funduscopic examination is mandatory in all cases to detect the presence of papilledema.

A complete blood count, blood chemistry including electrolytes, blood urea nitrogen (BUN), creatinine as well as a urinalysis should be obtained in all patients presenting with hypertensive crises. A peripheral blood smear should be obtained to detect the presence of a microangiopathic hemolytic anemia. In addition, a chest X-ray, electrocardiogram and head computed tomography (CT) are useful in patients with evidence of shortness of breath, chest pain, or neurological changes respectively. An echocardiogram should be obtained to assess left ventricular function and evidence of ventricular hypertrophy. In many instances, these tests are performed simultaneously with the initiation of antihypertensive therapy.

▌ Therapeutic Approach

Patients with hypertensive emergencies require immediate control of the blood pressure to terminate ongoing end-organ damage, but not to return blood pressure to normal levels. In patients with hypertensive urgencies blood pressure can be lowered gradually over a period of 24 to 48 hours usually with oral medication. The elevated blood pressure in patients with hypertensive emergencies should be treated in a controlled fashion in an intensive care unit (ICU). Intra-arterial blood pressure monitoring is generally useful in patients with hypertensive emergencies.

The use of sublingual nifedipine must be strongly condemned; this agent may result in a precipitous and uncontrolled fall in blood pressure. Given the seriousness of the reported adverse events and the lack of any clinical documentation attesting to a benefit, the use of nifedipine capsules for hypertensive emergencies and 'pseudo-emergencies' should be abandoned [6, 7]. Similarly, intravenous hydralazine may result in severe, prolonged and uncontrolled hypotension and it is, therefore, not recommended. Rapid and uncontrolled reduction of blood pressure may result in cerebral, myocardial, and renal ischemia/infarction.

The immediate goal of intravenous therapy is to reduce the diastolic blood pressure by 10–15% or to about 110 mmHg. In patients with a dissecting aneurysm this goal should be achieved as quickly as possible. In the other patients, this end point should be achieved within 30–60 min. Once the end points of therapy have been reached the patient can be started on oral maintenance therapy.

▌ Pharmacological Management

A growing number of pharmacologic agents are available for management of hypertensive crises. The appropriate therapeutic approach will depend upon the clinical presentation of the patient. However, agents which can be administered intravenously, are rapidly acting, easily titratable, and have a short half-life, are recommended (Table 2).

▌ Anti-Hypertensive Drugs Used in Hypertensive Crises (listed alphabetically)

Clonidine

Clonidine is available as an oral and transdermal formulation. Oral clonidine (0.1 mg PO every 20 min) has been used for the treatment of hypertensive urgencies. The onset of action is within 30 min to 2 hours with a duration of action of 6 to 8 hours. In a randomized, double-blind study, comparing the effects of oral nifedipine versus oral clonidine in 51 patients, clonidine was found to produce a more a gradual decrease in blood pressure than nifedipine. Sedation was observed in those patients taking clonidine. This medication is an excellent choice for those patients in whom rapid control of blood pressure is not required.

Diazoxide

This drug relaxes arteriolar smooth muscle and has been used in the treatment of severe hypertension. When given intravenously, the onset of action is within 1 min with a peak action at 10 min, and a total duration of action ranging from 3 to

Table 2. Dosages of intravenous antihypertensive medications

Drug	Dosage
Diazoxide	Intravenous injection of 1–3 mg/kg to maximum of 150 mg given over 10 to 15 min, may be repeated if inadequate response
Enalaprilat	Intravenous injection of 1.25 mg over 5 min 6 hourly, titrated by increments of 1.25 mg at 12–24 hour intervals to a maximum of 5 mg 6 hourly
Esmolol	Loading dose of 250 to 500 µg/kg over 1 min, followed by an infusion at 25 to 50 µg/kg/min which maybe increased by 25 µg/kg/min every 10 to 20 min until desired response to a maximum of 300 µg/kg/min
Fenoldopam	An initial dose of 0.1 µg/kg/min, titrated by increments of 0.05 to 0.1 µg/kg/min to a maximum of 1.6 µg/kg/min
Labetalol	Initial bolus 20 mg, followed by boluses of 20–80 mg or an infusion starting at 2 mg/min. Maximum cumulative dose of 300 mg over 24 hours
Nicardipine	5 mg/h, titrate to effect by increasing 2.5 mg/h every 5 min to a maximum of 15 mg/h
Nitroprusside	0.5 µg/kg/min, titrate as tolerated to maximum of 2 µg/kg/min.
Phentolamine	1–5 mg boluses. Maximum dose 15 mg
Trimethaphan	0.5–1 mg/min, titrate by increasing by 0.5 mg/min as tolerated. Maximum dose 15 mg/min

18 hours. The dose of administration of diazoxide is a minibolus of 1–3 mg/kg to maximum of 150 mg (single dose) injected over 10 to 15 min. If the response is inadequate, repeated doses at 10–15 min intervals may be given. Diazoxide has significant side effects. Salt and water retention are commonly seen and hyperglycemia and hyperuricemia may also occur.

Enalaprilat

The use of angiotensin-converting enzyme (ACE) inhibitors for the treatment of hypertensive crises has been studied over the last two decades [8, 9]. While sublingual captopril has been used in the treatment of hypertensive crises, enalaprilat, which is available in an intravenous formulation, has gained popularity for use in some hypertensive emergencies. Enalaprilat has an onset of action within 15 min with a duration of action of 12 to 24 hours. No adverse side effects or symptomatic hypotension have been reported with intravenous enalaprilat; however, ACE inhibitors are contraindicated in pregnancy.

Esmolol

Esmolol is a cardioselective, β-adrenergic blocking agent that has an extremely short duration of action. The metabolism of esmolol is via rapid hydrolysis by red blood cells and is not dependent upon renal or hepatic function. The onset of action is within 60 seconds with a duration of action of 10 to 20 min. The pharmacokinetic properties of esmolol, make it the 'ideal β-adrenergic blocker' for use in critically ill patients. This agent is available for intravenous use both as a bolus and as an infusion. It is of particular value for some supraventricular dysrhythmias and recently has been used in patients with hypertensive crises and postoperative hypertension [10, 11]. Esmolol has proven safe in patients with acute myocardial infarction; even those who have relative contraindications to β-blockers [12]. The recommended initial dosage is 0.5–1 mg/kg followed by an infusion of 50–200 µg/kg/min.

Fenoldopam

Fenoldopam is a dopamine agonist (DA1-agonist) that is short acting and has the advantages of increasing renal blood flow and sodium excretion. It represents a new category of antihypertensive medication and is highly specific for only DA1 receptors. Fenoldopam is ten times more potent than dopamine as a renal vasodilator [13].

Fenoldopam activates dopaminergic receptors on the proximal and distal tubules, inhibits sodium reabsorption, and results in diuresis and natriuresis. Fenoldopam is rapidly and extensively metabolized by conjugation in the liver, without participation of cytochrome P-450 enzymes. The onset of action is within 5 minutes, with the maximal response being achieved by 15 min. The duration of action is between 30 to 60 min, with the pressure gradually returning to pretreatment values without rebound once the infusion is stopped. No adverse effects have been reported. The dose rate of fenoldopam must be individualized according to body weight and according to the desired rapidity and extent of the pharmacodynamic effect. An initial starting dose of 0.1 µg/kg/min is recommended.

Fenoldopam has been under clinical investigation since 1981 and has been administered intravenously to more than 1000 patients. In a prospective, randomized, open-label, multicenter clinical trial, Panacek and co-workers compared fenoldopam with nitroprusside in the treatment of acute hypertension concluding that both agents had equivalent efficacy [14]. However, fenoldopam has been demonstrated to improve creatinine clearance, urine flow rates, and sodium excretion in severely hypertensive patients with both normal and impaired renal function, whereas these parameters fall in patients treated with nitroprusside [15–17]. Fenoldopam may therefore be the drug of choice in severely hypertensive patients with impaired renal function [18].

Labetalol

Labetalol is a combined blocker of α- and β-adrenergic receptors. Given intravenously, the α- to β-blocking ratio is 1:7. Labetalol's hypotensive effect begins within 2 to 5 min after an intravenous dose, reaches its peak at 5 to 15 min, and persists for about 2 to 4 hours. Heart rate is maintained or slightly reduced due to the β-blocking effect. Unlike pure β-blockers which decrease cardiac output, labetalol maintains cardiac output [19]. Labetalol reduces peripheral vascular resistance without reducing peripheral blood flow; cerebral, renal and coronary blood flow are maintained [19].

Labetalol has been shown to be effective and safe in the management of hypertensive emergencies, as well as in patients with acute myocardial infarction with systemic hypertension. A loading dose of 20 mg is recommended followed by repeated incremental doses of 20 to 80 mg given at 10 min intervals until the therapeutic goal is achieved. Alternatively, after the initial loading dose, an infusion commencing at 1–2 mg/min and titrated up until the desired hypotensive effect is achieved may be particularly effective. Once the target blood pressure has been achieved oral therapy can be initiated. Large bolus injections of 1 to 2 mg/kg have been reported to produce precipitous falls in blood pressure and should therefore be avoided.

Nicardipine

Nicardipine is a dihydropyridine derivative calcium channel blocker. Nicardipine is one hundred times more water soluble than nifedipine and, therefore, it can be administered intravenously. The onset of action of intravenous nicardipine is between 5 to 15 min with a duration of action of 4 to 6 hours.

Several studies have examined the acute effects of nicardipine when administered to patients with severe hypertension [20, 21]. There have also been several studies published comparing the effects of nicardipine with sodium nitroprusside. Halpern and coauthors conducted a multicenter, prospective, randomized study comparing the effect of this agent with nitroprusside in patients with severe postoperative hypertension [22]. These authors reported nicardipine to be as effective as sodium nitroprusside. Intravenous nicardipine, however, has been shown to reduce both cardiac and cerebral ischemia [23]. Its dosage is independent of the patient's weight. The current recommended dosage for rapid blood pressure control is 5 mg/h increasing the infusion rate by 2.5 mg/h every 5 min (to a maximum of 15 mg/h) until the desired blood pressure reduction is achieved.

Nifedipine

Oral/sublingual therapy with short-acting nifedipine has been widely used in the management of hypertensive emergencies, severe hypertension associated with chronic renal failure, perioperative hypertension, and PIH. Nifedipine is not absorbed through the buccal mucosa, but is rapidly absorbed from the gastrointestinal tract after the capsule is broken/dissolved [7]. Nifedipine causes direct vasodilatation of arterioles reducing peripheral vascular resistance. A significant decrease in blood pressure is observed 5 to 10 min after nifedipine administration, with a peak effect at between 30 to 60 min and a duration of action of about 6 hours [24]. This form of therapy, however, is not 'benign'. Sudden reductions in blood pressure accompanying the administration of nifedipine may precipitate cerebral, renal and myocardial ischemic events which have been associated with fatal outcomes. Elderly hypertensive patients with underlying structural vascular disease and target organ impairment tend to be more vulnerable to the rapid and uncontrolled reduction in arterial pressure. Because the hypotensive effects of nifedipine cannot be closely regulated, this drug *should not be used* for blood pressure control in patients with hypertensive crises.

Nitroprusside

Sodium nitroprusside is an arterial and venous vasodilator that decreases both afterload and preload. When using this agent, cerebral blood flow (CBF) may decrease in a dose-dependent manner. Furthermore, both clinical and experimental studies demonstrate that nitroprusside increases intracranial pressure (ICP).

Nitroprusside is a very potent agent. The onset of action of this drug is within seconds, with a duration of action of 1 to 2 min and a plasma half-life of 3 to

4 min. If the infusion is stopped abruptly, the blood pressure begins to rise immediately and returns to the pre-treatment level within 1 to 10 min. In patients with
coronary artery disease a significant reduction in regional blood flow (coronary
steal) can occur [25]. In a large randomized, placebo-controlled trial, nitroprusside
was shown to increase mortality when infused in the early hours after acute myocardial infarction (mortality at 13 weeks, 24.2 vs. 12.7%) [26].

Sodium nitroprusside is metabolized into cyanogen, which is converted into
thiocyanate by the enzyme thiosulfate sulfurtransferase. Nitroprusside contains
44% cyanide by weight. Cyanide is released non-enzymatically from nitroprusside,
the amount generated being dependent on the dose of nitroprusside administered.
Cyanide is metabolized in the liver to thiocyanate. Thiosulfate is required for this
reaction. Thiocyanate is 100 times less toxic than cyanide. The thiocyanate generated is excreted largely through the kidneys. Cyanide removal, therefore, requires
adequate liver function, adequate renal function and adequate bioavailability of
thiosulfate.

Sodium nitroprusside has been demonstrated to cause cytotoxicity through the
release of nitric oxide (NO), with hydroxyl radical and peroxynitrite generation
leading to lipid peroxidation. Nitroprusside may also cause cytotoxicity due to the
release of cyanide with interference of cellular respiration. Cyanide toxicity has
been documented to result in 'unexplained cardiac arrest', coma, encephalopathy,
convulsions, and irreversible focal neurological abnormalities [27, 28]. The current
methods of monitoring for cyanide toxicity are insensitive. Metabolic acidosis is
usually a preterminal event. In addition, a rise in serum thiocyanate levels is a late
event and not directly related to cyanide toxicity. Red blood cell cyanide concentrations (although not widely available) may be a more reliable method of monitoring
for cyanide toxicity [29]. A red blood cell cyanide concentration above 40 nmol/ml
results in detectable metabolic changes. Levels above 200 nmol/ml are associated
with severe clinical symptoms and levels greater than 400 nmol/ml are considered
lethal [29]. Data suggest that nitroprusside infusion rates in excess of 4 µg/kg/min,
for as little as 2–3 hours, may lead to cyanide levels which are in the toxic range
[29]. The recommended doses of nitroprusside of up to 10 µg/kg/min results in
cyanide formation at a far greater rate than human beings can detoxify.

Considering the potential for severe toxicity with nitroprusside, this drug should
only be used when other intravenous anti-hypertensive agents are not available and
then only in patients with normal renal and hepatic function. The duration of
treatment should be as short as possible and the infusion rate should not exceed
2 µg/kg/min. An infusion of thiosulfate should be used in patients receiving higher
dosages (4–10 µg/kg/min) of nitroprusside [30]. It has also been demonstrated that
hydroxocobalamin (vitamin 12a) is safe and effective in preventing and treating
cyanide toxicity associated with the use of nitroprusside. This may be given as a
continuous infusion at a rate of 25 mg/h. Hydroxocobalamin is unstable and should
be stored dry and protected from light. Cyanocobalamin (B12), however, is ineffective as an antidote and is not capable of preventing cyanide toxicity.

Phentolamine

Phentolamine is an a-adrenergic blocking agent which is frequently used for management of catecholamine-induced hypertensive crises (i.e., pheochromocytoma).
This medication is given intravenously in 1–5 mg boluses. The effect is immediate
and may last up to 15 min. Continuous intravenous infusions have also been used

with variable effects. This agent may cause tachydysrhythmias or angina. Once the initial blood pressure is under control, oral phenoxybenzamine, a long acting α-adrenergic blocking agent, may be given.

Other Agents

Nitroglycerin and hydralazine are sometimes used in the treatment of hypertensive crises and nitroglycerin may play a significant role in those patients with cardiac ischemia. However, it is important to emphasize that nitroglycerin is not an effective vasodilator. Nitroglycerin is a potent venodilator, and only at high doses affects arterial tone. Nitroglycerin reduces blood pressure by reducing preload and cardiac output; undesirable effects in patients with compromised cerebral and renal perfusion. In addition, it requires special tubing for administration.

Hydralazine has been used as an antihypertensive agent for over 40 years. Following an intramuscular or i.v. dose there is an initial latent period of 5 to 15 min followed by a progressive (often precipitous) fall in blood pressure lasting for up to 12 hours. Although the drug's circulating half-life is about 3 hours, the half-time of its effect on blood pressure is about 100 hours. Hydralazine has been demonstrated to bind to the walls of muscular arteries. This may explain the drug's prolonged pharmacologic effect. Because of hydralazine's prolonged and unpredictable anti-hypertensive action and the inability to effectively titrate the drug's hypotensive effect, hydralazine should be avoided in the management of hypertensive emergencies.

Other regimens utilizing medications such as reserpine, methyldopa, or guanethidine have largely been replaced by the agents described above.

▌ Treatment in Special Situations (see Table 3)

Acute Aortic Dissection

The aim of antihypertensive therapy is to lessen the pulsatile load or aortic stress by lowering the blood pressure. Reducing the force of left ventricular contractions and consequently rate of rise of aortic pressure retards the propagation of the dis-

Table 3. Recommended antihypertensive agents for hypertensive crises

Condition	Preferred treatment
▌ Acute pulmonary edema	Nitroprusside or fenoldopam in combination with nitroglycerin (up to 200 µg/min) and a loop diuretic
▌ Acute myocardial ischemia	Labetalol or esmolol in combination with nitroglycerine (up to 200 µg/min). Nicardipine or fenoldopam may be added if pressure is controlled poorly with labetalol/esmolol alone
▌ Hypertensive encephalopathy	Labetalol, nicardipine or fenoldopam
▌ Acute aortic dissection	Labetalol or combination of nitroprusside and esmolol
▌ Eclampsia	Hydralazine (traditional). In the ICU, labetalol or nicardipine are preferred
▌ Acute renal failure/ microangiopathic anemia	Fenoldopam or nicardipine
▌ Sympathetic crisis	Nicardipine, verapamil or fenoldopam

section and aortic rupture. The combination of a vasodilator and a β-blocker is the standard antihypertensive regimen used in these patients; a vasodilator alone may cause an increase in the velocity of ventricular contraction and lead to propagation of dissection. Esmolol is the β-adrenergic antagonist of choice. Metoprolol is a suitable alternative. While sodium nitroprusside has traditionally been used in patients with aortic dissection, nicardipine or fenoldopam are less toxic alternatives. Labetalol, an α- and β-adrenergic antagonist is an alternative to the combination of nitroprusside and β-blocker.

Cardiovascular surgical consultation is required in all patients with suspected aortic dissections. Surgery is indicated for all dissections involving the ascending aorta (type A dissection) with the exception of only a few patients with serious associated conditions contraindicating surgery. Patients with hypotension suggesting aortic rupture are candidates for emergency surgical repair. Complications of type B dissections, such as leakage of blood from the aorta, impairment of blood flow to an organ or limb, or persistent pain despite adequate medical regimen are best treated by surgery. Younger patients with Marfan's syndrome may benefit from surgery in the subacute phase and avoid rupture of a residual saccular aneurysm in the future.

Patients with uncomplicated distal dissections are best managed medically in the acute phase with antihypertensive therapy, as survival rate is around 75% whether patients are treated medically or surgically. Also, these patients are generally in the older age group with a history of cardiac, pulmonary, or renal diseases.

Treatment of Post Cerebrovascular Accident Hypertension

In healthy humans, cerebral autoregulation maintains constant CBF between a mean systemic arterial pressure of 60 and 120 mmHg. However, in patients with chronic hypertension, autoregulation is set at a higher level (approximately 120 to 160 mmHg), presumably to protect the brain from the effects of persistent hypertension [5]. After a stroke, the normal mechanisms of cerebral autoregulation are impaired. Perfusion in the ischemic penumbra becomes pressure dependent. A rise in systemic arterial pressure may be an adaptive response to maintain the blood flow to this vulnerable area. In a series of 334 patients with acute stroke admitted to hospital, Wallace and Levy found that over 80% had elevated blood pressure on the day of admission [31]; the blood pressures fell spontaneously and gradually over the next ten days. By the tenth day post-stroke only one-third of patients remained hypertensive. The mechanisms underlying post-stroke hypertension have not been fully elucidated. Activation of the sympathetic nervous system may be involved as part of a global metabolic response to cerebral infarction, cerebral hemorrhage, or associated edema.

There is no evidence that hypertension has a deleterious effect on the outcome of ischemic strokes during the acute phase [32–34]. Lowering the blood pressure in patients with cerebral ischemia may reduce cerebral blood flow, which, because of impaired autoregulation, may result in further ischemic injury. The common practice of 'normalizing' blood pressure is potentially dangerous. When a proximal arterial obstruction results in a mild stroke, a fall in blood pressure may result in further infarction involving the entire territory of that artery.

The current recommendation of the American Heart Association is that hypertension in the setting of acute ischemic stroke should only be treated "rarely and cautiously" [35, 36]. It is generally recommended that antihypertensive therapy be reserved for patients with a diastolic pressure greater than 120 to 130 mmHg aiming to reduce the pressure by no more than an arbitrary figure of 20% in the first 24 hours.

There are no data regarding the comparative effects of different antihypertensive drugs on CBF in ischemic stroke. In order to prevent a rapid reduction in blood pressure short-acting intravenous agents are preferred. These should be administered in an ICU under close blood pressure monitoring. While nitroprusside is commonly used in this situation, this drug increases ICP and has a very narrow therapeutic index, particularly in patients with renal dysfunction (cyanide poisoning). Labetalol is an effective agent, however, nicardipine or fenoldopam are suitable alternatives. Intravenous or oral ACE inhibitors, oral or sublingual nifedipine and hydralazine should be avoided due to their unpredictable and poorly titratable anti-hypertensive effects.

In patients with intracerebral hematomas there is almost always a secondary rise in ICP and 'reflex systemic hypertension.' Hypertension may serve to protect CBF, because it preserves cerebral perfusion in the face of high ICP. In patients admitted in the first few hours after intracerebral hemorrhage, systolic blood pressure and diastolic blood pressure average approximately 190 mmHg and 100 mmHg respectively. The natural history of this hypertensive response is for the blood pressure to decrease toward habitual levels over 7 to 10 days, with the greatest decline occurring in the first 24 hours. There is no good evidence that hypertension provokes further bleeding in patients with intracranial hemorrhage. However, a precipitous fall in systemic blood pressure will compromise cerebral perfusion. This problem is exacerbated in patients with chronic hypertension whose lower limits of autoregulation are set at higher levels than normotensive patients. Furthermore, the hematoma impairs the responsiveness of autoregulation in the surrounding area of marginal ischemia. However, severe hypertension can lead to worsening vasogenic edema. The current recommendation is that 'cautious' lowering of the blood pressure should be instituted when the systolic blood pressure is greater than 200 mmHg or the diastolic is greater than 110 mmHg [32, 33, 37]. This recommendation is supported by a recent study which demonstrated that rapid decline in blood pressure within the first 24 hours after presentation was associated with increased mortality in patients with intracranial hemorrhage. The rate of decline in blood pressure was independently associated with increased mortality [38]. The effect was independent of other variables known to correlate with outcome after intracranial hemorrhage, including hematoma volume, initial Glasgow Coma Scale (GCS) score and presence of ventricular blood.

Hypertensive Urgencies and Sympathetic Crises

Abrupt discontinuation of a short-acting sympathetic blocker (such as clonidine or propranolol) can lead to severe hypertension. Control of blood pressure can be achieved in this setting by readministration of the discontinued drug. Should evidence of pulmonary edema of coronary ischemia be present the patients should be treated as outlined in Table 3.

In addition to drug withdrawal, increased adrenergic activity can lead to severe hypertension in a variety of other clinical settings. These include the use of sympathomimetic drugs such as cocaine, amphetamines, phencyclidine or the combination of a monoamine oxidase inhibitor and the ingestion of tyramine-containing foods, pheochromocytoma, and autonomic dysfunction as in Gillain-Barré syndrome.

β-blockers should be avoided in these patients, since inhibition of β-receptor induced vasodilation results in unopposed α-adrenergic vasoconstriction and a further rise in blood pressure. β-blockers have been demonstrated to enhance cocaine-induced coronary vasoconstriction, increase blood pressure, fail to control the heart rate, increase the likelihood of seizures, and decrease survival [39, 40]. Although some patients have been treated with labetalol without adverse consequences, controlled experiments in animals and humans do not support its use [41]. In studies of cocaine intoxication in animals, labetalol increased seizure activity and mortality [42]. Furthermore, experimental studies have demonstrated that labetalol does not alleviate cocaine-induced coronary vasoconstriction [43]. Labetalol has been reported to have a hypertensive response in patients with pheochromocytoma. Control of blood pressure in these patients is best achieved with nicardipine, verapamil or fenoldopam. Phentolamine and nitroprusside are alternative agents.

Treatment of Hypertensive Crises in End-Stage Renal Disease

The most important cardiovascular complication of chronic renal failure is hypertension. The cause of hypertension in chronic renal failure is an increase in extracellular volume secondary to sodium retention by the diseased kidney as well as vasoconstriction due to increased activity of the renin-angiotensin system. Hypertensive crises may exacerbate renal failure and, therefore, need to be treated promptly. Intravenous calcium channel blockers have been used for these patients with some success. Patients may require emergent ultrafiltration in order to control the blood pressure. Bilateral nephrectomy has been reported to 'cure' malignant hypertension in hemodialysis patients.

▍ Conclusion

Hypertensive crises are a group of distinct clinico-pathological entities, which require the controlled reduction of the elevated blood pressure to limit end organ damage. This is best achieved in an ICU with the use of titratable intravenous hypotensive agents. Several antihypertensive agents are available including labetalol, fenoldopam, nicardipine and sodium nitroprusside. Understanding of the pathophysiology and the pharmacology will allow the practitioner to prescribe rationale treatment regimens for these patients.

References

1. Calhoun DA, Oparil S (1990) Treatment of hypertensive crisis. N Engl J Med 323:1177–1183
2. Anonymous (1997) The sixth report of the Joint National Committee of Prevention, Detection, Evaluation, and Treatment of High Blood Pressure. Arch Intern Med 157:2413–2446
3. Rey E, LeLorier J, Burgess E, Lange IR, Leduc L (1997) Report of the Canadian Hypertension Society Consensus Conference: 3. Pharmacologic treatment of hypertensive disorders in pregnancy. CMAJ 157:1245–1254
4. Prys-Rroberts C (1984) Anaesthesia and hypertension. Br J Anaesth 56:711–724
5. Strandgaard S, Olesen J, Skinhoj E, Lassen NA (1973) Autoregulation of brain circulation in severe arterial hypertension. Br Med J 1:507–510

6. Haft JI, Litterer WE (1984) Chewing nifedipine to rapidly treat hypertension. Arch Intern Med 144:2357–2359
7. van Harten J, Burggraaf K, Danhof M, van Brummelen P, Breimer DD (1987) Negligible sublingual absorption of nifedipine. Lancet 2:1363–1365
8. Strauss R, Gavras I, Vlahakos D, Gavras H (1986) Enalaprilat in hypertensive emergencies. J Clin Pharmacol 26:39–43
9. Komsuoglu SS, Komsuoglu B, Ozmenoglu M, Ozcan C, Gurhan H (1992) Oral nifedipine in the treatment of hypertensive crises in patients with hypertensive encephalopathy. Int J Cardiol 34:277–282
10. Balser JR, Martinez EA, Winters BD, et al (1998) Beta-adrenergic blockade accelerates conversion of postoperative supraventricular tachyarrhythmias. Anesthesiology 89:1052–1059
11. Platia EV, Michelson EL, Porterfield JK, Das G (1989) Esmolol versus verapamil in the acute treatment of atrial fibrillation or atrial flutter. Am J Cardiol 63:925–929
12. Mooss AN, Hilleman DE, Mohiuddin SM, Hunter CB (1994) Safety of esmolol in patients with acute myocardial infarction treated with thrombolytic therapy who had relative contraindications to β-blocker therapy. Ann Pharmacother 28:701–703
13. Tiberi M, Caron MG (1994) High agonist-independent activity is a distinguishing feature of the dopamine D1B receptor subtype. J Biol Chem 269:27925–27931
14. Panacek EA, Bednarczyk EM, Dunbar LM, Foulke GE, Holcslaw TL (1995) Randomized, prospective trial of fenoldopam vs sodium nitroprusside in the treatment of acute severe hypertension. Fenoldopam Study Group. Acad Emerg Med 2:959–965
15. Shusterman NH, Elliott WJ, White WB (1993) Fenoldopam, but not nitroprusside, improves renal function in severely hypertensive patients with impaired renal function. Am Heart J 95:161–168
16. Elliott WJ, Weber RR, Nelson KS, et al (1990) Renal and hemodynamic effects of intravenous fenoldopam versus nitroprusside in severe hypertension. Circulation 81:970–977
17. White WB, Halley SE (1989) Comparative renal effects of intravenous administration of fenoldopam mesylate and sodium nitroprusside in patients with severe hypertension. Arch Intern Med 149:870–874
18. Reisin E, Huth MM, Nguyen BP, Weed SG, Gonzalez FM (1990) Intravenous fenoldopam versus sodium nitroprusside in patients with severe hypertension. Hypertension 15:I59–I62
19. Pearce CJ, Wallin JD (1994) Labetalol and other agents that block both α- and β-adrenergic receptors. Cleve Clin J Med 61:59–69
20. Clifton GG, Cook ME, Bienvenu GS, Wallin JD (1989) Intravenous nicardipine in severe systemic hypertension. Am J Cardiol 64:16H–18H
21. Clifton GG, Wallin JD (1990) Intravenous nicardipine: an effective new agent for the treatment of severe hypertension. Angiology 41:1005–1009
22. Halpern NA, Sladen RN, Goldberg JS, et al (1990) Nicardipine infusion for postoperative hypertension after surgery of the head and neck. Crit Care Med 18:950–955
23. Schillinger D (1987) Nifedipine in hypertensive emergencies: A prospective study. J Emerg Med 5:463–473
24. Huysmans FT, Sluiter HE, Thien TA, Koene RA (1983) Acute treatment of hypertensive crisis with nifedipine. Br J Clin Pharmacol 16:725–727
25. Mann T, Cohn PF, Holman LB, Green LH, Markis JE, Phillips DA (1978) Effect of nitroprusside on regional myocardial blood flow in coronary artery disease. Results in 25 patients and comparison with nitroglycerin. Circulation 57:732–738
26. Cohn JN, Franciosa JA, Francis GS, et al (1982) Effect of short-term infusion of sodium nitroprusside on mortality rate in acute myocardial infarction complicated by left ventricular failure: results of a Veterans Administration cooperative study. N Engl J Med 306:1129–1135
27. Robin ED, McCauley R (1992) Nitroprusside-related cyanide poisoning. Time (long past due) for urgent, effective interventions. Chest 102:1842–1845
28. Vesey CJ, Cole PV, Simpson PJ (1976) Cyanide and thiocyanate concentrations following sodium nitroprusside infusion in man. Br J Anaesth 48:651–659
29. Pasch T, Schulz V, Hoppenshauser G (1983) Nitroprusside-induced formation of cyanide and its detoxication with thiosulphate during deliberate hypotension. J Cardiovasc Pharmacol 5:77–85

30. Hall VA, Guest JM (1992) Sodium nitroprusside-induced cyanide intoxication and prevention with sodium thiosulphate prophylaxis. Am J Crit Care 2:19–27
31. Wallace JD, Levy LL (1981) Blood pressure after stroke. JAMA 246:2177–2180
32. Lavin P (1986) Management of hypertension in patients with acute stroke. Arch Intern Med 146:66–68
33. O'Connell J, Gray C (1994) Treating hypertension after stroke. Br Med J 308:1523–1524
34. Prisant LM, Carr AA, Hawkins DW (1990) Treating hypertensive emergencies. Controlled reduction of blood pressure and protection of target organs. Postgrad Med 93:92–96
35. Emergency Cardiac Care Committee and Subcommittees, American Heart Association (1992) Guidelines for cardiopulmonary resuscitation and emergency cardiac care. Part IV, special resuscitation situations: stroke. JAMA 268:2242–2244
36. Adams HP, Brott TG, Crowell RM, et al (1994) Guidelines for the management of patients with acute ischemic stroke. A statement for the healthcare professionals from a special writing group of the stroke council, American Heart Association. Circulation 90:1588–1601
37. Hirschl MM (1995) Guidelines for the drug treatment of hypertensive crises. Drugs 50:991–1000
38. Qureshi AI, Bliwise DL, Bliwise NG, Akbar MS, Uzen G, Frankel MR (1999) Rate of 24-hour blood pressure decline and mortality after spontaneous intracerebral hemorrhage: A retrospective analysis with a random effects regression model. Crit Care Med 27:480–485
39. Lange RA, Cigarroa RG, Flores ED, et al (1990) Potentiation of cocaine-induced coronary vasoconstriction by β-adrenergic blockade. Ann Intern Med 112:897–903
40. Pitts WR, Lange RA, Cigarroa JE, Hillis LD (1997) Cocaine-induced myocardial ischemia and infarction: pathophysiology, recognition, and management. Prog Cardiovasc Dis 40:65–76
41. Gay GR, Loper KA (1988) The use of labetalol in the management of cocaine crisis. Ann Emerg Med 17:282–283
42. Catravas JD, Waters IW (1981) Acute cocaine intoxication in the conscious dog: studies on the mechanism of lethality. J Pharmacol Exp Ther 217:350–356
43. Boehrer JD, Moliterno DJ, Willard JE, Hillis LD, Lange RA (1993) Influence of labetalol on cocaine-induced coronary vasoconstriction in humans. Am J Med 94:608–610

Cardiac Arrest in Children

R. Berg

∎ Introduction

Cardiac arrest and cardiopulmonary resuscitation (CPR) in children and adults differ in many ways. Children are anatomically and physiologically different than adults and the underlying etiologies and pathophysiologies of cardiac arrests in children are quite different. In contrast to adults, children rarely suffer sudden ventricular fibrillation (VF) cardiac arrest due to atherosclerotic heart disease. The causes of pediatric arrests are more diverse and are usually secondary to profound hypoxia or asphyxia due to respiratory failure or circulatory shock [1, 2]. Prolonged hypoxia and acidosis impair cardiac function and ultimately lead to cardiac arrest. By the time the arrest occurs, all organs of the body have generally suffered significant hypoxic-ischemic insults [3–5].

Perhaps most different is the devastation that the death of a child wreaks on a family [3]. Coping with a sudden unexpected death is always difficult. When the victim is a child, the loss tends to be even more devastating. Although we know that each life is temporary, we do not expect children to die and are not prepared for it. Even health care providers, who are otherwise able to deal with devastating problems, often become very emotional, and occasionally dysfunctional, when faced with a dying child. The experience for the family is naturally much more intense and long lasting. Children are the family's future. Many families never overcome the grief associated with the premature death of a child.

This chapter addresses various aspects of pediatric basic life support and pediatric advanced life support. In particular, this chapter focuses on the four phases of cardiac arrest and resuscitation, the determinants of myocardial blood flow during CPR, the use of the pulse check as evidence of cardiac arrest, two thumb-encircling hand chest compressions versus two fingers on sternum chest compressions, bystander basic life support with rescue breathing alone vs chest compressions alone vs chest compressions plus rescue breathing for pediatric asphyxial cardiac arrest in the prehospital setting, intraosseous vascular access, vasopressors during CPR, effectiveness of CPR, and the use of mechanical cardiopulmonary support (e.g., extracorporeal membrane oxygenation (ECMO).

∎ The Four Phases of Cardiac Arrest and Resuscitation

It is increasingly clear that there are four distinct phases of cardiac arrest and resuscitation: the pre-arrest phase, the 'no flow' phase of untreated arrest, the 'low flow' phase of CPR, and the post-resuscitation phase (Table 1). The pre-arrest

Table 1. Four phases of cardiac arrest

Phase	Appropriate Intervention
▌Prearrest	Prevention
▌'No flow' – untreated arrest	Prompt CPR±defibrillation
▌Low flow – CPR	'Push hard, Push fast'
	Minimize interruptions
	Epinephrine IV prn
▌Post-resuscitation	Hemodynamic support
	Hemodynamic monitoring
	?Hypothermia

CPR: cardiopulmonary resuscitation; IV: intravenous; prn: as required

phase includes the premorbid state (preexisting acute and chronic diseases) and the acute pathophysiologic process resulting in cardiac arrest. The treatment and outcome of an adolescent with a witnessed drug-induced VF in the intensive care unit (ICU) is quite different from that of an infant in cardiac arrest after a severe traumatic injury. Animal models clearly demonstrate that successful resuscitation from cardiac arrest depends on the duration of the cardiac arrest before CPR is provided (duration of 'no flow'), duration of CPR (duration of 'low flow'), the ability to establish adequate myocardial and cerebral blood flow (CBF) with CPR (quality of 'low flow'), and early defibrillation in the case of VF [1, 3]. For asphyxial cardiac arrests, the duration of untreated asphyxia and early re-establishment of adequate oxygenation and ventilation are also quite important [4, 5]. Ventricular arrhythmias immediately post-resuscitation, and post-resuscitation myocardial dysfunction, are substantial contributors to poor outcomes [1, 6, 7].

Disturbingly, bystander CPR is only provided to 30% or less of prehospital pediatric cardiac arrest victims in most studies [1, 2]. Basic life support is often poorly performed in hospital as well as prehospital settings [1, 9, 10]. Moreover, interruptions in chest compressions are common (e.g., for tracheal intubation, transportation to the ambulance, attainment of vascular access), resulting in substantial further hemodynamic compromise [11]. Conversely, post-resuscitation inotropic support is commonly provided in pediatric ICUs [6].

▌ Determinants of Myocardial Blood Flow During CPR

The primary determinants of myocardial blood flow during CPR are: adequate preload, quality of chest compressions, and peripheral vascular tone (Table 2). Although preload is generally adequate in the pre-arrest phase for adults in VF or children with asphyxial arrests, children in cardiac arrest after acute traumatic injuries or septic shock often have inadequate preload. Not surprisingly, these children have a poor initial successful resuscitation rate and are rarely long-term survivors [1, 2, 12, 13]. The quality of compressions is generally described by depth of compressions and rate of compressions. In infants and children the sternum should generally be compressed ∼1/3 of the antero-posterior diameter of the chest, and the compression rate should be at least 100/minute. For the patient with indwelling arterial and central venous catheters, the goal is to attain an adequate coronary

Table 2. Determinants of myocardial blood flow during cardiopulmonary resuscitation

▌Adequate preload
▌Quality of chest compressions
  – Adequate depth and rate
  – Minimize interruptions
▌Adequate peripheral vascular tone

perfusion pressure (e.g., an aortic relaxation pressure minus right atrial relaxation pressure greater than 20–30 mmHg). For the child without vascular pressure monitoring, adequate compressions generally result in palpable femoral pulses. As noted above, compelling animal data suggest that interrupting chest compressions adversely affects CPR hemodynamics promptly and substantially [11]. Therefore, 'push hard, push fast', and minimize interruptions. When CPR is initiated, plasma concentrations of epinephrine, norepinephrine, and vasopressin are quite high, and autonomic tone promotes vasoconstriction. However, peripheral vascular tone decreases during CPR (and is lower after longer duration of untreated cardiac arrest), so vasoconstricting agents such as epinephrine or vasopressin may be needed to attain adequate coronary perfusion pressure.

▌ Pulse Check

The pulse check has been the 'gold standard' for evaluating the presence or absence of circulation. Traditionally, the American Heart Association has recommended the pulse check to identify pulseless patients in cardiac arrest who require chest compression. The carotid artery is generally palpated for the pulse check in adults and children, and brachial artery in infants [1]. The short, chubby neck of children under 1 year of age makes rapid location of the carotid artery difficult. In addition, one may compress the airway in attempting to palpate a carotid pulse in the neck of the infant [1, 14]. If the rescuer fails to detect a pulse within 5–10 seconds in an unresponsive non-breathing victim, cardiac arrest is presumed to be present and chest compressions are initiated.

Unfortunately, the pulse check is neither rapid nor reliable for detecting the presence or absence of circulation, based on adult manikin simulation, unconscious adult patients undergoing cardiopulmonary bypass, unconscious mechanically ventilated adult patients, and conscious adult 'test persons' [1, 15]. The most comprehensive study, performed by Eberle and colleagues, evaluated the ability of prehospital medical personnel to palpate a carotid pulse in an unconscious adult patient before and after placement on cardiopulmonary bypass (i.e., with and without pulsatile blood flow) [15]. When the pulse was truly absent, rescuers assessed the pulse as being present in about 10% of cases. When the pulse was truly present, the rescuers assessed the pulse as being absent in about 40% of cases. The pulse check is neither a sensitive nor specific indicator of true pulselessness.

Clearly, palpating a pulse in infants and children is a greater challenge than palpating the carotid pulse in an adult. Several studies have documented the inability of many lay rescuers to reliably find and count a pulse in healthy infants [1, 14, 16]. Although data are lacking regarding the pulse check in pulseless children, the sensitivity and specificity are surely worse in infants and small children than in adults.

Therefore, if a child has no signs of circulation (normal breathing, coughing, or movement), a layperson should assume cardiac arrest and provide chest compressions immediately. Although it is reasonable for the more skilled medical professional to attempt a pulse check, after 10 seconds of lifelessness and no palpable pulse, the healthcare professional should perform chest compressions rather than extending the attempts to palpate a pulse.

▌ Chest Compressions: Two Thumb-encircling Hand vs Two Finger on Sternum

Two chest compression techniques have been recommended for newborns and infants: the two finger sternal compression technique, and the two thumbs-encircling hand technique. There are three published human studies, a cadaver study and two case reports, suggesting that the two thumbs-encircling hand technique results in higher systolic blood pressures [1]. These data have been corroborated in swine models and mechanical models of CPR, and extended by demonstration of improved coronary perfusion pressures and fewer 'shallow' compressions with the two thumb-encircling hands technique. In addition, healthcare providers prefer the two thumb-encircling hands technique. Interestingly, there is not a single published report demonstrating an advantage to the two finger on the sternum technique. The dearth of data on all of these issues is humbling. For single rescuers, the two finger on the sternum technique may be easier to perform while providing rescue breathing.

▌ Bystander Basic Life Support for Pediatric Asphyxial Cardiac Arrest

Bystander CPR improves outcome of children in cardiac arrest [1, 4, 17–19]. Successful resuscitation techniques have included mouth-to-mouth rescue breathing alone, chest compressions alone, and chest compressions plus mouth-to-mouth rescue breathing. Interestingly, in Kouwenhoven's original description of closed chest cardiac massage, 17 of the 20 patients did not have VF, and 7 of the 20 did not receive any ventilatory support (no rescue breathing) [19]. Several of the patients were children, all 20 were initially successfully resuscitated and 14/20 survived to hospital discharge.

Because of the difficulties inherent in attempting to study bystander CPR prior to the arrival of medical personnel, we addressed the roles of chest compressions and rescue breathing for bystander CPR in two swine models of pediatric asphyxial cardiac arrests [4, 5]. In the first model, the endotracheal tube of these piglets was clamped until loss of aortic pulsations; the mean time until loss of aortic pulsations was 9 minutes. Most of the animals (7/10) provided with chest compressions and rescue breathing for 8 minutes of 'bystander CPR' were normal 24 hours later versus only 1/14 treated with chest compressions only, 1/7 treated with rescue breathing only, and 0/8 receiving no bystander CPR during these 8 minutes prior to simulated emergency medical service arrival. This study clearly delineates the crucial importance of combined chest compressions and rescue breathing for successful resuscitation from an asphyxial cardiac arrest [4].

However, at an earlier stage of the asphyxial process, chest compressions and rescue breathing each independently improved outcome from an asphyxial, pulseless, apparent cardiac arrest [5]. In the latter experiment, the endotracheal tube was clamped until the aortic systolic blood pressure was <50 mmHg (simulating a 'pulseless' child), and simulated bystander CPR was again provided for 8 minutes until simulated emergency medical revival service arrival. The mean time until simulated pulselessness was 7 minutes. Twenty-four-hour survival was attained in 8/10 animals provided with chest compressions and rescue breathing, 5/10 animals with chest compressions only, 6/10 animals with rescue breathing only, and 0/10 animals with no bystander CPR. Outcomes were statistically superior in all three experimental groups compared to the control group. Nearly all of the surviving animals in both experiments attained return of spontaneous circulation during the first minutes of simulated bystander CPR (i.e., prior to simulated emergency medical service arrival). These findings support the recommendation that bystander CPR with chest compressions and rescue breathing is the treatment of choice for asphyxial cardiac arrest, but either alone is better than no resuscitation attempt [1].

Since oxygenation and ventilation are clearly important for survival from fibrillatory cardiac arrest, why is rescue breathing not necessary in VF models, yet quite important in the asphyxial models [20–24]? Immediately after an acute fibrillatory cardiac arrest, aortic oxygen and carbon dioxide concentrations do not vary from the pre-arrest state because there is no blood flow and aortic oxygen consumption is minimal. Therefore, when chest compressions are initiated, the blood flowing from the aorta to the coronary circulation provides adequate oxygenation at an acceptable pH. At that time, myocardial oxygen delivery is limited more by blood flow than oxygen content. Over the next several minutes, arterial oxygenation and pH become increasingly important for effective resuscitation. Adequate oxygenation and ventilation can continue without rescue breathing because of chest compression-induced gas exchange and spontaneous gasping ventilation during CPR [21–23]. Rescue breathing is not necessary in the VF arrests because arterial oxygenation and pH can be adequate with chest compressions alone. Most importantly, because interrupting chest compressions for rescue breathing during CPR adversely effects myocardial blood flow, myocardial oxygen delivery does not differ whether rescue breathing is provided or not (i.e., the improvement in arterial oxygen saturation with rescue breathing is counterbalanced by the worse myocardial perfusion during CPR for VF) [11, 22, 23].

During the asphyxia experiments, oxygen consumption and carbon dioxide and lactate production continued for many minutes after endotracheal tube clamping prior to 'pulselessness' or cardiac arrest. In addition, continued pulmonary blood flow after endotracheal tube clamping presumably depleted the pulmonary oxygen reservoir. Therefore, asphyxia resulted in severe arterial hypoxemia and acidemia prior to resuscitation, in contrast to VF [4, 5].

The outcomes in these swine experiments are consistent with epidemiologic studies of prehospital CPR for apneic, unresponsive, pulseless children. 'Bystander' CPR improves outcome, and many of the long-term survivors are successfully resuscitated by the bystanders before the paramedics arrive [1, 4, 5, 18, 19]. Moreover, some apneic, apparently pulseless children are probably not in cardiac arrest. Such children may be at an earlier point in the asphyxial process. They may have some blood pressure and perfusion despite the bystander's inability to appreciate a pulse [1, 5, 12, 13]. If so, rescue breathing alone or chest compressions alone may be adequate for successful resuscitation [5].

In conclusion, the optimal treatment for a pediatric asphyxial cardiac arrest is prompt and effective rescue breathing and chest compressions. However, chest compressions alone or rescue breathing alone are better than nothing, especially early in the asphyxial process. The importance of the latter issue is magnified by the fact that only 30% of children suffering a cardiac arrest in the prehospital setting receive any form of bystander CPR [2]. We must encourage rescuers, lay and healthcare provider alike, to provide CPR promptly. The public needs to know that: 'Something is better than nothing'.

▌ Intraosseous Vascular Access

In infants and children requiring emergent vascular access during CPR, intraosseous vascular access should be promptly established if reliable venous access cannot be achieved rapidly [1, 25, 26]. Because of the difficulty establishing vascular access in pediatric cardiac arrest victims, it may be preferable to attempt intraosseous access immediately. A practical approach is to pursue intraosseous access and peripheral or central venous access simultaneously.

Intraosseous vascular access provides access to a non-collapsible marrow venous plexus, which serves as a rapid, safe, and reliable route for administration of drugs, crystalloids, colloids, and blood during resuscitation [1, 25–27]. Intraosseous vascular access often can be achieved in 30 to 60 seconds [25]. Although a styleted specially designed intraosseous or Jamshidi-type bone marrow needle is preferred to prevent obstruction of the needle with cortical bone, butterfly needles and standard hypodermic needles have been successfully used. The intraosseous needle is typically inserted into the anterior tibial bone marrow; alternative sites include the distal femur, medial malleolus or the anterior superior iliac spine, and the distal tibia. This vascular access technique can be used in all age groups, from preterm neonates through adulthood; however, it is most commonly used for infants and toddlers [1].

The needle should be twisted into, rather than shoved through, the bone marrow. Evidence for successful entry into the bone marrow includes:
▌ the sudden decrease in resistance after the needle passes through the bony cortex,
▌ the needle remains upright without support,
▌ aspiration of the bone marrow into a syringe (this is not consistently achieved), and
▌ the fluid infuses freely without evidence of subcutaneous infiltration [27].

Resuscitation drugs, fluids, and blood products can be safely administered by the intraosseous route [1]. Continuous catecholamine infusions can also be provided by the intraosseous route [27]. Onset of action and drug levels following intraosseous infusion during CPR are comparable to those achieved following vascular administration, including central venous administration. Intraosseous vascular access may also be used to obtain blood specimens for chemistry, blood gas analysis, and type and crossmatch, although administration of sodium bicarbonate through the intraosseous cannula eliminates the close correlation with mixed venous blood gases [1].

Complications have been reported in fewer than 1% of patients following intraosseous infusion. Complications include tibial fracture, lower extremity compartment syndrome, severe extravasation of drugs, and osteomyelitis [1]. Most of these complications may be avoided by careful technique.

▌ Vasopressors During Cardiac Arrest: Epinephrine

Landmark animal studies by Redding and Pearson in the 1960s established that 1 mg epinephrine improved outcome from both asphyxial and VF cardiac arrest [28, 29]. Subsequent investigations have established that epinephrine improves myocardial and cerebral hemodynamics during CPR primarily due to the α adrenergic effects. Vasoconstriction results in higher aortic diastolic pressure, thereby improving myocardial perfusion pressure and myocardial blood flow. In addition, vasoconstriction in the extracerebral carotid arterial distribution redirects most of the carotid blood flow into the cerebral circulation [1]. In controlled animal studies, epinephrine administration during CPR improves resuscitation rates and survival [29, 30]. Human data demonstrating an outcome improvement with epinephrine administration are lacking.

A series of animal and human investigations from the mid-1980s through the mid-1990s established that coronary and cerebral perfusion during CPR improves further with 10-fold-higher doses of epinephrine. These studies, and uncontrolled clinical observations, led may clinicians to consider high-dose epinephrine as a major breakthrough for treatment of cardiac arrest. In particular, high-dose epinephrine (0.2 mg/kg) appeared to be life-saving in a prospective study of pediatric cardiac arrest [31]. The high-dose epinephrine was administered to 20 pediatric cardiac arrest victims who had failed to respond to two standard 0.01 mg/kg doses of epinephrine. Twelve children had return of spontaneous circulation and eight children survived to hospital discharge. All 20 historical controls who had failed to respond to two standard epinephrine doses ultimately could not be resuscitated. Nevertheless, eight prospective, randomized, controlled studies in adults consistently showed no improvement in survival to hospital discharge [1]. The initial enthusiasm for high dose epinephrine was replaced by disappointment.

Four retrospective pediatric studies have also addressed this epinephrine dosage issue [32–35]. High-dose epinephrine did not improve initial successful resuscitation rates or survival. Furthermore, a collective review of 44 pediatric cardiac arrest studies over 27 years, including over 3 000 arrests, failed to show any benefit, or harm, to high-dose epinephrine [2].

Other studies suggest that high-dose epinephrine can have toxic effects. Animal studies established that high-dose epinephrine can lead to a toxic hyperadrenergic state immediately after resuscitation with atrial and ventricular tachyarrhythmias and severe hypertension [7, 36–38]. Moreover, in animal and human studies higher epinephrine dosage has been associated with worse post-resuscitation myocardial function [38, 39].

A recent adult study suggests that higher epinephrine dosage results in worse neurological outcome [40]. This retrospective cohort study evaluated neurological outcome up to 6 months after resuscitation from VF cardiac arrest. The total amount of epinephrine was much higher in the patients with poor neurological function. As expected, poor neurological function correlated with longer duration of untreated cardiac arrest (no flow) and longer interval of CPR (low flow). However, even after controlling for duration of arrest and other confounding factors, higher epinephrine dosage was associated with worse neurologic outcome.

Vasopressin is another vasoconstrictor with great promise as an agent to improve myocardial and cerebral blood flow during CPR [1]. Because there is substantial animal data and limited adult data indicating that vasopressin is an effective vasopressor during CPR for VF (perhaps superior to epinephrine), vasopressin is now recommended as an alternative vasopressor for adults during CPR for VF. However, there are inadequate data regarding vasopressin usage during CPR in children [1].

In summary, high-dose epinephrine for the initial dose is not supported by pediatric data or extrapolated data from adults or animals. The recommended dose is 0.1 ml/kg of 1:10000 or 0.01 mg/kg. The scanty dosage data regarding rescue therapy with high-dose epinephrine in patients that fail to respond to a standard dose result in less secure recommendations. For second and subsequent doses in refractory pediatric cardiac arrest, high-dose epinephrine (0.1 ml/kg of 1:1000 or 0.1 mg/kg) is not recommended as the treatment of choice, but is considered an acceptable alternative to standard-dose [1].

Consideration of higher doses of epinephrine in individual patients is reasonable, based in part on the observation of great interpatient variability regarding catecholamine pharmacokinetics and hemodynamic response, both in the non-arrest state and during cardiac arrest [1, 41]. If the patient has continuous intra-arterial pressure monitoring during CPR, subsequent epinephrine doses can be titrated to effect. For example, continued standard epinephrine doses are rational if the aortic diastolic pressure is greater than approximately 25–35 mmHg (or coronary perfusion pressure, aortic relaxation minus right atrial relaxation pressure, is greater than 20–30 mmHg), whereas higher epinephrine doses are rational if the pressure is low. The rationale for this approach is that the benefits from epinephrine are derived from improvements in the coronary perfusion pressure. Once coronary perfusion is adequate, increases in epinephrine dosage are more likely to incur adverse effects than add any benefit. Perhaps, the clinician's dilemma is: a dangerous dose for one individual may be life-saving for another.

∎ Endotracheal Epinephrine

Although case reports indicate that endotracheal epinephrine can be life-saving, data from animals and adults indicate that absorption of epinephrine via this route is poor and unreliable. The recommended tracheal dose of epinephrine during pediatric resuscitation is 10 times the dose given via an intravascular route. After attainment of vascular access, if the patient remains in cardiac arrest, intravenous epinephrine should be administered immediately without regard to previous endotracheal epinephrine dosage. The absorption and bioavailability of the endotracheal dose is simply unreliable [1].

∎ Is CPR in Children Effective?

Outcomes from CPR in children are generally quite poor, suggesting that CPR is ineffective. The animal studies noted above indicate that simulated bystander CPR can be quite effective [4, 5]. Prehospital pediatric studies demonstrate very poor outcomes for children who continue to be in cardiac arrest when professionals arrive at the scene, yet excellent outcomes after bystander CPR when the child has had return of spontaneous circulation prior to arrival of the health care professionals [1, 2, 17, 18]. For example, Sirbaugh and colleagues observed a dismal outcome of only six survivors among 300 children who were in cardiac arrest when the prehospital emergency medical personnel arrived [18]. In contrast, all 41 chil-

Table 3. In-hospital pediatric cardiopulmonary resuscitation (CPR) outcomes

	n	ROSC	24-hour Survival	1-year Survival	Good neuro outcome*
Reis (Brazil) [12]	129	64%	33%	15%	83%
Suominem (Finland) [42]	118	63%	37%	18%	–
Torres (Arkansas) [13]	92	–	36%	10%	78%
Parra (Miami) [43]	32	63%	–	34%	72%

ROSC, return of spontaneous circulation

* Good Neuro Outcome indicates 'normal' or no change from pre-CPR status at 6 months or 1 year

dren who attained return of spontaneous circulation from bystander CPR before arrival of prehospital medical personnel were long-term survivors. Although it is possible that some of these children did not need CPR, most of them were initially quite obtunded and many had documented severe metabolic acidosis upon arrival in the emergency department [Pepe, personal communication].

Several well-designed, in-hospital, pediatric CPR investigations with long-term follow-up have established that pediatric CPR and advanced life support can be remarkably effective (Table 3) [12, 13, 42, 43]. Nearly 2/3 of these patients were initially successfully resuscitated (i.e., attained sustained return of spontaneous circulation). Survival progressively decreased with time, in large part due to the underlying disease processes. Most of these arrests/events occurred in pediatric ICUs due to progressive life-threatening illnesses that had not responded to treatment. The 1-year survival rates of 10–34% are superior to outcomes from out-of-hospital pediatric CPR, and substantially superior to the certain 0% survival rate if CPR and advanced life support were not provided. Most importantly, the vast majority of the survivors had good neurological outcomes (i.e., normal or no demonstrable change in neurological status compared to pre-arrest).

In summary, CPR is a remarkably effective intervention; most children in these studies were immediately 'brought back to life'. However, CPR is only a 'bridge' to provide adequate tissue perfusion until return of spontaneous circulation is possible. It is quite impressive that so many of these children were ultimately long-term survivors with such limited neurological residua.

▌ ECMO During CPR

In some patients, CPR cannot 'bridge' the gap to return of spontaneous circulation. There are several published studies with extraordinary results after various mechanical cardiopulmonary support systems (e.g., ECMO) as a rescue therapy for pediatric cardiac arrests, especially in the settings of potentially reversible acute postoperative myocardial dysfunction or arrhythmias [43–45]. In one study, 11 children who suffered cardiac arrest in the pediatric ICU after cardiac surgery were placed on ECMO during CPR after 20–110 minutes of CPR [44]. Prolonged CPR was continued until ECMO cannulae, circuits, and personnel were available. Six of these 11 children were long-term survivors without apparent neurological sequelae. More recently, two centers have reported an additional remarkable eight pediatric cardiac patients provided with mechanical cardiopulmonary support during CPR within 20 minutes of the initiation of CPR [43, 45]. All eight children survived to hospital discharge.

CPR and ECMO are not curative treatments. They are simply cardiopulmonary supportive measures that may allow tissue perfusion and viability until recovery from the precipitating disease process. As such, they can be powerful tools.

▌ Conclusion

Children are not little adults. They are physiologically and anatomically different, and the causes of sudden death are different from adults. Nevertheless, the four phases of cardiac arrest and resuscitation also pertain to pediatric arrests: pre-arrest, 'no flow', 'low flow', and postresuscitation. In addition, the main determinants of myocardial blood flow during CPR are preload, quality of compressions, and peripheral vascular tone. The pulse check lacks specificity and sensitivity in adults, and is even more problematic in infants and young children. The two thumb-encircling hand chest compression technique appears to be superior to the two finger sternal technique for infants. Prompt provision of rescue breathing and chest compressions is optimal for pediatric bystander CPR, but early in the asphyxial process 'something is better than nothing'. Immediate attempts at intraosseous vascular access are recommended for children in cardiac arrest without prior vascular access. Intravenous standard-dose epinephrine (0.1 ml/kg 1:10 000 dilution or 0.01 mg/kg) is still the vasopressor treatment of choice for first, and subsequent, vasopressor boluses during pediatric cardiac arrest. Pediatric CPR is remarkably effective in restoring spontaneous circulation when provided promptly; however, long-term survival is limited by the underlying disease processes. Finally, ECMO can be a life-saving rescue therapy from intractable cardiac arrest if the underlying disorder is reversible.

References

1. Subcommittee on Pediatric Resuscitation AHA (2000) Guidelines for cardiopulmonary resuscitation and emergency cardiac care, Pediatric advanced life support and pediatric basic life support. Circulation 102:I291–342
2. Young KD, Seidel JS (1999) Pediatric cardiopulmonary resuscitation: a collective review. Ann Emerg Med 33:195–205
3. Berg RA, Goetting MG (1996) Pediatric sudden death. Paradis NA, Halperin HR, Nowak, RM (eds) Cardiac Arrest: the Science and Practice of Resuscitation Medicine. Williams and Willcins, Baltimore, pp 671–694
4. Berg R, Hilwig R, Kern K, Babar I, Ewy GA (1999) Simulated mouth-to-mouth ventilation and chest compression improves outcome in a swine model of prehospital pediatric asphyxial cardiac arrest. Crit Care Med 27:1893–1899
5. Berg RA, Hilwig RW, Kern KB, Ewy GA (2000) 'Bystander' chest compressions and assisted ventilation independently improve outcome from piglet asphyxial pulseless 'cardiac arrest'. Circulation 101:1743–1748
6. Lucking SE, Pollack MM, Fields AI (1986) Shock following generalized hypoxic-ischemic injury in previously healthy infants and children. J Pediatr 108:359–364
7. Berg RA, Otto CW, Kern KB, et al (1994) High-dose epinephrine results in greater early mortality after resuscitation from prolonged cardiac arrest in pigs: a prospective, randomized study. Crit Care Med 22:282–290
8. Kern KB, Hilwig RW, Berg RA, et al (1997) Postresuscitation left ventricular systolic and diastolic dysfunction: treatment with dobutamine. Circulation 95:2610–2613
9. Berg RA, Sanders AB, Milander MM (1994) Efficacy of audio-prompted rate guidance in improving resuscitator performance on children. Acad Emerg Med 1:35–40

10. Kern KB, Sanders AB, Raife J, Milander MM (1992) A study of chest compression rates during cardiopulmonary resuscitation in humans: importance of rate-directed chest compressions. Arch Intern Med 152:145–149

11. Berg RA, Sanders AB, Kern KB, et al (2001) Adverse hemodynamic effects of interrupting chest compressions for rescue breathing during cardiopulmonary resuscitation for ventricular fibrillation cardiac arrest. Circulation 104:2465–2470

12. Rcis AG, Nadkarni V, Perondi MB, et al (2002) A prospective investigation into the epidemiology of in-hospital pediatric cardiopulmonary resuscitation using the International Utstein Reporting Style. Pediatrics (in press)

13. Torres Jr A, Pickert CB, Firestone J, et al (1997) Long-term functional outcome of inpatient pediatric cardiopulmonary resuscitation. Pediatr Emerg Care 13:369–373

14. Whitelaw CC, Goldsmith LJ (1997) Comparison of two techniques for determining the presence of a pulse in an infant. Acad Emerg Med 4:153–154

15. Eberle B, Dick WF, Schneider T, Wisser G, Doetsch S, Tzanova I (1996) Checking the carotid pulse: Diagnostic accuracy of first responders in patients with and without a pulse. Resuscitation 33:107–116

16. Cavallaro DL, Melker RJ (1983) Comparison of two techniques for detecting cardiac activity in infants. Crit Care Med 11:189–190

17. Sirbaugh PE, Pepe PE, Shook JE, et al (1999) A prospective, population-based study of the demographics, epidemiology, management, and outcome of out-of-hospital pediatric cardiopulmonary arrest. Ann Emerg Med 33:174–184

18. Hickey RW, Cohen DM, Strausbaugh S, Dietrich AM (1995) Pediatric patients requiring CPR in the prehospital setting. Ann Emerg Med 25:495–501

19. Kouwenhoven WB, Jude JR, Knickerbocker GG (1960) Closed-chest cardiac massage. JAMA 173:94–97

20. Berg RA, Kern KB, Sanders AB, Otto CW, Hilwig RW, Ewy GA (1993) Bystander cardiopulmonary resuscitation. Is ventilation necessary? Circulation 88:1907–1915

21. Berg RA, Wilcoxson D, Hilwig RW, et al (1995) The need for ventilatory support during bystander CPR. Ann Emerg Med 26:342–50

22. Berg RA, Kern KB, Hilwig RW, et al (1997) Assisted ventilation does not improve outcome in a porcine model of single-rescuer bystander cardiopulmonary resuscitation. Circulation 95:1635–1641

23. Becker LB, Berg RA, Pepe PE, et al (1997) A reappraisal of mouth-to-mouth ventilation during bystander-initiated cardiopulmonary resuscitation. Circulation 96:2102–2112

24. Hallstrom A, Cobb L, Johnson E, Copass M (2000) Cardiopulmonary resuscitation by chest compression alone or with mouth-to-mouth ventilation. N Engl J Med 342:1599–601

25. Glaeser P, Losek J, Nelson D, et al (1988) Pediatric intraosseous infusions: impact on vascular access time. Am J Emerg Med 6:330–332

26. Kanter RK, Zimmerman JJ, Strauss RH, Stoeckel KA (1986) Pediatric emergency intravenous access: evaluation of a protocol. Am J Dis Child 140:132–134

27. Berg R (1984) Emergency infusion of catecholamines into bone marrow. Am J Dis Child 138:810–811

28. Redding JS, Pearson JW (1963) Evaluation of drugs for cardiac resuscitation. Anesth 24:203–207

29. Pearson JW, Redding JS (1965) Peripheral vascular tone in cardiac resuscitation. Anesth Analg 44:746–752

30. Sanders AB, Ewy GA, Taft TV (1984) The prognostic and therapeutic importance of the aortic diastolic pressure in resuscitation from cardiac arrest. Crit Care Med 12:871–873

31. Goetting MG, Paradis NA (1991) High-dose epinephrine improves outcome from pediatric cardiac arrest. Ann Emerg Med 20:22–26

32. Kuisma M, Suominen P, Korpela R (1995) Paediatric out-of-hospital cardiac arrests: epidemiology and outcome. Resuscitation 30:141–150

33. Carpenter TC, Stenmark KR (1997) High-dose epinephrine is not superior to standard-dose epinephrine in pediatric in-hospital cardiopulmonary arrest. Pediatrics 99:403–408

34. Dieckmann RA, Vardis R (1995) High-dose epinephrine in pediatric out-of-hospital cardiopulmonary arrest. Pediatrics 95:901–913

35. Ronco R, King W, Donley DK, Tilden SJ (1995) Outcome and cost at a children's hospital following resuscitation for out-of-hospital cardiopulmonary arrest. Arch Pediatr Adolescent Med 149:210–214

36. Berg RA, Otto CW, Kern KB, et al (1996) A randomized, blinded trial of high-dose epinephrine versus standard-dose epinephrine in a swine model of pediatric asphyxial cardiac arrest. Crit Care Med 24:1695–1700

37. Hörnchen U, Christoph L, Schüttler J (1993) Potential risks of high-dose epinephrine for resuscitation from ventricular fibrillation in a porcine model. J Cardiothorac Vasc Anesth 7:184–187

38. Rivers EP, Wortsman J, Rady MY, Blake HC, McGeorge FT, Buderer NM (1994) The effect of the total cumulative epinephrine dose administered during human CPR on hemodynamic, oxygen transport, and utilization variables in the postresuscitation period. Chest 106:1499–1507

39. Tang W, Weil MH, Sun S, et al (1995) Epinephrine increases the severity of postresuscitation myocardial dysfunction. Circulation 92:3089–3093

40. Behringer W, Kittler H, Sterz F, et al (1998) Cumulative epinephrine dose during cardiopulmonary resuscitation and neurologic outcome. Ann Intern Med 129:450–456

41. Berg RA, Donnerstein RL, Padbury JF (1993) Dobutamine infusions in stable, critically ill children: pharmacokinetics and hemodynamic actions. Crit Care Med 21:678–686

42. Suominem P, Olkkola KT, Voipio V, et al (2000) Utstein style of reporting in-hospital paediatric cardiopulmonary resuscitation. Resuscitation 45:17–25

43. Parra DA, Bala R, Totapally BR, et al (2000) Outcome of cardiopulmonary resuscitation in a pediatric cardiac intensive care unit. Crit Care Med 28:3296–3300

44. del Nido P, Dalton HJ, Thompson AE (1992) Extracorporeal membrane oxygenator rescue in children during cardiac arrest after cardiac surgery. Circulation 86:300–304

45. Dalton HJ, Siewers RD, Fuhrman BP, et al (1993) Extracorporeal membrane oxygenation for cardiac rescue in children with severe myocardial dysfunction. Crit Care Med 21:1020–1028

The Etiology of Obstetric Critical Illness

B. J. Williams and S. J. Brett

▌ Introduction

With the increasing rarity of maternal death in the developed World, the use of mortality figures to assess the quality of obstetric care has become inadequate. This difficulty has been exacerbated by the disparity between the recorded causes of maternal death and of severe maternal illness, as recorded by intensive care unit (ICU) admission.

As mortality rates improve, attention is switching to morbidity, and as a marker of this, obstetric admissions to the ICU have been scrutinized. It had been hoped that by the early identification of risk factors for severe illness, the likelihood of an unfavorable outcome for both mother and child could be reduced by appropriate intervention. However, it is possible that the reduction in maternal mortality and morbidity rates achieved for much of the last century may have plateaued; changing maternal demographics and the general health of the population may reverse some of these improvements. The admission of new and expectant mothers to intensive or high dependency facilities may become a more frequent occurrence.

▌ Mortality Data

The United Kingdom (UK) Confidential Enquiry into Maternal Deaths (CEMD), is widely regarded as the 'gold standard' of maternal mortality reporting worldwide, and provides a complete record of mortality data from the beginning of the first enquiry in 1952. Reports are published triennially and constitute the work of a panel of cross specialty assessors, to whom the reporting of a death is mandatory. For the purposes of the report a maternal death is defined as "... death from any cause, of a woman who is either pregnant or within one year following the delivery, termination of pregnancy, ectopic pregnancy or miscarriage". The assessors also identify those cases in which care was considered substandard, and make recommendations for future clinical service improvements, audit and research.

The last published report (for the period 1994–1996) [1] recorded 268 maternal deaths. Of these, 134 were a direct result of the pregnancy and 134 were caused indirectly, by a pre-existing condition exacerbated by pregnancy. This gives a maternal mortality rate of 12.2 per 100,000 pregnancies in the UK. This is consistent with rates across the developed world. A further 36 deaths discussed in the report were classed as fortuitous, and another 72 as late (occurring between 42 days and one year *post partum*). These are excluded from the following analysis as they are not counted towards maternal mortality. Of interest, only 35% of recorded cases were ever admitted to an ICU.

Direct Causes (Fig. 1)

Examining the last published report [1] in detail, the largest single cause of death was thromboembolic disease, accounting for 46 fatalities (17% of total deaths). This represents a sustained increase within the last 10 years [1–3]. Many of those dying had significant risk factors that went unrecognized, and thrombo-prophylaxis was often not administered. The impact of the Royal College of Obstetrics and Gynaecology recommendations for thrombo-prophylaxis post-Cesarian section, introduced in 1995, is as yet unknown.

Hypertensive disorders of pregnancy were the next largest cause of death, being directly responsible for 20 (7.5%) deaths and contributing to eight more. This number is virtually unchanged from the previous report. Although the proportion in which substandard care was implicated fell from 80 to 59%. Recommendations for improving the care of these patients were in two areas. First, increasing the awareness in the community, both among women and the professionals caring for them, to aid in early recognition and referral. Second, the development of departmental protocols for detailed management of the acute disease.

Hemorrhage formed the next significant group of direct maternal deaths. The number of deaths directly due to hemorrhage has continued to fall from 9.2 to 5.5 per million maternities over the last three reports [1–3]. The potential for catastrophic hemorrhage in obstetric patients is well recognized and has been highlighted in a number of reports. The latest report specifically recommended the early involvement of experienced clinicians in the management of placenta previa, and in the obstetric review of patients presenting to the emergency department. The combination of placenta previa and a previous uterine scar was identified as a

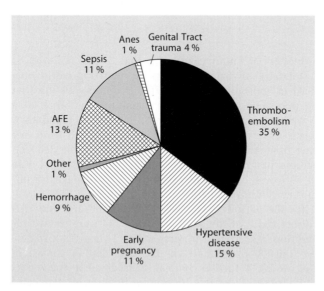

Fig. 1. Causes of direct maternal deaths in the UK: 1994–1996. (Data from [1])

specific hazard for surgery, mandating senior staff. The generation of departmental protocols for severe hemorrhage and 'fire drill' testing of these protocols, as suggested in previous reports was re-emphasized.

Amniotic fluid emboli (AFE) were responsible for 17 (6%) deaths in the 1994–96 report. Of these, 12 were aged 30 or over, and of 39 cases recorded since 1988 only one has been under 25 yrs old. In only one case did the AFE occur in an otherwise uncomplicated pregnancy. Associated complications included amniocentesis, polyhydramnios, placenta increta, fibroids, cervical suture, and intrauterine fetal death. The only recommendation possible, given the unpredictable nature and rapidly progressive course of this condition, was that the ICU care for the few patients surviving long enough to reach the ICU could possibly be improved.

Genital tract sepsis was responsible for 16 (6%) deaths; a number virtually unchanged from the previous two reports. In those cases with positive cultures, group A β-hemolytic *Streptococcus* was the commonest organism with group B β-hemolytic *Streptococcus, Clostridia species,* and coliforms accounting for the remainder. Case studies in the report emphasized the point that puerperal sepsis is a rapidly progressive condition and that early recognition and prompt institution of appropriate antibiotic therapy could have been life saving. Overcoming the assumption that this is a disease of the past, raising awareness, ensuring the use of prophylactic antibiotics in Cesarian section, and the early involvment of a microbiologist formed the recommendations for reducing the impact of this disease.

Indirect Causes

There were proportionally more indirect deaths than in the previous report. The 134 deaths in this category were divided into cardiac, of which there were 39 in the 1994–96 report, and "others", a broad and heterogeneous group encompassing all medical specialties.

In the first three reports from 1952–1960, 86% of the 277 reported deaths attributed to cardiac disease were thought to be due to rheumatic valve disease. The latest report was the first to record no deaths from rheumatic disease. The absolute number of cardiac deaths has declined from about 35 cases per year to around 13 per year since the fifties and in that time the pattern of disease has changed completely. Of the 39 (14.5%) cardiac deaths, 10 were due to congenital and 29 to acquired heart disease. The deaths from congenital pulmonary hypertension and Eisenmenger's syndrome made up the largest group in the congenital cardiac deaths. The care was generally of high standard, carried out in tertiary centers and illustrates the risks of pregnancy in these conditions. The impact of women surviving to reproductive age who have had surgical correction or palliation of previously lethal congenital defects has yet to become completely clear.

Acquired cardiac diseases accounted for 25 (9.3%) patients. Cardiomyopathy, puerperal or otherwise, and myocarditis were the largest group followed by thoracic aortic dissection and myocardial infarction. Two of those dying of puerperal cardiomyopathy weighed in excess of 110 kg; all of those dying of myocardial infarction were multigravid women in their thirties and, all bar one were known to be smokers. The 1988–90 report [3] noted only one death from thoracic aortic dissection. The next report recorded nine, and the latest report seven. While it is tempting to assign this increase to the increasing age of the maternal population, the 1991–93 report [2] noted that the age (29 years), of those dying with thoracic aortic dissection averaged only very slightly higher than that for the maternal population as a whole. In the cases of three patients in which substandard care was judged to have occurred, this was due to the diagnosis never being considered. The report recommended that the diagnosis of dissection should be considered in any woman with chest pain, and that a chest X-ray is safe in pregnancy and should always be performed in ill pregnant patients with chest pain.

The possibility of women becoming alienated from their specialists must be considered. This can occur when women with cardiac disease are advised not to become pregnant or proceed with pregnancy, and yet choose to continue, precipitating breakdown of relationships. Unless these difficult discussions are handled sensitively these patients may become separated them from their expert cardiology services at a time when they need them the most.

There were 86 (32%) "other" indirect maternal deaths in the 1994–96 report, an increase from 63 and 65 in the previous two reports. Twenty-nine separate causes were listed though intra-cranial hemorrhage and epilepsy accounted for half the cases in this group. Disseminating appropriate knowledge of the acute management of seizures to the families of epileptic patients, and improving cross specialty communication for patients with severe intercurrent illness, formed the primary recommendations for this group of patients.

▌ Obstetric Admissions to Intensive Care

There is no similar audit for maternal severe illness, although several studies have looked at the reasons for admission of obstetric patients to intensive care. The largest UK data set of obstetric ICU admissions has been collected by the Intensive Care National Audit and Research Centre (Rowen and Goldfrad, unpublished data), which has data from 91 UK ICUs. Of 342 obstetric admissions, 101 were for pregnancy-induced hypertension and 111 for hemorrhage. There were six deaths. From the UK studies published during the 1990s [4–10], the number of admissions varies between 0.1% and 0.75% of deliveries, giving an ICU admission rate of 8.2 to 61 admissions per maternal death in the Confidential Enquiry. The admitting diagnosis in these studies and the causes of maternal deaths as recorded in the CEMD for a similar period shows a considerable disparity.

Figure 2 compares the death rates and ICU admission rates for the principal subgroups of obstetric mortality/morbidity. In all published studies, pregnancy-induced hypertension and hemorrhage are the major causes of admission. However, pulmonary thrombo-embolic disease and AFE, two of the major causes of obstetric mortality in the CEMD, barely feature in the ICU admission data. This is partly accounted for by the fact that both these conditions may be rapidly fatal, but the failure to recognize the severity of the condition until too late may be an alternative explanation in some cases. An additional source of disparity may be early pregnancy deaths and those due to psychiatric disease.

Figure 3 demonstrates that the picture emerging from the studies in non-UK ICUs [11–19] is similar but with a few notable differences. Admission rates are broadly similar with pregnancy-induced hypertension and major hemorrhage being the single largest admission categories. In the North American studies [11–14, 16–18], admissions with pneumonia featured prominently, probably as a result of more generous ICU bed provision. In the French study [19] there was an increased incidence of pulmonary thrombo-embolic disease, although the reason for this is unclear. Figures 2 and 3 demonstrate the importance of the 'other' category. This re-

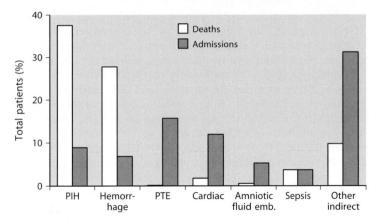

Fig. 2. Comparison of deaths versus admissions to the ICU. (Aggregated data from UK studies [1–10]).
PIH: pregnancy-induced hypertension; PTE: pulmonary thromboembolism

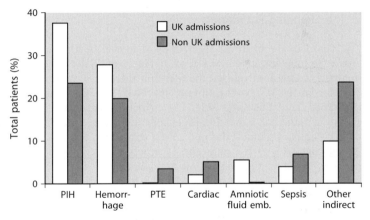

Fig. 3. Comparison of UK versus non-UK admissions to the ICU. (Aggregated data from [4–19] and Rowen and Goldfrad, unpublished data).
PIH: pregnancy-induced hypertension; PTE: pulmonary thromboembolism

presents a heterogeneous group of conditions of which we know little, but appear over-represented in the mortality figures compared with ICU admissions.

The majority of the studies in this field are simple retrospective data analyses of obstetric admissions to ICU. Two groups however, have performed large case-control studies looking at the incidence and predictors of severe obstetric morbidity. Bouvier-Colle et al. [20] used ICU admission for direct or indirect obstetric reasons as their marker for morbidity across three regions in France for a period of 6 months or a year. In total, 375 obstetric patients were identified. For each of these patients, two controls were recruited matched for type of maternity unit and pregnancy outcome and chosen by date of outcome. An extensive questionnaire was completed for all cases and controls, enquiring into socio-demographic characteristics, medical and obstetric histories, pregnancy surveillance, hospitalizations and transfers, procedures and treatments carried out at any stage of their pregnancy. The investigators found that a positive medical history, lack of antenatal care, non-European nationality and multiple pregnancy were most strongly linked to ICU admission. High parity also increased risk, but age (in this study >35yrs) did not.

Waterstone et al. [21] used severe morbidity defined by broadly accepted parameters, but they excluded those cases with diagnostic uncertainty (which included pulmonary and amniotic fluid emboli). Looking at the South-East Thames Region of the UK for a period of one year, these investigators found 588 cases of severe illness out of a total of 48,865 deliveries with five maternal deaths. The controls were women from the same region who delivered without problems. They found that age over 34, non-white ethnic group, hypertension, emergency Cesarian section, antenatal admission, multiple pregnancy, social exclusion, and the use of iron or antidepressant therapy at antenatal booking were all independently associated with morbidity. From their data, the authors propose the use of defined morbidity and morbidity to mortality ratios (in their study 118:1) or morbidity to delivery rates (12/1000) as useful indices both of care, and of the influence of measures taken to improve it.

■ The Changing Population

The trend in the absolute number of maternal deaths is likely to continue to decrease in the developed world as a result of a decrease in the total number of births. This figure disguises the fact that the rate of maternal mortality stopped decreasing in the UK by the time of the 1988–90 CEMD, and has in fact been rising in France since this time [22]. The principal reason for this is the age-related increase in maternal mortality, especially for the ages of 30 and over. On both sides of the English Channel, the percentage of women aged 30–49 as a proportion of all women aged 15–49 is rising and is expected to continue to do so until 2005. Predictions based on the population forecasts for 1995, 2000, 2005 and 2010 published by Eurostat [23, 24], combined with the fertility rates and mortality rates for these age groups, (calculated from 1990 figures), suggest an increase in the maternal mortality of around 0.5/100,000 live births by 2005. This, combined with the steadily increasing fertility rates (as defined by number of live births per unit of population in a certain age group) among women in their thirties and forties, means that the proportion of births to women aged over thirty is growing. The continuing increase in the fertility of the over thirties is likely to be linked to a further rise in the proportion of women who delay childbearing for social/professional reasons. In the 1988–90 CEMD, 49% of women having their first child were under 25. By the 1994–96 report this had fallen to 39%. Parity is a factor in maternal death and is closely associated with increasing maternal age. It can be expected that the proportion of primiparae over the age of thirty will continue to rise, further increasing the mortality and morbidity rates. In addition to the effect of increasing age, there is an increase in independent risk factors for respiratory, cardiovascular, and metabolic disease in the maternal population. The 1994–96 CEMD reported the prevalence of obesity (BMI > 30) increasing by 1.6% to 17% in the age group 16–64; this increase being highest in the age group 25–34. Four percent of these women were hypertensive compared with 1% of women with a BMI < 30. The long-term downward trend in womens' cigarette smoking has also halted, and indeed smoking prevalence actually increased by 0.5% from 1993–1996.

Data in the 1994–96 CEMD report seemed to suggest an increase in mortality among some minority ethnic groups compared with the general population. Though this has yet to be confirmed, if may become more important as the migrant population increases. This population also represents the most economically and socially deprived. Such factors have been shown in a recent World Health Organization (WHO) publication [25] to affect maternal mortality. Examination of figures from among the most deprived and vulnerable in the USA, revealed a mortality rate ten times the national average. For the purposes of the WHO, vulnerability was defined as insufficient financial and social support, poor diet and/or housing, substance misuse and poor access to healthcare.

▌ Conclusion

Maternal mortality is very rare in the developed world and its use as a statistical tool in improving obstetric services is now limited. The incidence of maternal severe illness, however, may be as much as 118 times higher. If each of these cases is viewed as a mortality near-miss then maternal safety on the labor ward should not be taken for granted. The declining birth rate and changing maternal demographics hint that there may be an increasing proportion of women becoming severely ill during pregnancy and labor; although total numbers are difficult to predict and may be falling. Because older mothers are at greater risk of both direct and indirect problems, their admission to ICU/high dependency facilities will become more frequent.

The obstetric patient on ICU continues to present a challenge. Altered physiology, certain unique disease states, and the presence of the fetus may necessitate changes in management strategies. Close co-operation between critical care, obstetric, and neonatal health care professionals is required. In global terms, however, maternal mortality rates in many countries are still above 1% and this discussion is a luxury few can afford.

References

1. Department of Health (1998) Why Mothers Die. Report on Confidential Enquiries into Maternal Deaths in the United Kingdom 1994–1996. HMSO, London
2. Department of Health (1996) Report on Confidential Enquiries into Maternal Deaths in the United Kingdom 1991–1993. HMSO, London
3. Department of Health (1993) Report on Confidential Enquiries into Maternal Deaths in the United Kingdom 1988–1990. HMSO, London
4. Graham SG, Luxton MC (1989) The requirement for intensive care support for the pregnant population. Anaesthesia 44:581–584
5. Hughes RL (1990) The requirement for intensive care support for the pregnant population. Anaesthesia 45:65
6. Yau EHS, Groves PA, Wathen NC, et al (1990) The requirement for intensive care support for the pregnant population. Anaesthesia 45:65–66
7. DeMello WF, Restall J (1990) The requirement for intensive care support for the pregnant population. Anaesthesia 45:888
8. Wheatley E, Farkas A, Watson D (1996) Obstetric admissions to an intensive therapy unit. Int J Obstet Anaesth 5:221–224
9. Hazelgrove JF, Price C, Pappachan J, et al (2001) Multicenter study of obstetric admissions to 14 intensive care units in southern England. Crit Care Med 29:770–775

10. Umo-Etuk J, Lumley J, Holdcroft A (1996) Critically ill parturient women admitted to intensive care: a 5 year review. Int J Obstet Anaesth 5:79–84
11. Lewinsohn G, Herman A, Leonov Y et al (1994) Critically ill obstetrical patients: Outcome and predictability. Crit Care Med 22:1412–1414
12. Cohen J, Singer P, Kogan A, et al (2000) Course and outcome of obstetric patients in a general intensive care unit. Acta Obstet Gynecol Scand 79:846–850
13. Mahutte NG, Murphy-Kaulbeck L, Le Q, et al (1999) Obstetric admissions to the intensive care unit. Obstet Gynecol 94:263–266
14. Baskett TF, Sterndahl J, (1998) Maternal intensive care and near-miss mortality in obstetrics. Br J Obstet Gynaecol 105:981–984
15. Ryan M, Hamilton V, Bowen M (2000) The role of a high dependency unit in a regional obstetric unit. Anaesthesia 55:1155–1158
16. Hogg B, Hauth JC (2000) Intensive care utilisation during pregnancy. Obstet Gynecol 95:62S (Abst)
17. Kilpatrick SJ, Mathay MA (1992) Obstetric patients requiring critical care. Chest 101:1407–1412
18. El-Solh AA, Grant BJB (1996) A comparison of severity of illness scoring for critically ill obstetric patients. Chest 110:1299–1304
19. Bouvier-Colle M-H, Salanave B, Ancel P-Y, et al (1996) Obstetric patients treated in intensive care units and maternal mortality. Eur J Obstet Gynecol Reprod Biol 65:121–125
20. Bouvier-Colle M-H, Varnoux N, Salanave B (1997) Case control study of risk factors for obstetric patients' admission to intensive care units. Eur J Obstet Gynecol Reprod Biol 74:173–77
21. Waterstone M, Bewley S, Wolfe C (2001) Incidence and predictors of severe obstetric morbidity: case-controlled study. Br Med J 322:1089–1093
22. Salanave B, Bouvier-Colle MH (1996) The likely increase in maternal mortality rates in the United Kingdom and France until 2005. Paediatr Perinat Epidemiol 10:418–422
23. Shaw C, Cruijsen H, de Beer J, de Jong A (1997) Latest population projections for the European Union. Population Trends 90:18–30
24. Pearce D, Bovagnet FC (2001) The demographic situation in the European Union. Population Trends 104:6–11
25. WHO (1998) World Health, 51st year. Number 1, Jan–Feb 1998 IX. (ISSN 0043-8502)

Severity of Illness

Measuring Organ Dysfunction

D. A. Zygun and C. J. Doig

▌ Introduction

Multiple organ dysfunction syndrome (MODS) is a clinical pattern of progressive organ dysfunction complicating the post-resuscitative phase of acute illnesses such as shock and severe infection, and is a frequent precursor of death in critically ill patients [1]. MODS is an important clinical entity in the intensive care unit (ICU), as approximately one-third of patients admitted to the ICU will have, or develop, organ failure. Further, mortality is directly correlated to the number of failing organ systems. For those patients with one organ failure, mortality is 16–42% and for those with three or more organ system failure, mortality is 55–100% [2–5]. Many organ dysfunction scales have been developed to measure the severity and course of organ dysfunction. With rare exception, these scales were developed on an ad-hoc basis, without formal validation, and often for single observational or therapeutic studies, to qualitatively describe clinical improvement or deterioration.

Ideal variables for describing organ dysfunction should possess several important characteristics. These variables should be objective, simple and easily available but reliable. They should be specific for the organ system being considered and of a continuous nature. In addition, they should be independent of patient type and therapeutic intervention. In the mid 1990s, at relatively the same time, four organ dysfunction scores were developed that met these 'optimal' characteristics for a variable, used rigorous albeit disparate methodology in variable/score development, and included or had subsequent attempts to assess the validity and operating characteristics of the scores. The Sequential Organ Failure Assessment (SOFA) score, Multiple Organ Dysfunction (MOD) Score, and the Logistic Organ Dysfunction (LOD) score have received the most attention in the literature while the Brussels Score remains only in abstract form. This article will review the methodology of creation and characteristics of each score, the validation of each score, and a brief comparison of two scores: the MOD and SOFA.

▌ SOFA

The SOFA score was developed by consensus conference of the European Society of Intensive Care Medicine (ESICM) in Paris in 1994 [6]. The purpose behind development was 2-fold: to improve the understanding of the natural history of organ dysfunction and be able to assess the effects of new therapies on the course of organ dysfunction. The SOFA score consists of six organ systems each scored from 0 to 4 with 0 representing normality and 4 representing the most severe dysfunction

Table 1. The SOFA score [6]

Organ System	Score				
	0	1	2	3	4
▌**Respiratory** PaO$_2$/FiO$_2$	> 400	≤400	≤300	≤200	≤100
▌**Renal** Creatinine (μmol/l)	≤110	110–170	171–299	300–440 Urine output ≤500 ml/d	> 440 Urine output < 200 ml/d
▌**Hepatic** Bilirubin (μmol/l)	≤20	20–32	33–101	102–204	> 204
▌**Cardiovascular** Hypotension	No hypotension	MAP < 70 mmHg	Dopamine ≤5[a], Dobutamine (any dose)	Dopamine > 5[a] or epinephrine ≤0.1[a] or norepinephrine ≤0.1[a]	Dopamine > 15[a] or epinephrine > 0.1[a] or norepinephrine > 0.1[a]
▌**Hematologic** Platelet count	> 150	≤150	≤100	≤50	≤20
▌**Neurologic** Glasgow Coma score	15	13–14	10–12	6–9	< 6

[a] Adrenergic agents administered for at least 1 h (doses given are in μg/kg/min)

(Table 1). The cardiovascular, respiratory, coagulation, hepatic, central nervous, and renal systems were chosen for inclusion with the worst physiological value for each day recorded. J.L. Vincent et al., on behalf of the working group on "sepsis-related problems" of the ESICM, published the first prospective evaluation of the SOFA score [7]. This international cohort study described organ dysfunction as measured by the SOFA in 1449 patients admitted to one of 40 ICUs during May 1995. Using a subset of patients staying at least a week in the ICU (544 patients), they found 44% of non-survivors increased their SOFA score compared to 20% of survivors. Further, 33% of survivors decreased their total score compared with 21% of non-survivors. Infected patients had more severe organ dysfunction compared with those without infection. Supporting the validity of the SOFA score as a surrogate ICU outcome measure, mortality was correlated with SOFA. Mortality was 9% for patients without organ failure and 83% for those with four or more organs failing (organ failure defined as ≥3). A maximum SOFA of >15 was associated with a 90% mortality rate. A proportional hazards analysis suggested the values within the cardiovascular, neurological and renal systems contribute the most to the risk of death.

Several issues regarding the analysis warrant discussion. The data presented suggest infection status is an important determinant of the course of organ dysfunction. Therefore, it is possible other factors related to case-mix such as age, gender, diagnostic category, co-morbid illness, and surgical status, among others, could potentially alter the course of organ dysfunction over time. The contribution of case-mix to the discriminant properties of SOFA or other scoring systems should be further described prior to acceptance of any of these scores as a surrogate outcome measure. Further, the restriction of the analysis to those staying at least a week in the ICU limits generalizability of the results of this study. Those staying at least 7 days in the ICU had higher admission respiratory, cardiovascular, and neurological scores. Therefore, it remains uncertain whether the predictive mortality for SOFA scores applies to a patient with an ICU length of stay (LOS) <7 days. The restriction of patients is a technique often used to deal with the difficult statistical situation of unbalanced, correlated data (a highly variable number of observations per patient). However, newer statistical techniques have been developed and are discussed below.

Two further analyses of this dataset examining the characteristics of the SOFA score have been published. The first examined the development of organ dysfunction in the subset of 181 trauma patients [8]. Those trauma patients who did not survive were significantly older and had significantly higher mean SOFA scores during the first week of ICU care. A higher SOFA score was independently associated in multiple regression analysis with a longer ICU LOS. Evaluation of these regression coefficients revealed the contribution of SOFA to ICU LOS decreased over the first 5 days. The additive coefficient for each SOFA point on day 0 was 0.85 days compared to 0.66 days at day 4. Non-survivors had more severe admission respiratory, coagulation, cardiovascular, and neurological scores than survivors. A SOFA score of greater than or equal to 5 was associated with a death rate 2.7 times greater than a SOFA score less than 5. After the first 4 days, only respiratory dysfunction has significant prognostic value in the trauma patient.

The second publication analyzed the association of total maximum SOFA score and delta SOFA score to ICU mortality [9]. A patient's total maximum SOFA score was calculated by summing the worst scores for each of the 6 component scores. The delta SOFA score was defined as the difference between the total maximum SOFA score and the admission SOFA score. The mean total maximum SOFA score was significantly higher for non-survivors than survivors (13.6 ± 4.8 vs 6.7 ± 4.5). The discriminative power, the ability of the scores to discriminate between survivors and non-survivors, for each maximum component SOFA score, total maximum SOFA score, admission SOFA score, and the delta SOFA score was determined using the area under the receiver operating characteristic (ROC) curve. Of the component scores, the cardiovascular score had the best discriminative power (area under the ROC = 0.802). However, when compared with the individual component scores, delta SOFA score, and admission SOFA scores, the total maximum SOFA score performed the best in terms of discriminative power (area under the ROC = 0.847). In logistic regression analysis, the cardiovascular component score was found to have the highest relative contribution to outcome (odds ratio (OR) = 1.683, 95% confidence interval (CI) = 1.488–1.905] while the hepatic component did not significantly contribute to the prediction of outcome (p = 0.192). Further logistic regression analysis revealed the degree of organ dysfunction at admission (admission SOFA score) and the degree of organ dysfunction developing during the ICU stay (delta SOFA score) significantly and independently contributed to the prediction of outcome with a similar weight (admission SOFA OR = 1.361, 95% CI = 1.303–1.421; delta SOFA OR = 1.367, 95% CI = 1.303–1.432).

The use of total maximum SOFA score has several advantages and disadvantages. The total maximum SOFA score captures the overall amount of dysfunction during the patient's ICU stay and its discriminative power is very good. In addition, because this single value can be calculated for each patient, no restriction based on the patient's ICU LOS is necessary for analysis. However, the total maximum SOFA score may be calculated using one to as many as six day's data. Thus, data which may contribute to the understanding of any observed association between SOFA and mortality is excluded from the analysis. It is also possible that individuals whose total maximum SOFA score is comprised of 6 days of observations are somehow different from those whose score is composed of only a single day of data. This method of analysis also lacks consideration of the timing of organ dysfunction. It is probable that the timing of the maximum organ dysfunction is an important predictor of outcome. Work from our group suggests a significant interaction between the daily SOFA score and the timing of measurement in the prediction of outcome (unpublished data).

The total maximum SOFA score has been further validated in 303 consecutive patients admitted to a medical ICU in Germany [10]. In this study, the total maximum SOFA score again showed very good discriminative power (area under the ROC 0.86) despite the fact that the patients were significantly different when compared with the multicenter trial described above; this study was comprised primarily of medical patients with an overall hospital mortality of 14.5% while the multicenter study included a large proportion of surgical patients and described a 26% overall hospital mortality. The SOFA score has also been scrutinized in other patient populations. In a sample of critically ill patients with cirrhosis, Wehler et al. [11] found day 1 SOFA score to have excellent discriminative power (area under the ROC = 0.94), which was superior to the APACHE II and Child-Pugh systems. Recently, Ferreira and colleagues [12] published a study of 352 consecutive patients admitted to a medicosurgical ICU in Belgium. They found mean SOFA score (sum of all daily SOFA scores divided by the ICU LOS) correlated best with mortality in univariate analysis (OR = 3.06 95% CI = 2.36–3.97) and had a very good discriminative power (area under the ROC curve = 0.88). However, the variable with the best discriminative power was the highest (highest, not maximum) SOFA score (area under the ROC 0.90). Supporting previous work, the change in SOFA score during the patient's ICU stay was independently predictive of outcome. For those with an initial SOFA of >11, a mean SOFA that increased or stayed the same was associated with a 91% mortality rate.

In summary, several studies have now described the use of the SOFA score. Increasing organ dysfunction as measured by the SOFA score consistently correlates with increasing mortality. SOFA is a reliable measure of organ dysfunction at admission during ICU stay in balanced datasets. The total maximum SOFA score and highest SOFA score hold promise as surrogate outcomes in the ICU.

∎ MOD Score

The MOD score was developed and validated on a cohort of 692 patients admitted to a tertiary Canadian surgical ICU [13]. The creation of the MOD score was methodologically sound. The principles of validity (construct, content, and criterion), reproducibility, and responsiveness guided an extensive literature search, which served as the basis for the selection and evaluation of variables. The first 336 patients served as a development set for the calibration of variables. The six organ systems chosen for the inclusion are the same as in the SOFA score. Each organ system was scored from 0 to 4. Thresholds were determined based on mortality rate. A score of 0 represented a mortality rate of <5% while a score of 4 repre-

Table 2. The MOD score [13]

Organ system	Score				
	0	1	2	3	4
▌**Respiratory** PaO$_2$/FiO$_2$	>300	226–300	151–225	76–150	≤75
▌**Renal** Creatinine (µmol/l)	≤100	101–200	201–350	251–500	>500
▌**Hepatic** Bilirubin (µmol/l)	≤20	21–60	61–120	121–240	>240
▌**Cardiovascular** PAR[a]	<10.0	10.1–15	15.1–20.0	20.1–30.0	>30.0
▌**Hematologic** Platelet count	>120	81–120	51–80	21–50	≤20
▌**Neurologic** Glasgow Coma Score	15	13–14	10–12	7–9	≤6

[a] Pressure-Adjusted Heart Rate: product of the heart rate multiplied by the ratio of the right atrial pressure to the mean arterial pressure

sented a mortality of >50%. Intermediate intervals were established so the ranges for each point were approximately equal and a given score in one system would predict an equivalent mortality for the same score in another system. The subsequent 356 patients served as a validation set to test the reproducibility of the intervals derived from the development set. The MOD score is presented in Table 2.

An increasing MOD score, calculated similarly to the total maximum SOFA score, correlated with ICU mortality. Patients with scores >20 had a mortality rate of 100%. A mortality rate of 25% was observed for patients with a score of 9–12, 50% for a score of 13–16, and 75% for a score of 17–20. In logistic regression analysis, the neurological and renal component had the largest contribution to predictive capacity while the hepatic component did not significantly contribute to the prediction of mortality. This logistic regression model (component scores as independent variables and ICU mortality as the dependent variable) had excellent discriminative power in both the development set (area under the ROC=0.936) and the validation set (area under the ROC=0.928). Like the SOFA score, the MOD score at admission and delta MOD score independently predicted ICU mortality in a logistic regression analysis (admission MOD score OR=1.47, delta MOD score OR=1.59). However, unlike the SOFA score, the delta MOD score contributed slightly more than the admission MOD score to the predictive capacity of the model.

Other investigators have described the use of the MOD score. Barie and colleagues measured daily MOD scores in a large prospective cohort of surgical ICU patients [14, 15]. The MOD score was significantly correlated with ICU length of stay. The MOD score also significantly predicted mortality in their multiple logistic regression analysis. Jacobs et al. [16] compared the MOD score to the APACHE II score in a prospective cohort of 39 patients with septic shock admitted to a medicosurgical ICU. The MOD score at admission was not statistically different between survivors and non-survivors. This was also true for the admission APACHE II score. However, the maximum MOD score calculated during the ICU stay was significantly higher in non-survivors than survivors. The corresponding value for APACHE II was not statistically different between survivors and non-survivors. Obviously, the relatively small number of patients limits the interpretation of this study. Recently, a Canadian group studied the MOD component scores in a cohort of 1200 patients admitted to 16 multi-system ICUs [17]. The goal of the study was to examine the relationship between the six components of the MOD score with time to death in the ICU. Cox regression analysis determined that only four organ systems were associated with ICU mortality: cardiovascular, respiratory, renal, and neurological. The relative risk of mortality was found to be time-dependent for the respiratory system (baseline and serial components) and the serial component of the hepatic system. Baseline hepatic score was not related to mortality. Unfortunately, the characteristics of the maximum MOD score were not described in this study. Further, the MOD score in this study utilized a different cardiovascular variable than described above. Instead of the pressure-adjusted heart rate, the cardiovascular component was scored as follows: 0 = heart rate <120; 1 = heart rate >120, <140; 2 = heart rate >140; 3 = need for inotropes > dopamine 3 µg/kg/min; 4 = lactate >5 mmol/l.

To summarize, the MOD score was developed using rigorous methodology and has been validated in a surgical ICU population. Like the SOFA score, it can be used to represent organ dysfunction at baseline and during the ICU stay. The MOD score significantly contributes to the prediction of ICU mortality. Its use as a surrogate outcome awaits further validation in other patient populations.

▌ SOFA or MOD Score?

Both the SOFA score and the MOD scores are now being reported as measures of organ dysfunction in clinical trials. Although they evaluate the same six organ systems, several important differences exist between the two scores. Although arguably, the MOD score was developed by a more rigorous methodology, the validation set was relatively small and consisted only of surgical ICU patients from a single center. Further, the study was performed from May 1988 to February 1990, and some intensivists may argue that the practice of critical care medicine has significantly changed in the last 10 years. Perhaps, a disadvantage in the MOD score is the calculation of the pressure-adjusted heart rate, a variable not intuitive to most clinicians. This value cannot be calculated in a significant proportion of ICU patients due to the absence of a central venous monitor. In fact, approximately one half of the patients in the original study describing the MOD score could not have a cardiovascular component calculated. Consensus conference creation of the SOFA score portends face validity and the SOFA score has been described in both surgical and medical patients. Although not ideal due to therapy dependence, the cardiovascular SOFA component score, which is based on degree of inotropic support, is readily available in virtually all patients. The two scores are also different with respect to the timing of measurement. It is recommended that the MOD score be measured at the same point in time every day (first morning values). However, the SOFA score incorporates the worst physiological value during the previous 24 hours in its calculation. The use of measurements at one particular time avoids capturing momentary physiological changes unrelated to patient condition. However, the choice of any particular time is arbitrary and the effect of the timing of measurement on validity has not yet been investigated. The MOD score arbitrarily assigns a maximum score to each component if the patient dies, to attempt to deal with the confounding that occurs due to the relatively large proportion of patients who do not survive to the end of the period of study. This is based on the assumption that multiple organ dysfunction increases in severity in non-survivors and death represents the most severe state of organ dysfunction. However, preliminary analysis on 1400 adult multisystem ICU patients from our health region does not support this assumption (Zygun et al., unpublished data).

Given the relative similarities of the MOD and SOFA scores, do they provide different results? Data from our institution indicate the total SOFA and MOD scores are in fact quite similar. In a cohort of consecutive multi-system ICU patients admitted to one of three ICUs in our health region over a 6 month period in 1999, daily SOFA and MOD scores were significantly correlated (Pearson correlation coefficient=0.89, p<0.0001). Least-squares linear regression revealed SOFA score=1.04 (MOD score)+1.10 (r^2=0.80, p<0.0001) (Fig. 1) [18]. Residual analysis revealed no obvious evidence against the assumption of homogeneity of variance. Examination of the scatterplot and normal quantile plot of the residuals did not suggest evidence against the assumption normality. Therefore, one can conclude that daily SOFA score is related to daily MOD score in a linear fashion with a slope of approximately one. However, this is not true for the component scores. Residual analysis and examination of the normal quantile plots for each component score indicates variations from the assumptions of linear regression for all components especially the cardiovascular score. Thus, although changes in total daily SOFA and MOD score are similar, individual component scores do not appear to be linearly related.

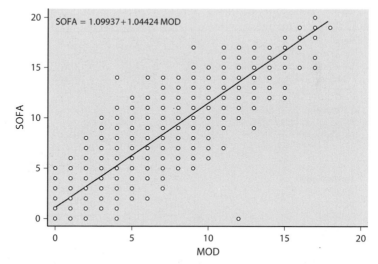

Fig. 1. Relationship of daily SOFA and MOD scores in a cohort of 1400 adult ICU patients admitted to one of three intensive care units in the Calgary Health Region. This graph demonstrates that the relationship between scores is linear, and over the entire population, the scores are closely associated

LOD Score

The LOD score was developed with rigorous statistical methodology [19]. The data set from the North American Study of Severity Systems was used and included values from 14745 ICU admissions in 137 medical, surgical or mixed ICUs in 12 countries. Eighty percent of the sample formed the developmental sample and the rest composed the validation sample. An involved complex process utilizing the LOWESS procedure and logistic regression techniques eventually resulted in the scoring system depicted in Table 3. The LOD score consists of 6 organ systems and twelve variables with a maximum score of 22. The variables had been recorded as the worst value in the first 24 hours of ICU admission. In the developmental sample, the resultant model based on the LOD score performed well. In the validation sample, the calibration was excellent with a Hosmer-Lemeshow statistic of 9.32

Table 3. The LOD score [19]

Organ System	LOD Points						
	Increasing severity/ decreasing values			Organ dysfunction free		Increasing severity/ increasing values	
	5	3	1	0	1	3	5
Neurologic Glasgow Coma Score	3–5	6–8	9–13	14–15			
Cardiovascular Heart rate (min) Systolic blood pressure (mmHg)	<30 or <40	40–69	70–89	30–139 and 90–239	≥140 or 240–269	≥270	
Renal Serum urea (g/l) Serum urea nitrogen (mM) Creatinine (µM) Urine output (l/d)	<0.5	0.5–0.74		<6 <6 and <106 and 0.75–9.99	6–9.9 6–9.9 or 106–140	10–19.9 10–19.9 or ≥141 or ≥10	≥20 ≥20
Pulmonary PaO$_2$/FiO$_2$ on MV or CPAP PaO$_2$ [kPa]/FiO$_2$		<150 (<19.9)	≥150 (≥19.9)	No ventilation, no IPAP or no CPAP			
Hematologic White blood cell count (×10^9/l) Platelets (×10^9/l)		<1.0	1.0–2.4 or <50	2.5–49.9 and ≥50	≥50.0		
Hepatic Bilirubin (µM) Prothrombin tine, seconds above standard (% of standard)				<34.2 and ≤3 (<2.5%)	≥34.2 or >3 (≥25%)		

FiO$_2$: Fraction of inspired oxygen: IPAP: inspiratory positive airway pressure; CPAP: continuous positive airway pressure

(p = 0.50) and very good discrimination (area under the ROC curve = 0.85). The LOD score was strongly correlated with hospital mortality. A LOD score of 0, 11, and 22 was associated with a probability of hospital mortality of 3.2%, 76% and 99.7%, respectively.

A recently published study whose primary goal was to investigate the association between pulmonary catheter use and mortality also analyzed the serial assessment of the LOD score [20]. In this cohort of 751 ICU patients, first day LOD score and worst LOD score were significantly different between survivors and non-survivors. In a multivariate logistic regression model, worst LOD score independently predicted mortality (OR = 1.368, 95% CI = 1.257–1.488). It should be noted the daily assessment of LOD score and, thus, the worst LOD score was not included in the initial description of the LOD score. Carson and Bach investigated the usefulness of the LOD score in a cohort of patients with prolonged critical illness [21]. Unfortunately, the discriminative power of the LOD score was poor with an area under the ROC of just 0.65. Calibration was also poor as demonstrated by a Hosmer-Lemeshow C-statistic of 49.5 (p < 0.0001). Admittedly, the acute physiology and chronic health evaluation (APACHE) II, mortality prediction model (MPM) II, and simplified acute physiology score (SAPS) II scoring systems also performed poorly in this cohort. An Austrian study of 3536 medicosurgical ICU patients from 13 ICUs found the original LOD score was not well calibrated in the prediction of hospital mortality (C statistic = 37.2, p < 0.001) [22]. Further, discrimination was good, but not as high as previously reported (area under the ROC = 0.80). However, a new model that integrated LOD score after day 1 was created. Accounting for the time course of the LOD score improved discrimination (area under the ROC = 0.86 for hospital mortality, 0.90 for ICU mortality), but calibration deteriorated. Timsit et al. [23] also demonstrated the added usefulness of the LOD score subsequent to day 1.

The LOD score measures organ dysfunction and can discriminate between survivors and non-survivors. Although not originally described as a serial measure, it appears this may hold the most promise for the LOD score as a surrogate outcome. However, this aspect warrants further investigation. The first day assessment of the LOD score predicts mortality, but the added benefit of assessing LOD score to the previously described and well validated severity scoring systems such as SAPS or APACHE is uncertain.

▌ Brussels Score

The Brussels score was developed through a series of consensus conferences [24]. Six organ systems are scored with 5 gradations of severity (Table 4). There is little published evidence supporting its validity. An abstract published in 1995 described the Brussels score measured on day 1 using large ICU dataset. Patients with organ dysfunction classified as normal/mild had lower mortality than those with more severe organ dysfunction for each organ system [25]. However, the concept of organ failure free (OFF) days, the number of days a patient is alive and free of clinically significant organ failure, arose from the Brussels score. This variable is attractive as it is a single value that can be calculated for all ICU patients creating balanced datasets. However, the use of OFF days removes the continuity of organ dysfunction creating a dichotomous view of organ failure. Further, it obscures the variable time course of organ dysfunction. Despite the lack of published validation, it has already been used as a surrogate outcome in clinical trials [26].

Table 4. The Brussels score [24]

Organs	Normal	Abnormal			
		Mild	Clinically significant organ dysfunction		
			Moderate	Severe	Extreme
Cardiovascular sBP (mmHg)	>90	≤90 responsive to fluid	≤90 unresponsive to fluid	≤90 & pH ≤7.3	≤90 & pH ≤7.2
Pulmonary PaO_2/FiO_2	>400	400–301	300–201 Acute lung injury	200–101 ARDS	≤100 Severe ARDS
CNS Glasgow Coma Score	15	14–13	12–10	9–6	≤5
Coagulation Platelets ($\times10^3/mm^2$)	>120	120–81	80–51	50–21	≤20
Renal Creatinine (mg/dl)	<1.5	1.5–1.9	2.9–3.4	3.5–4.9	≥5.0
Hepatic Bilirubin (mg/dl)	<1.2	1.2–1.9	2.0–5.9	6.0–11.9	≥12

Statistical Considerations

Data derived from the daily assessment of organ dysfunction poses a statistical challenge for two main reasons. Firstly, it is correlated. Thus, if one wants to be inclusive of all data collected, the analysis must take into account the repeated measurements taken on a single individual. Secondly, because patients can stay a dramatically different number of days, the datasets are significantly unbalanced. Thus, between individual error estimation is of unequal variance because each individual provides a variable number of data points. To overcome the statistical challenges, some investigators have restricted analysis to those with a minimum length of ICU stay. Obviously, this affects the generalizability of the conclusions drawn. Limiting analysis to specific days or maximum values excludes significant amounts of data and ignores the time course of organ dysfunction. Another commonly used method of analysis is Cox regression. This powerful method allows investigators to determine the relative contribution of organ dysfunction at admission, organ dysfunction developing during ICU, and organ dysfunction of each specific organ system to overall mortality. However, the instantaneous hazard ratio it produces gives little information on the course of organ dysfunction over time. Recently, newer statistical methods have been developed to deal with longitudinal datasets of this nature. Extensions of the general linear model are robust, validated methods of analyzing correlated data. Fixed effects, random effects, and population-averaged models are now available. Importantly, these models are not confined to the linear model. Use of these extensions has yet to enter the critical care literature, but are perfectly suited to help describe the natural history of organ dysfunction in the ICU as they allow for unbalanced, correlated datasets. Finally, each scoring system deals with missing data differently. The MOD score records a score of zero if the data is missing. The SOFA score averages the adjacent values if there is one missing value and records the value as missing if adjacent values are not present. The ideal method of dealing with missing data has yet to be scrutinized despite the potential that this can significantly affect conclusions.

∎ Conclusion

Four organ dysfunction scoring systems have now been developed to describe the natural history of organ dysfunction in the ICU. The SOFA and Brussels score were developed by consensus conference while the LOD score and MOD score were developed through meticulous statistical methodology. As the literature surrounding these scores develop, clinicians will become comfortable with their specific operating characteristics and eventually be able to confidently use these scores as surrogate outcomes. However, prior to acceptance, these scores must be further validated in different patient populations and the contribution of case-mix explored. These scoring systems will undoubtedly lead to a better understanding of MOD and hopefully to improvement in patient outcome.

References

1. Sibbald W, Martin C, Piper R (1998) Multiple organ dysfunction syndrome. In: Bone R (ed) Pulmonary & Critical Care Medicine. Mosby Inc, St. Louis, pp 1–23
2. Tran DD, Groeneveld AB, van der Meulen J, et al (1990) Age, chronic disease, sepsis, organ system failure, and mortality in a medical intensive care unit. Crit Care Med 18:474–479
3. Knaus WA, Draper EA, Wagner DP, Zimmerman JE (1985) Prognosis in acute organ-system failure. Ann Surg 202:685–693
4. Fry DE, Pearlstein L, Fulton RL, Polk HC Jr (1980) Multiple system organ failure. The role of uncontrolled infection. Arch Surg 115:136–140
5. Faist E, Bauer AE, Dittmer H, Heberer G (1983) Multiple organ failure in polytrauma patients. J Trauma 23:775–787
6. Vincent JL, Moreno R, Takala J, et al (1996) The SOFA (Sepsis-related Organ Failure Assessment) score to describe organ dysfunction/failure. On behalf of the Working Group on Sepsis-Related Problems of the European Society of Intensive Care Medicine. Intensive Care Med 22:707–710
7. Vincent JL, de Mendonca A, Cantraine F, et al (1998) Use of the SOFA score to assess the incidence of organ dysfunction/failure in intensive care units: results of a multicenter, prospective study. Working group on "sepsis-related problems" of the European Society of Intensive Care Medicine. Crit Care Med 26:1793–1800
8. Antonelli M, Moreno R, Vincent JL, et al (1999) Application of SOFA score to trauma patients. Sequential Organ Failure Assessment. Intensive Care Med 25:389–394
9. Moreno R, Vincent JL, Matos R, et al (1999) The use of maximum SOFA score to quantify organ dysfunction/failure in intensive care. Results of a prospective, multicentre study. Working Group on Sepsis related Problems of the ESICM. Intensive Care Med 25:686–696
10. Janssens U, Graf C, Graf J, et al (2000) Evaluation of the SOFA score: a single-center experience of a medical intensive care unit in 303 consecutive patients with predominantly cardiovascular disorders. Sequential Organ Failure Assessment. Intensive Care Med 26:1037–1045
11. Wehler M, Kokoska J, Reulbach U, Hahn EG, Strauss R (2001) Short-term prognosis in critically ill patients with cirrhosis assessed by prognostic scoring systems. Hepatology 34:255–261
12. Ferreira FL, Bota DP, Bross A, Melot C, Vincent JL (2001) Serial evaluation of the SOFA score to predict outcome in critically ill patients. JAMA 286:1754–1758
13. Marshall JC, Cook DJ, Christou NV, et al (1995) Multiple organ dysfunction score: a reliable descriptor of a complex clinical outcome. Crit Care Med 23:1638–1652
14. Barie PS, Hydo LJ, Fischer E (1996) Utility of illness severity scoring for prediction of prolonged surgical critical care. J Trauma 40:513–518

15. Barie PS, Hydo LJ (1996) Influence of multiple organ dysfunction syndrome on duration of critical illness and hospitalization. Arch Surg 131:1318–1323
16. Jacobs S, Zuleika M, Mphansa T (1999) The Multiple Organ Dysfunction Score as a descriptor of patient outcome in septic shock compared with two other scoring systems. Crit Care Med 27:741–744
17. Cook R, Cook D, Tilley J, Lee Ka K, Marshall J (2001) Multiple organ dysfunction: Baseline and serial component scores. Crit Care Med 29:2046–2050
18. Doig CJ, Sandham JD, Boiteau PJE, Rosenal T (2001) A description of SOFA and Marshall MODS in a regional critical care system. Am J Respir Crit Care Med 163:A801 (Abst)
19. Le Gall JR, Klar J, Lemeshow S, et al (1996) The Logistic Organ Dysfunction system. A new way to assess organ dysfunction in the intensive care unit. ICU Scoring Group. JAMA 276:802–810
20. Afessa B, Spencer S, Khan W, et al (2001) Association of pulmonary artery catheter use with in-hospital mortality. Crit Care Med 29:1145–1148
21. Carson SS, Bach PB (2001) Predicting mortality in patients suffering from prolonged critical illness: an assessment of four severity-of-illness measures. Chest 120:928–933
22. Metnitz PG, Lang T, Valentin A, et al (2001) Evaluation of the logistic organ dysfunction system for the assessment of organ dysfunction and mortality in critically ill patients. Intensive Care Med 27:992–998
23. Timsit JF, Fosse JP, Troche G, et al (2001) Accuracy of a composite score using daily SAPS II and LOD scores for predicting hospital mortality in ICU patients hospitalized for more than 72 h. Intensive Care Med 27:1012–1021
24. Bernard GR (1997) The Brussels Score. Sepsis 1:43–44
25. Bernard GR, Doig G, Hudson LD, et al (1995) Quantification of organ failure for clinical trials and clinical practice. Am J Respir Crit Care Med 151:A323 (Abst)
26. Bernard G, Wheeler A, Russell J, et al (1997) The effects of ibuprofen on the physiology and survival of patients with sepsis. N Engl J Med 336:912–918

Severity of Illness Scoring Systems

J. A. S. Ball, J. W. Redman, and R. M. Grounds

"partial truths serve as more effective instruments of deception than lies"
attributed to Christopher Lasch (b. 1932), U.S. historian, educator [1]

▌ Introduction

Despite at least 20 years of evolution and with an ever-increasing number of systems, severity of illness quantification remains an imperfect and misused art. To many practicing clinicians the subject remains difficult and is often misinterpreted. Significant discrepancies exist between what these systems actually tell us and what we would like to know. Our aim in this chapter is to highlight these discrepancies and suggest, as have others, that new systems, developed in novel ways, are required if we want reliable answers to certain questions.

▌ A Brief History

The 1970s saw the publication of three of the forerunners to the general intensive care unit (ICU) severity of illness scoring systems: the first of these were the Therapeutic Intervention Scoring System (TISS) [2] (since revised [3–5]), a prognostic respiratory failure score [6], and the physiological stratification of postoperative ICU patients [7].

▌ Acute Physiological and Chronic Health Evaluation (APACHE) – 1981

The first severity of illness scoring system for general ICU patients was published by Knaus and colleagues in 1981 [8]. The APACHE system was designed to stratify patients prognostically by risk of in-hospital death. It utilizes 34 physiological variables assigned a value of 0–4 based on the degree of derangement from normal. The total numerical score, termed the acute physiology score (APS), is then assigned a premorbid health status category, A–D, based on a simple questionnaire. A panel of experts selected the elements of the numerical score and their weighting. The scoring values of physiological variables are the most deranged observed in the first 32 hours of ICU admission. The developers tested APACHE on 805 successive ICU admissions from two general ICUs in the US, excluding patients with acute myocardial infarction, burns, and total ICU stay < 16 hours. The data were collected between April and November 1979. The authors found a degree of correlation between the numerical score of these patients and both the probability of in-hospital death and the TISS score. They combined the numerical score, premorbid health category, age, sex, primarily organ system failure and operative status to calculate the predicted number of patients in their test population who would die in hospital, setting the cut off point as a >50% risk. Their method demonstrated a high sensitivity (97%) but a low specificity (49%). The authors state that APACHE was developed specifically to stratify patients into groups with an associated risk of mortality, not predict individual patient outcome. Knaus et al. also expressed the opinion that previous efforts at determining the efficacy of new therapies had been frustrated by the lack of an adequate ability to control for severity of illness and compare the outcomes from individual ICUs. They felt that their broad based severity of illness index could be used to improve the ability of non-randomized study designs to produce convincing evidence of efficacy. However, APACHE was criticized because unmeasured variables were considered to be normal and because the number of variables was excessive and could result in over fitting [9] (an error which reduces the performance of a scoring system because some of the variables will be correlated with the outcome by chance alone [10]).

▌ Simplified Acute Physiology Score (SAPS) – 1984

In 1984, Le Gall and colleagues published the SAPS [11]. This was designed to overcome some of the perceived problems inherent in the APS by simplifying the process. The authors selected the 13 most 'easily measured' physiological variables available in 90% of patients from a previous survey employing the APS score that they had conducted [12]. SAPS scores these variables (0–4) in an identical manner to the APS, adds a score for age (0–4), and replaces respiratory rate with a fixed score of 3 for patients receiving mechanical ventilation or continuous positive airways pressure (CPAP). The most abnormal values from the first 24 hours of ICU admission are taken as the scoring values. The authors tested SAPS on 679 unselected patients from eight French ICUs. Of note 30% of these patients were hospital transfers, which may have been usual at that time for French ICUs, but was far greater than UK and US ICUs. The authors compared the SAPS to the APS and a number of SAPS permutations. Using the Youden index (a method to establish the cut off point setting that gives the fewest false positives for the most true positives [13]) the authors determined the optimal cut off score to employ for in-hospital mortality for APS (14) and SAPS (12) in their data set. The summary statistics of their results are shown in Table 1.

Le Gall et al. concluded that SAPS performed at least as well if not better than APS but was more useful as it was much simpler. They stressed that SAPS is appli-

Table 1. Summary statistics of SAPS development data [11]

In-hospital Mortality Prediction	APS	SAPS	
Sensitivity	0.56	0.69	
Specificity	0.82	0.69	
126 prediction disagreements from 679 patients: Correct prediction	45	81	p<0.001

cable to a wide range of pathologies but that its predictive performance can only be applied to groups of patients, not individuals.

▌ APACHE II – 1985

In 1985, Knaus and colleagues refined their severity of illness scoring system with the publication of APACHE II [14]. They reduced the number of physiological variables from 34 to 12 by employing a multivariate analysis of the APS [15] utilizing a database of 5030 patients from 13 US ICUs (data collection 1979–82). Unlike the APS, all 12 variables must be scored in APACHE II. The total physiological derangement score is the sum of the individual scores (0–4) for each variable, except the Glasgow Coma Scale (GCS) where the score is 15 minus the GCS (see 'Neurological system failure' below). The most deranged value in the first 24 hours of ICU admission is used as the scoring value for each variable. The total physiological derangement score is added to a score for age (0–6 derived from [16, 17]) and a chronic health score for patients with severe organ insufficiency (2 or 5 dependant upon admission surgical status). The authors combined the resulting total APACHE II score with a list of 49 principal admission diagnoses to give a disease specific risk of hospital mortality. APACHE II performed well when tested on the developmental patient database, as judged by an area under the receiver operator characteristic (ROC) curve of 0.863 which compared favorably to the performance of APACHE on the same database, whose area under the ROC curve (AUROC) was 0.851 (AUROC is discussed below). However, when tested in a large population of ICU patients in the UK and Ireland (8796 patients from 26 ICUs, data collected 1992) the calibration statistic (the measure of how accurately the severity of illness scoring system predicts in-hospital mortality) demonstrated a significant difference between the model and test populations [18]. Since that study, a number of further investigations have demonstrated a similar phenomenon in a diverse number of ICU sub-populations including: elderly trauma patients [19], postoperative surgical patients [20], patients with myocardial infarction [21], patients with respiratory failure due to cardiogenic pulmonary edema [22], patients with cirrhosis [23], obstetric patients requiring intensive care [24], ICU patients treated with renal replacement therapies [25], patients receiving total parenteral nutrition [26], aquired immunodeficiency syndrome (AIDS) patients with respiratory failure [27] and a large cohort of medical ICU patients [28]. The explanations for these findings are discussed below.

▌ Mortality Probability Model (MPM) – 1985/8

In 1985, Lemeshow and colleagues published their first attempt at an outcome prediction model [29] based upon multiple logistic regression [30]. The authors had already published a precursor to this model in 1982 [31]. They repeated and extended the exercise three years later, deriving the MPM [32]. They collected up to 377 historical, demographic, physiological and other variables on 2644 consecutive ICU patients admitted to a single US ICU between 1983–85. They collected variables at ICU admission, and after 24 and 48 hours if the patient remained on ICU. They excluded coronary care, cardiac surgery, burns patients, and those < 14 years of age. Hospital mortality was chosen as the outcome variable. The authors devel-

Table 2. Development statistics for mortality prediction model [32]

Model	No. of patients model based on	No. of variables to calculate	Sensitivity	Specificity	Correct classification rate	p-value of C statistic
MPM_0	2644	11	44.8%	96.6%	86.5%	0.53
MPM_{24}	1666	14	56.1%	94.2%	84.9%	0.82
MPM_{48}	994	11	52.0%	90.3%	77.8%	0.35
MPM_{OT}	–	3*	58.7%	90.2%	80.1%	0.202

* MPM_{OT} is determined by the values of MPM_0, MPM_{24} and MPM_{48}

Table 3. Validation statistics for 948 ICU patients whose LOS was >48 hours [32]

Model	Sensitivity	Specificity	Correct classification rate	p-value of C statistic
MPM_0	42.0%	93.2%	76.7%	<0.001
MPM_{24}	56.4%	89.9%	79.1%	0.207
MPM_{48}	54.8%	90.2%	78.8%	0.285
MPM_{OT}	58.7%	90.2%	80.1%	0.202

oped four models: MPM_0 (probability of death from data collected at ICU admission), MPM_{24} (probability of death from data collected at 24 h), MPM_{48} (probability of death from data collected at 48 h), and MPM_{OT} (probability of death 'over time' based on MPM_0 and the change in probability between MPM_0 and MPM_{24}, and between MPM_{24} and MPM_{48}). The summary statistics from the development data and validation data of these models on the cohort of patients whose ICU length of stay (LOS) was greater than 48 hours are shown in Tables 2 and 3.

The authors enhanced the predictive value of MPM_{OT} by examining the direction of change between the successive MPM models. Patients whose probability of mortality started high and stayed high, or increased by >10% had a very high actual mortality. MPM, in common with APACHE, APACHE II and SAPS, has a low sensitivity (ability to predict those patients who are going to die) but a high specificity (ability to predict those who will live). Unsurprisingly, all bar one of the goodness of fit statistics have p values >0.05 (see calibration/goodness of fit section below). However, given the ~40% reduction in patient numbers between successive MPM models, the applicability of the MPM models, as judged by goodness of fit statistics, is likely to be poor where the case mix differs markedly from this single center US sample.

▋ Riyadh Intensive Care Program (RIP) – 1988

This program [33, 34] tries to define changes in physiology (obtained from daily APACHE II data) that reflect organ failure or dysfunction and then uses the organ failure score by employing a series of algorithms to recognize changes incompatible with survival. This is a conceptually different scoring system in that it tries to recognize organ system failure and link this to outcome. However, in a validation study in the UK [35] this demonstrated a sensitivity of only 23.4% with a specificity of 99.8. In a second study conducted to assess this severity of illness scoring system, Rogers et al. were unable to avoid a false prediction of death with any useful sensitivity [36]. Some of the reasons for the failure of the RIP system are addressed in the APACHE III section below.

▌ APACHE III – 1991

In 1991, Knaus and colleagues published a further refinement to their severity of illness scoring system, termed APACHE III [37]. The authors started by assembling a much larger database of 17 440 patients' data, from 42 US ICUs, in 40 hospitals, between 1988–90. The hospitals were chosen by complex random selection to avoid geographical bias. Each unit contributed roughly the same number of patient datasets (299–449) in order that the database be a truly representative sample of US ICU patients. They excluded patients admitted to the ICU for < 4 h, burns patients, patients aged less than 16 yrs of age, and patients admitted with chest pain for coronary care. They collected data on coronary artery bypass graft (CABG) patients but analyzed these separately [38]. They rigorously ensured the accuracy of data collection. They then analyzed this database using multivariate logistic regression [39]. Turning first to the physiological derangement component of their score, their analysis resulted in the addition of 5 variables to the APACHE II set, taking the total to 17. The weighting of these variables was dramatically altered with a marked increase in complexity. The most deranged value in the first 24 hours remains the value of each variable scored. The authors re-weighted age and derived an extended chronic health/co-morbidity score. They also found that the origin and timing of patient selection for ICU admission had a major prognostic influence (see 'Lead time bias' section below) and thus these variables became incorporated into the final score. As with APACHE II, patients were assigned to a disease category based upon their perceived primary diagnostic reason for ICU admission. The number of categories was increased from 49 to 78. The authors' claim that the coefficients generated by this allocation permits calculation of a group or individual risk of hospital mortality. However, critics of this approach suggest that specifying a single 'most important' diagnosis for a complex patient relies too heavily on information that cannot be collected with acceptable reliability [40]. In addition, developing, in effect, a separate model for each primary diagnosis reduces the performance of the model as a whole by basing each co-efficient on data from a comparatively small number of patients. That the APACHE approach is superior to a more general model (see MPM II below) for patients within a disease category has yet to be demonstrated [40].

Using a complex development and validation protocol in which a random selection of the database was used for the development of the system and the resulting model then tested on the remainder [41], the authors determined the sensitivity, specificity, and percentage correct classification to be 50.4, 96.3 and 88.1%, respectively (with the cut off threshold set at a predicted risk of mortality of 50%). As discussed in the MPM section above, the low sensitivity of this model must limit its application. Despite this, the authors found the model equally effective when applied across the range of their sampled ICUs individually, despite mortality rates varying from 6 to 42%. The authors also stress the discriminatory performance of APACHE III whose AUROC for their dataset was 0.90. Of note, the authors give no calibration statistics for their model. Interestingly, they compare this to four studies in which physician estimates of outcome prediction achieve AUROCs of 0.84–0.89 [42–45] yet they try to defend the greater value of APACHE III by claiming its superior reliability and credibility. The authors do stress the limitations of the APACHE III model, which warrant repetition. First, an APACHE III score can be used alone (i.e., without defining the primary disease) only within homogeneous disease categories and then, for severity stratification, not hospital mortality prediction. Second, mortality prediction must control for the origin and timing of patient selection for ICU admission. Third, an APACHE III score can only be predictive of mortality if the scoring variables are taken from the first 24 hours of ICU admission. To address the issue of response to treatment, the authors developed a re-weighted equation for second and later ICU days that, when compared to the first day score, can predict hospital mortality for the day of measurement. As with the MPM model, the trend of changing probability is itself prognostic.

Independent validation of APACHE III has been undertaken by a number of studies looking at large cohorts of general ICU patients in the southern UK [46, 47], Scotland [48], Spain [49], Brazil [50], and the US [51, 52]. All of these studies found APACHE III discrimination performance to be acceptable (AUROC > 0.8) but all also found calibration to be inadequate with the p value of the C statistic to be < 0.01, with predicted mortality consistently less than observed (for a fuller explanation of this see the 'Statistical considerations' section below).

▌ SAPS II – 1993

In 1993, Le Gall and colleagues published a refined version of their severity of illness scoring system, termed SAPS II [53]. As with the development of APACHE III, the authors first constructed a large database. They collected 37 variables from 12,997 ICU patients, from 137 hospitals, in 10 European and two North American Countries. The scoring value of these variables was the most deranged recorded in the first 24 hours of ICU admission. All consecutive ICU admissions, ≥18 years of age, over a 4 month period (1991–92), were included, with the exception of cardiac surgical, coronary care and burns patients. They randomly selected 65% of this database (8,396 patients) to be used to develop the SAPS II model, leaving the remaining 35% (4,628 patients) to be used to validate the model. The 37 variables were reduced down to 17 (12 physiological, age, type of admission and three chronic health diagnoses) three more than SAPS. The weighting for each variable was calculated using the LOWESS method [54]. Multiple logistic regression analysis was performed to derive an equation for converting the SAPS II score into a probability of hospital mortality. The resulting model was tested on the development and validation groups, the discrimination and calibration statistics are shown in Table 4. Le Gall et al. argue that the main advantage of SAPS II over APACHE III is the ability to accurately predict mortality in stratified groups of patients without recourse to defining a single diagnosis, which is often only possible in a minority of patients [55] (see also further discussion below). The authors also council great caution in interpreting failure of the SAPS II model in predicting mortality as a number of explanations, most especially an inadequate calibration to the test data, may render it inapplicable. They clearly state that SAPS II is incapable of predicting outcomes for individual patients.

Table 4. Discrimination and calibration statistics for SAPS II [53]

	Development AUROC	Validation AUROC	Development Calibration	Validation Calibration
SAPS II	0.88	0.86	$p = 0.883$	$p = 0.104$

Independent Validation Studies

Despite the impressive discrimination and calibration statistics achieved by the SAPS II model on the original development and validation data, tests on independent validation data have almost universally shown poor calibration. Of 12 large studies only two [56, 57] were well matched to the SAPS II model, the remainder were not [58–67]. Of note, seven of these studies also found poor calibration with APACHE II [48, 60, 63–67] and four found poor calibration with MPM II [62, 64, 65, 67].

▌ MPM II – 1993/4

In 1993, Lemeshow and colleagues published a revision of their MPM model termed MPM II [40]. They employed a near identical method to that they had used in developing MPM. However, they applied this to the SAPS II development/validation database to which they added a data set from six US ICUs. They excluded patients ≤18 years of age, with burns, requiring coronary care or cardiac surgery, or who were ICU re-admissions. Data collection took place in 1990-92 with quality controls. As in APACHE III, the authors randomly split their database using 12 610 patients' data to construct MPM II_0 leaving 6514 patients' data for the resulting model to be validated on. The authors initially developed an MPM II_0 and MPM II_{24} deciding to temporarily abandon the MPM_{48} and MPM_{OT} from their previous model. MPM II_0 was determined by 15 variables measured at ICU admission, three physiology (two cardiovascular, one neurological), three chronic disease, five acute diagnoses, age, cardiopulmonary resuscitation (CPR) prior to admission, mechanical ventilation and non-elective surgery. The discrimination and calibration statistics of the development and validation data are shown in Table 5. Using their method, the authors found that patients alive but still requiring to be on ICU at 24 hours differed markedly in the odds ratios of their MPM II_0 variables from patients who had either died or been discharged. They therefore developed MPM II_{24} using the reduced data set of 10,357 patients still on ICU at 24 hours, 312 patients having died and 1,941 discharged. MPM II_{24} was determined by five of the variables collected for MPM II_0 with the addition of eight new variables collected at 24 hours. MPM II_{24} was validated on a sample of 5568 patients, the discrimination and calibration statistics are shown in Table 5. The authors propose that MPM II utilizes 15/23 variables that are clearly and objectively defined and routinely evaluated on most ICU patients. They emphasize that MPM II_{24} is a companion model to MPM II_0 and represents a different population of patients. This approach, they argue, exposes one of the main weaknesses of the APACHE and SAPS models, which take the worst data from the first 24 hours of ICU admission but fail to differentiate between the two populations observed by Lemeshow and colleagues. The authors also demonstrate a clarity in the assessment and presentation of their model's perfor-

Table 5. Discrimination and calibration statistics for MPM II [40, 69]

	Development AUROC	Validation AUROC	Development Calibration	Validation Calibration
MPM II_0	0.837	0.824	p=0.623	p=0.327
MPM II_{24}	0.844	0.836	p=0.764	p=0.231
MPM II_{48}	0.812	0.796	p=0.308	p=0.591
MPM II_{72}	0.794	0.752	p=0.311	p=0.408

mance (Table 5) following the consensus research and devlopment (RAND) guidelines [68]. These support the complimentary roles of calibration and discrimination statistics (see 'Statistical considerations' section below). Of note, when the authors tested the original MPM on their validation database they found the calibration p values to be <0.001. The explanation for the lack of fit almost certainly rests with the developmental data for MPM, which was derived from only a single US ICU.

The following year, Lemeshow and colleagues published two further models based upon their data set, MPM II_{48} and MPM II_{78} [69]. Both these models use the same 13 variables as MPM II_{24}. The co-efficients for these variables in the logistic regression equation are essentially unchanged with only the constant in need of re-calculation. As with the earlier MPM II models, the available data were split into development and validation cohorts. The values of the discrimination and calibration statistics are shown in Table 5. Lemeshow et al. re-enforce the point that the probability of dieing changes with time, such that an APACHE or SAPS score is only valid at 24 hours of ICU admission. They also emphasize that an ICU patient whose condition fails to change day after day is in fact deteriorating and has an increasing risk of dieing. This well recognized clinical phenomenon is accurately modeled over the first 72 hours of their ICU stay by MPM II. The same cannot be said for sequential APACHE II as amply demonstrated by the RIP model (see above). The authors describe an on-going process to develop MPM II models for successive time points beyond 72 hours though currently these are not available.

▌ First 7 ICU days serial APACHE III – 1994

In 1994, the APACHE group published the next phase of their developing severity of illness scoring system [70]. Using the original APACHE III development/validation database (see above for details) they examined the nature and effect of daily changes in the APS component of their score on the risk of ICU and hospital mortality. They developed a series of multiple logistic regression equations based on the premise that the changes in the APS would reflect the patient's response (or lack of it) to therapy, which is clearly of critical prognostic importance. They hypothesized that the daily APS component of the risk equation would be given by the formula:

daily risk = day 1 APS + current day APS + change in APS since yesterday

When added to the remaining patient variables included in the APACHE III score, the coefficients of each variable were established, resulting in prediction equations for days 1–7 of ICU admission. In view of the fact that these equations had not undergone stepwise variable selection (employed in the development of the day 1 APACHE III model), a grouped jackknife approach [71] was employed to avoid statistical over fitting [10]. This complex process involves dividing patients into subsets by randomization and by performing multivariable analysis on 9 out of every 10 to predict the outcome from the tenth. This analysis demonstrated that day 1 APS remains a significant predictor of hospital mortality, but its relative influence decreases dramatically over time (for example by day 3 its relative contribution to risk is only 5%). The current day APS (which must be measured retrospectively as scoring values are the most deranged in any 24 hour period) is by far, the single most important variable (for example its relative contribution to risk is 54.2% on day 3 with primary disease contributing 15%, age 13.3%, and so on). The relative relationship of these variables remains fairly constant over time. The discriminatory power of the resulting predictions when applied to this developmental/validation dataset, as measured by the AUROC, deteriorate from 0.90 for day 1 scores to 0.84 for day 6 and 7 scores. Although a calibration curve is presented in the paper, which appears to demonstrate good calibration, no goodness of fit statistics are quoted. This model agrees with the clinical finding that not only worsening APS but also constant APS scores over time are associated with an increased risk of hospital mortality. The authors acknowledge that the performance of their model requires independent validation before widespread clinical acceptance is achieved, to our knowledge this has not been performed and published. They also acknowledge that periodic recalculation of the regression equations on future population samples will be necessary to maintain the accuracy of the model. Despite its apparent performance and no doubt the ability of the authors to extend the model beyond day 7, daily APACHE III scoring remains in the research arena only. Due to the financial nature of this scoring system, its complexity, and apparent lack of independent validation, corrected daily scoring using this model is likely to remain outside mainstream practice for the foreseeable future.

▌ Multiple Organ Dysfunction (MOD) Score – 1995

It has long been recognized that the hallmark of critical illness is the evolution of multiple organ dysfunction syndrome. Although this may be the presenting complaint of a patient admitted to ICU it is often seen to develop in the days following admission. Serial estimates of disease severity have much broader application than mortality prediction and yet none of the above models is capable of accurately performing this task (with the possible exception of the first 7 days APACHE III model described above). Indeed, as was demonstrated by the MPM authors, the population of patients who require ICU for several days are poorly modeled by severity of illness scoring systems taken only once, after the first 24 hours. Despite this, serial measurements of APACHE II and SAPS II are widespread in the literature and clinical practice. Serial organ failure scores share a parallel history with the severity of illness scoring systems described above with at least six published methodologies prior to 1995 [72–77] though none have gained the widespread use of the severity of illness scoring systems. In 1995, Marshall and colleagues published the MOD score [78]. They performed a systematic search of the literature in order to identify a panel of the best variables for describing dysfunction in each of the major organ systems. They then prospectively collected patient data from a single surgical ICU with all consecutive admissions of >24 h included. They developed their scoring system on 336 patients whose data was collected 1988–89. They then validated their model on a further sample collected 1989–90. They statistically determined one optimal variable for each of the six major organ systems (neurological, cardiovascular, respiratory, renal, hepatic and hematological) by examining the differences between survivors and non-survivors in their development data set. They then weighted values of these variables by examining the correlation between individual organ dysfunction and ICU mortality, with each variable scoring 0–4. The chosen variables were GCS, pressure adjusted heart rate (HR×CVP/MAP), PaO_2/FiO_2, serum creatinine, serum bilirubin, and platelet count. Scoring values for the first 3 continuous variables were taken at a fixed time point on a daily basis. The scores for each organ are summed to produce the total MOD score (0–24). When tested on their validation sample, the authors found that both the number and severity of organ dysfunction, at any time point, as measured by their model, correlated closely with ICU mortality. In common with MPM, neurological failure had by far, the largest effect on predictive capacity. The admission score, maximum score and upward trend of the sequential score all correlated with ICU mortality. Logistic regression determined that an increasing MOD score after ICU admission is a more important determinant of outcome than admission MOD score. In addition, the admission MOD score demonstrated better predictive power than the APACHE II score in these patients. The AUROCs for the MOD score in the development and validation samples were 0.936 and 0.928 respectively, demonstrating the excellent discriminatory ability of this model in this population, though of note, no goodness of fit measure was performed. The authors stress that the MOD score is designed to be used as an outcome measure for patients with the multiple organ dysfunction syndrome rather than a predictive index. There are a number of significant weaknesses in this model: the development and validity samples were small and taken from a single surgical ICU; and the resulting case mix has a significantly lower mortality and lower median MOD score than a general ICU population. However, the principle and method are robust and the resulting model has clear advantages over the severity of scoring systems described above.

In a small independent validation study, Jacobs et al. compared daily MOD scores to daily APACHE II scores in 39 septic shock patients from one Saudi Arabian ICU [79]. Though methodologically flawed, as daily APACHE II scoring has previously been demonstrated to perform very poorly, the authors found that maximum MOD score and the maximum change in score from admission both discriminated very well between survivors and non-survivors whereas APACHE II did not.

The original authors have just published a minor revision to their system following application of the MOD score to 1200 patients, mechanically ventilated for >48 hours from 16 Canadian ICUs [80]. They have abandoned the pressure-adjusted heart rate in favor of a mixed cardiovascular score based on heart rate, use of inotropes and serum lactate. Their detailed analysis of the results of daily scoring demonstrate the prognostic insights gained by adopting their system. Whether this improvement in the understanding of the evolution of the multiple organ dysfunction syndrome can be translated into improvements in therapies/outcomes remains to be seen, but at least we appear to have a valid and simple monitoring tool.

■ The Logistic Organ Dysfunction (LOD) System – 1996

In response to the development of the MOD score, the SAPS group developed the LOD score [81]. Taking the SAPS II patient database, they examined the predictive capacity of 12 variables from the same six organ systems as the MOD score. They took the worst values from the first 24 hours of ICU admission. They applied the same exclusion criteria and undertook an identical methodology as they had for the development of SAPS II. Their derived model uses 12 variables from which a score of 0, 1, 3 or 5 (neuro, cardiac and renal only) is attributed to each of the six organ systems, the sum of which represent the LOD score (0–22). A reference table converts the score to a probability of hospital mortality, the relationship being sigmoid. The discrimination and validation statistics for the developmental and validation groups are shown in Table 6.

The LOD score aims to achieve similar goals to the MOD score, namely, to qualitatively and quantitatively describe organ dysfunction. The goal is to provide a tool that can itself provide a useful outcome measure (e.g., improvement/resolution of organ dysfunction) rather than merely predicting mortality. The strengths of the LOD score over the MOD score rest in the significantly larger developmental database, whose case mix, as evidenced by the proportion of patients with ≥2 organ failures (LOD 62%, MOD 17%), was far more representative of the general ICU population. This, coupled with the statistical method employed to derive the weighting of the variables, should result in the LOD score fitting (statistically) a larger proportion of ICU patients. However, the LOD score was developed using only data from the first 24 hours of ICU admission from all patients, which has been shown not to be representative of patients who require >24 hours of ICU care, whereas the MOD score developmental database was establish on patients who were admitted for >24 hours. The authors council that the LOD score model requires validating as a daily measure before it can be appropriately used as a prediction/assessment tool. They also suggest that the optimal timing for the recording of continuous variables (fixed time of day vs. worst in a defined 24 hour period) must be established. Finally, the authors emphasize the need for the weighting calculations to be periodically updated to ensure the validity of the LOD model.

Metnitz and colleagues tested the LOD score on 2893 consecutive ICU admissions to 13 Austrian ICUs [82]. They excluded patients <18 yrs of age, those missing vital data, and all re-admissions. LOD score on the first ICU day (LOD_1) they found was highly predictive of hospital mortality. They found the model as a whole had good discrimination but poor calibration. Accordingly, they customized the model by performing multiple logistic regression, which resulted in a satisfactory fit. The authors also measured LOD scores on some patients on some successive days. They then integrated and weighted these scores to see if this improved the predictive value. However, despite the customization of the model, the calibration remained poor though apparent discriminatory performance improved. In essence,

Table 6. Discrimination and calibration statistics for the LOD score [81]

	Development AUROC	Validation AUROC	Development Calibration	Validation Calibration
LOD score	0.843	0.850	p = 0.21	p = 0.50

all this study proves is that like SAPS II, the calibration of the LOD score for mortality prediction is problematic. No useful conclusions can be drawn regarding the utility of sequential LOD score measurement.

▌ Sequential (Formerly Sepsis-related) Organ Failure Assessment (SOFA) Score – 1996

In 1996, a working group of the ESICM met and published a consensus scoring system very similar to the MOD score [83]. They chose to use the same six organ systems and variables with the exception of the cardiovascular system, failure of which they defined by the requirement for, and dose of, adrenergic drugs. They copied the 0–4 weighting for the variables but modified the ranges based upon a literature review. They elected to use the most deranged value in a defined 24-hour period as the scoring value for each variable instead of the values at a fixed time point. To validate their system, the group prospectively collected daily SOFA scores on all ICU admissions >12 years of age, during May 1995, in 40 European ICUs in 16 countries. In addition they recorded the proven presence of infection. The only exclusions were patients who stayed in ICU <48 hours after uncomplicated surgery. Analyses of this data set were published between 1998–2000 [84–87]. Analysis of daily SOFA scores in this sample of patients found a statistically significant difference between survivors and non-survivors (at ICU discharge), in the mean score for each organ system and total score. The number of failing organs (defined as any organ system scoring ≥3) and/or severity of organ dysfunction all correlated with mortality. The presence of infection increased the mean score both for each organ and the total score. Maximum SOFA score also correlated with mortality and exhibited the best discriminative accuracy (AUROC 0.847). Overall, the SOFA score exhibited poor sensitivity but excellent specificity, like all of its predecessors. Of note, analysis of the relative contributions of the individual organ systems found the cardiovascular system to have the highest relative contribution, suggesting perhaps that the SOFA definition is superior to the original MOD score variable of pressure adjusted heart rate. The authors conclude that SOFA is a valid tool whose simplicity is a clear advantage over the other severity of illness scoring systems.

There are at least five published studies that have since examined the utility and accuracy of the SOFA score [88–92]. All have found that maximum SOFA score and increasing SOFA score are highly prognostic. In the only study to compare systems, Janssens and colleagues graphically demonstrate the value of SOFA over SAPS II [89]. Given that there is little to differentiate between SOFA and the newly modified MOD score, the unification of this approach would appear both sensible and timely.

▌ Composite SAPS II and LOD Score – 2000

In 2000, a further attempt to improve the performance of SAPS II/LOD score was undertaken by Timsit and colleagues [93]. They set out to produce a severity of illness scoring system that would accurately predict mortality in ICU patients who acquire nosocomial infections following admission to ICU (by definition >72 h following admission). They prospectively collected chronic health status, admission diagnosis and type, in addition to SAPS II and LOD scores on days 1, 2 and 3 of

Table 7. Discrimination and calibration statistics for composite SAPS II/LOD score [93]

	Development AUROC	Validation AUROC	Development Calibration	Validation Calibration
Composite score	0.794	0.826	p = 0.70	p = 0.55

ICU admission from 893 patients (10 French ICUs). They performed multivariable logistic regression on this data employing a highly complex protocol. Most notably, to avoid statistical over fitting [10] only the directions of change between scores on successive days were used as independent variables in the regression process, not the scores themselves. They derived a predictive equation, which they then tested on 312 patients from 24 separate French ICUs. The discrimination and calibration statistics for the developmental and validation data sets are shown in Table 7.

Although extremely complex, the authors' approach appears to deliver a model with a good fit in an independent validation dataset. The discrimination however is borderline (see statistics section below). They also performed MPM II$_{72}$ scoring on their datasets and found a similar discriminatory performance but a significantly worse calibration. Sadly, serial APACHE III scoring was not performed so no comparison can be made. The authors comment that they could have employed the MOD or SOFA scores (see below) but did not as neither of these are designed for predicting mortality. It remains unclear, to us at least, how Timsit et al. can justify the use of their complex model over the comparatively simplistic MOD or SOFA scores given that the discriminatory ability of their model is far too weak for it to be usefully employed for any other means than group stratification.

▌ Statistical Considerations

The development of scoring systems involves a complex combination of clinical acumen and advanced statistical techniques. Before they can be introduced into clinical practice they must be rigorously assessed in terms of accuracy, reliability, content validity, and methodological rigor [9]. Most of the scoring systems are first derived from a database of patients and their various physiological measurements during their ICU stay. This database is retrospectively analyzed (stepwise regression analysis) to find which of the selected variables are the most predictive of a chosen outcome, usually hospital mortality. However, although easily measured, hospital mortality can be highly misleading as discharge practices vary between hospitals and regions, and can all too easily be manipulated to influence assessment [52, 94, 95]. Having identified the physiological variables that appear to be the most predictive, their reference ranges and relative contribution, when combined, are quantified to produce weighting. The weighted variables are then combined to give a composite score. The accuracy of the model must then be tested prospectively against an independent cohort of patients. In many of the above models the original data set is randomly split into developmental and validation cohorts. The testing of a model on such a validation cohort cannot be considered to represent independent validation as the sample size and the randomization process used to select this cohort from the starting database make it inevitable that the developmental and validation samples perform interchangeably.

Accuracy is determined by two measures, calibration and discrimination. Calibration (goodness of fit) examines the scoring systems ability to predict mortality over the entire range of its values whilst discrimination determines how well the model differentiates survivors from non-survivors. Calibration is most often tested using a goodness of fit method, most commonly the Hosmer-Lemeshow C statistic [96]. The lower the value of the C statistic and hence the higher the p value (which represents the probability that the model and the test data are different) the better the model fits the data. Discrimination is usually tested using the AUROC. This ranges from 0.5 (no discrimination other than by chance alone) to 1.0 (perfect discrimination). For survival prediction models, most medical statisticians consider that the AUROC must be greater than 0.9 for the model to possess reliable discrimination. If the AUROC is greater than 0.8 but less than 0.9 then the model should only be interpreted in the light of additional clinical information. Any model with a AUROC of less than 0.8 has little or no discriminating value and certainly should not be used to make life or death decisions on individual patients (Bland J.M., personal communication). While most of the ICU scoring systems have an AUROC of > 0.8 when tested on their original database, none has an AUROC of greater than 0.9. Furthermore, the AUROC of all of these scoring systems falls when they are tested on patient populations other than those used to derive the original database. As alluded to above, calibration and discrimination are complementary such that a model whose AUROC is 0.90 but calibration p value is < 0.05 cannot be assumed to be a good model [40]. Comparison can be made between the AUROCs of two systems tested on the same data, however this requires the confidence intervals to be stated [97, 98]. Unfortunately, the majority of papers describing the above scoring systems omit one or more of the vital statistics needed to assess their performance. This had led editorialists to call for the establishment of consensus guidelines for the development and validation of scoring systems [99]. Regrettably, action is still awaited on this matter.

In addition to accuracy, reliability (both inter and intra observer variability) needs to be assessed in any new scoring system [9]. Although many authorities suggest that a coefficient of reliability of 0.7 (implying that up to 30% of scores may be inaccurate) is acceptable, most medical statisticians agree that the coefficient of reliability should be > 0.9 for any scoring system to be employed as a reliable guide to the appropriate initiation or termination of treatment [100], a claim made for a number of the severity of illness scoring systems whose performance has been shown to often fall below this level.

▌ Standardized Mortality Ratios (SMRs)

The SMR is the ratio of observed deaths to the number of deaths predicted by a severity of illness scoring system and has been recommended, and employed, as a method for comparing outcomes between two or more groups or ICUs. If your SMR is 1 then your outcome is as the severity of illness scoring system predicts, if it is greater than 1 then you have excess mortality and by implication, worse performance. Similarly if your SMR is less than 1, you exhibit a reduced mortality and by implication better performance. Thus to be useful, the SMR relies upon the accuracy of the severity of illness scoring system's prediction. However, the paradox of SMR is that the more accurate the scoring system, the more accurate will be the prediction of outcome and the more the SMR will tend towards 1. Take the most extreme example, that of a patient in ICU who is murdered by his doctor. If the scoring system is always accurate it will predict this death and thus the SMR will still be 1. It is also essential to consider the confidence intervals of any given SMR, as no conclusions can be drawn from SMR comparison if these overlap.

The SMR generated by the APACHE II system was reputed to equate with independent measures of performance and quality of care [101]. However, comparison by Boyd and Grounds [102] of the SMR for the 13 hospitals that contributed to the original APACHE II database demonstrated that SMRs >1 were generated by both level I and level III hospitals and that there was no clear relationship between supposed quality units (Teaching Hospitals) and SMR. Zimmerman and colleagues [103] later showed that there was no difference in SMR between 20 ICUs in 18 Teaching Hospitals and 17 ICUs in non-teaching hospitals. In the same year, Zimmerman et al. [104] performed a much more detailed study comparing SMRs from 9 of 42 hospitals in the APACHE III database with a quality care ranking performed by an experienced clinical investigation team. Once again there was no data to suggest that SMR was able to quantify performance. These data suggested that either the assessment team was unable to assess ICU performance or that SMR was not able to quantify performance or that neither method was of any use [105].

▌ Known Problems Associated with Current Scoring Systems in the ICU

There are a number of problems associated with ICU severity of illness scoring systems that may lead to inaccuracies and possible misinterpretations. Some of the main issues will be highlighted below.

Inaccuracy of Data Collection

All of the severity of illness scoring systems require the accurate collection and interpretation of the physiological and demographic data. Most of the developmental studies have expended considerable effort to ensure and measure data accuracy. However, the assumption that the data collection process in the real world would achieve the levels of accuracy demonstrated in the development studies of the severity of illness scoring systems is extremely optimistic. For example, in one of the independent APACHE III validation studies, Pappachan et al. [47] audited 20% of all data on their database for accuracy of entry and interpretation by reference to the patients original case notes and ICU records. The authors showed that between 9 and 18% of all data collected was inaccurate.

A study into the effects of minor inaccuracies in data recording was conducted by Goldhill and Withington [106]. They showed very clearly that small changes in the score obtained for APACHE II could lead to very significant differences in the predicted outcome of their ICU patients. From their database of 11,348 patients, they showed that their SMR, compared with that of the APACHE II database, was 1.13. However by increasing the APACHE II score by 2 or 4 points they showed that their SMR would decrease to 1.0 and 0.89 respectively. Conversely, by decreasing the APACHE II score by 2 or 4 increased the SMR to 1.27 and 1.44. They pointed out that relatively minor and frequent physiological abnormalities make a significant contribution to APACHE II score. For example if the mean arterial blood pressure falls below 70 mmHg, the heart rate below 70 beat per min, or the hemoglobin below 10 g/dl at least two points are scored.

The Effects of Automated Charting and High Sampling Frequencies

To add further insult to injury, automated charting of most physiological variables is now possible and increasingly used. This creates the problem of outlying data point handling. For example, what happens to the blood pressure values when the arterial line is occluded to permit blood sampling, or the central venous pressure (CVP) values when the transducer falls to the floor? This was examined in a study by Bosman et al. [107], who showed that using automated charting to acquire the most abnormal physiological values for severity of illness scores resulted in a 15% increase in the predicted mortality using APACHE II, a 25% increase using SAPS II, and a 24% increase using MPM_0. This finding has been confirmed more recently in a study by Suistomaa et al. [108] showing that increasing the sampling rate for physiological variables results in higher scores and lower SMRs.

Neurological System Failure

In addition to the above points regarding the accuracy of data collection, special consideration of the neurological system assessment in severity of illness scoring systems, is warranted. Most scoring systems use the GCS [109] or include data from the GCS to assess the degree of neurological system failure. Furthermore, the GCS frequently makes up a large component of the APS or equivalent. For example, GCS constitutes 25% of the physiological score in APACHE II, 20% in APACHE III and 22% in SAPS II. The explanation for this factor, is that in multivariant analysis of admission physiological variables, GCS is often the most highly predictive of hospital mortality [29]. It is vitally important therefore that the score is performed accurately and consistently. It has been recognized [110] that the reliability of the GCS scoring is quite variable, largely due to difficulties in interpreting level of consciousness when patients are sedated. The Scottish Intensive Care Society Audit Group [58] has assessed measurement of GCS and the effect of scoring GCS on the performance of APACHE II and APACHE III. They showed that for many of the patients in their study the APACHE II and/or the APACHE III score changed markedly, dependent on whether the patient's GCS was scored prior to sedation and artificial ventilation or once the patient was sedated and ventilated. Of note, two studies, one in patients with acute head injury [111], the other in patients with non-traumatic coma [112], demonstrated that GCS performed better as a predictor of hospital mortality than APACHE II or APACHE III.

Lead-time Bias

Lead-time bias refers to the effect on outcome prediction caused by appropriate treatment and resuscitation prior to ICU admission [113]. Bion et al. showed that patients who were stabilized and resuscitated prior to transfer to a tertiary center ICU had significantly lower APACHE II scores than patients, who had not been properly prepared. As a consequence, those patients who had been properly prepared for transfer, had a higher than expected SMR. Bion et al. argue that the treatment prior to admission reduces the APACHE II score but cannot alter the severity of the acute precipitating insult, thus causing an increase in the SMR. In 1989, Dragsted and colleagues reported on the admission of 432 patients to Danish ICUs [114]. They found that the mortality rate for hospital 1 was 28.7% (predicted 25.7%) and that the mortality rate for hospital 2 was 39.8% (predicted 26.6%). On investigation, they discovered that in hospital 2, 35% of the patients admitted to the ICU were transfers in from other ICUs. They suggested that this caused an adverse selection and lead-time bias for the patients at hospital 2. This conclusion is supported by the findings of Tunnell et al. [115], who measured the APACHE II, APACHE III, and the SAPS II scores in 76 ICU patients. Their study showed that the inclusion of data collected in the period prior to admission significantly increased the severity of illness score and estimated risk of death for all three scoring systems; the biggest effect being seen in medical patients, who had languished on the wards prior to ICU admission. It must be assumed that treatment before admission can affect outcome and it outlines the importance of establishing zero-time. Clearly, the second and third generation severity of illness scoring systems make some allowance for this phenomenon, in particular, APACHE III, however, whether this offers sufficient compensation remains to be proved.

Cross Cultural Application, the Accuracy of Predictions for Specific Disease Groups, and the Effect of Changes in Practice over Time

Can a severity of illness scoring system, developed and validated on data sampled from a general ICU population in the US in 1988, be accurate when applied to a UK, European, or other national population group in 2002? Equally, can severity of illness scoring system models developed from a general ICU population be accurate when applied to a group of patients with a specific disease. As alluded to above, these questions come down to calibration. As described above, in the vast majority of published studies that have aimed to test these questions using one or more of the severity of illness scoring systems, the calibration of models has been unacceptably poor, hence any meaningful comparisons cannot be made.

Treatment Effects

The whole aim of intensive care is to maintain the patient in a state of normal physiology while treatment can be commenced and the body effects healing. Thus for example, we institute mechanical ventilation in a patient with pneumonia to maintain normal oxygenation and thereby facilitate tissue oxygen delivery whilst the combination of antibiotics and the body's immune system control and eradicate the bacteria causing the pneumonia and then heal the underlying lung tissue damage. The aim of intensive care during this period is to maintain normal physiological function as judged by the measured physiological indices. It is intuitively obvious however, that a patient who has normal blood gas measurements when being artificial ventilated with 100% oxygen and 20 cmH$_2$O of positive end-expiratory pressure (PEEP) is considerably more likely to die than a patient with normal blood gases who is breathing air spontaneously. Similarly, a patient who is receiving an epinephrine infusion of 1 µg/kg/min to maintain a normal blood pressure is quite clearly more likely to die a patient who has can maintain normal blood pressure without one. However, many of the severity of illness scoring systems are deliberately designed to ignore all treatment effects and hence cannot discriminate between such patients. In both examples, any member of the public could probably guess who was most likely to die but certain of the scoring systems that are currently in use would give them roughly the same probability of death. Daily scoring with validated systems overcomes much of this problem [70, 80, 86].

▌ Conclusion

At present, APACHE II and SAPS II scoring systems are widely used and frequently considered accurate. Indeed they are considered by some to have "revolutionized intensive care" [9]. However, the case for continuing to use them and the other severity of illness scoring systems, whose accuracy is in fact at best questionable, especially when applied beyond the first 24 hours of ICU admission, is, we believe, on the basis of the above arguments, unjustifiable. That leaves us with the choice between the complexity of the serial APACHE III or the composite SAPS II/LOD score or the simplicity of the SOFA/MOD scores (now almost indistinguishable from each other). In the absence of good independent validation of either of the complex systems and the fact that, although not tested head to head on the same data, the apparent predictive ability of the simplistic scores is close if not equal to that of the complex scores, the justification for using serial APACHE III or the composite SAPS II and LOD score is not apparent, at least not to us. However, neither the SOFA nor the MOD score are accurate enough to answer all of the questions we want answers to, namely: How well is my ICU performing, what could I do to improve the performance, and what are the most efficacious treatments for my patients? Given the vast amount of time and effort that has already been poured into the pursuit of the perfect severity of illness scoring system it would appear far too few lessons have been learned. Two recent editorials [116, 117] suggest that those of us disenchanted with the available severity of illness scoring systems are not alone. To take a case in point, the experience of the Cleveland Health Quality Choice Coalition initiative [52, 94], which employed both standard and customized APACHE III scoring to evaluate the performance of 38 ICUs in 28 Cleveland hospitals, stands as a testament to the hazards of employing severity of illness scoring systems. This experience demonstrated that using hospital mortality as an outcome measure could be subverted by changes in discharge practice; the confidence intervals around the generated SMRs were too wide to facilitate the identification of better performing ICUs because, despite its complexity, APACHE III was insufficiently accurate. Thus, after expending a massive amount of resources on what we believe was already known to be a flawed methodology, this initiative was abandoned without any clear benefit having been gained [94].

Both of these editorials [116, 117] suggest ways forward, in essence starting from scratch and developing complex multidimensional models. However, the insightful question is also raised as to whether we possess the knowledge, and perhaps more importantly, the will to do this? If we do, then surely the time has come to abandon the flawed models and concentrate on such development. If not, then at least we should publicize the weaknesses of the current models and limit their use to the few applications to which they are valid.

References

1. Lasch C (1979) The Culture of Narcissism: American Life in an Age of Diminishing Expectations, WW Norton, New York
2. Cullen DJ, Civetta JM, Briggs BA, Ferrara LC (1974) Therapeutic intervention scoring system: a method for quantitative comparison of patient care. Crit Care Med 2:57–60
3. Keene AR, Cullen DJ (1983) Therapeutic Intervention Scoring System: update 1983. Crit Care Med 11:1–3
4. Cullen DJ, Nemeskal AR, Zaslavsky AM (1994) Intermediate TISS: a new Therapeutic Intervention Scoring System for non-ICU patients. Crit Care Med 22:1406–1411

5. Miranda DR, de Rijk A, Schaufeli W (1996) Simplified Therapeutic Intervention Scoring System: the TISS-28 items – results from a multicenter study. Crit Care Med 24:64–73

6. Bartlett RH, Gazzaniga AB, Wilson AF, Medley T, Wetmore N (1975) Mortality prediction in adult respiratory insufficiency. Chest 67:680–684

7. Shoemaker WC, Chang P, Czer L, Bland R, Shabot MM, State D (1979) Cardiorespiratory monitoring in postoperative patients: I. Prediction of outcome and severity of illness. Crit Care Med 7:237–242

8. Knaus WA, Zimmerman JE, Wagner DP, Draper EA, Lawrence DE (1981) APACHE-acute physiology and chronic health evaluation: a physiologically based classification system. Crit Care Med 9:591–597

9. Ridley S (1998) Severity of illness scoring systems and performance appraisal. Anaesthesia 53:1185–1194

10. Harrell FE, Califf RM, Pryor DP (1984) Regression models for prognostic prediction: advantages, problems and suggested solutions. Stat Med 3:143–152

11. Le Gall JR, Loirat P, Alperovitch A, et al (1984) A simplified acute physiology score for ICU patients. Crit Care Med 12:975–977

12. Le Gall JR, Loirat P, Nicolas F, et al (1983) [Use of a severity index in 8 multidisciplinary resuscitation centers]. Presse Med 12:1757–1761

13. Youden WJ (1950) Index for rating diagnostic tests. Cancer 3:32

14. Knaus WA, Draper EA, Wagner DP, Zimmerman JE (1985) APACHE II: a severity of disease classification system. Crit Care Med 13:818–829

15. Gustafson DH, Fryback D, Rose J, et al (1981) A decision theoretic methodology for severity index development. Med Decis Making 6:27–35

16. Kenney RA (1982) Physiology of Aging: A Synopsis. Year Book Medical Publishers Inc, Chicago

17. Wagner DP, Knaus WA, Draper EA (1983) Statistical validation of a severity of illness measure. Am J Public Health 73:878–884

18. Rowan KM, Kerr JH, Major E, McPherson K, Short A, Vessey MP (1993) Intensive Care Society's APACHE II study in Britain and Ireland–II: Outcome comparisons of intensive care units after adjustment for case mix by the American APACHE II method. Br Med J 307:977–981

19. Horst HM, Obeid FN, Sorensen VJ, Bivins BA (1986) Factors influencing survival of elderly trauma patients. Crit Care Med 14:681–684

20. Cerra FB, Negro F, Abrams J (1990) APACHE II score does not predict multiple organ failure or mortality in postoperative surgical patients. Arch Surg 125:519–522

21. Moreau R, Soupison T, Vauquelin P, Derrida S, Beaucour H, Sicot C (1989) Comparison of two simplified severity scores (SAPS and APACHE II) for patients with acute myocardial infarction. Crit Care Med 17:409–413

22. Fedullo AJ, Swinburne AJ, Wahl GW, Bixby KR (1988) APACHE II score and mortality in respiratory failure due to cardiogenic pulmonary edema. Crit Care Med 16:1218–1221

23. Wehler M, Kokoska J, Reulbach U, Hahn EG, Strauss R (2001) Short-term prognosis in critically ill patients with cirrhosis assessed by prognostic scoring systems. Hepatology 34:255–261

24. Hazelgrove JF, Price C, Pappachan VJ, Smith GB (2001) Multicenter study of obstetric admissions to 14 intensive care units in southern England. Crit Care Med 29:770–775

25. Schwilk B, Wiedeck H, Stein B, Reinelt H, Treiber H, Bothner U (1997) Epidemiology of acute renal failure and outcome of haemodiafiltration in intensive care. Intensive Care Med 23:1204–1211

26. Hopefl AW, Taaffe CL, Herrmann VM (1989) Failure of APACHE II alone as a predictor of mortality in patients receiving total parenteral nutrition. Crit Care Med 17:414–417

27. Chu DY (1993) Predicting survival in AIDS patients with respiratory failure. Application of the APACHE II scoring system. Crit Care Clin 9:89–105

28. Eapen CE, Thomas K, Cherian AM, Jeyaseelan L, Mathai D, John G (1997) Predictors of mortality in a medical intensive care unit. Natl Med J India 10:270–272

29. Lemeshow S, Teres D, Pastides H, Avrunin JS, Steingrub JS (1985) A method for predicting survival and mortality of ICU patients using objectively derived weights. Crit Care Med 13:519–525

30. Kleinbaum DG, Kupper LL, Morgenstern H (1982) Epidemiological Research. Principles and Quantitative Methods. Lifetime Learning Publications, Belmont, pp 419–491
31. Teres D, Brown RB, Lemeshow S (1982) Predicting mortality of intensive care unit patients. The importance of coma. Crit Care Med 10:86–95
32. Lemeshow S, Teres D, Avrunin JS, Gage RW (1988) Refining intensive care unit outcome prediction by using changing probabilities of mortality. Crit Care Med 16:470–477
33. Chang RW, Jacobs S, Lee B (1988) Predicting outcome among intensive care unit patients using computerised trend analysis of daily Apache II scores corrected for organ system failure. Intensive Care Med 14:558–566
34. Chang RW, Jacobs S, Lee B, Pace N (1988) Predicting deaths among intensive care unit patients. Crit Care Med 16:34–42
35. Atkinson S, Bihari D, Smithies M, Daly K, Mason R, McColl I (1994) Identification of futility in intensive care. Lancet 344:1203–1206
36. Rogers J, Fuller HD (1994) Use of daily Acute Physiology and Chronic Health Evaluation (APACHE) II scores to predict individual patient survival rate. Crit Care Med 22:1402–1405
37. Knaus WA, Wagner DP, Draper EA, et al (1991) The APACHE III prognostic system. Risk prediction of hospital mortality for critically ill hospitalized adults. Chest 100:1619–1636
38. Becker RB, Zimmerman JE, Knaus WA, et al (1995) The use of APACHE III to evaluate ICU length of stay, resource use, and mortality after coronary artery by-pass surgery. J Cardiovasc Surg (Torino) 36:1–11
39. Durrleman S, Simon R (1989) Flexible regression models with cubic splines. Stat Med 8:551–561
40. Lemeshow S, Teres D, Klar J, Avrunin JS, Gehlbach SH, Rapoport J (1993) Mortality Probability Models (MPM II) based on an international cohort of intensive care unit patients. JAMA 270:2478–2486
41. Daley J (1994) Validity of risk-adjustment methods. In: Iezzoni LI (ed) Risk Adjustment for Measuring Health Care Outcomes. Health Administration Press, Ann Arbor, pp 239–262
42. Kruse JA, Thill-Baharozian MC, Carlson RW (1988) Comparison of clinical assessment with APACHE II for predicting mortality risk in patients admitted to a medical intensive care unit. JAMA 260:1739–1742
43. Brannen AL, 2nd, Godfrey LJ, Goetter WE (1989) Prediction of outcome from critical illness. A comparison of clinical judgment with a prediction rule. Arch Intern Med 149:1083–1086
44. McClish DK, Powell SH (1989) How well can physicians estimate mortality in a medical intensive care unit? Med Decis Making 9:125–132
45. Poses RM, Bekes C, Winkler RL, Scott WE, Copare FJ (1990) Are two (inexperienced) heads better than one (experienced) head? Averaging house officers' prognostic judgments for critically ill patients. Arch Intern Med 150:1874–1878
46. Beck DH, Taylor BL, Millar B, Smith GB (1997) Prediction of outcome from intensive care: a prospective cohort study comparing Acute Physiology and Chronic Health Evaluation II and III prognostic systems in a United Kingdom intensive care unit. Crit Care Med 25:9–15
47. Pappachan JV, Millar B, Bennett ED, Smith GB (1999) Comparison of outcome from intensive care admission after adjustment for case mix by the APACHE III prognostic system. Chest 115:802–810
48. Livingston BM, MacKirdy FN, Howie JC, Jones R, Norrie JD (2000) Assessment of the performance of five intensive care scoring models within a large Scottish database. Crit Care Med 28:1820–1827
49. Rivera-Fernandez R, Vazquez-Mata G, Bravo M, et al (1998) The Apache III prognostic system: customized mortality predictions for Spanish ICU patients. Intensive Care Med 24:574–581
50. Bastos PG, Sun X, Wagner DP, Knaus WA, Zimmerman JE (1996) Application of the APACHE III prognostic system in Brazilian intensive care units: a prospective multicenter study. Intensive Care Med 22:564–570
51. Zimmerman JE, Wagner DP, Draper EA, Wright L, Alzola C, Knaus WA (1998) Evaluation of acute physiology and chronic health evaluation III predictions of hospital mortality in an independent database. Crit Care Med 26:1317–1326

52. Sirio CA, Shepardson LB, Rotondi AJ, et al (1999) Community-wide assessment of intensive care outcomes using a physiologically based prognostic measure: implications for critical care delivery from Cleveland Health Quality Choice. Chest 115:793–801
53. Le Gall JR, Lemeshow S, Saulnier F (1993) A new Simplified Acute Physiology Score (SAPS II) based on a European/North American multicenter study. JAMA 270:2957–2963
54. Cleveland WS (1979) Robust locally weighted regression and smoothing scatterplots. J Am Stat Assoc 74:829–836
55. Bahloul F, Le Gall JR, Loirat P, Alperovitch A, Patois E (1988) [Prognostic factors in resuscitation]. Presse Med 17:1741–1744
56. Auriant I, Vinatier I, Thaler F, Tourneur M, Loirat P (1998) Simplified acute physiology score II for measuring severity of illness in intermediate care units. Crit Care Med 26:1368–1371
57. Capuzzo M, Valpondi V, Sgarbi A, et al (2000) Validation of severity scoring systems SAPS II and APACHE II in a single-center population. Intensive Care Med 26:1779–1785
58. Livingston BM, Mackenzie SJ, MacKirdy FN, Howie JC (2000) Should the pre-sedation Glasgow Coma Scale value be used when calculating Acute Physiology and Chronic Health Evaluation scores for sedated patients? Scottish Intensive Care Society Audit Group. Crit Care Med 28:389–394
59. Apolone G, Bertolini G, D'Amico R, et al (1996) The performance of SAPS II in a cohort of patients admitted to 99 Italian ICUs: results from GiViTI. Gruppo Italiano per la Valutazione degli interventi in Terapia Intensiva. Intensive Care Med 22:1368–1378
60. Moreno R, Morais P (1997) Outcome prediction in intensive care: results of a prospective, multicentre, Portuguese study. Intensive Care Med 23:177–186
61. Metnitz PG, Valentin A, Vesely H, et al (1999) Prognostic performance and customization of the SAPS II: results of a multicenter Austrian study. Simplified Acute Physiology Score. Intensive Care Med 25:192–197
62. Moreno R, Miranda DR, Fidler V, Van Schilfgaarde R (1998) Evaluation of two outcome prediction models on an independent database. Crit Care Med 26:50–61
63. Sikka P, Jaafar WM, Bozkanat E, El-Solh AA (2000) A comparison of severity of illness scoring systems for elderly patients with severe pneumonia. Intensive Care Med 26:1803–1810
64. Fiaccadori E, Maggiore U, Lombardi M, Leonardi S, Rotelli C, Borghetti A (2000) Predicting patient outcome from acute renal failure comparing three general severity of illness scoring systems. Kidney Int 58:283–292
65. Patel PA, Grant BJ (1999) Application of mortality prediction systems to individual intensive care units. Intensive Care Med 25:977–982
66. Tan IK (1998) APACHE II and SAPS II are poorly calibrated in a Hong Kong intensive care unit. Ann Acad Med Singapore 27:318–322
67. Nouira S, Belghith M, Elatrous S, et al (1998) Predictive value of severity scoring systems: comparison of four models in Tunisian adult intensive care units. Crit Care Med 26:852–859
68. Hadorn DC, Keeler EB, Rogers WH, Brook RH (1993) Assessing the Performance of Mortality Prediction Models. RAND, Santa Monica
69. Lemeshow S, Klar J, Teres D, et al (1994) Mortality probability models for patients in the intensive care unit for 48 or 72 hours: a prospective, multicenter study. Crit Care Med 22:1351–1358
70. Wagner DP, Knaus WA, Harrell FE, Zimmerman JE, Watts C (1994) Daily prognostic estimates for critically ill adults in intensive care units: results from a prospective, multicenter, inception cohort analysis. Crit Care Med 22:1359–1372
71. Miller RG (1974) The jackknife – A review. Biometrika 61:1–15
72. Fry DE, Pearlstein L, Fulton RL, Polk HC, Jr (1980) Multiple system organ failure. The role of uncontrolled infection. Arch Surg 115:136–140
73. Stevens LE (1983) Gauging the severity of surgical sepsis. Arch Surg 118:1190–1192
74. Marshall JC, Christou NV, Horn R, Meakins JL (1988) The microbiology of multiple organ failure. The proximal gastrointestinal tract as an occult reservoir of pathogens. Arch Surg 123:309–315

75. Knaus WA, Draper EA, Wagner DP, Zimmerman JE (1985) Prognosis in acute organ-system failure. Ann Surg 202:685–693
76. Fagon JY, Chastre J, Novara A, Medioni P, Gibert C (1993) Characterization of intensive care unit patients using a model based on the presence or absence of organ dysfunctions and/or infection: the ODIN model. Intensive Care Med 19:137–144
77. Hebert PC, Drummond AJ, Singer J, Bernard GR, Russell JA (1993) A simple multiple system organ failure scoring system predicts mortality of patients who have sepsis syndrome. Chest 104:230–235
78. Marshall JC, Cook DJ, Christou NV, Bernard GR, Sprung CL, Sibbald WJ (1995) Multiple organ dysfunction score: a reliable descriptor of a complex clinical outcome. Crit Care Med 23:1638–1652
79. Jacobs S, Zuleika M, Mphansa T (1999) The Multiple Organ Dysfunction Score as a descriptor of patient outcome in septic shock compared with two other scoring systems. Crit Care Med 27:741–744
80. Cook R, Cook D, Tilley J, Lee K, Marshall J (2001) Multiple organ dysfunction: baseline and serial component scores. Crit Care Med 29:2046–2050
81. Le Gall JR, Klar J, Lemeshow S, et al (1996) The Logistic Organ Dysfunction system. A new way to assess organ dysfunction in the intensive care unit. ICU Scoring Group. JAMA 276:802–810
82. Metnitz PG, Lang T, Valentin A, Steltzer H, Krenn CG, Le Gall JR (2001) Evaluation of the logistic organ dysfunction system for the assessment of organ dysfunction and mortality in critically ill patients. Intensive Care Med 27:992–998
83. Vincent JL, Moreno R, Takala J, et al (1996) The SOFA (Sepsis-related Organ Failure Assessment) score to describe organ dysfunction/failure. On behalf of the Working Group on Sepsis- Related Problems of the European Society of Intensive Care Medicine. Intensive Care Med 22:707–710
84. Vincent JL, de Mendonca A, Cantraine F, et al (1998) Use of the SOFA score to assess the incidence of organ dysfunction/failure in intensive care units: results of a multicenter, prospective study. Working group on "sepsis-related problems" of the European Society of Intensive Care Medicine. Crit Care Med 26:1793–1800
85. Antonelli M, Moreno R, Vincent JL, et al (1999) Application of SOFA score to trauma patients. Sequential Organ Failure Assessment. Intensive Care Med 25:389–394
86. Moreno R, Vincent JL, Matos R, et al (1999) The use of maximum SOFA score to quantify organ dysfunction/failure in intensive care. Results of a prospective, multicentre study. Working Group on Sepsis related Problems of the ESICM. Intensive Care Med 25:686–696
87. de Mendonca A, Vincent JL, Suter PM, et al (2000) Acute renal failure in the ICU: risk factors and outcome evaluated by the SOFA score. Intensive Care Med 26:915–921
88. Hantke M, Holzer K, Thone S, Schmandra T, Hanisch E (2000) [The SOFA score in evaluating septic illnesses. Correlations with the MOD and APACHE II score]. Chirurg 71:1270–1276
89. Janssens U, Graf C, Graf J, et al (2000) Evaluation of the SOFA score: a single-center experience of a medical intensive care unit in 303 consecutive patients with predominantly cardiovascular disorders. Sequential Organ Failure Assessment. Intensive Care Med 26:1037–1045
90. Oda S, Hirasawa H, Sugai T, et al (2000) Comparison of Sepsis-related Organ Failure Assessment (SOFA) score and CIS (cellular injury score) for scoring of severity for patients with multiple organ dysfunction syndrome (MODS). Intensive Care Med 26:1786–1793
91. Ferreira FL, Bota DP, Bross A, Melot C, Vincent JL (2001) Serial evaluation of the SOFA score to predict outcome in critically ill patients. JAMA 286:1754–1758
92. Moreno R, Miranda DR, Matos R, Fevereiro T (2001) Mortality after discharge from intensive care: the impact of organ system failure and nursing workload use at discharge. Intensive Care Med 27:999–1004
93. Timsit JF, Fosse JP, Troche G, et al (2001) Accuracy of a composite score using daily SAPS II and LOD scores for predicting hospital mortality in ICU patients hospitalized for more than 72 h. Intensive Care Med 27:1012–1021
94. Sivak ED, Rogers MA (1999) Assessing quality of care using in-hospital mortality: does it yield informed choices? Chest 115:613–614

95. Burton TM (1999) Examining table: Operation that rated hospitals was success, but the patience died. Cleveland Clinic found fault with program of CEOs, whose ardor faded, too. Low grades spurred reforms. Wall Street Journal, New York, A1

96. Hosmer DW, Lemeshow S (1989) Applied Logistic regression. Wiley and Sons, New York, pp 140–145

97. Hanley JA, McNeil BJ (1982) The meaning and use of the area under a receiver operating characteristic (ROC) curve. Radiology 143:29–36

98. Hanley JA, McNeil BJ (1983) A method of comparing the areas under receiver operating characteristic curves derived from the same cases. Radiology 148:839–843

99. Angus DC, Pinsky MR (1997) Risk prediction: judging the judges. Intensive Care Med 23:363–365

100. Brazier JE, Harper R, Jones NM, et al (1992) Validating the SF-36 health survey questionnaire: new outcome measure for primary care. Br Med J 305:160–164

101. Knaus WA, Draper EA, Wagner DP, Zimmerman JE (1986) An evaluation of outcome from intensive care in major medical centers. Ann Intern Med 104:410–418

102. Boyd O, Grounds RM (1993) Physiological scoring systems and audit. Lancet 341:1573–1574

103. Zimmerman JE, Shortell SM, Knaus WA, et al (1993) Value and cost of teaching hospitals: a prospective, multicenter, inception cohort study. Crit Care Med 21:1432–1442

104. Zimmerman JE, Shortell SM, Rousseau DM, et al (1993) Improving intensive care: observations based on organizational case studies in nine intensive care units: a prospective, multicenter study. Crit Care Med 21:1443–1451

105. Boyd O, Grounds M (1994) Can standardized mortality ratio be used to compare quality of intensive care unit performance? Crit Care Med 22:1706–1709

106. Goldhill DR, Withington PS (1996) Mortality predicted by APACHE II. The effect of changes in physiological values and post-ICU hospital mortality. Anaesthesia 51:719–723

107. Bosman RJ, Oudemane van Straaten HM, Zandstra DF (1998) The use of intensive care information systems alters outcome prediction. Intensive Care Med 24:953–958

108. Suistomaa M, Kari A, Ruokonen E, Takala J (2000) Sampling rate causes bias in APACHE II and SAPS II scores. Intensive Care Med 26:1773–1778

109. Teasdale G, Jennett B (1974) Assessment of coma and impaired consciousness. A practical scale. Lancet 2:81–84

110. Chen LM, Martin CM, Morrison TL, Sibbald WJ (1999) Interobserver variability in data collection of the APACHE II score in teaching and community hospitals. Crit Care Med 27:1999–2004

111. Cho DY, Wang YC (1997) Comparison of the APACHE III, APACHE II and Glasgow Coma Scale in acute head injury for prediction of mortality and functional outcome. Intensive Care Med 23:77–84

112. Grmec S, Gasparovic V (2001) Comparison of APACHE II, MEES and Glasgow Coma Scale in patients with nontraumatic coma for prediction of mortality. Acute Physiology and Chronic Health Evaluation. Mainz Emergency Evaluation System. Crit Care 5:19–23

113. Bion JF, Edlin SA, Ramsay G, McCabe S, Ledingham IM (1985) Validation of a prognostic score in critically ill patients undergoing transport. Br Med J 291:432–434

114. Dragsted L, Jorgensen J, Jensen NH, et al (1989) Interhospital comparisons of patient outcome from intensive care: importance of lead-time bias. Crit Care Med 17:418–422

115. Tunnell RD, Millar BW, Smith GB (1998) The effect of lead time bias on severity of illness scoring, mortality prediction and standardised mortality ratio in intensive care – a pilot study. Anaesthesia 53:1045–1053

116. Angus DC (2000) Scoring system fatigue...and the search for a way forward. Crit Care Med 28:2145–2146

117. Moreno R, Matos R (2001) Outcome prediction in intensive care. Solving the paradox. Intensive Care Med 27:962–964

Quality of Care

Discharging the Critically Ill Patient

R. Moreno, P.G.H. Metnitz, and R. Matos

▍ Introduction

Created 50 years ago, the intensive care unit (ICU) is now an essential part of hospital care. After a couple of decades in which ICU research was more concerned with technical issues, a significant number of research groups are now focusing their attention on ways to improve the organization of the ICU and its place in the continuum of care. An essential part of this process is the evaluation of ICU discharge policies and their consequences.

The magnitude of the problem was highlighted some years ago when several European multicenter outcome studies presented data on vital status both at ICU discharge and at hospital discharge. These studies showed that, on average, approximately 30% of all deaths occurred in hospital after ICU discharge [1–6] (Table 1). Although, according to the study by Wallis et al. [7], approximately 25% of all deaths after ICU discharge could be foreseen, this means that 75% of the deaths were unexpected. Recent data suggest that at least some of these deaths were due to inappropriate early ICU discharge and thus could have been prevented.

Current guidelines for discharging patients from the ICU focus mainly on the qualitative evaluation of the overall physiologic status of the patient [8]. Consequently, the discharge decision is to be made "when a patient's physiologic status has stabilized and the need for ICU monitoring and care is no longer necessary". This advice, although conceptually clear, is difficult to put into practice, for at least two reasons: first, because it does not call for the quantification of residual organ dysfunction/failure still present at ICU discharge, and, second, because it does not match the level of care required by the patient after ICU discharge with the level of care that can be provided in the ward.

Table 1. Proportional post-ICU mortality in several European multicenter studies

First author	Country/Region	Proportional post-ICU mortality (%)
Apolone [1]	Italy	26
Moreno [2]	Portugal	23
Moreno [3]	Europe	30
Goldhill [4]	United Kingdom	27
Valentin [5]	Austria	27
Rowan [6]	United Kingdom	35

∎ Evaluating ICU Discharge Practices

Smith et al. [9] studied the relationship between the use of nursing workload resources before ICU discharge and the post-ICU outcome in a university teaching hospital without intermediate care facilities. The patients were discharged directly to in-hospital wards. The investigators found that 11% of discharged patients died in hospital and that those patients who needed a higher level of care on the last ICU day (as measured by the Therapeutic Intervention Scoring System [TISS] [10]) had a greatly increased risk of in-hospital death. Patients with a TISS score of ≥ 20 on the last ICU day had 21.4% mortality, compared with 3.7% in patients with a TISS score of < 10. Other factors associated with an increased risk of in-hospital death after ICU discharge were increased age, higher Acute Physiology and Chronic Health Evaluation II (APACHE II) scores, and male sex. Smith et al. [9] concluded that the level of nursing workload resources required by these patients at discharge from the ICU could not be provided in the general ward and that patients with a high TISS score at ICU discharge should instead be transferred to a high dependency unit.

Another view of the problem was presented in a study of the relationship between the amount of residual organ dysfunction/failure still present at ICU discharge and the post-ICU mortality [11]. Using the database of the EURICUS-II study (BMH4-CT96-0817), data on 2,958 patients discharged to the general wards were evaluated. The predischarge status of the patients was characterized by the Sequential Organ Failure Assessment (SOFA) score [12] and by the Nine Equivalents of Nursing Manpower Use Score (NEMS) [13]. Death after ICU discharge occurred in 8.6% of the patients and accounted for 32.8% of all in-hospital deaths. Patients who died in hospital after ICU discharge presented a higher Simplified Acute Physiology Score II (SAPS II) [2], were more frequently nonoperative, were admitted from the ward, and exhibited a longer length of stay (LOS) in the ICU. The degree of organ dysfunction/failure in these patients was higher, as interpreted by a higher admission SOFA score, a higher maximum SOFA score, and a higher delta SOFA score. These patients also required more nursing workload resources while in the ICU. In an analysis of the last 24 hours in the ICU, both the amount of organ dysfunction/failure (especially cardiovascular, neurological, renal, and respiratory) and the amount of nursing workload used were higher in those patients who subsequently died before hospital discharge. Residual central nervous system and renal dysfunction/failure were ominous prognostic factors at ICU discharge.

Although a significant relationship between the TISS score on the last day in the ICU and post-ICU outcome was present in univariate analysis, the contribution to post-ICU outcome of last-day NEMS did not reach significance in the multivariate analysis when the presence and amount of organ dysfunction/failure were simultaneously taken into account. This implies that the main determinant of post-discharge mortality is not the amount of nursing workload resources required by the patient but rather the underlying degree of organ dysfunction/failure, for which the former is just a surrogate marker.

These results are in agreement with data presented by Fieux et al. [15]. Studying a cohort of 17,476 patients from 30 Austrian ICUs, from which 780 required a second admission to the ICU, Fieux et al. analyzed the main determinants of readmission. Readmission occurred in 4.5% of all admitted patients (5.1% of all patients who were discharged after the first ICU stay) and was associated with a significant effect on outcome (hospital mortality of 21.7% versus 5.2% in non-readmitted patients). Readmitted patients were older, had a higher severity of illness, presented more organ failures at the first ICU admission, and had a higher risk of in-hospital death. On the day of their first discharge from the ICU, readmitted patients showed a significant increase in the use of nursing workload resources as measured by the TISS-28 [16], compared with non-readmitted patients: 26 (18–32) vs. 22 (16–26) TISS-28 points; $p < 0.001$. Readmitted patients needed significantly more organ support for the respiratory, cardiovascular, and renal systems. Patients who were readmitted were, for example, mechanically ventilated more than twice as often and significantly more often received supplementary ventilatory support as well as cardiovascular therapeutic measures. This provides evidence that, despite the decision to discharge these patients, there were still unresolved problems with their cardiorespiratory functions. This is also supported by the fact that, for mechanically ventilated patients, the time between extubation and discharge was significantly shorter for patients who were later readmitted: At least 25% of them had their tracheal tube removed on the day of ICU discharge.

These data from the last day of the first ICU stay show that these patients still needed a high level of observation and, to some extent, intervention. General wards, however, have a lower nurse-to-patient ratio than ICUs, which makes time-consuming activities very difficult or sometimes even impossible to carry out. Also, the ability to monitor impending organ failure is certainly lower in general wards. For these reasons, residual organ dysfunction may worsen and lead to readmission of the patient to the ICU.

The discharge of the patient should always be a planned and coordinated act. It has been demonstrated that the precipitate discharge of a patient, for example at night, can have a negative effect on outcome [17]. Night-time discharge, when the number of medical and paramedical personnel is lower than during the day, is presumably due to an emergency situation in which ICU beds are urgently needed and patients who seem not to be at acute risk are discharged to the ward. Several of these patients, however, still have underlying organ dysfunction which are, in turn, associated with an increased risk for a negative outcome.

▌ Using the Information to Improve the Effectiveness of Intensive Care

Recent studies highlight the importance of the timing of ICU discharge. Daly et al. [18], studying 13,924 patients from 20 ICUs in the United Kingdom, developed a multivariate model to predict mortality after ICU discharge. They found that age, end-stage disease, LOS, cardiothoracic surgery, and acute physiology score were associated with an increased risk for death after ICU discharge. On the basis of a simulation study, they concluded that the discharge mortality of at-risk patients might be reduced by 39% if they remain in the ICU for another 48 hours. They concluded, moreover, that up to 16% more ICU beds would be necessary in the United Kingdom if this algorithm were applied – thus obviously perceiving a longer LOS as an economic problem. However, the real magnitude of changing discharge practices according to the recommendations of Daly et al. cannot be estimated, since no prospective data were presented. Moreover, from their model, only LOS and physiologic status of the patients are eventually prone to changes.

Another recent study evaluated readmissions to a tertiary care center ICU in Switzerland over a period of 5 years [19]. In the group of early readmitted patients (defined as readmissions occurring within 4 days), it was concluded that, depending on the primary reason for readmission, between 13% (cardiocirculatory problems) and 86% (respiratory problems) of readmissions could be classified as potentially preventable. These data suggest that several patients could benefit from having their organ functions optimized before discharge. Although keeping these patients in the ICU longer will certainly increase ICU costs, such a strategy could well reduce the readmission rate as well as the post-ICU LOS, which could decrease overall hospital costs.

If we look at the factors that possibly influence post-ICU discharge mortality, some, such as age or the presence of chronic diseases, are not susceptible to intervention. However, the data show that providing the attending clinician with objective information about the presence and amount of residual organ dysfunction/failure is useful. This information can and should be complemented by data on the type and amount of nursing workload resources needed, since this can affect the destination of the patient after transfer (i.e., ward or high dependency unit). Objective data for well-coordinated ICU discharge policies are also needed to avoid overcrowding of the ICU because of an inadequate number of backup beds in the ward or high dependency unit [20].

▌ Conclusion

The decision to discharge a patient from the ICU is not always an easy one. The clinician who makes this decision needs to consider both clinical and economic constraints; i.e., he or she has to weigh the need to keep the patient in the ICU to optimize the patient's physiological status, with the need to open up beds for new admissions. Clearly, the presence or absence of post-ICU resources, such as intermediate care facilities, influences ICU discharge policies. Current data suggest, however, that if intermediate care facilities are present, the decision about where to discharge the patient should be made on the basis of the type and amount of nursing workload resources needed by the patient during the last day of the ICU stay.

Moreover, although no validated discharge scoring system yet exists, we recommend that for patients at high risk of in-hospital death after ICU discharge, a system of follow-up by ICU medical personnel (doctors and nurses) should be instituted.

Although it will certainly be difficult to create an appropriate balance between scientifically based recommendations, economic pressure, and ethical problems, the subject of ICU discharge practices and policies should be treated in an objective way to improve our performance of what society expects us to do: to get the patients back to their families and back to work.

References

1. Apolone G, D'Amico R, Bertolini G, et al (1996) The performance of SAPS II in a cohort of patients admitted in 99 Italian ICUs: results from the GiViTI. Intensive Care Med 22:1368–1378
2. Moreno R, Morais P (1997) Outcome prediction in intensive care: results of a prospective, multicentre, Portuguese study. Intensive Care Med 23:177–186
3. Moreno R, Reis Miranda D, Fidler V, Van Schilfgaarde R (1998) Evaluation of two outcome predictors on an independent database. Crit Care Med 26:50–61
4. Goldhill DR, Sumner A (1998) Outcome of intensive care patients in a group of British intensive care units. Crit Care Med 26:1337–1345

5. Valentin A, Lang T, Hiesmayr M, Metnitz PG (2001) Post ICU mortality contributes substantially to standardised mortality ratio and monitoring of ICU performance: results from 21.616 ICU admissions. Intensive Care Med 27 (suppl 2):A410 (Abst)
6. Rowan KM, Kerr JH, Major E, McPherson K, Short A, Vessey MP (1994) Intensive Care Society's Acute Physiology and Chronic Health Evaluation (APACHE II) study in Britain and Ireland: a prospective, multicenter, cohort study comparing two methods for predicting outcome for adult intensive care patients. Crit Care Med 22:1392–1401
7. Wallis CB, Davies HT, Shearer AJ (1997) Why do patients die on general wards after discharge from intensive care units? Anaesthesia 52:9–14
8. Task Force of the American College of Critical Care Medicine, SCCM (1999) Guidelines for intensive care unit admission, discharge, and triage. Crit Care Med 27:633–638
9. Smith L, Orts CM, O'Neil I, Batchelor AM, Gascoigne AD, Baudouin SV (1999) TISS and mortality after discharge from intensive care. Intensive Care Med 25:1061–1065
10. Cullen DJ, Civetta JM, Briggs BA, Ferrara LC (1974) Therapeutic intervention scoring system: a method for quantitative comparison of patient care. Crit Care Med 2:57–60
11. Moreno R, Miranda DR, Matos R, Fevereiro T (2001) Mortality after discharge from intensive care: the impact of organ system failure and nursing workload use at discharge. Intensive Care Med 27:999–1004
12. Vincent J-L, Moreno R, Takala J, et al (1996) The SOFA (Sepsis-related organ failure assessment) score to describe organ dysfunction/failure. Intensive Care Med 22:707–710
13. Reis Miranda D, Moreno R, Iapichino G (1997) Nine equivalents of nursing manpower use score (NEMS). Intensive Care Med 23:760–765
14. Le Gall JR, Lemeshow S, Saulnier F (1993) A new simplified acute physiology score (SAPS II) based on a European / North American multicenter study. JAMA 270:2957–2963
15. Fieux F, Lang T, Le Gall J-R, Metnitz P (2001) Prognosis in patients readmitted to the intensive care unit. Intensive Care Med 27:A410 (Abst)
16. Miranda DR, De Rijk A, Schaufeli W (1996) Simplified Therapeutic Interventions Scoring System: The TISS-28 items – Results from a multicenter study. Crit Care Med 24:64–73
17. Goldfrad C, Rowan K (2000) Consequences of discharges from intensive care at night. Lancet 355:1138–1142
18. Daly K, Beale R, Chang RW (2001) Reduction in mortality after inappropriate early discharge from intensive care unit: logistic regression triage model. Br Med J 322:1274–1276
19. Schriber P (2001). Does the readmission rate to the intensive care unit tell us anything about the quality of the care process? Doctoral Thesis, University of Geneva Medical School (in press)
20. Levin PD, Sprung CL (2001) The process of intensive care triage. Intensive Care Med 27:1441–1445

Patient Examination in the Intensive Care Unit

K. Hillman, G. Bishop, and A. Flabouris

"More is missed by not looking than by not knowing ..."
Anonymous

▌ Introduction

There is often a false sense of security when a patient is surrounded by all the paraphernalia of modern technology – a sense that physical examination and history in the presence of so much information and technology may be redundant. While we may intimidate the general public and impress our 'low tech' medical colleagues with our technology; it is only the indifferent critical care clinician who does not rely on thorough history taking and physical examination in the intensive care unit (ICU).

The examination of critically ill patients has created its own framework and knowledge. While this framework is based on traditional patient history taking and physician examination, it also has different challenges. For example, the history usually has to be taken from relatives/friends in order to obtain a picture of the patient's pre-existing health or from bystanders in order to reconstruct the sudden event which may have lead to hospital admission. The examination is based on that conventionally described in all medical textbooks. However, certain patterns of signs have emerged in the critically ill as a result of our ability to keep patients alive longer, e.g., critically ill polyneuropathy. The physical examination must include invasive lines and tubes as well as all the equipment supporting and monitoring the patient. The equipment must be looked at for the information that it provides, as well as how that equipment interacts with and causes complications in patients, e.g., observing pressure measurements from a central line as well as examining the skin at the site of the central line insertion for signs of infection.

The 'numbers' generated by a pulmonary artery catheter may create a common language for junior medical staff to communicate with critical care specialists in the middle of the night. However, most senior specialists remain anxious until they personally examine the patient. That involves thoroughly exposing and turning the patient, and thinking about what every sign may mean. For all the thousands of articles and books published around the subtleties of invasive support machines and monitoring, there are less than a handful published on the equally important issue of examination of the critically ill. This chapter will attempt to redress that balance.

❚ Standing at the End of the Bed

An ICU examination requires a 'focused' and enquiring mind. As an exercise in observation, attempt to diagnose a 'new' patient from the end of the bed, or summarize in your mind the changes in those patients you have seen before.

For example, what brings young adults to an ICU – it is commonly conditions such as trauma, poisoning, asthma, serious acute infections, or peripartum catastrophes. Trauma patients often have evidence of recent surgery or intracranial monitoring; poisoned patients may have the remnants of charcoal in the nasogastric tube; asthmatics have complex ventilatory patterns and an array of intravenous infusions. These are first impressions.

Before approaching the patient, it is important to acknowledge the nurse in charge of the patient. Second, have someone in the team briefly summarize the story of each patient, even if it has been done three times a day for the last six months. The story, including the initial problem and current hospital course, focuses you on where we have been, and where we are now. Then the handover occurs. Intensive care is about multiple handovers and maintaining continuity and focus during those handovers. The handover should include what happened during the last shift and where the focus should now be. It often helps to end the handover by starting: "in summary the problems are ... and our direction is ..." Handovers should always be at the patient's bedside and not in a separate room, concentrating on results and 'numbers'. This emphasizes the importance of the physical examination and the fact that the patient is a person and not only a series of numbers.

❚ The History

A unique approach to history taking is necessary for patients in the ICU and differs from the approach used for conscious patients in an ambulant setting. Patients are usually packaged before arrival – resuscitated and stabilized in another setting. An initial history has usually been taken somewhere else – e.g., the Emergency Room (ER), before surgery, or in the general wards; this will include ambulance notes, transfer details and information from bystanders. The patient is often incapable of giving a history, either as a result of their underlying illness or because of sedative drugs. Usually a diagnosis has already been made, but this must, of course, be questioned by ICU staff. Other important aspects of the history include the course of the illness since hospital admission, the severity of underlying co-morbidities, and the patient's quality of life before hospital admission.

This information will shed some light on the physiological reserve of the patient and how this in turn will interact with the severity of the current acute illness. As well as giving information on how to manage the illness, pre-hospital admission status will offer understanding about issues such as ultimate prognosis. For example, if the patient's pre-existing respiratory function limited them to being chair bound and on home oxygen, even relatively minor acute lung problems could make successful weaning from the ventilator impossible. The history should also include information about the patient's attitudes and beliefs towards end of life treatment. Similarly the history should also include the carer's opinions about these issues.

In summary, history taking in the ICU is complex and not confined to subtle clues concerning the current diagnosis (Table 1). The history is essential to recon-

Table 1. Components of history-taking in intensive care

▌ Pre-existing co-morbidities and functional status in the community
▌ Past history of medical and surgical conditions
▌ Pre-admission medications
▌ History of pre-admission current illness
▌ History of hospital, including intensive care, course
▌ History from previous shift to ensure continuity
▌ History of patient and carer's wishes with regard to end of life decisions

structing the patient's pre-admission health status, as well as details about the patient's course in hospital, up to the point of the current examination.

▌ The Initial Examination

The history overlaps with the initial examination. The monitoring and support surrounding patient can often provide a diagnosis without any history: drug infusions; the monitoring display; the ventilator settings; devices such as an intra-aortic balloon pump (IABP) and dialysis machines; urine color; the type and amount of drainage from body cavities; and the nature of operations, often reveal a lot about the underlying diagnosis and complications. For example, an oximeter on the ear rather than finger can be a sign of poor perfusion and obesity can warn you of pressure areas, difficulty inserting central lines, poor healing and collapsed lung bases.

Most clinicians these days wear protective gloves and possibly glasses and gowns for the physical examination.

The first step is to take in all the information provided by monitoring and support technology, including drug infusions and their rates and concentration. Next, look around the bed and observe what is draining, e.g., urine (Table 2), abdominal drains, pleural drains and whether they are bubbling. Look at the color of the secretions and the volume. Most hospitals empty drainage containers at 12 midnight, but ask the nurse if you are not sure. Ask the nurse for clarification about changes in drainage rates. Check for daily trends.

Table 2. Urine color

▌ Myoglobin – light brown, 'port wine', or 'machine oil' as the concentration increases
▌ Hemoglobinuria – opalescent pink urine without sediment
▌ Hematuria – cloudy urine with red-brown sediment
▌ Sulphonamides or phosphates/sulphates – pink
▌ Porphyria – red

▌ The Physical Examination

The information gained thus far should direct you to areas of special concern. Nonetheless, each physical examination in the ICU should be thorough. Symptoms are rare and signs become even more important. Moreover the seriously ill patient is often 'sign rich' because of multiorgan involvement and invasive procedures.

It is important before touching the patient to introduce yourself, using the patient's first name. Explain that you are about to examine them, even if you suspect they are deeply unconscious. This reminds us that we are dealing with a human being whose needs are almost totally in our hands. While ensuring the patient's privacy and dignity it is important to expose as much of the body as possible in order not to miss any abnormal signs. Some prefer to interact with results of investigations as they go through the physical examination. Others like to separate the two and refer to investigations at the end of their examination.

Examine all the operation sites; remove dressings or ask if you can be informed when routine dressing changes are being made. It is important to understand exactly what operation has been done and where all the drains are sited, in order to understand the significance of the drainage, especially from the thorax and abdomen. Ask the surgeons to draw clear diagrams of complex operations and leave them in a prominent position at the end of the bed. Attending the operation, especially with complex abdominal procedures, can give you a clearer understanding of what is happening, what the potential complications could be and what the drains mean. Check that the transducers for the monitoring devices are all correctly placed. Note invasive tubes and lines, that they are secured and that there are no signs of local inflammation or infection. Finally, there may be signs around the patient's bed regarding the language they speak, or reminders about important features of the patient such as an arm fistula for dialysis.

Neurological

The three major neurological assessments are the level of consciousness, brain stem signs, and any evidence of focal lesions. The level of consciousness is measured by the Glasgow Coma Scale (GCS). The trend in GCS is more important than a single measurement. Obviously the GCS has to be assessed in the light of sedation as well as renal/hepatic function. The brain stem is assessed by testing reflexes such as breathing, reaction to pain, pupil reaction, corneal reflexes, gag reflex, and vestibulo-occulo reflex. Focal signs are usually seen in the limbs. Power and sensation are difficult to assess in the unconscious patient, but tone and reflexes provide accurate and repeatable evidence of focal signs. Nursing staff should be asked about spontaneous movement of all four limbs. As the patient becomes more conscious after a prolonged stay in the ICU, problems such as polyneuropathy of the critically ill can become apparent.

Airway

Note the type of airway and, if it is artificial, its diameter, as this is usually the site of greatest resistance and the cause of increased work of breathing. Note how the artificial airway is secured, whether the securing bandage is causing ulcers at the corners of the mouth or contributing to raised intracranial pressure (ICP). Check the position of the artificial airway on chest X-ray. Check cuff pressures and enquire from the nursing staff about the nature and amount of airway secretions. Finally, enquire about the strength of the patient's cough.

Breathing

You should have observed ventilator settings, patient interaction with the ventilator, saturation and pattern of respiration, e.g., co-ordinated with the ventilator and no excessive work of breathing.

Check for surgical emphysema and position of trachea. Percussion is difficult to perform in the ICU and of little value. For example, a pneumothorax is usually more accurately detected by other signs in the ICU and definitively by a rapidly performed chest X-ray. However, auscultation remains important. Ronchi can not be seen on the chest X-ray and there are blind spots when reviewing the chest X-ray, especially in the lung bases posteriorly. Basal collapse and consolidation are common, especially in association with high abdominal pressures, after abdominal or thoracic surgery; and in association with conditions such as pancreatitis or obesity. Bronchial breathing is an accurate indication of pneumonia or collapse, rather than acute respiratory distress syndrome (ARDS) or pulmonary edema, probably related to the density of fluid around the bronchi. It is difficult to sit the patient up to auscultate the lung bases; sometimes auscultation can be achieved by holding the stethoscope bell in the palm of your hand and sliding it under the patient, pushing the back of your hand into the bed. The chest X-ray is a crucial part of the respiratory system examination and should be available at all times alongside the patient [1].

Note the position of the patient when assessing oxygenation, e.g., one side down, lying prone, or sitting up. The site of the lung pathology will influence the level of oxygenation, depending on the patient's position.

Table 3. Effect of challenges on functional reserve and pathophysiology of underlying disease

Airway	Positional changes on airway obstruction
Breathing	Effect on oxygenation due to: ▮ FiO$_2$ ▮ Patient position ▮ PEEP ▮ Ventilator patterns ▮ Recruitment maneuvers ▮ Drugs ▮ Fluids
Circulation	Effect on tissue perfusion due to: ▮ Fluid challenge ▮ Inotrope and vasopressor change ▮ Respiratory cycle affecting monitored blood pressure ▮ Increased abdominal pressure
Neurology	Effect on intracranial pressure of bilateral internal jugular compression as an indication of intracranial compliance
Liver/Kidney	Length of time to metabolize drugs

Intermittent hypotension and hypertension is also a strong indicator of hypo-volemia, especially on a background of chronic hypertension or in diseases with autonomic dysfunction such as Guillain-Barre or tetanus.

Also note the effect of 'challenges' other than position, on oxygenation, e. g., fluid boluses, PEEP and recruitment maneuvers. Challenging a physiological system can give information on the underlying reserve or nature of the pathophysiology on that system (Table 3).

Cardiovascular System

There is a tendency to be swamped and distracted by numbers in the assessment of the cardiovascular system. Concentrate on the important information first – arte-rial blood pressure, urine output, peripheral temperature as well as the pulse rate and rhythm. A crucial question always in the ICU is the status of the intravascular volume. Assess the peripheral pulses and auscultate the precordium for new sounds. Examine for site and extent of peripheral edema. Note whether the moni-tored display of blood pressure is swinging with respiration, indicating possible hy-povolemia. There are signs peculiar to the seriously ill such as a bounding precor-dium and neck, associated with a high cardiac output, as commonly found in sep-sis (Table 4). Then check this information against numbers, such as those gener-ated from the pulmonary artery catheter. Check the electrocardiogram (EKG) – par-ticularly in the elderly. Some would say that echocardiography is becoming the car-diovascular equivalent of the chest X-ray complementing the respiratory system.

Gastrointestinal System

The gastrointestinal (GI) system can be a primary source of admission to the ICU or be a source of secondary complications. The key to examination of the GI sys-tem is thorough inspection and palpation. First look at the general nutritional state. Then the head, examining the mouth, especially the sclera for signs of jaundice, teeth, as well as sinuses, ears and cervical nodes. Look for complications of artifi-cial tubes inserted through the nose or mouth. Inspect the abdomen for distension, wounds and drains. Palpate for tenderness, tenseness and abnormal masses. Older people in the ICU often suffer from gaseous distension or pseudo-obstruction, pre-senting as tympanic abdominal distension, often requiring early aggressive treat-ment. If you suspect the intra-abdominal pressure is raised, always measure it, as clinical assessment is not always accurate [2]. Auscultate for bruits and bowel sounds, enquire about bowel actions, and whether nasoenteral feeds are being tol-

Table 4. Signs peculiar to the critically ill. (From [4] with the permission of Cambridge University Press)

▌ Bounding in the neck and precordium often indicates sepsis
▌ An indentation ring in the skin on the anterior abdominal wall, left after listening for bowel sounds with a stethoscope, indicates extensive peripheral edema
▌ The silhouette of the head seen over the mediastinum on an upright chest X-ray is a poor prognostic sign and is usually followed by intubation within the next 24 hours
▌ Attempts to breathe against the ventilator, despite what appears to be an adequate minute volume, is of-ten due to severe metabolic acidosis
▌ Rapid deterioration in cardiorespiratory signs can indicate a pneumothorax

erated. Examine the perineum during examination of the back for perineal excoriation and pressure areas.

Renal System and Fluids

Examination of the cardiovascular system will give some indication of the adequacy of intravascular filling [3]. A fluid challenge, with the rapid infusion of 200–300 mls is often the best way of determining adequacy of intravascular fluid volume. The state of hydration, in terms of body water content, will be indicated by signs such as skin turgor and dry mouth, as well as serum sodium. Fluid balance charts, especially losses from drains, are important in assessing fluid status.

Renal function is roughly assessed by hourly urine volume. However, biochemical markers such as electrolytes, acid-base status, and levels of urea and creatinine are more accurate determinants of renal function

Limbs

The skin is the largest organ in the body. Rashes are difficult to diagnose in the ICU but can give important information about the underlying diagnosis, drug effects, and complications such as ischemia from inadequate perfusion. Hands, feet, and nails should be inspected. Fractures and their exact management need to be understood. Signs of compartment syndrome need to be looked for.

A mnemonic is presented to assist in remembering the major areas to be covered in the examination (Table 5).

▌ Other Factors Associated with Patient Examination in the ICU

▌ Just before you examine the patient, it is helpful to focus on what is the single most important feature that may indicate patient progress, e.g., the urine output, level of inotrope support, the GCS, the FiO_2 or oxygen saturation.

▌ In order to manage the ICU patient, continuity is essential. For example, medical specialists become familiar and confident about a complicated patient's course

Table 5. Guidelines for daily recording of patient's clinical status

A	Airway
B	Breathing
C	Circulation
D	Disability – GCS and focal neurology
E	Electrolytes – results
F	Fluids – are they appropriate?
G	Gut – examine and nutritional assessment
H	Hematology – results
I	Infection – latest microbiology and white cell count
L	Lines – are the sites clean? How long have they been in?
M	Medications – review and interactions
R	Relatives – what is the common message?

and direction if they are on duty for several days at a time, rather than changing each day. There may also be a reluctance to make major decisions if specialists change each day, as there is a tendency to just steer the patient through that 24 hours, focusing on processes rather than the bigger picture.

▌ Doctors and nurses need to meticulously handover problems and directions at the change of each shift.

▌ When assessing a patient, focus on the discrepancy between the patient's actual clinical state and what you had expected it to be. While patients have various levels of illness, they usually follow predictable clinical courses. Alarm bells ring when you are confronted, for example, with a patient who is not recovering as fast as you had expected; or when you are confronted with abnormal laboratory tests or clinical signs which you had not expected. It is at this point that contemplation and deliberation should replace routine care. Another way of looking at patients in the ICU is the analogy of aircraft. Imagine each patient cruising at certain altitudes – some very sick at dangerously low altitudes and some less sick at higher altitudes. You need to be alert when the patient moves suddenly or unpredictably from one of those anticipated flight paths.

▌ The final and crucial task is to distil all of the information and then construct a plan for the next 24 hours.

▌ Conclusion

This review has not focused on the numbers generated from patient monitoring nor the results of the many investigations patients have in the ICU. Intensive care journals and textbooks have abundant information on those aspects of our specialty. However, as in other medical specialties the 'numbers' and investigations are only there to supplement, not to replace, a thoughtful and thorough physical examination and history. The history usually comes from non-patient sources and needs to take into account the course of the acute illness during the hospital stay. Conventional medical textbooks have little information on the challenge of examining a seriously ill patient, as opposed to the usual signs found in ambulant patients. The signs found in the ICU may be as a result of the primary underlying illness, or complications of that illness, or as a result of the many monitoring and support strategies we use to maintain life. More is missed about the patient's illness in the ICU by not looking at these signs than by not knowing intricate details of disease pathophysiology.

Acknowledgement. To Dr. Bob Wright, an intensive care physician who carved out the art of examining the critically ill when there were no textbooks or guidelines and became the inspiration for many Australasian intensivists. If examination of the seriously ill in intensive care was an Olympic Games event, Bob would be a strong contender for the gold medal.

References

1. Kox W, Boultbee J, Hillman K (1988) The interpretation of the portable chest film and the role of complementary imaging techniques. In: Kox W, Boultbee J, Donaldson (eds) Imaging and Labelling Techniques in the Critically Ill. Springer, London, pp 45–65
2. Sugrue M, Hillman KM (1998) Intra-abdominal hypertension and intensive care. In: Vincent JL (ed) Update in Intensive Care and Emergency Medicine. Springer, Heidelberg, pp 667–676
3. Hillman K, Bishop G, Bristow P (1997) The crystalloid versus colloid controversy: Present status. In: Halkjamae H (ed) Baillier's Clinical Anaesthesiology. International practice and research. Plasma volume support. Bailliere Tindall, London, pp 1–3
4. Hillman K, Bishop G (1996) Clinical Intensive Care. Cambridge University Press, New York, pp 16

Are Autopsies still Useful in the Intensive Care Unit?

G. Dimopoulos

Introduction

As early as 1912, autopsy was noted by Cabot to be a medical procedure to obtain a diagnosis in complex cases, to provide quality assessment of clinical practice, and to improve understanding of medical limitations [1, 2]. Anderson et al. [3] defined quality assessment as the quantitative evaluation of results or outcomes ranged within predefined acceptable limits. Although in the United States, the institutional requirements of the Accreditation Council for Graduate Medical Education stated that a sufficient number of autopsies should be performed to maintain quality of patient care and for educational purposes, the autopsy rate has fallen over recent decades, from 50% in the 1940s to 10% in the 1980s [4]. This decline has been attributed to a number of factors, including:

- the fear of diagnostic errors being detected at autopsy;
- heary work for the pathologists;
- the high non-reimbursable cost involved in the procedure;
- difficulties in obtain consent from the family; and
- the greater sensitivity and specificity of modern diagnostic techniques [5, 6].

Autopsy in Non-Intensive Care Unit (ICU) Patients

In non-ICU patients a number of studies have evaluated the correlation of autopsy with clinical diagnoses, presenting a discrepancy rate ranging between 6 and 40% [7–12]. The discrepancies or 'missed diagnoses' reported by these studies included mainly infections (bacterial, fungal, viral), pulmonary embolus, acute myocardial infarction, tumors, and unsuspected postoperative hemorrhage. A discrepancy was considered to have occurred if the diagnosis was not listed on the death certificate, was not mentioned in the patient notes, or specific treatment was not started despite a high suspicion based on the medical records [13].

Goldman et al. [13] was the first to use a classification system to categorize autopsy diagnoses. According to this classification, uncovered discrepancies are divided into major diagnoses including the primary underlying diseases and the primary causes of death, and minor diagnoses including related diagnoses, contributing causes of death, and co-existing diseases. The major diagnoses are divided into Class I und II, while the minor diagnoses are divided into Classes III and IV (Table 1) [13].

Table 1. Goldman's criteria for the classification of discrepancies detected by autopsy. Modified from [13]

Missed Major Diagnoses	
▌**Class I**	Major diagnosis for which detection before death would have led to a change in management that might have resulted in cure or prolonged survival
▌**Class II**	Missed major diagnosis for which detection before death would probably not have led to a change in the management, because: – no good therapy was available at that time – the patient had presented with an acute cardiopulmonary arrest that was appropriately treated – the patient had already received appropriate therapy even though the diagnosis was not known, or – the patient refused further evaluation or therapy
Missed Minor Diagnoses	
▌**Class III**	Diseases that were related to the terminal disease process and not directly related to death
▌**Class IV**	Unrelated diagnoses that might eventually have affected prognosis, or processes that contributed to death in a terminally in patient

▌ Autopsy in ICU Patients

ICU patients are characterized by the rapid changes in their clinical situation and their inability to give details concerning their prior medical history. However, in these patients the primary diagnosis and the cause of death are usually already known due to improved diagnostic and monitoring techniques, and frequently multiple organ dysfunction syndrome causes the death in a similar fashion in these patients, minimizing the intensivist's interest in the autopsy procedure.

Over the last two decades, six studies have been conducted on adult ICU patients and two studies in the pediatric ICU population, evaluating the relationship of autopsy findings with clinical diagnoses [14–21].

Fernadez-Segoviano et al. [14] in a prospective study including 100 autopsies from 196 deaths (autopsy rate 51%) in a multidisciplinary ICU, reported a 7% discrepancy rate for major missed diagnoses, and no relation between the length of ICU stay and the detected discrepancies [14].

In a retrospective review of patients who died in a medico-coronary ICU, Blosser et al. found an autopsy rate of 31% (41 autopsies from 132 deaths) and reported a 27% discrepancy rate of major missed diagnoses [15]. In the same study only 19 of the autopsies were done on the complete body.

The autopsy rate reported by Mort et al. [16] in a surgical ICU was 29% compared with the hospital average of 18% [16]. In this study, the discrepancy rate for the major unexpected findings was 23%. The authors also reported that patients with a longer ICU stay (>48 hours) presented a significantly greater discrepancy rate than patients with a length of ICU stay <48 hours. The authors [16] suggested that these differences were due to the fact that patients who died during the first two days of ICU stay were unlikely to have developed a 'missed' infection because they would not have had time to be colonized by nosocomial strains.

Roosen et al. [17] studied 100 autopsies from 140 deaths (autopsy rate 93%) in a medical ICU, reporting a major missed diagnosis discrepancy rate of 16% and a shift in the type of missed major diagnoses toward opportunistic infections [17]. Recently, two other studies [18, 19] in medical ICUs have reported autopsy rates of 22.7 and 46.9%, respectively, and major missed diagnosis discrepancy rates of 44.4

and 8.7%, respectively. These studies noted that the autopsy rate is higher in younger than in older patients, and that there was a relation of discrepancies with patient age and the length of ICU stay [18, 19].

Goldstein et al. [20] conducted an autopsy study in a pediatric ICU, reporting an autopsy rate of 73% and a discrepancy rate of 12% for major missed diagnoses. The commonest unexpected findings in this study were undiagnosed infections, cardiac malformations, and unrecognized syndrome and malformations.

Autopsy Rates

The reported autopsy rates from the above mentioned studies ranged between 29 and 93%. These differences can be attributed to variations in the routine autopsy policies among ICUs, various legal constraints and regulations among different countries facilitating presumed consent and autopsy consent from relatives. An autopsy is requested in cases of diagnostic difficulty, and for educational or forensic reasons. Resistance from relatives and a negative approach by the medical staff are the most important factors for the failure to obtain consent for the autopsy [21]. The autopsy yield was similar among cases for which clinicians obtained an autopsy normally and those where an autopsy was obtained because of a program to increase the autopsy rate, suggesting that case selection presents a small effect on the number of missed diagnoses [21].

Discrepancy Rates

The reported discrepancy rates ranged between 18 and 61%, the differences being attributed to the different ICU populations evaluated. The major discrepancies uncovered by the autopsy included undiagnosed infections (mainly opportunistic), pulmonary embolus, and acute myocardial infarction. Developments in life-support systems, chemotherapy, organ transplantation, and anti-rejection chemotherapy has caused the prolongation of life, but has also caused an extreme change in the epidemiology of opportunistic infections. In addition, many modern diagnostic tests still have low sensitivity and/or specificity (e.g., despite the development of spiral computed tomography, the diagnosis of pulmonary embolism is notorioulsy difficult; the diagnosis of endocarditis is often not straightforward in the ICU patient; the available diagnostic methods for fungal infections are not able to differentiate colonization from systemic infection; the diagnosis of VAP [ventilator-associated pneumonia] remains difficult despite bronchoscopy and the use of quantitative cultures of bronchial secretions) [22–25].

Prior to 1970, undiagnosed malignancies ranged between 18–35%; since 1980 this rate has decreased to less 4%. Importantly, between 1912 (the first reported autopsy) and 1980 the type and not the percentage of missed diagnoses has altered because of developments in diagnostic techniques and different distributions of diseases [2, 26].

The relation of the length of ICU stay and patient age with the presence of missed diagnoses is not well recognized. Two studies (one in a pediatric ICU) have suggested there is no relationship between the discrepancies and the length of ICU stay, and two other studies have correlated a short ICU stay with increased missed diagnoses [14, 16, 19, 20]. Recently, Dimopoulos et al. reported in a study in multidisciplinary ICU patients, that the major discrepancies detected were related with the ICU stay (<40 days), while in patients who died after a prolonged ICU stay

(>10 days), the unexpected findings usually regarded coexisting diseases (mainly non-metastatic malignancies) which did not directly affect the cause of death [27]. However, Cameron et al. [21] in a non-ICU autopsy study, reported that even if the clinicians are certain or fairly certain of their ante-mortem diagnosis, in one fourth of the cases the postmortem diagnosis was different, and that these discrepancies probably indicate a close relationship with patient age and the duration of hospital stay. Ahronheim et al. [28] in a study conducted in non-ICU patients, reported that the detected discrepancies occurred twice as often in patients >70 years than in patients >70 years of age.

The limited available data regarding autopsies in ICU patients creates a need for further investigation, as a number of questions must be answered. Should patients be selected for autopsy? Should the autopsy be on the complete body or be limited to specific organs? Randomized studies including all hospital deaths might be an ideal protocol, but difficulties include the high cost and obtaining consent from the relatives.

▌ Conclusion

Although the autopsy rate has decreased worldwide, the autopsy remains an important educational procedure in critically ill patient, despite the use of sophisticated modern diagnostic techniques. Autopsy is useful independent of the length of ICU stay and patient age, promotes an improved understanding of the pathophysiological mechanisms of disease and causes of death, facilitates clinical research protocols, provides epidemiologic information, and aids in the monitoring of public health care. The so-called 'missed diagnosis' does not necessarily indicate medical malpractice but rather an increased incidence of complicated diseases in critically ill patients.

References

1. Cabot RC (1912) Diagnostic pitfalls identified during a study of 3000 autopsies. JAMA 59:2295–2298
2. Goldman L (1984) Diagnostic advances vs the valve of the autopsy. Arch Pathol Lab Med 108:501–505
3. Anderson RE (1984) The autopsy as an instrument of quality assessment: Classification of postmortem and premortem diagnostic discrepancies. Arch Pathol Lab Med 108:490–493
4. Accreditation Council for Graduate Medical Education (1996) Revised essentials of accredited residencies in graduate medical education. Part I, Institutional Requirements. ACGME Bulletin. ACGME, Chicago
5. Landefeld CS, Chren MM, Myers A, Geller R, Robbins S, Goldman L (1988) Diagnostic yield of the autopsy in a university hospital and a community hospital. N Engl J Med 318:1249–1254
6. McPhee SJ, Bottles K (1985) Autopsy: Moribund art or viral science? Am J Med 78:107–113
7. Hasson J, Gross H (1974) The autopsy and quality assessment of medical care. Am J Med 56:137–140
8. Battle R, Pathack D, Humble CC, et al (1987) Factors influencing discrepancies between premortem and postmortem diagnosis. JAMA 258:339–344
9. Cameron HM, McCoogan E (1981) A prospective study of 1152 hospital autopsies. II. Analysis of inaccuracies in clinical diagnoses and their significance. J Pathol 133:285–300
10. Gibinski K, Hartleb M, Koturbasz D (1985) Comparison between pre- and post-mortem diagnoses in a consecutive series of patients. Scand J Gastroenterol 20:370–372

11. Stephanovic G, Tucakovic G, Dotlic R, Kanjuh V (1986) Correlation of clinical diagnoses with athopsy findings: A retrospective study of 2145 consecutive autopsies. Hum Pathol 17:1225–1230
12. Landefeld CS, Goldman L (1989) The autopsy in clinical medicine. Mayo Clin Proc 64: 1185–1189
13. Goldman L, Sayson R, Robbins S, et al (1983) The value of autopsy in three medical eras. N Engl J Med 308:1000–1005
14. Fernandez-Segoviano P, Lazaro A, Esteban A, et al (1988) Autopsy as quality assurance in the intensive care unit. Crit Care Med 16:683–685
15. Blosser SA, Zimmerman HE, Stauffer JL (1998) Do autopsies of critically ill patients reveal important findings that were clinically undetected. Crit Care Med 26:1332–1336
16. Mort TC, Yeston NS (1999) The relationship of pre-mortem diagnoses and post-mortem findings in a surgical intensive care unit. Crit Care Med 27:299–303
17. Roosen J, Frans E, Wilmer A, Knockaert DC, Bobbaers H (2000) Comparison of postmortem clinical diagnoses in critically ill patients and subsequent autopsy findings. Mayo Clin Proc 75:562–657
18. Tai D, El-Bilbeisi H, Tewari S, et al (2001) A study of consecutive autopsies in a medical ICU. A comparison of clinical cause of death and autopsy diagnosis. Chest 119:530–536
19. Podbregar M, Voga G, Krivec B, Skale R, Porežnik R, Gabrešček L (2001) Should we confirm our clinical diagnostic certainty by autopsies. Intensive Care Med 27:1756–1761
20. Goldstein B, Metlay L, Cox C, Rubenstein JS (1996) Association of pre mortem diagnosis and autopsy findings in pediatric intensive care unit versus emergency department versus ward patients. Crit Care Med 24:683–686
21. Cameron HM, McCoogan E, Watson H (1980) Necropsy: a yardstick for clinical diagnoses. Br Med J 281:985–988
22. Ferretti GR, Bosson JL, Buffaz PD, et al (1997) Acute pulmonary embolism: Role of helical CT in 164 patients with intermediate probability at ventilation-perfusion scintigraphy and normal results at duplex US of the legs. Radiology 205:453–458
23. Gouello JP, Asfar P, Brenet O, et al (2000) Nosocomial endocarditis in the intensive care unit: An analysis of 22 cases. Crit Care Med 28:377–382
24. Geha DJ, Roberts GD (1994) Laboratory detection of fungemia. Clin Lab Med 14:83–97
25. Niederman MS, Torres A, Summer W (1994) Invasive diagnosis testing is not needed routinely to manage suspected ventilator-associated pneumonia. Am J Respir Crit Care Med 150:565–574
26. Goldman L (1986) Autopsy: seventy-five years after Gabot. J Am Geriatr Soc 34:897–898
27. Dimopoulos G, Piagnerelli M, Berrè J, Salmon I, Vincent JL (2000) Post mortem examination in the ICU. Still useful? Crit Care Med 28:78a (Abst)
28. Ahronheim JC, Bernholc AS, Clark WD (1983) Age trends in autopsy rates: striking decline in late life. JAMA 250:1182–1186

Subject Index

W

X